ESSENCE OF
ANESTHESIA PRACTICE

ESSENCE OF ANESTHESIA PRACTICE

EDITION 3

LEE A. FLEISHER, MD

Dripps Professor and Chair
Department of Anesthesiology and Critical Care Medicine
Professor of Medicine
University of Pennsylvania School of Medicine
Philadelphia, Pennsylvania

MICHAEL F. ROIZEN, MD

J. Gorman and Family Chair
Wellness Institute
Professor of Anesthesiology
Chief Wellness Officer
The Cleveland Clinic
Cleveland, Ohio

ELSEVIER
SAUNDERS

ELSEVIER
SAUNDERS

1600 John F. Kennedy Blvd
Ste 1800
Philadelphia, PA 19103-2899

Library of Congress Cataloging-in-Publication Data

Essence of anesthesia practice / [edited by] Lee A. Fleisher, Michael F. Roizen. – 3rd ed.
    p. ; cm.
    Includes bibliographical references and index.
    ISBN 978-1-4377-1720-4 (pbk. : alk. paper)   1. Anesthesia--Handbooks, manuals, etc.
2. Anesthesiology–Handbooks, manuals, etc.   I. Fleisher, Lee A.   II. Roizen, Michael F.
    [DNLM: 1. Anesthesia–Handbooks.   2. Anesthetics–Handbooks. WO 231]
    RD82.2.E87 2010
    617.9'6–dc22   2010041122

Executive Publisher: Natasha Andjelkovic
Developmental Editor: Brad McIlwain
Publishing Services Manager: Anne Altepeter
Team Manager: Radhika Pallamparthy
Project Managers: Cindy Thoms and Vijay Antony Raj Vincent
Senior Book Designer: Ellen Zanolle

Printed in the United States of America

Last digit is the print number: 9 8 7 6 5 4 3 2 1

Dedication from Lee A. Fleisher and Michael F. Roizen:
To Renee and Nancy, thanks for the inspiration

Contributors

Sanjib Adhikary, MD

Assistant Professor
Department of Anesthesiology
Penn State College of Medicine
Hershey, Pennsylvania
Magnesium Sulfate

Jorge Aguilar, MD

Fellow
Department of Neuroanesthesiology
University of Texas Medical School at Houston
Houston, Texas
Soy

Charles Ahere, MD

Assistant Professor
University of Mississippi Medical Center
Jackson, Mississippi
Sleep Apnea, Obstructive

Moustafa Ahmed, MD

Clinical Assistant Professor
Anesthesia and Critical Care Medicine
University of Pennsylvania
Philadelphia, Pennsylvania
Lumbar Laminectomy
Rotator Cuff Repair
Transurethral Resection of Bladder Tumor

Jane C. Ahn, MD

Assistant Professor
Department of Anesthesiology
and Perioperative Care
University of California
Irvine, California
Neurofibromatosis (NF)
Schizophrenia
Systemic Lupus Erythematosus

Shamsuddin Akhtar, MD

Associate Professor
Department of Anesthesiology
Yale University School of Medicine
New Haven, Connecticut
Diabetic Ketoacidosis (DKA)

David B. Albert, MD

Administrative Vice Chair and Director
Outpatient Anesthesia
Department of Anesthesiology
NYU Hospital for Joint Diseases;
Clinical Associate Professor of
Anesthesiology
Department of Anesthesiology
New York University
New York, New York
Osteoporosis

Nasrin N. Aldawoodi, MD

Resident
Department of Anesthesiology
University of North Carolina
Chapel Hill, North Carolina
Ventricular Tachyarrhythmias

John T. Algren, MD, FAAP

Professor and Vice Chair for Educational
Affairs
Department of Anesthesiology
Vanderbilt University School of Medicine
Nashville, Tennessee
Cystic Fibrosis

Gracie Almeida-Chen, MD, MPH

Assistant Professor of Clinical
Anesthesiology
Columbia University Medical Center
New York, New York
Imperforate Anus Repair

David Amar, MD

Director of Thoracic Anesthesia
Department of Anesthesiology and Critical
Care Medicine
Memorial Sloan-Kettering Cancer Center;
Professor of Anesthesiology
Weill Medical College of Cornell University
New York, New York
Paroxysmal Atrial Tachycardia

Zirka H. Anastasian, MD

Assistant Professor
Department of Anesthesiology
Columbia University
New York, New York
Cerebrovascular Transient Ischemic Attack (TIA)

Stephen Aniskevich, MD

Instructor
Department of Anesthesia
Mayo Clinic Florida
Jacksonville, Florida
Cholecystectomy, Laparoscopic

Solomon Aronson, MD

Professor
Executive Vice Chairman
Duke Medicine
Durham, North Carolina
Myxoma
Renal Function Testing

Harendra Arora, MD

Associate Professor
Department of Anesthesiology
University of North Carolina
Chapel Hill, North Carolina
Liver Function Tests (LFTs)

Amit Asopa, MD, FRCA

Department of Anesthesia, Critical Care and
Pain Medicine
Beth Israel Deaconess Medical Center
Boston, Massachusetts
Digitalis (Digoxin)

Joshua H. Atkins, MD, PhD

Assistant Professor
Department of Anesthesiology
and Critical Care

University of Pennsylvania
Philadelphia, Pennsylvania
Neuroprotection

John G. Augoustides, MD

Assistant Professor of Anesthesiology and
Critical Care
Hospital of the University
of Pennsylvania
Philadelphia, Pennsylvania
Sildenafil Citrate

Mohammad Fareed Azam, MBBS

Associate Professor
Department of Anesthesiology
University of Colorado–Denver
Aurora, Colorado
Multisystem Organ Failure, Lung
Dysfunction In

Catherine R. Bachman, MD

Assistant Professor
Department of Anesthesia
and Critical Care
University of Chicago
Chicago, Illinois
Rett Syndrome

Douglas R. Bacon, MD, MA

Professor of Anesthesiology and History
of Medicine
Mayo Clinic College of Medicine
Rochester, Minnesota
Sarcoma

Andrew D. Badley, MD

Professor of Medicine
Director, HIV Immunology Laboratory
Associate Director
Translational Program in Immunovirology
and Biodefense
Associate Director
Research Resources Mayo Clinical and
Translational Science Award
Mayo Clinic
Rochester, Minnesota
Cytomegalovirus Infection

Emily Baird, MD, PhD

Assistant Professor
Department of Anesthesia
Hospital of the University
of Pennsylvania
Philadelphia, Pennsylvania
Eclampsia
Retained Placenta, Removal of

Alethia Baldwin, MD

Instructor
Department of Anesthesiology and Pain
Medicine
University of Alabama School
of Medicine
Birmingham, Alabama
Pyruvate

Ryan Ball, MD

Chief Resident
Department of Anesthesiology
University of Pittsburgh
Pittsburgh, Pennsylvania
Craniosynostosis

Amir Baluch, MD

Anesthesiologist
Anesthesia and Perioperative Medicine
University of Miami
Miller School of Medicine
Miami, Florida
Dehydroepiandrosterone (DHEA)
Hepatitis, Alcoholic
Hypopituitarism
Lipidemias
Nutraceuticals
Nutritional Support
Tertracylines

David Bandola, MD, DMD

Assistant Clinical Professor
Department of Anesthesiology
Division of Pain Medicine and
Palliative Care
Columbia University Medical
Center, New York, New York
*Reflex Sympathetic Dystrophy (Complex Pheriph-
eral Pain Syndrome)*

Shawn Banks, MD

Assistant Professor of Clinical
Anesthesiology
Department of Anesthesiology
University of Miami
Miller School of Medicine
Miami, Florida
Burn Injury, Chemical
Burn Injury, Flame

Paul G. Barash, MD

Professor
Department of Anesthesiology
Yale University
New Haven, Connecticut
Aortic Regurgitation

Kathleen E. Barrett, MD

Resident
Department of Anesthesiology
University of Pittsburgh
Pittsburgh, Pennsylvania
Ulcerative Colitis, Chronic

Shawn T. Beaman, MD

Assistant Professor
Department of Anesthesiology
University of Pittsburgh School of Medicine
Pittsburgh, Pennsylvania
Hypokalemia
Ureteral Stent Placement

Jonathan C. Beathe, MD

Director of Training Programs
Assistant Attending Anesthesiologist
Department of Anesthesiology
Hospital for Special Surgery;
Clinical Instructor of Anesthesiology
Department of Anesthesiology
Weill Cornell Medical College
New York, New York
Knee Arthroscopy

Christopher D. Beatie, MD

Assistant Clinical Professor of
Anesthesiology
University of California – Los Angeles
School of Medicine
Los Angeles, California
Extracorporeal Shock Wave Lithotripsy (ESWL)

W. Scott Beattie, MD, PhD, FRCP

Professor,
University of Toronto;
R. Fraser Elliot Chair in Cardiac Anesthesia
University Health Network
Toronto General Hospital
Toronto, Ontario, Canada
Calcium-Channel Blockers

Perry S. Bechtle, DO

Assistant Professor of Anesthesiology
Mayo Clinic College of Medicine
Jacksonville, Florida
Central Neurogenic Hyperventilation

G. Richard Benzinger, MD, PhD

Assistant Professor
Department of Anesthesiology
Washington University in St. Louis
St. Louis, Missouri
Intraoperative Recall

Lauren Berkow, MD

Associate Professor
Departments of Anesthesia
and Critical Care Medicine
Johns Hopkins School of Medicine
Baltimore, Maryland
Transsphenoidal Surgery

Jeffrey M. Berman, MD, FAAP

Professor of Anesthesiology
University of North Carolina
Chapel Hill, North Carolina
Procainamide (Procan, Procanabid, Pronestyl)
Ventricular Tachyarrhythmias

Wendy K. Bernstein, MD

Associate Professor
Director Cardiothoracic Anesthesiology
Fellowship Program
Director Intraoperative Transesophageal
Echocardiography
Department of Anesthesiology
University of Maryland
School of Medicine
Baltimore, Maryland
Isoproterenol (Isuprel, Medihaler-ISO)
Off Pump and Minimally Invasive Cardiac
Procedures
Splenectomy

Arnold J. Berry, MD, MPH

Professor of Anesthesiology
Department of Anesthesiology
Emory University School of Medicine
Atlanta, Georgia
Hepatitis A
Hepatitis B
Hepatitis C

Frederic Berry, MD

Emeritus Professor of Anesthesiology
and Pediatrics

University of Virginia Medical Center
Charlottesville, Virginia
Foreign Body Aspiration

Ulrike Berth, MD

Englewood Hospital and Medical Center
Englewood, New Jersey
Pyloric Stenosis Repair

Walter Bethune, MD

Fellow in Cardiothoracic Anesthesiology
Department of Anesthesiology
and Critical Care
University of Pennsylvania
Philadelphia, Pennsylvania
Exercise Stress Testing
Pacemaker Implantation for Sick Sinus Syndrome

Sumita Bhambhani, MD

Assistant Professor
Department of Anesthesiology
Temple University Hospital
Philadelphia, Pennsylvania
Epidermolysis Bullosa

Shobana Bharadwaj, MBBS

Assistant Professor
Department of Anesthesiology
University of Maryland School of Medicine
Baltimore, Maryland
Preeclampsia

Neil Bhatt, MD

Resident
Department of Anesthesiology
Louisiana State University
Health Sciences Center
New Orleans, Louisiana
Atropine

Frederic T. Billings IV, MD, MSc

Assistant Professor of Anesthesiology
and Critical Care Medicine
Vanderbilt University
Nashville, Tennessee
Statins

Wendy B. Binstock, MD

Associate Professor
Department of Anesthesia
and Critical Care
Department of Pediatrics
Comer Children's Hospital
University of Chicago
Chicago, Illinois
Omphalocele Surgery

David J. Birnbach, MD, MPH

Professor of Anesthesiology, Obstetrics and
Gynecology, and Public Health
University of Miami
Miller School of Medicine
Miami, Florida
HELLP Syndrome

Michael Bishop, MD

Professor
Department of Anesthesiology
University of Washington and
Puget Sound Veterans Affairs Health Care
System
Seattle, Washington
Asthma Drugs, New

Stephanie Black, MD

University of Pennsylvania, Philadelphia,
Pennsylvania
Down Syndrome
Duchenne Muscular Dystrophy (Pseudohypertro-
phic Muscular Dystrophy)

Mary A. Blanchette, MD

Assistant Professor of Anesthesiology
and Perioperative Medicine
Oregon Health and Science University
Portland, Oregon
Multiple Endocrine Neoplasia (MEN) Type I and II
Parathyroidectomy

James M. Blum, MD

Department of Anesthesiology
and Critical Care
University of Michigan Health Systems
Ann Arbor, Michigan
Cigarette Smoking

**Krishna Boddu, MBBS, MD, DNB,
FANZCA**

Associate Professor
Department of Anesthesiology
Director, Acute Pain Medicine
University of Texas Medical School at Houston
Memorial Hermann Hospital
Houston, Texas
Monoamine Oxidase Inhibitors; Reversible Inhibi-
tors of Monoamine Oxidase
Pyridostigmine Bromide

Lara Bonasera, MD

University of Chicago
Chicago, Illinois
Garlic (Allium sativum)

Richard L. Boortz-Marx, MD, MS

Associate Professor
Department of Anesthesia and Pain
Medicine
Director of Pain Medicine
University of North Carolina
Chapel Hill, North Carolina
Amyotrophic Lateral Sclerosis
Spasmodic Torticollis

Cecil O. Borel, MD

Professor
Department of Anesthesiology
Associate Professor
Department of Surgery (Neurosurgery)
Duke University
Durham, North Carolina
Myasthenia Gravis

Gregory H. Botz, MD, FCCM

Professor of Anesthesiology
and Critical Care
Department of Critical Care
University of Texas MD Anderson
Cancer Center
Houston, Texas
Cardiomyopathy, Alcoholic

Charles D. Boucek, MD

Associate Professor of Anesthesiology
University of Pittsburgh
Pittsburgh, Pennsylvania
Bone Marrow Transplantation
(Harvest Procedure)

William Bradford, BS, MD

Department of Anesthesia
University of North Carolina Hospitals
Chapel Hill, North Carolina
V/Q Scan (Nuclear Ventilation-Perfusion
Scintigraphy)

Jason C. Brainard, MD

Anesthesiologist
University of Pennsylvania Hospital
Philadelphia, Pennsylvania
Acute Respiratory Distress Syndrome (ARDS)

Michelle Braunfeld, MD

Clinical Professor
Department of Anesthesiology
University of California–Los Angeles David
Geffen School of Medicine
Los Angeles, California
Diarrhea, Acute and Chronic
Drug Overdose, Rat Poison (Warfarin Toxicity)

Ferne R. Braveman, MD, CM

Professor of Anesthesiology and Obstetrics
and Gynecology
Vice Chair of Clinical Affairs
Department of Anesthesiology
Yale University School of Medicine
New Haven, Connecticut
Total Abdominal Hysterectomy

Caridad Bravo-Fernandez, MD

Assistant Professor
Department of Anesthesiology
Medical College of Wisconsin
Milwaukee, Wisconsin
Amputation, Above-Knee (AKA)

Peter H. Breen, MD, FRCPC

Associate Professor
Department of Anesthesiology and
Perioperative Care
University of California
Irvine Medical Center
Orange, California
Carbon Monoxide (CO) Poisoning
Cyanide Poisoning

Marjorie Brennan, MD

Assistant Professor of Anesthesiology
and Pediatrics
Children's National Medical Center/
George Washington University Medical
Center
Washington, DC
Carnitine Deficiency

Tricia Brentjens, MD

Associate Clinical Professor
Department of Anesthesiology
Section of Critical Care
College of Physicians and Surgeons
Columbia University
New York, New York
Wolff-Parkinson-White (WPW) Syndrome

Megan A. Brockel, MD

Instructor
Department of Anesthesiology
Washington University School of Medicine
St. Louis, Missouri
Mucopolysaccharidoses

Jay B. Brodsky, MD

Professor
Department of Anesthesia
Stanford University School of Medicine
Medical Director – Perioperative Services
Stanford University Medical Center
Stanford, California
Guillain-Barré Syndrome

Todd A. Bromberg, MD

Pain Management Fellow
Department of Anesthesiology
University of North Carolina
Chapel Hill, North Carolina
Amyotrophic Lateral Sclerosis
Spasmodic Torticollis

Adam J. Broussard, MD

Resident, Department
of Anesthesiology
Louisiana State University
Health Sciences Center
New Orleans, Louisiana
Myotonia Dystrophica (Myotonic Dystrophy,
Steinert's Disease)

Chris Broussard, MD

Resident
Department of Anesthesiology
Tulane University
New Orleans, Louisiana
Red Yeast Rice (Cholestin)

Carmen Labrie-Brown, MD

Assistant
Department of Anesthesiology
Louisiana State University
Health Sciences Center
New Orleans, Louisiana
Cerebral Palsy

Robert H. Brown, MD, MPH

Professor
Department of Anesthesiology and Critical
Care Medicine
Division of Pulmonary Medicine and
Radiology
Johns Hopkins School of Medicine
Environmental Health Sciences
Division of Physiology
Johns Hopkins School of
Public Health
Johns Hopkins University
Baltimore, Maryland
Latex Allergy

Charles S. Brudney, MB, ChB, FRCA

Assistant Professor
Department of Anesthesiology
Assistant Professor
Department of Medicine
Duke University
Durham, North Carolina
Cardiomyopathy, Ischemic

Sorin J. Brull, MD

Professor
Department of Anesthesiology
Mayo Clinic College of Medicine
Jacksonville, Florida
Cholecystectomy, Laparoscopic
Cholecystectomy, Open

Claude Brunson, MD

Assistant Professor
Department of Anesthesiology
University of Mississippi
School of Medicine
Jackson, Mississippi
Sleep Apnea, Obstructive

Trent Bryson, MD

Resident
Department of Anesthesiology
University of Colorado
Denver, Colorado
Blebs and Bullae

Jacob M. Buchowski, MD, MS

Assistant Professor of Orthopaedic and
Neurological Surgery
Director,
Center for Spinal Tumors
Washington University in St. Louis
St. Louis, Missouri
Scoliosis and Kyphosis Surgery

Stefan Budac, MD

Acting Assistant Professor
Department of Anesthesiology
Seattle Children's Hospital
University of Washington
School of Medicine
Seattle, Washington
Jeune Syndrome (Asphyxiating Thoracic Dystrophy)

Zachary D. Bush, MD Intern Pharmacist

Doctor of Pharmacy Candidate 2012
Mercer University
College of Pharmacy and Health Science
Atlanta, Georgia
Clopidogrel Bisulfate

John Butterworth, MD

R. K. Stoelting Professor and Chairman
Department of Anesthesia
Indiana University School of Medicine
Indianapolis, Indiana
Hypothyroidism

Lisbeysi Calo, MD

Anesthesiology Resident CA-2
Yale New Haven Hospital
New Haven, Connecticut
Labor, Epidural Block

Christopher Canlas, MD

Assistant Professor of Clinical
Anesthesiology
Department of Anesthesiology
Vanderbilt University
Medical Center
Nashville, Tennessee
Burr Hole

Ayana Cannon, MD

Chief Resident
Department of Anesthesiology
University of Maryland School of Medicine
Baltimore, Maryland
Isoproterenol (Isuprel, Medihaler-ISO)

Shawn M. Cantie, MD

Department of Anesthesiology, PGY-2
Jackson Memorial Hospital

University of Miami
Medicine Miller School of Medicine
Miami, Florida
Respiratory Distress Syndrome

Lisa Caplan

Pediatric Cardiovascular Anesthesia Fellow
Texas Children's Hospital
Houston, Texas
Valerian (Valeriana officinalis)

Marco Caruso, MD

Assistant Professor
Department of Anesthesiology
Temple University School of Medicine
Philadelphia, Pennsylvania
Alpha-2 Adrenergic Agonists

Davide Cattano, MD, PhD

Assistant Professor
Department of Anesthesiology
University of Texas Medical School
at Houston
Houston, Texas A
Angiotensin II Receptor Blocking Drugs
Phencyclidine (PCP)

Charles B. Cauldwell, PhD, MD

Clinical Professor of Anesthesia
Department of Anesthesia
and Perioperative Care
University of California, San Francisco
San Francisco, California
Pierre Robin Syndrome

Laura Cavallone, MD

Assistant Professor
Department of Anesthesiology
Washington University in Saint Louis
St. Louis, Missouri
Endoscopic Sinus Surgery (ESS)
Radical Neck Dissection

Maurizio Cereda, MD

Assistant Professor
Department of Anesthesiology
and Critical Care
University of Pennsylvania
Philadelphia, Pennsylvania
Acute Respiratory Distress Syndrome (ARDS)

Thomas M. Chalifoux, MD

Postdoctoral Scholar
Department of Anesthesiology
University of Pittsburgh
School of Medicine
Attending Anesthesiologist
Children's Hospital of Pittsburgh of UPMC
Pittsburgh, Pennsylvania
Coarctation of the Aorta

Susan Chan, MD

Clinical Professor
Department of Anesthesiology
University of California–Los Angeles
Medical Center
Los Angeles, California
Laparoscopy, Gynecologic

Theodore G. Cheek, MD

Associate Professor
Departments of Anesthesia and Obstetrics
and Gynecology

Director Obstetric Anesthesia
Hospital of the University of Pennsylvania
Pennsylvania, Philadelphia
Labor, Peripheral Blocks
Pregnancy, Intra-Abdominal
St. John's Wort (Hypericum Perforatum)

Alexander Chen, MD

Department of Anesthesiology and Critical Care
Hospital of the University of Pennsylvania
Philadelphia, Pennsylvania
Tracheal Resection

Samuel A. Cherry, III, MD

Assistant Professor of Anesthesiology
and Pathology
Birmingham VA Medical Center
University of Alabama at Birmingham
Medical Center
Birmingham, Alabama
Blood Components

Albert T. Cheung, MD

Professor
Department of Anesthesiology and Critical Care
University of Pennsylvania
Philadelphia, Pennsylvania
Mitral Stenosis
Mitral Valve Prolapse
Syndrome of Inappropriate Antidiuretic Hormone
Secretion (SIADH)

Grace L. Chien, MD

Chief, Anesthesiology Service
Co-Clinical Director, Operative Care
Division
Portland VA Medical Center
Clinical Professor of Anesthesiology
Department of Anesthesiology and
Peri-Operative Medicine
Oregon Health and Science University
Portland, Oregon
Bypass Graft Procedure, Infrainguinal

Peter T. Choi, MD, MSc, FRCPC

Associate Professor
Department of Anesthesiology
Pharmacology and Therapeutics,
University of British Columbia
Vancouver, British Columbia, Canada
Extracorporeal Shock Wave Lithotripsy (ESWL)

Christopher Ciarallo, MD

Department of Anesthesiology
Denver Health Medical Center
Pediatric Anesthesiology
The Children's Hospital
University of Colorado Denver
Assistant Professor
Department of Anesthesiology
University of Colorado Denver
Denver, Colorado
Cromolyn Sodium

Franklyn Cladis, MD

Assistant Professor of Anesthesiology
Department of Anesthesiology
The Children's Hospital of Pittsburgh
of UPMC
Pittsburgh, Pennsylvania
Craniosynostosis
Kasai Procedure
Hirschsprung's Disease

CONTRIBUTORS

Anthony J. Clapcich, MD

Assistant Professor of Anesthesiology
and Pediatrics
Children's Hospital of New York-
Presbyterian
Columbia University
New York, New York
Double Aortic Arch

Richard B. Clark, MD

Professor Emeritus
Department of Anesthesiology
University of Arkansas for Medical Sciences
Little Rock, Arkansas
*Diabetes, Type III (Gestational
Diabetes Mellitus)*

Mindy Cohen, MD

Pediatric Anesthesiology Fellow
Department of Anesthesiology
Children's Hospital Denver
Aurora, Colorado
Cleft Lip Repair

Neal H. Cohen, MD, MPH, MS

Vice Dean
School of Medicine
Professor
Department of Anesthesia and Perioperative
Care
Director, International Services
University of California San Francisco
San Francisco, California
Pneumocystis Carinii Pneumonia (PCP)

Robert I. Cohen, MA(Education), MD

Assistant Professor
Department of Anesthesia
Harward Medical School
Attending Anesthesiologist
Department of Anesthesia
Critical Care and Pain Medicine
Beth Israel Deaconess Medical Center
Boston, Massachusetts
Benzodiazepines (Midazolam, Lorazepam, Diazepam)
Conversion Disorder

Stephan J. Cohn, MD

Assistant Professor
Department of Anesthesia
and Critical Care
University of Chicago
Chicago, Illinois
Raynaud's Phenomenon

Aisling Conran, MD

Director of Office Based Anesthesia
West Central Anesthesia
Staff Anesthesiologist
Central Dupage Hospital
Winfield, Illinois
Tacrolimus (FK-506)

Richard I. Cook, MD

Associate Professor
Department of Anesthesia and Critical Care
University of Chicago
Chicago, Illinois
*Doxorubicin (Adriamycin) Daunorubicin (Ceru-
bidine)*
*Duchenne Muscular Dystrophy (Pseudohypertro-
phic Muscular Dystrophy)*

Randall F. Coombs, MD

Associate Professor
Anesthesia Department
University of North Carolina at Chapel Hill
Chapel Hill, North Carolina
AV Graft for Hemodialysis

David M. Corda, MD

Instructor
Department of Anesthesia
Division of Cardiothoracic Anesthesia
Mayo Clinic Florida
Jacksonville, Florida
Cholecystectomy, Open

Daniel Cormican, MD

Resident
Department of Anesthesiology
University of Pittsburgh Medical Center
Pittsburgh, Pennsylvania
Hypokalemia

Darren Cousin, MD

Assistant Professor
Department of Anesthesia
Louisiana State University
New Orleans, Louisiana
Cephalopelvic Disproportion

Vincent S. Cowell, MD

Associate Professor
Department of Anesthesiology
Temple University School of Medicine
Philadelphia, Pennsylvania
Cancer, Breast
Hemophilia

Lyndsey Cox, MD

Anesthesiology and Critical Care
Children's Hospital of Philadelphia
Philadelphia, Pennsylvania
Testicular Torsion Surgery

Paula A. Craigo, MD

Assistant Professor
Department of Anesthesiology
Mayo Clinic
Rochester, Minnesota
*Aspiration, Perioperative: Prevention and
Management*
Pneumonectomy

Richard C. Cross, MD

Associate Professor
University of Alabama Birmingham
Department of Anesthesiology
Birmingham, Alabama
Brain Death

Roy F. Cucchiara, MD

Professor of Anesthesiology
Mayo Clinic College of Medicine
Jacksonville, Florida
Central Neurogenic Hyperventilation

William H. Daily, MD

Assistant Professor
Department of Anesthesiology
University of Texas Health Science
Center-Houston
Houston, Texas
Hypophosphatemia

Gaurang Dalal, MBBS, MS, DORL

Researcher
Penn State Hershey Medical Center
Hershey, Pennsylvania
*Tracheotomy/Tracheostomy and
Cricothyrotomy*

Priti Dalal, MBBS, DA, MD, FRCA

Assistant Professor
Department of Anesthesiology
Penn State Hershey Medical Center
Hershey, Pennsylvania
*Tracheotomy/Tracheostomy and
Cricothyrotomy*

Michael Danekas, MD

Pediatric Anesthesiologist
Department of Anesthesiology
San Antonio Military Medical Center
San Antonio, Texas
Steroids

Ahmed M. Darwish, MD

Assistant Professor
Department of Anesthesiology
Keck School of Medicine
University of Southern California
Los Angeles, California
Lyme Disease

Ribal Darwish, MD

Assistant Professor of Anesthesiology
and Critical Care Medicine
Department of Anesthesiology
University of Maryland School of Medicine
Baltimore, Maryland
Pericarditi's Constrictive

Suanne M. Daves, MD

Associate Professor
Department of Anesthesia and Pediatrics
Director,
Division of Pediatric Cardiac Anesthesia
Medical Director
Perioperative Clinical Operations
The Pediatric Heart Institute
Monroe Carell Jr. Children's Hospital
at Vanderbilt
Nashville, Tennessee
*Extracorporeal Membrane Oxygenation
(ECMO)*

Kathleen Davis, MD

Assistant Professor
Department of Anesthesiology
University of Maryland School of Medicine
Baltimore, Maryland
Flow-Volume Loops
Spirometry

Peter J. Davis, MD, FAAP

Anesthesiologist-in-Chief
Department of Anesthesiology
Children's Hospital of Pittsburgh
Professor of Anesthesiology
and Pediatrics
Department of Anesthesiology
University of Pittsburgh
School of Medicine
Pittsburgh, Pennsylvania
Wilms' Tumor
Gastroschisis Surgery

Bracken J. De Witt, MD, PhD

Assistant Professor
Department of Anesthesia
Louisiana State University
New Orleans, Louisiana
Ephedra (Ma-Huang)

Ellise Delphin, MD, MPH

Department of Anesthesiology
University of Medicine and Dentistry
of New Jersey
New Jersey Medical School
Newark, New Jersey
Antithrombin III Deficiency

Seema Deshpande, MBBS

Assistant Professor
Department of Anesthesiology
University of Maryland School
of Medicine
Baltimore, Maryland
Parkinson's Disease (Paralysis Agitans)

Dawn P. Desiderio, MD

Attending
Department of Anesthesiology and Critical
Care Medicine
Memorial Sloan Kettering
Cancer Center;
Professor Clinical Anesthesia
Department of Anesthesiology
Weill Medical College of Cornell University
New York, New York
Cancer, Esophageal

Laura K. Diaz, MD

Attending Cardiac Anesthesiologist
Children's Hospital of Philadelphia
Assistant Professor of Anesthesiology
and Critical Care Medicine
University of Pennsylvania
School of Medicine
Philadelphia, Pennsylvania
Transposition of the Great Arteries (TGA)
Transposition of the Great Arteries, L Form
(L-TGA)

Christian Diez, MD

Assistant Professor of Clinical
Anesthesiology
Department of Anesthesiology
University of Miami
Miller School of Medicine
Miami, Florida
Burn Injury, Electrical
Carotid Sinus Syndrome
Encephalopathy, Hypertensive

Sanjay Dixit, MD

Associate Professor
Cardiovascular Division
Department of Medicine
Hospital of The University
of Pennsylvania;
Director
Cardiac Electrophysiology
Philadelphia Veterans Affairs Medical
Center
Philadelphia, Pennsylvania
Atrial Fibrillation Ablation
Implantable Cardioverter Defibrillators (ICDS),
Implantation

Karen B. Domino, MD, MPH

Professor of Anesthesiology
and Pain Medicine
Department of Anesthesiology
University of Washington
Seattle, Washington
Silicosis

Kathryn Dorhauer, MD

Department of Anesthesiology
Tulane University
New Orleans, Louisiana
Quinidine

Todd Dorman, MD

Associate Dean and Director
Continuing Medical Education
Professor and Vice Chair
Department of Anesthesiology
and Critical Care Medicine
Professor,
Department of Medicine and Surgery
Johns Hopkins University School of
Medicine
Professor
Department of Nursing
Johns Hopkins University School of
Nursing;
Baltimore, Maryland
Deep Vein Thrombosis

Don D. Doussan, MD

Anesthesiologist
East Jefferson General Hospital
Metairie, Louisiana
Shy-Drager Disease

James Duke, MD, MBA

Associate Director
Department of Anesthesiology
Denver Health Medical Center
Denver, Colorado
Associate Professor
Department of Anesthesiology
University of Colorado Denver
School of Medicine
Aurora, Colorado
Buerger's Disease: Thromboangiitis Obliterans
Gold (Auranofin, Aurothioglucose,
Aurothiomalate)
Hyperaldosteronism (Secondary)

Ann C. Duncan, RN, BSN

Clinical Informatics Specialist
Tanner Medical System
Carrollton, Georgia
Clopidogrel Bisulfate

Frank W. Dupont, MD

Assistant Professor
Department of Anesthesia and Critical Care
University of Chicago
Chicago, Illinois
Dilated Cardiomyopathy (DCM)
Epsilon-Aminocaproic Acid (EACA) (Amicar)

L. Jane Easdown, MD

Associate Professor
Department of Anesthesiology
Vanderbilt University Medical Center
Nashville, Tennessee
Cerebral Arteriovenous Malformations (AVMs)
Trigeminal Neuralgia (TIC Doloureux)

R. Blaine Easley, MD

Assistant Professor
Department of Anesthesiology
and Critical Care Medicine
Johns Hopkins Hospital
Baltimore, Maryland
Creatine
Licorice (Glycyrrhiza Glabra)

Thomas J. Ebert, MD, PhD

Professor and Vice-chair for Education
Program Director
Department of Anesthesiology
Medical College of Wisconsin;
Staff Anesthesiologist
Department of Anesthesiology
VA Medical Center
Milwaukee, Wisconsin
Autonomic Function
Familial Dysautonomia (Riley-Day
Syndrome)

David M. Eckmann, PhD, MD

Horatio C. Wood Professor of
Anesthesiology and Critical Care
Professor of Bioengineering
University of Pennsylvania
Philadelphia, Pennsylvania
Gastric Bypass Stapling for Morbid
Obesity

Talmage D. Egan, MD

Professor and KC Wong Presidential
Endowed Chair Holder
Department of Anesthesiology
University of Utah
Salt Lake City, Utah
Cigarette Smoking Cessation

Seth Eisdorfer, MD

Resident Physician
Department of Anesthesiology,
Perioperative Medicine and Pain
Management
University of Miami
Jackson Memorial Hospital
Miami, Florida
Gonorrhea

Nabil M. Elkassabany, MD

Assistant Professor
Department of Anesthesiology
and Critical Care
University of Pennsylvania
Staff Anesthesiologist
Department of Anesthesiology
Philadelphia VA Medical Center
Philadelphia, Pennsylvania
Atrial Fibrillation Ablation
Delirium (Postanesthetic)
Implantable Cardioverter-Defibrillators (ICDS),
Implantation

Ryan P. Ellender, MD

Resident Physician
Department of Anesthesiology
Louisiana State University
Health Sciences Center - New Orleans
New Orleans, Louisiana
Amputation, Lower Extremity (LEA)

Logan S. Emory, BA, MD
Director of Neuroanesthesia
Department of Anesthesiology
Ochsner Clinic Foundation
New Orleans, Louisiana
Multiple Sclerosis
Cerebral AVM Repair

Monique Espinosa, MD
Chief Resident
Department of Anesthesiology
Jackson Memorial Hospital
Miami, Florida
Metformin (Glucophage)

Lucinda L. Everett, MD
Associate Professor
Harvard Medical School
Chief, Pediatric Anesthesia
Department of Anesthesiology, Critical
Care, and Pain Medicine
Massachusetts General Hospital
Boston, Maryland
Inguinal Herniorrhaphy

Nauder Faraday, MD
Associate Professor
Department of Anesthesiology and Critical
Care Medicine
Johns Hopkins University School of Medicine
Baltimore, Maryland
Thrombocytopenia

James J. Fehr, MD
Associate Professor
Departments of Anesthesiology and Pediatrics
Director
Pediatric Simulation Center
Washington University
St. Louis, Missouri
Mucopolysaccharidoses

James M. Feld, BS, MD
Professor of Anesthesiology
Department of Anesthesiology
University of Illinois at Chicago
Chicago, Illinois
Hypomagnesemia

Lynn A. Fenton, MD
Assistant Professor
Department of Anesthesiology
and Perioperative Medicine
Oregon Health and Science University
Portland, Oregon
Riboflavin (Vitamin B₂)
Goldenseal (Hydrastis Canadensis)

Laura H. Ferguson, MD
Instructor
Department of Anesthesiology
University of Pittsburgh Medical Center
Mercy Hospital
Pittsburgh, Pennsylvania
Glaucoma, Open-Angle

Matthew Fiegel, MD
Assistant Professor
Department of Anesthesiology
University of Colorado Denver
Denver, Colorado
Uterine Rupture

Aaron M. Fields, MD
Associate Program Director
Anesthesiology Critical Care Fellowship
Wilford Hall Medical Center
San Antonio, Texas
Pickwickian Syndrome

Gordon N. Finlayson, BSc, MD, FRCP
Anesthesiologist and Intensivist
Anesthesiology Division of Critical Care
University of British Columbia VGH Site
Vancouver, British Columbia, Canada
Guillain-Barré Syndrome

A lan Fin ley, MD
Assistant Professor
Department of Anesthesia and Perioperative
Medicine
Medical University of South Carolina
Charleston, South Carolina
*Coronary Artery Disease (Left Main and Non-Left
Main Disease)*

Gregory W. Fischer, MD
Associate Professor Anesthesiology
Associate Professor Cardiothoracic Surgery
Mount Sinai Medical Center
New York, New York
*Ventricular Septal Rupture (Defect), Post
Myocardial Infarction*

Gary Fiskum, PhD
Professor and Vice-Chair Research
Department of Anesthesiology
University of Maryland School of Medicine
Baltimore, Maryland
Ginkgo

Molly Fitzpatrick, MD
Assistant Professor
Department of Anesthesiology
University of Maryland School of Medicine
Baltimore, Maryland
Parkinson's Disease (Paralysis Agitans)

Russell Flatto, MD
Fellow in Regional Anesthesia and Acute
Pain Medicine
Hospital for Special Surgery
New York, New York
Knee Arthroscopy

Lee A. Fleisher, MD
Dripps Professor and Chair Department of
Anesthesiology and Critical Care Medicine
Professor of Medicine
University of Pennsylvania School of Medicine
Philadelphia, Pennsylvania
Angina, Chronic Stable
Aspirin (Acetylsalicylic Acid)
Cherubism
Chromium
Clopidogrel Bisulfate
Dipyridamole Thallium Imaging
Nitroglycerin
Phytosterols
Radical Prostatectomy (Retropubic)
Renal Failure, Chronic
Scleroderma
Sildenafil Citrate
Splenectomy
Varicella-Zoster Virus

Ronda Flower, MD
Associate Professor of Clinical Anesthesia
Department of Anesthesiology
Louisiana State University
School of Medicine
New Orleans, Louisiana
Bulimia

Annette G. Folgueras, MD, JD
Assistant Professor
Department of Anesthesiology
University of Maryland
School of Medicine
Baltimore, Maryland
Hysteroscopy

Patrick J. Forte, MD
Assistant Professor
Department of Anesthesiology
University of Pittsburgh
Pittsburgh, Pennsylvania
Ulcerative Colitis, Chronic

Joseph F. Foss, MD
Staff
Director of Clinical Research
Department of General Anesthesiology
Cleveland Clinic
Cleveland, Ohio
Cisplatin

Charles J. Fox, MD
Associate Professor
Department of Anesthesiology
Tulane School of Medicine
New Orleans, Louisiana
Hyponatremia
Red Yeast Rice(cholestin)
Tranexamic Acid

William R. Furman, MD
Professor and Vice Chair
for Clinical Affairs
Department of Anesthesiology
Vanderbilt University School of Medicine
Nashville, Tennessee
Emphysema

Robert Gaiser, MD, MSEd
Professor
Anesthesiology and Critical Care
Hospital of the University
of Pennsylvania
Philadelphia, Pennsylvania
Split-Thickness Skin Graft

David R. Gambling, MB, BS, FRCPC
Staff Anesthesiologist
Department of Anesthesiology
Sharp Mary Birch Hospital for Women
and Newborns;
Associate Clinical Professor
Anesthesiology,
University of California San Diego
San Diego, California
Hypermagnesemia

Scott Gardiner, MD
Assistant Professor of Anesthesia
Department of Anesthesiology
Tulane University School of Medicine
New Orleans, Louisiana
Red Yeast Rice (Cholestin)

Matthew L. Garvey, MD

Resident Physician
Department of Anesthesiology
University of North Carolina
Chapel Hill, North Carolina
Kartagener's Syndrome

Abraham C. Gaupp, MD

University of Chicago – Anesthesia
Chicago, Illinois
*Psyllium, Bulk-Forming Laxatives (Plantago
Isphagula, Plantago Ovata)*

Steven Gayer, MD, MBA

Professor of Anesthesiology and
Ophthalmology
University of Miami Miller School
of Medicine
Miami, Florida
Retinal Buckle Surgery

Jeremy M. Geiduschek, MD

Clinical Professor
Department of Anesthesiology and Pain
Medicine
University of Washington
School of Medicine;
Director of Clinical Anesthesia Services
Director of Cardiovascular Anesthesiology
Seattle Children's Hospital
Seattle, Washington
*Mitochondrial Myopathy
Muscle Biopsy for Undiagnosed Myopathy*

Frank Gencorelli, MD

University of Pennsylvania
Philadelphia, Pennsylvania
Mediastinal Masses

Eric Gewirtz, MD

Assistant Professor
Department of Anesthesiology
Temple University
Philadelphia, Pennsylvania
Drug Abuse, Lysergic Acid Diethylamide (LSD)

Ghaleb A. Ghani, MD

Associate Professor of Anesthesiology
Emory University
Emory University Hospital
Atlanta, Georgia
Glomus Jugulare Tumors

Charles P. Gibbs, MD

Courtesy Clinical Professor
Department of Anesthesiology
University of Florida
Gainesville, Florida;
Professor Emiritus
Department of Anesthesiology
University of Colorado
Denver, Colorado
Abruptio Placentae

Jeremy L. Gibson, MD

Resident
Department of Anesthesiology and
Perioperative Medicine
Oregon Health and Science University
Portland, Oregon
*Histiocytosis
Mastocytosis*

Lori Gilbert, MD

Assistant Professor Clinical Anesthesiology
and Critical Care
Department of Anesthesiology
Hospital of the University of Pennsylvania
Philadelphia, Pennsylvania
Ludwig's Angina

Kevin J. Gingrich, BS, MD, MEngr

Associate Professor
Department of Anesthesiology
New York University School of Medicine
New York, New York
Intracranial Hypertension (ICH)

Gregory Ginsburg, MD

Instructor in Anesthesia
Harvard Medical School
Boston, Massachusetts
Inguinal Herniorrhaphy

Christopher Giordano, MD

Assistant Professor of Anesthesiology
University of Florida College of Medicine
Gainesville, Florida
Diuretics

Christine E. Goepfert, MD

Visiting Professor
Department for Anesthesiology
Division of Neuroanesthesia
Washington University
Barnes-Jewish Hospital
St. Louis, Missouri
*Carbamazepine
Stereotactic Neurosurgery*

Hernando Gomez, MD

Critical Care Medicine
University of Pittsburgh
Pittsburgh, Pennsylvania
Necrotizing Fasciitis

Santiago Gomez, MD

Assistant Professor of Clinical Anesthesiology
Department of Anesthesiology
Tulane University School of Medicine
New Orleans, Louisiana
Herpes, Type II

Alanna E. Goodman, MD

Assistant Professor
Department of Anesthesiology
Vanderbilt University
Nashville, Tennessee
*Appendicitis, Acute
Do Not Resuscitate (DNR) Orders*

Stephanie R. Goodman, MD

Associate Clinical Professor
Department of Anesthesiology
Columbia University
New York, New York
Pregnancy, Maternal Physiology

Alexandru Gottlieb, MD

Associate Professor
Anesthesia Institute
Cleveland Clinic
Cleveland, Ohio
*Bypass, Femoral-Femoral
Endovascular Aortic Stent Repairs*

Ori Gottlieb, MD

Assistant Professor
Department of Anesthesia
and Critical Care
University of Chicago
Chicago, Illinois
*Dexmedetomidine (Precedex)
Melatonin (N-Acetyl-5-Methoxytryptamine,
Bevitamel, Vitamist, Melatonex)*

Allan Gottschalk, MD

Associate Professor Anesthesiology and
Critical Care Medicine
Johns Hopkins Medical Institutions
Baltimore, Maryland
Aneurysm Coiling

**Basavana Gouda Goudra, MD, FRCA,
FCARCSI**

Assistant Professor
Department of Anesthesiology
Hospital of the University of Pennsylvania
Philadelphia, Pennsylvania
Transurethral Resection of Prostate (TURP)

Harry J. Gould, III, MD, PhD

Professor
Neurology and Neuroscience
Louisiana State University Health Sciences
Center
New Orleans, Louisiana
Headache, Migraine

Nikolaus Gravenstein, MD

Professor of Anesthesiology
University of Florida College of Medicine
Gainesville, Florida
Diuretics

Megan Graybill, MD

Department of Anesthesiology
University of North Carolina
Chapel Hill, North Carolina
Liver Function Tests (LFTs)

William J. Greeley, MD

Anesthesiologist-in-Chief
Children's Hospital of Philadelphia
Professor of Anesthesiology and Pediatrics
University of Pennsylvania
School of Medicine
Philadelphia, Pennsylvania
*Marfan's Syndrome
Total Anomalous Pulmonary Venous Return
Correction*

Patrick Guffey, MD

Pediatric Anesthesiology
Children's Hospital
University of Colorado, Denver
Denver, Colorado
Office-Based Anesthesia

Ala Sami Haddadin, MD, FCCP

Assistant Professor
Division of Cardiothoracic Anesthesia
Yale University School of Medicine;
Co-Director
Cardiothoracic Intensive Care Unit
Yale New Haven Hospital
New Haven, Connecticut
*Dopamine
Epinephrine*

John G. Hagen, MD

Resident
Department of Anesthesiology
Mount Sinai School of Medicine
New York, New York
Hip Fracture Repair

Karim Abdel Hakim, FRCA

Research Fellow in Anaesthesia
Division of Anaesthesia
and Intensive Care
University of Nottingham
Nottingham, Great Britain
Hypertension

Michael Hall, MD

Resident
Department of Anesthesiology and
Perioperative Medicine
Oregon Health and Science University
Portland, Oregon
Cardioversion

N. James Halliday, MB, ChB, FCARCS(I)

Director of Pediatric Anesthesia
Department of Anesthesiology
University of Miami
Miller School of Medicine
Miami, Florida
Diaphragmatic Hernia (Congenital)

Raafat S. Hannallah, MD

Professor of Anesthesiology and Pediatrics
Children's National Medical Center/George
Washington University Medical Center
Washington, DC
*Anhidrosis (Congenital Anhidrotic Ectodermanl
Dysplasia)*
Carnitine Deficiency

Jeremy Hansen MD

Resident
Department of Anesthesiology
University of Colorado, Denver
Aurora, Colorado
Buerger's Disease: Thromboangiitis Obliterans
*Gold (Auranofin, Aurothioglucose, Auro-
thiomalate)*

C. William Hanson III, MD

Professor of Anesthesiology and Critical
Care, Surgery and Internal Medicine
University of Pennsylvania
Philadelphia, Pennsylvania
Bronchitis, Chronic

Charles B. Hantler, MD

Professor
Department of Anesthesiology
Washington University School of Medicine
St. Louis, Missouri
Adrenal Insufficiency, Acute or Secondary

Andrew P. Harris, MD, MHS

Associate Professor
Department of Anesthesiology and Critical
Care Medicine
Johns Hopkins University
School of Medicine
Baltimore, Maryland
Cesarean Section, Planned

Jonathan Hastie

Fellow
Department of Anesthesiology
Columbia University
New York City, New York
Lung Transplantation

Henry A. Hawney, MD

Chief Resident
Department of Anesthesiology
Tulane University
New Orleans, Louisiana
Chloramphenicol (Chloromycetin)

Stephen O. Heard, MD

Chairman
Department of Anesthesiology
Professor of Anesthesiology and Surgery
University of Massachusetts
Medical School
Worcester, Massachusetts
TMJ Arthroscopy

James E. Heavner, DVM, PhD

Professor
Department of Anesthesiology and Cell
Physiology and Molecular Biophysics
Director
Department of Anesthesia and Pain
Research
Texas Tech University Health Sciences
Center
Lubbock, Texas
Dibucaine Number (Atypical Cholinesterase)

James G. Hecker, PhD, MD

Assistant Professor
Department of Anesthesia and
Critical Care
University of Pennsylvania
Philadelphia, Pennsylvania
Neuroprotection

Elizabeth A. Hein, MD

Assistant Professor
Departments of Anesthesia and Clinical
Pediatrics
Cincinnati Children's Hospital Medical
Center
Cincinnati, Ohio
Cleft Palate Repair

Eugenie Heitmiller, MD

Associate Professor
Vice Chairman for Clinical Affairs
Department of Anesthesiology and Critical
Care Medicine
Johns Hopkins School of Medicine
Baltimore, Maryland
Patent Ductus Arteriosus (PDA), Ligation of

Mark Helfaer, MD

Professor Anesthesiology and Critical Care
Pediatrics and Nursing
University of Pennsylvania
Philadelphia, Pennsylvania
Friedreich's Ataxia

Lori B. Heller, MD

Medical Director
Swedish Blood Management Program

Department of Anesthesiology
Division of Cardiac Anesthesia
Clinical Instructor
University of Washington
Seattle, Washington
Atorvastatin (Lipitor)
Pseudoephedrine

Andrew Hemphill, PhD

Associate Professor
Institute of Parasitology
Vetsuisse Faculty
University of Berne
Berne, Switzerland
Echinococcosis

Adrian Hendrickse, BM, FRCA

Assistant Professor
Department of Anesthesiology
University of Colorado Denver
Aurora, Colorado
*Disseminated Intravascular Coagulation
(DIC)*
Liver Resection

Frederick A. Hensley, Jr., MD

Vice Chair and Director
Division of Cardiothoracic
Anesthesiology
Benjamin Monroe Carraway Professor
Department of Anesthesiology
University of Alabama at Birmingham
Birmingham, Alabama
Atrial Septal Defect, Ostium Secundum

Ian A. Herrick, MD, FRCPC

Associate Professor of Anesthesiology and
Clinical Pharmacology
University of Western Ontario
London, Ontario, Canada
Occlusive Cerebrovascular Disease

Douglas Hester, MD

Assistant Professor
Department of Anesthesiology
Vanderbilt University Medical Center
Nashville, Tennessee
Cervical Spine Fusion

Eric J. Heyer, MD, PhD

Professor of Clinical Anesthesiology
and Clinical Neurology
Department of Anesthesiology
Columbia University
New York, New York
*Cerebrovascular Transient Ischemic
Attack (TIA)*

Michael S. Higgins, MD, MPH

Professor of Anesthesiology, Surgery,
and Biomedical Informatics
Department of Anesthesiology
Vanderbilt University
Nashville, Tennessee
Ileostomy

Roberta Hines, MD

Nicholas M. Greene Professor
Department of Anesthesiology
Yale University School of Medicine
New Haven, Connecticut
Lesch-Nyhan Syndrome
Opitz-Frias Syndrome (The G Syndrome)

Charles W. Hogue, Jr. MD

Professor of Anesthesiology and Critical
Care Medicine
Chief
Division of Adult Anesthesia
Johns Hopkins University School of Medicine
Johns Hopkins Hospital
Baltimore, Maryland
Atrial Flutter
Atrial Septal Defect, Repair of
Chagas' Disease

Kenneth J. Holroyd, MD, MBA

Assistant Vice Chancellor for Research
Associate Professor of Anesthesiology
and Medicine
Vanderbilt University School of Medicine
Nashville, Tennessee
Amyloidosis

Natalie F. Holt, MD, MPH

Assistant Professor
Department of Anesthesiology
Yale University School of Medicine
New Haven, Connecticut;
Attending Physician
Department of Anesthesiology
VA Connecticut Healthcare System
West Haven, Connecticut
Diabetes Insipidus

Simon J. Howell, FRCA, MD

Senior Lecturer in Anaesthesia
Section of Translational Anaesthetic
Surgical Sciences
University of Leeds
Leeds, Great Britain
Hypertension

Faisal Huda, MD

Resident
Department of Anesthesiology
University of Miami
Jackson Memorial Hospital
Miami, Florida
Amphetamines

Keith E. Hude, MD

Department of Anesthesiology
Tulane University School of Medicine
New Orleans, Louisiana
Glycine

Hayden R. Hughes, JD, MD

Assistant Professor
Department of Anesthesia
University of Alabama at Birmingham
Birmingham, Alabama
Anemia, Chronic Disease/Inflammation

James M. Hunter, Jr., MD

Assistant Professor of Anesthesiology
and Surgery
Department of Anesthesiology
University of Alabama at Birmingham
Birmingham, Alabama
Hypernatremia

Brad J. Hymel, MD

Resident
Louisiana State University Health Sciences
Center Anesthesiology

Louisiana State University Health Sciences
Center- New Orleans
New Orleans, Louisiana
Shy-Drager Disease

James W. Ibinson, MD, PhD

Resident
Department of Anesthesiology
University of Pittsburgh
Pittsburgh, Pennsylvania
Glaucoma, Open-Angle

Karen E. Iles, PhD

Assistant Professor
Department of Anesthesiology
University of Alabama at
Birmingham
Birmingham, Alabama
Folic Acid

Robert M. Insoft, MD

NICU Medical Director
Newborn Medicine
Brigham and Women's Hospital
Boston, Massachusetts
Necrotizing Enterocolitis

Shiroh Isono, MD

Associate Professor
Department of Anesthesiology
Graduate School of Medicine
Chiba University
Chiba, Japan
Swallowing Disorders

Yulia Ivashkov, MD

Assistant Professor
Department of Anesthesiology
University of Washington
Harborview Medical Center
Seattle, Washington
Asthma Drugs, New

Bozena R. Jachna, MD

Instructor, Harvard Medical School
Department of Anesthesia, Critical Care
and Perioperative Medicine
Beth Israel Deaconess Medical Center
Boston, Massachusetts
Phenytoin

Anna Jankowska, MD

Anesthesiologist
Langone Medical Center
New York, New York
Thalassemia

Norah Janosy, MD

Assistant Professor
of Anesthesiology
University of Colorado
School of Medicine
Children's Hospital
Aurora, Colorado
Tetralogy of Fallot (TOF)
Tetralogy of Fallot (TOF), Correction of

Arun L. Jayaraman, MD, PhD

Resident
Department of Anesthesiology
University of Pittsburgh
Pittsburgh, Pennsylvania
Kidney Transplantation

Nathalia Jimenez, MD, MPH

Acting Assistant Professor
Department of Anesthesiology and Pain
Medicine
Seattle Children's Hospital
University of Washington
School of Medicine
Seattle, Washington
Muscle Biopsy for Undiagnosed Myopathy

Judy G. Johnson, MD

Assistant Professor and Program Director
Department of Anesthesiology
Louisiana State University
Health Sciences Center
New Orleans, Louisiana
Atropine

Lyndia Jones, MD

Assistant Professor
Department of Anesthesiology
Tulane University
New Orleans, Louisiana
Urticaria, Cold

Edmund H. Jooste, MB, ChB

Assistant Professor
Children's Hospital of Pittsburgh
University of Pittsburgh
Pittsburgh, Pennsylvania
Coarctation of the Aorta

Zeev N. Kain, MD, MBA

Professor of Anesthesiology and Pediatrics
and Psychiatry
Chair,
Department of Anesthesiology and
Perioperative Care
Associate Dean for Clinical Operations
University of California, Irvine
Irvine, California
Cocaine
Neurofibromatosis (NF)

Maudy Kalangie, DO

Cardiac Anesthesiology Fellow
Department of Anesthesiology
University of Maryland
Baltimore, Maryland
Off Pump and Minimally Invasive Cardiac Procedures

Philip L. Kalarickal, MD, MPH

Clinical Assistant Professor
Department of Anesthesiology
Tulane University School of Medicine
New Orleans, Louisiana
Tranexamic Acid

Ihab Kamel, MD

Assistant Professor
Department of Anesthesiology
Temple University
Philadelphia, Pennsylvania
Pregnant Surgical Patient
Spinal Fusion

Mia Kang, MD, MHS

Assistant Professor of Anesthesiology
Department of Anesthesiology
University of North Carolina
Chapel Hill, North Carolina
*Procainamide (Procan, Procanabid,
Pronestyl)*

Ivan Kangrga, MD, PhD

Associate Professor
Department of Anesthesiology
Washington University School of Medicine
St. Louis, Missouri
  Carotid Endarterectomy
  Abdominal Aortic Aneurysm Repair

Ravish Kapoor, MD

Resident
Department of Anesthesiology
Penn State Milton S. Hershey Medical
Center
Hershey, Pennsylvania
  Blue Cohosh (Caulophyllum Thalictroides)

Helen W. Karl, MD

Associate Professor of Anesthesiology
Department of Anesthesiology
and Pain Medicine
University of Washington School of Medicine;
Attending Anesthesiologist
Department of Anesthesiology and Pain
Medicine
Seattle Children's Hospital
Seattle, Washington
  Tonsillectomy and Adenoidectomy

Christopher Karsanac, MD

Assistant Professor
Pediatrics and Anesthesiology
Monroe Carell Jr. Children's Hospital
at Vanderbilt
Nashville, Tennessee
  Liver Transplantation, Pediatric

Swaminathan Karthik, MD

Instructor, Harvard Medical School
Department of Anesthesia,
Critical Care and Pain Medicine,
Beth Israel Deaconess Medical Center
Boston, Massachusetts
  Digitalis (Digoxin)
  Ginseng
  Lung Volume Reduction Surgery (LVRS)

Jeffrey A. Katz

Professor of Clinical Anesthesia
Department of Anesthesia
and Perioperative Care
University of California, San Francisco
San Francisco, California
  Pemphigus

Alan Kaye, MD, PhD

Professor and Chair
Department of Anesthesiology
Professor Department of Pharmacology
LSU School of Medicine
New Orleans, Louisiana
  Androstenedione
  β-Sitosterol
  Cerebral Palsy
  Dehydroepiandrosterone (DHEA)
  Fish Oil
  Headache, Migraine
  Hepatitis, Alcoholic
  Hypertension, Uncontrolled with Cardiomyopathy
  Hyponatremia
  Hypopituitarism
  Lipidemias
  Lithium Carbonate (Lithobid)
  Multiple Myeloma
  Myotonia Dystrophica (Myotonic Dystrophy, Steinert's Disease)
  Nutraceuticals
  Nutritional Support
  S-Adenosyl-L-Methionine (SAMe)
  Tetracyclines
  Tissue Plasminogen Activator

Adam M. Kaye, PharmD, FASCP, FCPhA

Associate Clinical Professor
Department of Pharmacy Practice
Thomas J. Long School of Pharmacy and
Health Sciences
University of the Pacific
Stockton, California
  Androstenedione
  β-Sitosterol
  S-Adenosyl-L-Methionine (SAMe)
  Red Yeast Rice (Cholestin)
  Tranexamic Acid

A. Murat Kaynar, MD

Assistant Professor
Critical Care Medicine;
Assistant Professor
Department of Anesthesiology
University of Pittsburgh, School of Medicine
Pittsburgh, Pennsylvania
  Necrotizing Fasciitis

Nancy B. Kenepp, MD

Clinical Associate Professor
Department of Anesthesiology
Temple University School of Medicine
Philadelphia, Pennsylvania
  Epidermolysis Bullosa

Miklos D. Kertai, MD, PhD

Instructor in Anesthesiology
Department of Anesthesiology
Washington University School of Medicine
St. Louis, Missouri
  Congestive Heart Failure

Mary A. Keyes, MD

Clinical Professor of Anesthesiology
Department of Anesthesiology
David Geffen School of Medicine
University of California–Los Angeles
Los Angeles, California
  Bronchiopulmonary Dysplasia
  Reye's Syndrome

Sarah Khan, MBBS

Assistant Professor
Department of Anesthesiology
Yale University School of Medicine
New Haven, Connecticut
  Atrial Septal Defect, Ostium Primum

Swapnil Khoche, MD

Senior Resident
Department of Anesthesiology
Temple University Hospital
Philadelphia, Pennsylvania
  Hypercholesterolemia

David Y. Kim, MD

Associate Professor
Department of Anesthesiology
Temple University
Philadelphia, Pennsylvania
  Complement Deficiency

Jerry H. Kim, MD

Acting Instructor
Department of Anesthesiology
and Pain Medicine
University of Washington;
Acting Instructor
Department of Anesthesiology
and Pain Medicine
Seattle Children's Hospital
Seattle, Washington
  Mitochondrial Myopathy

Kimberly M. King, MD

Department of Anesthesiology
Johns Hopkins University
School of Medicine
Baltimore, Maryland
  Dandelion

Jeffrey Kirsch, MD

Professor and Chair
Department of Anesthesiology
and Perioperative
Oregon Health and Science University
Associate Dean for Veterans and Clinical
Affairs
Portland, Oregon
  Vitamin K Deficiency

Matthew A. Klopman, MD

Assistant Professor
Division of Cardiothoracic
Anesthesiology
Department of Anesthesiology
Emory University School of Medicine
Atlanta, Georgia
  Aortic Valve Replacement

Paul R. Knight III, MD, PhD

Professor of Anesthesiology and
Microbiology and Immunology
Executive Vice Chair for Research
Department of Anesthesiology
Director
Medical Scientist Training Program
University at Buffalo
State University of New York and VA
Medical Center
Buffalo, New York
  IgA Deficiency
  Immune Suppression
  Q Fever
  Rocky Mountain Spotted Fever

Donald D. Koblin, MD, PhD

Staff Anesthesiologist
Anesthesiology Service
Department of Veterans Affairs Medical
Center
San Francisco, California
  Vitamin B$_{12}$/Folate Deficiency
  Fluoxetine (Prozac)
  Haloperidol (Haldol)

W. Andrew Kofke, MD, MBA, FCCM

Professor
Director of Neuroanesthesia
Co-Director Neurocritical Care
Departments of Anesthesia
and Neurosurgery
University of Pennsylvania
Philadelphia, Pennsylvania
  Seizures, Epileptic

Vincent J. Kopp, MD

Associate Professor
Department of Anesthesiology
School of Medicine
University of North Carolina at Chapel Hill
Chapel Hill, North Carolina
Otitis Media

Joseph R. Koveleskie, MD

Clinical Assistant Professor
Department of Anesthesiology
Tulane University Medical Center
New Orleans, Louisiana
Chloramphenicol (Chloromycetin)

Valeriy V. Kozmenko

Assistant Professor of Clinical
Anesthesiology
Department of Anesthesiology
Louisiana State University
Health Sciences Center
New Orleans, Louisiana
*Hypertension, Uncontrolled with
Cardiomyopathy*

Kaylyn Krummen, MD

Pediatric Anesthesiology Fellow
Pediatric Anesthesiology
Children's Hospital
Aurora, Colorado
Asthma, Acute

Sapna R. Kudchadkar, MD

Clinical Fellow
Department of Anesthesiology
and Critical Care Medicine
Johns Hopkins University
Baltimore, Maryland
Subclavian Steal Syndrome

Nathan Kudrick, MD

Assistant Professor
Department of Anesthesiology and
Perioperative Care
University of California Irvine
Orange, California
Rheumatoid Arthritis

Adrienne Kung, MD

Instructor, Harvard Medical School
Department of Anesthesia,
Critical Care and Pain Medicine
Beth Israel Deaconess Medical Center
Boston, Massachusetts
Vaginal Delivery, Normal

C. Dean Kurth, MD,

Anesthesiologist-in-Chief
Department of Anesthesia
Cincinnati Children's Hospital Medical Center
Cincinnati, Ohio
Cleft Palate Repair

Robert Kyle, DO

Associate Professor
Department of Anesthesiology
University of North Carolina
at Chapel Hill
Chapel Hill, North Carolina
*V/Q Scan (Nuclear Ventilation-Perfusion
Scintigraphy)*

J. Lance LaFleur, MD, MBA

Department of Anesthesiology
University of Texas Medical School
at Houston
Houston, Texas
*Monoamine Oxidase Inhibitors; Reversible
Inhibitors of Monoamine Oxidase
Pyridostigmine Bromide*

Jason G. Lai, MD

Chief Resident
Department of Anesthesiology
University of Maryland School
of Medicine
Baltimore, Maryland
Tubal Ligation

Kirk Lalwani, MD, FRCA, MCR

Associate Professor of Anesthesiology
and Pediatrics
Department of Anesthesiology
and Perioperative Medicine
Oregon Health and Science University
Portland, Oregon
*Anemia, Hemolytic
Echinacea (American Coneflower, Purple
Coneflower: E. Angustifolia, E. Purpurea,
E. Pallida)
Tetanus*

William L. Lanier, MD

Professor of Anesthesiology
Mayo Clinic College of Medicine
Rochester, Minnesota
Hyperglycemia

Dawn M. Larson, MD

Fellow
Oregon Health and Science University
Portland, Oregon
Mitral Valve Replacement

Richard M. Layman, MD

Assistant Professor
Department of Anesthesiology
University of Texas Medical School
at Houston
Houston, Texas
*Soy
Hypertriglyceridemia
Valerian (valeriana officinalis)*

Chris C. Lee, MD, PhD

Assistant Professor
Department of Anesthesiology
Washington University School of Medicine
St. Louis, Missouri
*Scoliosis and Kyphosis
Scoliosis and Kyphosis Surgery*

Mark J. Lema, MD, PhD

Professor and Chair
Department of Anesthesiology
University at Buffalo, SUNY;
Professor of Anesthesiology and
Oncology
Chair
Department of Anesthesiology
Roswell Park Cancer Institute
Buffalo, New York
*Alkylating Agents
Bleomycin*

W. Casey Lenox, MD

Department of Anesthesiology
Phoenix Children's Hospital
Phoenix, Arizona
Orchiopexy

Jacqueline M. Leung, MD, MPH

Professor
Department of Anesthesia
and Perioperative Care
University of California, San Francisco
San Francisco, California
*Atherosclerotic Disease
Peripheral Vascular Disease*

Roy C. Levitt, MD

Clinical Professor
Director of Translational Research and
Academic Affairs
Department of Anesthesiology
University of Miami
Miami Veterans Healthcare Center
Miami, Florida
Bronchiolitis Obliterans Syndrome

Jerrold H. Levy, MD, FAHA

Professor and Deputy Chair for Research
Department of Anesthesiology
Emory University School of Medicine
Atlanta, Georgia
*Allergy
Anticoagulation, Preoperative*

J. Lance Lichtor, MD

Professor
Departments of Anesthesiology
and Pediatrics
University of Massachusetts
Medical School
Worcester, Massachusetts
Pyloric Stenosis Repair

Charles Lin, MD

Resident
Department of Anesthesiology
University of Pittsburgh Medical Center
Pittsburgh, Pennsylvania
Hysterectomy, Vaginal

Sharon L. Lin, MD

Assistant Clinical Professor
Department of Anesthesiology
and Perioperative Care
University of California
Irvine School of Medicine
Orange, California
*Schizophrenia
Systemic Lupus Erythematosus cocaine*

Karen S. Lindeman, MD

Associate Professor
Department of Anesthesiology
Johns Hopkins University
Baltimore, Maryland
Placenta Previa

Lesley Lirette, BS, MD

Resident
Department of Anesthesiology
Tulane University School of Medicine
New Orleans, Louisiana
Urticaria, Cold

Ronald S. Litman, DO

Professor of Anesthesiology and Pediatrics
University of Pennsylvania School of
Medicine
Anesthesiology and Critical Care
Children's Hospital of Philadelphia,
Philadelphia, Pennsylvania
Imperforate Anus Repair
Strabismus Repair
Thalassemia
Testicular Torsion Surgery
Kuppel-Feil syndrome

Qianjin Liu, MD, PhD

Assistant Professor
Department of Anesthesiology
Washington University School of Medicine
St. Louis, Missouri
Abdominal Aortic Aneurysm Repair

Renyu Liu, MD, PhD

Assistant Professor
Director of Preoperative Medicine
Department of Anesthesiology
and Critical Care
University of Pennsylvania
Philadelphia, Pennsylvania
Carnitine

Wen-Shin Liu, MD

Professor
Department of Anesthesiology
Northeastern Ohio University
College of Medicine
Rootstown, Ohio
Cancer, Prostate

Justin Lockman, MD

Department of Anesthesiology and Critical
Care Medicine
Johns Hopkins School of Medicine
Baltimore, Maryland
Patent Ductus Arteriosus (PDA), Ligation of

Stanley L. Loftness, MD

Pediatric Anesthesiologist
Department of Anesthesia
University of Colorado
Health Sciences Center
Aurora, Colorado
Myringotomy and Tympanostomy

Martin J. London, MD

Professor of Clinical Anesthesia
Department of Anesthesia
and Perioperative Care
University of California, San Francisco
San Francisco, California
Diagnostic 12-Lead ECG

Philip D. Lumb, MB, BS, FCCM

Professor and Chairman
Department of Anesthesiology
Keck School of Medicine of the University
of Southern California
Los Angeles, California
Lyme Disease

M. Concetta Lupa

Assistant Professor of Anesthesiology
University of North Carolina
Chapel Hill, North Carolina
Hypercalcemia

Anne Marie Lynn, MD

Professor
Department of Anesthesiology and Pain
Medicine and Pediatrics (adj.)
University of Washington School of
Medicine
Seattle Children's Hospital
Seattle, Washington
*Jeune Syndrome (Asphyxiating Thoracic
Dystrophy)*

Devi Mahendran, MD

Department of Anesthesia,
Critical Care and Pain Medicine
Beth Israel Deaconess Medical Center
Boston, Massachusetts
Ginseng

Jeffrey Mako, MD

Resident
Department of Anesthesiology and
Perioperative Medicine
Oregon Health and Science University
Portland, Oregon
Acidosis, Lactic/Metabolic

Anuj Malhotra, MD

Clinical research Fellow
Department of Anesthesia
and Critical Care
University of California, San Francisco
San Francisco, California
Nephrectomy/Radical Nephrectomy

Vinod Malhotra, MD

Professor of Clinical Anesthesiology
Professor of Anesthesiology in Clinical
Urology
Weill Medical College
of Cornell University;
Vice Chair for Clinical Affairs
Department of Anesthesiology and Clinical
Director of Operating Rooms
New York Presbyterian Hospital- Weill
Cornell Medical Center, New York
New York, New York
Nephrectomy/Radical Nephrectomy

Andrew M. Malinow, MD

Professor of Anesthesiology
and Obstetrics,
Gynecology and Reproductive Sciences
Director - Obstetric Anesthesiology
Vice Chair - Academic Affairs
Department of Anesthesiology
University of Maryland
School of Medicine
Baltimore, Maryland
Preeclampsia
Tubal Ligation

Mark G. Mandabach, MD

Assistant Professor
Department of Anesthesiology
University of Alabama at Birmingham
School of Medicine
Birmingham, Alabama
Hepatitis, Halothane

Dennis T. Mangano, MD, PhD

Director and Founder, McSPI Research
Group, San Francisco, California
Myocardial Ischemia (MIsch)

Sobia Mansoor, MBBS

Fellow
Department of Anesthesia
Children's Hospital of Pittsburgh
Pittsburgh, Pennsylvania
Hirschsprung's Disease

Inna Maranets, MD

Attending Anesthesiologist
Woodland Anesthesia Associates, PC.
Hartford, Connecticut
Eisenmenger's Syndrome
Pyloric Stenosis
Treacher Collins Syndrome

Jonathan B. Mark, MD

Professor of Anesthesiology
Duke University;
Chief
Anesthesiology Service
Veterans Affairs Medical Center
Durham, North Carolina
Cardiomyopathy, Ischemic

Sinisa Markovic, MD

Clinical Assistant Professor of
Anesthesiology University at Buffalo
Attending Anesthesiologist Buffalo Veterans
Administration HospitalBuffalo, New York
Rocky Mountain Spotted Fever

H. Michael Marsh, MB, BS, BSc(Med)

Professor and Chair
Department of Anesthesiology
Wayne State University
Detroit, Michigan
Bronchiectasis
Methemoglobinemia

Choendal Martin, MD

Instructor
Department of Anesthesiology
Washington University School of Medicine
St. Louis, Missouri
Scoliosis and Kyphosis

Nicole D. Martin, BSCHM, MD

Resident
Department of Anesthesiology
University of Miami/Jackson Memorial
Hospital
Miami, Florida
Hormone Replacement Therapy (HRT)

Douglas Martz, MD

Associate Professor of Anesthesiology
University of Maryland School of Medicine
Baltimore, Maryland
Narcolepsy

Veronica A. Matei, MD

Clinical Fellow of Cardiothoracic
Anesthesia
Department of Anesthesiology
Yale New Haven Hospital
New Haven, Connecticut
Cardiopulmonary Bypass (CPB)

Letha Mathews, MBBS, FFARCS(I)

Associate Professor
Department of Anesthesiology
Vanderbilt University
Nashville, Tennessee
Craniotomy, Awake

Lynne G. Maxwell, MD

Associate Professor of Anesthesiology
and Critical Care
University of Pennsylvania;
Senior Anesthesiologist
The Children's Hospital of Philadelphia
Philadelphia, Pennsylvania
Duodenal Atresia

Philip McArdle, MB, BCh, BAO, FFARCSI

Associate Professor
Department of Anesthesiology
University of Alabama at Birmingham
Birmingham, Alabama
Hepatic Encephalopathy (HE)

John P. McCarren, MD, MBA

Clinical Professor of Anesthesiology
Medical Director of Perioperative
Services
Thornton Hospital
University of California, San Diego
San Diego, California
Cancer, Bronchial

Brenda C. McClain, MD

Associate Professor
Department of Anesthesiology
Adjunct Associate Professor
Pediatrics
Yale University School of Medicine;
Director of Pediatric Pain Management
Services
Department of Anesthesiology
Yale University School of Medicine
New Haven, Connecticut
Cleft Palate

Brian McClure, BS, MD

Clinical Assistant Professor
Department of Anesthesiology
Tulane University Hospital and Clinic
New Orleans, Louisiana
Quinidine

William A. McDade, MD, PhD

Associate Professor of Anesthesia
and Critical Care
Associate Dean for Multicultural Affairs
University of Chicago Pritzker
School of Medicine
Chicago, Illinois
Sickle Cell Disease

Kathryn E. McGoldrick, MD

Professor and Chairman
Department of Anesthesiology
New York Medical College;
Director
Department of Anesthesiology
Westchester Medical Center
Valhalla, New York
Blowout Orbital Fracture
Cataract ± Iol

Brian J. McGrath, MD, MPH

Associate Vice President for Faculty
and Educational Resources
George Washington University Medical Center;
Associate Professor of Anesthesiology
and Critical Care Medicine
George Washington University
School of Medicine and Health Sciences
Washington, DC
Fat Embolism

Gregory L. McHugh, MD

Resident
Department of Anesthesiology
University of Pittsburgh Medical Center
Pittsburgh, Pennsylvania
Ureteral Stent Placement

David McIlroy, MD, MClinEpi, FANZCA

Assistant Professor
Department of Anesthesiology
Columbia University College of Physicians
and Surgeons
New York, New York
Lung Transplantation

Jason McKeown, MD

Assistant Professor
Department of Anesthesiology
University of Alabama School of Medicine
Birmingham, Alabama
Capsaicin

Thomas M. McLoughlin, Jr., MD

Associate Chief Medical Officer, Chair
Department of Anesthesiology
Lehigh Valley Health Network
Allentown, Pennsylvania;
Professor of Surgery
Division of Surgical Anesthesiology
University of South Florida College of Medicine
Tampa, Florida
Coagulopathy, Factor IX Deficiency
von Willebrand's Disease

R. Yan McRae, MD

Staff Anesthesiologist
Portland Veterans Affairs Medical Center;
Assistant Professor
Department of Anesthesiology
and Perioperative Medicine
Oregon Health and Science University
Portland, Oregon
Bypass Graft Procedure, Infrainguinal

William L. Meadow, MD, PhD

Department of Pediatrics
The University of Chicago
Chicago, Illinois
Apnea of the Newborn

Sameer Menda, MD

Resident Physician
Department of Anesthesiology
Oregon Health and Science University
Portland, Oregon
Vitamin K Deficiency

William T. Merritt, MD

Associate Professor
Department of Anesthesiology
and Critical Care Medicine
Johns Hopkins Medicine

Baltimore, Maryland
Jaundice

David G. Metro, MD

Associate Professor
Department of Anesthesiology
University of Pittsburgh School of Medicine
Pittsburgh, Pennsylvania
AV and Bifascicular Heart Block

Berend Mets, MB, ChB, PhD, FRCA, FFASA

Eric A. Walker Professor and Chair
of Anesthesiology
Penn State Milton S. Hershey Medical
Center
Hershey, Pennsylvania
Blue Cohosh (Caulophyllum Thalictroides)

Hosni Mikhaeil, MD

Assistant Professor
Department of Anesthesiology
Yale New Haven Hospital
New Haven, Connecticut
Labor, Epidural Block

David W. Miller, MD

Assistant Professor
Department of Anesthesiology
University of Alabama at Birmingham
Birmingham, Alabama
Abdominoperineal Resection
Folic Acid
Gastrectomy

Jessica Miller, MD

Assistant Professor
Department of Anesthesiology
and Peri-operative Medicine
Oregon Health and Science University
Portland, Oregon
Physiologic Anemia and the Anemia of Prematurity
Preterm Infant

Mohammed Minhaj, MD

Assistant Professor
Associate Chair for Residency Education
Department of Anesthesia
and Critical Care
University of Chicago Medical Center
Chicago, Illinois
Amniotic Fluid Embolism
Terbutaline

Marek A. Mirski, MD, PhD

Professor and Vice-Chair
Department of Anesthesiology
and Critical Care Medicine
Professor
Department of Neurosurgery
Professor
Department of Neurology
Johns Hopkins Medicine
Baltimore, Maryland
Seizures, Grand Mal (Tonic-Clonic)
Seizures, Petit Mal (Absence)

Nanhi Mitter, MD

Assistant Professor
Department of Anesthesiology
and Critical Care Medicine
Johns Hopkins Hospital
Baltimore, Maryland
Chagas' Disease

CONTRIBUTORS

Alexander J.C. Mittnacht, MD

Associate Professor Anesthesiology
Mount Sinai Medical Center
New York, New York
Ventricular Septal Defect (Congenital)

Raj K. Modak, MD

Department of Anesthesiology
Yale University School of Medicine
New Haven, Connecticut
Mitral Regurgitation
Pertussis (Whooping Cough)

Pierre Moine, MD

Associate Professor
Department of Anesthesiology
University of Colorado Denver
Aurora, Colorado
Cryptococcus Infection
Diphtheria

Constance L. Monitto, MD

Assistant Professor
Department of Anesthesiology and Critical
Care Medicine
Johns Hopkins University
Baltimore, Maryland
Ureteral Reimplantation

Richard C. Month, MD

Instructor in Anesthesia
Hospital of the University of Pennsylvania
Philadelphia, Pennsylvania
Labor, Peripheral Blocks

**Richard E. Moon, MD, CM, FRCPC,
FACP, FCCP**

Professor of Anesthesiology
Professor of Medicine
Medical Director
Center for Hyperbaric Medicine and
Environmental Physiology
Duke University Medical Center
Durham, North Carolina
Gas Embolism

Laurel E. Moore, MD

Clinical Assistant Professor
Department of Anesthesiology
University of Michigan
Ann Arbor, Michigan
Anterior Cervical Discectomy and Fusion (ACDF)
Electroconvulsive Therapy (ECT)

Roger A. Moore, MD

Chair Emeritus
Department of Anesthesiology
Deborah Heart and Lung Center
Browns Mills, New Jersey
Anomalous Pulmonary Venous Drainage
Cancer, Lung Parenchyma

Thomas A. Moore, II, MD

Professor of Anesthesiology and Neurosurgery
Department of Anesthesiology
University of Alabama School of Medicine
Birmingham, Alabama
Ventriculoperitoneal Shunt

Debra E. Morrison, MD

HS Clinical Professor
Director of Neonatal and Pediatric Anesthesia

Anesthesiology and Perioperative Care
Medical Director for Sedation
UC Irvine Medical Center:
University of California Irvine
Orange, California
Botulism

Jonathan Moss, MD, PhD

Professor of Anesthesia and Critical Care
University of Chicago
Chicago, Illinois
Anaphylaxis

John R. Moyers, MD

Professor
Department of Anesthesia
Carver College of Medicine
University of Iowa
Iowa City, Iowa
Mesothelioma

Jesse J. Muir, MD

Consultant Anesthesiologist
Assistant Professor
Department of Anesthesiology
Mayo Clinic Arizona
Phoenix, Arizona
Insulinoma

Adam J. Munson-Young, MD

Department of Anesthesiology
University of Pittsburgh School of Medicine
Pittsburgh, Pennsylvania
Pancreas Transplantation

Stanley Muravchick, MD, PhD

Professor of Anesthesiology
and Critical Care
Department of Anesthesiology
Hospital of the University of Pennsylvania
Philadelphia, Pennsylvania
Geriatric Surgery

John M. Murkin, MD, FRCPC

Professor of Anesthesiology
Department of Anesthesiology
and Perioperative Medicine
Director of Cardiac Anesthesiology
Research
Schulich School of Medicine
University of Western Ontario
London, Ontario, Canada
Thyroid Supplements

Peter Nagele, MD, MSc

Assistant Professor
Department of Anesthesiology
Washington University School of Medicine
St. Louis, Missouri;
Associate Professor
Department of Anesthesiology and General
Critical Care
Medical University of Vienna
Vienna, Austria
Trauma

Peter A. Nagi, MD

Assistant Professor of Anesthesiology
and Pain Medicine
Department of Anesthesiology and Critical
Care
University of Alabama at Birmingham,
Birmingham, Alabama
Urinary Lithiasis

Daniel A. Nahrwold, MD

Critical Care Fellow
Department of Anesthesia and Perioperative
Care
University of California
San Francisco, California
Hyperparathyroidism

Michael L. Nahrwold, MD

Adjunct Professor
Department of Anesthesiology
Vanderbilt University School of Medicine
Nashville, Tennessee
Hyperparathyroidism

Madhavi Naik, MBBS, MD, DA, FFARCS

Assistant Professor
Department of Anesthesiology
University of Maryland Medical Center
Baltimore, Maryland
Laparoscopic Adrenalectomy

Manchula Navaratnam, MBBS, FRCA

Instructor
Pediatric Anesthesia
Stanford University Medical Center
Stanford, California
Truncus Arteriosus

Stephan P. Nebbia, MD

Clinical Assistant Professor of
Anesthesiology
State University of New York at Buffalo
School of Medicine and Biomedical Sciences
Buffalo, New York
Sarcoma

Priscilla Nelson, MD

Department of Anesthesiology and Critical Care
University of Pennsylvania School
of Medicine
Philadelphia, Pennsylvania
Bicarbonate Sodium

Thai T. Nguyen, MD, PhD

Assistant Professor
Department of Anesthesiology and Critical
Care Medicine
Johns Hopkins University
Baltimore, Maryland
ACE Inhibitors

Viet Nguyen, MD

Resident
Department of Anesthesiology
Louisiana State University-New Orleans
School of Medicine
New Orleans, Louisiana
Lithium Carbonate (Lithobid)

Stavroula Nikolaidis, MD

Assistant Professor
Department of Anesthesiology
Temple University Hospital
Philadelphia, Pennsylvania
Cardiomyopathy, Hypertrophic (HCM)

Zoulfira Nisnevitch, MD

Assistant Professor
Department of Anesthesiology
University of Medicine and Dentistry
of New Jersey
Newark, New Jersey
Bleomycin Sulfate Toxicity

Dolores B. Njoku, MD

Associate Professor
Department of Anesthesiology and Critical
Care Medicine,
Pediatrics and Pathology
Johns Hopkins University
Baltimore, Maryland
Subclavian Steal Syndrome

Mary J. Njoku, MD

Associate Professor
Department of Anesthesiology
University of Maryland School of Medicine
Baltimore, Maryland
Encephalitis

Edward J. Norris, MD, MBA, FAHA

Clinical Professor and Vice Chairman
Department of Anesthesiology
University of Maryland School of Medicine;
Director,
Department of Anesthesiology
Baltimore VA Medical Center
VA Maryland Health Care System;
Adjunct Faculty
Department of Anesthesiology
and Critical Care Medicine
Johns Hopkins University School of Medicine
Baltimore, Maryland
*Whipple Procedure (Pancreatico
Duodenectomy)*

Omonele O. Nwokolo, MD

Assistant Professor
Department of Anesthesiology
University of Texas
Houston, Texas
Purpura, Thrombotic Thrombocytopenic (TTP)

Daniel Nyhan, MD

Professor
Vice Chair
Department of Anesthesiology and Critical
Care Medicine, Cardiac Anesthesiology
Johns Hopkins University
Baltimore, Maryland
Single (Including Common) Ventricle

William T. O'Byrne, III, MD

Assistant Professor of Anesthesiology
Division of Critical Care
Vanderbilt University Medical Center
Nashville, Tennessee
Emphysema

Edward A. Ochroch, MD

Associate Professor of Anesthesiology and
Critical Care
Hospital of University of Pennsylvania
Philadelphia, Pennsylvania
Tracheal Resection

Andrew Oken, MD

Assistant Chief of Service
Department of Anesthesiology
Operative Care Division Portland VAMC
Portland, Oregon
Cardioversion

Nathan Orgain, MD

Chief Resident
Department of Anesthesiology

University of Utah
Salt Lake City, Utah
Cigarette Smoking Cessation

Nancy E. Oriol, MD

Associate Professor
Department of Anesthesia,
Critical Care and Pain Medicine
Beth Israel Deaconess Medical Center;
Dean for Students
Harvard Medical School
Boston, Massachusetts
Vaginal Delivery, Normal

Pedro Orozco, MD

Clinical Instructor
Department of Anesthesiology
University of California Irvine
Orange, California
Rheumatoid Arthritis

Andreas M. Ostermeier, MD

Physician, Clinic for Anesthesiology
University of Munich
Munich, Germany
Sleep Apnea, Central and Mixed

†Andranik Ovassapian, MD

Professor
Department of Anesthesia and Critical Care
University of Chicago
Chicago, Illinois
*Bronchoscopy, Fiberoptic
Bronchoscopy, Rigid
Laryngoscopy*

Mehmet S. Ozcan, MD, FCCP

Assistant Professor
Department of Anesthesiology
University of Illinois at Chicago
Chicago, Illinois
Hypomagnesemia

Ira Padnos, MD

Assistant Professor
Department of Anesthesiology
Louisiana State University School of Medicine
New Orleans, Louisiana
Lithium Carbonate (Lithobid)

Sheela S. Pai, MD

Assistant Professor
Department of Anesthesiology
Temple University School of Medicine
Philadelphia, Pennsylvania
*Atrial Fibrillation
Transfusion-Related Acute Lung Injury (TRALI)
Ventricular Fibrillation*

Nirvik Pal, MD

Clinical Instructor
Department of Anesthesiology
(Cardiothoracic Division)
Washington University in St Louis
St. Louis, Missouri
Pulmonary Atresia

Dhamodaran Palaniappan, MD

Resident
Department of Anesthesiology
Perioperative Medicine and Pain
Management
University of Miami
Miami, Florida
Retinal Buckle Surgery

Susan K. Palmer, MD

Anesthesiologist
Oregon Anesthesiology Group
McKenzie-Willamette Medical Center
Springfield, Oregon
Pregnancy-Induced Hypertension

Howard D. Palte, MD

Assistant Professor
Department of Anesthesiology
Perioperative Medicine and Pain
Management
Miller School of Medicine
University of Miami
Miami, Florida
Eye Enucleation

Wei Pan, MD

Assistant Professor
Division of Cardiovascular
Anesthesiology
Baylor College of Medicine
Houston, Texas
Ginger (Zingiber Officinale)

Oliver Panzer, MD

Assistant Professor
Department of Anesthesiology
and Critical Care
Columbia University Medical Center
New York, New York
Wolff-Parkinson-White (WPW) Syndrome

Sibi Pappachan, DO

Pediatric Anesthesiology Fellow
Department of Anesthesiology
Children's Hospital of Pittsburgh
Lawrenceville, Pennsylvania
Kasai Procedure

Anthony Passannante, MD

Professor and Vice-Chair for Clinical
Operations
Department of Anesthesiology
University of North Carolina Hospitals
Chapel Hill, North Carolina
Glucosamine Sulfate

Dennis A. Patel, MD

Research Associate
Department of Anesthesiology
Louisiana State University
Health Sciences Center
New Orleans, Louisiana
Fish Oil

Dilipkumar K. Patel, MD

Associate Professor
Department of Anesthesiology
Temple University
Philadelphia, Pennsylvania
*Hypercholesterolemia
Leukemia*

Kirit M. Patel, MD

Assistant Professor
Department of Anesthesiology
Medical Center of Louisiana at New Orleans
New Orleans, Louisiana
Amputation, Lower Extremity (LEA)

†Deceased

Samir Patel, MD

Assistant Professor
Department of Anesthesiology
University of Alabama at Birmingham
Birmingham, Alabama
Hypernatremia

Shalin Patel

Anesthesiology Resident
Hospital of the University of Pennsylvania
Philadelphia, Pennsylvania
*Syndrome of Inappropriate Antidiuretic Hormone
    Secretion (SIADH)*

Sanup Pathak

Senior Medical Student
Baylor College of Medicine
Houston, Texas
Ginger (Zingiber Officinale)

Minda L. Patt, MD

Chief Resident
Department of Anesthesiology
Jackson Memorial Hospital
Miami, Florida
Encephalopathy, Hypertensive

Ronald W. Pauldine, MD

Clinical Associate Professor
Department of Anesthesiology
and Pain Medicine
University of Washington
School of Medicine
Seattle, Washington
Esophagectomy

Olga Pawelek

Assistant Professor
University of Texas Houston
Health Science Center
Houston, Texas
Purpura, Immune Thrombocytopenic (ITP)

Tim Pawelek, MD

Resident
Department of Anesthesiology
University of Texas-Houston
Houston, Texas
Hypertriglyceridemia

Kiarash Paydar, MD

Resident
Department of Anesthesiology
University of Maryland School of Medicine
Baltimore, Maryland
Ginkgo

Ronald G. Pearl, MD, PhD

Dr. Richard K. and Erika N. Richards
Professor and Chair of Anesthesia
Stanford University School of Medicine
Stanford, California
Pulmonary Embolism

Christine Peeters-Asdourian, MD

Assistant Professor
Harvard Medical School
Director
Pain Fellowship
Department of Anesthesia,
Critical Care and Pain Medicine
Beth Israel Deaconess Medical Center
Boston, Massachusetts
Herniated Nucleus Pulposus

Padmavathi R. Perela, MD

Associate Professor of Anesthesiology
University at Buffalo
State University of New York and VA
Medical Center
Buffalo, New York
Immune Suppression

Charise T. Petrovitch, MD

Clinical Professor
Department of Anesthesiology
and Critical Care Medicine
George Washington University Hospital
Chief
Anesthesia Section
VA Medical Center
Washington, DC
Warfarin (Coumadin)

Patricia H. Petrozza, MD

Professor of Anesthesiology and
Associate Dean for Graduate Medical
Education
Department of Anesthesiology
Wake forest University School
of Medicine
Winston Salem, North Carolina
Brain Cortex Resection (for Epilepsy)

Dennis Phillips, DO

Associate Chief Resident
Department of Anesthesiology
University of Pittsburgh
Pittsburgh, Pennsylvania
AV and Bifascicular Heart Block

Mark C. Phillips, MD

Assistant Professor
Department of Anesthesiology
University of Alabama at Birmingham
School of Medicine
Birmingham, Alabama
Bowel Resection
Crohn's Disease

Christine Piefer, MD

Department of Anesthesiology
University of Alabama at Birmingham
School of Medicine
Birmingham, Alabama
Gastrinoma

Edgar J. Pierre, MD

Associate Professor of Anesthesiology
and Surgery
Department of Anesthesiology
University of Miami
Miami, Florida
Amphetamines
Aortic Stenosis
Gonorrhea
Hormone Replacement Therapy (HRT)
Respiratory Distress Syndrome

S. William Pinson, MD

Resident
Department of Anesthesiology
Mount Sinai School of Medicine
New York, New York
Jehovah's Witness Patient

Evan G. Pivalizza, MBChB, FFASA

Professor
Department of Anesthesiology
University of Texas Health Science Center
Houston, Texas
Purpura, Immune Thrombocytopenic (ITP)
*Purpura, Thrombotic Thrombocytopenic
    (TTP)*

Raymond M. Planinsic, MD

Associate Professor of Anesthesiology
University of Pittsburgh School
of Medicine
Director of Hepatic, Intestinal,
Kidney and Pancreas Transplantation
Anesthesiology
University of Pittsburgh Medical Center
Pittsburgh, Pennsylvania
Pancreas Transplantation

Don Poldermans, MD, PhD, FESC

Professor of Medicine
Departments of Anaesthesiology / Surgery
Erasmus Medical Center
Rotterdam, The Netherlands
Dobutamine Echocardiography

Joel M. Pomerantz, MD

Instructor
Department of Anesthesiology
University of Pittsburgh
Pittsburgh, Pennsylvania
Herpes, Type I

Jason E. Pope, MD

Staff
Pain Medicine
Anesthesia Institute
Cleveland Clinic
Cleveland, Ohio;
Assistant Professor
Department of Anesthesiology
Vanderbilt University Medical Center
Nashville, Tennessee
Acetaminophen

Wanda M. Popescu, MD

Assistant Professor of Anesthesiology
Director Thoracic Anesthesia Section
Co-Director Grand Rounds
Yale University School of Medicine
New Haven, Connecticut
Heart Transplant, Adult

Vivian H. Porche, MD

Professor of Anesthesiology
Department of Anesthesiology and
Perioperative Medicine
University of Texas M.D. Anderson Cancer
Center
Houston, Texas
Neuroradiology

Jahan Porhomayon, MD, FCCP

Director of Critical Care Medicine
Assistant Professor of Anesthesiology and
Surgery
University at Buffalo
State University of New York and VA
Medical Center
Buffalo, New York
IgA Deficiency

Dmitry Portnoy, MD

Associate Professor
Department of Anesthesiology
The University of Texas Medical School at Houston
Houston, Texas
Constipation
Cranberry
Ephedrine
Ventricular Preexcitation Syndrome

Corinne K. Postle, MD

Resident
Department of Anesthesiology
New York Presbyterian Hospital-Weill
Cornell Medical Center
New York, New York
Joint Replacement Cementing (Methyl Methacrylate Cementing)

Paul J. Primeaux

Clinical Assistant Professor,
Director of Liver Transplant Anesthesia
Department of Anesthesiology
Tulane University School of Medicine
New Orleans, Louisiana
Hyponatremia

Donald S. Prough, MD

Rebecca Terry White Distinguished
Professor and Chair of Anesthesiology
Department of Anesthesiology
University of Texas Medical Branch
Galveston, Texas
Renal Failure, Chronic

Ferenc Puskas, MD, PhD

Associate Professor
Department of Anesthesiology
University of Colorado Denver
Aurora, Colorado
Coronary Artery Spasm (CAS)

Carlos A. Puyo, MD

Assistant Professor
Department of Anesthesia and Critical Care
Washington University in St. Louis
St. Louis, Missouri
Mycoplasma pneumoniae Infection

Forrest Quiggle, MD

University of Miami
Miller School of Medicine
Miami, Florida
Aortic Stenosis

Mary Rabb, MD

Professor of Anesthesiology
Director, Post Graduate Medical Education
University of Texas Medical School at Houston
Department of Anesthesiology
Houston, Texas
Cri Du Chat Syndrome (5p Syndrome)

Bronwyn R. Rae, FANZCA, DCH (Lond)

Attending Anesthesiologist
Department of Anesthesia
Children's Memorial Hospital
Chicago, Illinois
Congenital Methemoglobinemia

Muhammad B. Rafique, MD, FAAP

Assistant Professor
Department of Anesthesiology
University of Texas Medical School at Houston
Houston, Texas
Tuberculosis (TB)
Chest X-Ray

Jesse M. Raiten, MD

Assistant Professor of Anesthesiology and Critical Care
Department of Anesthesiology and Critical Care
University of Pennsylvania
Philadelphia, Pennsylvania
Hyperglycemic Hyperosmolar State (HHS)

Arvind Rajagopal, MBBS

Assistant Professor
Department of Anesthesiology
Rush University Medical Center
Chicago, Illinois
Phenylephrine (Neo-Synephrine)
Ventricular Tachycardia

Srinivasan Rajagopal, MD

Assistant Professor
Department of Anesthesiology
University of Iowa
Iowa City, Iowa
Mesothelioma

Gaurav Rajpal, MD

Fellow
Department of Anesthesiology
University of Pittsburgh
Pittsburgh, Pennsylvania
Rifampin

Chandra Ramamoorthy, MBBS, FRCA

Professor
Department of Anesthesiology
Stanford University Medical Center;
Director
Division of Pediatric Cardiac Anesthesia
Lucile Packard Children's Hospital
Palo Alto, California
Truncus Arteriosus

Ira J. Rampil, MS, MD

Professor of Anesthesiology and Neurological Surgery
Director of Clinical Research
University at Stony Brook
Stony Brook, New York
Laser Surgery of Airway
Pituitary Tumors

James G. Ramsay, MD

Professor of Anesthesiology
Emory University School of Medicine
Atlanta, Georgia
Aortic Valve Replacement

James A. Ramsey, MD

Assistant Professor
Department of Anesthesiology
Multi-Specialty Division
Vanderbilt University School of Medicine
Nashville, Tennessee
Syndrome X
Mastectomy

Vidya N. Rao, MD, FRCA

Department of Anesthesiology
Vanderbilt University
VA Hospital
Nashville, Tennessee
Prilocaine (Citanest)
Herniorrhaphy

Joana Ratsiu, MD

Fellow in Anesthesiology
University of Washington School of Medicine
Seattle, Washington
Tonsillectomy and Adenoidectomy

Selina Read, MD

Department of Anesthesiology
Penn State Medical Center
Hershey, Pennsylvania
Upper Respiratory Infections

Ronjeet Reddy, MD

Department of Anesthesiology
University of Miami
Jackson Memorial Hospital
Miami, Florida
Carotid Sinus Syndrome

Leila L. Reduque, MD

Assistant Professor
Division of Anesthesiology
Children's National Medical Center
Washington, DC
Evening Primrose

David L. Reich, MD

Horace W. Goldsmith Professor and Chair
Department of Anesthesiology
Mount Sinai Medical Center
New York, New York
Ventricular Septal Defect (Congenital)
Ventricular Septal Rupture (Defect), Post Myocardial Infarction

Karene Ricketts, MD

Assistant Professor
Pediatric Division
Department of Anesthesiology
University of North Carolina
Chapel Hill, North Carolina
Hypercalcemia
Otitis Media
Steroids

Cameron Ricks, MD

Clinical Instructor
Department of Anesthesiology and Perioperative Care
University of California, Irvine
Orange, California
Addison's Disease

Bernhard Riedel, MBChB, FCA, FANZCA, MMed, MBA, PhD

Director of Anesthetics
Division of Surgical Oncology
Peter McCallum Cancer Center
Melbourne, Australia;
Adjunct Professor
Vanderbilt University
Nashville, Tennessee
Statins

Jyotsna Rimal, MD

Assistant Professor
Department of Anesthesiology
UMDNJ-Newark
Newark, New Jersey
Oral Hypoglycemics

Joseph Rinehart, MD

Assistant Professor
Department of Anesthesiology
and Perioperative Care
University of California at Irvine
Orange, California
Malnutrition

James M. Riopelle, MD

Professor
Department of Anesthesiology
Louisiana State University
Health Sciences Center
New Orleans, Louisiana
Echinococcosis

Stacey A. Rizza, MD

Assistant Professor
Mayo Medical School
Mayo Clinic
Rochester, Minnesota
Cytomegalovirus Infection

Amy C. Robertson, MD, MMHC

Assistant Professor
Department of Anesthesiology
Vanderbilt University School of Medicine;
Department of Veterans Affairs
Tennessee Valley Healthcare System
Nashville, Tennessee
Waldenström's Macroglobulinemia

Stephen Robinson, MD

Clinical Professor of Anesthesiology
Department of Anesthesiology and
Perioperative Medicine
Oregon Health and Science University
Portland, Oregon
Mitral Valve Replacement
Trimethaphan

Peter Rock, MD, MBA, FCCM

Professor of Medicine, Surgery,
and Anesthesiology
Martin Helrich Professor and Chair
Department of Anesthesiology
University of Maryland
School of Medicine;
Anesthesiologist-in-Chief
University of Maryland Medical Center
Baltimore, Maryland
Flow-Volume Loops
Spirometry

Michael F. Roizen, MD

J. Gorman and Family Chair
Wellness Institute Professor of Anesthesiology
Chief Wellness Officer
The Cleveland Clinic
Cleveland, Ohio
Adrenalectomy for Pheochromocytoma
Chondroitin Sulfate
Cimetidine
Diabetes, Type I (Insulin-Dependent)
Diabetes, Type II (Noninsulin-Dependent)
Hyperthyroidism

Myocardial Ischemia (MIsch)
Phenoxybenzamine
Pheochromocytoma
Propylthiouracil—Antithyroid Drugs
Retropharyngeal and Peritonsillar Abscess
   Drainage in Adults
Sickle Cell Trait
Sleep Apnea, Central and Mixed
Sleep Apnea, Obstructive
Thyroidectomy (Open or Minimally Invasive) for
   Hyperthyroidism
Total Hip Arthroplasty

Daniel M. Roke, MD

Pediatric Anesthesiologist
Assistant Professor, Pediatrics and
Anesthesiology, Director of Resident Education
Monroe Carell Jr. Childrens Hospital at
Vanderbilt
Nashville, Tennessee
Cystic Fibrosis

Ryan Romeo, MD

Assistant Professor of Anesthesiology
Department of Anesthesiology
University of Pittsburgh School of Medicine
Pittsburgh, Pennsylvania
Hysterectomy, Vaginal

Joseph Rosa III, BA, MD

Associate Clinical Professor
Department of Anesthesiology
University of California–Los Angeles
Los Angeles, California
Appendectomy
Pregnancy, Ectopic

David A. Rosen, MD

Professor of Anesthesia and Pediatrics
Director of Pediatric Cardiac Anesthesia
West Virginia University
Morgantown, West Virginia
Intestinal Obstruction

Kathleen Rosen, MD

Pediatric Anesthesiology
Cleveland Clinic
Cleveland, Ohio
Intestinal Obstruction
Intussuscepted Bowel Repair

Stanley H. Rosenbaum, MD

Professor of Anesthesiology,
Internal Medicine and Surgery
Yale University School of Medicine
New Haven, Connecticut
Carcinoid Syndrome
Diabetes, Type II (Noninsulin-Dependent)

Andrew D. Rosenberg, MD

Chief of Service
Department of Anesthesiology
New York University Hospital for Joint Diseases;
Executive Vice-Chair
Department of Anesthesiology
New York University School of Medicine
New York, New York
Cervical Disk Disease (Cervical Spine Disease)
Sarcoidosis

Andrew L. Rosenberg, MD

Chief
Division of Critical Care
Department of Anesthesiology

Medical Director
Cardiovascular Intensive Care Unit
Associate Professor
Anesthesiology and Internal Medicine
University of Michigan Medical Center
Ann Arbor, Michigan
Myocardial Contusion (Blunt Cardiac Injury)

Henry Rosenberg, MD

Director
Department of Medical Education
and Clinical Research
Saint Barnabas Medical Center
Livingston, New Jersey;
President
Malignant Hyperthermia Association
of the United States
Sherburne, New York;
Adjunct Professor of Anesthesiology
Columbia University College of Physicians
and Surgeons
New York, New York
Malignant Hyperthermia (MH) and Other
   Anesthetic-Induced Myodystrophies (AIM)

Meg A. Rosenblatt, MD

Professor
Departments of Anesthesiology
and Orthopaedics
Mount Sinai School of Medicine
New York, New York
Hip Fracture Repair
Jehovah's Witness Patient

Steven Roth, MD

Professor of Anesthesia and Critical Care
University of Chicago;
Chief of Neuroanesthesia
University of Chicago Medical Center
Chicago, Illinois
Postoperative Encephalopathy, Metabolic

Brian Rothman, MD

Assistant Professor
Department of Anesthesiology
Director
Radiology/VUH1 Anesthesiology Services
Vanderbilt University School of Medicine
Nashville, Tennessee
GI Endoscopy/EGD, Non-Operating Room Anesthesia

Justin L. Rountree, MD

Department of Anesthesiology
University of North Carolina
Chapel Hill, North Carolina
Cushing's Syndrome

Matthew J. Rowan, MD

Oregon Health and Science University
Portland, Oregon
Autonomic Function

Marc Rozner, PhD, MD

Professor of Anesthesiology
and Perioperative Medicine
Professor of Cardiology
University of Texas MD Anderson Cancer
Center;
Adjunct Assistant Professor of Integrative
Biology and Pharmacology
Houston, Texas
Implantable Cardioverter-Defibrillators (ICDs)
Pacemakers

Ryan Rubin, MD, MPH

Assistant Clinical Professor
Department of Anesthesiology
Louisiana Health Sciences Center
New Orleans, Louisiana
Pickwickian Syndrome

Stephen M. Rupp, MD

Medical Director Perioperative Services
Department of Anesthesiology
Virginia Mason Medical Center
Seattle, Washington
Pituitary Resection, Transsphenoidal Approach

W. John Russell, MBBS, FRCA, FANZCA, PhD

Professor
Department of Anaesthesia
Royal Adelaide Hospital
Adelaide, Australia
Familial Periodic Paralysis (Hyperkalemic)
Familial Periodic Paralysis (Hypokalemic)

Thomas A. Russo, MD, CM

Professor of Medicine and Microbiology
and Microbiology and Immunology
Chief of the Division of Infectious Disease
University at Buffalo
State University of New York and VA
Medical Center
Buffalo, New York
Q Fever

Alecia L. Sabartinelli, MD

Louisiana State University Health Sciences Center
New Orleans, Louisiana
Multiple Myeloma

Tetsuro Sakai, MD, PhD

Assistant Professor
Department of Anesthesiology
University of Pittsburgh School of Medicine
Pittsburgh, Pennsylvania
Kidney Transplantation

Orlando J. Salinas, MD

Assistant Professor of Anesthesiology
Louisland State University Medical Center
New Orleans, Louisiana
Fish Oil

Paul L. Samm, MD

Assistant Professor
Co-Director of CV Anesthesia
Department of Anesthesiology
Louisiana State University Interim Hospital
New Orleans, Louisiana
Coronary Artery Bypass Graft (CABG)

Jibin Samuel, MBBS, MD

Pediatric Anesthesiology
Jackson Memorial Hospital
Miami, Florida
Diaphragmatic Hernia (Congenital)

Tor Sandven, MD

Resident
Department of Anesthesiology
and Perioperative Medicine
Oregon Health and Science University
Portland, Oregon
Trimethaphan

Ted J. Sanford, MD

Georgine M. Steude Professor
of Anesthesiology Education
Department of Anesthesiology
University of Michigan
Ann Arbor, Michigan
Hypoxemia

Joshua W. Sappenfield, MD

Resident
Department of Anesthesiology
University of Maryland School of Medicine
Baltimore, Maryland
Marijuana

Ponnusamy Saravanan, MBBS, PhD, MRCP

Associate Professor
Clinical Sciences Research Institute
University of Warwick
Coventry, Great Britain
Insulin Receptor Modifiers

Subramanian Sathishkumar, MBBS

Assistant Professor
Department of Anesthesiology
Penn State Milton S.
Hershey Medical Center
Hershey, Pennsylvania
Magnesium Sulfate

R. Alexander Schlichter, MD

Assistant Professor of Clinical
Anesthesiology and Critical Care
University of Pennsylvania
Philadelphia, Pennsylvania
Craniotomy

Eric Schnell, MD, PhD

Assistant Professor
Department of Anesthesiology and
Perioperative Medicine
Oregon Health and Science University;
Staff Anesthesiologist
Portland VA Medical Center
Portland, Oregon
Phenothiazines

David L. Schreibman, MD

Assistant Professor
Department of Anesthesiology
University of Maryland School of Medicine
Baltimore, Maryland
Encephalitis

Armin Schubert, MD, MBA

Professor and System Chair
Department of Anesthesiology
Ochsner Health System
New Orleans, Louisiana
Cerebral AVM Repair
Multiple Sclerosis

Peter Schulman, MD

Assistant Professor
Department of Anesthesiology
and Perioperative Medicine
Oregon Health and Science University
Portland, Oregon
Acidosis, Lactic/Metabolic
Septic Shock, Hyperdynamic; Systemic
  Inflammatory Response Syndrome (SIRS)

Todd A. Schultz, MD

Assistant Professor
Department of Anesthesia
University of Medicine and Dentistry
of New Jersey
Newark, New Jersey
Nonsteroidal Anti-Inflammatory Drugs
  (NSAIDs)

Alan Jay Schwartz, MD, MSEd

Professor of Clinical Anesthesiology and
Critical Care
University of Pennsylvania
School of Medicine;
Director of Education and Program
Director
Pediatric Anesthesiology Fellowship
Department of Anesthesiology
and Critical Care Medicine
Children's Hospital of Philadelphia
Philadelphia, Pennsylvania
Advanced Cardiac Life Support (ACLS)
Transposition of the Great Arteries
  (TGA)
Transposition of the Great Arteries, L Form
  (L-TGA)

Jamie McElrath Schwartz, MD

Assistant Professor
Departments of Anesthesiology
and Critical
Care Medicine and Pediatrics
Johns Hopkins School of Medicine
Baltimore, Maryland
Single (Including Common) Ventricle

Jeffrey J. Schwartz, MD

Associate Professor
Department of Anesthesiology
Yale University School of Medicine
New Haven, Connecticut
Pancreatitis, Acute
Pancreatitis, Chronic

Benjamin K. Scott, MD

Department of Anesthesiology
and Critical Care
Hospital of the University of
Pennsylvania Philadelphia,
Pennsylvania
Seizures, Epileptic

Joseph L. Seltzer, MD

Professor of Anesthesiology
Department of Anesthesiology
Jefferson Medical College
Philadelphia, Pennsylvania
Autoimmune Diseases, Cold

Tamas Seres, MD, PhD

Associate Professor
Department of Anesthesiology
University of Colorado Denver
Aurora, Colorado
Post Transplant Lymphoproliferative Disease

Daniel I. Sessler, MD

Professor and Chair
Department of Outcomes Research
Cleveland Clinic
Cleveland, Ohio
Hypothermia, Mild

Navil F. Sethna, MB, ChB, MD

Senior Associate in Anesthesia
Associate Professor of Anaesthesia
Harvard Medical School;
Department of Anesthesiology,
Perioperative and Pain Medicine
Children's Hospital Boston
Boston, Massachusetts
Prader-Willi Syndrome

Amar Setty, MD

Department of Anesthesiology
Johns Hopkins University School of Medicine
Baltimore, Maryland
Psyllium, Bulk-Forming Laxatives (Plantago Isphagula, Plantago Ovata)

Paul W. Shabaz, MD, PhD

Assistant Professor of Anesthesiology
University of Rochester Medical Center
Rochester, New York
Placenta Previa

Pranav Shah, MD

Resident
Department of Anesthesiology
University of Pittsburgh
Pittsburgh, Pennsylvania
Sick Sinus Syndrome (SSS)

Saroj Mukesh Shah, MBBS, MD

Assistant Professor of Clinical
Anesthesiology
Department of Anesthesiology
Louisiana State University School of Medicine
New Orleans, Louisiana
Myotonia Dystrophica (Myotonic Dystrophy, Steinert's Disease)

Milad Sharifpour, MS

4th year Medical Student
University of Michigan Medical School
Ann Arbor, Michigan
Anterior Cervical Discectomy and Fusion (ACDF)

Joanne Shay, MD, MBA

Assistant Professor
Department of Anesthesia and Critical Care
Medicine
Division of Pediatric Anesthesia
Johns Hopkins University School of Medicine
Baltimore, Maryland
Anemia, Aplastic

Jay Shepherd, MD

Resident
Department of Anesthesiology
Tulane University School of Medicine
New Orleans, Louisiana
Herpes, Type II

Jeffrey S. Shiffrin, MD

Associate Professor
Department of Anesthesiology
University of Colorado Denver
Aurora, Colorado
Physostigmine, Eserine

Marina Shindell, DO

Assistant Professor
Department of Anesthesiology
University of Colorado
Aurora, Colorado
Hereditary Hemorrhagic Telangiectasia (Osler-Weber-Rendu Disease)

Daniel Siker, MD

Staff Physician
Department of Pediatrics and
Anesthesiology
Medical College of Wisconsin
Milwaukee, Wisconsin
Cherubism

Richard Silverman, MD

Chief
Critical Care Medicine
Department of Anesthesiology
University of Miami
Miami, Florida
HIV Testing

Brett A. Simon, MD, PhD

Lowenstein Professor of Anaesthesia,
Harvard Medical School;
Chair
Department of Anesthesia,
Critical Care and Pain Medicine
Beth Israel Deaconess Medical Center
and Harvard Medical School
Boston, Massachusetts
Lung Volume Reduction Surgery (LVRS)

Nina Singh, MD

Assistant Clinical Professor
Department of Anesthesiology
University of Pennsylvania
Philadelphia, Pennsylvania
Bicarbonate Sodium
ORIF at Hip
Transurethral Resection of Prostate (TURP)

Ashish C. Sinha, MD, PhD, DABA

Assistant Professor
Department of Anesthesiology
and Critical Care
Department of Otorhinolaryngology and
Head and Neck Surgery
University of Pennsylvania
Philadelphia, Pennsylvania
Cancer, Bladder
Candidiasis
CREST Syndrome
Depression, Unipolar
Mediastinal Masses
Morbid Obesity

Robert N. Sladen, MBChB, MRCP(UK), FRCP(C), FCCM

Professor and Vice-Chair
Department of Anesthesiology
College of Physicians and Surgeons
of Columbia University;
Director
Cardiothoracic and Surgical Intensive Care
Units
Columbia University Medical Center
at New York Presbyterian Hospital
New York, New York
Renal Failure, Acute (ARF)

Kieran A. Slevin, MBBCh

Assistant Professor
Department of Anesthesiology
and Critical Care
University of Pennsylvania School of Medicine
Philadelphia, Pennsylvania
Autonomic Dysreflexia (AD)

Tod B. Sloan, MD, MBA, PhD

Professor
Department of Anesthesiology
University of Colorado Denver
Aurora, Colorado
Infratentorial Tumors
Supratentorial Brain Tumors

Kathleen Smith, MD

Assistant Professor
Department of Anesthesiology
University of North Carolina;
Assistant Professor
Department of Obstetrics and Gynecology
University of North Carolina
Chapel Hill, North Carolina
Cushing's Syndrome

Timothy E. Smith, MD

Associate Professor of Anesthesiology
and Pediatrics
Wake Forest University School
of Medicine
Winston-Salem, North Carolina
Hydrocephalus

Victoria Smoot, MD

Assistant Professor
Department of Anesthesiology
University of Maryland School of Medicine
Baltimore, Maryland
Breast Biopsy

Denis Snegovskikh, MD

Assistant Professor
Department of Anesthesiology
Yale University
New Haven, Connecticut
Cesarean Section, Emergent

Betsy Ellen Soifer MD, PhD

Anesthesiologist
Operative Care Division
Portland Veterans Affairs
Medical Center;
Associate Professor of Anesthesiology
and Perioperative Care
Oregon Health and Science University
Portland, Oregon
Subphrenic Abscess

Molly Solorzano, MD

Chief Resident
Department of Anesthesiology
Mayo Clinic
Scottsdale, Arizona;
University of Iowa
Iowa City, Iowa
Insulinoma

James M. Sonner, MD

Professor
Department of Anesthesia and
Perioperative Care
University of California
San Francisco, California
Pemphigus

Aris Sophocles

Department of Anesthesiology
Children's Hospital
Denver Colorado
Blalock-Taussig Shunt (BTS)
Carcinoid, Excision of
Patent Ductus Arteriosus
Ventricular Septal Defect, Repair of

James A. Sparrow, MD

Assistant Professor of Cardiothoracic
Anesthesia
Department of Anesthesiology
University of Alabama at Birmingham
Birmingham, Alabama
Atrial Septal Defect, Ostium Secundum

Joan Spiegel, BS, MD

Instructor, Harvard Medical School
Department of Anesthesia,
Critical Care and Pain Medicine
Beth Israel Deaconess Medical Center
Boston, Massachusetts
Chitosan
Conn's Syndrome
Saw Palmetto

Bruce D. Spiess, MD, FAHA

Professor of Anesthesiology
and Emergency Medicine
Director of Virginia Commonwealth University
Reanimation Engineering Shock Center
Virginia Commonwealth University
Health System
Richmond, Virginia
Pericardial Effusion

Ramprasad Sripada, MD, MMM, CPE

Associate Professor of Clinical
Anesthesiology
Vanderbilt University Medical Center
Nashville, Tennessee
Herniorrhaphy
Prilocaine (Citanest)
Transesophageal Echocardiography (TEE)

Stanley W. Stead, MD, MBA

CEO
Stead Health Group, Inc.
Encino, California;
Clinical Professor
Department of Anesthesiology and Pain
Medicine
University of California, Davis School of
Medicine
Sacramento, California
Blindness
Circumcision

Joshua D. Stearns, MD

Associate Professor Anesthesiology and
Critical Care Medicine
Johns Hopkins School of Medicine
Baltimore, Maryland
Atrial Septal Defect, Repair of

Kelly Stees, MD

Fellow in Pediatric Anesthesiology
Department of Anesthesia
Children's Hospital, Denver
Aurora, Colorado
Seizure Surgery
Bilirubinemia of the Newborn

Clinton Steffey, MD

Department of Anesthesiology
SUNY Downstate Medical Center
State University of New York
Brooklyn, New York
Pregnancy Testing

Christopher Stemland, MD

Assistant Professor of Anesthesiology
and Pediatrics
Department of Anesthesiology
University of Virginia
Charlottesville, Virginia
Foreign Body Aspiration

John Stene, MD, PhD

Department of Anesthesiology
Milton S. Hershey Medical Center
Hershey, Pennsylvania
Vitamin B_{12} (Cyanocobalamin)

Christopher T. Stephens, MD, MS

Director of Education, Trauma
Anesthesiology
R Adams Cowley Shock Trauma Center
Assistant Professor of Anesthesiology
University of Maryland School of Medicine
Baltimore, Maryland
Marijuana

Tracey L. Stierer, MD

Assistant Professor
Department of Anesthesiology
and Critical Care Medicine
Johns Hopkins Medical Institutions;
Medical Director Johns Hopkins Outpatient
Surgical Programs
Department of Anesthesiology and Critical
Care Medicine
Johns Hopkins Medical Institutions
Baltimore, Maryland
Oral Contraceptives

O. Jameson Stokes, MD, MS

Assistant Clinical Professor
Department of Anesthesiology
and Perioperative Care
University of California, Irvine
Orange, California
Carpal Tunnel Syndrome

Bryant W. Stolp, MD, PhD

Assistant Professor of Anesthesiology
Medical Instructor in the Department of Cell
Biology
Director
Anesthesiology Emergency Airway Services
Duke University Medical Center
Durham, North Carolina
Gas Embolism

David F. Stowe, MD, PhD

Professor of Anesthesiology and Physiology
Medical College of Wisconsin;
Adjunct Professor of Biomedical
Engineering
Marquette University;
Senior Staff Anesthesiologist
Zablocki Veterans Medical Center
Milwaukee, Wisconsin
Serotonin: Agonists, Antagonists, and Reuptake
Inhibitors

Ted Strickland, MD

Assistant Professor
Department of Anesthesiology
Tulane University
New Orleans, Louisiana
Glycine

Suzanne Strom, MD

Assistant Clinical Professor
Department of Anesthesiology
and Perioperative Care
University of California Irvine
Orange, California
Hyperkalemia

Erin A. Sullivan, MD

Associate Professor of Anesthesiology
Director
Division of Cardiothoracic Anesthesiology
Department of Anesthesiology
University of Pittsburgh Medical Center
Pittsburgh, Pennsylvania
Sick Sinus Syndrome (SSS)

Dajin Sun, MD

Professor
Department of Anesthesiology
Renji Hospital
Shanghai Jiaotong University
School of Medicine
Shanghai, China
Carnitine

Lena Sun, MD

E. M. Papper Professor of Anesthesiology
and Pediatrics
Vice Chairman
Department of Anesthesiology
Chief
Division of Pediatric Anesthesia
College of Physicians and Surgeons
Columbia University
New York, New York
Heart Transplant, Pediatric

Esther Sung, MD

Staff Anesthesiologist
Operative Care Department
(Anesthesiology)
Portland Veterans Affairs
Medical Center
Portland, Oregon
Nicotine Replacment Therapies (NRTs)

Veronica C. Swanson, MD

Associate Professor of Anesthesiology
and Perioperative Medicine
Associate Professor of Pediatrics
Oregon Health and Science University;
Director
Pediatric Cardiac Anesthesia
Doernbecher Children's Hospital
Portland, Oregon
Tetralogy of Fallot (TOF)
Tetralogy of Fallot, Correction of

Judit Szolnoki, MD

Assistant Professor
Department of Anesthesiology
Children's Hospital
University of Colorado
Aurora, Colorado
Seizure Surgery

Joe Talarico, DO

Assistant Professor of Anesthesiology
University of Pittsburgh School
of Medicine
Chair,
Evaluation and Competence Committee
Anesthesiology Residency Program
Pittsburgh, Pennsylvania
Calcium Deficiency/Hypocalcemia

**Gee Mei Tan, MB, BS,
MMED(Anesthesia)**

Assistant Professor
Department of Anesthesiology
Children's Hospital
University of Colorado Denver
School of Medicine
Aurora, Colorado
Hypospadias Repair

Darryl T. Tang, MD

Department of Anesthesiology and
Perioperative Medicine
Oregon Health and Science University
Portland, Oregon
Familial Dysautonomia (Riley-Day Syndrome)

Paul Tarasi, MD

Resident
Department of Anesthesiology
University of Pittsburgh
Pittsburgh, Pennsylvania
Calcium Deficiency/Hypocalcemia

René Tempelhoff, MD

Professor
Department of Anesthesiology
and Neurological Surgery
Washington University School
of Medicine
St. Louis, Missouri
Seizures, Intractable

John E. Tetzlaff, MD

Staff Anesthesiologist
Department of General Anesthesiology
Anesthesiology Institute
Cleveland Clinic;
Professor of Anesthesiology
Cleveland Clinic Lerner College
of Medicine
Case Western Reserve University
Cleveland, Ohio
Ankylosing Spondylitis
Degenerative Disk Disease

Alisa C. Thorne, MD

Director
Ambulatory Anesthesia
Memorial Sloan-Kettering Cancer Center
New York, New York
Lymphomas
Thyroid Neoplasms

Arlyne Thung, MD

Assistant Professor
Department of Anesthesiology
Yale University
New Haven, Connecticut
Beckwith-Wiedemann Syndrome
Treacher Collins Syndrome

Vasanti Tilak, MD

Assistant Professor
Department of Anesthesiology
University of Medicine and Dentistry
of New Jersey
New Jersey Medical School
Newark, New Jersey
Antithrombin III Deficiency

Kate Tobin, BA, MD

Assistant Clinical Professor
Department of Anesthesiology
and Perioperative Care
University of California Irvine,
Orange, California
Glaucoma, Closed-Angle

Joseph R. Tobin, MD

Professor and Chairman
Department of Anesthesiology
Wake Forest University School
of Medicine
Winston-Salem, North Carolina
Hydrocephalus

Michael J. Tobin, MD

Assistant Chief of Anesthesiology
Department of Anesthesiology
Shriners Hospitals for Children-Chicago
Chicago, Illinois
Tracheoesophageal Fistula Repair

R. David Todd, MD

Fellow
Interventional Pain Management
Vanderbilt University Medical Center
Nashville, Tennessee
Glossopharyngeal Neuralgia

Matthew Tomlinson, BS

4th Year Medical Student
Department of Anesthesiology
Oregon Health and Science University
Portland, Oregon
Anemia, Hemolytic

Thomas J. Toung, MD

Professor
Department of Anesthesiology
and Critical Care Medicine
Johns Hopkins University
School of Medicine
Baltimore, Maryland
Craniotomy, Sitting Position
Venous Air Embolism

Lien B. Tran, MD

Resident
Department of Anesthesiology
Louisiana State University
Health Sciences Center
New Orleans, Louisiana
*Hypertension, Uncontrolled, with
Cardiomyopathy*

Minh Chau Joe Tran, MD, MPH

Assistant Professor
Pediatric Anesthesia
University of Medicine and Dentistry
of New Jersey
Newark, New Jersey
Achondroplasia, Dwarfism

Kevin K. Tremper, PhD, MD

Robert B. Sweet Professor and Chair
Department of Anesthesiology
University of Michigan
Ann Arbor, Michigan
Cigarette Smoking

Sanyo Tsai, MD

Resident
Department of Anesthesiology
Louisiana State University
Health Sciences Center
New Orleans, Louisiana
Hashimoto's Thyroiditis

George S. Tseng, MD

Assistant Professor of Anesthesiology
and Critical Care Medicine
Department of Anesthesiology
and Critical Care Medicine
Washington University School
of Medicine
St. Louis, Missouri
Colostomy

Kenneth J. Tuman, MD

Professor and Chair
Department of Anesthesiology
Rush University Medical Center
Rush Medical College
Chicago, Illinois
Phenylephrine (Neo-Synephrine)
Ventricular Tachycardia

Avery Tung

Professor
Department of Anesthesia and Critical
Care
University of Chicago
Chicago, Illinois
Aminophylline

Cynthia Tung, MD

Assistant in Perioperative Anesthesia
Instructor of Anaesthesia
Harvard Medical School;
Department of Anesthesiology,
Perioperative and Pain Medicine
Children's Hospital Boston
Boston, Massachusetts
Meningomyelocele Repair

Rebecca Twersky, MD, MPH

Professor of Anesthesiology
Vice Chair, Research
Medical Director, Ambulatory Surgery
Unit
SUNY Downstate Medical Center
Brooklyn, New York
Pregnancy Testing

Mark Twite, MA, MB, BChir, FRCP

Director
Pediatric Cardiac Anesthesia
Department of Anesthesiology
Children's Hospital and University
of Colorado
Denver, Colorado
Blalock-Taussig Shunt (BTS)
Carcinoid, Excision of
Patent Ductus Arteriosus
Ventricular Septal Defect, Repair of

John A. Ulatowski, MD, PhD, MBA

Professor and Director
Anesthesiology and Critical Care Medicine
Johns Hopkins University
Baltimore, Maryland
Transverse Myelitis

Michael Urban, MD, PhD

Associate Professor of Anesthesiology
Weill Medical College of Cornell University;
Director
PACU/SDU
Hospital for Special Surgery
New York, New York
Total Knee Arthroplasty

Manuel C. Vallejo, MD, DMD

Professor
Department of Anesthesiology
University of Pittsburgh;
Director
Obstetric Anesthesia
Magee-Women's Hospital of UPMC
Pittsburgh, Pennsylvania
Herpes, Type I
Rifampin

Andrea Vannucci, MD

Assistant Professor
Department of Anesthesiology
Washington University School of Medicine
St. Louis, Missouri
Carotid Endarterectomy

Albert J. Varon, MD, MHPE, FCCM

Professor and Vice Chair for Education
Department of Anesthesiology
University of Miami Miller School of Medicine
Miami, Florida
Burn Injury, Chemical
Burn Injury, Electrical
Burn Injury, Flame
Metformin (Glucophage)

Anasuya Vasudevan, MD, FRCA

Instructor, Harvard Medical School
Department of Anesthesia
Critical Care and Pain Medicine
Beth Israel Deaconess Medical Center
Boston, Massachusetts
Chemotherapeutic Agents

Susheela Viswanathan, MD

Associate Professor of Clinical
Anesthesiology
Department of Anesthesiology
Louisiana State University
Health Science Center
New Orleans, Louisiana
Multiple Myeloma

Alexander A. Vitin, MD, PhD

Assistant Professor
Department of Anesthesiology
and Pain Medicine
University of Washington
Seattle, Washington
Silicosis

Wolfgang Voelckel, MD, MSc

Associate Professor of Anesthesiology
Department of Anesthesiology
and Critical Care Medicine

AUVA Trauma Center
Salzburg, Austria
Trauma

Ann Walia, MD

Chief of Anesthesiology
and Perioperative Care
Tennessee Valley Healthcare System
Professor of Clinical Anesthesiology
Department of Anesthesiology
Vanderbilt University Medical Center
Nashville, Tennessee
Liver Transplantation

Russell T. Wall III, MD

Vice Chair and Program Director
Department of Anesthesiology
Georgetown University Hospital;
Senior Associate Dean and Professor
of Anesthesiology and Pharmacology
Georgetown University School of Medicine
Washington, DC
Acromegaly
Anorexia Nervosa

Terrence Wallace, MD

Richmond, Virginia
Pericardial Effusion

Shu-Ming Wang, MD

Associate Professor
Department of Anesthesiology
Yale Medical School
New Haven, Connecticut
Dandelion

David C. Warltier, MD, PhD

Chairman
Department of Anesthesiology
Professor of Anesthesiology,
Pharmacology and Toxicology
Medical College of Wisconsin
Milwaukee, Wisconsin
Dobutamine

Lucy Waskell, MD, PhD

Professor of Anesthesiology
University of Michigan;
Professor of Anesthesiology
VA Medical Center
Ann Arbor, Michigan
Penicillins

Scott Watkins, MD

Assistant Professor
Pediatric Cardiac Anesthesia
Department of Anesthesiology
Vanderbilt University Medical Center
Nashville, Tennessee
Alcohol Abuse
Aortopulmonary Window

Denise Wedel, MD

Professor
Department of Anesthesiology
Mayo Clinic
Rochester, Minnesota
Osteoarthritis

Stuart J. Weiss, MD, PhD

Associate Professor
Department of Anesthesiology
and Critical Care

University of Pennsylvania
Philadelphia, Pennsylvania
Pacemaker Implantation for Sick Sinus Syndrome
Exercise Stress Testing

Charles Weissman, MD

Professor and Chair
Department of Anesthesiology and Critical
Care Medicine
Hebrew University - Hadassah School of
Medicine;
Hadassah - Hebrew University Medical Center
Jerusalem, Israel
Encephalopathy, Metabolic
Encephalopathy, Postanoxic
Protein C Deficiency

Nathaen Weitzel, MD

Assistant Professor
Department of Anesthesiology
University of Colorado Denver
Denver, Colorado
Endocardial Cushion Defect

Gregory Weller, MD

Anesthesiology and Critical Care Resident
University of Pennsylvania
Philadelphia, Pennsylvania
Strabismus Repair

Gina Whitney, MD

Assistant Professor of Anesthesiology
and Pediatrics
Pediatric Anesthesiology and Pediatric
Intensive Care
Vanderbilt Children's Hospital
Vanderbilt University Medical Center
Nashville, Tennessee
Supraventricular Tachycardia (Tacharrhythmias)

Robert A. Whittington, MD

Associate Professor of Clinical
Anesthesiology
Department of Anesthesiology
Columbia University-College of Physicians
and Surgeons
New York, New York
Dementia

Danny Wilkerson, MD

Associate Professor
Departments of Anesthesiology
and Obstetrics and Gynecology
University of Arkansas for Medical Sciences
Little Rock, Arkansas
Diabetes, Type III (Gestational Diabetes Mellitus)

Nancy C. Wilkes, MD

Professor of Anesthesiology
Department of Anesthesiology
Medical Director
Ambulatory Surgery Center
University of North Carolina Hospitals
Chapel Hill, North Carolina
Kartagener's Syndrome
Diverticulosis
Vitamin D Deficiency

Michael Williams, MD

Assistant Clinical Professor
Department of Anesthesiology
LSU Health Sciences Center
New Orleans, Louisiana
Hashimoto's Thyroiditis

Jimmy Windsor, MD

Assistant Professor of Clinical
Anesthesiology
Department of Anesthesiology
University of Miami
Miami, Florida
Tricuspid Atresia
Intra-Aortic Balloon Counterpulsation (IABCP)

Bernard Wittels, MD, PhD

Anesthesiologist
Department of Anesthesiology
Wheaton-Franciscan All Saints Hospital
Racine, Wisconsin
Gift Procedure

Gregory A. Wolff, BS, MD

Resident Physician
Department of Anesthesiology
University of Colorado, Denver
Aurora, Colorado
Cromolyn Sodium

Andrew K. Wong, MD

Assistant Professor
Department of Anesthesiology
University of Pennsylvania Health System
Philadelphia, Pennsylvania
Joint Replacement Cementing (Methylmethacrylate Cementing)

Stacie N. Woods, MD

Resident
Department of Anesthesiology
and Critical Care Medicine
Johns Hopkins University School
of Medicine
Baltimore, Maryland
Placenta Previa

A.J. Wright III, MLS

Associate Professor
Department of Anesthesiology
University of Alabama at Birmingham
Birmingham, Alabama
Hepatitis, Halothane

Zheng Xie, MD, PhD

Assistant Professor
Department of Anesthesia and Critical Care
University of Chicago
Chicago, Illinois
Transjugular Intrahepatic Portosystemic Shunt (TIPS)

Christopher C. Young, MD, FCCM

Associate Professor of Anesthesiology
Assistant Professor of Surgery
Chief - Division of Critical Care Medicine
Department of Anesthesiology
Duke University Medical Center
Durham, North Carolina
Thoracic Aortic Repair

Francine S. Yudkowitz, MD, FAAP

Associate Professor
Department of Anesthesiology
and Pediatrics
Mount Sinai School of Medicine;
Director of Pediatric Anesthesia
Department of Anesthesiology
Mount Sinai Hospital
New York, New York
Congenital Pulmonary Cystic Lesions/Lobar Emphysema
Gastroesophageal Reflux in Children
Moyamoya

James R. Zaidan, MD, MBA

Professor and Chair

Department of Anesthesiology
Associate Dean for GME
Emory University School of Medicine
Atlanta, Georgia
Mobitz I (Second Degree Atrioventricular Block)
Mobitz II (Second Degree Atrioventricular Block)

Paul Zanaboni, MD, PhD

Anesthesiologist
Western Anesthesiology Assoc, Inc.
St. Louis, Missouri
Cor Pulmonale

Warren M. Zapol, MD

Director
Anesthesia Center for Critical Care
Research
Department of Anesthesia,
Critical Care and Pain Medicine
Massachusetts General Hospital;
Reginald Jenney Professor of Anesthesia
Harvard Medical School
Boston, Massachusetts
Nitric Oxide (NO), Inhaled

Angela Zimmerman, MD

Department of Anesthesiology
and Perioperative Medicine
Oregon Health and Science University
Portland, Oregon
Chondroitin Sulfate

Maurice S. Zwass, MD

Professor of Anesthesia and Pediatrics,
Anesthesia and Perioperative Care
University of California, San Francisco
San Francisco, California
Croup (Laryngotracheobronchitis)
Epiglottitis

Foreword

Lee Fleisher and Michael Roizen have updated and expanded the second edition of *Essence of Anesthesia Practice*, which ingeniously encapsulated information important for any anesthesia consultant. Having been their associates at UCSF and Yale, we respect their clinical judgments, the fruit of years of experience in the practice of anesthesia. This book reflects the innovative yet comprehensive approach that they often take. They are no ivory tower practitioners—they work "in the trenches." We think that they have succeeded well in summarizing the pertinent aspects of the disease process, as well as the procedures, drugs, alternative medicines, and tests that are considered before a patient is anesthetized. Each chapter succinctly points the reader toward optimal care of a patient, by exploring the pathophysiology of a disease process and the management appropriate to specific conditions, clinical situations, and drug interactions. The intent is to help the physician rapidly and comprehensively plan perioperative management.

This is not a how-to-do-it book or "recipes" for perioperative care. Rather, it suggests that the pathophysiology of a disease or the physiologic imbalance caused by an operation should influence our thinking about therapeutic options. It offers a method for setting priorities to facilitate exemplary performance as a consultant in anesthesia. *Essence of Anesthesia Practice* has proven useful not only to anesthesiologists but also to our colleagues in other specialities who interface with the surgical patient.

The third edition expands on their previous success by including additional disease, drug, procedure, and laboratory testing topics and a section on alternative medicines. Interaction between herbal medicines and anesthetics is becoming increasingly important, and this text will serve as a handy reference.

The editors are to be congratulated for improving on their innovative clinical and educational format to serve both residents and practicing clinicians.

Paul G. Barash, MD
Professor, Department of Anesthesiology
Yale University School of Medicine
New Haven, Connecticut

Ronald D. Miller, MD
Professor, Department of Anesthesia
and Perioperative Care
University of California, San Francisco
San Francisco, California

Preface

It has been 9 years since the last edition of *Essence of Anesthesia Practice* was published and 14 years since the first edition. The goal of this text was, and continues to be, to provide a concise summary of the pathophysiology of both common and rare conditions seen in the perioperative period, medications used to treat these conditions, and the surgical procedures performed. These summaries are structured in a defined way to focus the clinician on the key facts and issues as well as the anticipated concerns regarding these conditions, medications, and procedures. Treatments, including medications for chronic conditions, continue to evolve, and it is difficult to keep up with the perioperative implications and the appropriate preoperative evaluation. Additionally, surgery has advanced and become more noninvasive over time. We therefore enrolled more than 500 authors, some of whom wrote the original chapters and many of whom are new and have either updated the original chapters or added new topics to address these concerns in the third edition of *Essence of Anesthesia Practice*.

This edition continues to improve and update the material that went before and to add the most up-to-date topics and new medications. We continue to include a large section on herbal medications, given their popularity and common use by our surgical patients. Mobile computing continues to advance and we are currently working on iPhone and Android applications that we hope will be available in the near future. We believe that the current format lends itself to quick review and orientation of the practitioner to perioperative implications at the point of care.

We wish to thank Natasha Andjelkovic, PhD, our publisher at Elsevier, and her editorial assistant, Brad McIlwain, for ensuring that our book received appropriate editing and development as well as providing the relentless support for this text to be published in a timely manner. We also wish to thank Eileen O'Shaughnessy, Lee's executive assistant, who managed the contributions of more than 500 authors, a herculean task.

Lee A. Fleisher, MD
Michael F. Roizen, MD

Contents

CONTENTS

SECTION II

Procedures

SECTION III

Drugs

Abbreviations

SYMBOLS

±	plus or minus
?	questionable
~	approximately
°C	degrees centigrade
°F	degrees Fahrenheit
1°	primary; first degree
2°	secondary; second degree
3°	third degree

A

A/G	albumin-globulin
a/w	associated with
A-a	alveolar-arterial
AA	arachidonic acid
AAA	abdominal aortic aneurysm
A-aDO$_2$	alveolar-arterial oxygen delivery
AAT	automatic atrial tachycardia
abd	abdomen; abdominal
ABF	aorto-bifemoral bypass
ABG	arterial blood gas
ABI	aorto-bi-iliac bypass
abn	abnormal; abnormality
ACAS	Asymptomatic Carotid Atherosclerosis Study
ACE	angiotensin-converting enzyme
ACG	angle-closure glaucoma
Ach	acetylcholine
AChE	acetylcholinesterase
ACL	anterior cruciate ligament
ACLS	advanced cardiac life support
ACOG	American College of Obstetricians and Gynae-cologists
ACS	acute confusional state
ACT	activated clotting/coagulation time
ACTH	adrenocorticotropic
ADH	antidiuretic hormone
ADHD	attention-deficit hyperactivity disorder
ADI	atlas-dens interval
ADL	activities of daily living
admin	administration; administered
ADP	adenosine diphosphate
AED	automated external defibrillator
AFIB	atrial fibrillation
AFLT	atrial flutter
A/G	albumin/globulin
AH	autonomic hyperreflexia
AI	aortic insufficiency
AICD	automatic implantable cardioverter defibrillator
AIDS	acquired immunodeficiency syndrome
AIMs	anesthetic-induced myodystrophies
AKA	above-knee amputation; also known as
alb	albumin
alk phos	alkaline phosphatase
ALL	acute lymphoblastic leukemia
ALT	alanine aminotransferase
Alv	alveolar
AM	morning
AML	acute myelogenous leukemia
AMP	adenosine monophosphate
ampl	amplitude

amt	amount
ANA	antinuclear antibody
angio	angiogram
ANS	autonomic nervous system
ant	anterior
anticoag	anticoagulation
AP	accessory pathway; action potential; anterior-posterior
API	alkaline protease inhibitor
apo B	apolipoprotein class B
approx	approximate; approximately
APTT	activated partial thromboplastin time
APUD	amine precursor uptake and decarboxylation
AR	aortic regurgitation
ARDS	acute respiratory distress syndrome
ARF	acute renal failure
art	arterial
AS	aortic stenosis
ASA	acetylsalicylic acid; Adams-Stokes attack; American Society of Anesthesiologists
ASAP	as soon as possible
ASCVD	atherosclerotic cardiovascular disease
ASD	atrial septal defect
assoc	associated
AST	aspartate aminotransferase
AT	antithrombin
AT1	angiotensin receptor 1
ATG	anti-thymus globulin
ATN	acute tubular necrosis
ATP	adenosine triphosphate; antitachycardia pacing
Au	gold
AV	atrioventricular
AVHB	atrioventricular heart block

B

β-hCG	beta human chorionic gonadotropin
BAER	brainstem auditory evoked response
BBB	bundle branch block; blood-brain barrier
BCNU	nitrosourea (carmustine)
BF	bifascicular; blood flow
BFHB	bifascicular heart block
bid	twice per day
BIG	botulism immune globulin
bilat	bilateral
BKA	below-knee amputation
bleo	bleomycin
BLS	basic life support
BM	bowel movement
BMI	body mass index
BMR	basal metabolic rate
BMT	bone marrow transplantation
BO	bronchiolitis obliterans
BOOP	bronchiolitis obliterans with cryptogenic organizing pneumonia
BP	blood pressure
BPD	bronchopulmonary dysplasia
BPH	benign prostatic hyperplasia/hypertrophy
bpm	beats per minute
BS	breath sounds
BSA	body surface area

BT	bleeding time; Blalock-Taussig (shunt)
BUN	blood urea nitrogen
Bx	biopsy

C

CA	cancer, cold agglutinins
ca.	about (L., circa)
Ca^{2+}	calcium
CAB	coronary artery bypass
CABG	coronary artery bypass graft
CAD	coronary artery disease
CAHS	central alveolar hypoventilation syndrome
cAMP	cyclic adenosine monophosphate
Cao_2	arterial oxygen concentration
cardiopulm	cardiopulmonary
CAS	coronary artery spasm
CASS	Coronary Artery Surgery Study
CATCH 22	cardiac defect; abnormal facies; thymic hypoplasia; cleft palate; hypocalcemia (syndrome)
cath	catheter; catheterization
CBC	complete blood count
CBF	cerebral blood flow
CBV	cerebral blood volume
CCNU	nitrosourea (lomustine)
CD4	antigenic marker on helper/inducer T cells
CD4+	presence of CD4
CDC	Centers for Disease Control and Prevention
CEA	carotid endarterectomy
CGL	chronic granulocytic leukemia
cGMP	cyclic guanosine monophosphate
C-GSF	granulocyte colony-stimulating factor
CHB	complete heart block
CHD	congenital heart disease; congenital heart defect
ChE	cholinesterase
ChemoRx	chemotherapy
CHF	congestive heart failure
CHO	carbohydrate
CI	cardiac index; confidence interval
CIN	cervical intraepithelial neoplasia
circ	circulation; circulatory
cis-DDP	cis-diamminedichloroplatinum
CK	creatine kinase
CK-MB	isoenzyme of creatine kinase with muscle and brain subunits
CLL	chronic lymphocytic leukemia
CLR	chlorambucil
CML	chronic myelogenous leukemia
$CMRO_2$	cerebral metabolic rate of oxygen
CMV	cytomegalovirus
CN	cranial nerve; cyanide
CNH	central neurogenic hyperventilation
CNS	central nervous system
CO	carbon monoxide; cardiac output
CO_2	carbon dioxide
coag	coagulation
COHb	carboxyhemoglobin
COM	chronic otitis media
COMT	catechol-o-methyltransferase
conc	concentration
COPD	chronic obstructive pulmonary disease
COX	cyclooxygenase
COX-2	cyclooxygenase-2
cP	centipoise
CP	cerebral palsy; cerebellopontine (angle)
CPAP	continuous positive airway pressure
CPB	cardiopulmonary bypass
CPD	cephalopelvic disproportion
CPP	cerebral perfusion pressure
CPR	cardiopulmonary resuscitation
CPT	carnitine palmityl transferase
CPZ	chlorpromazine
Cr	creatinine
CrCl	creatinine clearance
CRI	chronic renal insufficiency
cryo	cryoprecipitate
CS	chrondroitin sulfate
C-section	cesarean section
CSF	cerebrospinal fluid
CSH	carotid sinus hypersensitivity
CSM	carotid sinus massage
C-spine	cervical spine
CSS	carotid sinus syndrome
CT	computed tomography; connective tissue
CTX	cyclophosphamide (Cytoxan)
CV	cardiovascular
CVA	cerebrovascular accident
CVD	cerebrovascular disease
CVP	central venous pressure
CVS	cardiovascular status
CXR	chest x-ray
CYP	cytochrome P450
cysto	cystoscopy

D

2,3-DPG	2,3-diphosphoglyceric acid
2D	two-dimensional
d	day
D and T	diphtheria and tetanus
D&C	dilatation and curettage
D/C	discontinue(d)
D_5	dextrose 5% in water
DA	dopamine
DBP	diastolic blood pressure
DC	direct current
DCM	dilated cardiomyopathy
DDAVP	1-deamino(8-D-arginine) vasopressin; desmopressin acetate
DDT	dichlorodiphenyltrichloroethane
DEA	Drug Enforcement Agency
DEB	dystrophic epidermolysis bullosa
deriv	derivative(s)
derm	dermatology
DFA	direct immunofluorescent assay
DFT	defibrillation threshold
DGL	deglycyrrhized licorice
DGLA	dihomo-γ-linolenic acid
DHA	docosahexaenoic acid
DHEA	dehydroepiandrosterone
DHT	dihydrotestosterone
DI	diabetes insipidus
DIC	disseminated intravascular coagulation
diff	differential
Dig	digoxin
DJD	degenerative joint disease
DKA	diabetic ketoacidosis
DLco	carbon monoxide diffusion capacity in the lungs
DM	diabetes mellitus
DMD	Duchenne muscular dystrophy
DMT	dimethyltryptamine
DNR	do not resuscitate
Do_2	oxygen delivery
DOB	dobutamine

DOE	dyspnea on exertion
dP/dT	ratio of change in ventricular pressure to change in time
DPNB	dorsal penile nerve block
dSSEP	dermatomal somatosensory evoked potentials
DTIC	dimethyltriazenoimidazole carboxamide (dacarbazine)
DTPA	diethylenetriaminepenta-acetic acid
DTR	deep tendon reflex
DTs	delirium tremens
DVT	deep vein thrombosis
Dx	diagnosis; diagnostic

E

EACA	epsilon-aminocaproic
EBL	estimated blood loss
EBV	Epstein-Barr virus
EC	eclampsia
ECA	ethacrynic acid
ECC	extracorporeal circulation
ECD	endocardial cushion defect
ECFV	extracellular fluid volume
ECG	electrocardiogram
ECHO	echocardiogram
ECMO	extracorporeal membrane oxygenation
ECoG	electrocorticography
ECT	electroconvulsive therapy
ED_{50}	median effective dose
EDAS	encephalodural arteriosynangiosis
EDTA	ethylenediaminetetraacetic acid
EDV	end-diastolic volume
EEC	ectrodactyly-ectodermal dysplasia, cleft (syndrome)
EEG	electroencephalogram
EENT	eyes, ears, nose, throat
EF	ejection fraction
EGD	esophagogastroduodenoscopy
E-L	Eaton-Lambert
ELBW	extremely low birth weight
ELISA	enzyme-linked immunosorbent assay
EMD	electromechanical dissociation
EMG	electromyography
EMI	electromagnetic interference; electromechanical interference
EMLA	eutectic mixture of local anesthetics
endo	endocrine
ENT	ear, nose, and throat
EP	electrophysiologic
EPA	eicosapentaenoic acid
EPI	epinephrine
EPO	evening primrose oil
EPS	electrophysiologic study
ER	emergency room
ERCP	endoscopic retrograde cholangiopancreatography
ERV	expiratory reserve volume
ES	Eisenmenger's syndrome
es	estimated
ESM	ethosuximide
esp	especially
ESR	erythrocyte sedimentation rate
ESRD	end-stage renal disease
ESS	endoscopic sinus surgery
ESV	end-systolic volume
ESWL	extracorporeal shock wave lithotripsy
ET	endotracheal
$ETCO_2$	end-tidal carbon dioxide
ETN_2	end-tidal nitrogen
ETOH	ethanol

ETT	endotracheal tube; exercise tolerance test
eval	evaluation
Ex	exercise
exam	examination
ext	exterior

F

5-FU	5-fluorouracil
F	female(s)
Fa/Fi	fraction alveolar/fraction inspired
Fab	fragment, antigen-binding
FAD	flavin adenine dinucleotide
FBS	fasting blood sugar
FDA	food and Drug Administration
FDP	fibrin-degradation product
Fe	iron
Fe^{2+}	ferrous
Fe^{3+}	ferric
FEN_a	excreted fraction of filtered sodium
FES	fat embolism syndrome
FEV	forced expiratory volume
FEV_1	Forced expiratory volume in 1 second
FFA	free fatty acid
FFP	fresh frozen plasma
FHP	fulminant hepatic failure
FHR	fetal heart rate
FHT	fetal heart tone
FIO_2	fractional inspired oxygen
FIX	factor IX
FMN	flavin mononucleotide
FOB	fiberoptic bronchoscopy
FOI	fiber optic intubation
FRC	functional residual capacity
freq	frequent; frequency
FSBG	fingerstick blood glucose
FSH	follicle stimulating hormone
FSP	fibrin split products
FT_4E	free thyroxine estimate
FTT	failure to thrive
FUDR	floxuridine
FVC	forced vital capacity
FVIII	factor VIII
Fx	fracture

G

G	gauge
G6PD	glucose-6 phosphate dehydrogenase
GA	general anesthesia
GABA	γ-aminobutyric acid
GBL	gamma butyrolactone
G-CSF	granulocyte colony-stimulating factor
GDM	gestational diabetes mellitus
GE	gastroesophageal
GER	gastroesophageal reflux
GERD	gastroesophageal reflux disease
GETA	general endotracheal anesthesia
GFR	glomerular filtration rate
GGTP	gamma-glutamyl-transpeptidase
GH	growth hormone
GHB	gamma hydroxybutyrate
Gi	inhibitory G protein
GI	gastrointestinal
GIFT	gamete intrafallopian transfer
GLA	γ-linolenic acid
glu	glucose

GMP	guanosine monophosphate
Gn-RH	gonadotropin-releasing hormone
GRAS	generally recognized as safe
GTP	guanosine triphosphate
GTT	glucose tolerance test
GU	genitourinary
GVHD	graft vs. host disease
gyn	gynecologic

H

5-HIAA	5-hydroxyindoleacetic acid
5-HT	5-hydroxytryptamine
H & N	head and neck
H & P	history and physical
H_1	histamine receptor type 1
H_2	histamine receptor type 2
H_2O	water
HAF-PCM	hypoalbuminemic form of protein-calorie malnutrition
HAV	hepatitis A virus
HB	heart block
HbA_{1c}	glycosylated hemoglobin
HbAA	hemoglobin homozygous for A
HbM	hemoglobin Milwaukee
HbO_2	oxyhemoglobin
HbsAg	hepatitis B surface antigen
HbSS	homozygosity for hemoglobin S (sickle cell anemia)
HBV	hepatitis B virus
HCFA	Health Care Financing Administration
hCG	human gonadotropic hormone
HCM	hypertrophic cardiomyopathy
HCO_2	bicarbonate
Hct	hematocrit
HCV	hepatitis C virus
HD	heart disease; Hodgkin's disease
HDL	high-density lipoprotein
HDL-C	HDL cholesterol
He	helium
HEENT	head, eyes, ears, nose, throat
HELLP	hemolysis, elevated liver enzymes, and low platelet count (syndrome)
heme	hematology
Hg	mercury
Hgb	hemoglobin
HGPRT	hypoxanthine-guanine-phosphoribosyl-transferase
HHV-3-6	human herpes viruses
HIV	human immunodeficiency virus
HLA	human leukocyte antigen
hLH	hemophagocytic lymphohistiocytosis
HLHS	hypoplastic left heart syndrome
HMD	hyaline membrane disease
HMG CoA	3-hydroxy-3-methylglutaryl
HN_2	nitrogen mustard
hosp	hospitalization
HPV	hypoxic pulmonary vasoconstriction
hr	hour(s)
HR	heart rate
HSV	herpes simplex virus
HSV-1	HSV type 1
HSV-2	HSV type 2
ht	height
Htn	hypertension
HUS	hemolytic uremic syndrome
Hx	history

I

I & D	incision and drainage
I/O	intake-output
IABCP	intra-aortic balloon counterpulsation
IABP	intra-aortic balloon pump
IADH	inappropriate antidiuretic hormone
IBD	inflammatory bowel disease
ICA	internal carotid artery
ICD	implantable cardioverter defibrillator
ICGA	immunochromatographic assay
ICH	intracranial hypertension
ICMA	immunochemiluminometric assay
ICP	intracranial pressure
ICU	intensive care unit
ID	infectious disease
IDCM	idiopathic dilated cardiomyopathy
IDDM	insulin-dependent diabetes mellitus
IDL	intermediate-density lipoprotein
I:E	inspiratory:expiratory ratio
IFN	interferon
Ig	immunoglobulin
IGF	insulin-like growth factor
IGF-I	insulin-like growth factor I
IHD	ischemic heart disease
IHSS	idiopathic hypertrophic subaortic stenosis
IL	interleukin
IM	intramuscular
immuno	immunologic
in.	inch
incl	including
inf	inferior
info	information
INH	isoniazid
INR	International Normalized Ratio
insp	inspiratory
intox	intoxication
intraop	intraoperative
IOL	intraocular lens
IOP	intraocular pressure
IP	impedance plethysmography; intraperitoneal; intraperitoneally
IPPB	intermittent positive pressure breathing
IPPV	intermittent positive pressure ventilation
IQ	intelligence quotient
IRDS	infant respiratory distress syndrome
IRMA	immunoradiometric assay
ITP	immune thrombocytopenic purpura
I-V	interventricular
IV	intravenous
IVC	inferior vena cava
IVF	intravascular fluid; intravenous fluid
IVH	intracranial/intraventricular hemorrhage
IVP	intravenous pyelogram

J

JEB	junctional epidermolysis bullosa
JV	jugular vein
JVD	jugular venous distention
JVP	jugular venous pressure

K

K^+	potassium
Kr	krypton
KSS	Kearns-Sayre syndrome
KUB	kidney, ureter, bladder

L

L	left
L→R	left to right
LA	left atrial; left atrium; linoleic acid; local anesthetic
lab	laboratory
LAD	left anterior descending (coronary artery)
LAFB	left anterior fascicular block
LAO	left anterior oblique
LAP	left atrial pressure
lat	lateral
LBBB	left bundle branch block
LBO	large-bowel obstruction
LCAT	lecithin-cholesterol acyltransderase
LCH	Langerhans cell histiocytosis
LDH	lactate dehydrogenase
LDL	low-density lipoprotein
LDL-C	LDL cholesterol
LE	lower extremity
LEA	lower extremity amputation
LES	lower esophageal sphincter
LFT	liver function test
LGL	Lown-Ganong-Levine syndrome
LH	luteinizing hormone
LLQ	left lower quadrant
LMA	laryngeal mask airway
LMP	last menstrual period
LMW	low molecular weight
LMWH	low molecular weight heparin
LOC	level of consciousness; loss of consciousness
LOS	length of stay
LP	lumbar puncture
Lp(a)	lipoprotein(a)
L-PAM	melphalan (Alkeran)
LPFB	left posterior fascicular block
LPO	left posterior oblique
LR	lactated Ringer's (solution)
LRI	lower respiratory tract infection
LSB	lumber sympathetic block
LSD	lysergic acid diethylamide
LTB_4	leukotriene B_4
LUQ	left upper quadrant
LV	left ventricle
LVAD	left ventricular assist device
LVEDP	left ventricular end-diastolic pressure
LVEF	left ventricular ejection fraction
LVET	left ventricular ejection time
LVF	left ventricular failure
LVH	left ventricular hypertrophy
LVOT	left ventricular outflow tract
lytes	electrolytes

M

M	male(s)
M:F	male to female ratio
M2	muscarinic
MAC	minimum alveolar concentration; monitored anesthesia care
MALA	metformin-associated lactic acidosis
MAO	monoamine oxidase
MAOI	MAO inhibitor
MAP	mean arterial pressure
MAST	medical antishock trousers
MAT	multiform atrial tachycardia
max	maximum; maximal
MBC	maximal breathing capacity

MCA	middle cerebral artery
MD	muscular dystrophy
MEA	multiple endocrine adenomas
mech	mechanical; mechanism
med	medication
MEN	multiple endocrine neoplasia
MEN I	multiple endocrine neoplasia type I
MEN II	multiple endocrine neoplasia type II
MEP	motor/multimodality evoked potential
MET	metabolic equivalent
metab	metabolism; metabolic
metHb	methemoglobin
mets	metastases
MF-PCM	marasmic form of PCM
Mg^{2+}	magnesium
$MgSO_4$	magnesium sulfate
MH	malignant hyperthermia
MI	myocardial infarction
MIDCAB	minimally invasive direct coronary artery bypass
min	minimal; minimum; minute
MIsch	myocardial ischemia
mIU	milli-International unit
MIV	mivacurium
MLAP	mean left atrial pressure
MLD	median lethal dose
MMEFR	maximal midexpiratory flow rate
MMR	masseter muscle rigidity
mo	month
mo wt	molecular weight
MODS	multiorgan dysfunction syndrome
MP	mucopolysaccharide
MPAP	mean pulmonary artery pressure
MPD	mast cell proliferative disorder
MR	mitral regurgitation
MRA	magnetic resonance angiography
MRI	magnetic resonance imaging
MS	mental status; mitral stenosis; multiple sclerosis; musculoskeletal
ms	milliseconds
MSLT	Multiple Sleep Latency Test
MSOF	multisystem organ failure
MTX	methotrexate
MU	million units
mucocut	mucocutaneous
MUGA	multiple gated acquisition
musc	muscular
MVD	microvascular decompression
MVI	multiple vitamin infusion
Mvo_2	minute venous oxygen
MVP	mitral valve prolapse
MW	molecular weight
MYL	Myleran (busulfan)

N

N	nitrogen
n.	nerve
n-MPTP	1-methyl-4-phenyl-1,2,3,6-tetrahydropyridine
N/A	not applicable
N/S	normal saline
N/V	nausea/vomiting
N_2O	dinitrogen monoxide (nitrous oxide)
Na^+	sodium
NAC	N-acetyl-L-cysteine
NADH	nicotinamide adenine dinucleotide reduced form

NADPH	nicotinamide adenine dinucleotide phosphate, reduced form
NAPA	*N*-acetyl procainamide
NB	nota bene (note well)
NCV	nerve conduction velocity
Nd:YAG	neodymium:yttrium-aluminum-garnet
NE	norepinephrine
NEC	necrotizing enterocolitis
neg	negative
neuro	neurologic
NF	neurologic findings
NF-1	neurofibromatosis
NG	nasogastric
NH_3	ammonia
NHL	non-Hodgkin's lymphoma
NHR	non–hemodynamically related
NIBP	noninvasive blood pressure
NICU	neonatal intensive care unit
NIDDM	non–insulin-dependent diabetes mellitus
NIF	negative inspiratory force
NIH	National Institutes of Health
NK	natural killer (cell)
NM	neuromuscular
NMB	neuromuscular blockade
NMDA	*N*-methyl-D-aspartate
NMEPs	neuromuscular evoked potentials
NMJ	neuromuscular junction
nml	normal
NMS	neuroleptic malignant syndrome
NO	nitric oxide
no.	number
nondep	nondepolarizing
NP	nasopharyngeal
NPH	neutral protamine Hagedorn
NPO	nil per os (nothing by mouth)
NPPB	normal perfusion pressure breakthrough (syndrome)
NRI	nutritional risk index
NS	normal saline (solution)
NSAID	nonsteroidal anti-inflammatory drug
NSR	normal sinus rhythm
NT	nasotracheal
NTG	nitroglycerin
NTP	nucleoside triphosphate
NVD	nausea, vomiting, and diarrhea
NYHA	New York Heart Association

O

O/P	output
O_2	oxygen
OA	osteoarthritis
OB	obstetric
OB/GYN	obstetrics and gynecology
OC	oral contraceptive
OD	overdose
OG	orogastric
OKT3	Ortho Kung T cell (muromonab-CD3)
OLD	obstructive lung disease
OM	otitis media
OMIM	Online Mendelian Inheritance in Man
OPCAB	off-pump coronary artery bypass
ophthal	ophthalmologic
OPO	Organ Procurement Organization
OR	operating room
ORIF	open reduction internal fixation
Osm	osmole; osmolality
OTC	over-the-counter

P

P	phosphorus
$P(A-a)o_2$	alveolar-arterial oxygen difference
PA	plasma aldosterone; pulmonary artery
PAC	premature atrial contraction
$Paco_2$	partial pressure of carbon dioxide, arterial
PACU	postanesthesia care unit
PAF	platelet activating factor
PAIR	puncture-aspiration-injection-reaspiration
palp	palpation of
Pao_2	partial pressure of oxygen in arterial blood
PAOP	pulmonary artery occlusion pressure
PAP	pulmonary artery pressure
PAPVD	partial anomalous pulmonary venous drainage
PAT	paroxysmal atrial tachycardia
Paw	mean airway pressure
PAWP	pulmonary artery wedge pressure
PBF	pulmonary blood flow
PCA	patient-controlled analgesia
PCFS	posterior cranial fossa surgery
PCM	protein calorie malnutrition
PCO	polycystic ovary
Pco_2	partial pressure of carbon dioxide
PCP	phencyclidine
PCR	polymerase chain reaction
PCV	packed cell volume
PCWP	pulmonary capillary wedge pressure
PD	peritoneal dialysis
PDA	patent ductus arteriosus
PDE II	phosphodiesterase III (inhibitors)
PDI	pituitary diabetes insipidus
PDR	Physician's Desk Reference
PE	physical examination; preeclampsia; pressure equalization; pulmonary embolism
PEEP	positive end-expiratory pressure
PEF	peak expiratory flow
PEP	positive expiratory pressure
periop	perioperative
PET	positron emission tomography
$PETCO_2$	end-tidal partial pressure of carbon dioxide
PFO	patent foramen ovale
PFT	pulmonary function test
PG	prostaglandin
PGD_2	prostaglandin D_2
PGE_1	alprostadil (prostaglandin E_1)
pharm	pharmaceutical; pharmacy
pheo	pheochromocytoma
physiol	physiologic
P_i	inorganic phosphate
PID	pelvic inflammatory disease
PIH	pregnancy-induced hypertension
PIP	peak inspiratory pressure
pK_a	negative logarithm of the dissociation constant of an acid
plt	platelet
pM	picomolar
PMI	posterior myocardial infarction; point of maximal intensity
PMN	polymorphonuclear
PMS	premenstrual syndrome
PND	paroxysmal nocturnal dyspnea
PNS	peripheral nervous system
PO	per os
Po_2	oxygen partial pressure
PO_4	phosphate
POAG	primary open-angle glaucoma

pos	positive
poss	possible; possibly
postop	postoperative
PPAR	peroxisome proliferator-activated receptor
PPD	purified protein derivative (tuberculin)
PPH	persistent pulmonary hypertension
Pplat	plateau pressure
ppm	parts per million
PPV	positive predictive value; positive pressure ventilation
PR	per rectum
PRA	plasma renin activity
prb	problem
PRBCs	packed red blood cells
preg	pregnancy; pregnant
premed	premedication
preop	preoperative
prep	preparation
PRL	prolactin
prn	as needed
PS	pulmonary stenosis
PSA	prostate-specific antigen
PSVT	paroxysmal supraventricular tachycardia
psych	psychological
pt	patient
PT	physical therapy; prothrombin time
PTCA	percutaneous transluminal coronary angioplasty
PTH	parathyroid hormone
PTLD	post transplant lymphoproliferative disease
pts	patients
PTSD	posttraumatic stress disorder
PTT	partial thromboplastin time
PTU	propylthiouracil
PUD	peptic ulcer disease
pulm	pulmonary
PUVA	psoralens plus ultraviolet A
PVC	polyvinyl chloride; premature ventricular contraction
PVD	peripheral vascular disease
PVO_2	partial pressure of oxygen, venous
PVR	pulmonary vascular resistance

Q

Q	perfusion
q	every
q.a.m.	every morning
q.n.	every night
q.p.m.	every evening
qhs	every hour of sleep
qid	four times per day
Qp:Qs	ratio of pulmonary blood to systemic blood flow
QRS	Q wave, R wave, S wave

R

R	right
R/O	rule out
RA	rheumatoid arthritis; right atrial; right atrium
RAAS	renin-angiotensin-aldosterone system
RAD	reactive airway disease
RAE	right atrial enlargement
RAH	right atrial hypertrophy
RAI	resting ankle index
RAO	right anterior oblique
RAP	right atrial pressure
RAST	radioallergosorbent test
RBBB	right bundle branch block
RBC	red blood cell

RBF	renal blood flow
RCM	congenital methemoglobinemia of the recessive type
RDA	recommended daily allowance
RDS	respiratory distress syndrome
reg	regular
rehab	rehabilitation
REM	rapid eye movement
reprod	reproductive (system)
resp	respiratory
RH	releasing hormone
RHD	rheumatic heart disease
RHF	right heart failure
RIA	radioimmunoassay
RIJ	right internal jugular
RIMA	reversible inhibitor of monoamine
RIND	reversible ischemic neurologic deficit
RLD	restrictive lung disease
ROM	range of motion
ROP	retinopathy of prematurity
ROS	review of systems
ROSC	return of spontaneous circulation
RPO	right posterior oblique
RR	respiratory rate
R→L	right to left
RSD	reflex sympathetic dystrophy
RSV	respiratory syncytial virus
RT	radiation therapy
RTA	renal tubule acidosis
RUQ	right upper quadrant
RV	residual volume; right ventricle
RVE	right ventricular enlargement
RVEDP	right ventricular end-diastolic pressure
RVH	right ventricular hypertrophy
Rx	therapy; treatment; therapeutic

S

S	Svedberg unit
S/P	status post
SA	sinoatrial; beta S/beta A globin gene
SAH	subarachnoid hemorrhage
SAM	systolic anterior motion
SAMe	S-adenosyl-L-methionine
SaO_2	oxygen saturation in arterial blood
SAP	systematic arterial pressure
SAS	sleep apnea syndrome
sat	saturation
SBE	standard base excess; subacute bacterial endocarditis
SBO	small-bowel obstruction
SBP	systolic blood pressure
SCD	sudden cardiac death
SCH	succinylcholine
SD	standard deviation(s)
SEB	simplex epidermolysis
sec	second(s)
SEP	sensory evoked potential
seroneg	seronegative
SG	specific gravity
SGOT	serum glutamic-oxaloacetic transaminase
SGPT	serum glutamate pyruvate transaminase
SIADH	syndrome of inappropriate secretion of antidiuretic hormone
SICU	surgical ICU
SIDS	sudden infant death syndrome
SIRS	systemic inflammatory response syndrome

SL	sublingual
SLE	systemic lupus erythematosus
SMA	superior mesenteric artery
SMA-20	Sequential Multiple Analyzer
SNS	sympathetic nervous system
SOB	shortness of breath
soln	solution
SPECT	single-photon emission computed tomography
SPK	simultaneous pancreas-kidney
SpO_2	oxygen saturation as measured by pulse oximetry
spont	spontaneously
SQ	subcutaneous; subcutaneously
SSEP	somatosensory evoked potential
SSRI	selective serotonin reuptake inhibitor
SSS	sick sinus syndrome
STD	sexually transmitted disease
STP	2,5-dimethoxy-4-methylamphetamine
STSG	split-thickness skin graft
Stz	streptozocin
sup	superior
surg	surgery; surgical
SV	stroke volume
SVC	superior vena cava
SVO_2	mixed venous continuous oxygen saturation
SVR	systemic vascular resistance
SVT	supraventricular tachycardia
Sx	signs and symptoms
Sz	seizure

T

^{99m}Tc	technetium 99m
T	temperature
T&C	type and crossmatch
$T_{1/2}$	half-life
T_3	triiodothyronine
T_4	thyroxine
TA	tricuspid atresia
TAH	total abdominal hysterectomy
TAPVD	total anomalous pulmonary venous drainage
TB	tuberculosis
TCA	tricyclic antidepressant
TCD	transcranial Doppler
TDP	torsades de pointes
TEE	transesophageal echocardiography
TEF	transesophageal fistula
TEG	thromboelastography
temp	temperature
TENS	transcutaneous electrical nerve stimulation
tet	tetralogy of Fallot
TFA	trifluoroacetic acid
TFT	thyroid function test
TGA	transposition of the great arteries
TGV	transposition of great vessels
THC	delta-9-tetrahydrocannabinol
THR	total hip replacement
TIA	transient ischemic attack
tid	three times per day
TIPS	transjugular intrahepatic portosystemic shunt
TJC	The Joint Commission
TKR	total knee replacement
TLC	total lung capacity/compliance
Tm	maximal tubular excretory capacity (of kidney)
TM	temporomandibular
TMEP	telangiectasia macularis eruptive perstans
TMJ	temporomandibular joint
TMP/SMX	trimethoprim/sulfamethoxazole

TN	trigeminal neuralgia
TNF	tumor necrosis factor
TNM	tumor, nodes, and metastasis
TOF	train-of-4; tetralogy of Fallot
TP	total protein
t-PA	tissue plasminogen activator
TPN	total parenteral nutrition
TR	tricuspid regurgitation
TRH	thyrotropin-releasing hormone
TRUS	transrectal ultrasonography
TSH	thyroid stimulating hormone
TT	thrombin time
TTE	transthoracic echocardiography
T-TEPA	triethylene-thiophosphoramide (thiotepa)
TTP	thrombotic thrombocytopenic purpura
TURBT	transurethral resection of bladder tumor
TRUP	transurethral resection of the prostate
TV	tidal volume
TVH	total vaginal hysterectomy
Tx	transplant; transfusion
TXA_2	thromboxane A_2
TXA_3	thromboxane A_3
TXB_2	thromboxane B_2

U

UA	urinalysis
UE	upper extremity
UGI	upper gastrointestinal
UK	United Kingdom
U-lytes	urine electrolytes
UO	urine output
UP	urticaria pigmentosa
UPJ	ureteropelvic junction
URI	upper respiratory tract infection
urol	urology; urologic
US	ultrasound
USA	United States of America
UT	urinary tract
UTI	urinary tract infection
UV	ultraviolet

V

V	ventilation
V/Q	ventilation-perfusion
VACTERL	vertebral, anal, cardiac, tracheal, esophageal, renal, and limb
VAE	venous air embolism
VALI	ventilator-associated lung injury
VAS	Visual Analogue Scale
vasc	vascular
VATER	vertebral anomalies, anal atresia, tracheoesophageal fistula, esophageal atresia, radial dysplasia
VC	vital capacity; vocal cord
VCO_2	carbon dioxide consumption per unit time
V_d	volume of distribution
VD_{ss}	volume of distribution in a steady state
vent	ventilation
VFIB	ventricular fibrillation
VFP	ventricular filling pressure
VIPoma	vasoactive intestinal peptide-secreting tumors
vit	vitamin
VLBW	very low birth weight
VLDL	very low density lipoprotein
VM-26	teniposide
VMA	vanillylmandelic acid

VO_2	oxygen consumption per unit time
vol	volume
VP-16	etoposide
VPA	valproic acid
VR	venous return
VS	vital signs
vs.	versus
VSD	ventricular septal defect
VSM	vascular smooth muscle
VTach	ventricular tachycardia
VUR	vesicoureteral reflux
VVB	venovenous bypass
VVI	ventricular inhibited
vWF	von Willebrand factor

W

w/	with
w/o	without
WBC	white blood cell
wk	week(s)
WNL	within normal limits
WPW	Wolff-Parkinson-White syndrome
wt	weight

XYZ

Xe	xenon
XS	excessive
y	year(s)

SECTION I

Diseases

Abruptio Placentae

Charles P. Gibbs

Risk

- People within USA: 1:200 of the approximately 4 million births/y
- Races with highest prevalence: African-Americans and Caucasians vs. Asian and Hispanic
- Increased prevalence with preeclampsia, chronic hypertension, multiple gestations, LBW, hydramnios, thrombophilia, cocaine use, trauma, increased age and parity, smoking, premature rupture of membranes, and prior abruption

Perioperative Risks

- Maternal: Antepartum and postpartum hemorrhage, DIC, and death
- Fetal: Hypoxia due to maternal hypotension and/or decreased area for placental exchange; usually there is minimal bleeding from the fetus but it can occur

Worry About

- Concealed hemorrhage behind the placenta that does not manifest as vaginal bleeding, which may be considerable

- Postpartum hemorrhage refractory to usual oxytocic agents; some believe old blood can infiltrate into and between uterine muscle fibers and decrease the effectiveness of uterine contractions (Couvelaire uterus)
- Fetal distress and/or death
- Need for cesarean hysterectomy due to previous concerns

Overview

- Along with placenta previa, a major cause of antepartum hemorrhage, maternal mortality and perinatal mortality
- Maternal mortality: 1.8–2.8%
- Perinatal mortality: 30–40%
- Morbidity: ~20% of survivors have some form of neurologic deficit
- Abruptio placentae is the most common cause of DIC in pregnant patients; 20% with clinically significant abruption develop clotting defects. DIC is probably due to the release of thromboplastin by placenta and damaged tissues at abruption site.
- Postpartum hemorrhage correlates directly with severity of coagulopathy

- Blood and blood clots in muscle fibers may inhibit ability of uterus to contract, which leads to more blood loss

ICD-9-CM Code: 641.2

Etiology

- Separation of placenta from uterine wall along decidual plane between membranes and uterus

Usual Treatment

- Maintenance of volume status and fetal surveillance
- If fetus is premature and hemorrhage is not great, careful observation would be appropriate to allow for fetal growth
- If at term and volume status OK, labor with vaginal delivery is optimal
- If hemorrhage continues and/or fetal distress occurs, C-section is necessary. If fetus is at term and doing well, then may elect for ceserean section to prevent fetal harm or death from sudden increase in abruption process

ASSESSMENT POINTS

System	Effect	Assessment by Hx	PE	Test
CV	Hemorrhage	Vaginal bleeding and abdominal pain	Vaginal bleeding and firm, tender uterus; hypotension, tachycardia. low CVP and wedge pressures, decreased urine output	Hct
HEME	Hypovolemia; acute anemia	Bleeding diathesis	Hypotension, tachycardia, bleeding from puncture sites, easy bruisability	Hgb, Hct, clotting evaluation that includes platelets, fibrinogen, and fibrin split products
RENAL	Oliguria and/or acute renal failure	Urine output	Signs of hypovolemia	Urinalysis to include specific gravity and sodium excretion, possibly in addition to central hemodynamic monitoring values
UTERUS/ VAGINA	Abruption; hemorrhage	Painful vaginal bleeding	Tender, firm uterus; vaginal bleeding may be < CV signs and symptoms, indicating concealed hemorrhage	Hct and hemodynamic monitoring values
FETUS	Fetal distress and/or demise	Presence or absence of fetal movement	Fetal movement, heart rate	Electronic fetal monitoring

Key Reference: Mercier FJ, Van de Velde M. Major obstetric hemorrhage. *Anesthesiol Clin.* 2008;26(1):53–66.

Perioperative Implications—for Labor and Vaginal Delivery

Preinduction/Induction/Maintenance

- Epidural analgesia appropriate if volume status can be maintained and if hemorrhage controllable
- Optimize cardiovascular and fetal status and evaluate coagulation system
- Technique not different from that for normal labor and vaginal delivery except that the smallest effective doses should be used; combined spinal/epidural with narcotics and local anesthetic may be useful
- Electronic fetal monitoring is essential
- CV monitoring appropriate for volume and bleeding status

Perioperative Implications—for Cesarean Section

Preinduction/Induction/Maintenance

- Optimize CV and fetal status, usually by means of appropriate volume replacement

Monitoring

- All cases will require electronic fetal monitoring as well as intrauterine pressure monitoring
- Urine output
- Hct and clotting studies as above
- Consider CVP and/or PA catheter depending on severity of hemorrhage and decreased urine output not responsive to simple fluid challenges

General Anesthesia

- Probably required for massive hemorrhage and/or acute fetal distress
- Aspiration prophylaxis
- Rapid-sequence induction with cricoid pressure
- Consider ketamine 1 mg/kg and large-bore lines
- Watch for continued hemorrhage after delivery of infant. Uterus may not respond to usual tocolytic agents. For hemorrhage control:
  - Oxytocin 20–40 mU in 1 L of balanced salt solution
  - Methergine 0.2 mg IM; *not* in the presence of hypertension
  - Prostaglandin $F_2\alpha$ 250 μg IM or intramyometrial. May cause bronchospasm and decrease in SaO_2
    - Hypogastric artery ligation
    - Uterine, hypogastric artery embolization
    - Cesarean hysterectomy
- Awake extubation

Regional Anesthesia

- Appropriate in the absence of severe hemorrhage and/or acute fetal distress
- Aspiration prophylaxis
- Optimize volume status
- Epidural preferred over spinal because the level can be raised slowly, but could do same with continous spinal

- Treat hypotension early and vigorously, usually with ephedrine or phenylephrine
- Watch for continuing uterine hemorrhage

Postoperative Period

- Pt needs to be in an appropriately staffed and equipped recovery/SICU area
- Be alert for continuing uterine hemorrhage and/or development of coagulopathy
- Continue intraoperative monitoring

Anticipated Problems/Concerns

- Amount of bleeding may be considerably greater than what is evident per vagina. A significant amount of blood can be trapped behind the abrupted placenta.
- Be alert to the need for immediate cesarean section for fetal distress and/or dramatic increase in hemorrhage
- Best therapy for DIC is removal of the placenta by C-section or vaginal delivery
- Hemorrhage may continue postpartum from an atonic uterus that is refractory to the usual oxytocic agents
- C-section hysterectomy may be necessary, which may in itself be accompanied by large blood loss
- If multiple blood units are transfused, watch for dilutional thrombocytopenia.

Achondroplasia, Dwarfism

Minh Chau Joe Tran

Risk

- 1 per 15,000–40,000 births worldwide
- Females ≥ males
- No race predilection
- Most common type of dwarfism

Perioperative Risks

- Cervical spine instability
- Foramen magnum and cervical spine stenosis
- Restrictive pulmonary disease
- Thoracolumbar kyphosis

Worry About

- Central apnea
- Obstructive sleep apnea
- Cervicomedullary compression
- Cauda equina syndrome
- Paresthesia or paraplegia
- Nerve root compression

Overview

- Results from failure in development and premature ossification of bones that form from cartilage. This leads to the characteristic frontal bossing, short arms and legs, maxillary hypoplasia, depressed nasal bridge, and trident hands.
- Other major features incl cervicomedullary compression; foramen magnum stenosis; small, flattened chest; RVH; restrictive lung disease; pulmonary hypertension; apnea; thoracolumbar spinal stenosis; scoliosis; thoracolumbar kyphosis; and lumbar hyperlordosis
- Brainstem compression contributes to central apnea, whereas obstructive apnea is from midface structural abnormalities
- Mean adult male height is 131 ± 5.6 cm; the mean adult female height is 124 ± 5.9 cm (about 4 feet for both)
- Mean adult male weighs 120 lbs (55 kg); the mean adult female weighs 100 lbs (45 kg)
- Trunk length and intelligence are normal; life expectancy is normal
- Obesity is present in both sexes

ICD-9-CM Code: 756.4 Chondrodystrophy

Etiology

- Autosomal dominant trait with complete penetrance
- 80% of cases are from new mutations; 20% are familial
- An achondroplastic parent has a 50% chance of passing on the gene
- Homozygous form is incompatible with life due to resp failure
- Caused by a missense mutation in *FGFR3* (fibroblast growth factor receptor 3) on chromosome 4p
- Advanced paternal age (age >35 y) is a risk factor in de novo cases

Usual Treatment

- Distraction osteogenesis and various other orthopedic procedures
- Myringotomy and tube placement, tonsillectomy and adenoidectomy
- Suboccipital craniectomy, VP shunts, laminectomy
- Dental; tracheostomy, C-section

ASSESSMENT POINTS

System	Effect	Assessment by Hx	PE	Test
HEENT	Megalocephaly with frontal bossing, large mandible, chronic otitis media with hearing loss, choanal stenosis, narrow nasopharynx, cervical kyphosis with limited neck extension, cervical neck instability, foramen magnum stenosis, dental malocclusion and crowding	Recurrent otitis media Conductive hearing loss Apnea with cyanotic spells Speech problems	Limited neck ROM Limited ability to visualize glottic opening Nasopharyngoscopy	Cervical flexion/ extension neck films Hearing test
CV	Pulm Htn, RVH, RV strain	SOB with routine activities, fatigue, dizziness, syncope, supplemental oxygen use	JVD distention, lower extremity edema, hypoxia, cyanosis, arrhythmia	EKG, ECHO, heart catheterization
PULM	Restrictive lung disease, decreased FRC, OSA, hypoxemia, hypercapnia, apnea	Apnea with cyanotic spells, Daytime somnolence, SOB Recurrent respiratory infections Pneumothorax from positive pressure ventilation Loud snoring	Rib hypoplasia, pectus carinatum or excavatus	CXR, ABG, PFT, sleep study
GI	Obesity Gastric hypomobility	Reflux symptoms, recurrent aspiration, dysphagia, globus hystericus	BMI	EGD, CXR
CNS	Hydrocephalus, elevated ICP, hyperreflexia, hypertonia, clonus, hypotonia (in infancy and early childhood), central apnea from brainstem compression at the level of the foramen magnum, cervicomedullary compression	Headaches, vertigo, dizziness, paresis, pyramidal signs, cervical myelopathy, ataxia, incontinence, snoring, daytime somnolence, depression is common	Craniocervical stenosis, foramen magnum stenosis, kinking of the medulla, increased lateral ventricular size, hypoplasia of the corpus callosum	Axial head CT, MRI, MEP, SSEP, sleep study
MS	Pectus carinatum or excavatum, genu varum, narrow spinal canal, rhizomelic shortening of arms and legs, small thoracic cage	Delayed motor milestones, premature degenerative joint disease	Thoracolumbar kyphoscoliosis, proximal limbs < distal limbs, brachydactyly and trident hand configuration, hyperextensibility of most joints (knees in particular), limited elbow extension and rotation	Spine films Bone scans

Key Reference: Monedero P, et al. Is Management of anesthesia in achondroplastic dwarfs really a challenge? *J Clin Anesth.* 1997;9:208–212.

Perioperative Implications

Preoperative Preparation
- GI prophylaxis
- Review airway films and studies
- Assess pt using systems base approach
- Assume unstable cervical neck

Monitoring
- Standard ASA monitors
- Foley catheter; A-line; CVP; and frequent H/H checks for invasive cases with major fluid shifts
- MEP; SSEP for spinal cord surgeries

Airway
- Anticipate difficult mask ventilation and intubation
- Use oral airway, nasal airway will be more challenging with the choanal stenosis
- Consider AFOI; have LMA as rescue
- No guidelines for ETT size and depth placement; have different sized ETTs on hand
- Keep neck neutral and avoid hyperextension or hyperflexion

Induction
- Careful IV induction with controlled airway
- Prevent hypoxia, which can worsen pulm Htn

- Prevent sudden drops in SVR, which hypoperfuse the brain through the stenotic foramen magnum
- RA rarely indicated and can be anatomically challenging

Maintenance
- Pressure-controlled ventilation with careful attention to PAP
- MEP and SSEP with spinal surgeries
- Careful positioning

- OG tube for gastric decompression
- Increased sensitivity to muscle relaxants
- Use peripheral nerve stimulator

Postoperative Period
- Resp insufficiency with frequent ABG checks
- CXR
- Pain control
- ICU monitoring

Anticipated Problems/Concerns
- Difficult IV access
- SIDS: 2–5%
- Neurologic impairment
- Pain control and resp depression
- Postop ventilation

Acidosis, Lactic/Metabolic

Peter Schulman
Jeffrey Mako

Risk

- Incidence in USA: Unknown
- Present in a variety of disease states, from mild to severe systemic illness

Perioperative Risks

- Hemodynamic instability (due to arteriolar vasodilation and decreased cardiac output)
- Hyperkalemia
- Insulin resistance and hyperglycemia
- Acute respiratory failure

Worry About

- Decreased responsiveness to vasopressors and inotropes
- Decreased activity of local anesthetic agents
- Arrhythmias

Overview

- Physiologic disturbance resulting from excess acid production, failure of organic acid excretion, or inappropriate bicarbonate loss causing increased serum acidity
- Marker of an underlying disease process
- Severe when, in the presence of resp compensation, the serum $[HCO_3]$ is ≤8 mmol/L
- History, physical exam, and laboratory studies (basic metabolic panel, serum albumin, serum lactate, arterial blood gas) may be useful in diagnosing the underlying pathology

ICD-9-CM Codes: 276.2 (Acidosis; metabolic, mixed or lactic); 276.4 (Mixed acid-base disorder); 250.1 (Diabetic ketoacidosis)

Etiology

- Broadly differentiated by calculating the anion gap: $AG = [Na^+] - ([Cl^-] + [HCO_3^-])$. The anion gap (AG) corresponds to the presence of unmeasured anions in serum. The presence or absence of an elevated AG helps to determine the underlying cause and direct appropriate therapy. Normal AG is 7 ± 4 mEq/L and decreases 2.5 mEq/L for every 1 g/dL decreased in serum albumin. Corrected AG can be calculated as:
- **Corrected AG = Calculated AG − {2.5 × (4.0 − [albumin])}**
- High AG metabolic acidosis: Results from an accumulation of excess acid in the serum. Specific causes are due to production of lactate or ketones (diabetic, alcoholic, or starvation ketoacidosis), toxic ingestion (methanol, ethylene glycol, salicylates), uremia, or medication side effects (propofol infusion syndrome, lactic acidosis associated with metformin)
- Normal AG metabolic acidosis: Associated with excess HCO_3^- loss from the kidney or GI tract, failure of the kidney to excrete H^+, or rapid IV infusion of bicarbonate-free solutions (e.g., normal saline)
- Delta gap (ΔΔ): Used to determine the presence of concomitant metabolic derangements and calculated as: $\Delta AG / \Delta [HCO_3^-]$, where ΔAG = (calculated AG − expected AG) and $\Delta [HCO_3^-]$ = (24-$[HCO_3^-]$). ΔΔ<1 indicates AG metabolic acidosis *and* concurrent non-AG acidosis. ΔΔ>2 indicates AG metabolic acidosis and concurrent metabolic alkalosis. ΔΔ = 1-2 indicates a pure AG metabolic acidosis

Usual Treatment

- Centered on rapid identification and treatment of the underlying physiologic disturbance (e.g., DKA, sepsis, inadequate resuscitation, cardiovascular failure, abdominal ischemia)
- In high AG metabolic acidosis, alkali therapy may be indicated as a temporizing measure for acute, severe acidemia (pH <7.20). In normal AG metabolic acidosis, alkali therapy may be indicated to replace bicarbonate losses
- Sodium bicarbonate remains the most widely used buffer, however its use in correcting lactic acidosis is controversial because it may increase $Paco_2$ and paradoxically worsen intracellular acidosis. Other untoward effects of bicarbonate include hyperosmolarity and hypernatremia
- THAM (tromethamine) and CarbiCarb (equimolar combination of sodium bicarbonate and carbonate) are alternate buffers designed to limit CO_2 generation, offering theoretical benefits over bicarbonate. Only THAM is currently available for clinical use.
- Bicarbonate deficit: Calculate this value using the formula:
  Bicarbonate deficit (mEq) = 0.4 × body weight (kg) × (24−$[HCO_3^-]$). This can help guide appropriate dosing when alkali therapy is indicated.
- In some instances (hyperventilation syndromes, high altitude), acidosis may be compensatory and not require treatment

ASSESSMENT POINTS

System	Effect	Assessment by Hx	PE	Test
NEURO	Altered mental status, seizures	Level of consciousness, delirium, somnolence nausea/vomiting, seizures, toxic ingestion	Obtunded, confused, somnolent	Toxicology screen, osmolal gap, serum lytes
CV	Arteriolar vasodilation, hypotension, ↓ response to vasopressors & inotropes, arrhythmias, hypocontractility	Signs of end-organ hypoperfusion	Tachycardia, hypotension, poor peripheral pulses, cold extremities, poor capillary refill	Invasive hemodynamic monitoring, ECHO, ECG
PULM	Hypoxemia, hyperventilation, resp failure	Tachypnea, dyspnea	Rapid & shallow breathing, accessory muscle use, hypoxia, hypercarbia	CXR, ABG, pulse oximetry
RENAL	Oliguria, acute kidney injury, ATN	Urine output, chronic renal disease	Signs of hypo- or hypervolemia	UO, Cr, BUN, urine lytes, UA, serum lytes
GI		Nausea, vomiting, diarrhea, melena, abdominal pain	Abdominal pain to palpation	Serum lactate, radiographic imaging, upper/lower endoscopy
ID		Fever, rigors	Hyper- or hypothermia, signs of focal infection	WBC with differential, cultures, radiographic imaging
ENDO	Hyperglycemia, insulin resistance	DM, polyuria, polydipsia, hyperphagia	Signs of dehydration	Blood glucose, serum ketones

Key Reference: Morris CG, Low J. Metabolic acidosis in the critically ill: Part 1. Classification and pathophysiology and Part 2. Causes and treatment. *Anaesthesia*. 2008;63: 294–301, 396–411.

Perioperative Implications

Preoperative Preparation

- Pts with metabolic acidosis may be hemodynamically unstable and demonstrate decreased responsiveness to inotropes and vasopressors
- Consider postponing surgery until the underlying cause is corrected, unless treatment requires immediate surgical intervention
- If surgery is urgent or emergent, consider ways to optimize the pt preop

Intraoperative

- Invasive monitoring may be indicated, depending on the severity of illness
- Goal for induction is hemodynamic stability
- Inotropes and vasopressors should be readily available
- Consider the need for pt to remain intubated postop

Postoperative Period

- Pt may require postop ICU care and prolonged mechanical ventilation

Anticipated Problems/Concerns

- Hemodynamic instability with decreased responsiveness to inotropes and vasopressors
- Compensation for profound metabolic acidosis may lead to acute resp failure
- Treatment with bicarbonate may paradoxically increase $Paco_2$ and worsen intracellular acidosis and respiratory status

Acromegaly

Russell T. Wall III

DISEASES

Risk

- People within USA:
  - Prevalence is 40 cases/million; incidence is 3 new cases/million/y
  - Occurs with equal frequency in men and women and most frequently diagnosed in third to fifth decades of life (5–20 y lag between onset of symptoms and diagnosis)

Perioperative Risks

- Common conditions increasing periop risk incl airway abnormalities, cardiovascular dysfunction (Htn), resp impairment (obstructive sleep apnea), endocrine abnormalities (hyperglycemia)

Worry About

- Difficulty or inability to ventilate and/or intubate
- Extent of CV disease
- Postop airway obstruction

Overview

- Acromegaly is a slowly progressive, debilitating endocrinopathy resulting from excess secretion of growth hormone, usually from a benign macroadenoma of the pituitary gland, and characterized by overgrowth of soft tissues and bone and cartilage of skeleton (nose, jaw, hands, fingers, feet, toes). Excess growth hormone before puberty (epiphyseal closure) leads to gigantism (<5% of acromegalics)

ICD-9-CM Code: 253.0

Etiology

- >99% of cases result from primary pituitary adenoma

Usual Treatment

- Surgery—primary therapy
  - Transsphenoidal pituitary microsurgery versus transcranial; transsphenoidal more common and preferred, with less morbidity. Smaller tumors (<10 mm diameter) yield probable cure
- Pituitary radiation—reserved for persistent postsurgical disease or when surgery is contraindicated
- Medical—adjunctive therapy or for nonsurgical candidates, effective if adenoma cells have dopamine and/or somatostatin receptors
  - Dopamine agonists—bromocriptine and cabergoline
  - Somatostatin analogue—octreotide and lanreotide

ASSESSMENT POINTS

System	Effect	Assessment by Hx	PE	Test
HEENT	Bone and soft tissue overgrowth of head and neck	TMJ arthritis Hoarseness Deep voice	Enlarged frontal, nasal bones Enlarged sinuses Macroglossia with glossoptosis Prognathism Hypertrophy of larynx Vocal cord thickening & edema Subglottic narrowing Enlarged thyroid gland (25%) with possible tracheal compression/deviation	Indirect laryngoscopy Lateral neck x-rays CT of neck
CV	CAD PVD LV dysfunction Cardiomyopathy	Chest pain Htn CHF Dysrhythmias Diastolic dysfunction	Htn CHF Dysrhythmias Cardiomegaly Diastolic dysfunction	CXR ECG ECHO
RESP	Airway soft tissue overgrowth Upper airway and small airway narrowing	Obstructive sleep apnea (60% of patients)	Barrel chest with kyphosis	PFTs (if indicated) Sleep study
RENAL	↑ (GI) Ca²⁺ absorption Hypercalciuria ↑ Total body Na⁺	Urolithiasis	Peripheral edema	
ENDO	↑ BMR	Heat intolerance	Hyperhidrosis	To diagnose acromegaly: ↑ 24 h GH levels Best screening test: ↑ serum IGF I (insulin-like growth factor) Definitive test: Oral glucose tolerance test (GH levels do not ↓)
	Hyperprolactinemia (some adenomas secrete GH and prolactin) Hyperthyroidism (3–7%) Insulin resistance (80%) Glucose intolerance (30–45%) Overt DM (15–25%) Hypertriglyceridemia (20–45%) Hyperphosphatemia Colon polyps/malignancy	Men: ↓ Libido, impotence Women: Menstrual abnormalities	Enlarged thyroid (25%)	TFTs Glucose Cholesterol, triglycerides Phosphorus Colonoscopy
CNS	Pituitary mass effect	Headache Hypersomnolence Visual disturbances		CT MRI (with gadolinium) to determine tumor size +/– extrasellar expansion
PNS	Carpal tunnel syndrome	Paresthesias	Median nerve compression	EMG, NCVs
MS	Bone and soft tissue overgrowth Osteoporosis Myopathy	Arthralgias Osteoarthritis (knees, hips, shoulders, LS spine) Fatigue, weakness	Enlarged hands and feet Hip, knee, shoulder, low back pain Muscle weakness	X-rays

Key Reference: Schmitt H, Buchfelder M, Radespiel-Troger M, Fahlbusch R. Difficult intubation in acromegalic patients: Incidence and predictability. *Anesthesiology.* 2000;93:110–114.

Perioperative Implications

Preoperative Preparation
- Optimize hemodynamics—BP control, no CHF
- Somatostatin analogue (octreotide) may shrink large macroadenoma

Monitoring
- Pulse oximeter may be difficult to fit (large fingers, toes); recommend A-line, brachial or femoral preferable

Airway
- Large masks, airways, blades, intubating LMA, tracheostomy equipment available
- Consider awake fiberoptic endotracheal intubation

Induction
- If GA, anticipate airway obstruction
- If hypopituitarism from mass effect, then may need hydrocortisone

- Possible lumbar drain if suprasellar extension
- Prophylactic antibiotics

Maintenance
- For transsphenoidal approach—surgical use of cocaine or epinephrine. Beware of increased BP and dysrhythmias
- For transsphenoidal approach >15° head up tilt, caution for VAE
- If preop pneumoencephalography, do not use nitrous oxide
- Monitor serum glucose and treat hyperglycemia
- Pack pharynx before surgery to prevent bleeding into laryngeal area and post-extubation laryngospasm

Extubation
- Anticipate airway obstruction
- No nasal CPAP possible posttranssphenoidal surgery

Adjuvants
- If myopathy, cautious use of muscle relaxants
- If sleep apnea, cautious use of narcotics
- If peripheral neuropathy, document prior to regional

Postoperative Period
- Transient diabetes insipidus (20%), permanent 1-9 %
- CSF rhinorrhea <5% of patients
- Anterior pituitary insufficiency (ACTH, TSH, gonadotropins) (20%)—hormonal replacement with tapered cortisol therapy if necessary
- Meningitis, sinusitis, hematoma, cranial nerve palsy (III, IV, VI), nasal septal perforation, visual disturbances <1% each

Anticipated Problems/Concerns
- Airway management
- Hemodynamic stability

Acute Respiratory Distress Syndrome (ARDS)

Jason C. Brainard
Maurizio Cereda

Risk

- Incidence estimated at 15,000–140,000 cases per year in the USA. True incidence is unknown due to difficulty in defining the disease and making the diagnosis.
- Mortality rates vary from 25–40%. Mortality rate strongly influenced by associated conditions (e.g., higher when associated with sepsis, liver disease, and advanced age; lower with trauma, transfusion related lung injury, drug overdose, or other reversible conditions)

Perioperative Risks

- Increased risk of sudden and profound hypoxia secondary to loss of alveolar recruitment
- Worsening respiratory status due to effects of anesthesia and surgery
- Difficult balance between maintaining adequate intravascular volume and avoiding right ventricular dysfunction or worsening pulm edema leading to decreased oxygenation and ventilation

Worry About

- Maintaining required PEEP during pt transport with Ambu bag or Mapleson circuit. Transport with ICU ventilator may be necessary.
- Inability of standard OR ventilators to deliver required minute ventilation, high inspiratory pressures, and advanced modes of ventilation (bi-level, APRV, inverse ratio ventilation, high-frequency oscillatory ventilation)

Overview

- Defined as acute onset lung injury with Pao_2/FIO_2 ratio ≤ 200 mmHg (regardless of PEEP level), bilateral infiltrates on CXR, PCWP ≤ 18 when measured or no clinical evidence of cardiogenic edema. Criteria do not correlate well with lung histology and do not account for the effects of ventilator settings
- Though classically defined by severe hypoxia, also can be associated with profound hypercarbia due to elevated alveolar dead space
- Associated with low pulm compliance and lung volumes (due to alveolar edema and atelectasis) and, in certain pts, with abnormally low chest wall compliance
- Most deaths are from sepsis or multisystem organ failure (more rarely from refractory hypoxemia or hypercarbia)

ICD-9-CM Code: 518.81 (With respiratory failure)

Etiology

- Direct or indirect lung injury leading to acute inflammatory alveolar damage characterized by increased microvascular permeability with interstitial and alveolar edema and often progressing to fibrosis
- Precipitants incl aspiration, pneumonia, sepsis, massive transfusion, pancreatitis, trauma, ischemia-reperfusion, opiate or cocaine overdose, CNS injury, air embolism, cardiopulmonary bypass
- Mechanical ventilation may worsen lung injury through alveolar overdistention and shear forces from cyclic opening and closing of collapsed alveoli (ventilator-associated lung injury)

Usual Treatment

- ARDS net trial demonstrated reduced mortality in pts ventilated with lower tidal volumes and decreased airway plateau pressures. Aim for TVs 6–8 ml/kg (ideal body weight) and plateau pressure ≤ 30 cm H_2O. Maintain ventilation with increased respiratory rate.
- Do not attempt to correct hypercarbia. Instead, direct ventilation toward maintaining acceptable pH (>7.20). There is no evidence that moderate acidemia is harmful in pts who do not have specific contraindications (i.e., intracranial hypertension).
- Apply PEEP to maintain alveolar recruitment and achieve O_2 saturation ≥ 88–90%. No consistent evidence shows benefit from high versus moderate levels of PEEP. Higher PEEP is reasonable if pt remains hemodynamically stable. Watch out for auto-PEEP (air trapping).
- Choose the lowest tolerated FIO_2 (actual FIO_2 associated with oxygen toxicity is unknown)
- Decrease O_2 consumption through fever reduction and sedation. Consider paralysis only as last resort due to risk of diaphragm disuse atrophy.
- Advanced modes of mechanical ventilation (APRV, bi-level), inhaled vasodilators, and prone positioning are used frequently and appear to improve gas exchange, but they have no proven survival benefit
- Diagnose and treat precipitating and underlying conditions
- Prevent and treat fluid overload

ASSESSMENT POINTS

System	Effect	Assessment by Hx	PE	Test
CV	Pulm Htn RV and/or LV dysfunction Septic shock Fluid overload	Hypotension, $\downarrow$ renal and hepatic function, metabolic acidosis	Cool extremities, narrow pulse pressure, JVD, RV heave, peripheral edema, enlarged liver, abdominal distension	PA catheter, ECHO, mixed venous oxygen saturation
RESP	Ventilator-associated lung injury Pneumothorax	$\uparrow$ Airway pressures, impaired respiratory mechanics, worsening blood gases	Bilateral rhonchi, crackles decreased or absent breath sounds, tracheal deviation	CXR, CT chest
ID	Ventilator associated pneumonia Line sepsis	$\uparrow$ WBC/bandemia, new infiltrates, hypotension	Fever, purulent secretions	CXR, CT chest, blood and sputum culture
GI	Hemorrhage	$\downarrow$ Hct	Melena, bloody NG output	Esophagogastroduodenoscopy
GU	Acute kidney injury	Oliguria, increased creatinine	Peripheral edema	Serum creatinine
MS	Prolonged weakness Diaphragm atrophy	Pharmacologic paralysis, high-dose steroids, sepsis, prolonged ventilation	Polyneuropathy, myopathy	Electromyography, muscle biopsy

Key Reference: Bernard GR. Acute respiratory distress syndrome. *Am J Respir Crit Care Med.* 2005;172:798–806.

Perioperative Implications

Preoperative Preparation

- Assess current ventilator mode and settings in ICU and review last blood gas
- Assess pt preop hemodynamic and intravascular volume status
- Use PEEP valve for pt transport or consider transportation to OR on ICU ventilator
- Consider use of ICU ventilator intraop with concurrent total intravenous anesthesia, particularly when very high minute volumes and airway pressures are required
- Maintain comparable levels of mean airway pressure and minute volume when transitioning between modes or ventilators and when paralyzing the patient

Airway

- Avoid suctioning and unnecessary ETT disconnection. Even transient loss of PEEP may result in lung derecruitment and severe hypoxemia that is difficult to correct.

Monitoring

- CVP, PA catheter, or intraop TEE may be helpful in estimating intravascular volume status and ventricular function
- Closely monitor airway pressures (peak, plateau, mean airway), tidal volumes, minute ventilation
- Monitor oxygen saturation and obtain frequent blood gases. $ETCO_2$ may not be representative of arterial Pco_2 when dead space is high.

Preinduction/Induction

- Expect increased shunt with increased FIO_2 and/or PEEP requirements due to loss of hypoxic pulmonary vasoconstriction caused by anesthetics
- Prepare for worsening respiratory mechanics and decreased ventilation in spontaneously breathing pt given anesthetics, narcotics, or muscle relaxants
- Lying pt in full supine position associated with elevated mean airway pressures and increased risk of aspiration (suction stomach via NG/OG tube before lying supine)

Maintenance

- Attention to fluid management to avoid right ventricular dysfunction or worsening pulm edema from excessive fluid administration
- Avoid decreased oxygen delivery due to low cardiac output and anemia
- Treat worsened hypoxemia with recruitment maneuvers (apply continuous airway pressure of 40 to 50 cm H_2O for 40 seconds) followed by increased PEEP

Postoperative Period

- Continued careful monitoring of hemodynamic and volume status
- Reduce FIO_2 and airway pressures as tolerated

Anticipated Problems/Concerns

- Sudden and profound hypoxia can occur if lung recruitment is lost during transport, movement, positioning, or surgical retraction.

Addison's Disease

Cameron Ricks

Risk

- Incidence in USA: 60–110 cases/million
- Incidence 5 or 6/million/y
- M:F ratio: 1:1.5–3.5

Perioperative Risks

- Hypotension, distributive shock, hyperkalemia
- Muscle weakness, anorexia, vomiting, diarrhea, decreased level of consciousness

Worry About

- Acute adrenal insufficiency leading to hypotension and refractory distributive shock
- Cardiac dysrhythmia caused by hyperkalemia
- Hypovolemia, electrolyte imbalance

Overview

- Addison disease is adrenal insufficiency due to primary undersecretion of glucocorticoids and mineralcorticoids by the adrenal cortex or decreased ACTH secretion
- A normal adult will secrete 20 mg of cortisol daily and up to 100 mg/m² daily during stress. A normal adult will secrete 0.1 mg of aldosterone daily.
- Addison disease may be subtle or overlooked by the pt until the stress of surgery leads to adrenal crisis
- Diagnosis by the ACTH stimulation test
- Pts receiving chronic steroid therapy may develop adrenal insufficiency under surgical stress

ICD-9-CM Code: 255.4

Etiology

- Most frequently due to idiopathic adrenal insufficiency secondary to autoimmune destruction of the adrenal gland (80% of cases)
- Other causes incl bacterial, fungal and viral infection, TB, HIV, sepsis, hemorrhage into the adrenal gland, cancer, amyloid disease, and chronic corticosteroid therapy

Usual Treatment

- Glucocorticoid, mineralocorticoid and electrolyte replacement. For example, prednisone 5 mg q AM and 2.5 mg q PM or hydrocortisone 20 mg q AM 10 mg q PM for glucocorticoid replacement and fludrocortisones 0.05 mg–0.1 mg daily for mineralocorticoid replacement.
- Acute adrenal insufficiency treatment: Supportive treatment with rapid isotonic solution, hydrocortisone IV 100 mg q 8 hr and electrolyte replacement

ASSESSMENT POINTS

System	Effect	Assessment by Hx	PE	Test
CV	Hypotension	Low blood pressure	Pale, diaphoresis	BP
HEME	Low cortisol and aldosterone	Muscle weakness, anorexia, vomiting, diarrhea	Decreased level of consciousness, hypotension, shock	ACTH stimulation test
GI	Hypovolemia, electrolyte abnormalities	Anorexia, vomiting, diarrhea	Poor skin turgor, orthostatic vital signs, poor capillary refill, dry mucous membranes	Chemistry panel
ENDO	Hyperkalemia, hyponatremia, hypoglycemia	Weakness, cardiac disrhymia	Inability to stand from seated position	Chemistry panel
SKIN	Increased ACTH leading to increased melanocytes		Hyperpigmentation	ACTH stimulation test

Key Reference: Kohl BA, Schwartz S. Surgery in the patient with endocrine dysfunction. *Anesthesiol Clin.* 2009;27(4):687–703.

Perioperative Implications

Preinduction/Induction/Maintenance

- Glucocorticoid and mineralcorticoid levels should be checked
- Glucocorticoid and mineralcorticoid treatment should be optimized
- Potassium level should be checked and replaced as needed
- Glucose level should be checked and replaced as needed

Monitoring

- Standard ASA monitors
- Arterial line and central line may be necessary in acute adrenal insufficiency

General Anesthesia

- Pre-induction: Confirm that pt corticosteroid and mineralocorticoid levels are optimized. Elective cases should be postponed until levels are optimized.
- Induction: Avoid etomidate as it suppresses adrenal function
- Maintenance: Monitor for hypotension, cautious use of muscle relaxants as reduced dose may be necessary
- Emergence: Emergency can be prolonged

Postoperative Period

- Must monitor pts for adrenal insufficiency as there have been reports of signicant adrenal insufficiency into the postop period
- Continue steroid replacement for at least 24 hr postop
- Watch for complications of steroid use such as ulcers, infection, poor wound healing, glucose intolerance

Regional Anesthesia

- Effective in postponing the increase in cortisol

Anticipated Problems/Concerns

- The greatest danger comes from undiagnosed Addison disease. These pts may present with acute adrenal insufficiency intraop or postop secondary to surgical stress.
- Accurate diagnosis and treatment can be life saving. Refractory hypotension should alert clinicians to the possibility that the pt is adrenal insufficient.
- Glucocorticoid replacement and supportive care are the mainstays of treatment in the periop period

Adrenal Insufficiency, Acute or Secondary

Charles B. Hantler

Risk

- Risk of adrenal insufficiency: 1/1000–1/10,000 (if steroids used in prior year)
- With steroids >20 mg/d (cortisol equivalent), >7–14 d within 1 y (large variability in patient response to dose duration and timing of prior steroid use)
- Clinical signs worsen with stress, such as trauma, surgery, or infection

Perioperative Risks

- Increases CV instability, fever, CHF, electrolyte abnormalities
- High cardiac output failure, or low-output state (hypovolemia) with signs of tissue hypoperfusion
- Often evidence of systemic vasodilation with decreased reactivity to vasopressors

Worry About

- GI; N/V; dehydration
- Anemia, neutropenia with androgen deficiency: rare
- CV response; decreased SVR, decreased left ventricular stroke work index and decreased vascular responsiveness to maintain perfusion pressure; steroids necessary for blood vessel responsiveness to catecholamines
- Hyperkalemia with or without hyponatremia (usually aldosterone deficiency); hypoglycemia, acidosis, hypercalcemia, and anemia; cardiac conduction abnormalities

Overview

- Adrenal insufficiency results from inadequate production of glucocorticoids (cortisol), mineralocorticoids (aldosterone), and/or androgens
- Adrenal insufficiency can be acute or chronic, primary or secondary

- Primary adrenal insufficiency: Associated with >90% destruction of the adrenal glands and deficiency in both cortisol and aldosterone
- Secondary adrenal insufficiency develops from the hypothalamic-pituitary–adrenal axis dysfunction or failure
- May present without symptoms until stress
- Acute adrenal (addisonian) crisis may develop in periop period when another stress is present (infection, hemorrhage, or major or prolonged surgery), leading to hyponatremia, hyperkalemia, dehydration, and shock
- Adrenals secrete around 150 mg of cortisol in periop period, the production may increase up to 300 mg during the maximal stress
- Recovery of the adrenal function may take up to 9–12 m after withdrawal of exogenous steroids and the supplementation of the daily cortisol production is advised
- Critical illness–related corticosteroid insufficiency may develop from inadequate corticosteroid activity in relation to the severity of the patient's illness
- Pts with community-acquired pneumonia, severe pancreatitis, acute or chronic liver failure, post-liver transplantation, pts who underwent trauma with hemorrhagic shock or cardiac surgery, or pts who are being weaned from mechanical ventilation may benefit from glucocorticoid therapy, dosing recommendation requires further investigation
- Chronic adrenal insufficiency from use of steroids in prior year may manifest as weakness, fatigue, nausea, emesis, weight loss, and a variety of psychiatric disturbances
- Inadequate mineralocorticoid production can cause hyperkalemia, hyponatremia, and metabolic acidosis, with or without signs of dehydration

- Inadequate glucocorticoid production may cause signs of hemodynamic instability (hypotension) during stress
- See also Addison Disease in Diseases section

ICD-9-CM Code: 255.41

Etiology

- Primary adrenal insufficiency: Autoimmunity, infection (TB, HIV, CMV), hemorrhage (meningococcal sepsis, trauma, HIT, anticoagulants), drugs (etomidate, antifungals), infiltration (sarcoidosis, amyloidosis, histoplasmosis), metastatic disease (breast, lung, melanoma)
- Secondary adrenal insufficiency: Glucocorticoid therapy (systemic or topical), drugs (fluticasone, megestrol, medroxyprogesterone, ketorolac tromethamine), brain injury, pituitary or hypothalamic tumors

Usual Therapy

- Mild conditions (e.g., colonoscopy): 25 mg of hydrocortisone IV on day of surgery only
- Moderate stress (e.g., appendectomy, lobectomy): 50–75 mg or about 2× normal production on day of surgery, taper quickly to usual dose over 1–2 d
- Major stress (major trauma, major surgery): 100–200 mg of hydrocortisone on day of surgery, taper quickly to usual dose over 1–2 d
- Septic shock in pts who remain hypotensive despite adequate administration of fluids and vasopressors: 200–300 mg of hydrocortisone per day for at least 7 d, followed by taper to usual dose
- Early ARDS: 1 mg/kg methylprednisolone for more than 14 d, followed by taper to usual dose
- Aldosterone deficiency (manifested by abnormalities in Na⁺/K⁺ or dehydration): Fludrocortisone (Florinef), 50–200 µg/d

ASSESSMENT POINTS				
System	Effect	Assessment by Hx	PE	Test
CV	Dehydration, hypotension, high-output failure	Postural symptoms, fatigue; Wt loss, Hx of surgery on adrenals, pituitary	Low BP, postural drop, signs of dehydration	Hct BUN/Cr, adrenal, ACTH stimulation, insulin tolerance, metyrapone test
RESP	CHF (high or low output)	DOE, SOB	S_3, rales	CXR
GI	Dehydration, nausea, emesis	Appetite, HX of emesis	See CV	Lytes
HEME	Anemia, neutropenia		Hyperpigmentation (excess corticotropin)	Hct WBC
CNS	Depression, confusion, psychosis			Reverses with replacement
MS	Weakness, potentiation of neuromuscular blockage			Nerve stimulator

Key Reference: Marik P. Recommendations for the diagnosis and management of corticosteroid insufficiency in critically ill adult patients: Consensus statements from an international task force by the ACCCM. *Crit Care Med.* 2008;36:(6):1937–1949.

Perioperative Implications

Preoperative Preparation

- Consider periop steroid coverage if benefits outweigh risks if high index of suspicion of adrenal depression (e.g., supraphysiologic doses of steroids for >1 wk within last y)
- Correct electrolyte abnormalities, hypoglycemia, and dehydration prior to elective surgery
- Fludrocortisone with resistant aldosterone (K⁺ and Na⁺) abnormalities; glucose for hypoglycemia

Monitoring

- ECG for signs of abnormal conduction (QRS duration, u waves)
- Consider CVP, PCWP, or TEE if fluid/electrolyte and hemodynamic abnormalities
- Sodium, potassium, bicarbonate, and glucose

Airway

- None

Premedication/Induction

- Consider volume status with regard to hydration and choice of agents

Maintenance

- No hemodynamic instability: Follow electrolytes and glucose as needed
- Hemodynamic instability (hypotension)
  - R/O other causes, then consider hydrocortisone hemisuccinate, 25–100 mg IV, then 100 mg q 12–24 hr for 2 or 3 d
  - Fluid resuscitation as needed

Extubation

- Possible potentiation of nondepolarizing muscle relaxants with use of high-dose steroids; ensure adequate muscle relaxant reversal

Adjuvants

- Glucose, fluids, careful monitoring of temperature to avoid hyperthermia

Postoperative Period

- Stress steroids possibly required several days postop

- High steroid doses may be associated with decreased wound healing and immunosuppression with increased infection risk
- Consider prolonged steroid coverage if severe stress continues (e.g., severe trauma with multiple operations)
- Mineralocorticoid administration as needed; usually glucocorticoids have significant mineralocorticoid action

Anticipated Problems/Concerns

- Severe resistant hypotension, hyperthermia, and CNS abnormalities, such as confusion, coma, lethargy, may occur intraop or postop and may be unpredictable
- Syndrome may occur in severely traumatized pts without history of steroid use, with clinical picture of sepsis and associated abnormalities in adrenal function; Rx is life saving

Alcohol Abuse

Scott Watkins

Risk
- Incidence in USA: 10 percent of Americans, including physicians, will abuse alcohol at some point in their lives
- Third leading cause of death and disability, including 30% of traffic fatalities
- Male gender and family Hx major risk factors

Perioperative Risks
- Severe malnutrition as significant as ethanol-induced end-organ injury
- Risk of Htn, CVA, diabetes, GI disease
- Liver most severely affected organ
- Dilated cardiomyopathy
- Withdrawal symptoms can themselves be life-threatening

Worry About
- Concomitant use of other drugs: Amphetamines, cocaine, benzodiazepines
- Affects of chronic smoking, such as COPD and emphysema

- Vasopressor effect of ETOH may cause Htn
- Withdrawal symptoms, caused by sympathetic stimulation, leading to life-threatening Htn and tachycardia

Overview
- Disease characterized by addiction (compulsion and craving despite consequences) to alcohol
- Clinical syndromes related to direct effect of ETOH and secondary adaptive response to excess ETOH exposure
- ETOH rapidly absorbed and metabolized
- Hepatic dysfunction usually takes 10–15 y to develop
- Cirrhosis may develop after 1 or more acute episodes

ICD-9-CM Code: 303.0 (Acute)

Etiology
- Unknown: Likely mutifactorial with environmental, genetic, and psychosocial components

Usual Treatment
- Recovery involves some or all of the following:
  - Detoxification: Inpatient, residential, day treatment, or outpatient
  - Evaluation for comorbid psychiatric disorder
  - Referral to Alcoholics Anonymous or other alcohol programs
- Pharmacotherapy to help with withdrawal and prevent relapse
  - Disulfiram (Antabuse): Acetaldehyde dehydrogenase inhibitor
  - Naltrexone (Revia): Pure opioid receptor antagonist, blunts ETOH's pleasurable effects and reduces craving. Available as monthly IM depot.
  - Acamprosate (Campral): A synthetic derivative of homotaurine, a structural analog of gamma-aminobutyric acid (GABA). Decreases excitatory glutamatergic neurotransmission during alcohol withdrawal

ASSESSMENT POINTS

System	Effect	Assessment by Hx	PE	Test
CV	Cardiomyopathy, arrhythmias, hypertension	Orthopnea, nocturnal urination, coughing, and leg swelling	Dyspnea BP lying and standing HR	ECG, ECHO Electrolytes
GI	Erosive gastritis, hepatic cirrhosis, acute hepatitis, pancreatitis, fatty liver	Hx of bleeding, easily bruised, anorexia, N/V	Ascites, jaundice Hepatomegaly, "spider" angiomas Abd pain Abd pain, hepatomegaly	Upper endoscopy, stool guaiac LFTs LFTs Serum amylase Mg^{2+}; K^+
ENDO	Gynecomastia, testicular atrophy, irregular menses			
HEME	Leukopenia, anemia, thrombocytopenia			CBC with differential
CNS	Wernicke's syndrome Korsakoff's syndrome Peripheral polyneuropathy Cerebellar degeneration	Amnesia, impaired reasoning	Sixth nerve palsy, ataxia CNS exam Distal numbness and paresthesias Unsteady gait	MRI or CT scan

Key Reference: May JA, et al. The patient recovering from alcohol or drug addiction: special issues for the anesthesiologist. *Anesth Analg.* 2001;92(6):1601-1608.

Perioperative Implications

Preoperative Preparation
- Gastric prophylaxis
- Blood ETOH and toxicology screen if indicated

Monitoring
- Standard ASA monitors
- Consider invasive monitors for cardiomyopathy, hepatic dysfunction, and/or end-organ compromise

Airway
Consider full stomach in acute intoxication

Preinduction/Induction
- Consider long-acting benzodiazepine, barbiturate, or α_2-adrenergic agonist
- Anesthetic doses increased in chronic disease
- Decreased dose in acute intoxication

- Rapid sequence in acute intoxication
- Consider Rx of nutritional/metabolic deficiencies

Maintenance
- Requirements vary by age, general health, nutrition and hydration states, concomitant disease

Extubation
- Ensure return of airway reflexes

Postoperative Period
- Provide adequate analgesia in PACU
- Anxiety can worsen withdrawal symptoms
- Withdrawal syndrome may develop within 6–8 hr; treat with IV ETOH, β-adrenergic agonist, α_2-adrenergic agonist, benzodiazepines, PO ETOH
  - DTs develop in 5% of pts in withdrawal

- 10% mortality secondary to hypotension, arrhythmias; treat with diazepam, β-adrenergic agonist

Adjuvants
- Long-term consumption of ETOH impairs hepatic metabolism
- Short-term consumption inhibits drug metabolism
- Polyneuropathy a relative contraindication to regional anesthesia
- Consider periop clonidine patch

Anticipated Problems/Concerns
- Recognition and treatment of withdrawal important, as significant mortality occurs if inadequately treated

Allergy

Jerrold H. Levy

DISEASES

Risk

- Incidence in USA: 5% of adults in are allergic to one or more drugs
- During surgery, the risk of anaphylaxis is 1:3500–1:20,000, with a mortality rate of 4%
- Females > males (1.6:1)

Perioperative Risks

- Intensity of Sx variable: From an isolated cutaneous eruption to CV collapse and death
- CV, cutaneous, resp systems are mostly involved
- Increased morbidity and hospitalization time if intensive care required

Worry About

- Patient's Hx: Knowledge of prior allergic event leads to avoiding drugs or other components involved
- Hypotension, bronchospasm, and angioedema may become life-threatening events

Overview

- IgE anaphylaxis (type I immediate hypersensitivity reaction): Adverse response of host; mediated by antibodies, the antigen bridges with two IgE on the surface of basophils and mast cells; can be reproduced if foreign substance reinjected
- Anaphylactoid reactions or histamine release: Describes a clinically indistinguishable syndrome probably involving similar mediators but not mediated by IgE antibody and not necessarily requiring previous exposure to the inciting substance, associated with vancomycin, benzylisoquilinium-derived muscle relaxants, but term should be avoided.

ICD-9-CM Codes: 995.3 (Allergic reaction); 477.0–477.9 (Inhaled allergen)

Etiology

- Clinical history of allergy or perianesthetic allergic reaction considered to put patient at increased risk for a reaction from neuromuscular blocking agents and induction agents

Usual Treatment

- Preventive therapy with corticosteroids and antihistamines is of unproven value
- Severe allergic therapy: Stop antigen, maintain the airway with 100% O_2 and intubate if necessary; discontinue all anesthetic drugs, volume expansion, epinephrine (5–10 μg IV boluses as starting doses and titrate upward), antihistamines, β-sympathomimetic if bronchospasm, arginine vasopressin for refractory shock, phosphodiesterase inhibitors for RV dysfunction, airway evaluation prior to extubation, ICU observation

ASSESSMENT POINTS

System	Effect	PE	Test
CV	Hypotension, tachycardia, dysrhythmias Pulm Htn Cardiac arrest	BP	ECG PA pressure
RESP	Dyspnea, sneezing Coughing, wheezing Laryngeal edema Fulminant pulm edema Acute resp failure	Chest exam	CXR PA catheter ETCO$_2$ ABGs
DERM	Urticaria, flushing Perioral, periorbital edema	Skin exam	

Key Reference: Levy JH, Adkinson Jr NF. Anaphylaxis during cardiac surgery: implications for clinicians. *Anesth Analg.* 2008;106:392–403.

Perioperative Implications

Preoperative Preparation
- Prick tests, intradermal testing: Anesthetic drugs (neuromuscular blocking agents)
- Most of the allergic reactions are unexpected. In case of established allergy, those drugs or latex should be strictly avoided.

Monitoring
- Routine

- If major anaphylaxis occurs, consider pulm and radial arterial catheterization to guide therapeutic interventions.

Airway
- None, except specific care for the asthmatic patient

Preinduction/Induction/Maintenance/Extubation
- Slow injection of drugs. Avoid histamine-releasing drugs in high-risk pts.

Anticipated Problems/Concerns

- For each pt who has a periop allergic reaction, consider evaluation 1 mo after with skin testing, antigen-specific IgE level dosage (radioallergosorbent test, ELISA).
- Measure tryptase if anaphylactic reaction within 1–2 hr of reaction, then 24 hr later to support diagnosis.
- Latex allergy incidence is increasing. Healthcare workers at greater risk, and Hx has to be evoked at the preanesthetic evaluation.

Amniotic Fluid Embolism

Mohammed Minhaj

Risk

- True incidence is unknown but estimated to occur between 1:8000–80,000 deliveries

Perioperative Risks

- Amniotic fluid embolism accounts for approx 10% of maternal deaths in the USA
- Mortality has been reported to be as high as 61–86% but more recent registries have reported mortality between 27–37% of pts
- Morbidity is also high as it is suggested that only 15% of survivors are neurologically intact

Worry About

- Hypoxia
- Hypotension/cardiopulmonary collapse
- Heart failure (can have both right and left ventricular failure)
- DIC: Occurs in nearly all survivors of the initial catastrophic event
- Hemorrhage: 40% of amniotic fluid embolism-associated deaths are due to hemorrhage
- Altered mental status
- Seizures

Overview

- Amniotic fluid going to central circulation
- There are three necessary conditions:
  - Amniotomy (breach in the barrier between the intact fetal membranes that isolate amniotic fluid from the maternal circulation)
  - Laceration of endocervical or uterine vessels
  - Traditionally it was thought that a pressure gradient (intrauterine pressure > CVP or uterine venous pressure) was needed, but the presence of an electrochemical gradient can provide the means for mediators of AFE to inflict damage
- Immunological factors may also be involved as complement activation may play a role in the pathophysiology of AFE

ICD9-CM: 673.1

Etiology

- Postulated mechanism of action: Powerful contractions force amniotic fluid into the maternal circulation through a defect in the fetal membranes, placenta, or elsewhere
- Risk factors incl turbulent labor; cesarean delivery; advanced maternal age; multiparity; meconium (present in 75% of cases); intrauterine fetal demise (present in 40% of cases); male fetus, sudden fetal expulsion; meconium staining of the amniotic fluid; chorioamnionitis; and macrosomia.

Usual Treatment

- Usually supportive to maintain oxygenation, circulatory support, and correct coagulopathy
- Case reports of successful treatment with cardiopulmonary bypass (both thrombectomy and placement of ventricular assist devices) have been reported in the literature
- Employ left uterine displacement to prevent aortocaval compression
- Stop oxytocin infusion if present
- Cardiopulmonary resuscitation, often requiring intubation with 100% O_2/PEEP. Inhaled nitric oxide has also been described.
- Pressors and inotropes will often be required
- Delivery of fetus as soon as is practical; may require operative or cesarean delivery
- Replacement of clotting factors if pt develops DIC. Recent case reports describe use of recombinant factor VII (rfVIIa).

ASSESSMENT POINTS

System	Effect	Assessment by Hx	PE	Test
CV	Tachycardia			HR
	Hypotension			BP
RESP	Hypoxia	Dyspnea	Tachypnea	Pulse oximetry
	Pulm edema		Cyanosis	Aspirate blood from pulmonary artery or renal artery
			Frothy pink sputum	Stain buffy coat for cells and mucin
GI		Nausea	Vomiting	
HEME	DIC		Excessive bleeding	PT, PTT, plt, fibrinogen, FSP
			Thrombolysis (bleeding from IV sites)	
CNS		Anxiety	Convulsions	
			Shivering	
			Sweating	

Key Reference: Gist S, et al. Amniotic fluid embolism. *Anesth Analg*. 2009;108:1599–1602.

Perioperative Implications

- Most common presentation is hemodynamic collapse

Preoperative Preparation

- Maximize maternal oxygen delivery
- Place several large-bore IVs, consider central access for inotrope administration and fluid resuscitation
- Notify blood bank of anticipated coagulopathy and cross-match for several units of packed RBCs, FFP, platelets, and cryoprecipitate
- Consider preparing for cardiopulmonary bypass, if an option

Monitoring

- If amniotic fluid embolism is suspected, consider PA catheter to aspirate blood; hemodynamic management

Maintenance

- Usually resuscitative with support of breathing and circulation
- Case reports of use of CPB, inhaled nitric oxide, ventricular assist devices

Extubation

- If pt survives, keep intubated until stable

Anticipated Problems/Concerns

- Not all sudden deaths during the peripartum period are due to amniotic fluid embolism. The pathologic diagnosis is quite specific (finding hair, mucin, or nucleated squamous cells in the maternal circulation), but its sensitivity is unknown.
- Even with early and aggressive intervention, AFE carries a high maternal and fetal mortality. Given that an AFE can occur unpredictably and then has such a high risk for morbidity and mortality, it can be devastating for the pt's families and healthcare providers. Psychological counseling for all parties involved should be considered to deal with any posttraumatic stress.

Amyloidosis

Kenneth J. Holroyd

DISEASES

Risk

- Incidence in USA: 1:50,000
- Race with highest prevalence: Unknown

Perioperative Risks

- Increased risk of periop renal failure, CHF, bleeding from coagulopathy
- Autonomic neuropathy

Worry About

- Signs of CHF
- Decreasing urine output

Overview

- Extracellular deposition of amyloid-type proteins
- Congo-red stain of tissue reveals green birefringence in a polarizing microscope
- Associated end-stage renal, myocardial, and neuropathic disease
- Best diagnosed by subcutaneous abdominal fat pad aspirate or rectal biopsy

ICD-9-CM Code: 277.3

Etiology

- Both acquired and hereditary forms exist
- Major risk factors for acquired disease: multiple myeloma, chronic infectious or inflammatory disease (osteomyelitis, rheumatoid arthritis)
- Hereditary forms very rare

Usual Treatment

- Acquired: Treat underlying disease, stem cell transplant, Chem RX
- Hereditary: Colchicine, liver transplantation

ASSESSMENT POINTS

System	Effect	Assessment by Hx	PE	Test
HEENT	Macroglossia Tracheal stenosis	Enlarged tongue Dyspnea	Macroglossia Stridor	CT scan Flow-volume loop
CV	Restrictive myopathy LV and RV dysfunction Conduction abnormalities	Exercise tolerance Dyspnea Syncope	S_3 Bradycardia	ECHO ECG
RESP	CHF Lung nodules	Cough Chest wall pain	Rales	CXR
GI	Autonomic dysfunction	Wt loss Diarrhea	Biopsy	
HEME	Factor X deficiency	Bruising	Periorbital bruises	Factor X assay
RENAL	Decreased renal perfusion Nephrotic syndrome			BUN/Cr urine
CNS	Autonomic neuropathy	Inability to sweat; hoarseness; early satiety; postural dizziness	Orthostasis	Biopsy

Key Reference: Noguchi T, Minami K, Iwagaki T, Takura H, Sata T, Shigematsu A. Anesthetic management of a patient with laryngeal amyloidosis. *J Clin Anesth.* 1999;11:339–341.

Perioperative Implications

Preoperative Preparation

- Optimize treatment of heart failure
- Avoid dehydration (renal failure)

Monitoring

- Consider PA catheter for large fluid shift operations or patients with severe LV dysfunction

Airway

- Macroglossia or tracheal stenosis
- Increased risk of bleeding into airway from capillary fragility and possible coagulopathy

Preinduction/Induction

- May develop reduced CO and hypotension
- Coagulopathy may contraindicate regional anesthesia

Maintenance

- No agent or technique shown superior
- Maintain adequate urine output

Extubation

- Patient fully awake to minimize risk of reintubation
- Use caution with nasal airway—may cause hemorrhage

Postoperative Period

- Close monitoring of CV and renal status
- Consider ICU setting for postop care

Adjuvants

- Avoid digoxin: not usually helpful in treating amyloid CHF, associated with increased arrhythmias

Anticipated Problems/Concerns

- Difficult airway
- CHF
- Hypotension
- Renal failure

Amyotrophic Lateral Sclerosis

Todd A. Bromberg
Richard L. Boortz-Marx

Risk

- Estimated incidence of 1 to 3 per 100,000
- Mean age of onset is in the sixties, but ALS can occur as early as the twenties
- Disease duration is approximately 3 y from the time of diagnosis to death
- Slight male predominance of sporadic spinal ALS; slight female predominance of bulbar ALS
- Most cases are sporadic but 5–10% are familial
- The risk of anesthesia increases as the FVC falls below 50% such that ALS patients can be stratified as low risk if the FVC is greater than 50%, moderate risk if the FVC is 30–50%, and high risk if the FVC is less than 30%

Perioperative Risks

- Aspiration
- Resp depression
- Inability of pt to communicate secondary to bulbar weakness

Worry About

- Succinylcholine induced hyperkalemia
- Prolonged resp depression with inability to extubate, even without use of muscle relaxants
- Hypersensitivity to non-depolarizing neuromuscular blockers
- Disease exacerbation with use of regional anesthesia

Overviw

- Disease of unclear etiology that leads to progressive degeneration of the upper and lower motor neurons causing amyotrophy (muscle wasting) and lateral sclerosis (gliosis of the corticospinal tracts)
- ALS has a relenting course that leads to weakness of all skeletal muscles in the body
- Typically, ALS is asymmetric involving the distal extremities first followed by bulbar muscle weakness as the disease progresses
- Pts are usually wheelchair bound by 18 mo and die after 3–5 y from resp suppression
- Upper motor neuron signs incl spasticity, hyperactive reflexes, and upgoing plantar response; lower motor neuron signs incl muscle atrophy and fasciculations
- Disease does not affect ocular muscles, bladder, bowel, and sensation
- ALS variants include:
  - Primary lateral sclerosis: Progressive degeneration of upper motor neurons
  - Progressive muscular atrophy: Progressive degeneration of lower motor neurons
  - Progressive bulbar palsy: Progressive motoneuron loss from lower cranial nerve nuclei and cervical spine

ICD9-CM: 335.20

Etiology

- Familial ALS caused by gene mutations: 14 mutations described. Most studied occurs in the gene encoding superoxide dismutase: forms aggregates leading to mitochondria and muscle complex dysfunction.
- Etiology of sporadic ALS remains uncertain, but autoimmune, infectious, and neurotoxic mechanisms likely contribute. An interaction between a genetic susceptibility and environmental exposure likely leads to the disease.

Usual Treatment

- Care is mainly supportive consisting of psychological therapy, symptom management, physical therapy, and palliative care
- Care in a multidisciplinary clinic is associated with prolonged survival and improved quality of life
- Riluzole, which inhibits glutamate release, is the only drug shown to improve survival. On average, patients live 2–3 mo longer on riluzole versus a placebo.

ASSESSMENT POINTS

System	Effect	Assessment by Hx	PE	Test
HEENT	Dysarthria, dysphagia, siallorrhea	Slurred speech, coughing with eating, drooling	Decreased gag reflex	Swallow study
CV	Reduced sympathetic tone Vagal dysfunction	Syncope Cardiac arrest		Prolonged QTc Tachycardia
PULM	Aspiration; nocturnal apnea; weak cough	Recurrent pneumonia; nighttime arousals; lethargy	Decreased breath sounds; coarse breath sounds	PFTs Nocturnal oximetry CXR ABG
GI	Malnourished	Caloric intake Food journal	BMI	Albumin
CNS	Motor neuron loss in spinal cord and brain	Weakness Pseudobulbar affect	Weakness Fasciculations Atrophy	EMG/NCS

Key Reference: Brambrink AM, Kirsch JR. Perioperative care of patients with neuromuscular disease and dysfunction. *Anesthesiol Clin.* 2007;25:483–509.

Perioperative Implications

Preinduction/Induction/Maintenance

- Succinylcholine is contraindicated as it can cause hyperkalemia
- Non-depolarizing agents may be used, but anticipate prolonged weakness
- Short-acting muscle relaxants should be used when necessary

Preoperative Considerations

- Preop pulm function tests may help to predict anesthetic risk
- Consider aspiration prophylaxis
- Avoid opioids and benzodiazepines if possible

Monitoring

- Routine
- Anesthesia should be performed in an inpatient setting

General Anesthesia

- Avoid if possible
- May cause significant postop resp depression
- Diaphragmatic pacing stimulation may improve resp compliance and stimulate respirations
- Extubate when pt is fully awake

Regional Anesthesia

- May be preferred compared to general anesthesia
- Case reports have documented successful use of epidural anesthesia
- Minimize neuraxial extent of blockade to reduce risk of resp depression

Postoperative Period

- Anticipate prolonged postop ventilation
- Use nonsedating medications for pain control

Anticipated Problems/Concerns

- Anticipate hospitalization secondary to prolonged weaning from ventilator
- Communication with ALS pts may be difficult because pts have weakened oropharyngeal muscles. Prior to anesthesia, determine the best way to communicate with pts (i.e., letter boards) and have family members available to assist
- Close resp monitoring is essential following anesthesia. Exacerbation of apnea may result from supplemental oxygen.

Anaphylaxis

Risk

- Approximately 1 in 5000 anesthetic procedures
- Females outnumber males 3:1
- No prospective data to suggest an increased risk of generalized allergy, although Hx of atopy is overrepresented in several series of life-threatening anaphylaxis to anesthetic agents

Perioperative Risks

- Significant risks of life-threatening airway compromise, CV collapse, and bronchospasm—particularly severe in patients on β-blockers

Worry About

- Pts with pre-existing ASCVD tolerate CV sequelae poorly
- Pts with Hx of allergy to anesthetics
- Antibodies (and potentially anaphylaxis) to muscle relaxants may persist for >25 y

Overview

- The body's response to what is perceived to be a foreign substance

- Although itching, cutaneous manifestations, and a feeling of doom are present in the awake pt, CV collapse is the most common and serious presentation under general anesthesia
- Bronchospasm occurs in <50% of life-threatening cases of anaphylaxis
- Usually occurs during induction of anesthesia or within 10 min of drug administration
- Often confused with anaphylactoid reactions (e.g., vancomycin) that involve chemically mediated histamine release. These are common, related to drug dose and speed of injection, blocked by H_1/H_2 antihistamines.

ICD-9-CM: 995.0

Etiology

- IgE binds to mast cells and causes a degranulation, releasing many vasoactive substances, incl histamine. Although pts may not have been exposed to anesthetics, there may be common epitopes between cosmetics and myorelaxants.

- Risk factors for latex allergy incl meningomyelocele and other congenital defects. Also allergy to figs, papayas, or avocados.
- Is most commonly associated with administration of muscle relaxants, particularly SCH. Can be caused by all muscle relaxants, even those that do not release histamine chemically (e.g., rocuronium, vecuronium). Second most likely are antibiotics.
- The second most common cause appears to be latex allergy
- Rarely due to opiates or local anesthetics (more likely intravascular injection or epinephrine)

Usual Treatment

- IV fluids (put in large-bore IV), often to 7 L in adults
- Epinephrine even in the face of significant tachycardia
- O_2 and supportive measures
- Possible H_1 and H_2 antagonists

ASSESSMENT POINTS				
System	Effect	Assessment by Hx	PE	Test
HEENT	Head and neck swelling, and potential glottic edema	Will occur suddenly	Swelling	Clinically obvious
CV	↑ HR, ↓ BP and SVR, ↑ ectopy, change in PR interval, coronary vasospasm		Hypotension, tachycardia	ECG may reveal PVCs or change in P-R interval, CV collapse may ensue
RESP	Bronchospasm		Wheezing	↑ Peak insp pressure, ↓ O_2 saturation
SKIN	Urticaria or other cutaneous manifestations, generalized edema with fluid leakage		Body rash	Not needed, CVP or PA pressures or TEE

Key References: Moss JM. Allergic to anesthetics. *Anesthesiology.* 2003;99:521–523; Mertes PM, Laxenaire M-C, Alla F: Groupe d-etudes des réactions anaphylactoïdes peranesthésiques: Anaphylactic and anaphylactoid reactions occurring during anesthesia in France in 1999–2000. *Anesthesiology.* 2003;99:536–545.

Perioperative Implications

Monitoring

- It is important to distinguish from drug effects or mechanical problems
- CV collapse with or without associated bronchospasm or cutaneous manifestations during induction, but without evidence of mechanical problems, suggest anaphylaxis
- Prophylactic H_1 and H_2 antagonists may attenuate the severity, although not the incidence
- The airway may swell, making intubation very difficult

Induction

- Reactions usually occur during induction. Consider administering antibiotics in the preop holding area or after rather than during induction.

Maintenance

- Perpetuation of reaction can occur, particularly if due to latex
- Significant cross-reactivity between myorelaxants (approaching 80%)
- Avoid all muscle relaxants in pts with prior reactions

Extubation

- Ensure stable from a cardiorespiratory viewpoint
- Assess for airway edema

Adjuvants

- Epinephrine is drug of choice in true anaphylaxis, even in the face of tachycardia

Postoperative Period

- Blood should be drawn for possible tryptase levels. Although histamine measurements during

the acute event can assist in Dx, they can be difficult to perform. Tryptase can be drawn up to 2 hr afterward and may be positive in anaphylaxis, but is not elevated in chemically mediated reactions.
- Skin testing may be done several weeks after initial event to assess etiologic agent

Anticipated Problems/Concerns

- Early aggressive treatment may be critical
- Advise pts exactly what drugs they have received for future anesthetics

Anemia, Aplastic

Joanne Shay

Risk

- Incidence in USA: 2000 new cases/y
- 1.1 per million up to age 9
- Southeast Asia and South Africa have 10–20 times higher incidence
- Within USA, related to agricultural areas or petrochemical industry and chemical exposures

Perioperative Risks

- Infection
- Hemorrhage
- LV dysfunction due to high-output state and fluid overload

Worry About

- Sepsis
- Co-existing congenital anomalies, especially renal and cardiac
- Concomitant GI and intracranial hemorrhage
- Difficulty cross-matching blood products after previous multiple transfusions

Overview

- Self-perpetuating disorder resulting in pancytopenia due to a congenital or acquired loss of hemopoietic pluripotent stem cells

- Fanconi anemia is congenital familial marrow hypoplasia associated with mental retardation, kidney, spleen, and skeletal hypoplasia
- Estren-Dameshek anemia is inherited marrow hypoplasia without physical abnormalities
- Pathophysiology: Reduction or dysfunction of pluripotent stem cells or their microenvironment from toxic or immunologic causes
- Prognosis for long-term survival has increased to 40–75% in those treated with antilymphocyte serum and 60–80% in those treated with bone marrow transplantation (BMT)
- Two forms of drug-induced aplastic anemia are possible:
  - Hypersensitivity: Not related to dose or duration
  - "Reversible" reaction: Often resolves with discontinuation; severity proportional to dosage

ICD-9-CM Code: 284

Etiology

- 50–75% of cases idiopathic
- Fanconi anemia demonstrates autosomal recessive inheritance with heterozygote frequency of 1 in 300,000–600,000 in the USA

- Drug-induced: Chloramphenicol, NSAIDs, anti-epileptics, gold and sulfa group-containing compounds
- Environmental toxins incl aromatic hydrocarbons (benzene, naphthalene, toluene, glue), pesticides (DDT, lindane), and radiation
- Infectious causes incl hepatitis C, CMV, EBV, HIV, TB, and toxoplasmosis
- Sequelae of other processes such as pancreatitis, pregnancy, and lupus erythematosus, paroxysmal nocturnal hemoglobinemia, thymoma, thymic CA

Usual Treatment

- Pts <55 y are managed with HLA-matched BMT or hematopoietic stem-cell transplant
- Pts >55 y or those unable to find HLA-matched donor receive immunosuppression and immunomodulation Rx incl ATG, cyclosporine, steroids, androgens, and G-CSF
- Hematopoietic growth factors such as G-CSF and GM-CSF may improve the short-term hematological recovery at the risk of long-term clonal evolution to myelodysplastic syndrome and AML.

ASSESSMENT POINTS

System	Effect	Assessment by Hx	PE	Test
HEENT	Epistaxis Oral/mucosal friability	Headache	Stomatitis	CBC, differential, plt PT, PTT, CT scan
RESP	Pulm embolism Pneumonia Interstitial pneumonitis Pulm edema	Dyspnea	Tachypnea Lung field consolidation Wheezing	CXR, V/Q scan CT scan ABGs, bronchoscopy ± Bronchoalveolar lavage, biopsy
CV	LV failure ASD/VSD	Dyspnea Lethargy	Tachycardia, S_3 Displaced posterior MI	ECG
GI	GI bleeding GI GVHD Hepatic veno-occlusive disease	N/V, diarrhea Melena	Acute abdomen Hypoactive bowel sounds Jaundice	Endoscopy, bleeding scan Selective angiography Albumin, transferrin LFT, liver biopsy
CNS	Microcephaly, meningitis, intracranial hemorrhage	Irritability, lethargy Headache, seizures	Meningismus Papilledema	Lumbar puncture after coagulopathy treated, head CT, MRI
HEME	Pancytopenia Leukemia Paroxysmal nocturnal hemoglobinuria	Bleeding gums, infections Easy bruisability Fatigue	Petechiae Retinal hemorrhage Pallor	CBC, differential Reticulocyte count BM biopsy Ham's test
METAB	Electrolyte abnormalities Glucose intolerance Hypoproteinemia	Long-term hyperalimentation GI GVHD		Electrolytes Ca^{2+}, Mg^{2+}, phosphate, albumin, transferrin

Key Reference: Kojima S, Nakao S, Tomonaga M, et al. Consensus Conference on the Treatment of Aplastic Anemia. *Int J Hematol.* 2000;72:118–123.

Perioperative Implications

Preoperative Preparation

- Reverse isolation precautions
- Adequacy of blood products
- Severe neutropenia, co-existing congenital heart disease (HD) may warrant prophylactic antimicrobial therapy
- Avoid IM and rectal sedation
- Concomitant steroid therapy and necessity of stress doses should be considered

Monitoring

- Arterial line if indicated
- Consider CVP or PA catheter as indicated
- Urine output for new-onset hemoglobinuria as first sign of transfusion reaction

Airway

- Avoid nasal manipulation

- Use extreme caution with friable oral and pharyngeal mucosal surfaces

Preinduction/Induction

- May exhibit hypotension and excessive fluid requirements to maintain adequate CO
- Central neuraxial blockade contraindicated in ongoing thrombocytopenia requiring transfusion
- Peripheral neural blockade may be approached cautiously if coagulation status is judged adequate

Maintenance

- PEEP assures adequate tissue oxygenation at lower FIO_2 as hyperoxia depresses normal erythropoietin synthesis and marrow function
- Nitrous oxide depresses bone marrow function even after brief exposure; best to use O_2-air mixture
- Normothermia promotes coagulation

- Chronically anemic pts may tolerate lower Hct; adequacy of tissue O_2 must be addressed if CV decompensation ensues
- Avoid induced hypotension in anemic pts

Extubation

- Period with greatest O_2 demands

Postoperative Period

- Continued monitoring of coagulation status
- Transfusion requirements > normal
- Increased susceptibility to infection
- Pain management improves pulm toilet

Anticipated Problems/Concerns

- Age of RBC in pts with aplastic anemia is older than usual, with lower 2,3-DPG levels inside cells resulting in increased O_2 binding by Hgb (shift to the right) and decreased delivery of oxygen to tissues for same SaO_2

Anemia, Chronic Disease/Inflammation
Hayden R. Hughes

Risk
- Incidence in USA: All anemia, 8%; ACD/I second most common form
- Having chronic infectious, inflammatory, or malignant conditions
- >130 million Americans living with chronic diseases

Perioperative Risks
- Risks related to underlying diseases
- Transfusion related risks; e.g., TRALI, hemolytic reactions, immunosuppression
- Risks related to compensatory mechanisms for increasing O_2 delivery; e.g., angina, heart failure, dysrhythmias

Worry About
- Underlying diseases and their periop complications
- Impaired tissue O_2 delivery and compensatory mechanisms aimed at correcting it
- Delayed wound healing and infection

Overview
- WHO definition of anemia: Children 6 mo–6 y: Hgb <11 g/dl; 6–14 y: Hgb <12 g/dl; nonpregnant females: Hgb <12 g/dl; pregnant females: Hgb <11 g/dl; males: Hgb <13 g/dl
- Normochromic, normocytic with low reticulocyte count
- ACD/I due to disturbances of Fe homeostasis due to diversion of Fe from the circulation into storage sites within the reticuloendothelial system
- Usually mild with Hgb 8–11 g/dl

ICD-9-CM Code: 285.21 Anemia in chronic kidney disease

Etiology
- Relative Fe deficiency
- Certain treatments for chronic conditions

Usual Treatment
- Treatment of underlying disease
- Fe, folic acid, cobalamin supplementation
- uman recombinant erythropoietin
- Allogeneic blood transfusion

ASSESSMENT POINTS

System	Effect	Assessment by Hx	PE	Test
CV	Hyperdynamic circulation Myocardial ischemia CHF	Palpitation Pounding pulse Angina Sx, dyspnea Exercise intolerance	Tachycardia Wide pulse pressure	ECG Exercise ECG
RESP		Dyspnea		
GI	Chronic blood loss Hypoperfusion	Blood in stool Angina equivalent (pain, nausea, indigestion)		Occult blood in stool See CV
HEME	Hgb below WHO definition level (see Overview)	↓ In exercise tolerance		Hgb
RENAL	Chronic renal failure	↓ Urine output Dialysis	Shunt	Cr K+
CNS	Decreased cerebral O_2 delivery	Dizziness Headache Transient cerebral ischemia		
MS	Low exercise capacity	Fatigue		

Key Reference: Shander A. Anemia in the critically ill. *Crit Care Clin*. 2004;20(2):159–178. Review.

Perioperative Implications

Preoperative Preparation
- Standard monitoring
- Warm the room
- CVP, Hgb, electrolytes
- ST-segment analysis in pts with signs of CAD
- PA catheter for large fluid shifts or pts with signs of LV dysfunction or advanced renal failure
- ABG

Airway
- None

Preinduction/Induction
- Prehydrate liberally if CV status will tolerate
- Avoid CO reduction
- Avoid hypoxemia
- Choose drugs according to underlying conditions

Maintenance
- Avoid hypoxemia
- Maintain CO
- Avoid hypovolemia
- Keep pt warm
- Maintain Hgb above critical level for pt taking comorbities into account

Extubation
- Keep pt warm
- Maintain high Pao$_2$
- In pt with CAD, this is the period of greatest risk for ischemia

Postoperative Period
- Keep pt warm, prevent shivering
- Maintain high Pao$_2$

Adjuvants
- According to underlying disorder

Anticipated Problems/Concerns
- Myocardial ischemia/infarction or CHF in pts with concomitant CAD
- Deterioration of renal function in pts with CRI
- Prolonged effects of drugs in pts with impaired renal and/or hepatic function

Anemia, Hemolytic

Matthew Tomlinson
Kirk Lalwani

Risk

- Autoimmune disorders (SLE, RA, scleroderma, cold agglutinin disease)
- Lymphoproliferative disorders (CLL, NHL)
- Prosthetic heart valves (ball-and-cage, and bileaflet valves). Usually subclinical, but can be severe in up to 15% of pts
- Family history of hemoglobinopathies or RBC membrane defects (thalassemia, sickle cell disease, G6PD deficiency, spherocytosis)
- Exposure to drugs (cephalosporins, penicillins, NSAIDs) or other chemicals (naphthalene, fava beans)

Perioperative Risks

- Anemia, hypoxia
- Underlying CV compromise
- Splenomegaly in pts with extravascular hemolysis (within the reticuloendothelial system). Splenectomy is a common surgical procedure in pt with sickle cell disease due to hemolysis and sickling.
- Renal failure due to massive hemolysis (cold agglutinin hemolysis, sickling, drug reaction, etc.)

- Varying levels of liver disease depending on type of hemolytic anemia. Synthetic function of liver is usually normal, but in severe cases can be compromised.

Worry About

- Uncompensated anemia in pts with sub-acute hemolysis
- Periop hemolysis and/or hypoxia
- Need for transfusion and/or fluids

Overview

- Pts with hemolytic anemia may present with any of the following: fatigue, angina, SOB, tachypnea, tachycardia, or jaundice. The hemolysis can lead to changes in blood viscosity, gallstone production, splenomegaly, and renal failure in severe cases. Many pts will be both iron and folate deficient.
- Epidemiology varies by pt population. For example, G6PD is an X-linked condition and its prevalence is near 50% in Kurdish Jews, but around 1:1000 in North American and European populations
- Other things to consider incl monitoring periodic Hct levels, and administering prophylactic

antibiotics/vaccinations to pts who have had a splenectomy.

ICD-9-CM Code: 282.#, 283.#

Etiology

- Multiple causes; see Risk section (RBC structural abnormalities, autoimmune reaction, enzyme deficiency, hemoglobinopathies, mechanical heart valves, drugs, etc.)

Usual Treatment

- Treatment depends on etiology
  - Autoimmune: corticosteroids, plasmapheresis, packed RBC transfusion for symptomatic pts, supportive care
  - Drug induced: Discontinuation of offending medication, corticosteroids, supportive care
  - Prosthetic valve: Cardiology consult and transfusion if symptoms rapidly worsen
  - RBC membrane defect: Splenectomy and supportive care
  - Enzyme deficiency: Avoidance of triggers, splenectomy, supportive care

ASSESSMENT POINTS

System	Effect	Assessment by Hx	PE	Test
CV	Dehydration	Fatigue, dizziness	Hypotension, weak pulses, increased capillary refill	CBC, BNP
HEME	Anemia	Fatigue, SOB, dizziness	Jaundice, pallor, splenomegaly	Hgb, Hct, reticulocyte count, indirect bilirubin, LDH
RENAL	Hemoglobinuria, acute renal failure	Dark urine (episodic)	Possible Htn, resp rate changes	Urine analysis, BUN, Cr
GI	Liver disease		Hepatosplenomegaly	LFTs

Key Reference: Firth Paul G. Anesthesia and hemoglobinopathies. *Anesthesiol Clin.* 2009;27(2):321–336.

Perioperative Implications

Preinduction/Induction/Maintenance

- Preop management and treatment of underlying cause of hemolytic anemia
- The test obtained periop depends on the etiology, severity, and chronicity of the hemolytic anemia.
- Avoidance of hypoxia, hypercarbia, acidosis, low-flow conditions, and hypothermia
- Optimize CV status with adequate hydration; consider IV fluid treatment the day before surgery if hypovolemic
- RBC transfusion may be considered to improve O_2 carrying capacity depending on etiology (most common in patients with sickle cell disease)

- Normothermia should be strictly maintained in any pt requiring transfusion(s)

Monitoring

- Standard monitors and urine output, CV status, O_2 saturation (pulse oximetry), and temp regulation (avoiding hypothermia)

General Anesthesia

- Choice of anesthetic technique can vary, but all approaches should have the goal of avoiding hypoxia, hypercarbia, acidosis, stasis, low-flow conditions, and hypothermia
- Avoidance of hypoventilation

Regional Anesthesia

- Goals for regional anesthesia are the same as for general anesthesia. No specific contraindications.

Postoperative Period

- Supplemental O_2 therapy
- Adequate hydration
- Early ambulation
- Continued temp regulation
- Active pulm toilet

Anticipated Problems/Concerns

- Acute periop hemolysis; may warrant transfusion
- Periop sickling event due to hypoxia, acidosis, hypothermia, or low flow. Sickling can be decreased by increasing arterial oxygen tension.
- Hypothermia-induced cold agglutinin hemolysis; decreased by maintaining normothermia
- Hypoxia and end-organ damage

Angina, Chronic Stable

Lee A. Fleisher

Risk

- Incidence in USA: 3 million
- Annual rates per 1000 new episodes of angina for non-black men are 28.3 for ages 65–74, 36.3 for ages 75–84, and 33.0 for age 85 and older. For non-black women in the same age groups, the rates are 14.1, 20.0 and 22.9, respectively. For black men, the rates are 22.4, 33.8 and 39.5, and for black women, the rates are 15.3, 23.6 and 35.9, respectively
- African Americans have highest death rates

Perioperative Risks

- Increased risk of periop MI and death varies, depending on study (3–12%)
- Risk of LV dysfunction, hypotension, MI

Worry About

- Increasing frequency of symptoms
- Signs of LV dysfunction with ischemia
- Silent myocardial ischemia

Overview

- Chronic stable angina identifies pts at risk for developing myocardial ischemia and MI
- Angina is present in <25% of episodes of myocardial ischemia
- Symptoms should be stable for previous 60 d for "stable" diagnosis
- Can result from:
  - Inadequacy of myocardial O_2 supply in pts with critical coronary artery stenosis
  - Coronary vasospasm
  - Inadequacy of myocardial O_2 supply 2° to increased demand from ventricular hypertrophy
  - Endothelial cell-mediated vasoconstriction

- Thrombosis overlying unstable plaque can lead to unstable angina/MI

ICD-9-CM Code: 413

Etiology

- Acquired disease with genetic predisposition
- Pts with diabetes have higher incidence of CAD, frequently silent
- Other risk factors incl Htn, hyperlipidemia, advanced age, tobacco use, homocystinemia

Usual Treatment

- Medical therapy: β-adrenergic receptor antagonist, Ca^2-channel antagonists, nitrates, aspirin, clopidogrel, folate, lipid-reducing agents, combination agents
- Percutaneous coronary interventions
- CABG

ASSESSMENT POINTS

System	Effect	Assessment by Hx	PE	Test
CV	Myocardial ischemia LV dysfunction	Angina Sx Angina-equivalent Sx Dyspnea Exercise tolerance	Displaced posterior maximal impulse S_3	ECG Exercise ECG Exercise radionuclide scintigraphy Pharmacologic stress testing ECHO Coronary angiography Coronary CT
RESP	CHF	Dyspnea Nighttime cough Orthopnea Chest tightness	S_3 Rales Wheezing	CXR
GI		Angina-equivalent Sx LUQ pain Nausea, indigestion		See CV assessment
RENAL	↓ Renal perfusion	↑ UO at night		Cr
CNS	Syncope	Syncope with chest pain		Exercise stress test
MS	Angina-equivalent Sx Arm pain/neck pain			See CV assessment

Key Reference: Fleisher LA, Beckman JA, et al. 2009 ACCF/AHA focused update on perioperative beta blockade incorporated into the ACC/AHA 2007 Guidelines on Perioperative Cardiovascular Evaluation and Care for Noncardiac Surgery: A Report of the American College of Cardiology Foundation/American Heart Association Task Force on Practice Guidelines. *Circulation.* 2009;120(21):e169–e276.

Perioperative Implications

Preoperative Preparation

- Continuation of chronic anti-anginal medications associated with a lower incidence of myocardial ischemia/infarction, especially beta blockers, statins, and antiplatelet agents

Monitoring

- ST-segment analysis
- PA catheter for large fluid shift operations or pts with signs of LV dysfunction, although RCT unable to document benefits of routine monitoring
- TEE most sensitive, but technical issues of real-time interpretation

Airway

- None

Preinduction/Induction

- May develop reduced CO and hypotension with ischemia
- Avoid tachycardia, hypotension

Maintenance

- Myocardial ischemia may manifest as
  - CV instability
  - Intraop myocardial ischemia
  - Reduced CO, increased PCWP
- No one agent or technique shown superior
- Maintain normothermia, adequate hematocrit (≥28%)

Extubation

- Period at greatest risk for developing ischemia

Postoperative Period

- Pain management may be critical

Adjuvants

- β-adrenergic receptor antagonist, nitroglycerin, Ca^{2+}-channel blockers

Anticipated Problems/Concerns

- Pts with angina who develop dyspnea on exertion are at greatest risk for developing periop cardiac complications
- Exercise tolerance may be the best predictor of periop risk. Pts with a good exercise tolerance may not require further evaluation for less-invasive procedures.
- Pts who develop periop MI are at increased risk of periop death and long-term morbidity/mortality. Elevated troponin also associated with worse long-term outcomes.

Anhidrosis (Congenital Anhidrotic Ectodermanl Dysplasia)

Raafat S. Hannallah

Risk

- Rare, 1:125,000,000
- Clusters in Japan and Israel

Perioperative Risks

- Impaired thermoregulation (risk of hyperthermia in infants)
- Postop chest infections

Worry About

- Absence of sweat leads to impaired thermoregulation
- Insensitivity to superficial and deep painful stimuli with intact tactile perception. Still require considerable amounts of inhalational anesthetics to maintain hemodynamic stability.

Overview

- Innervation of the eccrine sweat glands is lacking; heat loss by evaporation is impaired
- Absent mucous glands from resp tract and esophagus; frequent resp infections
- Partial or complete absence of teeth
- Hypotrichosis (absent hair)
- Self-mutilating behavior and mental retardation
- Characteristic facies: Prominent supraorbital ridges, depressed bridge and root of nose, large deformed ears, thick lips, underdeveloped maxilla and mandible

ICD-9-CM Code: 705.0

Etiology

- Sex-linked recessive disorder
- Human *TRKA* (*NTRK1*) encodes the receptor tyrosine kinases (RTKs) for nerve growth factor (NGF) and is the gene responsible
- Full expression only in males; carrier females may be mildly affected

Usual Treatment

- Protect from risks of hyperpyrexia due to infection, hot weather, vigorous exercise

ASSESSMENT POINTS

System	Effect	Assessment by Hx	Test
HEENT	Airway anomalies	Snoring Difficult breathing	
RESP	Decreased mucus	Repeated infections	
OPHTHAL	Decreased lacrimation	Dryness, ulceration	
METAB	Hyperpyrexia		Record/monitor temp

Key Reference: Rozentsveig V, Katz A, Weksler N, et al. The anaesthetic management of patients with congenital insensitivity to pain with anhidrosis. *Pediatr Anesth.* 2004;14:344–348.

Perioperative Implications

Preoperative Preparation

- Avoid anticholinergic premedication; however atropine has been used to treat bradycardia

Monitoring

- Routine
- Temp

Airway

- Awkward mask fit

- Laryngoscopy and intubation may be difficult

Maintenance

- Regional anesthesia may be preferable when possible
- Humidify anesthetic gases
- Controlled room temp to avoid hyperthermia

Extubation

- Vigorous postop chest physical therapy

Adjuvants

- Protect eyes with tape and ophthalmic ointment (lacrimation is reduced)

Anticipated Problems/Concerns

- Difficult airway (mask and/or intubation)
- Hyperthermia
- Postop chest infections
- High incidence of CV events (hypotension and bradycardia) reported

Ankylosing Spondylitis

John E. Tetzlaff

Risk

- 1:2000 incidence in Caucasians, rare in non-Caucasians
- M:F: 10:1; more severe in males
- 18–50% incidence in Native Americans

Perioperative Risks

- Difficult airway, atlantoaxial instability
- "Bamboo spine" with potential for fracture during airway manipulation
- Rigid chest with difficult ventilation
- Myocarditis, myocardial conduction defects
- Increased blood loss due to abnormal chest structure, mechanics

Worry About

- Inability to intubate, spine fracture, arrhythmia, inability to ventilate, massive blood loss
- Airway edema after extubation

Overview

- An arthritic process, seronegative for rheumatoid factor, that attacks ligamentous attachments of the spinal column
- Characterized by low back pain, sacroiliitis, multiplane rigidity of spine, chest stiffness, uveitis, and insidious onset at <40 y of age
- Autosomal dominant and strongly prevalent among first-degree relatives

ICD-9–CM Code: 720.00

Etiology

- Unknown
- Genetic transmission led to discovery of a genetic marker, HLA-B27. Also involved are the major histocompatability complex, numerous HLA-B27 subtypes, and IL23R (also associated with ulcerative colitis) and ERAP-1.
- Infectious origin speculated; one species of *klebsiella* reported to be associated with some cases

Usual Treatment

- Symptomatic, with exercise, NSAIDs, immunosuppression can be tried in severe cases
- Wedge osteotomy is a drastic surgical intervention
- Infliximab—monoclonal antibody specific for tumor necrosis factor (TNF)
- Enanercept—anti TNF protein
- Adalimumab—monoclonal antibody specific for tumor necrosis factor (TNF)

ASSESSMENT POINTS

System	Effect	Assessment by Hx	PE	Test
HEENT	Uveitis TMJ arthritis Arytenoid deviation	Visual disturbance Limited mouth opening, jaw pain, voice abnormality	Funduscopic exam Airway exam, indirect laryngoscopy	Fiberoptic nasopharyngoscopy
CV	Cardiomyopathy, conduction defects	SOB, chest pain, palpitation	Distant heart sounds, rales, arrhythmia	ECG, CXR, ECHO
RESP	Pleuritic inflammation, chest rigidity	Chest pain, limited exercise tolerance	Decreased breath sounds, chest excursion	Pulm function tests, CXR
GI	Irritable bowel syndrome Ulcerative colitis	Abdominal pain, bowel dysfunction	Abdominal pain	
GU	Chronic prostatitis	Pain with urination	Rectal exam	
CNS	Atlantoaxial subluxation, occult spine fracture	Long tract signs, sphincter abnormality Sometimes no symptoms	Basic neurologic exam	Cervical spine x-ray with flexion-extension, MRI
PNS	Radiculopathy	Radiating pain in extremities	ROM of the extremity	EMG (medicolegal use)
MS	Back pain, sacroiliitis, joint ankylosis, kyphosis ("chin on chest"), "bamboo spine," spondylodiskitis	Review of skeletal function	Spine, skeleton	Radiologic studies

Key Reference: Van der Linden S. Ankylosing spondylitis. In Kelly WN, Harris Jr ED, Ruddy S, Sledge CB, eds. *Textbook of rheumatology*, 7th ed, Philadelphia: Elsevier Saunders; 2005.

Perioperative Implications

Preoperative Preparation
- Airway evaluation, pulm function assessment; consider positioning difficulties
- Antisialagogue for awake intubation
- Review MRI of the spine

Monitoring
- ST-segment analysis; pulm artery catheter if severe myocardial dysfunction
- Arterial line, central venous access for extensive osteotomy secondary to blood loss

Airway
- Inability to intubate possible, owing to cervical spine fusion, distortion. Fiberoptic intubation may be necessary. Cervical spine instability possible. Spine fracture possible with airway manipulation. Occult spine fracture may already be present.
- Increasing role for videolaryngoscopy

Induction
- If general anesthesia, any approach acceptable. If limited cardiac reserves, avoid depressants of myocardial contractility.
- If regional, skeletal abnormality can make the block difficult to perform, and response to injection is unpredictable. In some cases, epidural space is obliterated and cannot be completely accessed. Strongly consider paramedian approach to central block. If local anesthetic toxicity, airway management can be difficult.

Maintenance
- With positive pressure ventilation, decrease tidal volume and increase rate
- High ventilating pressure may predict large blood loss

Extubation
- Awake is preferable
- Airway edema possible after extensive anterior osteotomy, decompression and/or fusion. Compression of the airway from retropharyngeal hematoma is possible. Consider leak test prior to extubation, or maintaining the pt intubated and sedation for 12–24 hr postop

Adjuvants
- Ischemic optic neuropathy with prolonged procedures in the prone position

Postoperative
- Comfortable position, pain control without airway embarrassment

Anticipated Problems/Concerns

- Airway control
- The extreme distortion of the spine, esp. the neck, may make intubating trachea and ventilating pt very difficult
- Any airway compromise or depression of ventilation can result in catastrophe
- Depression of ventilation with opiate analgesics can be dangerous
- Pulm function
  - Because of abnormal mechanics of the thorax and neck, the ability to ensure normal oxygenation during surgery and in the postop period can be a potential problem
- Regional anesthesia
  - Placement of spinal, epidural, or caudal block could be technically very difficult. Action of local anesthetics in the central axis could be unpredictable.
- Prolonged postop intubation
  - Substantial blood loss, fluid/blood product administration, and the prone position make airway edema likely, requiring extended postop intubation necessary. Pt should be informed preop to avoid postop panic.

Anomalous Pulmonary Venous Drainage
Roger A. Moore

Risk

- 1% of all congenital heart defects
- Total anomalous pulm venous drainage (TAPVD), the severe form, or partial anomalous pulm venous drainage (PAPVD), the less severe form, exists when pulm veins drain into the venous circulation
- M:F 4:1 in infradiaphragmatic type

Perioperative Risks

- Rapid CV deterioration secondary to hypercapnia and resultant acidosis
- Sudden pulm Htn and RHF during hypoventilation
- Periop mortality: 2–20% depending on preop status

Worry About

- Air bubbles entering the venous circuit
- Endocarditis risk

- Polycythemic hyperviscosity attack with:
  - Periop dehydration
  - Cold OR environment

Overview

- TAPVD incompatible with life unless an ASD allows adequate R→L shunting of blood. TAPVD pts with small ASDs are more critically ill and often require balloon septostomy as a bridge to surgery. Some cyanosis, usually with O_2 saturations of 85–95%.
- Increased flow through pulm vascular beds, resulting in pulm Htn
- Four types of TAPVD:
  - Supracardiac: Pulm veins connect to the left innominate vein via an anomalous "vertical vein" or connect to right SVC via an anomalous "short connecting vein," or connect to the left SVC (45%)
  - Cardiac: Pulm veins drain into coronary sinus or directly into the right atrium (23%)

- Infracardiac: Pulm veins drain into IVC, portal veins, hepatic veins, or ductus venosus (21%)
- Mixed: Combined supracardiac, cardiac, and infracardiac connections (11%)

ICD-9–CM Code: 747.41

Etiology

- Embryologic atresia or malformation of the common pulm venous system resulting in persistence of abnormal connections

Usual Treatment

- Severe TAPVD with little systemic shunt needs immediate cardiac correction after birth. Most children with TAPVD require cardiac correction before 1 y of age.
- Cardiac correction of PAPVD may be postponed into childhood.

ASSESSMENT POINTS

System	Effect	Assessment by Hx	PE	Test
HEENT	Hypoxemia	Snoring	Airway class	
CV	CHF Hypoxemia Monitoring problems	Decreased activity level Dyspnea Anomalous peripheral vessels	Rales Cyanosis Pulses and blood pressures in all four extremities	ECG—RVH, RAH ECHO; catheterization Cardiac consultation
RESP	Hypoxemia	Bronchospasm SOB Pulmonary edema Exertional cyanosis	Wheezing Tachypnea Clubbing	CXR Granular lung fields
HEME	Sludging DIC	Polycythemia Bleeding or bruising	Clubbing Bruises	Hgb PT PTT, bleeding time
CNS		Previous stroke	Complete neurologic evaluation	CT scan if neurologic findings
MS		Feeding difficulty Failure to thrive	Ht, wt, head circumference	Plot of growth curves

Key Reference: Caldarone CA, Najm HK, Kadletz M, et al. Surgical management of total anomalous pulmonary venous drainage: Impact of coexisting cardiac anomalies. *Ann Thorac Surg.* 1998;66:1521–1526.

Perioperative Implications

Preoperative Preparation

- Desired hemodynamics: Preload—normal (CVP 10–12 mmHg); afterload—low; PVR—normal; HR—normal to high; contractility—normal
- Liberal oral fluids preop
- Avoid premedication causing hypoventilation
- Subacute bacterial endocarditis prophylaxis

Monitoring

- Absolute air bubble precaution
- Arterial catheter
- CVP catheter—know specific anatomy, incl SVC variations
- TEE
- Others as per ASA routine

Airway

- Associated congenital syndromes with airway anomalies
- Cricoid ring limiting diameter of airway
- Primary need to maintain airway and avoid increased $Paco_2$
- PEEP, with pulm edema or elevated pulm blood flow

Induction

- If IV in place use fentanyl or ketamine with pancuronium or vecuronium.
- If no IV
  - If unstable, ketamine IM
  - If stable, slow inhalational induction with sevoflurane (avoid high sevoflurane levels until IV placed)
- Actively avoid hypoventilation and agents that produce myocardial depression

Maintenance

- Use fluids judiciously to avoid RV overload
- Positive pressure ventilation usually improves oxygenation
- Use narcotics in conjunction with inhalational agents as tolerated
- Avoid nitrous oxide
- Use high FIO_2
- Capnographic $ETCO_2$ will not accurately reflect $Paco_2$
- Prepare for hypothermic cardiac arrest during TAPVR repair
- Avoid hypothermia before and after bypass

Extubation

- Do not attempt deep or early extubation
- Prior to extubation assess adequacy of ventilation with insp pressures of at least -20 mmHg and adequate tidal volumes

Postoperative Period

- Close monitoring of ventilation and pulse oximetry
- Active warming with avoidance of shivering
- Be prepared for immediate reintubation

Adjuvants

- Inotropic support with dopamine or dobutamine

Anticipated Problems/Concerns

- If pulm hypertensive crisis occurs
  - Hyperventilate
  - 100% inspired O_2
  - Consider prostaglandin E_1, tolazoline, amrinone, isoproterenol, or nitric oxide

Anorexia Nervosa

Russell T. Wall III

Risk

- Primarily in white adolescent females from middle- or upper-class families, 4–10% are males
- More common in models, ballet students, professions demanding high achievement
- 0.4–1.5/100,000 population
- Bimodal peak age of onset: 14 and 18 years

Perioperative Risks

- Predisposing conditions incl:
  - Cardiovascular dysfunction (bradycardia, hypotension, dysrhythmias)
  - Acid-base abnormalities (both metabolic acidosis and alkalosis are possible), electrolyte abnormalities (decreased K, decreased Mg, decreased Na, decreased P),
  - Hematologic abnormalities (decreased Hgb, decreased WBC, decreased fibrinogen, decreased plt)
  - Hypothermia, delayed gastric emptying, and renal dysfunction (prerenal azotemia)

Worry About

- Degree and duration of malnutrition (excess protein depletion = impaired cellular function)
- Degree of organ dysfunction
- Greater weight loss = greater risk

Overview

- Anorexia nervosa
  - Obsessive fear of obesity, obsessive pursuit of thinness
  - Refusal to maintain weight above 85% IBW
  - Distorted body image
  - Amenorrhea for >3 mo
  - Radical restriction of caloric intake
  - Appears cachectic
  - Risk of death high if wt loss >40% of IBW
  - 40–50% recover with treatment, 20–30% improve with treatment
- Bulimia
  - Means "ox hunger" or voracious appetite
  - Obsessive fear of obesity, over-concern with body shape and weight
  - Appears well nourished
  - Averages two binge-eating episodes each week for at least 3 mo
  - Irresistible urge to overeat, loss of control in desire to eat
  - Wt control by self-induced vomiting, diuretic and laxative use, strict dieting/fasting, vigorous exercise
  - Greater percent of alcohol use, illicit drug use, stealing, self-mutilation, and suicide attempts than anorexia
  - 30–60% recover with treatment

ICD-9–CM Code: 307.1

Etiology

- Unknown, possibly hypothalamic dysfunction or psychiatric cause

Usual Treatment

- No specific/definitive treatment
- Therapies offered
  - Psychotherapy (individual, group, family)
  - Behavior modification
  - Antidepressants (tricylics, MAO inhibitors, serotonin uptake inhibitors) often prescribed but not consistently effective
  - Nutrition counseling (1500–2500 calories/d, metoclopramide or bethanechol for gastric emptying, benzodiazepine before meals)
  - Relaxation exercises
- If severe: Hospitalization stressing wt gain, with tube feedings or hyperalimentation as last resort

ASSESSMENT POINTS

System	Effect	Assessment by Hx	PE	Test
CV	↓ Response to SNS		Bradycardia	ECG
	Hypovolemia		Hypotension (<70 mmHg systolic)	
	LV dysfunction (myocardial atrophy)	CHF symptoms		
	↓ LV wall thickness		CHF	CXR
	↓ LV cavity size			ECHO
	MV prolapse		Murmur	
	Cardiomyopathy 2° ipecac			
	Conduction abnormalities		Dysrhythmias (tachydysrhythmias, AV blocks, nonspecific ST-T changes)	ECG
	Hypercholesterolemia			Cholesterol, triglycerides
	Anemia			Hct
	Thrombocytopenia			Platelets
	Hypofibrinogenemia			Fibrinogen
RESP	Aspiration pneumonia	Vomiting with ↓ consciousness	Hypoxia, tachypnea	CXR
	Respiratory insufficiency	Dyspnea	Bradypnea (<15/min)	
		Muscle weakness		↓ P
GI	Delayed gastric emptying, ↓ motility	Early satiety, abdominal pain		
	Esophagitis, esophageal/gastric rupture	Vomiting with bulimia	Pneumomediastinum	CXR
			Pneumoperitoneum	Abdominal x-rays
	Hepatic insufficiency		Fatty infiltration of liver	↑ LFTs
RENAL	Prerenal azotemia 2° to ↓ volume	Starvation		BUN 60–70 mg/dl
		Dehydration, vomiting		Electrolytes (K, Na, P, Mg)
	Renal insufficiency	↓ GFR		Serum creatinine
	Renal calculi			
	Polyuria	XS caffeine and water ingestion		
	Acid-base abnormalities (metabolic acidosis / alkalosis)	Vomiting		ABGs
				Electrolytes
	Electrolyte abnormalities (↓ K, ↓ Na, ↓ Mg, ↓ P)	Diuretics, laxative abuse		<3 grams/dl is evidence of severe protein malnutrition
	Hypoalbuminemia		Peripheral edema	
	ATN	Rhabdomyolysis		CPK, LDH, aldolase

(Continued)

System	Effect	Assessment by Hx	PE	Test
ENDO	↓ BMR		Vasoconstriction	
	Hypothermia (<96.6°F rectally)			
	Estrogen deficiency	Amenorrhea		
	Depressed immune function			↓ WBC (leukopenia)
	Hypophosphatemia			
	Hypomagnesemia			
	Hypoglycemia			
	Euthyroid sick syndrome		Bradycardia	
			Hypothermia	Serum P
			Cold intolerance	Serum Mg
			Dry skin and hair	Serum glucose
			Slow DTRs	TFTs
CNS	Brain atrophy with dilated ventricles	Starvation		
	Depression	Illicit drug, alcohol use		
PNS	Peripheral neuropathy			EMG changes
MS	Osteoporosis	Estrogen, IGF-I deficiency	Vertebral compression fractures	X-rays of back, extremities
			Stress fractures	
	Cachexia (if anorexic)	Dieting		
	Myopathy			

Key Reference: Seller CA, Ravalia A. Anaesthetic implications of anorexia nervosa. *Anaesthesia*. 2003;58(5):437–443.

Perioperative Implications

Preoperative Preparation
- Evaluate degree and duration of malnutrition
- Assess degree of organ damage (esp. cardiac, pulm, renal, hepatic)
- Severely malnourished for emergency surgery have significant increased morbidity and/or mortality
  - Delay elective surgery until pt is medically stable and nutritional status is improved
  - Optimize hemodynamics, volume status, acid-base status, electrolytes (Na, K, P, Mg) and glucose
- Treat severe anemia if present
  - Consider metoclopramide to promote gastric emptying

Monitoring
- ABGs, lytes
- A-line, CVP, PA catheters may be indicated

Airway
- Induction
  - Consider rapid-sequence induction (decreased GE sphincter tone, decreased gastric emptying)
  - Cautious dosing because of possible LV dysfunction and hypovolemia
  - Antibiotics

Maintenance
- Aggressively avoid hypothermia
- Cautious use of potent inhalation agents to avoid hemodynamic depression
- Excess fluids may precipitate pulm edema, CHF

Extubation
- Consider awake extubation

Adjuvants
- Cautious use of muscle relaxants (decreased muscle mass, electrolyte and acid-base abnormalities)

Anticipated Problems/Concerns
- Temp control
- Hemodynamic stability
- Acid-base and electrolyte management
- Metabolic reserve adequate to accommodate intraop and postop surgical stress and/or demands of wound healing and combating infection?

Anticoagulation, Preoperative

Jerrold H. Levy

DISEASES

Risk

- Pts with mechanical heart valves, atrial fibrillation, pulm embolism, recent venous thrombosis
- Oral anticoagulant therapy (warfarin, oral Xa inhibitor, dabigatran) and use of LMW heparin, pentasaccharide may increase potential risks in elective or emergency surgery
- Other populations are pts who receive heparin IV before vascular or cardiac surgery and pts undergoing cardiac surgery with extracorporeal circulation

Perioperative Risks

- Balance between risk of bleeding versus thromboembolic complication is major periop risk
- Risk increases with major and emergency versus elective surgery

Worry About

- Excessive allogeneic transfusions, either to correct effects of anticoagulation or for risk of excessive bleeding
- In pts with valvular heart disease, concomitant hepatic dysfunction due to HF may produce abnormal PT and/or thrombocytopenia
- Heparin-induced thrombocytopenia can be associated with heparin therapy due to acute administration or prolonged use (~5 d)

Overview

Heparin (Standard Unfractionated)

- For preventive therapy and acute management, binds to antithrombin III and factor X to inhibit their effects
- Variability in response to heparin depends on
  - Prep of heparin administered
  - Individual characteristics of pts
  - Duration of therapy (due to decreased antithrombin III levels)
- Duration of action depends on dose and method of administration
  - 100U/kg: $T_{1/2}$ 56 min
  - IV: 60 min
  - 400U/kg: $T_{1/2}$ tripled
  - SQ: 3 hr
- Depolymerized in endothelial cells
- Eliminated in urine
- Heparin resistance (many proteins neutralize anticoagulant therapy; prolonged therapy can lower antithrombin III levels)
- Monitoring of the anticoagulant effect: PTT

Heparin (LMW)

- $T_{1/2}$ 4–7 hr
- Higher and more predictable bioavailability: 100%
- Removed by renal filtration
- Not reversed with protamine, no current reversal therapy except time

Heparin Reversal Treatment

- Protamine reversal according to the ratio heparin:protamine 1:1.3 (or start with 50–100 mg and check the ACT)
- Monitoring: ACT in cardiac surgery

Warfarin

- Oral anticoagulant
- Member of the coumarin family
- Vitamin K antagonist causing inactivation of factors II, VII, IX, X and anticoagulants C, S
- Used for thromboembolic complication prevention
- Peak plasma concentration reached 1–4 hr after ingestion
- $T_{1/2}$: 36–42 hr
- International normalized ratio (INR) required: 2–3
- Stop for surgery and replace with heparin

Warfarin Reversal Treatment

- Vitamin K: 10–20 mg PO, IM, or IV, but takes several days for normalization of INR
- Fresh frozen plasma starting with 2U but higher doses required
- Purified protein concentrates of II, VII, IX, X with protein C and AT III (Beriplex and Octaplex) are used outside of USA and under investigation here.

Novel Agents Approved in Other Countries not yet Available in the United States

- Rivaroxaban and apixiban are oral Xa inhibitors
- Dabigatran is an oral thrombin inhibitor
- These agents studied in periop DVT prophylaxis and AF treatment; no current reversal therapy except time

ASSESSMENT POINTS

System	Effect	Assessment by Hx
ENDO	Risk of protamine reactions is 10- to 30-fold higher in diabetics receiving protamine-containing insulin	Hx of insulin use

Key Reference: Levy JH, Tanaka KA, Dietrich W. Perioperative hemostatic management of patients treated with vitamin K antagonists. *Anesthesiology*. 2008;109:918–926.

Perioperative Implications

Preoperative Preparation

- Elective surgery/warfarin therapy
  - Stop warfarin 5 d before surgery
  - Replace with heparin in checking INR, PTT, platelet count
  - Stop heparin 60–90 min before surgery
- Reversal for emergency surgery

- Warfarin therapy can be acutely reversed with PCC, and heparin therapy can be reversed with protamine
- Consider avoiding regional anesthesia
- Approach anticoagulation reversal cautiously in the anticoagulated patient

Postoperative Period

- Restart heparin therapy immediately after surgery (PTT, plt count, blood cell count, bleeding)

Anticipated Problems/Concerns

- Introduction of epidural or spinal anesthesia requires minimum 60–120 min between stopping and restarting heparinization; consider removing catheter at least 120 min after stopping heparinization and complete restoration of normal clotting time. Longer times are required with other longer-acting anticoagulation agents.

Antithrombin III Deficiency

Ellise Delphin
Vasanti Tilak

Risk

- Incidence in USA: 1 in 2000–5000 (may be higher)
- Men and women equally affected, no racial or ethnic difference

Perioperative Risks

- Risk of postop thromboembolic phenomena; 40–70%, most common (in descending order): DVT, pulm embolus, mesenteric thrombosis, cerebral venous and retinal thrombosis, highest risk in those with antithrombin III (AT III) levels <50% of normal
- Risk of pregnancy-related venous thromboembolism may be >50% in untreated pts
- Heparin resistance is common

Worry About

- Hypercoagulable state periop
- Thrombus formation on indwelling catheters
- Pulm emboli or DVT with immobility

- Mesenteric, inferior vena cava, or CNS thrombosis
- Withdrawal of warfarin sodium preop, as pts may be heparin-resistant
- Timing of neuraxial anesthesia in anticoagulated pts

Overview

- AT III is an α_2-globulin and a serine protease inhibitor, capable of inactivation of thrombin and factor Xa in blood
  - It has anti-inflammatory properties via interactions with the endothelium
  - AT III deficiency results in an unusual susceptibility to thromboembolic disease
- Heparin resistance may be problematic during surgery
- Massive thromboembolism can occur periop with AT III levels <50

ICD-9-CM Code: 286.5

Etiology

- Genetic: Reduced AT III synthesis inherited as an autosomal dominant trait, manifests as thromboembolism in late teens to early 30s
- Acquired: Secondary to consumption of AT III due to massive thromboembolic disease, disseminated intravascular coagulation, renal disease with proteinuria (esp. nephrotic syndrome), chronic liver disease, prolonged heparin therapy, increased protein catabolism
- Conflicting data about role of oral contraceptive use, pregnancy, and CAD

Usual Treatment

- Medical therapy: LMW heparin, unfractionated heparin, sodium warfarin or combination of oral anticoagulants and plt suppression (aspirin or dipyridamole)
- Periop: Fresh frozen plasma, cryo-precipitate, AT III concentrate (plasma derived or recombinant), heparin; heparin resistance can be treated with FFP

ASSESSMENT POINTS

System	Effect	Assessment by Hx	PE	Test
CV	CAD		Angina, dyspnea	ECG, CXR, angiography
PERIPHERAL VASC	DVT Arterial occlusion		Gangrene, absent pulses	
RESP	Pulm embolus	Dyspnea Exercise tolerance decreased	SOB	CXR V/Q scan
GI	Mesenteric artery/vein occlusion Decreased AT III	Abdominal pain Chronic liver disease symptoms	Rectal bleeding, jaundice, hepatomegaly	Serum albumin, AT III level
HEME	Bleeding and thrombosis	DIC	Petechiae, purpura, thrombosis	FDP, PT, PTT, plt count, AT III level
GU	Decreased albumin and AT III levels	Nephrotic syndrome, proteinuria	Edema	Urinalysis, serum albumin
CNS	CVA	Sudden onset, Hx of other embolic disease	Seizure, loss of vision, loss of motor function	CT scan, angiogram

Key Reference: Maclean PS, Tait RC. Hereditary and acquired antithrombin deficiency: Epidemiology, pathogenesis and treatment options. *Drugs.* 2007;67:1429–1440.

Perioperative Implications

Preinduction/ Induction/Maintenance
- Assess whether congenital or acquired; if acquired, treat primary disease if possible
- Stop oral anticoagulation and substitute FFP or AT III concentrate to bring AT III level to 80–120% normal
- Heparin to provide PTT of >1.5 times control
- Provide mechanical and pharmacological thromboprophylaxis

Monitoring
- Careful attention to temp
- Volume status, resp variables
- PTT, AT III levels

General Anesthesia
- No special concerns with airway, induction, or adjuvant drugs
- Maintain normothermia to avoid hyperviscosity

- Maintain intravascular volume
- IV heparin effect should be monitored
- Careful evaluations of hypotension or change in $ETCO_2$

Regional Anesthesia
- Neuraxial techniques require meticulous attention to the timing of
  - Neuraxial anesthesia in relation to the last dose of anticoagulant
  - First postop dose of anticoagulant in relation to the placement of neuraxial block and/or removal of indwelling catheter
- Plexus and peripheral blocks risks in anticoagulated patients remain undefined

Postoperative Period
- Consider ICU for monitoring
- Continue anticoagulation
- Early mobilization

- Remove indwelling catheters as soon as possible
- Oral anticoagulation might be reintroduced ASAP

Anticipated Problems/Concerns

- Embolic phenomena can occur intraop
- Monitoring lines may be foci for thrombus formation
- Periop thromboembolic events major concern; continuous anticoagulation is required, as is operative prophylaxis with, AT III concentrate (plasma derived or recombinant), FFP, and heparin

Aortic Regurgitation

Paul G. Barash

Risk

- 100,000 aortic valve operations/y
- 20–30% of aortic valve replacements have AR
- 12–30% of aortic valve replacements have combined AR and stenosis
- M:F ratio: 3:1
- Racial predominance: None known

Perioperative Risks

- LVF
- RVF
- Subendocardial ischemia
- Splanchnic ischemia

Worry About

- Aspiration pneumonitis (acute AR)
- Avoid htn, which increases AR and decreases cardiac output
- Avoid bradycardia, which increases AR and decreases cardiac output

Overview

- Long latency period between onset of hemodynamic changes and symptoms (~20–30 y)
- Myocardial ischemia uncommon
- Abdominal pain manifestation of splanchnic ischemia

ICD-9-CM Code: 424.1

Etiology

- Damage to leaflets
- Aortic root dilatation
- Loss of commissural support

Treatment

- Medical: Vasodilator, calcium channel blockers, ACE inhibitors, diuretic, digoxin
- Surgical: Prosthetic valve

ASSESSMENT POINTS

System	Effect	Assessment by Hx	PE	Test
CV	Aortic valve dysfunction		High-pitched, early diastolic, decrescendo blowing murmur Mid-diastolic low-pitched murmur (Austin Flint) Widened arterial pulse pressure (water-hammer) To and fro bobbing of head (de Musset's sign)	CXR ECHO
	LV dysfunction	Dyspnea with exercise Nocturnal dyspnea	Displaced posterior MI S_3	ECG CXR ECHO Cardiac catheterization
RESP	CHF	Dyspnea Nocturnal dyspnea	Rales S_3	CXR
GI	Splanchnic ischemia	Abdominal pain	Distended abdomen	

Key Reference: Otto CM, Bonow RO. Valvular heart disease. In Libby P, Bonow RO, Mann RL, Zipes DP, Braunwald E, eds. *Heart disease: A textbook of cardiovascular medicine*, 8th ed, Philadelphia: Saunders Elsevier; 2008:1635–1645.

Perioperative Implications

Preoperative Preparation

- Consider optimizing LV performance with vasodilators, inotropes, and diuretic
- Avoid reduction in aortic diastolic pressure
- Emergent procedures (acute AR): Full-stomach precautions

Monitoring

- Arterial catheter
- ECG leads II/V5 and ST-segment analysis
- Consider PA catheter or TEE

Preinduction/Induction

- Elective: Consider narcotic induction with inhalation supplement (0.25–50% MAC); nondepolarizing muscle relaxant devoid of bradycardic effects
- Emergency (acute AR with aortic dissection): Consider rapid-sequence technique with ketamine, etomidate, or low-dose narcotic plus amnestic agent
- Decreased aortic diastolic pressure and decreased coronary perfusion pressure and may lead to subendocardial ischemia

- Bradycardia and Htn increased regurgitant fraction and decreased cardiac output

Maintenance

- During period until institution of cardiopulmonary bypass, consider maintaining LV function with minimum of anesthetic interventions
- PCWP may underestimate LVEDP due to premature closure of mitral valve
- PCWP may overestimate LVEDP in pts with combined AR and MR

Extubation

- Consider extubation for pts undergoing valve replacement in ICU after respiratory and hemodynamic criteria are met

Postoperative Period

- Consider augmenting preload to maintain and preserve filling volume of still-dilated, hypertrophic LV
- Inotropic support may be required to maintain CO if inadequate intraop myocardial preservation
- Evaluation for neurologic injuries 2° to embolism during valve replacement

Anticipated Problems/Concerns

- Prolonged Trendelenburg position poorly tolerated during PAC insertion
- Intra-aortic balloon counterpulsation contraindicated before valve replacement
- Atrial fibrillation or other supraventricular tachycardias poorly tolerated and require aggressive treatment
- Retrograde cardioplegia (not anterograde) may be required for myocardial protection
- Associated diseases may present difficult intubation, e.g., rheumatoid arthritis, Marfan's syndrome, trauma (acute aortic dissection)

Aortic Stenosis

Edgar Pierre
Forrest Quiggle

Risk

- Incidence: In persons older than 65 years, 25% have calcific aortic valve disease
- 1%–2% of the population has a bicuspid aortic valve; 5%–15% may become stenotic

Perioperative Risks

- Hypotension from impaired ability to augment cardiac output, (stenosed valve creates fixed cardiac output), in response to stress or hypovolemia
- Increased risk for myocardial ischemia due to LVH, high intraventricular pressures, and decreased diastolic time
- Increased risk of infective endocarditis when undergoing noncardiac surgical procedures

Worry About

- HD instability due to
  - Decreased SVR; decreases coronary perfusion causing hypotension-induced ischemia, subsequent ventricular dysfunction, and worsening hypotension
  - Decreased preload and subsequent stroke volume

- Tachycardia; decreases diastolic filling time and increases myocardial oxygen demand
- Myocardial ischemia
- Diastolic dysfunction
- Atrial fibrillation; loss of atrial kick, can precipitate acute HD instability

Overview

- Stenosis of the aortic valve creates an obstruction to LV ejection
- Intraventricular systolic pressure increases to preserve forward flow
- Chronic pressure overload results in concentric LV hypertrophy
- Hypertrophy decreases LV compliance and diastolic dysfunction may ensue
- Atrial contraction is often critical for maintaining adequate LV filling and stroke volume
- The ability to increase CO in response to a drop in SVR is impaired
- Decreased aortic root pressure decreases myocardial perfusion gradient
- Angina, dyspnea, and syncope are common presenting symptoms

- Diagnosis is made echocardiographically
- AS is graded as mild for a valve area greater than 1.5 cm^2, moderate for areas between 1.0 and 1.5 cm^2, and severe for a valve area less than 1.0 cm^2
- Mean and peak pressure gradients across the valve also are used to classify severity

ICD-9-CM Code: 424.1

Etiology

- Congenital bicuspid aortic valve
- Rheumatic aortic stenosis
- Calcific degenerative disease

Usual Treatment

- Surgical aortic valve replacement (AVR) is the definitive treatment
- Percutaneous aortic valve replacement is a new and evolving technology
- Balloon vavuloplasty as a bridge to surgical repair

ASSESSMENT POINTS

System	Effect	Assessment by Hx	PE	Test
CV	Progression of stenosis	Angina, dyspnea, syncope	Systolic murmur	ECHO
	Myocardial ischemia	Angina	Rales, edema, wheeze	ECG, coronary angiography
	Diastolic dysfunction	Dyspnea		CXR, ECHO
	Arrhythmias	Palpitations, syncope		ECG, Holter
CNS	Syncope	Syncope		ECG, Holter, ECHO

Key Reference: Zigelman CZ, Edelstein PM. Aortic valve stenosis, *Anesthesiol Clin.* 2009;27:519–532.

Preoperative Preparation

- Premedication is indicated to avoid anxiety-induced tachycardia
- Replace any preop fluid deficit, ensure adequate ventricular preload
- Pts with severe symptomatic AS may benefit from postponement of elective surgery until AVR is performed

Monitoring
- ECG for ST segment analysis
- Invasive arterial pressure monitoring
- Consider pulm artery catheter
- Transesophageal ECHO when blood loss or volume shifts are anticipated

Airway
- None

Preinduction/Induction
- Phenylephrine or norepinephrine prepared, since hypotension can cause myocardial ischemia

- Slow titration of induction agent to avoid a ↓ in SVR with reflex tachycardia
- Laryngoscopy only after sufficient sympathetic attenuation

Maintenance
- Volatile agents may improve diastolic relaxation due to their intrinsic myocardial depression
- Consider beta blockade for tachycardia-induced ischemia
- Caution with agents that decreased preload and afterload (e.g., nitroglycerin, nitroprusside), or any agent with significant histamine release
- Caution with agents that directly or indirectly increased HR (e.g., pancuronium, atropine)
- Consider pharmacologic rate manipulation or artificial pacing for severe bradycardia
- Hypotension treated with
  - Volume expansion
  - Alpha agonists
- Blood loss replaced expeditiously

- Consider early electrical cardioversion for atrial fibrillation
- Neuraxial anesthesia associated hypotension from sympatholysis may precipitate HD instability

Extubation
- Minimize sympathetic stimulation

Postoperative Period
- Aggressive pain control

Anticipated Problems/Concerns
- Myocardial ischemia
- Diastolic dysfunction
- Dysrhythmias

Apnea of the Newborn

William L. Meadow

Risk

- Full-term infants with neurologic disorders
- Premature infants, with or without neurologic disorders

Perioperative Risks

- More prone to apnea during local or epidural anesthesia
- More prone to apnea postop

Worry About

- Unexpected apnea in recovery room
- Unexpected apnea in hours after outpatient procedures
- Unexpected apnea on ward hours after inpatient procedures

Overview

- Apnea in term infant never physiologic
- Apnea in preterm infants may signal central nervous system disorder or developmental immaturity
- Sudden onset of apnea in any infant may also reflect sepsis or hypoglycemia
- Relationship to subsequent SIDS unclear
- Utility of pneumogram screening controversial
- Indications for home apnea monitoring controversial

ICD-9-CM Code: 770.8

Etiology

- Term or preterm infants:
  - CNS disorders (seizures, bleeds, structural changes)
  - Systemic disorders (hypoglycemia, sepsis, GE reflux)
- Preterm infants:
  - Same as term infants
  - If full evaluation is negative, physiologic apnea of prematurity diagnosed

Usual Treatment

- Theophylline or caffeine
- O_2
- Transfusion
- CPAP

ASSESSMENT POINTS

System	Effect	Assessment By Hx	PE	Test
CV	Congenital heart disease leads to desaturation PDA may cause CHF	CHD, PGE_1 treatment	Murmur; cyanosis	ECHO
RESP	Children with bronchopulmonary dysplasia may be prone to apnea	Hx of hyaline membrane disease or other parenchymal lung disorder	Abnormal pulm compliance or O_2 requirement	CXR; ABGs; O_2 sat
GI	GE reflux may cause vagal overload	Hx of reflux	None obvious	pH study; barium swallow
CNS	Seizures may cause apnea; structural abnormalities may create ineffective respiratory drive	Hx of seizures or change in neurologic development	Exam for seizures or neurologic change	EEG, head ultrasound; CT; MRI

Key Reference: Henderson-Smart DJ, Steer P. Postoperative caffeine for presenting apnea in preterm infants. *Cochrane Database Syst Rev.* 2000;CD000048.

Perioperative Implications

Monitoring
- Routine

Airway
- Not usually a problem; obstructive apnea may occur but is rare
- Bronchospasm may occur in infants with bronchopulmonary dysplasia

Maintenance
- Usually no problem during procedure; vigilance required postop

Extubation
- Watch for intermittent inadequate resp effort for hours

Adjuvants
- No special concerns

Anticipated Problems/Concerns

- Periop not complex; vigilance regarding care and assessment in postop period

Appendicitis, Acute

Alanna E. Goodman

Risk

- Life time risk: Men 8.6%, women 6.7%
- Peak incidence 2nd and 3rd decades, but all age can be affected
- > 250,000 cases/y Dx in the USA
- More challenging diagnosis in the young and elderly as well as pregnant women

Perioperative Risks

- Mortality: <1% for nonperforated, ≈ 3% for perforated, ≈ 15% elderly patients, 4% pregnant women with perforation
- Fetal mortality: 3–5% nonperforated, 20–35% perforated
- Increased morbidity and mortality due to delay in diagnosis and treatment for young children, pregnant women, and the elderly
- Risks increase with perforation: Peritonitis, sepsis, and other complications
- Clinical diagnosis, approxi 15% negative appendectomies, improved accuracy with imaging studies (US, CT, MRI)

Worry About

- Aspiration (full stomach, delayed gastric emptying, oral contrast for CT scan)
- Antibiotic coverage
- Sepsis

- Carcinoid of the appendix
- Pregnancy: Pregnant women tend to have more advanced illness as symptoms and signs often overlap with those of pregnancy, causing a delay in diagnosis and treatment.
  - Must consider the fetus
  - Increased complication of pregnancy if appendectomy in first and second trimesters
  - Incorrect diagnosis—possible conversion to more extensive procedure

Overview

- One of the most common causes of surgical acute abdomen
- The most common reason for non-obstetric surgery in pregnant women
- Presentation varies depending on anatomic location of the appendix and stage of disease
- Pts often present with abdominal pain, anorexia, and N/V
- Mild dehydration and fever are common

ICD-9-CM Code: 540.9 (Acute appendicitis without peritonitis)

Etiology

- Appendiceal obstruction: Fecalith (majority), hypertrophied lymphoid tissue (esp children), tumors, stones, infection, and parasites

- Obstruction causes mucus accumulation and distention. This in turn results in elevation of luminal and intramural pressure ultimately leading to thrombosis/occlusion of vessels and lymphatic stasis (schemia). There is inflammation as well as bacterial proliferation and neutrophilic infiltration of the wall of the appendix. Ultimately there may be necrosis, gangrene, and perforation.
- Perforation results in a local abscess or diffuse peritonitis

Usual Treatment

- Urgent procedure, to the operating room as soon as possible
- Laparoscopic versus open appendectomy: Controversy in the literature
- Laparoscopy often used if uncertain diagnosis, female of childbearing age, or obesity
- Perforated appendicitis
  - Free perforation: Emergent laparotomy, appendectomy, and I&D (skin may be partially closed or left open if gross contamination)
  - Contained perforation/abscess in non-toxic pt: Conservative, nonoperative treatment with antibiotics, IVF, bowel rest, possible percutaneous drainage, and interval appendectomy

ASSESSMENT POINTS

System	Effect	Assessment by Hx	PE	Test
CV	Tachycardia	Fever, dehydration emesis, infection/sepsis	Resting pulse Orthostatic signs	
RESP	V/Q mismatch	Dyspnea, tachypnea	Splinting Observation	Pulse oximetry, RR
GI	Ileus	Anorexia, vomiting	Abdominal auscultation	Electrolytes (if protracted) Imaging studies
	Perforation			Higher WBC and temp, more likely perforation
RENAL	Dehydration	Oliguria	Skin turgor Orthostatic signs	Urine specific gravity, BUN/Cr (rarely needed)
	UTI vs. local effects of appendicitis, vs. both	Pyuria, hematuria		U/A
CNS	Somnolence/confusion	Rule out sepsis, side effect of narcotics	Mental status exam	WBC
	Pain	Visceral afferents T8-T10 with obstruction and distention of appendix	Classic periumbilical pain	
		Somatic nerve stimulation with peritoneal irritation	Peritoneal signs: Rebound tenderness, guarding	

Key Reference: Vissers RJ, Lennarz WB. Pitfalls in appendicitis. *Emerg Med Clin North Am.* 2010;(28):103–118.

Perioperative Implications

- Replace fluid deficits and correct electrolyte abnormalities (ideally prior to surgery)
- All women of childbearing age should have a pregnancy test
- Antibiotic coverage (gram negative and anaerobic coverage: A beta-lactam/beta-lactamase inhibitor, third generation cephalosporin plus metronidazole, fluoroquinalone plus metronidazole, or a carbapenem)
- Aspiration prophylaxis: Nonparticulate antacid and H₂ blocker
- Avoid metoclopramide if bowel obstruction

Monitoring
- Routine, unless septic

Airway
- Assume full stomach: Rapid-sequence induction versus awake intubation
- Secure airway with cuffed ETT

Induction
- Intravenous, rapid-sequence induction
- Anticipate hemodynamic instability if not sufficiently resuscitated or sepsis
- Consider nasogastric/orogastric tube and Foley catheter (esp if laparoscopic)
- Neuraxial anesthetic possible if non-septic, appropriately resuscitated, cooperative pt and limited likelihood of high abdominal exploration

Maintenance
- Balanced technique
- Requires muscle relaxation for dissection, but quick closure (consider intermediate duration non-depolarizing neuromuscular blocker)
- Laparoscopic procedure: Time depends on surgeon experience, skill, and intraop findings

Extubation
- Extubate when pt is fully awake
- Vomiting common, use antiemetic prophylaxis

Postoperative Period
- Pain control with local anesthetic infiltration (SQ and deeper) by surgeon, opioids, and NSAIDs
- Laparoscopic procedures tend to be less painful, result in shorter length of stay, but may be associated with higher complications and readmission rate than open procedures

Adjuvants
- Antibiotic interaction with nondepolarizers
- Fever in postop period (postop sepsis versus malignant hyperthermia)

Anticipated Problems/Concerns
- Concern for aspiration
- Complications of appendicitis: Wound infections, abscesses, bowel obstruction, fistulae, pyelophlebitis, and portal venous thrombosis

Aspiration, Perioperative: Prevention and Management

Paula A. Craigo

Risk

- Risk of aspiration: ~3 per 10,000 anesthetics; ~11 per 10,000 emergency and/or afterhours cases
- Loss of protective reflexes and sphincter function
- Obstructed or abnormal GI motility
- Increased GI contents, decreased pH
- Trauma, emergency/night surgery, pregnancy, difficult airway, ASA status > 2

Perioperative Risks

- Mortality after aspiration: 5%; higher if ASA > 2

Worry About

- 20% of pts who aspirated had no risk factor: of these, 66% had difficult intubation
- Rapid-sequence induction may have deleterious effects on heart rate, blood pressure
- Difficult intubation

Overview

- Prevention of aspiration best, as there is no definitive treatment
- Vast majority of pts with risk factor(s) do not aspirate
- Consider aspiration in differential diagnosis of bronchospasm with hypoxemia

ICD-9-CM Codes: 997.3 (Aspiration pneumonia after procedure); 668.0 (Aspiration, peripartum)

Etiology

- Loss of protective reflexes: Sedation, neuromuscular disorders/relaxants, altered mental status
- Obstructed or abnormal motility: Achalasia, gastroparesis, pain, opioids
- Increased GI contents: Bleeding, obstruction, feeds
- Other: Difficult airway, pregnancy, obesity, emergency surgery

Usual Treatment

- Suctioning: bronchoscopy if obstructing particles
- Lavage, steroids not helpful; surfactant investigational
- Empiric antibiotics may confuse cultures: Consider if compromised pt, fulminant course, high bacterial load

ASSESSMENT POINTS

System	Effect	Assessment by Hx	PE	Test
HEENT (airway)	Awake intubation in difficult airway; cricoid pressure may distort anatomy, obstruct ventilation	Hx difficult airway, head and neck surgery/radiation, diabetes	Airway exam	X-rays, CT scan, OR records as available
CV	Rapid-sequence intubation may lead to ischemia with tachycardia, hyper/hypotension; myocardial depression	Anginal Sx, exercise intolerance, Hx CHF, CAD Age, sex, risk factors	S_3, rales, displaced PMI	ECG, ECHO in selected patients
RESP	Rapid-sequence intubation may lead to bronchospasm	Hx pulm disease, wheezing with URI, smoking	Wheezing, prolonged expiratory phase	CXR
GI	Abnormal sphincters, motility, acidity	Hx peptic ulcer disease, reflux Sx, diabetes, scleroderma		
NM	↑ ICP leads to vomiting; depressed protective reflexes; muscle weakness		Neurologic exam	

Key Reference: Marik P. Aspiration pneumonitis and aspiration pneumonia. *N Engl J Med.* 2001;344(9):665–671.

Perioperative Implications

Preoperative Preparation
- NPO status
  - Generally, no solids for 6 hr, clear liquids allowed up to 2 hr preop
- Prophylaxis in selected patients:
  - Increase Gastric pH: Nonparticulate antacid, H_2 blockers, proton pump inhibition
  - Decrease GI contents: Prokinetics, NG suction

Monitoring
- Routine

Airway
- Protect airway with ETT or maintain protective reflexes
- Awake intubation in difficult airway
- LMA not protective against aspiration

Preinduction/Induction
- Regional associated with aspiration if seizures or hypotension decrease alertness
- GA: Risk at induction, extubation
- Denitrogenation with 100% O_2
- Check optimal pt position, table height, drugs and tools available, suction at hand
- Rapid-sequence induction; cricoid pressure until ETT placement assured by $ETCO_2$

Maintenance
- Care with level of sedation during sedation/regional cases

Extubation
- Return of muscular strength/coordination/consciousness adequate to protect airway if emesis occurs
- If emesis, head-down or right-side tilt, thoroughly suction oropharynx and trachea

Postoperative Period
- If no symptoms in 2 hr, significant aspiration extremely unlikely
- If pneumonitis occurs, initial postop CXR may be normal, proceeding to white-out in a few to 24 hr
- PEEP redistributes lung water, improves oxygenation; higher PEEP may decrease cardiac output and ventilation
- Maintaining low filling pressures may limit lung fluid accumulation, but may worsen negative effects of PEEP

Adjuvants
- Muscle relaxants must be dependably rapid-acting
- Regional drugs—avoid oversedation, hypotension
- Drug interactions between anesthetic drugs and 1 or 2 doses of aspiration prophylaxis not significant

Anticipated Problems/Concerns

- Must balance concern for aspiration risk against airway quality, cardiopulmonary reserve, and feasibility of regional techniques

Asthma, Acute

Kaylyn Krummen

Risk

- Incidence in USA: 10 million, incidence nearly 5% for persons age 5–34 y
- Greatest incidence of new cases in persons less than 5 y old
- Increased prevalence and severity in African Americans, adult females, and atopic individuals

Perioperative Risks

- Risk related to preop control
- Symptomatic pts: Morbidity due to bronchospasm and laryngospasm

Worry About

- Bronchospasm due to mechanical stimulation of hyperreactive airways
- Resp resistance following tracheal intubation/extubation
- Medication side effects (e.g., β-agonists causing tachycardia and hypokalemia)
- Adrenal insufficiency (chronic corticosterioid use)

Overview

- Characterized by bronchial wall inflammation, reversible expiratory airflow obstruction, airway hyperreactivity, wheezing, dyspnea, and cough)
- Types: Allergen-induced, exercise-induced, nocturnal, aspirin-induced, occupational, and infectious
- Airway obstruction from airway inflammation, intraluminal mucus, and bronchoconstriction
  - Reversibility of obstruction is characteristic
  - Severe airway obstruction may lead to dynamic hyperinflation
- Intubation frequently increases airway resistance

ICD-9-CM Code: 493.9 (Asthma, unspecified)

Etiology

- Allergen-induced immunologic: Repeated antigen exposure causes specific IgE antibodies, thus release of inflammatory mediators
- Abnormal autonomic nervous system regulation of airway function: Imbalance between excitatory and inhibitory neural input, thus responsive to β-agonist

Usual Treatment

- Bronchodilator drugs inhaled β-agonists albuterol, anticholinergics ipratropium
- Antiinflammatory drugs (corticosteroids, cromolyn, and leukotriene inhibitors)
- Treatment of status asthmaticus: Supplemental oxygen, repeated administration of inhaled β-agonists, IV corticosteroids, SQ epinephrine, terbutaline in pregnancy
- Mechanical ventilation indicated for arrest, obtundation, impending ventilatory failure; high peak airway pressures, prolonged expiratory phase, lower PEEP, and permissive hypercapnia

ASSESSMENT POINTS

System	Effect	Assessment by Hx	PE	Test
CV	Tachyarrhythmias, possible pulm HTN	Palpitations, HR	Tachycardia, irregular rhythm, loud P_2	EKG, ECHO
RESP	Airflow obstruction decreased lung elastance, hyperinflation, hypoxemia, hypercapnia, variations in peak flow	Dyspnea, cough, wheeze, chest tightness, nighttime awakenings, symptoms induced by exercise, allergens, etc.	Prolonged I:E, decreased breath sounds, wheezing, pulsus paradoxus	PFT, CXR, ABG
ENDO	Steroid-induced hyperglycemia, adrenal insufficiency (prior <1 y steroid users)	Polyuria, polydipsia, weakness	Hypotension in adrenal insufficiency	Glucose, electrolytes, cortisol, ACTH, stimulation test
MS	Steroid myopathy, steroid-paralytic myopathy	Difficulty climbing stairs or rising from chair, difficulty weaning mechanical ventilation	Proximal muscle weakness in steroid myopathy, possible quadriplegia in steroid-paralytic myopathy	Measurement of inspiratory muscle force, CPK, EMG, muscle biopsy

Key Reference: Woods BD, Sladen RN. Perioperative considerations for the patient with asthma and bronchospasm. *Br J Anaesth.* 2009;103(suppl 1):i57–i65. Review.

Perioperative Implications

Preinduction/Induction/Maintenance

- Assess severity and characteristics of disease, review PFTs (reversibility with bronchodilators), blood eosinophil count, chest auscultation, CXR, ABG
- Consider chest physiotherapy, systemic hydration, antibiotics, and bronchodilators preop
- Goal of maintenance: Depress airway reflexes
- Consider alternatives to ETT (e.g., LMA, regional)
- Volatile anesthetics, propofol, ketamine cause bronchodilation

Monitoring

- Airway peak-to-plateau gradient (as determined by an inspiratory pause) is a useful measure of airway resistance at a constant flow for time-to-time comparison
- Plateau pressure (P_{plat}) serves as a measure of lung hyperinflation and may be best predictor of complications of hypotension and barotrauma. Peak pressure does not predict complications
- Aim for P_{plat} <30 cm H_2O by prolonging expiratory time (e.g., decreased minute ventilation and/or increased inspiratory flow; use square flow waveform)

General Anesthesia

- Postintubation hypotension may result from lung hyperinflation, hypovolemia, and sedation. Significant lung hyperinflation mimics tension pneumothorax. A trial of hypoventilation improves cardiopulmonary status within 30–60 sec in former. Volume challenge is indicated for hypotensive pts.
- Rising peak-to-plateau pressure gradient suggests increased airway resistance
- Rising P_{plat} suggests worsening lung hyperinflation
- Consider keeping P_{plat} <30 cm H_2O by prolonging expiratory time. May need to accept hypercapnia
- Extubation may precipitate exacerbation. Inhaled β-agonists may be needed more frequently post extubation.
- Muscle relaxants in addition to systemic corticosteroids may cause acute myopathy
- Volatile anesthetics, propofol, and ketamine are bronchodilators

Regional Anesthesia

- Excellent alternative to avoid airway instrumentation
- Neuraxial blockade improves postop lung function due to improved pain therapy and diaphragmatic function
- Neuraxial blockade may reduce vital capacity and FEV_1 (negligible under lumbar or low thoracic block and benefits of pulm function prevail)
- Concern for bronchial constriction due to sympathetic blockade is not significant and unproven
- Overall pulm function and pain control are improved with neuraxial blockade in pts with reactive airway disease.

Postoperative Period

- Consider deep extubation or lidocaine IV to suppress hyperreactive airway reflexes
- Observe for postop bronchospasm

Anticipated Problems/Concerns

- Hypokalemia from β_2-agonist administration
- Hypotension or pneumothorax from lung hyperinflation
- Increased risk of tension pneumothorax. Clinical features of lung hyperinflation mimic tension pneumothorax. If trial of hypoventilation does not quickly achieve hemodynamic stability, consider chest tube placement.

Atherosclerotic Disease

Jacqueline M. Leung

Risk

- Incidence in USA: 2 million
- 56,000,000 persons have some form of CV disease

Perioperative Risks

- CAD increases the risk of developing postop myocardial ischemia
- Presence of CAD in vascular surgical pts increases operative and long-term mortality

Worry About

- Increased risk of periop myocardial ischemia and periop cardiac complications
- Increased risk of CVA not evident after non-vascular surgery
- Aortic dissection in cases of aneurysm requiring emergency surgery
- Co-existing diseases such as DM, tobacco smoking, and Htn

Overview

- Thickening and hardening of the medium and large arteries accounts for large proportion of heart attacks and cases of IHD
- Also leads to strokes, PVD, and aneurysm of lower abdominal aorta
- Blood vessels affected incl coronary, carotid, basilar, and vertebral arteries, as well as aorta and iliac arteries

ICD-9-CM Code: 414.0 (Atherosclerotic heart disease)

Etiology

- Multifactorial
- Risk factors: Hyperlipidemia, Htn, cigarette smoking, male sex, DM

Usual Treatment

- Primary prevention incl modification of risk factors, esp in high-risk individuals, and prophylaxis with aspirin and statins
- Atherosclerotic heart disease: Antianginal Rx is employed for symptomatic persons; other treatment incl angioplasty and CABG surgery
- Carotid artery disease: Carotid endarterectomy or carotid stenting
- Other cerebrovascular insufficiency: Extracranial-intracranial bypass sometimes performed
- Peripheral vascular insufficiency: Angioplasty or revascularization of lower extremities
- AAA: Abdominal aortic aneurysmectomy or endovascular stent

ASSESSMENT POINTS

System	Effect	Assessment by Hx	PE	Test
CV	Htn Coronary artery stenoses MI	Usually asymptomatic Angina, may be asymptomatic	Normal if treated S_3 and/or S_4 Cardiomegaly	Vital signs ECG exercise treadmill Pharmacologic stress test, coronary angiography, ECHO, radionuclide studies
	Ventricular dysfunction (systolic and/or diastolic)	Exercise intolerance Sx of heart failure	S_3 and/or S_4 Cardiomegaly	LV ejection fraction and function by ECHO, radionuclide studies, diastolic function by Doppler ECHO (if indicated)
RESP	COPD (many are smokers)	Dyspnea on exertion	Decreased breath sounds, prolonged expiration, wheezes	ABGs PFTs (if indicated)
CNS	Cerebrovascular insufficiency Cerebral infarct	TIAs Syncope Strokes	Carotid bruits Focal neurologic deficits	Doppler or angiogram (if indicated)
Peripheral arteries	Occlusive lesions Abdominal aortic aneurysm	Claudication Abdominal pain, may be asymptomatic	Decreased pulses Pulsatile abdominal mass	Angiogram (if indicated) Aortogram (if indicated) MRI (if indicated)
GI	Intestinal ischemia	Abdominal pain Occult blood in stool or gastric contents Leukocytosis Serum amylase may be elevated	Abdominal exam may be paradoxically normal	Mesenteric angiography

Key Reference: Lauer MS. Cardiovascular medicine update 2007: Perioperative risk, carotid angioplasty, drug-eluting stents, stronger statins. *Cleve Clin J Med.* 2007;74:505–511.

Perioperative Implications

Preoperative Preparation

- Stabilize cardiac Sx medically
- Continue antianginal Rx (B-blockade, aspirin and statins)
- Attention to and stabilization of co-existent diseases
- Consider periop β-blockade to ↓ myocardial ischemia

Monitoring

- Cardiovascular
  - ECG with appropriate lead placement, ST trending
  - Consider CVP catheterization to monitor preload, esp in pts with Hx of CHF
  - Consider TEE, esp in pts with uninterpretable ECG (e.g., ventricular pacemaker or LBBB)
- Cerebrovascular
  - In carotid endarterectomy, measurement of stump pressure, EEG, and SEPs have been used
  - CSF pressure monitoring and drainage in thoracoabdominal aneurysmectomy

Airway

- None

Preinduction/Induction

- Preventing tachycardia (use of short-acting β-blockers desirable)
- Treat BP changes aggressively

Maintenance

- No one anesthetic agent or technique superior; maintaining HR at low level and hemodynamic stability more important
- For peripheral vascular surgery, regional anesthesia in combination with postop epidural analgesia may decrease incidence of graft thrombosis (see also Peripheral Vascular Disease)
- For carotid endarterectomy, maintaining cerebral perfusion pressure important goal
- For abdominal aortic surgery, optimizing loading conditions, detecting and treating myocardial ischemia and ventricular dysfunction are important, particularly during and after aortic clamping

Extubation

- Same concerns as during induction

- Rapid awakening to allow neurologic assessment after carotid endarterectomy

Adjuvants

- β-blocking agents and other antihypertensives useful in hyperdynamic situations
- Prophylactic nitroglycerin and Ca^{2+}-channel blockers to treat myocardial ischemia not conclusively proved effective
- Caution in use of vasoconstrictors, such as α-adrenergic agonists, to increase BP in cases of heart failure

Anticipated Problems/Concerns

- Postop myocardial ischemia and other cardiac complications
- Graft occlusion (with peripheral revascularization procedures)
- Heart failure (with a history of CHF)
- Paraplegia, particularly after surgery for thoracoabdominal aneurysms
- Renal dysfunction in cases of aortic surgery

Atrial Fibrillation

Sheela S. Pai

Risk

- Affects >1% of those > 60 y
- 0.4% of adult population overall
- In the postcardiac surgical population, the incidence is as high as 27–40%
- Racial predominance: None
- Increased prevalence with older age
- In pts presenting for cardiac surgery, the incidence increases with increasing left atrial size as well as in the presence of valvular abnormalities

Perioperative Risks

- Rapid ventricular response in CHF
- May be a sign of impending or ongoing myocardial ischemia
- Embolization if persists beyond 48 hr without anticoagulation

Worry About

- Decreased cardiac output due to loss of atrial kick esp in the presence of left ventricular hypertrophy, aortic stenosis, or diastolic dysfunction
- Myocardial ischemia secondary to increased myocardial O_2 demand
- Embolization risk increases with increased duration.

Overview

- Develops over 2 decades in 2% of pts >30 y
- Related to left atrial size, underlying heart disease, and abnormal electrophysiology
- Incidence increases with age
- Most affected people have underlying cardiac disease
- Common after cardiac surgery, particularly valve surgery

ICD-9-CM Code: 427.31

Etiology

- CAD
- RHD (Rheumatic heart disease)
- Cardiomyopathy, heart failure
- Mitral stenosis, mitral regurgitation esp with left atrial enlargement
- Htn and associated left ventricular hypertrophy
- Pericarditis
- Resp insufficiency incl hypoxia and hypercarbia
- Hypercatecholamine states such as hyperthyroidism
- Subarachnoid hemorrhage
- Sarcoidosis/amyloidosis
- Idiopathic

Usual Treatment

- Cardioversion for hemodynamic instability in the first 48 hr
- Digitalis
- β-blockers
- Calcium antagonists
- Quinidine (with digitalis)

ASSESSMENT POINTS

System	Effect	Assessment By Hx	PE	Test
CV	CHF Angina Stroke	Palpitations Chest pain Dyspnea Orthopnea	Variation in intensity of first heart sound; absence of A waves in jugular venous pulse; irregularly irregular ventricular rhythm	ECHO (if indicated)
RESP	CHF Pulm embolism	Dyspnea Orthopnea Chest pain Tachypnea	S_3 Rales Wheezing	CXR V/Q scan (if suspicion of pulmonary embolism)
GI	Ischemic bowel from low flow or embolization	Abdominal pain	Acute abdomen	ABGs/electrolytes
RENAL	↓ Renal perfusion	↓ Urine output		BUN/Cr
CNS	Syncope, fatigue	Stroke	Neurologic deficit	Head CT

Key Reference: Anter E, Jessup M, Callans DJ. Atrial fibrillation and heart failure: Treatment considerations for a dual epidemic. *Circ.* 2009;119:2516–2525.

Perioperative Implications

Preoperative Preparation

- Search for precipitating causes—new onset may signify acute disease process, which may delay surgery
- Control ventricular response or perform synchronized cardioversion to normal sinus rhythm if unstable

Monitoring

- ECG with ST-segment analysis
- Additional monitoring such as use of arterial line or pulm artery catheter should be predicated on type of surgery, additional co-morbidities, or hemodynamic instability.

Airway

- None, consider intubation if shock present

Preinduction/Induction

- Avoid excessive sympathetic stimulation
- Maintain oxygenation/ventilation

Maintenance

- Monitor oxygenation, maintain normocarbia, correct electrolyte imbalances
- Control ventricular response

Extubation

- Avoid excessive sympathetic stimulation

Adjuvants

- Digitalis has little effect on anesthetic agents
- Ca^{2+} antagonists can decrease AV conduction; can increase NM blockade
- β-blocker agents can cause decreased AV conduction
- Quinidine (with digitalis) can increase NM blockade

Postoperative Period

- Maintain adequate analgesia
- New onset may require prompt treatment

Anticipated Problems/Concerns

- Rapid ventricular response may result in significant fall in cardiac output.
- Direct current (DC) synchronized cardioversion establishes sinus rhythm in >90%.
- Pretreatment with amiodarone increases chances of remaining in sinus rhythm.

Atrial Flutter

Charles W. Hogue

Risks

- Uncommon in children and young adults
- More common in the elderly
- Usually occurs in pts with structural heart disease (those with left ventricular dysfunction, right ventricular dysfunction, pulm vascular disease, RHD, and CHD)
- Occurs relatively frequently after cardiac surgery but seldom after noncardiac surgery

Perioperative Risk

- Circulatory insufficiency or myocardial ischemia from extremes of heart rate esp in pts with CHD
- Cerebral, coronary, or systemic embolism from left atrial thrombus
- Associated disease, esp adequacy of CV and pulm function
- Accelerated ventricular rates

Worry About

- Increased proarrhythmia risk with drugs for pharmacologic cardioversion particularly in high risk groups such as those with CAD, impaired left ventricular function, left ventricular hypertrophy, acquired or congenital long QT-syndromes, or history of proarrhythmia

Overview

- Mechanism is atrial re-entry, usually in right atrium
- Type I or typical atrial flutter: most common form characterized by regular atrial rates 240–340 bpm with fixed (often 2:1) atrioventricular (AV) conduction
- Type II or atypical atrial flutter: Less common presents with regular atrial rates 340–450 bpm with variable or fixed atrioventricular (AV) conduction that may result in irregular, irregular QRS complex and pulse

ICD9-CM: 427.32

Etiology

Usual Treatment

- Goals incl control of ventricular rate, restoring normal sinus rhythm, maintenance of sinus rhythm after cardioversion, and anticoagulation to prevent systemic embolization if sinus rhythm not restored.
- Cardioversion can be accomplished with direct current cardiovesion, pharmacologically (amiodarone, ibutilide, procainamide, sotalol), or with overdrive atrial pacing (for type I flutter).
- Consider early cardioversion if pt is hemodynamically unstable.
- Drugs for ventricular rate control incl β-blockers and Ca²⁺-channel blockers such as diltiazem and verapamil.
- Anticoagulation should be considered for atrial flutter lasting more than 48 hrs or sooner if low cardiac output.
- Choice of anticoagulant determined by perceived embolic risk (aspirin for low risk or coumadin for higher risk)
- Prophylactic amiodarone and β-blockers lowers the risk for atrial flutter after cardiac surgery.
- For type 1 atrial flutter atrial pacing at 10% above the flutter rate (rate <350 bpm) for 15–30 sec using atrial or esophageal atrial pacing leads, frequently converts atrial flutter to sinus rhythm
- Radiofrequency ablation of the atrial flutter re-entrant pathway can prevent recurrence but this therapy is for chronic atrial flutter and it is not an acute treatment.

ASSESSMENT POINTS

System	Effect	Assessment by PE	Ex	Test
CARDIAC	Atrial flutter, left ventricular function, coronary disease severity	Palpitations, dizziness, weakness, lethargy, orthopnea, cough dyspnea, exercise intolerance, symptoms of angina	Irregular pulse/pulse deficit, S_1–S_2 intensity rales, wheezes	ECG, Holter monitoring, EP studies, ECHO, exercise ECG, MRI, cardiac catheter, stress ECG, dipyridamole scintigraphy, angiography
RESP	CHF COPD	Dyspnea, orthopnea, cough Dyspnea, wheezing	S_3, rales wheezes	CXR, pulm function testing
GI	↓ Perfusion	GI distress, diarrhea		
RENAL	↓ Perfusion	Polyuria (nocturnal)		BUN/Cr
NEURO	Ischemia or stroke	Syncope, mental changes, paresis/paralysis, dementia	Mental deficits Neurologic exam	See CV assessment

Key Reference: Kastor JA. *Arrhythmias.* 2nd ed. Philadelphia: Saunders; 2000. pp 131–163.

Perioperative Implications

Preoperative Preparation

- Adequate ventricular rate control (80–100 bpm) with β-blockers or Ca²⁺-channel blockers with AV conduction slowing properties
- Treat CHF if present; otherwise, optimize cardiopulmonary function
- If acute onset (< 48 hr), consider cardioversion
- When atrial flutter is of >48 hr duration, intra cardiac thrombus must be excluded before cardioversion or the pt should receive course of anticoagulation before and after cardioversion

Monitoring

- ECG with ST–T trending and strip-chart recorder for documentation of new arrhythmias or myocardial ischemia
- Consider direct arterial and pulm artery catheter monitoring in the presence of concomitant left ventricular dysfunction depending on the type of procedure

Anesthesia Induction

- Left ventricular dysfunction and atrial flutter increase risk for hypotension during induction with agents such as thiopental or propofol.
- Desflurane, ketamine, and pancuronium may accelerate ventricular rate.

Maintenance

- Expect increased circulatory instability and less tolerance of large fluid shifts or blood loss.
- No anesthetic drugs are esp contraindicated; caution should be used with drugs that speed conduction.

Tracheal Extubation

- Possibly at increased risk for thromboembolism with hyperdynamic circulatory state
- Sympathomimetic or antimuscarinic drugs may accelerate ventricular rate.

Atrial Septal Defect, Ostium Primum

Sarah Khan

Risk

- Ostium primum ASD is also known as partial AV canal defect. Classified as an ASD, it is actually an endocardial cushion defect
- Less common than secundum ASDs, it comprises 0.5–1% of all congenital heart defects
- Gender prevalence: Female > male, 2:1
- Greater incidence in Down syndrome

Perioperative Risks

- Periop mortality rate: 3%, lower mortality if repair is before onset of pulm Htn.
- Late in course, CHF with left to right shunt
- Increased risk of atrial dysrhythmias, heart block, and air embolus with surgical repair
- Significant risk of mortality if Eisenmanger's syndrome has occurred.

Worry About

- Defect frequently involves mitral and tricuspid valves, requiring repair

Overview

- Failure of inferior atrial septum to close at the level of tricuspid and mitral valves
- Symptoms present earlier and are more severe than in secundum pts. These incl dyspnea, fatigue, recurrent resp infections and failure to thrive.
- Left to right shunt increases pulm blood flow
- Late in course: CHF, also more common than in secundum pts and shunt reversal
- Frequently associated with mitral regurgitation with a cleft in the anterior mitral leaflet present in 50% of the patients and/or tricuspid regurgitation
- Diagnosis is by ECHO, appearing as an absence of the lower atrial septum.
- Cardiac catheterization may be required to assess PVR and pulm Htn in large shunts

ICD-9-CM Code: 745.61

Etiology

- Failure of septum primum to fuse with endocardial cushion to close ostium primum

Usual Treatment

- Asymptomatic pts require no medications. Diuretics are used for CHF.
- Ace inhibitors may be used for afterload reaction in the presence of mitral regurgitation
- Antiarrhythmics are occasionally needed for atrial dysrhythmias
- Percutaneous closure is not possible as it is in secundum defects because there is inadequate rim of inferior atrial tissue to prevent the device from impinging on the valves
- Surgery is the definitive management, usually between 2–5 y. May be earlier if there is mitral regurgitation, CHF or failure to thrive. Incision is median sternotomy or right thoracotomy.
- Endocarditis prophylaxis is indicated for 6 mo after repair. Persistent AV valve abnormalities may require long-term prophylaxis.

ASSESSMENT POINTS

System	Effect	Assessment by Hx	PE	Test
HEENT	Difficult intubation	Down syndrome	Down syndrome facies	
CV	Atrial dysrhythmias, right-sided heart failure L→R shunting, hypertrophic RA and RV Mitral regurgitation	Palpitations SOB, frequent fatigue Cyanosis if shunt reversal	Irregular rate and rhythm Right heart enlargement Normal S_1, fixed splitting of S_2, and crescendo-decrescendo systolic murmur	ECG (RBBB + RVH) CXR—cardiomegaly ECHO—standard angiography Dye dilution study
RESP	↑ Pulmonary blood flow ↑ PVR	SOB, frequent URIs	Rales, wheezing	CXR- ↑ pulm vascular markings
GI	Hepatic dysfunction if severe CHF	Jaundice	Hepatomegaly	LFTs, PT
CNS	Embolic stroke from chronic AFIB	Various neurologic changes		Head CT, cardiac ECHO if emboli suspected
MS			Enlarged left costal cartilage	
RENAL	Renal dysfunction if severe CHF			Cr, BUN

Key Reference: Shannon M, Rivenes MD. *Atrial septal defect, ostium primum: treatment and medication.* Nov 7, 2008.

Perioperative Implications

Preoperative Medications
- Midazolam 0.5–0.7 mg/kg po 30 min before the procedure
- Antibiotic prophylaxis

Monitoring
- Routine monitors, arterial line, CVP; TEE to assess anatomy before CPB, AV valve regurgitation and function, ventricular function and to check for air and residual shunt after CPB; central and peripheral temp monitoring

Induction
- IV induction theoretically slowed by left to right shunt because of increased pulm blood flow; inhalational induction not significantly affected
- May place an epidural with loss of resistance to saline technique to avoid air embolism. Must be placed 1 hr prior to heparinization.

Maintenance
- Avoid nitrous oxide to minimize size of air bubbles; any other techniques appropriate; watch for shunt reversal with hypoxemia, hypercarbia, and hypothermia

Extubation
- If intraop course is smooth pt may be extubated at the end of the procedure.
- Control BP with milrinone, nitroprusside or nitroglycerin.
- Keep mechanically ventilated if the repair has been complex or arrythmias are present.

Adjuvants
- Watch for supraventricular dysrhythmias and AV conduction defects, must have pacing wires.

Postoperative Period
- Adequate analgesia for sternotomy or thoracotomy pain; pacemakers available for transient heart block

Anticipated Problems/Concerns

- Air emboli with vascular access
- Dysrhythmias: SA node or AV node dysfunction
- Heart failure
- Third degree AV block with repair of low lying defects
- Residual pulm Htn which can lead to tricuspid regurgitation and RV failure
- Residual mitral valve insufficiency may remain or worsen
- Endocarditis esp with a residual cleft mitral valve
- Discrete subaortic stenosis may be present which can progress after operation

Atrial Septal Defect, Ostium Secundum

James A. Sparrow
Frederick A. Hensley, Jr.

Risk

- Incidence in USA: 140,000 with ostium secundum ASD (70–80% of ASDs)
- Accounts for 7% of all congenital cardiac defects; 30–40% of congenital cardiac defects in pts over 40 y
- Gender prevalence: Female > male, 2:1 in isolated ASDs
- Familial incidence: Significant if associated with P-R prolongation or forearm and hand abnormalities (Holt-Oram syndrome)
- Increased incidence in high altitude

Perioperative Risks

- Periop mortality rate: 1%
- Late in course, associated with atrial dysrhythmias, pulm hypertension and right heart failure
- Increased risk of atrial dysrhythmias, heart block (rare), and air embolus with surgical repair

Worry About

- Risk of infectious endocarditis and paradoxical air embolization with IV access

Overview

- Failure of closure of midseptal fossa ovalis
- Usually asymptomatic early in life
- 15% incidence of associated noncardiac anomalies
- Associated with mitral valve prolapse (10–20%)
- Left to right shunt increases pulm blood flow (shunt fraction is proportional to ASD size)
- Late in course: Pulmonary Htn, right heart failure with possible shunt reversal; supraventricular arrythmias
- Uncorrected defect carries a mortality rate of 6% per year over the age of 40
- Diagnosis by echocardiography and Doppler color flow echocardiography
- >80% spontaneous closure in the first year of life for small defects

ICD-9-CM Code: 745.5

Etiology

- Failure of septum secundum to fuse with septum primum secondary to defective formation or resorption of the septum primum, shortening of the septum secundum or a combination of the three

Usual Treatment

- Digitalis and diuretics for child with CHF
- Antiarrhythmics occasionally needed for atrial dysrhythmias
- Surgery or transcatheter closure is indicated when Qp:Qs ratio ≥1.5:1 in pts between 3 and 5 y
- Surgery indicated if ASD >25 mm diameter or if anomalous pulm venous return is present
- Endocarditis prophylaxis: Not indicated after successful simple surgical closure, indicated for 6 mo after repair using a prosthetic device

ASSESSMENT POINTS

System	Effect	Assessment by Hx	PE	Test
CV	Atrial dysrhythmias Right-sided heart failure L→R shunting	Palpitation, SOB, DOE	Irregular rate and rhythm, right heart enlargement, loud S_1, fixed S_2, and crescendo-decrescendo systolic murmur	TEE w/ color Doppler flow, four chamber view, bicaval view Angiography Dye dilution study
RESP	↑ Pulm blood flow ↑ PVR	SOB, frequent URIs	Rales, wheezing	CXR
GI	Hepatic dysfunction if severe CHF	Jaundice	Hepatomegaly	LFTs, PT
RENAL	Renal dysfunction if severe CHF			Cr, BUN
CNS	Embolic stroke from chronic AFIB	Various changes		Head CT, cardiac ECHO if suspected emboli
MS			Holt-Oram syndrome Large left costal cartilage	

Key Reference: Findlow D, Doyle E. Congenital heart disease in adults. *Br J Anaesth.* 1997;78:416–430.

Perioperative Implications

Preoperative Medications

- Narcotics and anticholinergics
- Antibiotic prophylaxis
- Continue digoxin if used for rate control

Monitoring

- Routine monitors, arterial line, CVP; TEE indicated for assessing anatomy before CPB, evaluating for air and residual shunting after CPB; central and peripheral temp monitoring

Induction

- IV induction theoretically slowed by left to right shunt; inhalational induction not significantly affected

- Epidural with loss of resistance to saline technique to avoid air embolism

Maintenance

- Avoid nitrous oxide to minimize size of air bubbles; inhalational, TIVA or a combination of techniques are appropriate; watch for shunt reversal with hypothermia, hypercarbia, hypoxemia

Extubation

- In isolated lesions, patients can be extubated at the end of case if hemodynamically stable

Adjuvants

- Watch for dysrhythmia from hypokalemia if pt is on digoxin and diuretics, maintain potassium of 4.0 or higher

Postoperative Period

- Adequate analgesia for sternotomy or thoracotomy pain

Anticipated Problems/Concerns

- Paradoxical air emboli with vascular access
- Dysrhythmia (5–10% if no prerepair dysrhythmia)
- Heart failure
- Heart block after CPB (rare)
- Sternal infection (rare)
- Endocarditis (rare)

Autoimmune Diseases, Cold

Risk

- Rare
- Autoimmune hemolytic anemias occur in 1 of 80,000 persons; of these, 17.3% are due to cold antibodies

Perioperative Risks

- Acute hemolysis due to cold
- Hemoglobinemia
- Hemoglobinuria
- Rarely, vascular occlusion

Worry About

- Cooling to 28–31°C will cause hemolysis

- These temps can be reached in extremities during cardiopulmonary bypass.

Overview

- In two circumstances antibodies will react in the cold to produce hemolysis:
  - IgG antibodies associated with mononucleosis, *Mycoplasma* pneumonia
  - IgM antibodies are found in the idiopathic form of the disease and in lympho-proliferative disease.
- Hemolysis usually occurs at temp below 31°C.

ICD-9-CM Code: 283.0

Etiology

- Idiopathic
- Lymphoid malignancy
- Infections: *Mycoplasma* pneumonia, mononucleosis, cytomegalovirus, varicella

Usual Treatment

- Keep warm, folic acid
- For severe cases, chlorambucil or cyclophosphamide
- Plasmapheresis
  - Rituxmab
  - Prednisone

ASSESSMENT POINTS

System	Effect	PE	Test
HEME	Mild to moderate anemia		Hgb, blood bank antiglobulin tests
GU	Hemoglobinuria		
CV	Dyspnea on exertion if anemia is severe		
SKIN	Agglutination of red cells in cold	Acrocyanosis	

Key Reference: Young S, Haldane G. Major colorectal surgery in a patient with cold agglutinin disease. *Anaesthesia*. 2006;61:593–596.

Perioperative Implications

Perioperative Preparation
- Plasmaphersis—may be used (no more than two d before surgery)

Monitoring
- Temp
- Urine output

Maintenance
- Keep warm, incl extremities
  - Consider forced air warming
  - Warm all fluids
- Normothermic cardiopulmonary bypass
- No preferred agent or technique
- Consider hemodilutional autologous transfusion or other techniques to avoid homologous transfusion and formation of new antibody.

Anticipated Problems/Concerns

- Hemolysis if temp falls
- Renal dysfunction due to hemoglobinuria
  - May see molting or cyanosis of the skin

Autonomic Dysreflexia (AD)

Kieran A. Slevin

Risk

- AD esp occurs in pts with SCI at T6 or above.
- The higher the injury level, the greater clinical manifestations of CV dysfunction
- Risk of AD greater with complete (91%) vs. incomplete (27%) cord transections.
- AD occurs more often in chronic SCI; some clinical evidence seen in first days-weeks.

Perioperative Risks

- AD most commonly triggered by irritation and/or manipulation of urinary bladder, colon and in labor
- Severe increased BP and increased or decreased HR associated with stimulation below level of transection
- Objectively, increased SBP >20–30 mmHg considered a dysreflexic episode. However, be aware usual resting ABP in these pts is 15–20 mmHg less than non SCI subjects.
- Awake pts may complain of HA, anxiety, sweating, piloerection and flushing above and dry, pale skin below the injury level. In anesthetized pts, SBP rising to up to 300 mmHg heralds the onset of severe, life-threatening AD.

Worry About

- Untreated episodes can lead to intracranial hemorrhage, retinal detachment, seizures, and death.

Overview

- Physiologically, AD is caused by a massive sympathetic discharge triggered by a noxious or nonnoxious stimulus originating below the level of the SCI.
- Specifically, destruction of the vasomotor pathways results in a loss of inhibitory and excitatory supraspinal input to the sympathetic preganglionic neurons thus causing labile BP.
- Also, changes in spinal sympathetic neurons and primary afferents underlie abnormal CV Δs.
- Symptoms are usually short-lived because of treatment or self-limiting nature of episode.

ICD-9-CM Code: 337.3

Etiology

- Most common cause is traumatic interruption of the spinal cord
- Can also occur due to infectious or oncologic processes causing destructive spinal lesions

Usual Treatment

- STOP initiating stimulus when possible.
- Can decrease or prevent AD by use of neuraxial blockade (spinal >> epidural)
- When signs of AD are evident, administer ganglionic blockers (trimethaphan), direct vasodilators (nitroprusside) or α-antagonists (phentolamine), GA or spinal anesthesia
- Level 1 evidence that intrasphincteric anal block with lidocaine limits the AD response in pts undergoing anorectal procedures. Level 1 evidence that topical lidocaine does not.
- Level 1 evidence that prazosin is superior to placebo in prophylactic management of AD
- Level 2 evidence that nifedipine can prevent BPΔ's during cysto in SCI pts with AD
- Level 4 evidence that epidural anesthesia may be effective in pts with AD during labor and delivery.
- Centrally acting hypotensive agents (e.g., clonidine) are not effective in treating AD
- Treat tachyarrhythmias with β-blockers in combination with antihypertensives
- Complete bladder deafferentation does not abolish AD during bladder urodynamic studies.

ASSESSMENT POINTS

System	Effect	Assessment by Hx	PE	Test
HEENT	Difficult airway	C-spine trauma/surgery H/O difficult intubation	↓ C-spine ROM ↓ Mouth opening	Airway exam
CV	Orthostatic hypotension Baseline relative hypotension (15–20 mmHg)	H/O dizziness when going from supine to upright position	↓ BP, orthostasis, tachycardia, bradycardia A/fib	Orthostatic BPs ECG
RESP	↓ Resp volumes, atelectasis, pneumonia, hypoxemia Impaired cough reflex	SOB Difficulty w/secretions	Tachypnea Cyanosis ↓/unequal BS	CXR ABG evaluation
GI	Full stomach status due to GI atonicity	Complaints of reflux		
RENAL	UTI, renal stone disease, renal failure	Flank pain	Chronic Foley catheter	UA, BUN/Cr
CNS	Bowel and bladder dysfunction Chronic and central pain states Altered MS (if severe head trauma)	Incontinence Chronic opioid therapy Adjuvant pain meds	Hyperreflexic below level of transection Babinski's sign positive	Hyperalgesia Allodynia
PNS	Insensate below level of transection Pain at level of transection	Skin color changes	Flushing/piloerection above Dry, pale skin below	
MS	Paralysis, muscular atrophy below Sacral decubiti	Paraplegia or quadriplegia	Muscle atrophy Sacral decubiti	

Key Reference: Krassioukov A. A systematic review of the management of autonomic dysreflexia after spinal cord injury. *Arch Phys Med Rehabil*. 2009;90:682–695.

Perioperative Implications

Preoperative Preparation

- Nifedipine can be used for prophylaxis, given 30 min prior to procedure likely to trigger AH
- Attention to CV and pulm function, volume status, and airway exam.

Monitoring

- Consider pre-induction invasive monitoring (arterial, CVP/PA catheters) if volume changes are expected and in setting of poor cardiac reserve (high lesions) and renal insufficiency

Airway

- Be prepared for fiberoptic intubation

Induction

- Use nondepolarizing muscle blockers when relaxation is necessary.

- Succinylcholine can cause severe K+ release and hyperkalemia in chronic lesions.
- Consider nitroprusside prior to induction.

Maintenance

- GA with volatile agent superior to nitrous-narcotic technique for prevention/treatment of AD

Regional Anesthesia

- Anesthetic technique of choice when possible
- Spinal anesthesia highly effective in preventing AD precipitated by surgery
- Ensure careful assessment of level of spinal blockade in SCI pts due to sensory deficits below injury—avoid unnecessarily high or inadequate blocks

- Epidural anesthesia effective in preventing AD in laboring pts

Extubation

- May be difficult due to resp insufficiency in pts with high level spinal lesions

Adjuvants

- Muslce relaxants required in abdominal surgery due to diffuse increase in muscle tone

Postoperative Period

- AD can occur postop in setting of unrecognized or untreated distended bladder or rectum.
- Consider intracerebral hemorrhage protocol in the setting of unexplained delayed emergence with increased BP.

AV and Bifascicular Heart Block

Dennis Phillips
David G. Metro

Risk

• Prevalence: First degree (0.65–1.6%); second degree (0.003% in young adults, higher in organic heart disease); third degree (overall 0.02%; congenital 1:20,000 live births); increases with age presumed due to small vessel disease
• Inferior MI: Carries low mortality even if associated with high degree AV block
• Anterior MI: If high degree AV block results then mortality approaches 80%

Perioperative Risks

• Progression of benign heart block to second degree type II or third degree
• Heart failure, myocardial and global ischemia, shock, pacemaker failure

Worry About

• Autonomic changes influencing the degree of blockade
• Pacemaker failure, electrocautery interference
• Intracardiac wire or PA catheter placement leading to third degree block
• Beta blockers, calcium channel blockers, digoxin, and anticholinergic influencing degree of heart block

Overview

• AV blocks: First degree: PR interval >0.20 sec. Block site = AV node. Usually benign. If pt has structural heart disease this block type becomes more significant. Associated with anterior MI, digitalis, certain neuromuscular diseases
• Second degree type I (mobitz I or wenckebach): Increasingly prolonged PR interval until QRS dropped. Block site = AV node (normal QRS). Usually benign. Elderly pts and those with structural heart disease make this block type more significant. Usually does not progress over time to second degree type II or third degree. May progress acutely with anesthesia, autonomic influences, or intracardiac catheters/wires
• Second degree type II (mobitz II): Fixed PR interval with occasional dropped QRS. Block site = usually infranodal (wide QRS), permanent. The more infranodal block site yields a slower ventricular rate and symptoms. High mortality. Common progression to third degree.
• Bifasicular block: Three 'fascicles'/'bundles' of nerves conduct via the ventricles. Right bundle branch, left anterior fascicle, left posterior fascicle. When 2 of 3 are blocked it is termed 'bifasicular'. When third fascicle is blocked, the pt is in third degree heart block.
• Third degree: Atria and ventricles have separate pacemakers. Any atrial rhythm (afib/flutter, etc). Ventricular rate/rhythm depends on site of blockade. More infranodal block yields slower ventricular rate. If only upper AV node blocked pt may have junctional rhythm (normal QRS) and be more stable. If entire AV node blocked then ventricular rate 20–40 bpm and perfusion is compromised.

ICD-9-CM Code: Complete: 426.0; First degree: 426.11; Second degree type II: 426.12; Other second degree AV block: 426.13; bifasicular block RBBB+LPFB: 426.51; bifasicular block RBBB+LAFB: 426.52; other bilateral BBB: 426.53

Etiology

• First degree: Usually benign or associated with anterior MI, digitalis
• Second degree type I: Benign (athletes and children) from high vagal tone or from myocarditis, mononucleosis, Lyme disease, amyloidosis, sarcoidosis, beta blockers, calcium channel blockers, digitalis, and volatile anesthetics
• Second degree type II and bifascicular blocks: Anterior MI
• Third degree: Inferior MI (usually more stable HR >40); anterior MI with necrosis of bundle branches (unstable HR <40); severe hyperkalemia, hypermagnesemia; concurrent use of calcium channel and beta blockers; digitalis; high doses of volatile anesthetics, opiates, anticholinesterases; increased vagal input (laryngoscopy, esophagoscopy/TEE, peritoneal retraction, ocular pressure); or congenital

Usual Treatment

• First degree: Asymptomatic no tx. If symptomatic = permanent pacemaker (2008 ACC/AHA/HRS Class IIa recommendation). If associated with neuromuscular disease even without symptoms = pacemaker (Class IIb recommendation)
• Second degree type I and II: If symptomatic bradycardia = pacemaker (Class I recommendation)
• Second degree type II: Asymptomatic with wide QRS = pacemaker (Class I recommendation); with narrow QRS = pacemaker (Class IIa recommendation). If associated with neuromuscular disease = pacemaker (Class I recommendation). Atropine usually ineffective
• Bifasicular: With transient second degree type II or third degree, or alternating BBB = pacemaker (Class I recommendation); with syncope = pacemaker (Class IIa recommendation). Third degree and symptomatic = pacemaker (Class I recommendation).

ASSESSMENT POINTS

System	Effect	Assessment by HX	PE	Test
CV	Heart failure	Syncope, SOB, DOE, 'skipped beats', last pacemaker battery replacement, fatigue	Bradycardia, JVD	EKG, ECHO, BNP
PULM	Pulm edema, hypoxia	Cough, pink sputum, orthopnea	Rales, tachypnea, wheezing, cough	CXR, pulse ox
RENAL	Pre-renal failure, fluid retention	Oliguria, edema, fatigue, N/V	Edema, impaired mentation	BUN, Cr, FeNa, lytes
NEURO	Poor cerebral perfusion	Lightheadedness, N/V	Impaired mentation	CT head

Key Reference: Olgin JE, Zipes DP. Specific arrhythmias: diagnosis and treatment. In: Libby, ed. *Braunwald's heart disease: A textbook of cardiovascular medicine.* 8th ed. Philadelphia: Saunders; 2008 [Chapter 35].

Perioperative Implications

Preinduction/Induction/Maintenance
• Ascertain indication for and type of pacemaker as well as functionality.
• Consider changing pacemaker to asynchronous mode if electrocautery to be used.
• Have external and/or intravenous pacemaker and magnet available.
• Consider preinduction arterial catheter.
• Anticipate medication influences on autonomic nervous system balance (i.e., vagolysis from pancuronium, glycopyrrolate, etc).
• Avoid intracardiac placement of central line wire.
• Consider using bipolar electrocautery; ensure proper electrocautery return pad placement away from pacer.

Monitoring
• Low SaO$_2$ and high peak airway pressures can signify pulm edema.
• Low ETCO$_2$ may indicate low cardiac output.
• Arterial waveform: Diminished rate of rise may indicate poor cardiac output.

• Ensure adequate and constant ECG tracing with special attention to PR interval, QRS width and AV association.

General Anesthesia
• Anticipate the effects of laryngoscopy, intubation, TEE placement.
• Avoid rapid increases in volatile anesthetic concentration.
• Avoid high-dose opiates.
• Use beta-blockers or calcium channel blockers carefully; use short acting agents.
• Retraction or insufflation of vagal mediated structures can worsen bradycardia.
• Surgeon may need to stop offending maneuver until pt stabilized.
• Monitor and maintain normal serum electrolyte concentration.

Regional Anesthesia
• High thoracic spinal block will result in bradycardia even without pre-existing heart block.
• Pre-existing heart block may worsen after sympatholysis
• Atropine ineffective if heart block is below the AV node; use direct acting agents.
• Utilize epinephrine without delay.

• Verify or induce euvolemia.

Postoperative Period
• Obtain EKG to verify preop baseline, cardiology consult.
• Pacemaker interrogation by electrophysiology, return to previous mode.
• Perform physical exam looking for signs of heart failure.

Anticipated Problems/Concerns

• If heart block is at AV node then:
  • AV conduction is worsened by: Increased vagal input, peritoneal insufflation, esophageal manipulation (intubation, TEE, esophagoscopy); beta blockers, calcium channel blockers, high dose opiates, anticholinesterases.
  • AV conduction is improved by: Vagolysis (antimuscarinics), exercise, isoproterenol.
• If heart block is infranodal then autonomic influences are opposite of above.
• Development of slow ventricular response rate <40–50 bpm.
• Transcutaneous and/or transvenous pacemaker availability and practitioner knowledge.
• Have direct-acting sympathomimetics available.

Beckwith-Wiedemann Syndrome

Arlyne Thung

Risk

- 1:13,700
- No gender predilection although with monozygotic twins seen more with females than males

Perioperative Risks

- Acute airway obstruction, difficult mask ventilation and intubation secondary to macroglossia
- Hypoglycemia due to islet cell hyperplasia and hyperinsulinemia
- Cardiac malformations

Worry About

- Persistent hypoglycemia, which may cause CNS damage and therefore necessitates intraop infusion of glucose containing solution and frequent glucose checks
- Difficult airway management

Overview

- Commonly known for EMG triad (exomphalos, macroglossia, gigantism)
- Other clinical features incl anterior earlobe creases, posterior helical pits, facial nevus flammeus, hemihyperplasia, renal anomalies, embryonal tumors, cardiac malformations and hypoglycemia

- 7.5% estimated risk for embryonal tumor development, which occurs in the first 10 y of life. Most common tumors are Wilms tumor and hepatoblastoma but may also incl rhabdomyosarcoma, adrenocortical carcinoma and neuroblastoma
- Cardiac involvement often limited to mild cardiomegaly although other cardiac defects have been reported (atrial and ventricular septal defects, tetralogy of Fallot, hypoplastic left ventricle, cardiomyopathy, cardiac tumors, and valvular disease)
- Hypoglycemia due to islet cell hyperplasia and hyperinsulinemia occurs in 50% of BWS pts, is often responsive to medical therapy and usually regresses during the first 4 mo of life. Persistent hypoglycemia refractory to medical management may require pancreatectomy

Etiology

- Clinically and genetically heterogeneous
- May be genetically transmitted (15%) or occur sporadically (85%)
- Variety of mutations in chromosome 11p15.5 region
- Mutation near gene for IGF-II

Usual Treatment

- Prenatal detection of polyhydramnios, omphalocele, placentomegaly, macrosomia, macroglossia and renal anomalies on fetal ultrasound may prompt genetic testing and counseling if BWS is suspected
- Screening for hypoglycemia in the first few days of life if BWS is suspected. Surgical intervention if hypoglycemia persists despite medical management
- Surgical repair of omphalocele
- Possible reduction of macroglossia in the first year of life to avoid complications of airway obstruction, feeding and speech difficulties
- Infants with hypoglycemia and severe oral intolerance due to macroglossia may require gastrostomy tube placement as a temporizing measure until regular feeds are possible following glossal resection
- Orthopedic follow up to monitor leg length discrepancies due to hemihyperplasia
- Tumor surveillance (abdominal ultrasound, alpha-fetoprotein)
- Surgical resection of operative tumors

ASSESSMENT POINTS

System	Effect	Assessment by Hx	PE	Test
HEENT	Macroglossia	Hx of difficult mask ventilation and intubation	Determine extent by physical inspection and oral palpation, previous anesthesia Hx	No testing
CV	VSD, ASD, TOF, valvular disease, hypoplastic LV, cardiac tumor and cardiomegaly (most common) possible	SOB, DOE	Cardiac exam for murmurs	ECHO CXR
ENDO	Hypoglycemia Hypothyroidism	Shaking, lethargy		Glucose Thyroid function tests
RENAL	Renal medullary dysplasia Nephrolithasis	Hx of renal tumors/previous resections; chronic UTIs	Palpate for masses Flank pain	US BUN/Cr

Key Reference: Weksberg R, Shuman C, Beckwith JB. Beckwith-Wiedemann syndrome. *Eur J Hum Genet.* 2009;June:1–9.

Perioperative Implications

Preparation

- Coordinated care with endocrinology and ENT to assist in the management of hypoglycemia and difficult airway
- Discussion with ENT for planned tracheostomy if significant airway edema and swelling is anticipated following glossal resection
- Review of lab results (hypothyroidism, polycythemia, hypocalcemia and hyperlipidemia have been reported in pts with BWS in addition to hypoglycemia)
- Review cardiac work-up if available
- Pretreatment with antisialogogue (glycopyrrolate or atropine) if intubation is planned

Monitoring

- Standard monitoring appropriate for surgical procedure
- Frequent glucose checks

Airway

- Assume difficult mask ventilation due to macroglossia
- Nasal > oral intubation may be more performed more easily in pts with significant macroglossia. Pre-treat with a nasal decongestant and dilate with nasal trumpets if nasal intubation is considered.
- Assistance with glossal manipulation if direct laryngoscopy is performed
- Backup airway devices (e.g., fiberoptic, glidescope, LMA) and surgical support (ENT) if conventional laryngoscopy fails
- Age-appropriate ETT

Induction

- Inhaled induction with sevoflurane versus awake intubation with sedation/topicalization
- Clinicians should be aware that administration of IV anesthetics and muscle relaxants may cause tongue to fall backward causing acute airway obstruction

Postoperative Period

- After meeting strict extubation criteria, pts should be monitored in ICU or recovery area with immediate backup for management of airway issues and hypoglycemia

Anticipated Problems/Concerns

- Difficult airway
- Hypoglycemia

Bilirubinemia of the Newborn

Kelly Stees

DISEASES

Risk

- Common and mostly benign problem in neonates
- Observed during first week of life in 60% of term and 80% preterm infants
- Clinical, epidemiologic, and genetic risk factors associated with significant hyperbilirubinemia incl preterm gestational age, exclusive breastfeeding, glucose-6-phosphate dehydrogenase deficiency, Rh/ABO incompatibility, East Asian or Native American ethnicity, any jaundice observed in the first 24 hr of life (hemolysis until proven otherwise), cephalohematoma or significant bruising after delivery, and Hx of a previous sibling treated with phototherapy

Perioperative Risks

- Must consider pathophysiologic conditions present in premature or LBW and ill-term infants (e.g., RDS, sepsis, hemolysis, hypoxemia and acidosis)
- Increased risk of CNS injury with elevated levels of unconjugated bilirubin and compromised blood-brain barrier. Neurotoxic effects are directly related to permeability of BBB and nerve cell membranes (all are adversely influenced by asphyxia, prematurity, hyperosmolality, and infection)

Worry About

- Factors that increase blood-brain barrier permeability to unconjugated bilirubin: Hypoxia, hypercarbia, acidosis, hyperosmolality, Htn, seizure activity, sepsis
- Drugs (e.g., sulfonamides, ceftriaxone, ampicillin, salicylates, furosemide, and contrast dye) and physiologic states (dehydration, hypercarbia, and acidosis) that displace bilirubin from albumin can increase free fraction of unconjugated bilirubin in the blood.
- Binding of some drugs to albumin may be altered in the presence of hyperbilirubinemia in the neonatal period.
- Surgically induced increases in heme degradation (e.g., hematoma absorption)
- Liver dysfunction
- Hemolytic anemia

Overview

- Bilirubin is derived from the catabolism of proteins that contain heme; usually from the breakdown of hemoglobin from RBCs.
- Heme is oxidized to biliverdin and then reduced to bilirubin which is unconjugated, nonpolar, and lipid-soluble (indirect-reacting).
- Unconjugated bilirubin circulates bound to albumin in equilibrium with its unbound fraction that readily crosses the blood brain barrier and can cause neurotoxicity.
- Bilirubin is conjugated in the liver cell microsome by the enzyme (UDP)–glucuronyl transferase to form the polar, water-soluble glucuronide of bilirubin (direct-reacting).
- Most of the conjugated bilirubin is excreted as bile which is metabolized by intestinal flora and excreted in the feces.
- The danger of unconjugated hyperbilirubinemia is kernicterus (yellow staining of brain affecting the basal ganglion, hippocampus and cerebral and bulbar nuclei).
- Bilirubinemia peaks in term infants between 3–5 d; preterm infants 5–6 d
- Clinical features of hyperbilirubinemia are lethargy, anorexia, nausea, vomiting, icteric skin and sclera.
- Clinical features of kernicterus (very rare):
  - *Acute*: Opisthotonic posturing, muscle rigidity, seizure, oculogyric crisis
  - *Chronic*: Clinical tetrad of choreoathetoid cerebral palsy, high-frequency central neural hearing loss, palsy of vertical gaze, and dental enamel hypoplasia as the result of bilirubin-induced cell toxicity
- The ability of anesthetic agents to displace bilirubin from albumin has not been well studied.

ICD-9-CM Code: 774

Etiology

- Physiologic jaundice due to immature hepatic glucuronyl transferase
- Excess bilirubin production from RBC breakdown (intravascular–hemolysis or polycythemia, extravascular–bruising or cephalohematoma)

- Decreased removal of bilirubin through gut (decreased meconium evacuation–increased enterohepatic recirculation, decreased bile flow due to liver disease or cholestasis)
- Sepsis and/or viral infection
- Breastfeeding jaundice (occurs in first wk after birth and implies inadequate hydration or caloric intake)
- Breast-milk jaundice (unidentified factors in normal mature human milk that cause increased reabsorption of UB from gut) can last for 3–4 w up to 3 mo

Usual Treatment

- Goal of therapy is to prevent indirect-reacting bilirubin related neurotoxicity while not causing undo harm.
- Phototherapy and, if unsuccessful, exchange transfusion remain the primary treatment modalities used to keep the maximal total serum bilirubin below the pathologic levels.
- Phototherapy works by bypassing the hepatic system and produces photoisomers of bilirubin that are more water soluble and can be cleared directly in bile or urine without conjugation in the liver.
- Exchange transfusion removes infants' sensitized and destroyed RBCs and circulating antibodies; double-volume exchange replaces 85% of circulating RBC volume and decreases biilrubin level by 50% and corrects anemia.
- AAP guidelines for healthy term infant: Phototherapy when serum bilirubin >12–15 mg/dL, Exchange transfusion >20–25; premature or ill term infants have lower threshold for starting therapy.
- Several factors are important when determining the bilirubin level above which kernicterus is possible (gestational age, degree of illness, evidence of hemolysis, rate of rise, albumin level and physiologic stress).

ASSESSMENT POINTS

System	Effect	Assessment by Hx	PE	Test
DERM	Jaundice resulting from accumulation of unconjugated, nonpolar, lipid-soluble bilirubin pigment in the skin		Jaundice progresses in cephalocaudal direction (face~5 mg/dL; abdomen ~15 mg/dL)	
RESP	Pleural effusion, pulm edema	Maternal prenatal history	Resp distress	CXR
HEME	Hemolysis	Rh/ABO maternal-fetal incompatibility	Anemia, bruising, cephalohematomas hepatosplenomegaly, jaundice	Maternal ABO, Rh typing Cord blood type, Rh and direct Coombs' CBC, diff, retic and blood smear Fractionated bilirubin, LFTs, ammonia, PT/PTT, blood and urine cultures
CNS	Bilirubin toxic to CNS cells	High levels of bilirubin	Abnormal posture, tonicity, and reflexes	

Key Reference: Piazza AJ, Stoll BJ: Digestive system disorders. In Kliegman RM, Behrman RE, Jenson HB, Stanton BF (eds): Nelson Texbook of Pediatrics, 18th edition.

Perioperative Implications

Preoperative Preparation
- Assess and correct hydration status
- Active efforts to lower bilirubin levels
- Address co-existing disease states
- Consider atropine 0.1 mg IV to help prevent bradycardia

Monitoring
- Arterial blood sampling may be indicated

Airway
- Neonatal airway concerns

Induction
- Maintain normal hemodynamics

Maintenance
- No one agent or technique preferred
- Few data reflecting effects of anesthetic agents on bilirubin levels
- Adjust for FIO$_2$ to SaO$_2$ 90–95%
- Supplemental glucose and calcium
- Maintain normothermia

Extubation
- Maintain intubation if infant ill or premature or for extensive surgical procedure

Adjuvants
- Chloral hydrate and pancuronium associated with hyperbilirubinemia
- Maternal epidural bupivacaine associated with neonatal jaundice

Postoperative Period
- Apnea/bradycardia risks
- Monitor bilirubin levels

Anticipated Problems/Concerns
- Ultimate goal of therapy and management is to prevent kernicterus

Blebs and Bullae

Trent Bryson

DISEASES

Risk

- Prevelance of blebs as high as 6% of young, healthy adults, although spontaneous rupture occurs only in 7.4–18 per 100,000
- Incidence of ruptured bulla is 26 per 100,000
- Increased incidence of primary disease in young males
- Increased prevelance with smoking Hx–incl cigarettes and illicit substances, COPD, chronic bronchitis, cystic fibrosis, lung cancer, staphylococcal pneumonia, tuberculosis, Marfan's syndrome, Ehlers-Danlos syndrome, alpha-1 antitrypsin deficiency, sarcoidosis, fiberglass pneumocosis and BMI < 22

Perioperative Risks

- Pneumothorax
- Bronchopleural fistulae
- Caval compression of non-ruptured giant bulla
- Pulm Htn and RV failure
- COPD

Worry About

- CV collapse from tension pneumothorax
- Expanded dead space ventilation

- Inability to adequately ventilate due to bronchopleural fistula
- Inadequate venous return from caval compression
- Expansion of bulla leading to compressive effects or rupture

Overview

- "Bleb" usually refers to a collection of air caused by ruptured aveoli within the visceral pleura without any other lining that is <1 cm in size
- Bulla are >1 cm in size and arise from various sources, which cause destruction of lung parenchyma
- Nitrous oxide is contraindicated and positive pressure ventilation should be avoided if possible
  - Nitrous oxide is 35 times more soluble than nitrogen in blood. Because of this, nitrous oxide readily diffuses into any gas-filled cavity much more rapidly than nitrogen is absorbed, which leads to rapid expansion of pneumothoraces.
  - In spontaneous ventilation, bullae are more compliant than normal lung tissue and preferentially fill. At higher pressures and volumes bullae are much less compliant than normal lung and therefore have much higher peak pressures than normal tissue and are prone to rupture.

ICD-9-CM Code: 492.0

Etiology

- Primary: Unknown but may be genetic. More common in young males
- Secondary: Emphysema, smoking, lung cancer, cystic fibrosis, pneumonia, tuberculosis

Usual Treatment

- No treatment for asymptomatic, incidental blebs
- First time rupture of a bleb is treated conservatively depending on size of pneumothorax. Varies from 100% O_2 to chest tube placement.
- Surgical treatment indicated for ruptured blebs in those in high-risk occupations which involve frequent changes in barometric pressure or recurrent spontaneous pneumothorax
- Surgical treatment of bullae done for increasing SOB or recurrent pneumothorax
- Surgical approach usually is VATS, but may require thoracotomy or median sternotomy. Laser ablation and mechanical pleurodesis may be utilized.

ASSESSMENT POINTS

System	Effect	Assessment by Hx	PE	Test
CV	CAD, pulm Htn, RV failure	Angina, DOE	Signs of RV failure (palpable PA, peripheral edema)	ECG, stress test, ECHO
RESP	Expiratory obstruction, air trapping V/Q mismatch Hypoxia, hypercarbia Pneumothorax	Exercise tolerance Cough	Pursed-lip breathing, tachypnea	CXR, ABGs, chest CT, V/Q scan
ENDO	Possible steroid use			Glucose
MS	Barrel-chested			

Key Reference: Kim H, Kim HK, Choi YH, Lim SH. Thoracoscopic bleb resection using two-lung ventilation anesthesia with low tidal volume for primary spontaneous pneumothorax *Ann Thorac Surg.* 2009;87(3):880–885.

Perioperative Implications

Preinduction/Induction/Maintenance

- Optimize oxygenation and deliver bronchodilators if necessary.
- Regional or neuraxial anesthesia is preferential to general endotracheal anesthesia.
- Some associated conditions may have significant mucus plugging; fiberoptic bronchoscope with suction and irrigating capabilities may be useful.
- Careful attention to hemodynamic monitors and ventilator peak pressures and volumes is essential.
- Should have surgical team available during induction as this is most common time for pneumothorax to occur.
- Recent chest x-ray evaluation for severity of disease and progression is also essential.

Monitoring

- Routine
- Consider arterial line to more rapidly recognize signs of CV collapse from pneumothorax or caval compression.

General Anesthesia

- Maintaining spontaneous ventilation through induction can minimize complications. Avoid the use of paralytics or consider mask induction or awake fiberoptic intubation techniques.

- Consider ketamine induction to maintain ventilation for IV induction.
- If positive pressure ventilation needed, pressure control ventilation at low pressures with higher rate may be useful, but beware of breath-stacking.
- Allow adequate exhalation times to avoid breath stacking (auto-PEEP) by appropriately setting I:E ratio.
- Do not use nitrous oxide under any circumstance.
- Consider use of isoflurane as it is the most bronchodilating inhalation agent and may decrease pressure requirements or obstruction in COPD pts.
- Careful attention to spontaneous ventilatory rate and volumes prior to extubation.
- Avoid high airway pressures from fighting the ventilator.
- If paralyzed for case, assure full reversal before attempt to extubate.
- COPD pts may retain CO_2 so be careful not to drive $ETCO_2$ too low and prolong emergence.

Regional Anesthesia

- Preferred technique if possible for most cases
- Optimize volume status
- Watch for resp distress from loss of accessory resp muscles from neuraxial anesthesia.

- Epidural may be preferable to spinal to avoid loss of accessory muscles by slowly raising level by interval dosing.
- Pleurodesis is exquisitely painful and often requires a thoracic epidural to control pain and assure adequate chest excursion during recovery.

Postoperative Period

- Beware of CO_2 narcosis in those who retain CO_2.
- Spontaneous rupture can occur at any time. Continue adequate monitoring and watch for sudden dyspnea, desaturation, and loss of unilateral breath sounds.

Anticipated Problems/Concerns

- Rupture of bleb or bulla will cause a pneumothorax, which may rapidly progress to tension.
- Treatment of choice for tension pneumothorax is needle thoracostomy in second to third intercostal space in midclavicular line (in line with the nipple of a male pt). Most failures of needle thoracostomy occur from placement of needle too medial into the mediastinum.
- Obstructive pulmonary pathology incl bronchoconstriction and accessory muscle use even in the spontaneously breathing pt.
- Positive pressure ventilation is to be avoided and nitrous oxide is absolutely contraindicated.

Bleomycin Sulfate Toxicity

Zoulfira Nisnevitch

Risk

- Pts with a Hx of germ cell tumors, squamous cell carcinomas, lymphomas, treated with bleomycin (BLM)
- Incidence of BLM lung toxicity (BLT) is 10–40%. The mortality is 1–2%.
- Risk of BLT increases with total dose >400 units, Creatinine clearance <50% or prior or concurrent chest radiation therapy
- Age older than 70 y
- O_2 exposure, smoking

Perioperative Risks

- Exposure to high FIO_2 can cause pneumonitis and potentially lethal ARDS.
- Pre-existing pulm fibrosis in combination with low FIO_2 can lead to intraop hypoxia.
- Risk higher if pulm injury on PFTs, BLM exposure within 2 mo
- Pulm adverse events rarely related to the intrapleural administration of BLM for pleurodesis

Worry About

- Periop exposure to FIO_2 >30%
- Periop hypoxia
- Carefully monitor fluid replacement, focusing on colloid rather than crystalloid.
- Intrapleural administration of BLM has been associated with local pain and hypotension requiring symptomatic treatment.

Overview

- Antitumor antibiotic from a family of natural glycopeptides isolated from fungus *Streptomyces verticillus* used predominantly in treatment of germ cell testicular cancers, Hodgkin's and non-Hodgkin's lymphoma, squamous cell carcinoma of the head and neck.
- BLM is effective as a sclerosing agent for the treatment of malignant and recurre nt pleural effusions.
- BLM is inactivated by the enzyme bleomycin hydrolase. Lungs and skin have the lowest level of BLM hydrolase and thus are the predominant sites of injury.

- Cleared by renal excretion. Elimination half time ($T\frac{1}{2}$) 4 hr

ICD-9-CM Code: E930.7 (Bleomycin-therapeutic)

Etiology

- The toxicity is unpredictable. In the presence of Fe^{2+} and O_2, BLM causes DNA damage. Injury to double-stranded DNA is thought to be the major source of cytotoxicity.
- The event sequence to lung injury is: (1) endothelial and interstitial capillary edema; (2) pneumocytes type II proliferation and necrosis with surfactant release; (3) surfactant phagocytocis by alveolar macrophages with mediator release and stimulus to fibroblast production.
- Pts who had previously received BLM and needed O_2 support during surgery were susceptible to development of lung toxicity and ARDS, even with low inspired FIO_2. O_2-free radicals may inactivate antioxidant enzymes leading to genetic injury, cell death, and resulting in alveolar injury.

ASSESSMENT POINTS

System	Effect	Assessment by Hx	PE	Tests
RESP	Pulm fibrosis ARDS with O_2 exposure	Dyspnea, dry cough	Frequently normal Earliest sign is fine rales	CXR- nonspecific patchy opacities Decreased O_2 sat PFTs—decrease in total lung volume and a decrease in vital capacity and DLCO
MUCOCUT	Inflammation, dermal fibrosis	Itching, burning, skin tenderness	Stomatitis, alopecia, scleroderma-like skin changes	
HEME	Minimal bone marrow toxicity			CBC

Key Reference: Azambuja E, et al. Bleomycin lung toxicity: Who are patients at risk? *Pulm Pharmacol Ther.* 2005;18:363–366.

Perioperative Implications

Preoperative Preparation

- In pts with a Hx of testicular, squamous cell cancer, or lymphoma, inquire about exposure to BLM, dose and time of the last dose.
- Any pt with abnormal pulm studies or who is clinically symptomatic should be considered high risk for development of ARDS.
- Exposure to BLM within 2 mo should be considered high risk for postop ARDS, although even with a longer interval between the last BLM dose and exposure to hyperoxia, pts still can develop ARDS.

Intraoperative Management

- Maintain FIO_2 at concentrations close to that of room air (30%) during surgery and the postop period. Accept SaO_2 above 90% if appropriate. Consider use of PEEP to reduce FIO_2.

- Carefully monitor fluid replacement, focusing more on colloid administration rather than crystalloid. Consider using intravascular monitoring when large fluid shifts are expected. Treat hypotension with vasopressors and decreasing the anesthetic concentration rather than fluid boluses if appropriate.
- In high-risk pts pretreatment with corticosteroids (1 mg/kg prednisone) may be helpful in limiting postop ARDS.

Postoperative Period

- Provide adequate oxygenation with the lowest possible inspired FIO_2.
- Observe carefully for 3–5 d after surgery for signs of dyspnea, hypoxia, cough, or rales.
- Obtain daily X-ray for 3–5 d after surgery.
- Use PEEP or CPAP to treat postop hypoxia.

- Add methylprednisolone up to 1 mg/kg d if developing ARDS, diuretics in the presence of excessive lung water.

Anticipated Problems/Concerns

- Pts who had previously received BLM and needed O_2 support during surgery, even with low inspired FIO_2 are susceptible to development of lung toxicity and ARDS.
- Maintaining adequate oxygenation with the lowest possible FIO_2 can be difficult.
- Restrictive goal-directed fluid management with invasive monitoring is preferred.

Blindness

Stanley W. Stead

Risk

- Eye injuries represent 4% of claims analyzed in the American Society of Anesthesiologists (ASA) Closed Claims Project.
- Majority of entries in the ASA Postoperative Visual Loss (POVL) Registry are associated with cardiac and spine cases, with a reported incidence as high as 4.5% and 0.2%, respectively. Other surgical procedures with POVL reported incl head and neck, liver transplants, thoracoabdominal aneurysm resections, peripheral vascular procedures and prostatectomies.
- In the Registry, POVL is most often associated with ischemic optic neuropathy (ION) 89% of the time and central retinal artery occlusion (CRAO) 11% of the time.
- Blindness can result from injury to the eye, its surrounding structures (eyelid and conjunctiva), blood supply and optic nerve.
- Blindness may be transient (glycine absorption), prolonged or permanent (ischemic optic neuropathy, central retinal artery occlusion, traumatic, central ischemic events).

Perioperative Risks

- ION: Bilateral blindness in spine procedures in the prone position, cardiopulmonary bypass, head and neck dissections, where there is significant facial swelling and venous hemodynamics may be altered.
- CRAO: Periocular trauma and rarely bilateral blindness.
- Procedure dependent factors: Anemia, blood loss greater than 1L, systemic hypotension and procedure duration greater than 6 hours.
- Intraocular procedures, procedures around the eye, prone position with padding around the face and eyes, exophthalmos or ophthalmic nerve blocks
- 1.5% glycine irrigation during TURP, transurethral bladder procedures and hysteroscopic procedures in women

Worry About

- Pressure on the globe or contact with eye by foreign objects or solutions
- Positioning of pt, esp prone
- Low blood flow states: Systemic hypotension, anemia, venous drainage impairment of the head and neck
- Operations in physical proximity to the eyes
- During ophthalmic surgery:
  - Movement of pt under either MAC or GA during intraocular surgery
  - Trauma to optic nerve, retinal artery, or vein during orbital or sinus surgery
  - Coughing or substantial Valsalva maneuvers by pt following intraocular surgery
- During ophthalmic nerve block:
  - Perforation of globe
  - Trauma to the optic nerve, retinal artery, and vein

Overview

- Unless associated with glycine irrigating solution, blindness is often an irreversible complication following anesthesia and surgery.
- Blindness is most often associated with injury to the eye, its surrounding structures (eyelid and conjunctive), blood supply, and optic nerve.

ICD-9-CM Codes: 362.3 (Retinal vascular occlusion), 362.84 (Retinal ischemia), 368.12 (Transient), 369.00 (Acquired); 377.41 (Ischemic optic neuropathy), 950.9 (Due to nerve injury)

Etiology

- Conditions that can result in blindness following anesthesia incl: Corneal abrasion, vitreous loss, hemorrhage, movement of pt while operating on or in the eye, chemical injury to the cornea or conjunctiva from cleaning materials on the anesthetic mask, spillage of prep solution into the eye, and direct trauma to the eye due to OR table padding, needle used in retrobulbar block, anesthetic mask pressure on the globe or foreign body falling into eye. Additionally, prone position, hypoxemia following cardiac arrest, prolonged hypotension, central retinal artery occlusion, increased intraocular pressure, and embolization, occlusion, thrombosis, or spasm of the retinal artery.
- Following absorption of glycine irrigating solution during TURP. Glycine distribution similar to that of γ-aminobutyric acid, an inhibitory neurotransmitter. Levels of glycine >143 mg/L associated with transient blindness.

Usual Treatment

- In the case of glycine, supportive treatment is indicated until plasma glycine levels <143 mg/L.
- ION: There is not effective treatment and most lost vision is not recovered.
- CRAO: Immediate lowering of intraocular pressure with acetazolamide and topical medications. Hyperbaric O_2 therapy may be beneficial if begun within 2–12 hrs of symptom onset.

ASSESSMENT POINTS

System	Effect	Assessment by Hx	PE	Test
OVERALL	Retinal artery occlusion	Migraines, coagulopathies, hemoglobinopathies, oral contraceptives ↑ IOP	Pale ischemic retina with pathognomonic cherry-red spot and afferent papillary defect	
HEENT	Ischemic retinopathy	Hypotension Hypoxemia Shock	Funduscopic: A normal retina but optic nerve head is swollen and ischemic. Eventual optic nerve pallor.	
	Orbital pressure		Funduscopic: An edematous retina with dilated arterioles and engorged veins.	
GU	Transient blindness during or after TURP	TURP with glycine irrigating solution	Normal papillary response to light and accommodation. Fundus normal.	Plasma glycine level (nml 13–17 mg/L)

Key Reference: Lee LA, Roth S, Posner KL, Cheney FW, et al. The American Society of Anesthesiology Postoperative Visual Loss Registry. *Anesthesiology.* 2006;105:652–659.

Perioperative Implications

Preinduction/Induction/Maintenance
- Proper positioning essential
- If prone, adequate padding so no pressure is transmitted to either globe or nasal bridge
- When the face is completely draped, consider use of a metallic Fox shield to protect eye from inadvertent pressure.

Monitoring
- Eye checks frequently during the procedure to ensure no pressure on the globe
- Ensure adequate venous drainage without increased venous pressure or increased intracranial pressure, particularly when venous outflow may be compromised by position or procedure.

General Anesthesia
- Anesthetic masks may injure eye, either through inadequate drying and application of cleaning solution to eye or through direct pressure.
- Hypotension and hypoxemia implicated in cases of CRAO.
- Hypotension, anemia, and prolonged procedures are implicated in ION.

Regional Anesthesia
- In ophthalmic nerve blocks, needle does not enter globe or retinal artery, vein, or nerve. Avoid excessive volume of local anesthetic, which increases IOP and may compromise vascular supply of globe.

Postoperative Period
- When recovered in prone position, ensure that there is no pressure on orbit or globe.

Anticipated Problems/Concerns
- Absorption of glycine from 1.5% glycine irrigation fluid may be significant.
- ION almost always occurs without any other evidence of vascular injury.
- Optic nerve may be very vulnerable to hemodynamic changes in the prone position.

Botulism

Debra E. Morrison

Risks

- Infant botulism
- Wound botulism
- Foodborne botulism
- Adult intestinal toxemia
- Injection botulism
- Biological warfare/inhalational botulism (Category A biological threat)

Perioperative Risks

- Dx late, incorrect or missed
  - Differential Dx: For adults, myasthenia gravis, Eaton-Lambert, Guillain-Barre, CVA, organophosphate exposure, tick paralysis. For infants, sepsis, failure to thrive, dehydration, encephalitis, metabolic disease
    - Non-specific history and physical findings
    - Laboratory result takes days-weeks and should be used only as confirmation; treat before confirmation
    - Triad: Bulbar symptoms, resp compromise and dilated pupils
- Prolonged weakness requiring prolonged support
- Enteral nutrition desired but problematic due to gastroparesis and bowel paralysis
- Aspiration risk
- Elevated potassium if immobile in ICU

Worry About

- Arrhythmias
- Hyperkalemia, arrhythmias, then cardiac arrest
- Prolonged weakness necessitating prolonged intubation and leading to nosocomial infection

Overview

- Botulism is a rare but serious neuroparalytic illness caused by a nerve toxin (BoNT) produced by the rod-shaped bacterium *Clostridium botulinum*, commonly found in soil. *C. botulinum* grows best in low oxygen conditions; spores survive in dormant state until exposed to conditions that support growth. Seven types of toxins (A-G), but only A, B, E, F cause illness in humans; three different intracellular protein targets; different durations.
- Infant: Between 2 w-1 y old; ingestion of spores which grow in intestine and release toxin, usually by honey ingestion; parent who works with soil; rural areas
- Wound: IV/skin popping drug users or organisms contaminating any traumatized tissue cause local infection and absorption of produced toxin—increased incidence over last several years in IV drug users (black tar heroin), esp in California
- Foodborne: Improperly preserved or cooked food allows germination and toxin production by contaminating spores; consumption of food with preformed toxin results in absorption of potent neurotoxin; with education and control of food industries, now uncommon in USA; ingestion of infected inadequately cooked wildlife poses at least potential risk.
- Intestinal: Spore colonization—possible in adults as well
- Injection: Cosmetic (Black market toxin, Botox® overdose or spread beyond injection site), cerebral palsy (Botox® overdose or spread beyond injection site)
- Inhalational: Genetically engineered toxin, development of biological warfare (at-risk locations). Concern is inadequate stocking of antidotes worldwide, inadequate preparation and medical support. Biological warfare in Iraq has led to organization of task forces such as Scorpio at the national/regional level to stockpile antidotes.

ICD-9-CM Code: 005.1: Botulism food poisoning, 040.01: Infant Botulism, 040.02: Wound Botulism

Etiology

- Botulinin toxin binds irreversibly to synaptic membrane of cholinergic nerves and prevents release of acetylcholine.

Usual Treatment

- Supportive, may be on ventilator for weeks, intense medical and nursing care
- Nutritional support; enteral preferred (basic maintenance plus need to keep bowels moving to eliminate spores), but parenteral also required
- Early antitoxin treatment shows better outcome, antitoxin blocks action of circulating toxin, prevents pts from worsening but recovery still takes many weeks
- Equine-derived antitoxin for adults (risk of serum sickness/anaphylaxis); skin testing and desensitization instructions provided with antitoxin; more broad spectrum antitoxins associated with increase in hypersensitivity
- Presently trivalent antitoxin preparation is available for adults (10 mL vial with 7500 IU type A, 5500 IU type B, 8500 IU type E)
- Baby BIG (human botulism immune globulin) used for infant botulism came out in 1990, more in use since 2003
- Botulism reportable to CDC or state health department, requires report to obtain antitoxin
- Antibiotics for secondary infections
- Avoid aminoglycosides and clindamycin, which may potentiate or exacerbate neuromuscular blockade
- Guanadine increases the release of acetylcholine from nerve terminals, appears to be useful in mild cases
- Modern clinical practice and early antitoxin treatment: mortality reduced from 60% to ≤10%

ASSESSMENT POINTS

System	Effect	Assessment by Hx	PE	Tests
RESP	Pharyngeal constrictor and genioglossal hypotonia, paralysis of resp musculature Infection Atelectasis	Drooling Poor feeding Decreased resp effort Increased secretions Tracheal secretions Poor resp effort Poor color	Poor head control Absent gag Weak cough Fever Rhonchi Rales Cyanosis	Diagnosis of elimination; electrophysiology studies are fastest diagnostic tool to rule out other causes; EEG and neuroimaging are normal as long as there is no hypoxic insult; edrophonium test to rule out myasthenia gravis shows no improvement
GI	Constipation	No bowel movement Irritability	Palpable stool Abdominal distention	Blood, urine, CSF analysis and culture, metabolic and hepatic profiles are generally within normal limits
RENAL	UTI	Foul-smelling urine		Stool samples are difficult to collect due to constipation, can use sterile water enema
CNS	SIADH Seizures Cranial neuropathies	Infrequent urination Twitching Altered consciousness Ptosis Expressionless face Feeble cry	Diminished urine flow Seizure activity Fixed and dilated pupils Facial palsy Poor cough and gag	Serum testing possible if stool unobtainable but low sensitivity compared to stool testing (negative serum test does not exclude possibility of infant botulism) Samples injected into mice, look for signs of botulism Laboratory result takes days-weeks and is used as confirmation
PNS	Spinal neuropathies	Limp limbs	Hypotonia	Tests only performed at some state health department labs and CDC; samples must be collected sterilely, refrigerated and shipped with cold packs

Key Reference: Robinson RF, Nahata MC. Management of botulism. *Ann Pharmacother*. 2003;37:127–131.

Perioperative Implications

- Early diagnosis, treatment, and optimization
- Continue supportive resp care
- Sepsis from secondary infections
- Avoid resp depressants, paralytics
- Aspiration risk
- Pts may require feeding tube and/or parenteral nutrition
- Likely to OR for wound debridement
- If possible, avoid airway manipulation, unnecessary medications and those that are resp depressants

Preoperative Preparation

- Recommend pt receives antitoxin prior to wound debridement so additional toxin release does not cause further paralysis
- Low threshold for treatment if suspecting botulism
- Manage preop electrolytes
- Continue antibiotics
- CXR to help assess status
- Aspiration prophylaxis

- If pregnant, parturient can safely be given antitoxin (intrathecally in severe cases); consider early tracheostomy to avoid sequelae of resp depression; botulism not known to cause direct fetal risks, only those associated with mother's ventilatory compromise, since molecule is too large to pass through placental barrier

Monitoring

- Standard ASA monitors
- If unstable in ICU, consider arterial cannulation for management of autonomic dysfunction (infants may see motor function return before autonomic system)

Airway

- Aspiration risk
- May already be intubated

Induction

- Avoid succinylcholine
- May not require paralytic

Maintenance

- May not require paralytic throughout case

Extubation

- Likely unable to extubate
- Continue supportive care postop

Adjuvants

- Avoid resp depressants if possible
- Consider regional procedures rather than narcotics for pain control in wounds

Postoperative Period

- Continued supportive care
- Manage electrolytes

Associated Problems/Concerns

- Aspiration pneumonia
- Sepsis from wound
- Missed diagnosis
- Malnutrition
- Biological warfare: Limited information on effectiveness of antitoxin success with inhalational botulism, amount of neutralizing antibody in presently available formulation may not be enough for treatment of genetically engineered toxin.

Brain Death

Richard C. Cross

Risk

- Shortage of organs for transplant persist despite utilization of expanded donor pool and living unrelated donors
- Inadequate donor organ function limits organ supply
- Optimizing donor management increases donor yield

Perioperative Risks

- CV instability
- Endocrine dysfunction
- Metabolic imbalance
- Coagulopathy
- Hypothermia

Worry About

- Organ loss secondary to CV collapse

Overview

- Brain death secondary to cerebral herniation from increased ICP
- Associated with autonomic storm, vasomotor instability and hormone deficiencies resulting in hypotension
- Criteria: Irreversible coma (no response to painful stimuli), absent brainstem reflexes, apnea and no confounding conditions (hypothermia <35° C, metabolic disturbances, intoxication incl neuromuscular blockade)

- Confirmatory test: No flow during cerebral angiography or absent activity on EEG

ICD-9-CM Code: 348.8

Etiology

- Traumatic brain injury and SDH

Usual Treatment

- Critical pathways promoted to enhance organs transplanted per donor

ASSESSMENT POINTS

System	Effect	Assessment by Hx	PE	Test
RESP	Neurogenic pulm edema ALI/ARDS			ABGs, CXR
CV	Hypovolemia Ventricular dysfunction Depletion of myocardial substrates Unstable vasomotor center Nonfunctional sympathetic system Arrhythmias	Need for inotropic support		BP Cardiac catherization TEE Atropine resistance (2 mg)
HEME	Coagulopathy Anemia			Coagulation studies Hct
GU	Diabetes insipidus Osmotic diuresis Hypernatremia			UO >3 mL/kg/hr Lytes Urine SG < 1.0005 Serum osmolality >310 mOsm
CNS	Lack of cerebral and brainstem function Poikilothermic	Hx of drug ingestion, metabolic encephalopathy, and/or hypothermia excluded		CT, EEG, cerebral angiograpy Toxicology screen Midsized pupils Absent brainstem reflexes Positive apnea test Temp monitor

Key Reference: Wood, Kenneth E, et al. Care of the Potential Organ Donor. *NEJM.* 2004;351:2730–2739.

Perioperative Implications

Monitoring
- Temp
- A-line
- CVP or PA catheter
- UO
- ABGs

Airway
- Low FIO$_2$ and PEEP (5 cm H$_2$O)
- Tidal volumes to keep peak pressure <30 mmHg

Maintenance
- Correct metabolic derangements (avoid acidosis, hypoxemia, and hypercarbia) and monitor for, and nudge toward correction of, electrolyte abnormalities (hypernatremia and hyperglycemia)

- Treat anemia to Hct >30% and keep coagulation studies normal (values <1.5X control)
- Dopamine or dobutamine for MAP >60 mmHg
- Hormonal resuscitation with insulin, steroids, vasopressin and thyroid hormone (Papworth cocktail) and pulm artery catheter placement for EF <45%
- Fluids and hemodynamic medications to minimize use of alpha-agonists
- Lung expansion ventilatory techniques, judicious colloid fluid resuscitation and steroids to preserve lung function
- Maintain UOP >100 mL/hr and treat DI with DDAVP or low dose AVP
- Keep normothermic

Extubation
- Not done
- Ventilation discontinued when cross-clamp:
  - Ascending aorta for heart-lung donors
  - Descending aorta for liver-kidney donors above SMA and celiac artery

Adjuvants
- Drugs per procurement team, e.g., heparin, chlorpromazine

Anticipated Problems/Concerns

- Anticipate increase in BP and HR with incision—does not obviate criteria for brain death
- Knowledge of sequelae of brain death

Bronchiectasis

H. Michael Marsh

Risk

- Incidence in USA: <1:10,000 hospital admissions
- Gender prevalence: None
- Socioeconomic or ethnic prevalence: Inbreeding and primitive health care, particularly lack of immunization and poor treatment of childhood bronchitides, increase the prevalence. Ciliary deformities have been shown in a Polynesian population.
- Occasionally seen in children:
  - Bronchial cartilage deficiency (Williams-Campbell syndrome)
  - Tracheobronchomegaly (Mounier-Kuhn's syndrome)
  - Inherited immunoglobulin deficiencies, impaired phagocytosis, complement deficiency
  - α_1-Antitrypsin deficiency
- Occasionally seen in adults with acquired γ-globulin deficiency:
  - Cystic fibrosis
  - RA
  - Pulm ciliary dyskinesias (Kartagener's syndrome)

Perioperative Risks

- Spillage of infected secretions from bronchiectatic regions to normal lung leads to pneumonitis, retention of secretions

- Risk from bacteremia, after manipulation
- Risk of secondary acute resp failure
- Massive hemoptysis
- Pneumothorax

Worry About

- Exacerbation of asthma
- Amount of sputum produced and its nature
- Fever, hemoptysis: Acute pulm infection
- Right heart function
- Check frequency of cough and daily sputum volume; culture and smear for composition; check body temp and WBC count for acute infection
- Exercise tolerance will indicate associated impairment or disability. Right heart function may need assessment.

Overview

- Abnormal widening or dilatation of one or more branches of the bronchial tree. Widened segments commonly filled with purulent secretions; mucosa is swollen and inflamed and may be ulcerated with granulation tissue exposed. Extensive collateral flow occurs in these chronically inflamed bronchi (3–12% of CO).

ICD-9-CM Codes: 494; 748.61 (Congenital); 011.5 (Tuberculous)

Etiology/Pathogenesis

- Exact etiology for acquired form remains unclear but often involves necrotizing infection in tracheobronchial wall. Five mechanisms may predispose:
  - Bacterial, viral, or fungal bronchopulmonary infections, incl TB, pertussis, and measles
  - Bronchial obstruction
  - Immunodeficiency states, incl IgG deficiency, IgA deficiency, and leukocyte dysfunction
  - Hereditary defects in ciliary-mucosal clearance, incl Kartagener's syndrome, α_1-antitrypsin deficiency, and cystic fibrosis
  - Miscellaneous disorders, incl recurrent aspiration, inhaled irritants, Young's syndrome, and bronchiolitis obliterans following heart-lung transplantation

Usual Treatment

- Medical therapy: Postural drainage, deep breathing and assisted coughing, antibiotics, bronchodilators, and fluids/humidity. Drainage of sinuses.
- Surgical therapy: Resection indicated for uncontrolled hemoptysis; or lobar closely confined disease, age >20 y. Bronchopulmonary lavage under GA with divided airway (double-lumen tube).

ASSESSMENT POINTS

System	Effect	Assessment by Hx	PE	Test
HEENT	Sinusitis	Postnasal drip Stuffiness, headache	Translucency	X-ray, ultrasound, bright lights
CV	Clubbing, cyanosis CHF (cor pulmonale) Kartagener's syndrome	Exercise tolerance Pulm Htn, edema Chronic sinusitis	Situs inversus	ABGs Loud P_2 Right heart studies Immotile spermatozoa
RESP	Bronchiectasis	Cough, sputum Hemoptysis Wheezing	Rhonchi CXR—93% tram lines, 7% normal	Smear, culture, high-resolution CT, bronchoeram Bronchoscopy PFTs
HEME	Immunodeficiency Infection			IgG, IgA, WBC
CNS	Brain abscess			CT/MRI

Key Reference: O'Brien C, Guest PJ, Hill SL, Stockley RA. Physiological and radiological characterization of patients diagnosed with chronic obstructive pulmonary disease in primary care. *Thorax.* 2000;55:635–642.

Perioperative Implications

Monitoring
- Routine: Consider PA catheter for cor pulmonale or CHF

Airway
- Careful frequent suctioning and humidification of inspired gases

Induction
- Avoid asthma exacerbation
- Consider regional anesthesia when possible

Maintenance
- Routine

Extubation
- Depends upon degree of pulm and cardiac dysfunction

Adjuvants
- Routine

Postoperative Period
- Use stir-up regimen; monitor for retained secretions and resp failure
- Check for platypnea, orthodeoxia if right atrial pressures become elevated

Anticipated Problems/Concerns

- Retained secretions, secondary resp failure
- Right heart decompensation if hypoxemia persists
- Bacteremia from airway manipulations

Bronchiolitis Obliterans Syndrome

Risk

- Incidence in USA: 1:40,000
- Racial predilection: None
- Occurs primarily after lung and bone marrow transplantation
- Industrial workers who have presented with bronchiolitis obliterans syndrome (BOS): Nylon-flock, battery workers, manufacturer of flavorings (diacetyl butter-like flavoring)

Perioperative Risks

- Hypoxemia and severe periop airway obstruction
- Pulm infection, sepsis, pulm edema posttransplant
- Injury to tracheal anastomosis due to ETT placement
- Prolonged intubation (increased sensitivity to medications incl muscle relaxants, pulm functions, renal impairment and pulm edema)
- Complications of immunosuppression (infection, hemorrhage, renal impairment)
- Preop focus must differentiate between active invasive pulm infection and ongoing chronic rejection with colonization; and maximizing medical condition and stratifying risk.

Worry About

- Pulm functions
- Differentiating BOS from untreated invasive pulm infection and other disorders
- Side effects of immunosuppression incl infection with invasive techniques, hemorrhage, and renal failure with cyclosporine

- Allograft denervation (physiologic and pharmacologic side effects)
- Other effects of etiologic agents

Overview

- Persistent airflow obstruction often associated with chronic inflammation and scarring that obliterates small airways resulting in progressive obstructive lung disease.
- Because bronchiolitis obliterans (BO) is difficult to confirm histologically (transbronchial biopsy of larger airways with sporadic involvement often provides insufficient samples and has a high false-negative diagnostic rate), the International Society for Heart and Lung Transplantation proposed a staged clinical definition of BO termed bronchiolitis obliterans syndrome (BOS; stages 0–3 defined by changes in pulm functions rather than histology).
- BOS clinical staging is important to the clinician because it indicates allograft function.

ICD-9-CM Code: 491.8

Etiology

- The mechanism involved in the etiology of BO remains poorly understood.
- Two forms of BOS with inflammation and fibrosis: Rejection-related and non-rejection related.
- After transplant, the syndrome reflects small airway obliterations due to "chronic rejection."
- Several risk factors incl: Transplantation; ischemia-reperfusion injury; alloimmunity, Hx of acute graft rejection, mismatches at human leukocyte antigen (HLA) loci, development of antibodies to class I HLA, GE reflux with resultant

aspiration; loss of cough reflex due to denervation, complication of prematurity (bronchopulmonary dysplasia); toxicant inhalation ("Popcorn lung"); exposure to infectious agents (bacterial, viral, and some atypical organisms incl mycoplasma, chlamydia and fungi) (BO with organizing pneumonia or BOOP).
- BOS is described after lung, heart-lung, bone marrow, renal, pancreas, liver and hematopoietic stem cell transplantation; BOS remains the leading causes of death after lung transplantation.

Usual Treatment

- Varies depending on whether or not BOS is rejection-related
- Rejection-related BOS is mainly treated with additional immunosuppression and supportive care incl O_2, bronchodilators, and chest physical therapy
- Non-rejection related BOS is treated with supportive care, anti-infective agents, and may respond to steroids (esp toxic fumes and other environmental exposures).
- Newer treatments for rejection-related: Azithromycin, aerosolized cyclosporine, augmentation of immunosuppression agents, statins, (IL-1 receptors antagonist, IL-2 receptor antagonists, and adenosine A_{2A} receptor agonists in posttransplant pts have been proposed recently)
- Severe cases often require lung transplant and even retransplant.

ASSESSMENT POINTS

Use previous classification to determine possible cause of BO including post-transplantation or environmental exposure(s).

System	Effect	Assessment by Hx	PE	Test
GENERAL	Active infection	Fever, non-rejection related change in status	↑ Temp, tachycardia with infection	↑ WBC
RESP	Loss of lung functions (% FEV_1)	Recent change in functional capacity, invasive lung infections, meds, lung colonization (resistant bacteria), risk factors, BOS staging; environmental exposure (e.g., diacetyl production)	Tachypnea, wheezes, cough, fever, cyanosis, pulm edema	CXR, PFTs (↓ FEV_1, ↓ O_2 saturation, hypoxia) bronchoscopy for endobronchial biopsy, culture, bronchoalveolar lavage, lung biopsy (diagnosis)
RENAL	Loss of function due to immunosuppression	Change in status, dialysis	A-V fistula (avoidance for procedures), fluid overload, pulm edema, ↑ weight	↓ Renal functions, tachycardia, peripheral edema, SOB
HEME	Thrombocytopenia due to medications	Prolonged bleeding	Bruising	CBC with ↓ platlets, ↑ bleeding time

Key Reference: Yoshihara S, et al. Bronchiolitis obliterans syndrome (BOS), bronchiolitis obliterans organizing pneumonia (BOOP), and other late-onset noninfectious pulmonary complications following allogeneic hematopoietic stem cell transplantation. *Biol Blood Marrow Transplant*. 2007;13:749–759.

Perioperative Implications

Preoperative Preparation

- PFTs for BOS staging and resp status, bronchoscopy for biopsy and culture
- Treat active infections aggressively
- Evaluate renal functions, adjust periop medications where appropriate
- Continue anti-infective and immunosuppressive therapy during the periop period and adjust dosing to keep within the indicated therapeutic range
- Strict aseptic techniques due to immunosuppression
- Premedication useful due to excessive secretions, but avoid excessive resp depression
- Corticosteroids supplementation esp for long, invasive, stressful procedures
- Watch for: Increased sensitivity to opioids, hypercarbia, resp acidosis, bronchial

hyperresponsiveness (bronchoconstriction), hyperkalemia and hypomagnesemia
- Most common side effect of immunosuppressive drugs: Cyclosporine and tacrolimus (HTN, diabetes, neurotoxicity, renal failure), OKT3 (leucopenia, fever, anaphylaxis), azathioprine (anemia, thrombocytopenia)

Monitoring

- Routine
- Consider arterial line placement if hypoxic, acidotic or O_2 saturation inadequate—invasive monitoring must be carefully weighed against possibility of infection from intravascular catheters
- TEE may be helpful in monitoring cardiac functioning in post heart-lung transplant pts, and when there is evidence of pulm edema and pulm Htn
- CVP insertion recommended (when necessary) on side of native lung (one lung transplant)

Airway

- ETT cuff placement should avoid tracheal anastomosis
- Oral intubation is preferred over nasal intubation (infection, thrombocytopenia)
- Increase FIO_2
- Use aseptic tracheal suction technique

Induction

- Short acting agents are preferred and adjust doses to pt status and to avoid prolonged CV depression

Maintenance

- Avoid fluid overload (disruption of lymphatic drainage in posttransplant cases can lead to pulm edema with fluid overload)
- **Significant reductions of cyclosporine or tacrolimus blood levels can be caused by dilution with IV fluids**

• Adjust neuromuscular blocking dosage due to interactions with immunosuppressive agents and adjust dosage if renal impairment. (Cyclosporine enhances the effect of muscle relaxants producing a prolonged block.)

• Prevent additional mechanical obstruction (ventilator-induced disease and excessive tidal volumes).

• **Hyperventilation during mechanical ventilation should be avoided because seizure threshold in pts taking immunosuppressive agents may be lowered.**

• Use shorter-acting agents to avoid prolonged CNS, CV, and resp depression to facilitate a swift recovery of functions and timely extubation.

Extubation

• Delay until adequate ventilation assured (sustained tetanus on monitoring).

• The lack of cough reflex below the tracheal anastomosis makes pts unable to clear secretions, unless they are awake, increasing the risk of silent aspiration.

Adjuvants

• Consider regional technique for anesthesia/periop analgesia.

Postoperative Period

• Monitor for and aggressively treat resp depression, infection, and fluid overload.

Anticipated Problems/Concerns

• Many pts with resting hypoxia and marginal compensated lung functions come to OR for diagnostic lung biopsy. A thoracoscopic technique may be impossible owing to adhesions post heart/lung transplantation or inability to tolerate one-lung ventilation.

• Anticipate further perioperative resp decompensation after open-lung biopsy.

• Arrange postop disposition (monitored bed and ventilator support) depending on preop functional status and the potential for periop complications.

Bronchitis, Chronic

C. William Hanson III

Risk

- Incidence in USA: 14 million
- Race with highest prevalence: Caucasian
- M:F ratio: 1:2
- Smoking, second-hand smoke, occupational exposure to pulm toxic substances (radon, coal, silicates, asbestos)

Perioperative Risks

- Bronchospasm

Worry About

- Airway stimulation at light levels of anesthesia
- Laryngospasm (due to secretions and hyperreactivity)
- Hypoxia
- Hypercarbia

Overview

- Chronic productive cough with periodic exacerbations (most d for at least 3 mo and for at least 2 consecutive y)
- Enlargement of the mucus-secreting glands in the airways with excessive sputum production
- Expiratory airways obstruction
- Derangement in V/Q relationships
- Chronic hypoxia with right heart failure
- Exacerbations with intercurrent bacterial or viral infections

ICD-9-CM Code: 491.9

Etiology

- Acquired, usually due to smoking
- May also be due to asthma or frequent childhood resp infections

Usual Treatment

- Avoidance of environmental irritants such as cigarette smoke (preferably >8–10 wk prior to elective surgery)
- Antibiotics for acute exacerbations; inefficacious for prophylactic treatment
- Oral glucocorticoids appropriate for acute exacerbations but not for maintenance therapy
- Short-acting bronchodilators, such as beta agonists or anticholinergics, for acute exacerbations; long-acting beta agonist bronchodilators plus inhaled steroids for long-term maintenance therapy

ASSESSMENT POINTS

System	Effect	Assessment by Hx	PE	Test
HEENT			Short, fat neck	
CV	Right heart failure	Exercise tolerance	RV heave Dependent edema	ECG ECHO
	Pulm Htn			PA catheter
RESP	Airways obstruction	Smoking Hx (current, recent, remote) Number and severity of recent exacerbations	Cyanosis	PFT, DLco, ABGs
MS			Clubbing of fingers	

Key Reference: Tamul PC, Peruzzi WT. Assessment and management of patients with pulmonary disease. *Crit Care Med.* 2004;32(suppl 4):S137–S145.

Perioperative Implications

Preoperative Preparation

- Smoking cessation
- Antibiotics to decrease sputum production
- Resp conditioning

Monitoring

- Consider arterial line to monitor blood gases
- Consider pulm artery catheter for large fluid shift operations

Airway

- Often, truncal obesity (esp with corticosteroids); may have redundant soft tissue in airway or short, fat neck

Preinduction/Induction

- Avoid stimulating the airway while in light levels of anesthesia; may precipitate bronchospasm (although less likely than with asthma)
- Regional anesthesia may be preferable

Maintenance

- Frequent suctioning of ETT
- Limit narcotic administration (danger of periop CO_2 retention)
- Adjuvant regional anesthesia for postop pain management in procedures that affect resp mechanics (e.g., intercostal nerve blocks, epidural analgesia)

Extubation

- Administer intratracheal bronchodilator in responsive pts prior to extubation
- Consider IV lidocaine prior to extubation

Anticipated Problems/Concerns

- Postop resp complications (secretions, mucus plugging, atelectasis, pneumonia, prolonged requirement for mechanical ventilation)

Bronchiopulmonary Dysplasia

Mary A. Keyes

Risk

- The at-risk group is largely comprised of infants born at 24–28 wks gestation who have very low birth weight (VLBW).
- Incidence of bronchopulmonary dysplasia (BPD) is inversely proportional to gestational age.
- Classic BPD occurs in infants with severe RDS requiring prolonged mechanical ventilation and O_2 therapy.
- Other VLBW infants require mechanical ventilation for apnea/poor resp effort likely due to immaturity of central respiratory control.

Perioperative Risks

- Adequate oxygenation and ventilation during intraop period and transport.
- NICU parameters are: Pao_2 50–70 mmHg, $Paco_2$, and pH about 7.3. Goals intraop are to avoid hyperoxia and hypocarbia without predisposing to hypoxemia. GERD common in VLBW infants, which improves with growth.
- Retinopathy of prematurity (ROP) in same at risk infants.
- Postop apnea following general anesthesia or sedation in infants <54 wks PCA.
- Occult RAD in formerly premature infants who otherwise appear well.

Worry About

- Endobronchial or accidental extubation during position changes and transport.
- ETT intubation may lead to airway reactivity and bronchospasm.
- Subglottic stenosis, tracheomalacia, or bronchomalacia may develop following prolonged intubation.
- A pulm exacerbation may be triggered by an upper resp tract infection. Elective procedures postponed 10–14 d following cessation of symptoms.

Overview

- BPD defined as chronic lung disease characterized by O_2 dependence at 36 wks PCA.
- Early use of CPAP and rapid extubation decrease risk of BPD.
- Recurrent infection and inflammation predispose infants to additional pulm injury.
- BPD results from a variety of toxic factors that injure small airways and interfere with alveolarization, leading to reduction in surface area for gas exchange.
- The developing pulm microvasculature can also be injured.
- Recovery is dependent on growth of lung tissue and pulm vasculature.
- Pulm function generally improves with age, but airway hyperreactivity may persist.

- Prolonged mechanical ventilation, pulm Htn, cor pulmonale, and prolonged O_2 dependence are poor prognostic indicators.
- Rehospitalization for pulm disease is most common in the first 2 y of life with gradual decrease in symptom frequency through childhood.

ICD-9-CM Code: 770.7

Etiology

- O_2 and/or O_2-free radicals
- Barotrauma from mechanical ventilation
- Inflammation and infection
- Patent ductus arteriosus leading to increased pulm blood flow
- Excessive fluid administration

Usual Treatment

- Ventilation strategies that limit volume and oxygen exposure
- Early extubation and use of nasal CPAP
- Bronchodilators: Albuterol and/or ipratropium bromide
- Nutritional support for growth and additional work of breathing
- Diuretics and fluid restriction
- Methylxanthines to increase resp drive and decrease apnea

ASSESSMENT POINTS

System	Effects	Assessment by Hx	PE	Test
CV	Cor pulmonale LV failure	Inability to wean from ventilator Poor feeding and weight gain Dyspnea in extubated infant	Tachypnea Sternal retractions Nasal flaring Hepatomegaly Cardiomegaly Pulm rales	CXR ECHO
RESP	↑ Airway reactivity ↑ FRC ↑ $Paco_2$ ↓ Pao_2	Inability to wean from supplemental O_2 or ventilator Poor feeding and weight gain Frequent URI associated with bronchospasm	Tachypnea Sternal retractions Nasal flaring Wheezing/rhonchi	CXR ABGs

Key Reference: Kliegman RM, Behrman RE, Jenson HB, Stanton BF. *Nelson textbook of pediatrics.* 18th ed. Chapter 101.4.

Perioperative Implications

Preoperative Preparation

- Optimal medical management achieved with bronchodilators and diuretics
- Electrolytes and Hg WNL for age
- GERD controlled with medication
- No active infection, if URI present, postpone elective surgery
- Inpatient postop apnea monitoring for infants <54 PCA wks for at least 12 hrs

Monitoring

- Routine
- ABG monitoring indicated if tenuous cardiac or pulm status or major surgery

Airway

- Expect reactive airway

Preinduction/Induction

- Ensure adequate anesthetic depth prior to instrumentation of the airway (once the cycle of bronchospasm and desaturation has been initiated, it is difficult to recover).

Maintenance

- Usually inhalational with sevoflurane
- Judicious use of narcotics

Extubation

- Awake with regular resp pattern during infancy
- Postop apnea monitoring

- Deep extubation as in pt with asthma may be appropriate in older child

Adjuvants

- Spinal anesthesia acceptable in suitable procedures, particularly premature infants

Anticipated Problems/Concerns

- Tenuous pulm status that is challenged during anesthesia and surgery
- Some infants may not fit extubation criteria and require additional mechanical ventilation postop
- Older child with Hx of BPD at risk for RAD.

Buerger's Disease: Thromboangiitis Obliterans

Jeremy Hansen
James Duke

DISEASES

Risk

- Current or recent chronic tobacco/nicotine exposure
- Ashkenazi Jewish ethnicity, prevalence much greater in Eastern Europe, Southeast Asia, Japan
- Age < 45, male gender (M:F ratio: 10–100:1)
- Incidence in the USA: Progressively decreasing in association with decreasing smoking prevalence: < 8–10/100,000

Perioperative Risks

- Similar to any pt with chronic tobacco exposure
- Risks to already compromised perfusion of distal extremities

Worry About

- Co-existing pulm disease as pts are tobacco smokers
- Abnormal Allen test result in young (<45 yr) male smoker with leg ulcerations (classic clinical scenario for Buerger's)
- All extremities as TAO is never confined to a single limb

Overview

- Inflammatory vasculitis of small and medium arteries and veins in extremities
- Classic distribution is infrapopliteal or distal to the brachial artery

- Results in extremity ischemia leading to claudication of calf, foot, forearm, or hands
- Severe ischemia results in ulcerations and gangrene progressing to necrosis and eventual amputation of ischemic extremity
- Olin (2000) criteria:
  - Age <45 years
  - Current or recent history of tobacco use
  - Presence of distal-extremity ischemia indicated by claudication, rest pain, ischemic or gangrenous ulcers, and documentation by non-invasive vascular testing
  - Exclusion of autoimmune diseases (scleroderma, CREST, sclerodactyly, telangectasia), hypercoaguable states (antiphospholipid syndrome or homocysteinemia), or DM
  - Exclusion of proximal embolic source by echocardiography or angiography
- Diagnosis confirmed with biopsy of active lesion showing a highly-cellular thrombus formation with neutrophils, giant cells, microabscesses but intact internal elastic lamina—differentiates from other vasculitis conditions
- Anti-endothelial antibody titers may allow tracking of disease progression and severity.
- Lesions occasionally occur in coronary, mesentaric, and cerebral vasculature, but always present initally in extremities.

ICD-9-CM Code: 443.1 (ICD-10 I73.1)

Etiology

- Autoimmune reaction against vascular endothelial cells potentiated by nicotine exposure
- Anti-endothelial antibodies trigger immune reaction, micro abscesses and thrombosis formation
- Impaired endothelium-mediated vasodilation in peripheral vasculature results in ischemia
- Angiographic evidence of disease exists prior to clinical presentation in unaffected limbs

Usual Treatment

- Complete tobacco and/or nicotine cessation, incl nicotine patches/gum and avoidance of passive smoking, all other treatments are palliative.
- Arterial revascularization is usually not possible given distal and diffuse nature of vascular lesions.
- Sympathectomy can provide palliative short-term pain relief, but no long-term benefit; spinal cord stimulators can provide pain relief.
- Prostaglandins (e.g., IV iloprost), vascular endothelial growth factor gene therapy trials show clinical promise.
- Ultimately, amputation of affected distal digit and/or extremity for nonhealing ulcerations or gangrene.

ASSESSMENT POINTS

System	Effect	Assessment by Hx	PE	Test
CV	Coronary lesions c/w ischemia	Angina, MI, CHF	Third heart sound, regular rhythm or no, rales	ECG, coronary angiography if high suspicion for coronary lesions
RESP	c/w Chronic tobacco exposure	SOB, cough, increased sputum	Findings c/w chronic smoker	PFT results c/w obstructive pattern
HEME	Carboxyhemogobin	Smoking Hx	N/A	Blood gases with co-oxymetry
CNS	Vascular lesions -> cerebral ischemia	Syncopal episodes, TIA, CVA	Carotid bruit	Carotid US, CT angiogram
GI	Mesenteric ischemia	"Intestinal angina"	Abdominal bruit	Mesenteric angiography
EXTREMITIES	Distal ischemia; gangrene	Claudication, rest pain, non-healing lesions, prior amputations	Cool extremities, poor capillary refill, hair loss, thrombosis migrans, ulcerations/gangrene	Allen test, Doppler ultrasound, angiography with e/o "corkscrew collateral" revascularization

Key Reference: Olin JW, Shih A. Thromboangiitis Obliterans (Buerger's Disease). *Curr Opin Rheumatol.* 2006;18(1):18–24.

Perioperative Implications

Preinduction/Induction/Maintenance

- Carefully document locations/extent of distal extremity ulcerations and thrombosis migrans.
- Optimize pre-induction pulmonary status.
- Pay special attention to padding and protection of distal extremities.
- Prevent hypothermia in the entire periop phase by keeping extremities warmed and covered.

Monitoring

- Consider risks vs. benefits of distal arterial, e.g., radial arterial catheterization.

- Femoral arterial line would be a viable option for invasive monitoring.
- Pulse oximetry may be more accurate in a proximal location, such as the ear lobe.

General Anesthesia

- OR ambient temperature should be increased.
- Maintain intravascular volume and avoid alpha agonists if possible.
- Regional anesthesia can be performed safely
- Avoid epinephrine in local anesthetic solutions to limit risk of vasospasm.

Postoperative Period

- Keep distal extremities warm; 40% of pts have concurrent Raynaud's phenomenon

Anticipated Problems/Concerns

- Excellent opportunity to reiterate importance of smoking cessation
- If no critical limb ischemia, smoking cessation will prevent amputation
- Long-term prognosis for major amputation: 11% at 5 y; 21% at 10 y; 23% at 20 y

55

Bulimia

Ronda Flower

Risk

- Affects 5–18% of adolescent girls and young women
- Bulimic symptoms can be part of anorexia nervosa syndrome

Perioperative Risks

- Increased risks (which have not been quantified) of hypotension, cardiac arrhythmias, hypothermia, aspiration of gastric contents, and metabolic abnormalities and their consequences

Worry About

- Reduced cardiac muscle mass with decrease in chamber size, impaired myocardial contractility with decreased cardiac output, and relative hypotension
- Mitral valve prolapse and its arrhythmogenic effects
- Starvation, dehydration and electrolyte abnormalities (hyponatremia, hypokalemia, hypoalbuminemia, hypomagnesemia, hypocalcemia, hypophosphatemia)
- Alterations (hypofunction) in autonomic nervous system function and a hypervagal state
- Abnormal temp regulation
- Decreased gastric emptying, gastric dilatation, diminished GE sphincter tone, aspiration of gastric contents, gastric rupture and accompanying peritonitis
- Mallory-Weiss tear or esophageal rupture leading to acute mediastinitis

Overview

- Eating disorder characterized by binge-eating episodes followed by self-induced vomiting, fasting, and abuse of diuretics or laxatives

- Greatest periop risks are associated with low cardiac output and cardiac arrhythmias
- Hx is characterized by denial and is often unreliable. Pts may report exercise intolerance, cold intolerance, weight fluctuation, syncope

ICD-9-CM Codes: 783.6; 307.51

Etiology

- Unknown; thought to be largely emotional

Usual Treatment

- SSRIs, such as fluoxetine (Prozac), have been found most effective pharmacotherapy. Second line of pharmacologic treatment is with tricyclic antidepressants.
- Cognitive behavioral therapy
- K+ supplements

ASSESSMENT POINTS

System	Effect	Assessment by Hx	PE	Test
CV	Cardiomyopathy, mitral valve prolapse, arrhythmia, ipecac cardiomyopathy	Exercise intolerance, syncope	Heart sounds, BP, pulse	ECG, ECHO
GI	Gastric dilatation, diarrhea Gastric rupture/peritonitis Hepatic dysfunction Inanition	Usually unreliable Projectile vomiting	Skin turgor, pulse, BP, abdomen	Lytes CT scan, ABG, CBC Hepatic enzymes Serum glucose
ENDO	Amenorrhea, "euthyroid sick," ↓ norepinephrine, ↓ vasopressin secretion, abn temp regulation	Cold intolerance		
HEME	Pancytopenia	Bruising, infections	Skin	CBC, plt
RENAL	↓ GFR on basis of dehydration			BUN/Cr
CNS	Depression, ↓ CSF norepinephrine			
MS	Muscle mass	Marked weight fluctuation	Thin	

Key Reference: Suri R, Poist ES, Hager WD, Gross JB. Unrecognized bulimia nervosa: A potential cause of perioperative cardiac dysrhythmias. *Can J Anaesth*. 1999 46(11):1048–1052.

Perioperative Implications

Perioperative Preparation

- Assess cardiac, lyte, hepatic enzymes, volume status, UPT
- Consider urine toxicology screen to rule out co-morbid substance abuse

Monitoring

- Routine
- Arrhythmia, volume status, myocardial function
- Temp monitoring important

Airway

- May have increased risk of aspiration of gastric contents

Induction

- Hypovolemia, myocardial dysfunction, ANS dysfunction may make for CV instability.

Maintenance

- CV instability, volume and lyte status, temp should dictate anesthetic regimen.

Extubation

- Awake due to GI motility dysfunction
- Autonomic hypofunction may lead to sudden postop collapse.

Adjuvants

- Vary if lyte, renal, or hepatic dysfunction exists.

Anticipated Problems/Concerns

- Gastric volume changes may increase risk of aspiration.
- Volume status, lyte, CV, and ANS changes increase risk of hypotension, arrhythmia, and sudden postop collapse
- Habitus and metabolic changes may predispose to hypothermia.
- Menstual irregularities. UPT advised.

Burn Injury, Chemical

Shawn Banks
Albert J. Varon

Risk

- 3% of all reported burn injuries from 1999–2008.
- Risk increases with age; 1% of burn injuries from birth to age 16, 3.7% from 20–30, and 5% from 30–50 according to the National Burn Repository Report on Data from 1999–2008.
- Majority of chemical exposures are occupational, occurring in men of working age. Assaults with caustic chemicals are more likely to occur against women.
- American Association of Poison Control Centers reports approximately 130,000 exposures to caustic substances in 2007.

Perioperative Risks

- Morbidity varies by exposure type and substance. Surface burns may be regarded like thermal burns after decontamination.
- Caustic ingestion may result in perforation and/or bleeding and resp compromise from upper airway edema.

Worry About

- Identify injury setting, chemical involved, areas of exposure, and duration before decontamination.
- Airway compromise may arise from face/ingestion exposures; develop an airway management plan early.
- Occupational exposures may have associated traumatic injuries from explosions, fire, falls, etc.
- Chemical burns may produce more tissue necrosis than their initial appearance would suggest.

Overview

- A large number of chemicals can potentially cause injury incl acids, bases, organic, and inorganic compounds.
- Acid burns generally produce coagulative necrosis; depth may be limited by formation of coagulated proteins at base of burn.
- Bases typically generate liquefactive necrosis; depth often much deeper than acid burns.
- Organic compounds cause direct heat production and chemical reactions that disrupt skin.
- Inorganic compunds bind directly to the skin and create salts that damage skin integrity.
- Severity of the burn is related to a variety of factors incl the pH, concentration, volume, physical form, and contact time duration of the offending agent.

ICD-9-CM Code 940-949; (Burns of internal organs from ingested chemicals: 947)

Etiology

- Surface burns: Most commonly work-related injury, accidental. Upper limbs more commonly injured as these substances are usually handled or carried. Injuries to the lower limbs and face can occur through splashing.
- Ingestions: Pediatric most commonly accidental; adult most frequently suicidal gesture.

Usual Treatment

- Remove contaminated clothes.
- Early decontamination with water or saline irrigation for surface exposures; elemental metals (K^+, lithium) should not be exposed to moisture due to strong exothermic reaction.
- Prevent contaminated irrigation solution from running onto unaffected skin.
- After initial decontamination pt is treated as a typical burn pt.
- Ensure adequate fluid resuscitation for large BSA burns.
- Take measures to prevent complications (e.g., hypothermia, infection, rhabdomyolysis).

ASSESSMENT POINTS

System	Effect	Assessment by Hx	PE	Test
HEENT	Face and airway burns, eye injuries	Dysphonia, odynophagia, dysphagia Visual changes	Denuded or inflamed oral mucosa, conjunctivits	Endoscopy; ophthalmologic evaluation
PULM	Chemical pneumonitis, ARDS	Dyspnea	Hypoxemia, possible rales or evidence of edema, auscultation may be normal	CXR, ABG
CV	Arrhythmias, hypovolemic shock	Palpitations, chest pain, dyspnea	Tachycardia or irregular rhythms	ECG, CXR
GI	Esophagogastritis, perforated viscus	Odynophagia/dysphagia; hematemsis; epigastic pain	Abdominal tenderness/ guarding	Endoscopy; contrast CT scan; x-ray.
RENAL	Electrolyte disturbances, ARF, acute tubular necrosis	Deep or large surface area burns, associated crush injuries	Myoglobinuria, oliguria	Basic metabolic profile (BUN/Cr), urine myoglobin
MS	Rhabdomyolysis, compartment syndromes	Deep or large surface area burns, associated crush injuries	Evolving loss of motor/senory function	Serum myoglobin, compartment pressure monitoring

Key Reference: Seth R, Chester D, Moimen N. A review of chemical burns. *Trauma.* 2007;9:81–94.

Perioperative Implications

Preinduction/Induction/Maintenance

- Review Hx of the current injury, incl the amount of associated TBSA burn, and elapsed time since injury.
- Reliable vascular access is essential for adequate fluid resuscitation.
- Normalization of electrolytes, if possible.
- Preop medication should be used to alleviate anxiety and reduce pain, and to facilitate pt comfort during transfer and transport.

Monitoring

- Adequate intraop monitoring is essential due to the potential for extensive blood loss, frequent changes of position, and duration of surgery.
- Placement of surface monitors can be difficult due to location of burns.
- Try to place invasive lines away from injury, not through damaged skin.
- Consider arterial line placement for extensive debridements/grafting to allow beat-to-beat monitoring and frequent sampling of arterial blood.
- Presence of an arterial line should not preclude placement of an NIBP cuff (backup if arterial line fails during procedure). Negotiate with surgeon best location for NIBP cuff.

General Anesthesia

- Most surface chemical burns that proceed to OR are extensive enough to be treated as thermal injuries.
- Choices for induction and maintenance of general anesthesia depend on associated hemodynamic instability and airway status.
- Muscle relaxants: Avoid succinylcholine after acute phase (first 24 hr), resistance to nondepolarizers may evolve after acute phase.
- Narcotic tolerance may be higher in the chronic phase.
- Transfusions may be required in extensive debridement procedures.
- Epinephrine-soaked pads may be applied by surgeon to decrease bleeding. This may result in tachycardia and a falsely stable BP that deteriorates after removal of pads.
- Thermoregulation is impaired. Warm OR as much as possible. Apply forced-air heating blankets. Administer warmed fluids and blood products.
- Extubation in the acute phase should be carefully considered if there is suspicion of airway edema or difficult reintubation.

Regional Anesthesia

- No contraindication in small or peripheral injuries.
- Preferrable to place block through intact skin.
- Excision and grafting procedures may be accompanied by large fluid shifts and blood loss, in which case the loss of sympathetic tone resulting from a neuraxial block may be undesirable.

Postoperative Period

- Acute, extensive injury may require ICU care.
- Pain management can be challenging in chronic phase.

Anticipated Problems/Concerns

- Early, goal-directed resuscitation and correction of electrolyte abnormalities.
- Careful monitoring of airway and early airway intervention, if needed.
- Maintain normothermia.

Burn Injury, Electrical

Christian Diez
Albert J. Varon

Risk

• 3–5% of all burns are electrical. Low-voltage burns (less than 1000 volts) commonly occur in children at the home.
• High-voltage burns (1000 volts or greater) are more common in adults and characteristically occur in outdoor environments near power sources and lines.
• Lightning electrical burns carry the highest rate of mortality and usually have energy greater than 30 million volts.

Perioperative Risks

• Pts with an acute burn or a Hx of burns may present an additional challenge to securing the airway. Fluid resuscitation in acutely burned pts may cause severe airway edema; pts with a history of burns, esp facial, may have limited mobility of mouth opening and neck extension.
• Difficult IV access is a common problem. Two large bore IVs are commonly needed for major burn surgery, however, depending on length of stay and surface area burn, central access and intra-arterial monitoring of BP may be necessary.

Worry About

• Arrhythmias and cardiac arrest.
• Resp failure and edematous airway. Resp failure may occur due to tetany of resp muscles or cerebral injury.
• Blunt injuries, fractures, and dislocations if pts were jolted from electrical shock or fell from high places.

• Compartment syndrome: Delayed exploration and decompression may result in increased amputation rates along with increased organ failure and mortality.
• Rhabdomyolysis and myoglobinuria from muscle injury leading to obstructive nephropathy and renal failure.

Overview

• Severity of electrical burn depends on current, route taken by the current, and the duration of contact with the electrical source.
• Entry wounds occur often in the hands with a leathery, charred appearance. Exit wounds are often explosive.
• Extent of injury may be misleading as visibly burned area is often small. Large amounts of destroyed tissue may be present under normal appearing skin leading to under resuscitation.
• Signs of electrical injury incl loss of consciousness, extremity mummification, loss of pulses in an extremity, myoglobinuria, elevated serum creatinine kinase, and cardiac arrest.
• The electrical current in most households is between 110–220V, which may produce a low-voltage burn and dysrhythmias. High-voltage burns often cause immediate cardiac arrest and/or resp paralysis.
• Direct lightning strikes are rarely survivable.

ICD-9-CM Code: 948 (Burns classified according to extent of body surface involved); 994.8 (Electrocution and nonfatal effects of electric current); 994.0 (Effects of lightning)

Etiology

• Causes vary greatly from electrical appliances in water, to work related accidents.
• Children may be involved in low-voltage burns at home. One frequent cause is chewing at electrical cords causing oral mucosa burns.

Usual Treatment

• If ventricular fibrillation or asystole is present, CPR must be immediately initiated. If initial dysrhythmias are present, continuous cardiac monitoring is required since most serious dysrhythmias occur within 24 hr. If dysrhythmia not present on arrival and no cardiac arrest at the scene, further cardiac monitoring is not necessary.
• Secure airway if needed and obtain appropriate IV access.
• If myoglobinuria present, maintain urine output over 100 cc/hr with generous hydration. Consider sodium bicarbonate infusion to alkalinize urine and mannitol to help maintain urine output.
• Escharotomy and fasciotomy may be required for vascular or nerve decompression.
• Indications for surgical decompression incl progressive neurologic dysfunction, vascular compromise, increased compartment pressure, and systemic clinical deterioration from suspected ongoing myonecrosis.

ASSESSMENT POINTS

System	Effect	Assessment by Hx	PE	Test
DERM	Burn injuries, edema, compartment syndrome	Prehospital information, mechanism of injury	Remove all clothing to determine nature and extent of injury, check peripheral pulses	Measurement of comparttment pressures (>30 mmHg, or within 10–20 mmHg of diastolic pressure)
CARDIO	Arrhythmias, hypovolemia	Arrest in the field, ventricular fibrillation, high voltage burn	Hypotension, bradycardia or tachycardia	EKG
RESP	Paralysis, edema	Lightning or high voltage injury	Signs of hypoxia	ABG, pulse oximetry
HEME	Hemolysis, vascular thrombosis, dehydration	Extensive tissue injury	Edema, extensive burns	Hematocrit
RENAL	Obstructive nephropathy, renal failure	High >> Low-voltage injury	Large muscle destruction and tissue necrosis	Urine myoglobin, BUN/Cr
NEURO	Peripheral and central neuropathies	Injury that crosses midline, limb compartment syndrome	Neurologic deficits	MRI

Key Reference: Lovich-Sapola JA. Anesthesia for burns. In: Smith CE, ed. *Trauma anesthesia*. Cambridge, New York: Cambridge University Press; 2008:322–342.

Preoperative Implications

Preinduction

• Burn pts have increased metabolic rate; NPO time should be kept to a safe minimum.
• Surgeon to anticipate extent of surgery and amount blood loss.
• Careful airway evaluation as an increased risk for airway edema and skin or muscle rigidity due to burns.
• Labs checked incl blood gases, K⁺, and type and cross.
• Large bore IV access may be needed in cases of complex debridement/grafting.

Perioperative Implications

General Anesthesia

• Selected for most large skin graft procedures.
• Many pts already receiving ventilation support.

• Recommended for cases in which large blood loss anticipated.

Monitoring

• Standard ASA monitors. May be difficult to place monitors on burned surfaces. Use of staples and/or sutures to secure ECG leads or catheters may be required.
• Arterial monitoring may be necessary for large procedures or for pts receiving prolonged ventilatory support. Ultrasound can facilitate arterial cannulation.
• Maintaining normothermia is a major challenge. Ambient temp in OR must be raised, fluid warmers used, and sterile forced-air warmers may be needed.

Induction

• Many pts are catecholamine depleted. Induction agents such as ketamine may be useful

in pts that are not already receiving ventilatory support.
• In burn pts succinylcholine is contraindicated after 24 hr from their injury. In addition, larger doses of non-depolarizing muscle relaxants may be required for adequate muscle relaxation.
• Larger doses of narcotics may also be needed since burn pts often develop tolerance to the narcotics. The analgesic properties of ketamine make it a good choice for induction.

Maintenance

• Choice of inhaled anesthetic does not alter outcome.
• Judicious use of crystalloids, RBCs, and fresh frozen plasma to maintain normal blood volume and composition, and to avoid worsening edema.

Regional Anesthesia
• Can be used for analgesia after determining cause and extent of any neurologic sequelae and excl possibility of a compartment syndrome.
• May be used for anesthesia during minor procedures.

Postoperative Period
• Standard extubation criteria should be followed paying special attention to total fluids given and the possibility of airway edema.

• Increased analgesic demands. Consider physical ability to activate pt-controlled anagelsia (PCA) before instituting it.
• Careful monitoring during transport, esp in critically ill pts.

Anticipated Problems/Concerns
• Minimize the possibility of renal failure by maintaining adequate urine output and alkalinizing the urine.

• Monitor edema during surgery as the ETT tape may become a facial tourniquet or the tube may migrate outside glottis.
• Pts that develop sepsis or multiorgan failure have worse outcome.
• Burn pts have an increased incidence of infection. Therefore, meticulous aseptic care during line placement, intubation, and all invasive procedures is essential.

Burn Injury, Flame

Shawn Banks
Albert J. Varon

Risk

- American Burn Association reports that flame injuries account for 40% of all burn cases from 1999–2008.
- Estimated 500,000 burn-injured pts sought medical attention in 2007.
- Approx 70% of injuries are accidental, nonwork related.
- Approx 70% of injuries occur at home.

Perioperative Risks

- Major predictors of mortality: BSA >40%, age > 60, presence of inhalation injury.
- Predicted mortality is 0.3%, 3%, 33%, or 90%, depending on whether zero, one, two, or three of the above risk factors are present.
- Up to ⅓ of pts with inhalation injury will develop acute airway obstruction.
- Other incidental traumatic injuries may be present.

Worry About

- Airway protection and ventilation.
- Hypovolemia: Early goal-directed volume resuscitation is the single-most important therapeutic intervention.
- Hypothermia.

Overview

- Direct thermal energy produces direct cellular destruction and coagulative necrosis.
- Systemic microvascular integrity is lost in massive inflammatory response; proteins are lost into interstitial space.
- Significant shift of fluids, electrolytes, and proteins into the interstitium with rapid equilibrium of intravascular and interstitial compartments.
- Changes reflected by massive edema formation and loss of circulating plasma volume, hemoconcentration, decreased urine output, and depressed CV function.
- Cardiac output is reduced due to hypovolemia, decreased contractility, and increased afterload.
- Most of the edema occurs at the burn site and is maximal at 24 hr after the injury. Edema results in tissue hypoxia and increased tissue pressure with circumferential injuries.

ICD-9-CM Codes: 940–949 (948—Burn classified by percent body affected)

Etiology

- American Burn Association stratifies thermal injury etiologies as: Fire, hot liquids, contact with hot objects, electrical sources. Flame burns are the most lethal of all thermal injuries.

Usual Treatment

- Most important points of initial phase are assessment of current (and prediction of subsequent) airway patency and documentation of the presence or absence of inhalation injury.
- Early intubation likely if face/inhalation injury or if BSA injured requires aggressive fluid resuscitation.
- Provide supplemental O_2 and monitor O_2 saturation in all burn pts with significant injury. Most pts with large burns will require prompt ET intubation and mechanical ventilatory support.
- Prompt establishment of large-bore IV access and rapid initiation of fluid resuscitation. Parkland or "Universal" formula is most commonly used (4 ml/kg/BSA% over 24 hr, first half given over first 8 hr).
- Insert urinary catheter early to monitor urine output as guide for volume status.
- Evaluate all extremities and chest wall for potential compartment requiring fasciotomy or escharotomy for urgent release.
- Multiple skin grafting procedures may be necessary during admission.
- Early debridement of eschar is performed to minimize infection; dead tissue readily supports bacterial growth.

ASSESSMENT POINTS

System	Effect	Assessment by Hx	PE	Test
HEENT	Face and airway burns	Dysphonia, dysphagia. Reports of fumes or extraction from enclosed space	Singed face or nose hair, carbonaceous sputum, facial burns	Oral inspection, laryngoscopy, bronchoscopy
CV	Arrhythmias, hypovolemic shock, myocardial depression	Palpitations, dyspnea. Loss of consciousness, depressed mental status	Tachycardia or irregular rhythms, hypotension	ECG
RESP	Pneumonitis, ARDS, restrictive disease from eschar, carboxyhemoglobinemia	Cough, dyspnea, stridor	Hypoxemia, circumferential chest eschar	ABG, co-oximetry, chest radiograph
RENAL	Acute renal failure, ATN, electrolyte disturbances	Large BSA burns, crush injuries	Myoglobinuria, oliguria	Electrolyte profile (BUN/Cr), urine myoglobin, urinalysis
CNS	Hypoxemia	Loss of consciousness, confusion	Focused neurologic exam	ABG, co-oximetry
MS	Tissue destruction, rhabdomyolysis, compartment syndrome	Large BSA burns, over-administration of fluids	Evolving loss of motor and/or sensory function	Serum myoglobin, compartment or bladder pressure monitoring

Key Reference: Latenser BA. Critical care of the burn patient: The first 48 hours. *Crit Care Med.* 2009;37(10), 2819–2826.

Perioperative Implications

Preoperative Preparation

- Thermoregulation is impaired. Warm OR as much as possible before pt arrives. Use forced-air warming blankets and fluid warmers intraop.
- Anesthesia services may be requested for bedside debridement and other procedures; adds the challenges of off-site care.
- Assess location and adequacy of venous access.
- Document presence of other invasive devices (arterial catheter, ET or tracheostomy tubes, feeding tubes, etc.) and ventilatory settings.

Monitoring

- Standard monitors may be difficult to apply to extensive burns.
- Arterial line is advisable for extensive grafting procedures that can be long and involve significant blood loss.
- Central venous access may be necessary if peripheral access sites are burned. Lines should preferentially be placed through intact skin.

Airway

- Intubate with largest feasible ETT to aid pulm toilet, minimize mucus plugging, and decrease work of breathing. Need for postop mechanical ventilation is common.

Preinduction/Induction

- Succinylcholine should be avoided after acute phase (first 24 hr after injury).
- Gastroparesis and high residual gastric volumes are common after injury; use aspiration precautions.
- Induction agent doses should be adjusted in the context of hypovolemic shock.

Maintenance

- Requirements for neuromuscular blockers usually increased. Attributed to increased binding sites at extrajunctional receptors.
- Pts may need significantly increased levels of narcotics.
- Keep the OR room temp at ≥ 85°F to minimize heat loss and decrease metabolic rate.
- Communicate decreases in core body temp to surgeons; case may be shortened to prevent severe hypothermia.

Extubation

- Cautiously consider extubation in early stages of management. Emergent reintubation may be very difficult due to edema.

Anticipated Problems/Concerns

- Most common complications: Pneumonia, UTI, resp failure, cellulitis, and sepsis.
- Ventilator-associated pneumonia may develop in 70% of pts with inhalation injury.
- Pain management is usually challenging. Opioid doses often significantly exceed recommended standard dosing guidelines. Autograft donor sites are very painful; regional analgesia may be useful.
- Abdominal compartment syndrome (ACS) is a life-threatening complication caused by high-volume resuscitation. Extremity compartment syndromes can also result from extensive edema formation.
- Incidence of DVT in burn pts is increased (1% to 23%). Therefore, DVT chemoprophylaxis is routinely used.

Calcium Deficiency/Hypocalcemia

Paul Tarasi
Joe Talarico

Risk

- Common in critically ill pts.
- Reported to range from 26% in hospitalized, non-ICU pts to 88% in critically ill ICU pts.

Perioperative Risks

- Neuromuscular instability leading to seizure, laryngospasm, bronchospasm, or resp arrest
- Impaired cardiac function: Heart failure, hypotension, and dysrhythmias

Worry About

- Symptomatic hypocalcemia

Overview

- Normal serum calcium content: 8.5–10.5 mg/dL
  - 40–50% bound to plasma proteins (albumin)
  - 45–50% ionized (physiologically active)
  - 10–15% non-ionized, bound to inorganic anions such as as phosphate, citrate, and sulfate
- Total calcium level can also be affected by albumin level, acid-base status.
- Ionized calcium level is the preferred measurement (normal: 4.75–5.3 mg/dL [1.19–1.33 mmol/L])
- Physiologic role of calcium:

- Muscle contraction
- Exocrine/endocrine/neurocrine hormone secretion
  - Cell growth
  - Transport and/or secretion of fluids

ICD-9-CM Code: 275.41

Etiology

- Acute
  - Severe, acute hyperphosphatemia (tumor lysis syndrome, acute renal failure, rhabdomyolysis)
  - Acute critical illness (sepsis, burns, pancreatits, fat embolism)
  - Large-volume transfusion with citrated blood (chelation) or albumin
  - Medications: Protamine, heparin, glucagon
  - Acute hypoparathyroidism after thyroidectomy/parathyroidectomy
  - Alkalosis (metabolic/respiratory): increased calcium binding to proteins
- Chronic
  - Hereditary/acquired hypoparathyroidism
  - Hypomagnesemia
  - Chronic renal failure
  - Hyperphosphatemia
  - Vitamin D deficiency

- Pseudohypoparathyroidism
- Osteoblastic metastatic disease (breast, prostate cancer)
- Most common causes of acute intraop hypocalcemia: Acute hyperventilation (resp alkalosis) and massive infusion of citrated blood products (>1.5mL/kg/min)

Usual Treatment

- No need to treat low total calcium level if ionized calcium level is normal.
- Asymptomatic hypocalcemia rarely requires treatment.
- Symptomatic hypocalcemia requires emergent treatment.
- 3–5 mL 10% calcium chloride (27.2 mg Ca^{2+}/mL) or 10–20 mL 10% calcium gluconate (9.3 mg Ca^{2+}/mL) over 10 min.
  - Follow with 0.3–2 mg/kg/hr elemental calcium if continuous replacement is needed.
  - Administer slowly as venous irritation can occur. Central venous admisistration is preferred as calcium chloride can cause tissue necrosis if extravasated from a peripheral vein.
  - Must rule out hypomagnesemia/hyperphosphatemia. Treat as needed.

ASSESSMENT POINTS

System	Effect	Assessment by Hx	PE	Test
CV	Calcium involved in generation of cardiac pacemaker activity and generation of cardiac action potential	Hx of dysrhythmia SOB (or other symptoms of heart failure)	Prolonged QT Hypotension Pulm vascular congestion	EKG Continuous cardiac monitoring Chest x-ray
HEME	Citrate in stored blood products chelates calcium	Massive transfusion of citrated blood products (>1.5 mL/kg/min)		Ionized calcium level
GASTRO	GI smooth muscle spasm	Abdominal cramping		
RESP	Resp smooth muscle contraction/tetany	SOB Laryngospasm Bronchospasm	Hypoxia Stridor Wheezing Resp arrest	Pulse oximetry
NEURO	Calcium is essential for all muscular movement. Calcium is involved in the muscular excitation/contraction coupling.	Muscle spasm Seizure Depression Psychosis Irritability Circumoral numbness Tingling in fingers/toes	Facial grimacing Seizure Papilledema (secondary to increased intracranial pressure) Irritability	Chvostek's sign (twitch of circumoral muscles with tapping of the facial nerve anterior to the ear) Trousseau's sign: Carpal spasm induced by inflation of a BP cuff to 20 mmHg above systolic BP for 3 min
INTEG			Dry scaley skin Brittle nails	

Key Reference: Barash PG, et al, ed. *Clinical Anesthesia*, 6th ed. Lipincott, 2009:315–317. Fauci AS, et al, ed. *Harrison's Principles of Internal Medicine* 17th ed. McGraw, 2008:2393.

Perioperative Implications

Preinduction/Induction/Maintenance

- Correct symptomatic hypocalcemia preop.
- Goal of treatment is to eliminate symptoms, not necessarily return calcium levels to normal range.

Monitoring

- Serial ionized calcium measurements.
- Continuous EKG monitoring.

General Anesthesia

- Negative inotropic effects of anesthetic medications may become more pronounced.

Regional Anesthesia

- Hypocalcemia results in increased neuronal membrane irritability/tetany.
- Parasthesia is a common finding.
- Thorough Hx and physical exam is essential.

Postoperative Period

- Acute hypocalcemia may develop after thyroidectomy/parathyroidectomy.

Anticipated Problems/Concerns

- Risk of hypocalcemia with massive transfusion of citrated blood products (>1.5 mL/kg/min).
- Alkalosis increases Ca^{2+} binding to proteins, therefore decreasing ionized calcium.

Cancer, Bladder

Ashish C. Sinha

Risk

- Primary risk factor is smoking (smokers are more than twice as likely to get bladder cancer as nonsmokers)
- Incidence: Males 37 per 100,000; females 9 per 100,000
- No associate increased risk with alcohol or caffeine consumption
- Median age of diagnosis: 73 y
- Caucasian > African-Americans
- Quitting smoking decreases risk over time (baseline in 5–8 y)
- Incidence on a decline since 1999

Perioperative Risks

- Risks varies based on surgical procedure and co-existing disease
- Chemotherapy: Pulm fibrosis, renal and cardiac dysfunction
- Fatty infiltration of liver in those with poor nutritional status
- Protein-calorie malnutrition due to the cancer, metabolism and anorexia: anemia, hypoalbuminemia; dehydration

Overview

- Transitional cell cancer generally systemic disease at time of Dx—60% will die of metastatic complications

- Pts are typically elderly with long Hx of smoking, thereby promoting concurrent diseases; COPD, lung CA, artherosclerosis, angina, CAD, CHF, Htn
- Chemotherapy/radiation therapy may be used preop, thus complicating periop period

Survival and Stage

- 5-y relative survival (%):
  - In situ (only in the layer of cells in which it began): 96.6
  - Localized (confined to primary site): 73.3
  - Regional (spread to regional lymph nodes): 36.1
  - Distant (cancer has metastasized): 5.6

Worry About

- Significant blood loss (type and cross blood products)
- Hyperextension of lumbar spine/pelvis and compression of iliac veins results in reduced venous return of blood volume
- Adequate padding of peripheral nerves (upper and lower extremities)
- Maintenance of neutral neck position in flexed body position
- Monitoring of UO difficult after ligation/division of ureters

ICD-9-CM Code 188.9

Etiology

- Exposure to aromatic amines (arylamines): β-naphthylamine in cigarette smoke causes bladder cancer in mice.
- Work-related exposure: β-naphthylamine and benzene in the manufacture of rubber products, arylamines in synthetic textile and hair dyes, paint pigments
- Drivers of diesel trucks
- "Slow acetylators" (homozygous, autosomal recessive) may be at higher risk; *N*-acetyltransferase may detoxify aromatic amines.

Usual Treatment

- Chemotherapy
- Doxorubicin/bleomycin/cyclophosphamide/cisplatin/methotrexate; 5-fluorouracil/vinblastine/teniposide
- Radiation therapy
- Transurethral fulgeration
- Radical cystectomy

ASSESSMENT POINTS

System	Effect	Assessment by Hx	PE	Test
CV	Doxorubicin (Adriamycin) toxicity; cardiomyopathy	>550 mg/m², prior or concurrent mediastinal radiation therapy	Signs of CHF	Endomyocardial biopsy, serial ECHO; radionuclide angiography, DL_{co}, ECG
	5- Fluorouracil Myocardial ischemia (rare)	Angina		ECG
	Cyclophosphamide Pericarditis with effusion	CHF	Signs of CHF	ECHO
RESP	Smoking-related injury	Cough, sputum, infections	Wheezes, rhonchi, barrel chest	CXR PFT
	Bleomycin or cyclophosphamide toxicity: pulm fibrosis	>500 mg (bleo), cough, dyspnea	Rales, fever	CXR
	Methotrexate: Inflammation		Pulm edema, effusions, infiltrates	CXR
RENAL	Cisplatin: ATN	Occurs 3–5 d after course		BUN, Cr, proteinuria, hyperuricemia
	Methotrexate: Renal failure			Hematuria, proteinuria
HEPATIC	Methotrexate: Fibrosis			SGPT
CNS	Methotrexate: Encephalopathy	Confusion, somnolence, ataxia, tremors, focal signs		

Key Reference: Whalley DG, Berrigan MJ. Anesthesia for radical prostatectomy, cystectomy, nephrectomy, pheochromocytoma, and laproscopic procedures. *Anesthesiol Clin North America*. 2000;18:899–917.

Preoperative Implications

Preoperative Preparation
- Consider rehydration after bowel preparation
- 2 large bore IVs or one peripheral IV plus a central line

Monitoring
- Considering arterial catheterization
- Renal perfusion difficult to judge after division of ureters: Consider CVP or PAC or TEE
- Anesthesia technique
- Consider combined general-epidural anesthesia to treat postop incisional pain, reduce blood

loss and fluid requirements for cystectomy as well as less risk of postop ileus
- Epidural placement ideally T9, T11

Induction
- Watch for hypotension due to volume depletion from prep and/or decreased systolic function from cardiotoxic chemotherapeutic agents

Maintenance
- Avoid high concentrations of O_2 in pulm fibrosis
- Consider avoiding N_2O (bowel surgery)
- Maximize efforts to prevent hypothermia

Postoperative Considerations
- Consider overnight ventilation if long procedure, significant blood loss/fluid resuscitation. Epidural catheter can optimize pulm toilet and recovery.
- Fluids shifts occur during first 48 hr
- EBL: TURBT about 200 mL; cystectomy between 500–1000 mL
- Pain score: 7–9 (cystectomy)

Cancer, Breast

Vincent S. Cowell

Risk

- 100 times more common in women than men
- 1 in 8 women develop breast cancer. Besides skin cancer, most common cancer in USA for women
- The chance of getting breast cancer goes up as women get older. About 2 out of 3 women with invasive breast cancer are 55 or older when the cancer is found
- Racial predilection: Caucasians > African-Americans > Asians, Hispanics, and Native Americans
- African-Americans are more likely to die of breast cancer because their cancers tend to be more aggressive.
- 10% of breast cancer cases are directly due to inherited mutations of the *BRCA1* and *BRCA2* gene
- Increased risk: Family Hx among close blood relatives, personal Hx increases the risk of developing a new cancer in the other breast.
- >70% of breast cancers are diagnosed in women with no family Hx
- Associated increased risk: Obesity, high-fat diets, aging, high alcohol consumption, and estrogen exposure

Perioperative Risks

- Mortality very rare
- Lymphedema of arm following axillary node dissection
- Ipsilateral brachial plexus injury from extensive abduction of the arm, or iatrogenic
- Injury to long thoracic and/or thoracodorsal n. during surgical dissection of axilla
- Rare incidence of unrecognized pneumothorax
- Breast surgery is associated with postop N/V, incidence as high as 60%

Worry About

- Systemic or regional impact of metastasis to lung, brain, or bones
- High incidence of postop N/V
- NMB and identification of major n.
- Access to an upper extremity may be restricted or limited
- Potential adverse effects of chemotherapeutic drugs and chest radiation therapy

Overview

- Abnormal growth of adenomatous tissue that results in systemic symptoms and metastasizes to liver, bone, lung, and brain
- Early detection of breast cancer increases time of survival
- There is controversy over the role of mammography in detection of breast cancer.
- Physical exam and mammography are complementary.
- Needle biopsies provide histological Dx.
- Presurgical needle localization may be necessary for nonpalpable lesions.
- Most breast biopsies yield benign diagno

ICD-9-CM Code: 174

Etiology

- Cause of most breast cancers is still not known
- BRCA genetic mutations

Usual Treatment

- Noninvasive breast cancer: Lumpectomy or partial mastectomy rarely with sentinel node Bx and/or axillary node dissection with radiation and/or hormonal therapy (e.g., tamoxifen)
- Invasive breast cancer: Lumpectomy, partial mastectomy with SLN Bx, possible ALND or radiation, possible chemotherapy, possible hormonal therapy
- Radical mastectomy rarely performed
- Reconstructive surgery integral part of management

Prognosis

- In the US about 40,410 women will die from breast cancer this year, making it the second most lethal cancer in women (lung cancer is the leading cancer killer in women).
- The 5-year survival rate for women diagnosed with cancer is 80%. About 88% of women diagnosed wih breast cancer will survive at least 10 years. Unfortunately, women in lower social and economic groups still have significantly lower survival rates than women in higher groups.

ASSESSMENT POINTS

System	Effect	Assessment by Hx	PE
CHEST	Lung lesions	Nipple discharge Chest pain or discomfort	Breast as Nipple di crusting Nipple re Skin dim
GI	Liver metastasis	Fatigue, abdominal pain	Enlarged
HEME	Bone metastasis	Lethargy, SOB	Anemia,
CNS	Brain metastasis	Change in mental status, seizures	Neurolog
MS	Bone metastasis Pathologic fractures	Severe pain Immobility Arm swelling	Deformit Pain on p Axillary a

Key Reference: Vila Jr H, Liu J, Kavasmaneck D. Paravertebral block: New benefits from an old procedure.

Handwritten notes:

CANCER ACs.

Think: (GENERAL)
1) MASS
2) Metabolic
3) Meds (i.e. chemo, rads)
4) Malnourished (i.e. ↑ risk post-operative pulm. edema)
5) Metastasis.

Perioperative Implications

Preoperative Preparation

- Optimal preop preparation, in response to associated anxiety, which can be achieved through both pharmacologic and nonpharmacologic means

Monitoring

- Routine with attention to placement of ECG leads
- IV site and BP cuff on contralateral arm

Airway

- Table arrangements may warrant a secure airway
- Nasal O_2 or LMA may be appropriate

Induction

- Thoracic epidurals, intercostal nerve blocks; and local infiltration have successfully been administered as primary anesthetics and adjuvants to GA

Maintenance

- Consideration for the high incidence of postop N/V
- Incision over operative breast that can also incl axilla
- Dissection can incl breast areolar tissue, muscle down to chest wall, and extension into axilla
- Identification of thoracodorsal and long thoracic n. often requires stimulation that contraindicates presence of NM blocking agents
- Surgical field will be in view and allow for monitoring of active blood loss
- Surgical team leaning on chest can affect ventilatory performance

Postoperative Considerations

- Pain score: 2–6
- Pain adequately managed with Torodol, narcotic PCA, or regional block
- Communicate with PACU that no venous sticks or BP measurements should be performed on arm of operative side when axillary lymph node dissection is involved.

Anticipated Problems/Concerns

- Anxiety associated with the fear of breast cancer and altered body image can be quite significant

Cancer, Bronchial

John P. McCarren

Risk

- Incidence in USA: 160, 000 cases/y
- Race: No difference among ethnic groups when >30 cigarettes/d smoked, but higher in people of Asian ancentry, African Americans, and Native Hawaiians when < 30 cigarettes/d smoked
- Tobacco cigarette consumption is the major risk factor; males slightly > females

Perioperative Risks

- Resp and cardiac complications: Atelectasis, pneumonia, pulm edema, resp insufficiency, right ventricular dysfunction, arrhythmias, and ischemia

Worry About

- Endobronchial obstruction, obstructive pneumonitis, consolidation, atelectasis, localized air trapping, and resp insufficiency

- Metastasis: Brain, bone, adrenal glands, pericardium, pleura, mediastinum, endobronchial
- Paraneoplastic syndromes: Cushing, SIADH, hypercalcemia, neuromuscular (Lambert-Eaton myasthenic syndrome (LEMS), cerebellar degeneration, myopathy, neuropathy, dermatomyositis), hematologic (migratory thrombophlebitis, marantic endocarditis, DIC).
- Desaturation during one lung ventilation (OLV)

Overview

- Histology: Squamous, adeno-, large cell, and small-cell carcinomas
- Leading cause of cancer deaths in USA for both men and women; 20% 1-y and 8% 5-y survival
- Severe COPD may limit lung resection and affects periop management
- Paraneoplastic syndromes occasionally affect management

ICD-9-CM Code 162.9

Etiology

- 85% related to cigarette smoking; other risk factors are passive smoking, ionizing radiation, asbestos, heavy metal exposure (arsenic, chromate), halo ethers, polycyclic aromatic hydrocarbons, vinyl chloride, formaldehyde, and genetic factors

Usual Treatment

- Surgical resection for localized non–small cell carcinoma
- Chemotherapy, radiation therapy for small-cell carcinoma
- Unresectable endobronchial or endotracheal tumors treated with external beam radiation and/or bronchoscopic laser resection

ASSESSMENT POINTS

System	Effect	Assessment by Hx	PE	Test
HEENT	Tracheal fixation or obstruction	Dyspnea, cough, stridor	Rhonchi	CXR, CT, PFT, FOB
CV	Pericardial effusion SVC syndrome	Dyspnea, cough Dyspnea, cough	Dilated neck veins Facial edema	ECHO CXR
RESP	Lung mass, consolidation, atelectasis, pleural effusion	Dyspnea, cough, fever	Rhonchi, fever, percussion dullness	CXR, ABG
GI	Rarely pancreatitis from ↑ Ca++	Anorexia, constipation		Serum, Ca++
CNS	Brain metastasis, paraneoplastic syndrome (optic neuritis, neuropathy, cerebellar degeneration, LEMS)	Headache, visual changes, unsteady gait, sensory or motor symptoms	Fundoscopic or neurologic findings	Head CT scan
MS	Bone metastasis Polymyositis	Bone pain Muscle soreness	Bone tenderness	↑ Alk phosphatase, PET/CT ↑ CK, EMG

Key Reference: Ranu H, Madden BP. Endobronchial stenting in the management of large airway pathology. *Postgrad Med J.* 2009;85(1010):682–687.

Perioperative Implications

Preoperative Preparation

- Adequate hydration, correct electrolyte abnormalities, bronchodilators, antibiotics, steroid coverage for adrenal insufficiency, and PFTs
- Incentive spirometry instruction

Monitoring

- Arterial line for lung resection and OLV

Airway

- Determine need for left- or right-sided double lumen ETT

Preinduction/Induction

- Bronchodilators
- Antibiotics
- Arrhythmia drugs if indicated

- Judicious use of neuromuscular blockers if LEMS

Maintenance

- No one agent or technique is superior
  - Volatile agents decrease bronchomotor tone and HPV minimally, but permit high FIO$_2$.
  - CPAP and PEEP as required, esp during OLV
  - Consider thoracic epidural

Extubation

- Change to single-lumen ETT if pt will remain intubated.

Adjuvants

- Consider bronchodilators and anti-arrhythmia medications

Postoperative Period

- Consider thoracic epidural, intrapleural catheters, paravertebral nerve blocks or cryoanalgesia for pain management.

Anticipated Problems/Concerns

- Potentially life-threatening problems: Bronchial disruptions, cardiac herniation, tension pneumothorax, cardiac dysrhythmias, and resp insufficiency
- Adequate analgesia is esp beneficial for pts with COPD

Cancer, Esophageal

Dawn P. Desiderio

DISEASES

Risk

- Incidence in USA: 7.7 in 100,000 white men, 2.0 in 100,00 white women, 12.7 in 100,000 in black men, 4.2 in 100,000 black women
- Incidence of adenocarcinoma has increased in white men, while incidence of squamous cell carcinoma is highest in black men
- Overall mortality rate: 8.8%

Perioperative Risks

- Reflux as a risk for aspiration
- Malnutrition with dehydration due to swallowing dysfunction
- Periop arrhythmias occur 20–60% of esophagectomies
- Anastomotic leak most frequent surgical complication

Worry About

- Pulm compromise due to lung injury from preop chemotherapy/radiation therapy, chronic aspiration, extensive tobacco Hx, and inflammatory response to mechanical ventilation
- Hydration status
- Airway protection at time of anesthesia induction and postop
- Alcohol withdrawal syndromes
- Arrhythmias

Overview

- Primarily either squamous cell from esophageal squamous epithelium or adenocarcinomas of gastric origin
- Usually 55–65 y, with a long-standing Hx of tobacco and alcohol intake
- Dysphagia and wt loss are initial symptoms, often present for 3–4 mo
- Characterized by extensive local growth and lymphatic involvement before becoming widely disseminated

ICD-9-CM Code: 150

Etiology

- Achalasia of 25 y or longer, tobacco use, excessive alcohol intake, lack of aspirin use are associated with an increased incidence of squamous cell cancer.
- Reflux esophagitis (Barrett's esophagus), GERD, and obesity are associated with adenocarcinoma.
- Nutritional factors and ingestion of hot liquids have been implicated.

Usual Treatment

- Treatment depends on extent of disease and pt's medical status.
- Surgery with or without chemotherapy the only possibly curative option.
- Pts who are unacceptable surgical risks or with advanced disease may benefit from radiation.
- Palliative placement of an internal esophageal stent allows for swallowing of liquids and secretions.

ASSESSMENT POINTS

System	Effect	Assessment by Hx	Pe	Test
CV	Alcohol abuse–induced cardiomyopathy and arrhythmias	DOE Exercise tolerance		ECG ECHO, stress test
RESP	Tobacco abuse Chronic aspiration Radiation/chemotherapy	Pneumonias; RV Htn Cough, dyspnea Sputum	Wheezing RV heave	CXR PFTs, diffusion capacity ABGs
GI	Obstruction Reflux Malnutrition	Difficulty swallowing, unable to sleep flat, wt loss	Debilitated	UGI Endoscopy
CNS	Alcohol abuse Delirium tremens	Last alcohol ingestion and amount		
MS	Weakness	Poor nutrition	Muscle wasting	Serum albumin
RENAL	Dehydration	Limited intake		Lytes, Cr, BUN

Key Reference: Ng JM. Perioperative Anesthetic Mangement for Esohagectomy. *Anesthesia Clinics.* 2008;26:293–304.

Perioperative Implications

Preoperative Preparation
- Premedication not to obtund a pt at risk for aspiration
- Antisialagogue (atropine 0.4 mg or glycopyrrolate 0.2 mg)
- Premedication with H_2 blocker for acid aspiration prophylaxis plus metoclopramide to promote gastric emptying
- Steroids given if recently used
- Consider β-blockade for prophylaxis
- Placement of thoracic epidural for postop pain control

Monitoring
- Central venous or PA catheter placement for volume assessment and replacement, and for volume loading prior to surgical compression of the mediastinal structures optional
- Arterial line for BP monitoring and ABGs

Airway
- Rapid-sequence induction or awake fiberoptic intubation
- The surgical need for one-lung ventilation if thoracoabdominal approach requires a double-lumen ETT, a bronchial blocker, or a Univent tube and proper positioning

Induction
- Hypovolemia often results in BP fluctuation
- Aspiration risk during intubation

Maintenance
- No one agent or technique shown superior
- Volume requirements due to mediastinal compression, blood loss, and initial dehydration status
- Oxygenation concerns during one-lung ventilation, the use of 100% O_2 and chemotherapy Hx (bleomycin, mitomycin), prior pulm compromise due to tobacco history, volutrauma during mechanical ventilation
- Lung-protection advocated during mechanical ventilation, lower tidal volumes 5–6 mL/kg recommended with/without peep, using either volume or pressure modes of ventilation to maintain adequate oxygenation with peak inspiratory pressures <30–35 cm of water
- Hypothermia is concern in long procedures
- Placement of NG tube with surgical guidance

Extubation
- Continuing risk of aspiration
- Aim for early extubation in the OR or within a few hours of surgery. Less need for postop sedation leading to less fluid requirements. Requires presence of functioning epidural.
- Caution with obsese and sleep apnea pts
- Pts with double-lumen ETT in place should be reintubated or bronchial blockers pulled back (Univent) or removed if postop ventilation is required.

- Reintubation difficult because of edema and fluid shifts. With solid paralysis and pharyngeal suctioning, and a tube exchanger (Cook airway exchanger catheter) is recommended. Double-lumen tube is withdrawn over the tube exchange and a single lumen tube is threaded over the exchanger with a laryngoscope used to help with soft tissue that may impede placement.

Adjuvants
- Pts who have received chemotherapy (mitomycin or bleomycin) might be administered an O_2 concentration of 28% or as low as possible (see Bleomycin in Drugs section)

Postoperative Period
- Epidural analgesia is beneficial
- Inceased risk for supraventricular tachycardia and atrial fibrillation. Rate control recommended by the AHA initially with IV diltiazem and/or β-blockers if BP can tolerate

Anticipated Problems/Concerns
- Airway management: Aspiration risk, reintubation problems, extubation criteria
- Volume status in a dehydrated pt undergoing a lengthy surgical procedure with mediastinal compression and a thoracic epidural
- Arrhythmias in the postop period, use of prophylatic β-blockade

65

Cancer, Lung Parenchyma

Roger A. Moore

Risk

- Lung cancer is primary cause of cancer death
- Asbestos exposure increases risk 5–fold
- Smoking increases risk 15–fold
- Radon exposure increases risk 2–fold

Perioperative Risks

- Associated CAD
- Pulm insufficiency following lung tissue resection

Worry About

- Optimization of preop pulmonary status
- Issues secondary to metastatic spread, such as superior vena caval syndrome
- Myasthenic syndrome (Eaton-Lambert) with oat cell carcinoma
- Massive hemoptysis with cancer invasion of bronchial arteries
- Active pneumonia in pulm parenchyma distal to obstructed bronchioles

Overview

- Four primary types of lung cancers: Squamous cell or bronchogenic; adenocarcinoma (most common); large cell carcinoma; small cell carcinoma
- 70% with COPD need extra postop pulm care
- Pts often nutritionally depleted
- Many have alcohol abuse history
- Preop pulm state may limit option of lobectomy
- Hormonal imbalances common due to hormone secreting tumors
  - 3% of pts are cushingoid
  - 70% of bronchogenic carcinomas have increased ACTH or pro-ACTH
  - Up to 60% with lung cancer have inappropriate ADH
- Myasthenic syndrome occurs owing to decreased release of nerve-ending acetylcholine leading to increased sensitivity to all muscle relaxants

ICD-9-CM Code: 162

Etiology

- Environmental factor important (smoking, asbestos exposure, radon exposure)
- Higher incidence in areas located near oil refineries

Usual Treatment

- Oat cell cancer frequently treated with radiation and chemotherapy (need good renal function)
- Lobectomy or pneumonectomy common approaches in other types of lung cancers; DLco of < 60% predicts 75% mortality; > 100% predicts 100% survival
- Lobectomy increasingly performed using a video-assisted thoracoscopic surgery (VATS), while pneumonectomy still primarily performed with a thoracotomy

ASSESSMENT POINTS

System	Effect	Assessment by Hx	PE	Test
CV	Myocardial ischemia, arrhythmia, cor pulmonale	Angina SOB Palpitations SOB	S_3 gallop Irregular pulse Distended neck veins	Exercise stress test ECG Catheterization ECHO
RESP	Pneumonia, bronchospasm, COPD	Productive cough, wheezing, SOB, dyspnea	Rhonchi-rales, wheezes, decreased BS Clubbing	CXR; PFTs: MBC, MMEFR, DLco; ABGs
ENDO	SIADH	Lethargy, ↑ weight, ↓ urine Thin skin, poor wound healing Weight gain, striae	Hypometabolic	Electrolytes Elevated urine sodium (rarely needed)
	↑ ACTH		Cushingoid, ↑ BP	Cortisone level (rarely needed)
NM	Eaton-Lambert (myasthenic)	↓ Muscle weakness	↓ Muscle strength with exercise	EMG (rarely needed)
NUTRITION	Wasting DTs	Wt loss, alcohol abuse	Cachexia, BMI change, ↑ Liver size	Liver function tests (esp albumin)

Key Reference: Heerdt PM, Park BJ. The emerging role of minimally invasive surgical techniques for the treatment of lung malignancy in the elderly. *Anesthesiol Clin.* 2008;26(2):315–324.

Perioperative Implications

Preoperative Preparation
- Resp optimization with bronchodilatation, antibiotics, pulm hygiene, and smoking cessation
- Correction of lyte imbalances

Monitoring and operative care
- Routine monitors
- Intra-arterial line and possible pulm catheter, but if a PA catheter is used, be alert to it being caught in the surgical pulm incision
- Neuromuscular blockade monitor
- Thoracic epidural

Airway
- Double-lumen tube or bronchial blocker needed—usually left-sided
- Fiberoptic bronchoscope should be available for positioning of endobronchial tube

Induction
- Anesthetic choice dependent on associated medical problems
- Light or no premedication to decrease CO_2 retention

- When right-sided double-lumen tube used, ensure right upper lobe ventilation (easiest with fiberoptic bronchoscope)

Maintenance
- Nerve damage with lateral position
  - Use axillary roll
  - Brachial plexus injury with arm hyperextension
  - Pad all pressure points
- Substantiate pulse oximetric and capnographic readings with ABGs
- If O_2 saturation falls during one-lung ventilation, PEEP on dependent lung may help. If not, CPAP on nondependent lung may help.
- Intraop fluid restriction, incl use of blood and blood products, can significantly decrease postop resp failure

Extubation
- If postop ventilation required and double lumen tube has been used, it needs to be switched to single-lumen tube
- Extubation should be determined by adequacy of resp variables

Adjuvants
- Bronchodilators for intraop use, inotropes for myocardial depression, antiarrhythmics for post lobectomy-pneumonectomy arrhythmias (some advocate prophylactic digoxin—but conflicting reported results)

Postoperative Period
- If pneumonectomy performed, there is a significant risk for postop ARDS
- Adequate pain management usual for recovery of pulm function
  - PCA or use of intercostal blocks can be effective
  - Thoracic epidural most efficacious
- Be watchful for DTs, inappropriate ADH, and decreased neuromuscular strength

Anticipated Problems/Concerns

- Intensive pulm toilet postop
- Careful suctioning of bronchial stump because of possibility of rupture
- Bronchopleural fistula or tension pneumothorax should be anticipated

Cancer, Prostate

Wen-Shin Liu

Risk

- The second leading cause of cancer death in men after lung cancer
- Estimated 192,280 new cases and 27,360 deaths from prostate cancer in the USA in 2009
- Screening with prostate-specific antigen (PSA) and digital rectal examination led to an increase in earlier-stage detection
- The incidence increases with age; more than 75% of cancers diagnosed are in men older than age 65
- Men who undergo prostatectomy have a very high chance of surviving at least 15 y

Perioperative Risks

- Periop mortality for open radical prostatectomy (ORP) is approximately 0.3%.
- Risks of ORP incl excessive blood loss, rectal laceration, ureteral injury, wound infection, DVT, pulm embolus, anastomotic leak, MI, and later lymphocele, incontinence, impotence, and anastomotic stricture.
- Laparoscopic radical prostatectomy (LRP)—less morbidity, less blood loss
- Robotic-assisted laparoscopic prostatectomy (RALP)—less blood loss and rare blood transfusion, a trend for symptomatic ileus to be more prevalent

Worry About

- Increased prevalence of age-related, multiple concomitant diseases and a decline in basic organ function in these elderly men

- Periop complications: Risks of blood loss, rectal injury

Overview

- Early Dx by the triad of elevated serum PSA, an abnormal digital rectal exam, and transrectal ultrasound (TRUS)-guided prostate biopsies
- Localized disease—rarely causes symptoms
- Locally advanced or metastatic disease—obstructive voiding and irritative voiding symptoms, bone pain
- TNM system is the most widely used clinical staging system. Briefly, in TNM system, T1 and T2 tumors are confined to the gland, whereas T3 and T4 tumors have local extension. The most prominent histologic grading system is the Gleason Scoring System.
- Heterogeneous tumors (usually acinar adenocarcinomas) composed of hormone-sensitive and hormone-insensitive cells

ICD-9-CM Code: 185

Etiology

- Genetic predisposition, hormonal influences, dietary and environmental carcinogenic influences, infectious agents

Usual Treatment

- Quality-of-life issues and co-morbid condition help to guide treatment choices
- Watchful waiting—esp if other diseases present or age >70 y with moderately differentiated, low-volume cancer, and a life expectancy of fewer than 10 y
- Open radical prostatectomy (ORP)—(retropubically or perineally)—in selected pts with clinically confined prostate cancer, usually for those < 70 y.
- Laparoscopic radical prostatectomy (LRP)—offers decreased blood loss and transfusion rate, and shorter length of hospital stay
- Robotic-assisted laparoscopic prostatectomy (RALP)—has following advantages: Robotics provides three-dimentional visualization, magnification, tremor filtration, expanded degrees of freedom and wrested instrumentation, less blood loss and postop pain, and shorter hospital stay. Demand for this procedure is increasing worldwide—more than half of all prostatectomy surgeries performed in the USA are robotic
- Radiation therapy and brachytherapy—external-beam radiotherapy or interstitial radioactive seed implantation, proton therapy
- Hormonal therapy—for locally advanced or metastatic cancer: Estrogens, bilateral orchiectomy, LH-RH agonists, anti-androgens, and combined androgen blockade
- Others—Cytotoxic chemotherapy; cryosurgery; high-intensity focused ultrasound; radiofrequency interstitial tumor ablation

ASSESSMENT POINTS

System	Effect	Assessment by Hx	PE	Test
RESP	Age-related changes	COPD, smoking Hx		CXR
CV	Age-related changes	HTN, CAD, exercise tolerance		ECG
HEME	In advanced stages: anemia, azotemia, uremia		Anemia in extensive metastases	Blood work, T & Screen or T & C
GU	Early—asymptomatic; late stages—hesitancy, intermittency, urgency, frequency, retention, infection, impotence, hematospermia	Pathologic finding in prostate tissue; renal function impairment	Rock-hard nodule on digital rectal exam	Renal function test
METAB	Increased incidence of DM; malnutrition	Malaise	Wt loss in extensive metastases	Blood work
CNS and eye	Age related changes, glaucoma, metastasis	Hx of CVA, Alzheimer's	Neurologic deficits in lower limbs	Documenting neurologic changes
MS	Arthritis Metastases to spine	Bone pain (commonly in lumbosacral area)	Pathologic fracture (uncommon)	Radionuclide bone scans if bone metastases present

Key Reference: Hernandez J, Thompson IM. Diagnosis and treatment of prostate cancer. *Med Clin North Am.* 2004;88:267–279.

Perioperative Implications

Preoperative Preparation
- Assess CV and pulm status
- Leg pumps or compression stockings or low-dose coumadin to reduce DVT
- Appropriate bowel preparation

Anesthetic Technique
- ORP: General, may use epidural, or spinal for some cases
- RALP and LRP: General
- Consider pt's concomitant diseases, position on the operating table, intraop blood loss, and possible thromboembolic events in choosing anesthetic technique

Monitoring
- Consider arterial line depending on surgery
- Consider CVP and/or PA catheter for expected excessive blood loss and/or severe co-existing disease

Adjuvants
- Increased risk of adverse drug effects in elderly pts

- Hormonal therapy causes abnormal liver metabolism

Surgical stages
- In RALP: Access to the pt is limited as soon as the robot is docked, place invasive monitors preop in high-risk pts; cushioned stirrups are used in modified lithotomy position; pt is well strapped to operating table to prevent pt sliding off table; arms and legs are properly position and adequately padded; decompression of stomach; fluid restriction minimizes facial edema and excessive urine output, complete muscle relaxation is essential; pneumoperitoneum with CO_2 insufflation is associated with adverse hemodynamic and resp effects, esp in pt with limited cardiac reserve or impaired resp function; occult blood loss may occur
- In ORP—higher intraop blood loss in retropubic group; higher risk for rectal injury in the perineal group

Anticipated Problems/Concerns

- Air embolism from prostatic fossa during surgery in Trendelenburg position
- Intraop hemorrhage—esp with ORP retropubic approach
- In open radical prostatectomy—injury to obturator nerve, ureter, or rectum; immediate postop DVT and pulm embolism; symptomatic pelvic lymphocele; wound or UTIs; periop main CV complications—MI and postop arrhythmias; long-term surgical complications—incontinence and impotence
- In LRP and RALP—possible complications resulted from steep Trendelenburg position (25-45 degree head down) incl post-extubation resp distress secondary to laryngeal edema, brachial plexus injury, serious ocular consequences secondary to increased intraocular pressure
- For nonprostate surgery—worry about effects of chemotherapeutic agents, hormones, or radiation on hematologic, liver, renal, and vascular systems

Candidiasis

Ashish C. Sinha

Risk

- Pts with suppressed immune system from diseases like AIDS; chemotherapy drugs; extended steroid therapy
- Current and recent broad spectrum antibiotic therapy
- Diabetes, leukemia, and neutropenia
- IV hyperalimentation and prolonged ICU stay
- Breaches of protective epithelial barrier: Surgical trauma, burn injury, long-term indwelling IV or bladder catheters
- Even in healthy individuals, candida can be cultured from the oral cavity in a third to more than half; this increases with chronic illness and duration of hospitalization.
- As systemic bacterial infections have declined with aggressive antibiotic use, systemic fungal infections have correspondingly increased.
- Candida is fourth most common organism recovered from blood cultures.

Perioperative Risk

- Candidemia with septic shock is infrequent in non immunocompromised pts but has a vey high mortality rate, ~30% higher than bacteremic septic shock, and a high likelihood of MOF along with delayed recovery from this organ failure
- Pts more likely to have compromised renal function at baseline

Worry About

- Disseminated candidemia and associated organ dysfunction
- Candidemic septic shock
- Side effects of –azole, nystatin, or amphotericin-B therapy

Overview

- Candidemia in 30 cases per 100,000 admissions (in USA), associated with ~14.5% increase in mortality, 10-day increase in hospital stay and ~$40,000 increase of charges

- ~50 cases per 1,000 pt-y; of these 10% develop Candidemia, with an attributable mortality of 25%
- ~1% pts colonized on wards
- Incidental culture positive to fatal Candidiasis

ICD-9-CM Code: 112.5 (Systemic)

Etiology

- Among isolated species: ~ 60% C. albicans, ~20% C. tropicalis, rest in decreasing order, incl C. glabrata, C. parapsilosis, C. krusei, and Candida spp.
- Follows antibiotic therapy because the normal flora that keeps fungal growth in check is eliminated with antibiotics

Usual treatment

- Oropharyngeal: Oral itraconazole and flucanozole
- Esophageal: Oral and IV flucanozole, oral itraconazole, low dose IV amphotericin B
- Vulvovaginal: Topical and oral -azole agents
- Systemic infections: IV amphotericin B, high dose flucanozole

ASSESSMENT POINTS

System	Effect	Assessment by Hx	PE	Test
HEENT	Thrush Endophthalmitis	Dysphagia Visual changes	White oral plaques Ophthalmic lesions	Bleed on scraping Fundoscopic and field of vision
CVS	Endocarditis Septic shock	SOB Refractory hypotension	Cardiac murmurs Fever	Auscultation CVP, CO, PCWP
RESP	Pneumonia ARDS	SOB, cough, tachypnea, dec exercise tolerance	Rapid shallow breathing, hypoxemia, consolidation	PFT, ABG, CXR
CNS	Meningitis Brain abscess	Altered mental status, signs of increased ICP, nausea, vomiting, headache, seizures, loss of appetite	Mental status exam, neck stiffness, photophobia, confusion	CT, MRI, blood cultures, CSF cultures
RENAL	Renal abscess Cystitis	Dysuria, polyuria, low back pain, hematuria	Costovertebral tenderness on affected side	Urine culture, cystoscopy, CT
SKELETAL	Fungal osteomyelitis	Tenderness over bone, skin breakdown over infected bone	Moderate to severe bone pain, limited range of motion	X-ray, culture and sensitivity, bone scan
GI	Inflammation through GI tract, intra-abdominal abscess	Dysphagia, abdominal pain, diarrhea	Abdominal tenderness, signs of peritoneal irritation, hepatomegaly, splenomegaly	CT or MRI, endoscopy, abdominal ultrasound

Key Reference: Marchena-Gomez J, Saez-Guzman T, Hemmersbach-Miller M, et al. Candida isolation in patients hospitalized on a surgical ward: Significance and mortality-related factors. *World J Surg.* 2009;33:1822–1829.

Perioperative Implications

Preoperative Preparation
- Continue antifungal therapy
- Evaluate for septic shock
- Rule out infected lines or catheters; change if indicated

Monitoring
- If septic, A-line, CVP ± PA catheter, along with standard monitoring

Airway
- Be careful not to aggravate oral lesion at intubation

Pre induction /Induction
- Choose drugs based on septic signs and symptoms
- Worry about hypotension and hypoxemia at induction

Maintenance
- Choose drugs based on hemodynamic status
- Choose ventilatory modes based on presence of ARDS

Extubation
- May have to be delayed if ARDS or septic state require hemodynamic support

Adjuvants
- In the presence of compromised renal or hepatic function modify anesthetic drugs accordingly

Anticipated Problems/Concerns

- Candidemia presents with a diverse clinical picture, from low-grade fever to fulminant septic shock. There is higher periop mortality in this group of pts.

Carbon Monoxide (CO) Poisoning

Peter H. Breen

Risk

- Most frequent toxic gas in smoke (COHb can reach 10% in smokers)
- Major cause of death
- CO produced by all internal combustion engines, incomplete oxidative combustion (e.g., house fires, charcoal and gas grills, malfunctioning butane/propane stoves), and endogenous sources (e.g., by liver from exogenous exposure to paint stripper)
- No odor, taste, color, or irritation
- Toxicity potentiated by low inspired O_2 concentration (e.g., smoke inhalation)
- To minimize CO in circle circuit carbon dioxide absorbers: Use fresh soda lime, use sevoflurane, and minimize drying (lower FGF and stop FGF during non-use)
- During GA, use semiclosed circuits, esp when machine has not been used for 2–3 d (e.g. Monday morning)

Perioperative Risks

- Main target organs: Heart and brain
- Heart: Can resemble ischemia; potentiated by CAD
- Brain: Acute loss of consciousness; after initial improvement, up to 30% risk of secondary syndrome: chronic psychiatric dysfunction and cerebral and cerebellar syndromes

Worry About

- Seek other smoke inhalation injury
- Consider concomitant cyanide poisoning that potentiates CO toxicity
- Be alert for CO poisoning in donor for organ transplantation

Overview

- CO, a colorless, nonirritating, and odorless gas, is a natural byproduct of combustion
- CO binds avidly to Hgb ($>200 \times O_2$) to form carboxyhemoglobin (COHb), which carries no O_2 and causes left shift in oxyhemoglobin dissociation curve (decreases O_2 off-loading to tissues)
- CO binds to intracellular hemoproteins such as myoglobin and cytochrome aa_3 (esp cardiac) to inhibit O_2 uptake and metabolism
- "Classic" cherry-red complexion rarely observed (need COHb >40%; may be obscured by co-existent hypoxia and cyanosis)
- COHb level correlates poorly with clinical condition
- Treatment should be guided by symptoms and signs, not by blood COHb concentration

ICD-9-CM Code: 986

Etiology

- CO produced by incomplete oxidative combustion (e.g., house fires, malfunctioning butane/propane stoves, home heaters, and all internal combustion engines)
- Suicide attempts

Usual Treatment

- Normobaric O_2: $T_{1/2}$ of COHb decreases from 3.5 hr (air-breathing) to 0.75 hr (O_2-breathing)
- Treat clinical symptoms, not just increased COHb
- General supportive care, esp for other aspects of smoke inhalation injury
- Hyperbaric O_2 (2.5 atm) decreases COHb $T_{1/2}$ to 20 min and has been shown to decrease probability of development of delayed neurologic complication; for pts with neurologic Sx (incl impaired consciousness), evidence of myocardial ischemia, fetal distress (if pregnant), poisoning in pediatric pt, or other Sx of significant exposure (e.g., COHb >25%), hyperbaric O_2 is recommended if feasible, within 6–8 hr of exposure

ASSESSMENT POINTS

System	Effect	Assessment by Hx	PE	Test
HEENT	Thermal/toxic upper airway injury	Fire exposure/smoke inhalation	Perioral burns Airway edema	Laryngoscopy/bronchoscopy
RESP	CO diffuses rapidly into blood → COHb	Dyspnea, tachypnea		Co-oximetric COHb: Po_2 usually normal
	Thermal/toxic airway and parenchymal injury		Bronchoconstriction and pulm edema	CXR Bronchoscopy
CV	↓ Blood O_2 content and ↓ Tissue O_2 unloading	Possibly angina or evidence of heart failure; tachycardia	Cardiac failure	ECG: Ischemic ST-T changes; CXR
METAB	Tissue hypoxia → acidosis			Lactic acidosis
CNS	Coma, cerebral edema	Temporal headache, N/V, restlessness	Muscle weakness, altered mental status	Abnormal neuropsychometric testing Can occur after initial recovery
	Neuropsychiatric syndrome	Cerebral, cerebellar		

Key Reference: Breen PH, Isserles SA, Westley J, Roizen MF, Taitelman UZ. Combined carbon monoxide and cyanide poisoning: a place for treatment? *Anesth Analg.* 1995;80:671–677.

Perioperative Implications

Preoperative Preparation
- Continuous 100% O_2
- Document CNS status
- Consider hyperbaric O_2 if mental status altered or pt has myocardial ischemia or is pregnant

Monitoring
- Routine monitors
- Standard pulse oximetry (SpO_2) does not distinguish between O_2Hb and COHb. Thus, SpO_2 overestimates O_2Hb during CO poisoning
- Newer SpO_2 monitors (Masimo Corp., Irvine, CA) can discriminate between O_2Hb and COHb (and metHb)
- Mixed venous oximeter catheters overestimate O_2Hb in presence of COHb
- Arterial cannula for frequent blood sampling
- Venous and arterial COHb levels are almost identical

Airway
- Airway injury and edema often occur during smoke inhalation, which may require emergent airway management

Induction
- Avoid cardiac depressant agents

Maintenance
- 100% O_2 (no N_2O)
- Assess muscle weakness to guide muscle relaxant dosage

Extubation
- Ensure CNS status permits natural airway maintenance and protection

Adjuvants
- Consider treatment for concomitant cyanide poisoning (see under Cyanide Poisoning in Diseases section)

Postoperative Period
- Maintain 100% O_2
- Consider hyperbaric O_2

Anticipated Problems/Concerns

- Heart and brain affected most
- Follow CNS function carefully
- Seek concomitant smoke inhalation injury and cyanide toxicity
- CO toxic in trace quantities (breathing 0.1% inspired CO for 1 hr results in significant toxicity, with COHb ~ 30%); CO not detectable with conventional gas analysis instruments (e.g., capnographs, mass spectrometers)
- Standard pulse oximeters do not specifically measure COHb, and SpO_2 measurements are only minimally affected, even by severe CO poisoning

Carcinoid Syndrome

Stanley H. Rosenbaum

Risk
- Most common GI endocrine tumor
- 15 cases/1 million population per year

Perioperative Risks
- Associated with pt's ability to tolerate abrupt hemodynamic change and/or bronchospasm

Worry About
- Abrupt Htn or hypotension with stress
- Right-sided valvular heart disease
- Bronchospasm

Overview
- Endocrinologically active tumor from GI mucosa
- May release histamine-like substances leading to hypotension and bronchospasm, or may release serotonin leading to hypertensive reactions (and hypovolemia)
- Commonly in ileum (esp appendix) or rectum, less so in pancreas and lung
- Systemically active when metastatic to liver, or when released substances avoid metabolism by liver (carcinoid syndrome)

ICD-9-CM Codes: 209.# (Tumor); 259.2 (Syndrome)

Etiology
- Acquired disease
- May be associated with other ectopic humoral tumors, such as MEN 1 syndrome

Usual Treatment
- Surgery or arterial embolization to reduce tumor burden
- Histaminic effects blocked only partially by H_1 and H_2 blockers
- Somatostatin analogues octreotide and lanreotide block humoral release
- Interferon α (alpha) may control symptoms
- No specific medical Rx for established valvular heart lesions
- Catecholamines may increase humoral release and worsen symptoms

ASSESSMENT POINTS

System	Effect	Assessment by Hx	PE	Test
HEENT	Cutaneous flushing, lacrimation Pellagra-like skin lesions	Episodic flushing induced by stress, eating, alcohol consumption	Hyperkeratosis, hyperpigmentation	
CV	Histamine-induced hypotension Serotonin-induced Htn Endomyocardial fibrosis, esp in right heart	Sx of right-sided CHF	Murmurs of pulmonic stenosis, tricuspid regurgitation, ascites, edema	ECHO Cardiac catheterization
RESP	Bronchospasm Endobronchial tumor with obstruction	Episodic asthma poorly responsive to medication Focal wheeze at site of obstructing tumor	Wheezing associated with episodes of flushing	
GI	Diarrhea Obstructing tumor	Episodic watery diarrhea		Bowel films, hepatic CT, ultrasound, angiograms
ENDO	Serotonin secretion			Urinary 5–HIAA levels elevated in most pts Occasionally need to measure plasma histamine
RENAL	Dehydration from chronic vasospasm or diarrhea			BUN/Cr, electrolytes
CNS	Hemodynamic instability, vasodilation	Hypertensive headache Syncope with flushing		
MS	Cutaneous flushing, lacrimation Pellagra-like skin lesions	Episodic flushing, induced by stress, eating, alcohol consumption	Hyperkeratosis, hyperpigmentation	

Key Reference: Ogunnaike BO, Whitten CW, Barash PG, et al., eds. *Clinical Anesthesia.* 6th ed. Philadelphia: Wolter Kluwer LWW; 2009:1227–1228.

Perioperative Implications

Preoperative Preparation
- Assess adequacy of fluid balance.
- Assess right-sided valvular status.
- Somatostatin analogue (octreotide) available; its use has dramatically decreased hazards of anesthesia for pts with carcinoid syndrome.

Monitoring
- Expect rapid fluctuation of BP.
- Central venous pressures may not correlate well with fluid volumes.

Airway
Risk of stress-induced wheezing (Rx: somatostatin analogue)

Induction
- Chronic vasoconstriction and diarrhea may cause hemodynamic instability.

Maintenance
- Volume assessments complicated by changing vascular tone
- Cardiac function limited by right-sided valvular lesions

Extubation
- Possible stress-induced hemodynamic instability (Rx: somatostatin analogue)

Adjuvants
- Caution! Catecholamines may increase humoral release and worsen symptoms.
- Somatostatin analogue for hypo- or hypertension or bronchospasm has dramatically decreased anesthesia risk for pts with carcinoid syndrome

Postoperative Period
- Humoral effects of hemodynamically active metastatic carcinoid usually not eliminated by surgery

↓ get fibrous deposits in heart
- usually involves the ventricular aspect of the tricuspid valve and associated chordae.

CARCINOID CRISIS
- can occur spontaneously or as a response to stress (ie. chemo, anesthesia)
- Symptoms → intense flushing, diarrhea, abdo pain, tachy, HYPER or HYPOTENSION, altered MS, and coma
- Rx c̄ somatostatin analog (ie. octreotide)
N.B. Catecholamines may worsen symptoms!

Cardiomyopathy, Alcoholic

Risk

- Incidence in USA: 15 to 20 million chronic heavy ethanol users
- As much as 50% of dilated cardiomyopathy may be ethanol related
- Population at risk: Unclear; likely incl chronic ethanol users with at least 90 g of daily ETOH for at least 5 y (1 standard drink = 12 grams ETOH)
- Gender: Male predominance

Perioperative Risks

- Alcohol withdrawal
- CHF
- Dysrhythmias common: AFIB, PAC, PVC

Worry About

- Myocardial ischemia: supply < demand (CAD rare)
- Abnormal systolic and diastolic function
- Chronic alcohol use alters myocardial response to inotropes
- Alcohol withdrawal symptoms

Overview

- Insidious onset; Sx uncommon unless severely stressed until late in course
- Dilated cardiomyopathy: ventricular hypertrophy early, chamber dilation later
- Low-output cardiac failure (as compared with high-output failure in cirrhosis and beriberi)
- Malnutrition often co-exists

ICD-9-CM Code: 425.5

Etiology

- Direct myocardial damage by ethanol and its metabolites
- Progressive chamber dilation and ventricular hypertrophy; microscopic fibrinoid deposition
- Possible intracellular calcium dysregulation
- Possible muscle excitation-contraction impairment

Usual Treatment

- Abstinence: Ventricular function improves markedly after abstinence
- Pharmacologic management: Digitalis, diuretics, beta-blockers, ACE inhibitors
- Address nutritional deficits: Thiamine, folate, multivitamin

ASSESSMENT POINTS

System	Effect	Assessment by Hx	PE	Test
HEENT	Plethora, reflux, esophageal varices, friable mucosa	Reflux Sx Hematemesis	Spider angiomata	Endoscopy
CV	LV dysfunction CHF Myocardial ischemia Dysrhythmia	Fatigue, orthopnea PND Rare angina Palpitations	Narrow pulse pressure Cardiomegaly S_3, S_4, murmur JVD, peripheral edema	ECG ECHO Stress testing
RESP	Pulm edema	Dyspnea Cough	Rales	CXR
GI	Hepatic congestion	Poor appetite, distention	Hepatomegaly	PT, albumin, LFTs
HEME	Coagulopathy, Anemia	Abnormal bleeding	Pallor Ecchymosis	CBC PT/PTT, plt
RENAL	↓ Renal perfusion	Oliguria		Cr, FENa
CNS	Poor perfusion	Confusion	Abn mental status	
MS	Proximal muscle weakness		Proximal limb weakness and muscle atrophy	

Key Reference: Piano MR. Alcoholic Cardiomyopathy. *Chest.* 2002;121:1638–1650.

Perioperative Implications

Preoperative Preparation
- Pharmacologic management of CHF

Monitoring
- ECG with ST-segment analysis
- Consider arterial pressure catheter, pulm artery catheter, TEE depending on surgery and ventricular function

Airway
- None

Preinduction/Induction
- May have intravascular volume depletion

Maintenance
- Avoid tachycardia, increased sympathetic activity
- Avoid depression of myocardial contractility

Extubation
- Routine

Postoperative Period
- Consider monitoring in critical care unit
- Observe for ethanol withdrawal

Adjuvants
- Multivitamins, thiamine, B_{12}, folate continued
- Consider benzodiazepines, α_2 agonists for prophylaxis against withdrawal symptoms
- Volume of distribution may be increased; consider adjusting drug dosages

Anticipated Problems/Concerns

- Postop ventricular dysfunction and CHF can occur.
- Alcohol withdrawal symptoms can develop.

Cardiomyopathy, Hypertrophic (HCM)

Risk

• Incidence: 0.2% (1/500) of general population; equally affects males and females, no racial group predominance; median age of 35 y (but can manifest in any age)
• Heterogeneous clinical presentation: Frequent cause of sudden cardiac death (SCD) in young athletes; elderly pts tend to be less symptomatic, reflecting diverse genetic background.
• May be asymptomatic (20–25%) or undiagnosed at the time a pt presents for general surgery (anesthesia may "unmask" HCM)

Perioperative Risks

• Dynamic left ventricular outflow obstruction (either at rest or provoked) present in approx 50% of pts with HCM
• Diastolic dysfunction, risk for heart failure from impaired relaxation of a hypertrophic and non-compliant LV
• Risk for myocardial ischemia even in the absence of obstructive CAD, due to increased myocardial O_2 demand (LVH, high intraventricular pressures) and limited supply (abnormal impaired coronary reserve, microvascular and subendocardial ischemia, intramyocardial coronary arteries)
• Supraventricular (atrial fibrillation) and ventricular dysrhythmias

Worry About

• Factors that can aggravate dynamic outflow obstruction and lead to hypotension and hemodynamic compromise: Decreased preload (hypovolumia), decreased afterload (vasodilation), Increased sympathetic activation (from pain, surgical stimulation), increased LV contractility
• Myocardial ischemia (even in a background of a "normal" coronary angiogram or thallium)
• Diastolic dysfunction; heart failure difficult to control with traditional diuresis (caution with volume depletion)
• Supraventricular (atrial fibrillation increases risk of embolic stroke) and ventricular dysrhythmias

Overview

• Definition: Hypertrophied, nondilated LV in absence of other cardiac or systemic causes for LVH.

• Variable clinical spectrum (from asymptomatic to severely symptomatic to sudden cardiac death)
• Although left ventricular outflow tract (LVOT) obstruction, clinical symptoms, family Hx or documented genetic mutation may be present, none of the above are considered mandatory criteria for the diagnosis of HCM.
• Myocardial disarray on histopathology (95%)
• The interventricular septum is usually (~70%) disproportionately "thicker" (> 15 mm). Less common variants (20–30%) involving the apex (often in Asian pts) or LV free wall have been described.
• Vigorous LV contractility and hypertrophied myocardium may physically obstruct left ventricular outflow tract (LVOT) during systole, resulting in dynamic outflow tract gradient.
• The gradient may be absent or minimal at rest in about 20–30% of pts, but increases with dynamic "provocation" manoeuvres (Valsalva, post-PVC, anything that increases contractility or promotes vasodilation).
• Associated mitral regurgitation (MR) is often present.
• Systolic anterior motion [SAM] of the mitral valve leaflet is considered the predominant mechanism of MR in HCM. The anterior leaflet of mitral valve may be "drawn" into the LVOT by Venturi effect during systole, contact the septum and contribute to dynamic obstruction
• Primary structural abnormalities of the mitral valve apparatus and/or papillary muscles have been described and may be present in at least 1/3 of HCM pts, independent of SAM.
• Clinical manifestations of HCM may relate to diastolic heart failure (dyspnea, fatigue), ischemia (angina, often in the absence of obstructive CAD) arrhythmias (palpitations, syncope, even sudden death) or hypotension associated with obstruction (dizziness, syncope).
• Rarely (~10%) advanced "burn out" stage with LV dilatation resembling dilated cardiomyopathy.
• Diagnostic modalities incl:
  • 12-lead ECG (LVH voltage criteria, arrhythmias, characteristic deep T-wave pattern in apical HCM)

• ECHO (LVH in non-dilated LV, LVEF > 60%, LVOT gradient at rest or with Valsalva, SAM, or other mitral valve abnormalities).
• Cardiac catheterization is not mandatory but frequently performed to exclude CAD and confirm the diagnosis or "localize" the gradient (differentiate from AS) when ECHO images are suboptimal.
• Cardiac MRI with gadolenium hyperenhancement demonstrates a characteristic pattern of HCM-related microvascular ischemia and can be helpful to plan surgical management.
• Other tests (HOLTER, exercise stress ECHO, biospsy) are rarely necessary.

ICD-9-CM Code: 425.1 (Hypertrophic obstructive cardiomyopathy)

Etiology

• Genetically heterogeneous: At least 400 mutations in 12 genes that encode for cardiac sarcomeric proteins (beta myosin heavy chain, myosin binding protein C, troponins T and I, tropomyosin) identified; the diversity in mutations and variability in penetrance account for the very wide spectrum in prognosis (from asymptomatic to sudden death). Certain mutations carry worse prognosis, esp regarding risk of SCD. Genetic testing is now widely available and offered to pts and their first degree relatives.

Treatment

• Medical: Negative inotropes (β-blockers, non-dihydropyridine Ca^{2+}-channel blockers, i.e., verapamil or diltiazem, the class Ia antiarrhythmic disopyramide)
• ICD in pts at high risk of sudden death based on clinical risk factors or family Hx or "high-risk" genetic mutations (DDD pacer alone rarely used)
• "Septal reduction" therapies to reduce LVOT gradient:
  • Surgical septal myectomy (produces LBBB), mitral valve replair or replacement if warranted
  • Percutaneous intervention: Septal ablation by alcohol injection (produces RBBB, risk of high-grade AV block)

ASSESSMENT POINTS

System	Effect	Assessment by Hx	PE	Test
CV	Myocardial ischemia	Angina	Worse with nitrates (avoid)	ECG, exercise tests, coronary angio (may be "normal"), cardiac MRI
	LVOT obstruction	Dyspnea, syncope, dizziness	Systolic murmur accentuated by Valsalva	ECHO
	Mitral regurgitation	Dyspnea	Holosystolic murmur	ECHO
	Dysrhythmias	Syncope, sudden death, palpitations		ECG, Holter
	Diastolic dysfunction	Dyspnea	Rales, wheeze, edema	ECHO, CXR
RESP	Pulm congestion	Dyspnea, orthopnea	Rales, wheeze	CXR
	Secondary pulm hypertension			Right heart catheterization
CNS	Syncope	Syncope, presyncope		Negative CNS work-up

Key Reference: Pollack LC, Barron ME, Maron BJ. Hypertrophic cardiomyopathy. *Anesthesiology*. 2006;104:183–192.

Perioperative Implications

Preoperative Preparation

• Avoid physiologic changes that reduce LV cavity size (maintain preload and afterload, avoid tachycardia)
• Ensure adequate preload, replace any preop volume depletion
• Optimize pre- and periop β-blocker or Ca^{2+}-channel blocker therapy
• Note: HCM pts often are on high doses of β-blocker preop (caution for withdrawal)

• Also note disopyramide (used preop in severe HCM) has anticholinergic activities
• Sedate adequately to prevent anxiety-induced sympathetic stimulation
• SBE prophylaxis recommended for HCM pts with severe MR or septal myectomy
• ICD/pacemaker evaluation (rarely pt may be pacer-dependant, esp postseptal ablation)

Monitoring

• Depending on nature of surgical procedure, consider invasive arterial pressure monitoring and/or pulm artery catheter

• Transesophageal ECHO can be invaluable, esp if major blood loss, volume shifts, or sympathetic stimulation are anticipated.

Airway

• None

Preinduction/Induction

• Avoid drug-induced vasodilation or sympathetic activation. When choosing an induction agent, etomidate may be advantageous over ketamine or propofol.
• Phenylephrine infusion (alternatives: vasopressin, norepinephrine) should be immediately

available, as worsening dynamic outflow tract gradient may be anticipated with any drop in SVR or sympathetic stimulation.
• Avoid prolonged laryngoscopy, as it may induce sympathetic stimulation.
• Insertion of CVP/PAC may induce atrial or ventricular dysrhythmias.

Maintenance

• Volatile agents that decrease LV contractility without dramatic vasodilation are desirable. Halothane is the classic example. Likewise, sevoflurane is preferable over isoflurane or desflurane.
• Avoid agents that decrease preload and afterload (e.g., nitroglycerin, nitroprusside) or increase contractility (inotropes) as well as agents associated with significant histamine release.
• Avoid agents that directly or indirectly increase HR and contractility (e.g., pancuronium, atropine, epinephrine, ephedrine).
• Hypotension treated with
  • Volume expansion (avoid anemia; promptly replete blood loss).

• Pure α-adrenergic agonist (e.g., phenylephrine).
• Spinal anesthesia may be associated with hypotension. Epidural analgesia may be considered to avoid sympathetic stimulation from pain, but with caution to avoid significant afterload reduction and hypotension.
• Consider early electrical cardioversion for atrial fibrillation. Defibrillator available in OR.
• Consider β-blockade or Ca^{2+}-channel blockade to prevent tachycardia, LVOT obstruction or ischemia.

Extubation

• Avoid sympathetic stimulation. Assure adequate analgesia.
• Anticipate subendocardial ischemia. Utilize β-blockade or Ca^{2+}-channel blockade.
• Pulm edema from diastolic dysfunction and MR is difficult to treat (use diuretics very judiciously if at all).
• Secondary pulm Htn from HCM and related MR worsens with "conventional" pulm vasodilators (increase LVOT obstruction).

• Advisable to maintain minute ventilation by using higher rates, lower tidal volumes (higher tidal volumes with lower rates will decrease venous return).

Postoperative Period

• Aggressive postop pain management: If neuraxial analgesia is considered, administration of intrathecal or epidural narcotics only is the preferred and better tolerated approach.

Anticipated Problems/Concerns

• Myocardial ischemia (usually subendocardial if conditions favor high O$_2$ demand)
• Profound hypotension in settings of hypovolemia, decreased preload/afterload, or increased contractility
• Dysrhythmias (ventricular, supraventricular, bradyarrhythmias in the setting of prior septal reduction procedures)
• Diastolic dysfunction with possibility of pulm edema (esp with prolonged mechanical ventilation) and secondary pulm Htn (exacerbated by significant MR)

Cardiomyopathy, Ischemic

Jonathan B. Mark
Charles S. Brudney

Risk

- Approximately 1:1000 incidence per year
- M:F ratio: 2:1

Perioperative Risks

- Most important periop risk factor for cardiac morbidity and mortality
- Risk of CHF, hypotension, pulm edema, myocardial ischemia and infarction, renal insufficiency, arrhythmias
- Left ventricular ejection fraction (LVEF) important for prognosis, periop complications. LVEF may not correlate with symptoms or exercise tolerance

Worry About

- CHF exacerbation, pulm edema, hypotension, myocardial ischemia and infarction, renal insufficiency, inability to tolerate fluid shifts associated with major surgery, arrhythmias

Overview

- Severe impairment of LVF leading to CHF; that arising from myocardial ischemia and infarction

has extremely poor prognosis, with 30–50% 2-y mortality.
- Pts may benefit from intensive medical therapy for underlying ischemia (nitrates, β-blockers, calcium antagonists, aspirin), CHF (ACE inhibitors, hydralazine, digoxin, diuretics, aldosterone antagonists, angiotension-II receptor blockers), prevention of cardiac thrombus formation (warfarin), and HR control for atrial fibrillation (digoxin, β-blockers).
- An implantable cardioverter-defibrillator (ICD) for secondary prevention of sudden cardiac death (SCD) will be present in many pts.
- Cardiac resynchronization therapy (CRT) with biventricular pacing improves symptoms in pts in prolonged QRS duration with low EF.
- Associated mitral regurgitation, left ventricular aneurysm, and ventricular arrhythmias may have specific periop considerations.

ICD-9-CM Code: 414.8

Etiology

- Acquired disease with genetic predisposition
- Risk factors incl associated Htn, diabetes, hyperlipidemia, cigarette smoking, advanced age, peripheral vascular disease.

Usual Treatment

- Medical therapy—Myocardial revascularization (percutaneous coronary angioplasty, atherectomy, stent or laser coronary bypass surgery, or transmyocardial laser revascularization)
- Cardiomyoplasty (generally experimental)
- Cardiac transplantation
- Associated cardiac surgery (mitral valve replacement/repair, left ventricular aneurysmectomy, implantation of AICD [automatic implantable cardioverter defibrillator])
- Data are limited on the relative efficacy of percutaneous coronary intervention (PCI)
- Possible future therapy: Stem cell and autologous myoblast transplantation

ASSESSMENT POINTS

System	Effect	Assessment by Hx	PE	Test
CV	Myocardial ischemia Arrhythmias CHF	Angina Dyspnea, PND palpitations	S_3, S_4, loud P_2 Narrow pulse pressure Displaced point maximal impulse	ECG Stress testing ECHO Stress ECHO MRI Myocardial contrast ECHO Cardiac catheterization
RESP	Pulm congestion/edema	Dyspnea on exertion Orthopnea Cough	Rales Wheezes	CXR
GI	Ascites	Abdominal distention	Shifting dullness Fluid wave Hepatomegaly	Liver function tests PT Albumin
CNS	Embolic stroke due to cardiac thrombosis	Weakness Vision problems Confusion	Altered mental status Focal deficits	CT or MRI
MS	Peripheral edema	Swollen ankles Weakness	Pitting edema	
RENAL	Insufficiency (prerenal)	Oliguria		Cr, BUN Excreted fraction of filtered sodium

Key Reference: Rahimtoola SH, La Canna G, Ferrari R. Hibernating myocardium: Another piece of the puzzle falls into place. *J Am Coll Cardiol*. 2006;47:978.

Perioperative Implications

Preoperative Preparation
- Pharmacologic control of myocardial ischemia and CHF

Monitoring
- ECG (V_5 or multilead) with ST-segment analysis
- Arterial catheter (close BP monitoring, ABGs)
- Consider PA catheter or TEE for major operations and/or poor medical condition

Airway
- None

Preinduction/Induction
- Avoid tachycardia and increased afterload to prevent ischemia and reduced cardiac output.

- Hypovolemia may result from diuretic therapy.

Maintenance
- Limited ability to increase cardiac output in response to stress
- Attention to fluid balance, monitor PAWP to avoid pulm edema or low cardiac output
- High doses of inhaled anesthetics may be poorly tolerated because of myocardial depression superimposed on cardiomyopathy

Extubation
- May be time of greatest stress for developing myocardial ischemia or LV dysfunction.
- Consider postop mechanical ventilation if a large fluid resuscitation was required intraop.

Adjuvants
- Extensive preop medical therapy may have circulatory consequences.
- Preop anticoagulation may preclude regional anesthesia.

Postoperative Period
- Epidural pain management techniques may limit stress if operation was major (beware of warfarin therapy).
- Intensive care and hemodynamic monitoring may prevent complications if operation was major.

Anticipated Problems/Concerns

- Periop myocardial ischemia and CHF remain paramount concerns.

Carnitine Deficiency

Raafat S. Hannallah
Marjorie Brennan

Risk

- Rare (1:40,000 in Japan)

Perioperative Risks

- Hypoglycemia triggered by fasting.
- Massive rhabdomyolysis and cardiac arrest described following GA and succinylcholine. The response may be confused with malignant hyperthermia.

Worry About

- Periop hypoglycemia: Avoid prolonged fast; IV glucose should be administered.
- Neurologic and cardiopulmonary status: Determine if a cardiomyopathy is present.

Overview

- Carnitine is essential cofactor in enzymatic transport of long-chain fatty acids into mitochondria, in which they are oxidized.
- When carnitine is deficient, peripheral tissues cannot use fatty acids for energy production and the liver cannot adequately make ketone bodies as an alternative substrate.
- The tissues become glucose dependent, and their metabolism exceeds liver's capacity for glucose production.
- This glucose dependency can lead to severe liver failure (↑ hepatic enzymes, lactic acidosis, hypoketotic encephalopathy) and hypoglycemia.

ICD-9-CM Code: 277.8

Etiology

- Mutations in the *SLC22A5* gene lead to the production of defective OCTN2 carnitine transporters.
- Differentiate from carnitine palmityl transferase (CPT) deficiency, which results in impaired transfer of fatty acids into mitochondria.
- CPT deficiency associated with rhabdomyolysis and higher incidence of renal insufficiency.

Usual Treatment

- Dietary supplementation with L-carnitine and high-carbohydrate diet to prevent hypoglycemia.

ASSESSMENT POINTS

System	Effect	Assessment by Hx	Test
CV	Cardiomyopathy		ECHO
HEPATIC	Hypoglycemia Hepatomegaly with fatty infiltration	Lethargy	Blood glucose Bilirubin Liver function tests
HEME	Coagulopathy	Bleeding	Hypoprothrombinemia
CNS	Encephalopathy	Vomiting, diarrhea	Hyperammonemia
RENAL	Renal insufficiency	Recurrent myoglobinuria	BUN/Cr

Key References: Lucas M, Hinojosa M, Rodriguez A, Garcia-Guasch R. Anaesthesia in lipid myopathy. *Eur J Anaesthesiol*. 2000;17:461–462; Lilker S, Kasodekar S, Goldszmidt E. Anesthetic management of a parturient with carnitine palmitoyltransferase II deficiency. *Can J Anaesth*. 2006;53:482–486.

Perioperative Implications

Preoperative Preparation

- Continue daily carnitine therapy
- Glucose infusion preop
- Avoid protracted preop fasting
- For emergency surgery while in metabolic crisis, rehydrate; correct glucose, acid-base, and electrolyte imbalances, use IV carnitine if necessary, treat hypoprothrombinemia with FFP

Monitoring

- Routine

Airway

- Best to avoid succinylcholine for intubation

Maintenance

- IV glucose infusion, frequent monitoring of serum glucose level
- Muscle weakness may be present and requires careful titration of muscle relaxant dosing

Extubation

- No unusual concerns

Adjuvants

- Consider antiemetic prophylaxis to speed resumption of oral intake

Anticipated Problems/Concerns

- Periop hypoglycemia, metabolic acidosis/decompensation
- In the presence of carnitine deficiency, propofol may theoretically result in mitochondrial dysfunction and cellular hypoxia

Carotid Sinus Syndrome

Ronjeet Reddy
Christian Diez

Risk

- Male > female
- 9% of pts with recurrent syncope
- Incidence increases with age
- Peripheral vascular disease/previous carotid endarterectomy
- Head and neck cancer

Perioperative Risks

- Presence of carotid sinus syndrome (CSS) does not increase rate of mortality, sudden death, or stroke when compared to pts with similar age and risk factors.
- CSS does increase morbidity, secondary to injuries sustained during syncopal episodes.

Worry About

- Presence of co-morbid conditions: Coronary artery disease, carotid stenosis, neck tumor
- Severity of CSS and frequency of syncopal episodes
- Hemodynamic compromise: Bradycardia and/or hypotension

Overview

- The carotid sinus reflex occurs with changes in transmural pressure of the baroreceptors at the carotid sinus.
- Reflex arc
  - Afferent signals are sent via glossopharyngeal and vagus nerves to the nucleus tractus solitarius.
- Efferent signaling occurs through sympathetic and vagus nerves to the heart and blood vessels.
- Carotid sinus hypersensitivity (CSH) is defined as an exaggerated response to baroreceptor stimulation.
- Carotid sinus syndrome (CSS) occurs in pts with CSH when direct carotid sinus massage (CSM) or accidental neck stimulation produces symptoms such as dizziness/syncope or bradycardia and/or hypotension.
- There are 3 types of CSS
  - Cardioinhibitory type comprises 70–75% of cases due to vagal stimulation of SA and AV nodes, resulting in sinus bradycardia and may be treated with atropine.
  - Vasodepressor type represents 5–10% of cases, resulting in hypotension due to inhibition of vasomotor sympathetic tone; differentiated with cardioinhibitory type by not responding to atropine treatment.
  - Mixed type occurs in 20–25% of cases and results in bradycardia and loss of vasomotor tone.
- Diagnosis: Perform carotid sinus massage (CSM) in supine position and massage each carotid individually for 5 sec. Test is positive if any of the 3 are true: asystole greater than three sec (cardioinhibitory type); decrease in systolic BP greater than 50 mmHg (vasodepressor type); and combination of previous (mixed type)

ICD-9-CM Code: 337.0

Etiology

- Unclear, several proposed theories
- Mechanical deformation of the carotid sinus from neck tumors or previous carotid endarterectomy may lead to an exaggerated response.
- Degenerative process of the nucleus tractus solitarius that occurs with age
- Possible association with dementia, esp dementia with Lewy body disease (DLB)

Usual Treatment

- Medication
  - Atropine or vasopressors for acute, symptomatic pt
  - Seratonin reuptake inhibitors and alpha 1-agonists (midodrine) have been used with moderate success.
- Permanent dual chamber cardiac pacing is effective for cardioinhibitory and mixed types of CSS in pts who are symptomatic (pacing is of no benefit in vasodepressor type)
- Surgical denervation of carotid sinus may be attempted to treat vasodepressor type or pts who remain symptomatic despite pacing.
- Blocking the afferent limb (glossopharyngeal nerve) of the reflex with ethanol ablation is controversial due to a high complication rate.
- Volume expansion and increased salt intake is beneficial in vasodepressor type.
- Surgical removal of neck mass causing carotid sinus compression

ASSESSMENT POINTS

System	Effect	Assessment by Hx	PE	Test
CNS	Syncope	Dementia, DLB	CSM	MRI brain
AIRWAY / HEENT	Potential difficult intubation/ventilation Bradycardia and/or hypotension	Neck mass, neck surgery, symptoms with neck movement	Airway exam, tracheal deviation, Carotid bruit	CSM with EKG monitoring and A-line Carotid duplex CT/MRI neck
CV	Bradycardia and/or hypotension	Syncope with head turning or neck stimulation, CAD, PVD	CSM	CSM with EKG monitoring, A-line

Key Reference: Kenny RA, et al. Carotid sinus syndrome: A modifiable risk factor for nonaccidental falls in older adults. *Journal of American College of Cardiology*. 2001;38(5).

Perioperative Implications

Preoperative
- EKG, increased workup if advanced CAD
- CXR and/or CT scan to r/o tracheal compression if neck mass present
- Interrogate pacemaker, convert to DOO mode if unipolar cautery is to be used.

Monitoring / lines
- Consider arterial line for symptomatic pts
- If no pacemaker is present, must have external pacer readily available.

Airway
- Minimize neck extension during laryngoscopy, inline immobilization may be used.
- Asleep fiberoptic if pt has frequent symptoms with neck movement.
- Awake fiberoptic if mediastinal mass may cause tracheal compression with loss of spontaneous ventilation.

Positioning
- Avoid turning of pts neck.
- Ensure that instruments or personnel are not causing pressure to pts neck.

General Anesthesia
- Emergency drugs may be required based on type of CSS.
- General anesthesia may be preferred since inhalational agents have been shown to attenuate baroreceptor reflexes.
- Avoid hypotension on induction if coronary or carotid disease is present.
- Avoid long-acting beta blockers or antihypertensive drugs.

Regional Anesthesia
- Glossopharyngeal nerve block for CSS treatment may be performed.
- As an adjuvant to general anesthesia, local anesthetic may also be injected around carotid sinus prior to ipsilateral neck dissection to attenuate the baroreceptor response.

Postoperative Period
- Strict postop orders in PACU outlining no head turning or neck compression.
- If intraop asystole has occurred, surgeon may have to place a temporary transvenous pacer.

Anticipated Problems/Concerns

- Potential difficult intubation
- Must assess pacemaker function if present
- Pt may undergo profound hypotension or asystole at any time in the periop setting; emergency drugs should be readily available.

  Goal: Avoid neck stimulation and maintain hemodynamic stability.

Central Neurogenic Hyperventilation

Roy F. Cucchiara
Perry S. Bechtle

Incidence

• True central neurogenic hyperventilation (CNH) is exceedingly rare; exact incidence unknown
• In pts with neurologic injury, it is not rare and most often associated with pulm dysfunction or shunting (aspiration, pneumonia, pulm edema, baseline disease)
• No association with age or gender

Overview

• A diagnosis of exclusion in neurologic disorders and hyperventilation; life-threatening causes of hyperventilation (hypoxemia, ischemic bowel, acidosis) must be sought and ruled out
• Primary diagnostic criteria are hyperventilation that persists during sleep; low $PaCO_2$, high PaO_2 and absence of drug or metastatic causes

• Associated primarily with brainstem tumors with inconsistent involvement of midbrain, pons, and/or medulla
• CNS lymphomas and astrocytomas are the most common tumor types with gliomas, lymphomatoid granulomatosis, medulloblastoma, metastatic tumors also reported
• Effects of GA unknown

ICD9-CM: 786.01 (Hyperventilation)

Etiology

• Exact etiology and level of brainstem dysfunction not known
• Probable etiology
  • Uninhibited stimulation of inspir and expir centers in the medulla and/or loss of descending inhibitory control of ventilation by cerebral cortex with brainstem lesion

• Ultimate control of respiration may lie in medulla (dorsal and ventral respiratory groups) with fine control from the pneumotaxic center of the pons with input from cerebral cortex, hypothalamus, chemo- and mechanoreceptors, and vagal nerve
• Stimulation of most areas of cerebral cortex except motor/premotor areas, which inhibit respiration
• Unlikely etiology
  • There are no reported cases with stroke.
  • Tumor pH: in vivo is alkalotic; does not appear to contribute to resp control
  • Destructive lesions of midbrain or pons in animal studies does not produce CNH, but animal models may not simulate the human brain

ASSESSMENT POINTS

System	Effect	Assessment by Hx	PE	Test
RESP	Tachypnea	Tachypnea that persists during sleep and is unpleasant to conscious pt	Resp rate Normal inspiratory and expiratory excursion	ABGs (all must be present to diagnose): Pco_2 (low) pH (alkalotic) Pao_2 (increased for age) Decreased bicarbonate Alveolar-to-arterial gradient not larger than normal
CNS		Pt cannot volitionally inhibit hyperventilation	Focal or nonfocal CNS findings	CSF pH may be normal CT/MRI

Key Reference: Tarulli AW, Lim C, Bui JD, et al. Central neurogenic hyperventilation. A case report and discussion of pathophysiology. *Arch Neurol.* 2005;62:1632–1634.

Differential Diagnosis for Hyperventilation

• Metabolic acidosis
• Bowel ischemia with acidosis
• Pulm pathology with hypoxemia (pneumonia, pulm embolus, pulm edema, restrictive or obstructive lung disease)
• Drug toxicity (salicylates, theophylline, cyanide, topiramate)
• Sepsis
• Encephalopathy/CNS lesions (glioblastoma, encephalitis, multiple sclerosis, brainstem lymphoma, brainstem glioma, liver dysfunction)
• Anxiety
• Psychogenic
• Cardiac (CHF, valvular disease)
• High altitudes
• Hyperthyroidism
• Pregnancy
• Must exclude other etiologies for resp alkalosis with appropriate lab/Dx testing

Adverse Effects

• Resp alkalosis shifts oxyhemoglobin curve to left
• Hypocapnia is a potent cerebral vasoconstrictor, subsequently decreasing cerebral blood flow and volume
• Hypocapnia in injured brains may result in ischemic insults
• Effect of severe hypocapnia in normal brains is less clear and may produce ischemia when combined with Bohr effect

Treatment

• No completely effective or consistent treatment
• Narcotics may attenuate resp rate and improve blood gases but will not correct rate or alkalosis.
• Increasing dead space ventilation, administration of supplemental oxygen and benzodiazepines are not effective.

• Treatment of tumor with steroids, chemotherapy, or radiation therapy; however, not always effective.
• Mechanical ventilation with neuromuscular blockade and sedation during treatment of tumor has been attempted.

Outcome

• Death from progressive neurologic deterioration or other complications (aspiration, pneumonia) likely
• Improvement with treatment of tumor or long-term narcotics

Cephalopelvic Disproportion

Darren Cousin

Risk

- 1% to 3% of pregnant population

Perioperative Risks

- Increased maternal and fetal morbidity and mortality
- Protracted labor
- Arrested labor
- Uterine rupture
- Increased rate of cesarean section
- Increased rate of forceps or assisted delivery

Worry About

- Increased need for surgical delivery

- Increased incidence of fetal distress and need for emergency intervention

Overview

- Leads to abnormal labor pattern with subsequent high incidence of operative delivery
- Operative delivery associated with higher incidence of morbidity and mortality to mother and fetus
- Anesthesia necessities: Complete system exam incl airway for possible emergency C-section and landmarks for regional anesthesia

ICD-9-CM Code: 653.4

Etiology

- Maternal causes incl abnormalities of the pelvis, Hx of scoliosis, previous pelvic trauma, Hx of poliomyelitis
- The primary fetal cause is macrosomia often secondary to gestational diabetes

Usual Treatment

- Obstetric: Proper evaluation prior to and during labor
- Anesthesia: Regional for pain relief during labor or operative delivery

ASSESSMENT POINTS

System	Effect	Assessment by Hx	PE	Test
GYN	CPD	Failure to adequately respond to oxytocin	Pelvic exam	Radiographic cephalopelvimetry

Key Reference: Glantz JC. Elective induction vs. spontaneous labor associations and outcomes. *J Reprod Med.* 2005;50(4):235–240.

Perioperative Implications

- *Labor* is usually more prolonged and painful in pts with CPD.
- Epidural or combined spinal epidural is adequate to cover pain without prolonging the course of labor.

Anesthetic Technique

- Epidural analgesia: Low concentration of bupivacaine .25% or ropivacaine .20% supplemented with an opioid of your preference
- Combined spinal and epidural analgesia. *In early labor:* 25mcg fentanyl combined with 1 mL of .20% ropivacaine or .25% bupivacaine intrathecally followed by continuous epidural at 8 to 10 mL

per hr. *In late labor:* The initial intrathecal injection of local anesthetic and opioid is often sufficient for the remainder of the first and second stages of labor.
- *C-section* (in all cases): Anesthesia machine checked. Left uterine displacement to maximize uterine blood flow. Apply ASA standard monitors.
- *Elective C-section:* Spinal anesthesia in usual fashion. Prehydration with 15mL/kg, followed by 1.4 cc of .75% bupivacaine injected at L4. Maintain BP within normal limits using ephedrine when necessary.
- *Emergency C-section:* Following labor without fetal distress (failure to progress): If pt has a reliable epidural block, epidural anesthesia is

extended using 3% chloroprocaine, 2% lidocaine, or .5% ropivacaine if time permits. If pt does not have an epidural catheter, then a spinal technique may be used.
- *Following labor with fetal distress:* If pt has an epidural catheter, dose with 3% chloroprocaine or 2% lidocaine if time permits. If pt doesn't have a catheter, GA may be necessary.

Anticipated Problems/Concerns

- If there is no epidural catheter in place and a difficult airway is suspected, then use spinal anesthesia or perform an awake intubation. A fast track LMA, a fiberoptic scope, or a video-enhanced laryngoscope should be available.

Cerebral Arteriovenous Malformations (AVMs)

L. Jane Easdown

Risk

- Rare: 1–2% cause of CVA in a younger population
- Symptomatic cases: 1/100,000 person-years
- 4.3% of population at autopsy

Perioperative risks

- Yearly risk of hemorrhage is 1–3%.
- 45–70% present with hemorrhage or seizures
- Postop "normal perfusion pressure breakthrough"

Worry about

- Massive intraventricular or intraparenchymal hemorrhage
- Seizure
- New neurologic deficits
- Cerebral edema, hyperemia postsurgery or endovascular embolization

ICD9-CM 747.81 (Anomalies of cerebrovascular system)

Overview

- Localized arteriovenous shunt comprised of a tangle or "nidus" of abnormally walled vessels which cause symptoms by rupture, ischemia, and diversion of flow or pressure on adjacent structures. Many are detected on routine scans.
- 70% are supratentorial, 4–10% are associated with aneurysms.
- AVMs usually present in the second to the fourth decade of life with a yearly risk of bleed of 3–4%. There is an increased risk of rebleed of 6% within the first year. The majority of AVMs will bleed at least once.
- Mortality from an initial hemorrhage is 10–30%.
- Vein of Galen malformations are rare congenital lesions with connections between the intracerebral vessels and the great vein of Galen. This disorder in neonates or infants may result in high output CHF or increased ICP from hydrocephalus.

Etioloy

- Although congenital in origin, no specific genetic defect has been determined. Sometimes associated with hereditary hemorrhagic telangiectasia.

Usual treatment

- Evidence-based neurosurgical management is predicated on the Spetzler-Martin grading scale. AVMs are graded 1–5 based on their size, location, and pattern of venous drainage.
- Smaller and more superficial AVMs (grade 1–2) might be surgically resected. Higher grade AVMs may be treated with neuroembolization, radiosurgery or conservative management. Combinations of therapy are common, esp embolization prior to surgical resection.

ASSESSMENT POINTS

System	Effect	Assessment by Hx	PE	Test
HEENT	Airway protection	Aspiration	Active gag reflex	
CVS	CHF in children with vein of Galen AVM		S3, CHF	CXR, ECHO, ECG
CNS	Seizures, focal deficits, CVA, raised ICP	Headaches, seizures, changes in mentation	Neurologic exam	MRI, MRA, CT, cerebral angiography

Key Reference: Avitsian R, Schubert A. Anesthetic considerations for intraoperative management of cerebrovascular disease in neurovascular surgical procedures. *Anesthesiol Clin.* 2007;25:441–463.

Perioperative considerations

Preoperative preparation

- Endovascular embolization procedures may require GA or MAC
- Craniotomy for resection requires preop preparation similar to aneurysm clipping.
- Neurologic exam with attention to focal deficits, raised ICP
- Prior embolization may have been performed.
- Careful assessment of size and location of AVM

Monitoring

- Invasive BP monitoring
- For craniotomy-preparation for extensive blood loss incl central assess if surgery will involve deep structures
- Precordial Doppler for detection of air
- Jugular bulb venous O_2 monitoring has been described.
- Intraop neuro monitoring may incl EEG, SSEPS

Airway

- ETT for craniotomy, LMA or intubation for airway management for embolization

Induction

- Careful management of BP to prevent Htn (increased ICP, hemorrhage) or hypotension (ischemia).

Maintenance

- Careful management of BP, ICP esp with intubation, pinning, and incision.
- Surgeons may request burst suppression with propofol or barbiturates for brain protection if temporary clips are used.
- Surgeons may request hypotension or hypercapnia.
- Blood glucose control
- Strict isotonic/hypertonic fluid management
- Angiography prior to emergence
- Plan for arousal and neurologic testing immediately postop

Extubation

- Careful BP control—labetolol, additional opioid
- Expect request for neurologic exam
- May elect to remain intubated

Adjuvants

- Cell saver
- BP control with nicardipine, NTG, NTP, beta blockers
- Phenylephrine infusion
- Propofol infusion for TIVA or burst suppression
- Steroids, mannitol
- Antiepilepsy medications

Postoperative period

- Complete obliteration of a large AVM will lead to redistribution of the CBF and hyperemia or 'normal perfusion pressure breakthrough" Until autoregulation returns, the pt may require lower BP and control of CO_2 by intubation and ventilation.
- Postop ICU neurologic monitoring will be required.

Cerebral Palsy

Carmen Labrie-Brown
Alan Kaye

Risk

- Leading cause of childhood motor disability1–2 per 1000 live births in developed countries
- Incidence has not decreased despite improved perinatal care because of increased survival in premature neonates

Perioperative Risks

- Dehydration
- Electrolyte imbalance
- Hypothermia
- Delayed recovery

Worry About

- Difficult intubation
- GE reflux and aspiration
- Associated resp impairment
- Drug interactions
- Latex allergy

Overview

- Any nonprogressive central motor deficit dating to events in the pre-, peri-, or postnatal periods
- Wide spectrum of symptoms
  - Cognitive impairment
  - Seizures
  - Sensory loss (visual, hearing)
  - Communication, behavioral disturbances
  - Resp, GI, orthopedic problems
- Often have normal intellect (esp dyskinetic group)
- Classified as spastic (70%), dyskinetic (10%), ataxic (10%), and mixed (10%)

ICD-9-CM Code: 343.9

Etiology

- Mostly unknown
- Antenatal cerebral events causing complications at time of delivery, e.g., periventricular hemorrhage and infection
- Postnatal events such as trauma and infection
- All causes result in damage to CNS during early brain growth.

Usual Treatment

- Anticonvulsants, antispasmodies (benzodiazepines, baclofen, dantrolene), antidepressants, antireflux agents, laxatives, anticholinergies
- Often intramuscular botulinum toxin injections and orthopedic procedures (tendon releases and osteotomies), fundoplication for reflux, and dental extractions

ASSESSMENT POINTS

System	Effect	Assessment by Hx	PE	Test
HEENT	Tongue thrusting Poor dentition Salivary drooling	Difficulty swallowing	Dental malocclusion Dental caries	Formal airway assessment usually difficult
RESP	Restrictive defect Aspiration pneumonia Recurrent chest infections	Cough Dyspnea (difficult to detect if mobilization limited)	Often normal Reduced air entry Bronchial breathing Wheeze	Pulm function tests ABGs CXR
CV	Right-sided heart failure from restrictive lung disease	Often normal Dyspnea	Tachycardia S_3 or S_4 Distended JVP Hepatomegaly	ECG ECHO
GI	GE reflux Esophageal dysmotility	Poor swallowing Night wakening	Dehydration Pallor Malnutrition	CBC Electrolytes ± Endoscopy
MS	Spasticity Dyskinesia Ataxia	Muscle pain and spasms	Increased muscle tone Contractures Tremor	Gait analysis performed before major orthopedic surgery
CNS	Epilepsy (30%) Visual and hearing defects	Tonic-clonic and complex-partial seizures	Myopia Visual field defects Strabismus	Not usually relevant
HEME	Iron-deficiency anemia	Fatigue	Pallor	CBC, differential
METAB	Electrolyte imbalance	Laxative use Fatigue	Dehydration Malnutrition	UA Albumin

Key Reference: Nolan J, Chalkiadis GA, Low J, Olesch CA, Brown TO. Anaesthesia and pain management in cerebral palsy. *Anaesthesia.* 2000;55:32–41.

Perioperative Implications

Preoperative Preparation

- Can have normal intellect
- Involve parents in management, as parents have good insight into periop care
- Avoid unfamiliar faces if possible
- Optimize resp status (bronchodilators, antibiotics, physical therapy)
- Optimize nutrition; fix lyte imbalance
- Continue medical Rx, esp anticonvulsants
- May need antireflux, antisialagogue, or sedative premed (cautious doses of sedatives)
- Topical local anesthetic for venipuncture
- Discuss periop analgesia (often regional technique for lower limb surgery)

Monitoring

- Core temp (susceptible to hypothermia)
- Neuromuscular blockade
- Airway pressures

Airway

- ETT is better sized to age, not wt
- Salivary secretions may make ventilation difficult
- Overbite may make intubation difficult

Induction

- Rapid-sequence may be required but often impractical
- IV access often difficult
- Inhalation sometimes favored (in semisitting position if concerns of reflux)

Maintenance

- Careful positioning, check frequently
- Consider antiemetics
- IV fluids
- MAC may be lower in cerebral palsy—as much as 20% and up to 30% if pt is on anticonvulsants
- Use warming devices
- Consider regional (epidural) techniques for lower limb surgery

Other Intraoperative Challenges

- Bleeding
  - Anectodal: Pts with neuromuscular scoliosis bleed > idiopathic scoliosis
  - Poor nutritional/nonambulatory status
  - Borderline low platelet count and function due to anticonvulsants
  - Subnormal clotting factor level
- Temp
  - Severe CP kids may be unable to regulate temp
  - Little subcutaneous fat
  - Some arrive to OR with temp <35°C
  - Warm room till pt draped, use warming blanket/gases/fluids

Extubation

- Awake if prone to reflux

Drug considerations

- Baclofen should not be stopped abruptly but may cause postop bradycardia and hypotension
- Resistance to nondepolarizing NMB (probably not clinically significant)
- Ketamine and methohexital may be avoided in epileptic pts
- N_2O and opiates may worsen nausea

Postoperative Period

- Aggressive resp care
- Maintain normothermia
- Susceptible to N/V
- Avoidance/treatment of muscle spasm (IV diazepam, epidural clonidine)
- Early mobilization

Anticipated Problems/Concerns

- Latex allergy
- Hypothermia
- Prolonged recovery time
- Postop NIV (worse with opiates)
- Postop muscle spasms
- Retention of secretions and postop chest infection

Cerebrovascular Transient Ischemic Attack (TIA)

Zirka H. Anastasian

Eric J. Heyer

Risk

- Overall risk in USA is approx 83/100,000
- Risk related to demographic factors of age, gender, race
- Age and gender: Estimated prevalence of TIA in men of 2.7% vs. 1.6 % in women for 65–69 y old, 3.6% in med vs. 4.1% in women for 75–79 y of age. The overall prevalence is estimated to be 0.4% among adults 45–64 y of age.
- Race: Blacks and men are at highest risk

Perioperative Risk

- Pts with Hx of TIAs at increased risk of postop stroke
- Increased risk of periop stroke in pts with medical Hx of cerebral vascular disease, peripheral vascular disease, Htn, diabetes, chronic renal insufficiency, COPD, and atrial fibrillation
- Pts with coronary artery disease for CABG have a high incidence of carotid stenosis (50% with some, 20% with stenosis >50%)
- Likewise, pts with carotid stenosis have high incidence of coronary artery disease (over 50%).
- Increased risk of periop stroke in pts with planned surgery: CABG (3%–6%), vascular (1%)

Worry about

- Crescendo TIAs
- Duration of symptoms >1 hr

- Symptomatic or critical internal carotid artery stenosis
- Known cardiac source of embolus such as atrial fibrillation
- Known hypercoagulable state

Overview

- Transient ischemic attack (TIA): A transient episode of neurologic dysfunction caused by focal brain, spinal cord, or retinal ischemia, without acute infarction. The endpoint is biologic (tissue injury) rather than arbitrary (24 hr).
- Risk of hospitalization for major cardiac event after TIA is 2.6% for first 90 d.
- ABCDD score for assessing risk of stroke after TIA:
  - A = Age (>60 y = 1 point)
  - B = Blood pressure elevation when first assessed after TIA (systolic ≥140 mmHg or diastolic ≥90 mmHg = 1 point)
  - C = Clinical features (unilateral weakness = 2 points; isolated speech disturbance = 1 point; other = 0 points)
  - D = Duration of TIA symptoms (≥60 min = 2 points; 10 to 59 min = 1 point; <10 min = 0 points)
  - Diabetes (present = 1 point)
- Score interpretation:
  - Score 6 to 7: High 2-d stroke risk (8.1 %)

ICD-9-CM Code: 435.9

- Score 4 to 5: Moderate 2-d stroke risk (4.1%)
- Score 0 to 3: Low 2-d stroke risk (1.0%)

Etiology

- Cerebral vessel disease: Atherosclerosis, lipohyalinosis, inflammation, amyloid deposition, arterial dissection, developmental malformation, aneurysmal dilation, or venous thrombosis
- Remote disease: Embolus forms from the heart or other circulation and lodges in a cerebral vessel.
- Blood-flow related: Inadequate cerebral blood flow due to decreased perfusion pressure or increased blood viscosity (hypotension, trauma, surgical compression, steal, coagulopathy)

Usual Treatment

- Determine causing factor
- Cerebral vessel disease: Antiplatelet therapy, anticoagulation, and revascularization (carotid endarterectomy, carotid stent, vertebral artery stent)
- Remote disease: Investigate and treat causing factor (atrial fibrillation, valvular disease, etc), antiplatelet therapy and anticoagulation.
- Blood flow related: Treat underlying cause, antiplatelet therapy, anticoagulation

ASSESSMENT POINTS

System	Effect	Assessment by Hx	PE	Test
HEENT	Neck trauma Compression			
CNS	CV disease dz	TIA Sx Previous stroke	Carotid bruit Bilat BP	Carotid Doppler Angio: Carotid, vertebral artery.
CV	CAD disease	Hx of MI, angina Arrhythmia Decreased exercise tolerance Risk factors for atherosclerosis	Murmur Irregular rate/rhythm	EKG Stress test Holter TEE/TTE
GI		N/V		
CNS	Transient focal neurologic deficit	Vision changes, changes in language, weakness, sensory changes, ataxia	Ischemic retina Often neuro exam normal	CT/MRI CV imaging

Source: Definition and evaluation of transient ischemic attack: A scientific statement for healthcare professionals from the American Heart Association/American Stroke Association Stroke Council; Council on Cardiovascular Surgery and Anesthesia; Council on Cardiovascular Radiology and Intervention; Council on Cardiovascular Nursing; and the Interdisciplinary Council on Peripheral Vascular Disease. The American Academy of Neurology affirms the value of this statement as an educational tool for neurologists. Easton JD, Saver JL, Albers GW, Alberts MJ, Chaturvedi S, Feldmann E, Hatsukami TS, Higashida RT, Johnston SC, Kidwell CS, Lutsep HL, Miller E, Sacco RL; American Heart Association; American Stroke Association Stroke Council; Council on Cardiovascular Surgery and Anesthesia; Council on Cardiovascular Radiology and Intervention; Council on Cardiovascular Nursing; Interdisciplinary Council on Peripheral Vascular Disease. *Stroke.* 2009 Jun;40(6):2276–93. Epub 2009 May 7. Review.

Perioperative Preparation

- Determine BP range that pt normally experiences
- Manage BP with both cerebral perfusion and CAD in mind
- Preop cardiac workup and medical stabilization if non-emergent surgery
- Preop neurologic exam
- Avoid excessive premedication (pt can be more sensitive)
- Avoid long-acting intraoperative agents that can obscure postop neuro exam

Monitoring

- EKG monitoring for ischemia and arrhthymia
- Consider arterial line and central line/PA catheter if extensive CV disease

Airway

- Avoid extreme neck manipulation and pressure on carotid artery during ventilation and intubation.

Preinduction/Induction

- Maintain pressure to allow for sufficient cerebral perfusion (rightward shift in cerebral autoregulation in Htn)
- Titrate medication as pt requirements can be decreased

Maintenance

- Pts can be more sensitive to medications
- Avoid long-acting agents if neurologic exam to be performed postop

- Isoflurane theoretically neuroprotective: Allows lowest cerebral flood flow prior to EEG symptoms of ischemia

Extubation

- Ensure pt is awake, following command, and able to protect airway
- Ensure pt does not have large neurologic deficit which would lead to swelling and resp insufficiency postop.

Postoperative Period

- Period of greatest risk for stroke after general surgery
- Resume antiplatelet therapy and anticoagulation as soon as possible.

Cervical Disk Disease (Cervical Spine Disease)

Andrew D. Rosenberg

Risk

- Incidence in the USA: 12,000 deaths /y; 70 million with cervical disk disease, spondylosis, or trauma
- Disk disease—a consequence of aging (third–fifth decades)
- Present in rheumatoid arthritis (RA), ankylosing spondylitis, other rheumatic disorders
- Trauma, esp motor vehicle accidents
- M:F ratio: 3:2

Perioperative Risks

- Mortality (acute) 1–5% (depending on associated injuries)
- Spinal cord damage with C-spine movement
- Difficulty intubating or reintubating postextubation
- After neck surgery, swelling or hematoma can cause obstruction of airway
- Steroid-induced complications

Worry About

- Airway management; C-spine movement during or after intubation

- Exacerbating or causing spinal cord damage with neck motion
- Osteoarthritis with osteophytes impinging on nerve roots

Overview

- Neck pain present in 30% of adults in the USA
- Can cause radiculopathy, which can be aggravated by neck extension
- Root
  - C3: Unusual
  - C4: Numbness rare, pain at root of neck
  - C5: Numb over shoulder to lateral aspect of upper arm ("epaulet" area)
  - C6: Second-most common radiculopathy; pain across top of neck, along biceps muscle into tips of thumb and index finger as well as biceps muscle weakness
  - C7: Most common herniation: pain across back of shoulder triceps, and into middle finger as well as loss of triceps reflex

- C8: Numb small finger, interossei weak

ICD-9-CM Codes: 952.0 (Cervical spine injury); 756.19 (Cervical spondylosis)

Etiology

- Disk disease is a process of aging
- Inflammatory arthropathy or trauma: In trauma, can have fractures, dislocations, or ligamentous damage causing spinal cord paralysis; can get swelling of soft tissues of neck

Usual Treatment

- Neck should be stabilized, not forced into position; any movement can cause damage
- In pts with atlantoaxial subluxation, avoid flexion. Can have superior migration of odontoid as well as subaxial subluxation.
- Stabilization and time to heal, repair
- Shoulder and strap muscle strengthening exercises
- Epidural steroids for recent disk disease
- Steroids for acute spinal cord injury

ASSESSMENT POINTS

System	Effect	Assessment by Hx	PE	Test
HEENT	Numbness and pain in RA: Superior migration of odontoid, atlantoaxial subluxation, atlas-dens interval (ADI) increased (> 4 mm unstable), subaxial subluxation, cricoarytenoid arthritis, airway abnormalities, trauma, swelling	Hoarseness, snoring	In RA: TMJ problems, hypoplastic mandible	In RA: Neck x-ray flexion and extension (measure ADD) Evaluate bones, ligament alignment, soft tissue swelling, motion
CV	Trauma: Possible cardiac contusion/injury, spinal shock		Heart sounds distant Unstable BP	ECG, ECHO
RESP	Rheumatologic disorders: Fibrosis, honeycombing Ankylosing spondylitis: Restrictive pattern Trauma: Diaphragm function (C3–C5), pneumothorax, hemothorax, contusion, aspiration, rib fractures	SOB	In trauma: Dyspnea, paradoxical ventilation, flail chest, breath sounds absent with pneumothorax	CXR, ABGs
GI	Ulcers 2° to aspirin for RA			
HEME	RA: Anemia 2° to medications		Trauma: Look for signs of bleeding	Hgb
CNS	Vertebral artery compression: Dizziness, vertigo, nausea, blurred vision			

Key Reference: MacDonald D. Intraoperative motor evoked potential monitoring: Overview and update. *J Clin Monit Comput.* 2006;20(5):347–377.

Perioperative Implications

- Assess neck in disk disease, rheumatic diseases, trauma
- Consider intubation with neck stabilized by assistant to avoid flexion or extension or awake fiberoptic intubation.
- Consider intubating with fiberoptic intubation, Glidescope, AirTraq, larygeal mask airway, light wand or other airway assistance device.
- Avoid medications (e.g., midazolam) incl muscle relaxants if they are used at all for initial intubation that might interfere with specialized spinal cord monitoring Somatosensory Evoked Potentials (SSEPs) or Transcranial Motor Evoked Potentials (TCMEPs)

Monitoring

- Acute spinal cord shock may require arterial and PA catheters or TEE to facilitate monitoring and treating hemodynamic disturbances

- When using intraop TCMEPs, protect the tongue and ETT from masseter and muscles of mastication contraction during stimulation. Remember, muscle relaxants cannot be used when TCMEPs are utilized.

Induction

- Consider not initiating irreversible steps (e.g., muscle relaxants) until airway is secured.

Extubation

- Consider not extubating until pt is able to maintain airway without threat of swelling or airway obstruction.

Adjuvants

- Steroids reduce injury in acute traumatic spinal cord injury.

Postoperative Period

- Observe for neck swelling, hoarseness, airway obstruction

- Assess neurologic status

Anticipated Problems/Concerns

- Anticipate difficulty intubating pts due to abnormal anatomy or limitation of motion. Prepare pt for fiberoptic intubation.
- Associated traumatic injuries—cardiac, brain, lung, abdomen, bladder, long bones—and their consequences
- ARDS from aspiration in preop traumatic event
- Injury to tongue or ETT from biting down as a result of muscle contraction from TCMEP stimulation.

Chagas' Disease

Charles Hogue
Nanhi Mitter

Risk

- 16–18 million infected worldwide
- Rare in Southern USA; chronic disease more likely in immigrants from endemic region (South America, central Brazil prevalence 6–8%)
- More than 50,000 die each year, mortality estimated at 50% at 4 y secondary to heart failure
- Laboratory workers and personnel exposed to blood products, travelers to endemic areas

Perioperative Risks

- Not defined
- Most important prognostic factor is degree of myocardial dysfunction
- Esophageal changes due to megaesophagus and reflux
- Associated with myasthenia gravis
- CNS symptoms—meningoencephalitis (particularly in immunocompromised pts)

Worry About

- LV dysfunction and CHF: Chagas' myocarditis, refractory heart failure. Most often biventricular in nature right > left. Sudden cardiac death associated with 55–65% deaths; precipitated by exercise, VT, Vfib, asystole, AVB
- Conduction abnormalities (complete AV block, right bundle branch block (RBBB), left anterior fascicular block (LAFB)
- Ventricular arrhythmias (VT, atrial fibrillation)
- Ventricular aneurysms (posterior-lateral, inferior basal, apical)
- Megaesophagus, achalasia, risk of pulm aspiration
- Blood transmission and infections
- Thromboemboslism, stroke

Overview

- Acute infection mostly in pediatric population, asymptomatic in $^2/_3$ of pts, followed by chronic disease after latency of > second and third decades
- In endemic areas, mild forms of disease common with benign course
- Pathogenesis to chronic, progressive end-organ disease poorly understood; autoimmunity, microvascular dysfunction, autonomic neuropathy implicated
- Cardiac involvement most serious end-organ manifestation; colon and esophagus also affected
- Mechanisms proposed for cardiac involvement unclear but incl neurogenic mechanisms, parasite-dependent inflammation, microvascular disease and immune-mediated injury.
- In USA, Dx usually not considered; presentation as CAD or dilated cardiomyopathy, or with AV heart block, CHF, ECG conduction abnormalities, sustained VTach.
- Serologic test for Dx, based on hemagglutination, immunofluorescence, ELISA, PCR, is usually negative during first week so Dx dependent on detection of circulating parasites.
- Continues to cardiac involvement—decapillarization of the myocardium.
- Downregulation of the nicotinic Ach receptors and associated myasthenia gravis symptomatology.

ICD-9-CM Code: 086.0

Etiology

- Protozoan infection: Trypanosoma cruzi
- Transmission to humans by reduviid bug, the "kissing bug".
- Transmission by blood transfusion, organ transplantation, vector, laboratory accident, reactivation of chronic disease during immunosuppression. Recently oral chagasic infection via food contamination (sugar and acai juices) also possible with more severe clinical course.
- Central and South America endemic areas.

Usual Treatment

- Nifurtimox (limited efficacy, poor oral bioavailability); for acute disease; usefulness for indeterminate phase or chronic disease not established.
- Benznidazole (similar efficacy as nifurtimox) second agent, not available in USA.
- Recent success with protriptyline in the acute and chronic form.
- Allopurinol for the cutaneous form
- No evidence trypanocide drug therapy cures disease.
- Other treatment related to symptomology: Amiodarone for arrhythmias related to LV dysfunction; sotalol. Invasive treatment modalities incl surgical excision, catheter ablation, aneurysmectomy, epicardial mapping.
- Pts at high risk for sudden cardiac death will have ICD placed.
- Heart transplant, bone marrow cell transplant uncertain.

ASSESSMENT POINTS

System	Effect	Assessment by Hx	PE	Test
CV	Conduction abnormalities LV dysfunction and aneurysm	Syncope, DOE, orthopnea, fatigue Atypical Angina	JVD, edema, rales, cardiomegaly Murmurs TR, MR, wide split S2, prominent diffuse apical thrust	ECG ECHO MUGA Cardiac catheter CXR: cardiomegaly
	Ventricular arrhythmias	Syncope, palpitations	Biventricular enlargement	Holter electrophysiologic study, TTE, TEE
GI	Megaesophagus, megacolon	Dysphagia, GE reflux, constipation	Abdominal distention	Barium studies CXR, endoscopy

Key Reference: Leckie RS, Leckie S, Mahmood F. Perioperative management of a patient with Chagas disease having mitral valve surgery. *J Clin Anesth*. 2009;21(4):282–285.

Perioperative Implications

Preoperative Preparation

- LV function optimization with diuretics, ACE inhibitors, consider β-blockers and Ca²⁺-channel blockers. Consider amiodarone in cases of VTach/VFIB.
- Prophylaxis against pulm aspiration.
- Assessment of conduction abnormalities, arrhythmias.

Monitoring

- Dictated by degree of LV dysfunction and proposed procedure; consider PA catheter or TEE. On TEE may see biventricular enlargement, thinning of ventricular walls, apical aneurysm, intramural thrombus.
- ECG during entire periop period. Often see long QT interval, AV block, bundle branch block. Can have VTach/VFIB.

Preinduction/Induction

- Consider temporary pacing if symptomatic AV block
- Caution with negative inotropic drugs
- Awake or rapid-sequence intubation
- Consider judicious use of muscle relaxants

Maintenance

- Technique dictated by preferences, procedure, degree of cardiac involvement
- Avoid hypoxemia (facilitates ischemic myocardial changes on capillary level, which can further progress to wall thinning and aneurysm formation)

Postoperative Period

- Continued monitoring depends on pre-existing LV dysfunction and operative procedure
- ECG monitoring for ventricular arrhythmias and AV conduction block

Cherubism

Daniel Siker
Lee A. Fleisher

Risk

- >250 cases in world literature
- Cherubs have a 40% chance of a cherub offspring

Perioperative Risks

- Swelling of lower face causing airway obstruction
- Displacement of ocular orbit and lower eyelid causing visual changes
- Excessive blood loss from curettage of vascular lesions
- Association with Noonan syndrome

Worry About

- Pulm valve stenosis (Noonan syndrome)
- Undiagnosed hyperparathyroidism
- Convex, V-shaped hypertrophied hard palate
- Small mouth opening and mild trismus

Overview

- Progressive symmetric fullness of cheeks and jaw, with retraction of lower eyelids exposing an inferior rim of sclera
- Onset age: 2–12 y
- These round-faced, upwardly gazing infants look like Renaissance art cherubs
- Diagnostic biopsy of mandible shows multinucleated giant cells
- Associated problems with speaking, breathing, swallowing, chewing
- Pathognomonic x-ray of jaw demonstrates radiolucent lesions

ICD-9-CM Code: 526.89

Etiology

- Mutations in the *SH3BP2* gene cause cherubism
- Familial: Autosomal dominant

- Penetrance: 100% for boys, 50% for girls
- Unknown but named alternatively familial fibrous dysplasia, bilateral giant cell tumors, familial multilocular cystic disease
- Multilocular cystic malformation of mandible and maxilla with painless submandibular lymphadenopathy

Usual Treatment

- Operative curettage, removal of displaced teeth, cortical reshaping of mandible
- Selective embolization with operative excision of vascular lesions
- Bone grafts

ASSESSMENT POINTS

System	Effect	Assessment by Hx	PE	Test
HEENT	Orbits shifted	Loss of binocular vision	Upward gaze	
	Enlargement	Photo review by age	Painless jaw swelling Lymphadenopathy	Jaw series
	Poor opening	Moderate trismus	Soft tissue swelling Concave palate	
	Malocclusion	Absence of third molar	Loose teeth	X-ray
CV	If associated with Noonan syndrome	Pulmonic valve disease	Pulm valve stenosis	ECHO
RESP	Generally unaffected	Obstructive airway		Sleep study
ENDO	Rule out hyperparathyroidism	Onset at older age		Normal Ca^{2+}, K^+
CNS	Midparental intelligence	No developmental delay, except with Noonan syndrome		
MS	Long bone lesions		Humerus, anterior ribs, femoral neck	

Key Reference: Monclus E, Garcés A, Artés D, Mabrock M. Oral to nasal tube exchange under fibroscopic view: A new technique for nasal intubation in a predicted difficult airway. *Paediatr Anaesth.* 2008;18(7):663–666.

Perioperative Implications

Preoperative Preparation

- Rule out parathyroid disease
- Available blood for curettage replacement

Monitoring

- Routine

Airway

- Difficult airway protocol
- Oral intubation using a laryngeal mask technique has been reported. Fiberscopic control of the exchange and the introduction of a Cook exchange catheter into the trachea through the oral tube before withdrawal permits oxygenation of the pt and acts as a guide for oral tube reintroduction if required.

Preinduction/Induction

- Spontaneous ventilation
- Laryngeal mask airway

Maintenance

- Consider hypotensive technique for minimizing blood loss

Extubation

- May require ICU admission for prolonged intubation

Adjuvants

- Routine

Postoperative Period

- Extubation awake with confirmation of no bleeding

Anticipated Problems/Concerns

- Nasal intubation for oral procedures may be problematic, similar to Pierre Robin, Goldenhar's, and Treacher Collins syndromes. As mandibular rami approach midline, no space for visualization of airway.

Cigarette Smoking

[handwritten: When to quit and what will it do for you ↓]

James M. Blum
Kevin K. Tremper

Risk
- Incidence in the USA: Estimated 43.4 million
- Native Americans have highest rate of smoking (36.4%)
- More common in impoverished individuals
- M:F ratio: 4:3; young females fastest-growing group

Perioperative Risks
- Increased risk of CAD × 2.0 of nonsmokers of same age
- Postop pulm complications up to × 6 of nonsmoker
- Carboxyhemoglobin (COHB) increased (up to 15%)
- Hyperreactive airway
- Does not increase risk of pulm aspiration
- Reduces risk of postop N/V

Worry About
- CAD, COPD, PVD, productive cough, reactive airway
- Increases physiologic age by 8 y (30 pack-y) relative to nonsmoker
- Decreased tolerance to pain, requiring increased doses of analgesics

Overview
- Addictive habit. Cigarette smoke contains > 4000 identifiable constituents, many of which are pharmacologically active, toxic, or have tumorigenic effects. Acute effects relate to CO and nicotine.
- 90% of tobacco smoke is gaseous, consisting of nitrogen, O_2, carbon monoxide along with gaseous irritants and carbon monoxide. Particulate matter consists of nicotine, tar, and other volitile organics.
- Nicotine stimulates the sympathetic ganglia, causing release of catecholamines from the adrenal medulla and sympathetic nerve endings, increasing BP, HR, and SVR, that persists for 30 min after one cigarette.
- Associated with decreased MAO and increased dopamine levels in brain
- Inhaled CO produces up to 5–15% COHb compared to 0.3–1.6% in nonsmokers. Combined effects of nicotine and COHb put diseased myocardium at risk.
- An irritant to pulm system, increasing mucus production while decreasing ciliary activity and mucus flow, markedly impairing tracheobronchial secretion clearance
- Chronic use associated with CAD, Htn, COPD, peripheral vascular disease, numerous cancers
- Smoking also increases all blood cell lines, increases platelet reactivity, and fibrinogen.
- Cessation for 3–4 hr results in insignificant hemodynamic side effects from nicotine and improves myocardial O_2 supply:demand.

- Cessation of smoking the night before surgery will reduce the COHb and nicotine levels to that of nonsmokers.
- Cessation 4–6 d will result in a return of ciliary activity.
- Cessation of smoking for ≤8 wk has controversial additional benefits; cessation of > 8 wk has demonstrated decreased incidence of postop pulm complications. Cessation for 2 y reduces risks of MI to that of the nonsmoking population.
- Considered to be the cause of 1 of every 6 deaths in the USA and is the leading cause of preventable mortality (400,000 preventable deaths/y).

ICD-9-CM Code: 305.1 (Tobacco abuse)

Etiology
- Habituation

Usual Treatment
- Nicotine patch and clonidine, varenicline, bupropion, Smokers Anonymous, or self-withdrawal

Treatment *[handwritten: (recommendations)]*
- Cessation for a minimum of 12–24 hr. Decrease in COHb and nicotine.
- Cessation for ≥8 wk will reduce postop pulm complications
- Cessation for ≥2 y decreases risk of MI

ASSESSMENT POINTS

System	Effect	Assessment by Hx	PE	Test
HEENT	Oral, pharyngeal, head and neck cancers		Lesions on exam or intubation	Usually not needed
CV	↑ Heart rate, SVR, coronary vascular resistance → Myocardial ischemia ↑ PVR ↑ Blood viscosity	Exercise tolerance, angina (see Coronary Artery Disease in Diseases section)	Two-flight walk	ECG
RESP	↑ COHb, COPD ↓ FEV_1FVC ↑ Secretion ↓ Clearance ↑ Airway reactivity	Exercise tolerance, chronic productive cough, character of sputum	Auscultation	CXR if symptomatic Hct, sputum (see COPD)

Key Reference: Moores LK. Smoking and postoperative pulmonary complications. *Clin Chest Med.* 2000;21:139–146.

Perioperative Implications

Preoperative Preparation
- Cessation overnight will decrease COHb and nicotine.
- Cessation for 8 wk will decrease postop pulmonary complications.
- If chronic productive cough, consider preop antibiotic treatment.

Monitoring
- Routine
- SpO_2 monitoring, may read higher SpO_2 than actual if COHb present (SpO_2 = % HbO_2 + % COHb)
- Consider invasive monitoring if symptomatic pulm or cardiac disease.

Airway
- Potential laryngeal hyperreactivity

Premedication/Induction
- Consider deep induction if Hx of reactive airway disease.

Maintenance
- Routine unless symptomatic cardiac or pulm disease
- Avoid light anesthesia and desflurane to reduce potential bronchospasm.

Extubation
- Consider deep extubation if severe reactive airway disease but is easy to intubate and ventilate, with no aspiration risk.

Adjuvants
- Routine; smoking increases metabolism of theophylline, decreases half-life from 265 to 180 min

Postoperative Period
- Epidural analgesia may be beneficial in decreasing complications of hypercoagulability, CAD, or COPD.

Anticipated Problems/Concerns
- Long-standing Hx of smoking with symptomatic pulm disease leads to high risk of developing postop pulm complications (pneumonia) due to increased mucus production and decreased ciliary function. Cessation for 8 wk is recommended.
- Airway reactivity significantly increased in smokers; abstinence for 24 hr does not change this reactivity. Reactivity starts reducing after 24–48 hr and reduces to near level of nonsmokers after 10 d of cessation.
- Risk of MI decreases to that of nonsmokers after several years of cessation.

Cigarette Smoking Cessation

Talmage D. Egan
Nathan Orgain

Risk

• Incidence in USA: Adults: ~20% smoke tobacco, higher among lower socioeconomic classes
• Minorities are more likely to smoke and less likely to quit.
• Prevalence among adults and teens declining.

Perioperative Risks

• Risk not well defined through controlled studies; 25 pack-year Hx increases physiologic age 8 y in those 40–65 y
• Increases perioperative morbidity and mortality related to smoking-associated diseases
• Increases risk of postop lung complications

Worry About

• Undiagnosed or poorly treated smoking-related disease that may require modification of the anesthetic plan (e.g. CAD, cerebral vascular disease, COPD)
• Propensity for bronchospasm, coughing, and mucus plugging
• Decreased O_2 content 2° to high carboxyhemoglobin (COHb) levels
• Increased autonomic activity (increased heart rate and BP) 2° to nicotine in pts who have smoked just prior to anesthesia

• Home exposure to second-hand smoke may increase risk of periop pulm complications in children (e.g. laryngospasm, asthma exacerbation)

Overview

• Smoking results in acute changes in cardiopulmonary function even in otherwise asymptomatic patients. With long-term use, smoking causes chronic changes in cardiopulmonary function that eventually culminate in irreversible cardiopulmonary disease.
• Acute changes include carbon monoxide-mediated decreases in O_2 content and nicotine-induced increases in heart rate and BP. Nicotine-mediated effects are relatively short-lived, whereas carboxyhemoglobin persists for many hours.
• Chronic changes include a gradual decline in lung function consisting of decreased FEV_1, decreased mucociliary activity, decreased gas exchange surface, and decreased pulmonary macrophage activity
• Associated diseases incl CAD, COPD, cerebrovascular disease, and numerous cancers (lung, laryngeal, oral, stomach, bladder, others)

ICD-9-CM Code: 305.1 (Nondependent tobacco use disorder)

Etiology

• Acquired behavior that is generally viewed as addiction (both physical to components of tobacco e.g. nicotine, and psychological/social)
• Highest risk factors are low education level, low socioeconomic status, age of smoking onset

Usual Treatment

• Counseling (both by physicians and other counselors
• Group therapy (e.g., "12-step" program)
• Pharmacologic adjuncts, e.g. nicotine replacement gum/patch/pill, bupropion, varenicline
• The perioperative period is a window during which patients may be more open to and successful in quitting, and supports anesthesiologist's role in urging pt to quit
• Referral to quitting resources (e.g. Quit Line phone resource, hospital counselors, state health programs) should be made if possible during perioperative visits

ASSESSMENT POINTS

System	Effect	Assessment by Hx	PE	Test
HEENT	Oral/laryngeal cancer	Hoarseness	Oral exam (and inspection during direct laryngoscopy)	
CV	CAD (± altered LV function)	Exertional chest pain, dyspnea, poor exercise tolerance, orthopnea, paroxysmal nocturnal dyspnea	S_3 gallop, dysrhythmia	ECG, stress test, ECHO, angiography
RESP	COPD	Dyspnea, poor exercise tolerance	Tachypnea, rales, wheezing, pursed lip breathing	CXR, ABGs
OTHER	↑ Carboxyhemoglobin (with recent smoking)	Dyspnea	Tachycardia, tachypnea	ABGs with co-oximetry (measure CoHb%

Key reference: Shi Y, Warner DO. Surgery as a teachable moment for smoking cessation. *Anesthesiology.* 2010;112(1):102–107.

Perioperative Implications

Preoperative Preparation

• Advise smoking cessation for at least 12 h before operation (so that carboxyhemoglobin levels fall to near-normal)
• Advise that a much longer period of cessation (i.e., ~2 mo) is necessary to achieve a decrease in postop pulmonary morbidity; may rarely be worthwhile in true pulmonary cripples undergoing major procedures and very worthwhile for long-term motivation
• Suggest that now is an excellent time to quit smoking (reduce future disease risk, improve postsurgical wound healing, recovery, reduce smoking-related aging)
• Evidence suggests that both the anesthesiologist's reinforcement and in-hospital tobacco cessation programs consisting only of a brief education and counseling visit, self-help take-home materials, and a follow-up phone call are cost-effective in promoting cessation.

• Employ "5 A's": Ask, Advise, Assess, Assist, Arrange for tobacco cessation

Monitoring

• Routine
• Most SpO_2 monitors do not distinguish between COHb and oxyhemoglobin. Significant levels of COHb may exist without decrease in SpO_2 reading (obtain ABG with co-oximetry if concern exists)

Airway

• Smokers vulnerable to bronchospasm or mucus plugging obstruction anytime
• Children with second-hand smoke exposure may be at increased risk of laryngospasm

Induction

• Avoid instrumentation of airway until deep level of anesthesia
• Provide complete preoxygenation since less tolerance of apnea

Maintenance

• Routine; ensure adequate depth of anesthesia to avoid bronchospasm

Extubation

• Consider deep extubation if other considerations permit in order to avoid bronchospasm (e.g., empty stomach, easy laryngoscopy)

Postoperative Period

• Monitor for respiratory complications (e.g., pneumonia, bronchospasm)
• Continue to encourage permanent smoking cessation
• Ensure patient does not attempt to smoke in presence of supplemental O_2

Anticipated Problems/Concerns

• Propensity for bronchospasm
• Decreased O_2 content secondary to high carboxyhemoglobin levels

Cleft Palate

Risk

- ~1/800 live births
- Racial predominance: Caucasian
- Frequently associated with cleft lip
- Gender predominance: Cleft lip/palate more common in males (2:1); isolated cleft palate more common in females (3:1)

Perioperative Risks

- Morbidity and mortality extremely low; only five life-threatening cases of postop airway obstruction described in literature

Worry About

- Difficult airway when associated with syndromes such as Mohr, Shprintzen, 4P, or Pierre Robin
- Submental obstruction of airway during mask ventilation; tongue obstructs view on direct laryngoscopy
- Laryngospasm on anesthetic induction and airway obstruction due to chronic URIs, chronic otitis media, and/or tongue becoming wedged in cleft
- Difficult intraop oxygenation due to chronic aspiration syndrome
- Increased risk for transfusion if anemic due to poor ability to feed
- Intraop airway obstruction and extubation by Dingman gag
- Intraoperative dysrhythmias caused by surgical infiltration of epinephrine
- Postop airway obstruction by forgotten pharyngeal packs and severe lingual edema
- Undiagnosed associated congenital heart and renal diseases

Overview

- Congenital condition occurs by 7th to 12th wk of intrauterine life and is multifactorial but can be associated with a single cause such as benzodiazepine usage
- Cleft palate repaired at 12–18 mo; cleft lip is closed at 3 mo, if also present; single to multiple stage methods employed dependent on type of defect(s)
- Usually not associated with severe blood loss
- Postop airway obstruction may occur more frequently in prolonged procedures
- A tongue stitch is often placed at end of surgery for management of possible airway obstruction and is removed the next day.

ICD-9-CM Code: 749.00

Usual Treatment

- If child is in otherwise good health, a palatoplasty is performed electively.
- All children with cleft palate should have repair by 18 mo to ensure:
  - Normal speech development
  - Appropriate social integration
  - Normal growth of maxilla

ASSESSMENT POINTS

System	Effect	Assessment by Hx	PE	Test
HEENT	Otitis media Clear rhinorrhea Difficult airway	Ear pain Snore, grunt	Temporomandibular exam Airway exam (micrognathia)	
CV	Associated congenital heart disease	SOB, cyanosis, poor growth	CV exam, club foot	ECG, ECHO
RESP	URI Aspiration	Cough, fever Congestion SOB, cyanosis	Chest exam Chest exam	CXR
GI	Impaired deglutition Malnutrition	Nasal regurgitation Poor growth		Observe feeding
HEME	Anemia	Malnutrition	Pallor	Hgb/Hct
RENAL	Associated congenital defects	UTI	Club feet	UA, BUN/Cr

Key Reference: Hodges SC, Hodges AM. A protocol for safe anesthesia for cleft lip and palate surgery in developing countries. *Anaesthesia* 2000;55:436–441.

Perioperative Implications

Preoperative Preparation
- Recognize possibility of multiple future procedures and attempt to minimize stress during induction; consider oral premedication

Anesthetic Technique
- GA usually induced via mask using increasing concentrations of volatile agent in O₂
- Oral airway or gauze packing of cleft may help manual ventilation by preventing tongue from lodging in cleft
- Intubation, often with RAE ETT secured to mandible, as access to airway may be severely limited

Monitoring
- Precordial stethoscope
- Maintain normocapnia if epinephrine injection and halothane inhalation

Postoperative Considerations
- Significant risk for airway obstruction due to edema
- Often obligate mouth breathers
- Transfusion usually not required for cleft palate repair
- Judicious use of opioids in a monitored setting; rectal acetaminophen frequently sufficient

Anticipated Problems/Concerns

- Airway difficulty during induction and intubation, esp when associated with other facial anomalies
- Postop airway obstruction due to forgotten pharyngeal pack, severe lingual edema, or obligate mouth breathing

Coagulopathy, Factor IX Deficiency

Thomas M. McLoughlin, Jr.

Risk

- Incidence in USA: 3000–4000 (15% of all hemophiliacs). Incidence = 1:25,000–50,000 males
- Race with highest prevalence: None
- Gender with highest prevalence: Overwhelmingly male
- Acquired factor IX deficiency associated with liver disease
- Adult levels may not be reached in healthy newborns until 6 mo of age

Perioperative Risks

- Increased risk of hemorrhagic complications from any and all operations

Worry About

- Excessive and/or uncontrollable hemorrhage
- Tendency for recurrent hemorrhage after initial control
- Expansive deep and soft tissue hematomas

- Increased risk if hepatic dysfunction present from prior plasma product transfusions

Overview

- Inherited disorder also called hemophilia B or Christmas disease
- Clinically indistinguishable from hemophilia A (classic hemophilia)
- Hemarthroses account for 75% of bleeding episodes; chronic debilitating arthritis is a common development
- Soft tissue hematomas and hematuria also common
- Intracranial hemorrhage is common fatal complication, accounting for death in 25%
- Severity of disease proportional to circulating factor IX activity (<1% normal activity = severe disease, >5% = generally mild disease)

ICD-9-CM Code: 286.1

Etiology

- Sex-linked recessive disorder

Usual Treatment

- Restoration of circulating factor IX activity, biological half-life is 18–24 hr
- Plasma-derived pooled factor IX concentrates (AlphaNine SD, Mononine, Profilnine SD, ProplexT, Bebulin VH)
- Recombinant factor IX concentrate now available (BeneFix, Genetics Institute, Cambridge, MA). Dose (IU) = body weight (kg) × desired factor IX activity increase (%) × 1.2 IU/kg
- Prothrombin complex concentrates and FFP are alternatives for life-threatening hemorrhage if concentrates unavailable

ASSESSMENT POINTS

System	Effect	Assessment by Hx	PE	Test
GI				LFTs if hepatitis Hx
HEME	Coagulopathy	Dental extractions, menses, lacerations, epistaxis	Ecchymoses, hematomas	Prolonged PTT; PT, plt count usually normal
RENAL	Hematuria; eventual clot formation can obstruct collecting system	Discolored urine		BUN/Cr, urine dipstick or microscopic exam
CNS	Intracranial hemorrhage	Headache	Neurologic exam	
PNS	Discrete peripheral neuropathies	Hx of compressive hematoma	Sensory and motor exam	
MS	Hemarthroses, chronic arthritis	Painful, warm joints	↓ ROM	X-rays usually not necessary

Key Reference: Lee JW: Von Willebrand disease, hemophilia A and B, and other factor deficiencies. *Int Anesthesiol Clin.* 2004;42(3):59–76.

Perioperative Implications

Preoperative Preparation

- Collaboration with consulting hematologist.
- Schedule surgery early in wk to allow optimal laboratory support of postop assessment of hemostasis; if multiple procedures are contemplated in near future, schedule simultaneously.
- Assess preop factor IX activity; determine goal as guided by magnitude of hemostatic challenge (15–30% factor IX activity for minor lacerations/hematomas; 30–50% for hemarthroses or major hemorrhage, 50–75% for periop coverage or life-threatening bleeding).
- Units factor IX needed = (2)(wt in kg) (plasma volume in mL/kg)(fractional increase in factor IX activity desired); once-daily dosing is sufficient for maintenance.

Monitoring

- Confirm expected increase in factor IX activity after preop dose but before incision.

Airway

- Laryngoscopy to avoid tissue trauma, consider mask ventilation
- Nasotracheal route best avoided

Maintenance

- Consider tourniquets and local cooling to minimize blood loss

Extubation

- Avoid coughing on ETT
- Cautious oropharyngeal suction, best done under direct vision

Adjuvants

- Regional anesthesia not absolutely contraindicated but consider with caution; successful brachial plexus blockade at the axilla has been described.
- Postop factor IX activity requirement: 15–40%

Anticipated Problems/Concerns

- Excessive periop blood loss, hematoma formation
- Potential for delayed or recurrent bleeding after initial control
- Increased likelihood of infectious blood-borne disease (HIV, hepatitis)

Coarctation of the Aorta

Thomas M. Chalifoux
Edmund H. Jooste

Risk
- Sixth most-common congenital heart defect
- Recognized in 5–8% of pts with CHD.

Perioperative Risks
- Perioperative mortality: 1% when associated with no other cardiac anomalies in neonates, 10% when associated with a VSD, and 50% when associated with HLHS; children and adults: <0.5%.
- Postop risk of paraplegia: 0.5–1.5% (risk even lower if younger than 1 y of age)

Worry About
- Closure of the ductus arteriosus in neonates and infants can lead to acute left ventricular failure and hypoperfusion distal to coarctation.
- Maintaining adequate perfusion to the lower portion of the body during cross-clamping of the aorta to provide adequate perfusion to spinal cord and abdominal vital organs.
- Intraop systemic Htn proximal to the aortic cross-clamp
- Acute hypotension and metabolic acidosis on release of aortic cross-clamp
- Postop systemic Htn

Overview
- Congenital narrowing of the aorta at or near the ductus arteriosus or ligamentum arteriosum, causing a hemodynamically significant pressure gradient
- Commonly associated defects in neonates and infants: Bicuspid aortic valve, mitral valve anomalies, PDA, aortic hypoplasia, VSD
- Usually an isolated defect in older children and adults

ICD-9-CM Code: 747.10

Etiology
- Several theories: Abnormal flow patterns in the developing fetal heart may cause decreased aortic flow resulting in aortic hypoplasia; ectopic ductal tissue in the aorta; or a combination of both
- May be a component of trisomy 13, trisomy 18, deletion of chr 22q11, Turner syndrome, or Kabuki syndrome

Usual Treatment
- Surgical repair for initial management using several techniques: Subclavian flap aortoplasty, resection and end-to-end anastomosis, prosthetic patch augmentation. Left thoracotomy common; but repair of associated defects may require sternotomy and CPB with or without DHCA.
- Transcatheter balloon angioplasty for initial management of native coarctation and for management of recoarctation. May incl endovascular stent placement.

ASSESSMENT POINTS

System	Effect	Assessment by Hx	PE	Test
General	Failure to thrive	Poor feeding	Poor growth	Growth chart
NEURO	Intracranial aneurysm (child and adult)			
HEENT	Upper body Htn (rare in neonate <5 d old)	Epistaxis Headache		Four extremity blood pressure measurement
CVS (General)			Systolic pressure and pulse gradient between upper and lower extremities (may not be present with PDA)	ECHO, ECG, CXR, MRI/MRA, cardiac catheterization with angiography
CVS (neonate/infant)	CHF	Poor feeding	Tachypnea, cyanosis, hepatomegaly, metabolic acidosis	ABG, CXR
CVS (child/adult)	Development of collateral circulation			CXR showing rib notching (a late finding)
PULM	CHF (neonate, infant)		Resp failure	CXR, ABG
RENAL	Renal failure secondary to poor perfusion (neonate, infant)			Electrolytes, BUN, creatinine, urine output and analysis
MS	Poor peripheral perfusion Spinal cord compression by dilated anterior spinal artery or branch compressing a nerve root	Claudication, lower extremity pain, paresthesia, muscle weakness	Diminished or absent femoral pulses	

Key Reference: Landsman IS, Davis PJ. Aortic coarctation: Anesthetic considerations. *Semin Cardiothorac Vasc Anesth.* 2001;5(1):91–97.

Perioperative Implications

Preoperative Preparation and Induction
- Neonate/infant: Maintain PDA with PGE_1. PDA closure can lead to CHF, upper body Htn, lower body hypoperfusion and shock.
- The presence of a VSD leads to significant left-to-right shunting and a further steal of the systemic blood flow. Do not decrease PVR further by hyperventilation or the use of 100% O_2.
- Right lateral decubitus position for left thoracotomy. Good padding important.
- Regular ETT for neonates and infants but consider bronchial blocker or double lumen ETT in older child and adult.

Monitoring
- Standard monitors, pulse oximeter × 2 (right upper and either lower extremity), urinary catheter.
- Right upper extremity arterial catheter (radial, ulnar, or axillary). Lower extremity arterial catheter if pressure gradient is high. Otherwise a combination of arterial and NIBP monitoring used in RUE and a lower extremity.
- Central venous access required for infusion of vasoactive medications.
- SSEPs may be used to motor spinal cord perfusion during aortic cross-clamping (particularly if aortic gradient is high or little collateral circulation).

Maintenance
- To prevent spinal cord ischemia: Passively cool to core temp 34–35 °C, maintain normocapnia and keep distal mean arterial pressure >40 mmHg.
- Control Htn with titratable agents: Inhalation agent, sodium nitroprusside, esmolol, nicardipine.
  - If mean arterial pressure <40 mmHg or significant change in SSEP signal with aortic cross-clamp application, institute left heart bypass.
  - Be prepared to treat a sudden drop in BP and acidosis following aortic cross-clamp release with fluids and sodium bicarbonate.

Postoperative
- Neonates and infants with CHF remain intubated and ventilated until condition improves.
- Children and adults may usually be extubated in the OR.
- Pain management: Opioids, dexmedetomidine, intercostal nerve block by surgeon, paravertebral catheter, epidural catheter (must consider risk of epidural hematoma).

Anticipated Problems/Concerns
- Paraplegia, likely secondary to spinal cord ischemia, particularly if clamp time >30 min
- Postcoarctectomy syndrome: Severe abdominal pain with tenderness, Htn, fever, vomiting, ileus, melena, leukocytosis (occurs 2–3 d postop)
- Pulm Htn in neonates and infants with CoA and VSD (Rx: NO, milrinone)
- Stridor/partial airway obstruction at extubation secondary to recurrent laryngeal nerve injury
- Ventilatory compromise at extubation secondary to phrenic nerve injury causing hemidiaphragmatic paralysis
- Postop bleeding
- Chylothorax from thoracic duct injury
- Recoarctation (late complication)

Complement Deficiency

David Y. Kim

Risk

- C1 esterase inhibitor deficiency incidence 1:50,000 to 1:150,000 of general population
  - Symptoms onset and Dx approx at 20 y, by 30 y approx 98% of pts have symptoms.
- C2 deficiency incidence: <0.1% of general population
  - M:F ratio: 1:6
  - Higher (6%) in pts with autoimmune disease (see Immune Suppression in Diseases section)
  - Pts with Hx of *Neisseria* meningitis have incidence of 15%
- C3 and C5–C8 deficiencies are noted to have increased risk for infections.

Perioperative Risks

- Life threatening airway compromise possible
- Increases risk of postop infection, particularly if the deficiency affects the early complement components.
- Risk for inflammatory complications, e.g., glomerulonephritis, vasculitis

Worry About

- Acute airway edema resulting from laryngeal or mucous membrane swelling can result in definitive airway obstruction. Abdominal pain from intestinal edema may be an associated finding on exam.
- Increased risk of nfection

Overview

- Hereditary angioneurotic edema is associated with a complement deficiency of the enzyme C1 esteraste inhibitor. This is a rare genetic deficiency that can lead to uncontrolled production of C2, C3, and C5 complement resulting in acute non-inflammatory, painless, non-puritic, non-pitting edema. Initial inciting events are often the result of trauma, but may even be attributed to emotional stress.
- May affect any component of classical pathway, alternate pathway, or terminal common pathway
- Virtually all deficiencies show some ↑ risk of infection and/or autoimmune disease
- Deficiencies in other complement components, C2 and C3, have also been associated with immunocompromise, resulting in recurrent life-threatening infections due to a variety of organisms.
- Increases risk of autoimmune diseases
- Deficiency in any of the terminal components C5–C8 show selective risk of recurrent neisserial infections, usually not life-threatening

ICD-9-CM Code: 279.8

Etiology

- C1 complement results from a heterozygous deficiency of C1 esterase inhibitor. The mediators of the angioedema response result from coagulation, complement, and the kinin pathway. C1 esterase inhibitor is key regulator for Hageman factor, coagulation, plasmin, and plasma kallikrein. More than 100 mutations on the C1 esterase gene, for pts without hereditary angioedema, 20% of those new mutations with no prior Hx.
- All complement proteins inherited in autosomal fashion, with possible exception of properdin, which appears to be X-linked

Usual Treatment

- Stanazolol, danazol, methyltestosterone, oxymetholone, aminocaproic acid, tranexamic acid, and cinnerazine. Mechansm of action for therapeutics being increased synthesis of C1 esterase inhibitor, for the steroids, and inhibition of plasmin activation, for the antifibrinolytics.
- Acute preop prophylaxis consist of fresh frozen plasma and epinephrine. But caution because plasma provides substrates which may aggravate the scenario and worsen the edema. Purified concentrates of C1 esterase inhibitor given IV have been used outside of the USA.
- Antibiotic treatment dictated by specific infection

ASSESSMENT POINTS

System	Effect	Test
IMMUNO	Infectious risk for all systems	CH50 screening test for complement-mediated lysis of sheep erythrocytes; tests for specific complement components available at reference laboratories. Assess other specific organs as indicated by autoimmune disease (renal for SLE, etc.)

Key Reference: Jensen NF, Weiler JM. C1 esterase inhibitor deficiency, airway compromise, and anesthesia. *Anesth Analg.* 1998;87:480–488.

Perioperative Implications

Preoperative Preparation

- In C1 deficiency consideration to preop administration of 2 units of fresh frozen plasma or C1 concentrate should be considered with appropriate consideration to risks and benefits of this therapy.
- Sterile technique strictly observed

Monitoring

- Routine
- Coagulation profile
- Minimize invasive lines

Airway

- Airway management should minimize trauma. Tracheal intubation is acceptable, but preparations for an emergency tracheostomy should be made. Laryngeal mask airway use should be tempered by the concerns for upper airway edema and resulting ineffective ventilation. Regional anesthesia is an acceptable alternative to prevent airway manipulation.

Induction

- Routine

Maintenance

- Routine

Extubation

- Extubate and remove all lines at earliest opportunity

Postoperative Period

- Maintain sterile techniques

Anticipated Problems/Concerns

- If an emergency intubation is required, an otolaryngologist is recommended, or surgical personnel, to be present for a possible tracheostomy or cricothyroidotomy.
- Meticulous sterile technique to minimize risk of infection

Congenital Pulmonary Cystic Lesions/Lobar Emphysema

Francine S. Yudkowitz

Risk

- Cause of cardiorespiratory compromise
- 10–15% associated with CHD

Perioperative Risks

- May develop worsening of cardiorespiratory status
- Contamination of unaffected lung by infected material from cyst

Worry About

- Associated congenital anomalies
- Tension pneumothorax
- Cardiorespiratory compromise

Overview

- There are two types of congenital pulmonary cystic lesions.
  - Bronchogenic: Abnormal budding and branching of tracheobronchial tree
  - Dermoid: Lined with keratinized, squamous epithelium
- Congenital Pulmonary Airway Malformation (CPAM): previously known as CCAM, similar to bronchioles but without alveoli, bronchial glands, and cartilage. Overdistension due to gas trapping leads to resp distress.
- Congenital lobar emphysema
  - Hyperinflation and air trapping result in expansion of affected lobe.
  - Most commonly occurs in the left upper lobe, followed in frequency by the right middle, and then the right upper lobe
  - Preterm infants on mechanical ventilation develop emphysema in the right upper lobe.
  - CXR shows emphysematous lobe crossing midline, mediastinal shift, atelectasis in other lobes and possibly contralateral lung. The presence of bronchovascular markings distinguishes this from pneumothorax and congenital cysts.

ICD-9-CM CODE: 748.4 (Congenital bronchogenic/Pulmonary cyst); 770.2 (congenital lobar emphysema)

Etiology

- Congenital pulmonary cystic lesions may be bronchogenic, alveolar, or a combination of both; anomalous development of bronchopulmonary system
- Congenital lobar emphysema have extrinsic bronchial obstruction from abnormal vessels or enlarged lymph nodes; intrinsic bronchial obstruction from deficient bronchial cartilage, bronchial stenosis, or redundant bronchial mucosa

Usual Treatment

- Surgical removal

ASSESSMENT POINTS

System	Effect	Assessment by Hx	PE	Test
RESP	↓ Lung volume	Cyanosis, dyspnea, grunting, coughing	Tachypnea, retractions, wheezing, ↓ BS, asymmetric chest expansion	CXR CT scan
CV	Mediastinal shift, ↓ CO VSD, PDA	Irritability, poor feeding	↓ Heart sounds Murmur	CXR, ECG, ECHO

Key Reference: Hammer G, Hall S, Davis PJ. Anesthesia for general abdominal, thoracic, urologic, and bariatric surgery. In: Motoyama EK, Davis PJ, eds. *Smith's anesthesia for infants and children*. 7th ed. Philadelphia: Mosby; 2006.

Perioperative Implications

Preoperative Preparation

- Assess the severity of cardiopulmonary compromise.
- Identify associated congenital anomalies.
- Optimize resp infection if pt is stable.
- Aspirate cyst prior to induction if there is cardiac compromise or airway obstruction.

Monitoring

- Arterial line for blood pressure monitoring and blood gas analysis.

Induction

- Avoid positive pressure ventilation until thorax is opened to avoid expansion of cyst or lobe.
- Avoid N_2O, which will expand the lobe or cyst.
- Inhalation induction with 100% O_2.
- Intubate without the use of muscle relaxants.
- May need to isolate the affected lung. In small infants and children this may be accomplished by using a bronchial blocker or doing a mainstem intubation.
- Surgeon should be available to open the chest immediately if deterioration should occur during induction of anesthesia.

Maintenance

- No one anesthetic preferred
- Maintain spontaneous ventilation or assist with low airway pressures until the thorax is opened.
- Once the pathology is removed, N_2O may be used.
- If Hx of repeated lung infections (cysts), there may be large blood losses.

Extubation/Postoperative Period

- May be extubated after uncomplicated surgery and when cardiopulmonary function is adequate

Anticipated Problems/Concern

- Pts with altered cardiopulmonary reserve before surgery may require postop intubation and ventilation.
- If pneumonectomy performed; there will be overinflation of the remaining lung with a decrease in vital capacity. These children may have significant exercise intolerance for a prolonged period after surgery.
- To avoid postop atelectasis, coughing, and early ambulation or increase in activity, important
- Altered pulm mechanics (decreased forced vital capacity and delayed forced expiration) may be present throughout childhood.

Congenital Methemoglobinemia

Bronwyn R. Rae

DISEASES

Risk

- Navajo Indians, Alaskan Indians, people of Puerto Rican and Cuban ancestry
- Normal life span (except for recessive congenital methemoglobinemia [RCM] type II)

Perioperative Risks

- Oxidizing agents may increase MetHB to dangerous levels
- Pregnancies not compromised

Worry About

- Measurement of SpO_2
- Oxidant drugs, e.g., prilocaine, benzocaine, nitroglycerin, sulfonamides, phenacetin, nitric oxide, contraindicated
- Myocardial ischemia due to decreased O_2 delivery
- Blood loss due to decreased O_2 carrying capacity

Overview

- Enzyme deficiency. Shift of O_2 dissociation curve to left leads to mild erythrocytosis. Normal RBC life span.
- Heterozygotes have increased susceptibility to metHb formation after exposure to oxidant drugs and chemicals.
- RCM type I defect restricted to red cell soluble cytochrome b5 reductase only. Cyanosis is sole clinical symptom.
- RCM type II: Defect in all tissues; involves both soluble and microsomal forms of cytochrome b5 reductase. Mental retardation, spasticity, opisthotonos, microcephaly, growth retardation. Death by 2–3 y.
- RCM type III: Nonerythroid enzyme deficiency, but CNS spared.
- HbM variations: Alpha chain variants affected from birth, beta chain variants by 3–6 mo of age. Mild hemolytic anemia.

ICD-9-CM Code: 289.7

Etiology

- RCM types I, II and III: Autosomal recessive inheritance. Due to deficient reducing capacity of oxidized heme due to NADH cytochrome b5 reductase (diaphorase) deficiency.
- HbM variants—autosomal dominant inheritance. Due to structural abnormality in globin moiety: Amino acid substitutions create abnormal environment for heme residues, displacing the equilibrium toward the ferric state.

Usual Treatment

- RCM types I, II and III: Reducing agents, e.g., riboflavin 20–60 mg orally, methylene blue 1 mg/kg IV. Effect lasts 10–14 d. Ascorbic acid used for chronic management.
- HbM variants: No chronic treatment available. In an emergency, hyperbaric O_2 therapy and exchange transfusion may be used.

ASSESSMENT POINTS

System	PE	Test
RESP	Look cyanosed but more "blue" than "sick"	15–30% MetHb
HEME	RCM types I and II: Mild erythrocytosis HbM variants: Mild hemolytic anemia	CBC
CVS	May be unable to meet increased metabolic demand	ECG

Key Reference: Maurtua MA, Emmerling L, Ebrahim Z. Anesthetic management of patient with congenital methemoglobinemia. *J Clin Anesth*. 2004;16:455–457.

Perioperative Implications

Preoperative Preparation

- Can give reducing agents to pts with RCM type I but no data on whether treatment is indicated prior to anesthesia

Monitoring

- Pulse oximeter overestimates at low SpO_2 and underestimates at high SpO_2. In practice reads between 80–85% regardless of true saturation.
- Use co-oximetry for SaO_2 and MetHB levels.
- Monitor ECG for ischemic changes.

Airway

- None

Preinduction/Induction

- Adequate preoxygenation with 100% O_2 as O_2-carrying capacity is already decreased.

Maintenance

- Prilocaine, benzocaine, EMLA cream contraindicated. Literature contradictory on lidocaine—use with caution.
- Nitrous oxide, propofol, volatile agents OK

Adjuvants

- None

Postoperative Period

- Avoid acetanilids for pain relief; narcotics OK

Anticipated Problems/Concerns

- Avoid oxidant drugs in both homozygotes and heterozygotes
- Pulse oximetry is inaccurate; use ABGs with co-oximetry
- May require supplemental O_2 postop

Congestive Heart Failure

Miklos D. Kertai

Risk

- Heart failure is a syndrome, not a disease
- Incidence in USA: about 4.8 million; 400,000 new cases diagnosed annually. Primary discharge diagnosis in 1 million pts.
- 1-y and 5-y survival rates are 57% and 25% in men and 64% and 38% in women; Median survival after onset is 1.7 y in men and 3.2 y in women

Perioperative Risks

- Heart failure occurs in 1 to 6% of pts after major surgery; between 6 and 25%, in pts with existing cardiac conditions
- EF <35% associated with increased operative risk
- Single greatest risk factor for cardiac surgery. Use congestive heart failure score (CASS): Hx of CHF = 1; Rx digitalis = 1; Rales = 1; Overt symptoms after treatment = 1; Total 0–4: If score = 4, operative risk is 8× greater.

Worry About

- Ventricular dysfunction preop; associated with increased operative mortality
- Pt with diastolic dysfunction may be asymptomatic at rest, but sensitive to increases in heart rate, which may result in flash pulm edema
- Dysrhythmias due to cardiac ischemia (sudden cardiac death)
- Associated acute or chronic mitral insufficiency
- Volume status
- Prolonged effect of ACE inhibitors

Overview

- Different types of failure (left versus right; acute versus chronic; systolic versus diastolic; low output versus high output)
- Reduced contractility, decreased stroke volume, increased heart rate, hypertrophy and ventricular dilatation
- Acute ischemia can lead to global diastolic dysfunction and CHF
- Papillary muscle ischemia may lead to severe mitral regurgitation and pulm congestion
- New York Heart Association classification: I: no limitation; II: slight limitation; III: marked limitation; IV: inability to carry out any physical activity. Overall 1-y mortality for classes III and IV; 34–58%.

ICD-9-CM Code: 428.0

Etiology

- Acquired, acute or chronic: CHD, MI; cardiomyopathy (idiopathic, hypertrophic, hypertrophic obstructive, congestive, alcoholic). Valvular heart disease: Arrhythmias, severe hypertension.
- Congenital: Congenital heart disease, left to right shunts; intracardiac (ASD, VSD, atrioventricular canal), extracardiac (PDA, anomalous pulm venous connection). Obstructive (coarctation of the aorta, aortic stenosis). Complex (Ebstein's anomaly).
- Multiple precipitating causes: Noncompliance with medications (digitalis, diuretics), excessive Na⁺; excessive IV fluids; drugs (doxorubicin, corticosteroids, disopyramide, nortriptyline, NSAIDs, thiazolidinediones, metformin, cilostazol, PDE-5 inhibitors [sildenafil, vardenafil]) androgens and estrogens). Pulm embolism: High-output states (pregnancy, fever, hyperthyroidism, sepsis, AV fistula, anemia).

Usual Treatment

- Chronic
  - Physical activity encouraged
  - Restriction of sodium intake
  - Chronic, well titrated β-blockade may lead to substantial clinical benefit (carvedilol, metoprolol)
  - Inhibit renin-angiotensin-aldosterone system (RAAS) (ACE inhibitors, angiotensin receptor blockers, aldosterone inhibitors)
  - Improvement in systolic heart failure (digitalis)
  - Diuretics (hydrochlorothiazide, furosemide, spironolactone)
  - Vasodilators
- Acute
  - Optimize pre- and afterload before starting inotropes and vasodilators
  - Inotropes (dobutamine, epinephrine, milrinone, amrinone)
  - Vasodilators (nitroglycerin, nitroprusside, and nesiritide)
  - Maintenance of beta-blocker therapy in acute exacerbation of systolic heart failure
- Special measures
  - Stimulation therapy (biventricular pacing + ICD)
  - Surgical correction (CABG, CHD, valvular surgery, cardiomyoplasty, cardiac transplantation)
  - Assist devices (IABP, LV assist, artificial heart)

ASSESSMENT POINTS

System	Effect	Assessment by Hx	PE	Test
CV	Inadequate cardiac output, congestion	Tachycardia, arrhythmias	Peripheral edema Facial edema (infants/young children), cardiomegaly, pulsus alternans, distended neck veins, Kussmaul's sign, abdominojugular reflex	Exercise testing ECG, CXR Circulation time
RESP	Pulm congestion, decreased lung compliance, VC, TLC, pulm diffusion capacity	Breathlessness (exertional dyspnea, orthopnea, paroxysmal nocturnal dyspnea) Frequent resp infections	Rales and wheezes Pleural effusions Expectoration: frothy blood-tinged sputum	PFT ABGs CXR
GI	Hepatic and intestinal congestion	Nausea, bloating, fullness	Congestive hepatomegaly, ascites, icterus, cachexia	Liver enzymes
RENAL	Decreased GFR, activation RAAS	Nocturia, oliguria	Ankle edema	BUN/Cr, K⁺, Na⁺, proteinuria, specific gravity
CNS	Hypoperfusion	Confusion, impairment of memory	Mental status exam	
PNS	Increased sympathetic tone	Cool extremities	Peripheral vasoconstriction, pallor, diaphoresis, tachycardia, clubbing	

Key Reference: Hammill BG, Curtis LH, Bennett-Guerrero E, et al. Impact of heart failure on patients undergoing major noncardiac surgery. *Anesthesiology.* 2008;108:559–567.

Perioperative Implications

Preoperative Preparation

- Stabilize pt by treating CHF before surgery
- Continue inotropic support
- Continue cardiac medications (ACE inhibitors may cause hypotension on induction)

Monitoring

- Consider arterial line
- Consider CVP, PA catheter, or TEE
  - CVP may be inaccurate in assessing volume

Airway

- Frothy secretions may lead to difficult visualization

Induction

- Preop therapeutic regimen (diuretics) causes hypovolemia, hypokalemia, and hyponatremia, which are potential problems before surgery
- Judicious volume replacement (avoid dehydration and overhydration)
- Avoid myocardial contractility depressants (e.g., barbiturates)

Maintenance
• Maintain myocardial contractility, reduce afterload, and normalize PVR

Extubation
• May be delayed owing to CV and pulm insufficiencies

Adjuvants
• Rx inotropes; digitalis, diuretics
  • May be less responsive to catecholamines

• Regional anesthesia debated and not recommended by some (sympathectomy, volume status) or preferred (reduce preload) by others

Postoperative Period
• Inotropic support and mechanical assistance may be needed
• Pulm edema develops in 2–16% of pts

Anticipated Problems/Concerns
• Pulm edema may necessitate prolonged ventilation with high FIO$_2$
• RV and/or LV failure in the postop period

Conn's Syndrome

Joan Spiegel

Risk

- Accounts for 0.05–1% of the population with Htn
- Twice as common in women as in men
- Peak incidence occurs in the third to sixth decades of life
- Morbidity and mortality are primarily related to Htn and hypokalemia

Perioperative risks

- Associated with hypokalemia and chronic Htn if not corrected preop

Worry About

- Hypokalemic effects from kaliuresis (arrhythmias, muscle weakness, tetany, and alkalosis) and worsening hypokalemia from hyperventilation
- Potentiation of neuromuscular blocking agent effect from hypokalemia
- Longstanding hypertensive effects on the CV system (CAD, CHF)

Overview

- Characterized by increased aldosterone secretion from the adrenal glands, suppressed plasma renin activity (PRA), Htn, and hypokalemia.

- Aldosterone promotes active reabsorption of sodium and excretion of K^+ through the renal tubules. Water is retained resulting in an increase in extracellular fluid volume of the order of 10–30%, and accounts for occasional refractory Htn. Increase in serum sodium concentration, despite a total body increase, is rarely more than 2–3%, because of the dilutional effect of the retained water. There is also tubular secretion of hydrogen ions and magnesium ions, resulting in a mild degree of metabolic alkalosis.
- Htn, esp if left untreated for many years, can lead to many complications, incl heart disease (e.g., CAD, CHF), and intracerebral hemorrhage (with very high blood pressure).
- Hypokalemia, esp if severe, causes cardiac arrhythmias, which can be fatal.

Etiology

- Present when there is excess secretion of aldosterone from a functional tumor (aldosteronoma) independent of a physical stimulus.
- Most common etiology of primary aldosteronism (50–60% of primary aldosteronism) cases.

The remainder is due to adrenal hyperplasia or carcinoma.
- May be associated with pheochromocytoma, primary hyperthyroidism, or acromegaly.
- Differential diagnosis: Any disorder that causes elevated mineralocorticoids—adrenal carcinoma, congenital disorders, glycyrrhizic acid (licorice or Chinese herbals), and renal tubular disorders.

Usual Treatment

- Surgical removal of the adenoma or antihypertensive therapy.
- Antihypertensives are a first-line agent, usually a K^+-sparing diuretic such as spironolactone or eplerenone, competitive aldosterone antagonists.

ASSESSMENT POINTS

	Effect	Assessment by Hx	PE	Test
ENDO	Abnormal glucose tolerance ($\uparrow$ Glucose)	Polyuria		Electrolytes
RENAL	$\downarrow$ Serum K+, total K^+ body depletion $\downarrow$ Mg++, $\uparrow$ urine K+	Nocturia, muscle weakness, and cramps	See MS	Serum and urine electrolytes, Suppressed renin level in untreated pts Aldosterone: Renin level, sodium challenge
CV	Htn	Headache	S4 gallop	ECG, 2-D ECHO
RESP	Muscle weakness	Exercise tolerance	Tachypnea	
MS	Weakness	Fatigue, muscle weakness	Decreased or absent DTRs	K^+ (serum electrolytes)

Key Reference: Gockel I, et al. Changing pattern of the intraoperative blood pressure during endoscopic adrenalectomy in patients with Conn's syndrome. *Surg Endosc.* 2005;19:1491–1497.

Perioperative Implications

Preoperative Preparation

- Treatment of Htn (ideally at least 6 wk of antihypertensive treatment prior to surgery)
- Correction of electrolyte imbalance (specifically K^+ and magnesium)
- Assessment of cardiac function (ECG, 2-D ECHO)

Intraoperative

Airway

- No change from normal

Induction

- Avoid etomidate, which causes adrenal suppression; hypokalemia may modify responses to nondepolarizing paralytics

Maintenance

- Avoid hyperventilation (this will decrease K^+); Pts may be sensitive to rapid blood loss if hypovolemic (?pre-op diuretic); with bilateral adrenalectomy, may need to replace mineralocorticoids (cortisol); follow electrolytes

Monitoring

- Excessive preop preparation (diuretic) may leave pt hypovolemic. A CVP or Swan-Ganz catheter may be useful in some cases to follow fluid status

Postoperative

- Should continue to monitor acid base status and plasma electrolytes postop

Anticipated Problems/Concerns

- Hypokalemia-induced arrhythmia, hypomagnesemia
- Adrenal insufficiency postop in bilateral adrenalectomy pts

Constipation

Dmitry Portnoy

Risk

- 12% of people worldwide, 17% in the Americas suffer from self-defined constipation
- Incidence in USA: 12–19% (depending on definitions and ascertainment methods)
- Prevalence in elderly 27–50% and as high as 74% in nursing home residents
- Occurs in 20–83% of ICU pts
- M:F ratio: 1:3

Perioperative Risks

- Increased risk of N/V, abd pain, headache
- Delayed weaning from mechanical ventilation in ICU pts
- Delayed discharge of ICU pts

Worry About

- Possible risk of pulm aspiration due to abd distension
- Risk of pseudo-obstruction of the intestine
- Increased PIP, decreases VC and decreased FRC if intra-abd pressure is significant

- Risk of intestinal perforation and pulm embolism in ICU pts
- Delayed enteral feeding and prolonged ICU stay

Overview

- Can cause N/V, abd pain and distension
- Excessive straining may effect cerebral and coronary circulation and lead to syncope
- Severe constipation may lead to fecal impaction, incontinence, and urinary retention
- No evidence that toxins from constipation harm the body
- Idiopathic form, if not complicated, does not usually affect life expectancy

ICD-9-CM Code: 564.00

Etiology

- Primary or idiopathic in most cases (types: functional, slow-transit, and outlet dysfunction)
- Secondary (or combined form): Due to underlying conditions; congenital (e.g., Hirschsprung's disease) or acquired diseases (e.g., DM, MS, depression). Also, as a result of diet, lifestyle, and

the use of certain medications (e.g., opioids, calcium channel blockers, beta-blockers, diuretics, antidepressants, anticonvulsants, antacids, anticholinergics)
- Imbalance of neurotransmitters (serotonin, somatostatin, peptide YY, and vasoactive intestinal peptide) may play a role in idiopathic form of constipation

Usual Treatment

- Lifestyle and diet modifications with increased water intake, which are not always sufficient
- Treatment depends on the etiology and underlying cause
- First line: Bulking agents, increase dietary fiber, increase physical activity, dietary adjustment
- Second line: Stimulant and osmotic laxatives, stool softeners, suppositories, and enemas
- Lactulose and polyethylene glycol are effective in critically ill pts
- Enteral naloxone: For the reversal of opiate-induced constipation in ICU pts
- Surgery is rare; outcomes of colectomy and ileorectostomy in elderly are uncertain

ASSESSMENT POINTS

System	Effect	Assessment by Hx	Test
RESP	Elevated diaphragm Increased airway pressure	Abd distention	CXR PIP
GI	Intestinal obstruction N/V Gastroparesis	Abd distention	Abd imaging
CNS	Headache		

Key Reference: Mostafa SM, Bhandari S, Ritchie G, Gratton N, Wenstone R. Constipation and its implications in the critically ill patient. *Br J Anaesth*. 2003;91(6):815–819.

Perioperative Implications

Monitoring

- PIP and other ventilatory parameters if increased intra-abd and intrathoracic pressure
- Electrolytes and/or intravascular volume status, if vigorous bowel preparation preceded anesthesia

Airway

- Vital capacity and FRC may be decreased.

Induction

- Rapid-sequence induction may be indicated if intestinal obstruction is present.

Maintenance

- Avoid using nitrous oxide if there is an obstruction of the intestine.
- Consider regional anesthesia, when feasible, to reduce the use of opioids.

Extubation

- Extubate after the airway reflexes have recovered.

Adjuvants

- Opioids and other μ-opioid agonists (e.g., loperamide) delay GI transit.
- Aspirin and other NSAIDs may insignificantly contribute to constipation in elderly.

- Agents with anticholinergic effect (e.g., atropine, antispasmodics, antipsychotics, TCA) may cause slow transit constipation.

Anticipated Problems/Concerns

- Distention of gut and elevated diaphragm may be present.
- Mechanical ventilation might require higher PIP.
- GI transit may be delayed.
- Discharge from ICU may be delayed if constipation is not managed effectively.

Conversion Disorder

Robert I. Cohen

Risk

- Reported prevalence varies widely (11–500/100,000); may account for as much as 1–14% of general medical/surgical pts
- Reported to be more common in rural populations, developing areas, lower socioeconomic groups, those less medically sophisticated and following physical and sexual abuse

Perioperative Risks

- Hx of conversion disorder may not increase periop morbidity or mortality per se although risk may increase for failure to diagnose if new symptom complexes are too quickly attributed to conversion disorder

Worry About

- Presence of undiagnosed cognitive, neurologic or general medical illnesses, drug or treatment adverse effect
- Periop appearance of conversion symptoms mimicking medical disturbances, drug effects, or anesthetic or surgically related complications
- Malingering, factitious disorder, dissociative disorder, addiction, pseudoaddiction and withdrawal

Overview

- DSM-IV TR (2000): In conversion disorder, a subclassification of somataform disorder, a pt generates symptoms suggestive of a medical condition that is not present.
- Following anesthesia, seizures, generalized or focal weakness or sensory loss, trouble with speaking, swallowing, or voiding have serious implication that require workup though may also be the presentation of conversion disorder. The amount of medical knowledge held by the pt may predict how closely presenting symptoms mimic known medical conditions and how accurately the symptoms are reproduced on serial evaluation.
- Different from malingering and factitious disorder, the pt is not consciously generating false symptoms. In isolation, neither report of pain nor sexual dysfunction is sufficient to meet criteria.
- Most common in the second through fourth decades, with initial symptom onset lasting up to two wk, according to the DSM-IV-TR, loss of body movement, sight, or speech have better long-term outcome than symptoms of seizure or tremor.
- **Coding:** In effect at the time of this writing, both DSM-IV-TR (2000) and ICD-9-CM code "conversion disorder" as 300.11. However in DSM-V and ICD-10 drafts, the term conversion is broadened to become synonomous with the dissociative disorders group, of which it is currently a distinct subdivision.

Etiology

- While unknown, symptoms may occur as an unconsious solution to trauma or unresolved neurotic coinflict.
- More common in pts with prior medical and psyciatric diagnoses
- Possible genetic predisposition suggested in twin and familial studies

Treatment

- Confirm Dx with psychiatric consultant while excluding possible medical conditions
- Reassure pt and family members that symptoms do not appear to represent a life threatening condition and that investigation and treatment will continue.
- Optimize treatment of co-existing psychiatric (esp anxiety and depression) and medical conditions
- Conversion disorder may respond to behavioral, psychodyamic therapy, or psychoanalysis and may also respond to psychopharmacologic treatment of co-morbid anxiety and depression.
- There is no specific psychopharmacologic intervention for conversion disorder. ECT is not indicated unless used to treat a co-morbid condition.

ASSESSMENT POINTS

System	Effect	Assessment by Hx	PE	Test
CNS	Four subtypes: 1. Motor: Impaired coordination or balance, paralysis or localized weakness, aphonia, difficulty swallowing or sensation of lump in the throat, urinary retention 2. Sensory: Loss of touch or pain sensation, double vision, blindness, deafness, hallucinations 3. Seizures or convulsions 4. Mixed presentation	Differential diagnosis incl almost any medical condition (e.g., myasthenia gravis, MS, porphyria, diabetic neuropathy, hyperparathyroidism, tumors, idiopathic or substance-abuse dystonias)	Findings may not conform to known anatomic pathways or physiologic mechanisms, symptoms may be inconsistent, (e.g., unacknowledged strength in antagonistic muscles; normal muscle tone, intact reflexes; equal difficulty swallowing solids and liquids; paralyzed extremity moves on own with dressing: arm held over patient's head by examiner and dropped will not fall on head; stocking-glove anesthesia without proximal to distal gradient; equal loss of touch, temperature, and pain at sharply demarcated anatomic landmarks rather than dermatomes)	Absence of expected findings (including EEG, EMG, lumbar puncture, CT, MRI, SPECT scan, nerve conduction velocity, drug screen) suggest and confirm diagnosis
GENDER		Gender tendencies: Men—antisocial personality, work-related or military injury Women—more common, esp on left side of body Children <10 y: seizures, gait disturbances		

Key Reference: American Psychiatric Association. *Diagnostic and statistical manual of mental disorders.* 4th ed. *Text revisions.* Washington DC: American Psychiatric Association; 2000.

Perioperative Implications

Perioperative Preparation

- Careful Hx and PE, carefully documenting normal function as well as any pre-existing neurologic deficits
- Confer with treating providers, (e.g., internist, neurologist, psychiatrist/psychotherapist)
- Consider possibility that reason for surgery in pt with multiple procedures may involve conversion symptom

Monitoring

- Routine

Airway

- None

Premedication/Induction/Maintenance

- Attempt to treat reported pain in holding area prior to titrating anxiolytic
- Regional anesthesia not contraindicated

Extubation

- None

Adjuvants

- Pt to take usual dose of psychiatric medications preop

Postoperative Period

- Consider conversion disorder when thorough work-up of medical condition does not explain symptoms, esp if a prior trauma or unresolved neurotic stressors can be readily identified.

- Caution: Apparent conversion symptoms may represent previously undiagnosed medical disease.

Anticipated Problems/Concerns

- As conversion disorder is more common among pts with other psychiatric and medical diseases, clear documentation of these during the preop clinic may prove of immeasurable value to the treating anesthesiologist in the postop period when new symptom complexes are reported and conversion disorder is considered within the differential diagnosis.

Cor Pulmonale

Paul Zanaboni

Risk

- Third most common cardiac Dx after age 50 y
- 10–20% of all CHF admissions have some aspect of right heart failure
- Gender predominance: Male > female

Perioperative Risks

- Increased risk for resp failure, severe right heart failure (≥10% if cor pulmonale Dx made preop)
- Risk of prolonged postop ventilatory support

Worry About

- Increased pulm vascular resistance (PVR) may cause systemic hypotension
- Hypoxia, hypoxemia, hypercarbia, and acidosis intraop or in early postop period, which increases PVR
- Underlying CAD, LV dysfunction

Overview

- Alteration in RV structure (hypertrophy) and function

- Common causes: Pulm embolic events resulting in RV outflow obstruction and COPD resulting in increased PVR (2° to chronic hypoxia and structural changes)
- Any disease that increases PVR chronically can induce RV changes, incl idiopathic and toxin-induced pulm Htn, pulm fibrosis, severe obstructive sleep apnea, congenital heart disease (CHD) with chronic RV overload or RV outflow obstruction
- Prognosis: Favorable for those who can maintain a near-normal Pao_2; unfavorable for those with structural changes

ICD-9-CM Code: 416.9

Etiology

- COPD: Smoking or severe asthma
- Longstanding untreated OSA
- Left ventricular heart failure
- Acute or chronic pulm embolus
- CHD with RV volume overload (L>R shunt, long-standing pulmonic insufficiency) or afterload increase (pulm outflow obstruction)

- Primary pulm Htn or severe pulm fibrosis

Usual Treatment

- Decreasing PVR toward normal levels by increasing Pao_2 to 60 mmHg (beware of depression of hypoxic drive to breathe; may have desensitized hypercarbic drive to breathe 2° to chronic increasing $Paco_2$); giving diuretics, digoxin to relieve symptoms of CHF (Caution: Diuretics may increase Hct by hemoconcentration; if Hct already increased 2° to decreasing Pao_2, this may further increase the viscosity of blood, increasing risk for sludging and microemboli)
- Vasodilators (only ⅓ of pts improve); inhaled nitric oxide or iloprost (stable prostacyclin analogue); phosphodiesterase-5 inhibitors (such as sildenafil) have shown promise; other vasodilators, such as calcium-channel blockers, have been tried; use caution because may decrease SVR in face of fixed increasing PVR, causing severe systemic hypotension (unable to increase CO); antibiotics for prompt treatment of infection

---

ASSESSMENT POINTS

System	Effect	Assessment by Hx	PE	Test
CV	RV failure ↑ PVR Tricuspid regurgitation	DOE Effort-related syncope Chest pain	Accentuated pulm S_2 Diastolic or systolic murmur Dependent edema	CXR ECHO Right heart catheterization
RESP	COPD	DOE Chronic cough, sputum	Hyperinflated lungs Wheezing, rhonchi	CXR PFTs
GI	Passive congestion of liver, spleen		Hepatosplenomegaly	LFTs Albumin PT
RENAL	Impaired ability to excrete Na^+, H_2O	Edema	Edema	Urinary Osm Urine specific gravity
CNS	Stimulation of sympathetic nervous system 2° to hypoxia		Tachycardia	

Key References: Haddad F, Coulture P, Tousignant C, Denault A. The right ventricle in cardiac surgery, A perioperative perspective: I. Anatomy, phyiology and assessment. *Anesth Analg.* 2009;108(2):407–421. Haddad F, Coulture P, Tousignant C, Denault A. The right ventricle in cardiac surgery, A perioperative perspective: II. Pathophysiology, Clinical Importance and Management. *Anesth Analg.* 2009;108(2):422–433.

Perioperative Implications

Preoperative Preparation

- Mortality risk in pts with primary pulm Htn and cor pulmonale high (7%)
- Treat underlying infections
- Maximize treatment of reversible airway disease
- Avoid preop medications that will depress ventilation
- Consider baseline ABG to assess PaO_2, $PaCO_2$

Monitoring

- Consider arterial line for beat-beat arterial pressure monitoring, noninvasive cardiac output measurement and ABG collection
- Consider intraop TEE to monitor RV function, RV dilation
- Consider pulm arterial catheter to monitor PA pressures, CVP monitoring for evaluation of RV function for large fluid shift reoperations

Airway

- Potential for bronchospasm

Induction

- Try to increase SVR in face of fixed increased PVR

- Deep anesthesia for intubation may decrease incidence of bronchospasm and sympathetic stimulation, which increases PVR; must use caution, however to avoid hypercarbia

Maintenance

- Potent inhalational agents for bronchodilation
- Consider avoiding nitrous oxide (which may increase PVR) and large doses of narcotics (which may cause postop hypoventilation and hypercarbia)
- Although positive pressure ventilation may increase PVR 2° to alveolar expansion, it can decrease PVR 2° to better oxygenation
- Aggresively prevent hypercarbia, hypoxemia, and hypothermia, all of which may cause an increase in PVR
- Consider the use of β-adrenergic agents such as dobutamine or epinephrine to support RV cardiac output if faced with hemodynamic instability
- Consider the use of inhaled NO or iloprost to treat increased PVR
- Can also consider use of IV prostaglandin E_1 to decrease PVR (beware of decreased SVR, which may require treatment with an α-adrenergic agonist)

Extubation

- Bronchospasm may occur during emergence
- Avoid hypoventilation and resultant hypercarbia

Adjuvants

- Regional anesthesia an option, but high level may decrease SVR in face of fixed increased PVR leading to CV collapse
- Inhaled nitric oxide or iloprost increasing in use
- Preop phosphodiesterase-5 inhibitors may be used routinely in future; may accenuate effects of intraop vasodilators

Postoperative Period

- Postop pain management with either low-dose epidural local anesthetics with low-dose opioids or low-dose intrathecal opioids can minimize resp depression

Anticipated Problems/Concerns

- Increased PVR and RV dysfunction from hypoxia/hypercarbia or hypothermia

Coronary Artery Disease (Left Main and Non-Left Main Disease)

Alan Finley

Risk

- Incidence in USA: 16.8 million
- ~1.5 million pts per year with CAD will have an acute MI; one third of these will die
- CAD responsible for ~ one of every five deaths in USA
- Male predominance <55 y, M = F >55 y
- Risk factors: Htn, diabetes, smoking, familial incidence, hyperlipidemia, and high cholesterol

Perioperative Risks

- Presence of disease by coronary anatomy is good predictor of survival with CAD
- Presence of left main disease with high degree of stenosis is life-threatening
- Recent MI increases risk, but revascularization interventions protect pt
- Impaired ventricular function, unstable anginal pattern, major surgery, and emergency surgery increases risk
- Increased risk if reoperation for bypass surgery
- Presence of a bare metal stent or drug eluting stent places pt at risk for a MI secondary to in stent thrombosis (esp <3 mo after bare metal stent and <12 mo after drug eluting stent)

Worry About

- Myocardial ischemia can lead to MI
- Postop MI carries very high mortality (>50%) in noncardiac surgical pts

- Atherosclerosis in other vascular beds (CNS, renal, mesentery)
- Increased bleeding during and after surgery if pt is taking an anticoagulant for prevention of MI
- In stent thrombosis with associated MI if pt discontinued antiplatelet medications with up to 50% mortality

Overview

- Atherosclerosis of vessels supplying blood to heart results in ↓ blood flow by limitation of flow due to anatomy or due to vasoactive dysfunction (spasm, etc.)
- Single greatest cause of death in USA population (~500,000 deaths/y)
- Most prevalent form of CV disease: >16.8 million in USA population has CAD
- Leading cause of death in major noncardiac surgery

ICD-9-CM Code: 414.0

See also Angina, Chronic Stable, in Diseases section

Etiology

- Atherosclerosis and obstructive deposits in coronary artery
- Interaction of genetics, diet, and environment: Htn, cigarette smoking, and diabetes are three common predisposing factors

- Myocardial O_2 delivery does not meet myocardial O_2 demands: causes myocardial ischemia
- Myocardial O_2 supply does not reach myocardium after thrombosis of coronary artery: causes MI

Usual Treatment

- Medical: Nitroglycerin, β-blockers, calcium-channel blockers (low dose and in vasospastic component), diet, antihyperlipidemia drugs, antiplatelet therapy, exercise, wt loss, antioxidants
- Catheter-based interventional cardiology (indicated in ≤2-vessel CAD: PTCA (has 30% 3-mo closure rate), intracoronary stent (has good angiographic result and lower closure rate, but event-free survival is little different from PTCA)
- CABG surgery (indicated in ≥2-vessel CAD, left main disease, diabetics)
- Coronary revascularization is indicated in pts with stable angina before noncardiac surgery in left main disease, 3-vessel disease and in pts with high-risk unstable angina
- If possible, delay surgery for 3 mo after bare metal stent implantation and 12 mo after drug eluting stent implantation. During the periop period, continue antiplatelet therapy if possible.

ASSESSMENT POINTS

Concern	Effect	Assessment by Hx	PE	Test
Noncardiac Surgery				
Ischemia	Causes ventricular dysfunction and arrhythmias Can herald and/or cause MI	Angina Dyspnea on exertion		Holter monitor, ECG exercise radionuclide, treadmill stress ECHO
Infarction	Indicates severe CAD Causes death	Unstable angina		ECG, CK-MB and troponin enzyme release
Impaired function	Heart failure, shock	Activity Hx Stair climbing Orthopnea	Orthopnea gallop Neck veins Rales Peripheral edema	Ejection fraction (cath, ECHO, radionuclide)
Stent thrombosis	Cardiogenic shock, death ↑ risk if bare metal stent implanted <3 mo or drug eluting stent <12 mo	Antiplatelet regimen Type of stent (bare metal vs. drug eluting) Stent(s) location and date implanted		
Cardiac Surgery				
Cardiac function	Best predictor of outcome	Activity Hx, stair climbing		Ventricular angiogram (EF >50% = good risk)
Coronary anatomy	Extent of disease and overall long-term survival			Coronary angiography
Renal function	↑ Risk if impaired			Cr ≥1.4 mg/dL denotes ↑ risk
CNS	↑ Risk of stroke Aortic atheromatous disease and prior stroke increase risk	Hx of TIA Amaurosis fugax	Carotid bruit	Carotid Doppler study, epiaortic ultrasound

Perioperative Implications

Preoperative Preparation

- Supportive preop interview to decrease stress and anxiety
- Consider analgesic (opioid) if pain or likelihood of pain prior to anesthesia
- Give morning cardiac medications, esp β-blockers, antiplatelets if pt has intracoronary stent

- Nitroglycerin at bedside

Monitoring

- Consider systemic arterial BP (invasive and continuous in unstable pts or in cases where BP swings are anticipated)
- Consider CVP and/or PA catheters; in cardiac surgical pts, EF ≤30% should trigger consideration of central line, or use of TEE

- Consider TEE if pt is hemodynamically unstable

Anesthesia

- Principle is to maintain O_2 supply and to minimize myocardial O_2 consumption
- Maintain cardiac output, O_2 sat and Hgb concentration (O_2 delivery)
- Maintain diastolic BP (perfusion pressure)

- Decrease HR, contractility, and wall tension (O$_2$ consumption)
- No outcome difference demonstrated among general anesthetics
- Regional and conduction anesthesia with postop analgesia may be beneficial
- Transient periods of Htn are well tolerated; prolonged periods of hypotension, tachycardia, and anemia are not well tolerated

Adjuvants

- Nitroglycerin, sublingual or (preferably) by continuous infusion (0.5–2.0 μg/kg/min), can treat myocardial ischemia.

- β-blockers by bolus or infusion decrease HR and myocardial contractility and can prevent and treat ischemia
- RBCs to maintain Hct ≥ 28%

Postoperative Period

- Second and third postop days are most common time for MI in noncardiac surgical pts; ischemia intraop, designate as high risk in postop period
- Maintain good analgesia to decrease stress response

- Maintain cardiac medications (esp β-blockers)
- Consider use of aspirin or other medications to decrease coronary thrombosis in high-risk non-cardiac surgical pts (esp in pts with intracoronary stents)

Coronary Artery Spasm (CAS)

Ferenc Puskas

Risk

- Mostly disease of middle and old-aged men and post-menopausal women
- Gender difference: Higher incidence in women
- Periop CAS is prevalent in elderly male pts with coronary risk factors
- Teenagers and young adults with illicit substance abuse, primarily cocaine
- Occurs in 1% to 5% of percutaneous coronary interventions
- Ethnic differences: Higher frequency in eastern populations
- Type A behavior pattern, severe anxiety, and panic disorder
- Age, smoking, high sensitivity C-reactive protein (marker of inflammation)

Perioperative Risks

- Change of sympathetic activity may trigger CAS
- CAS can lead to myocardial ischemia
- Chest pain, ischemic ST segment changes on ECG
- May result or associated with myocardial infarction
- Coronary thrombosis may trigger CAS, leading to acute MI, unstable angina, or ischemic sudden death

Worry About

- Cardiogenic shock: Decreased LV and RV compliance, decreased pump function

- Tachyarrhythmias: When CAS is associated with anterior ST segment elevations, ventricular arrhythmias and even ventricular fibrillation may occur
- Bradyarrhythmias: More frequent with inferior CAS, potentially resulting in complete atrioventricular block, associated with hypotension and syncope

Overview

- Classical CAS (Prinzmetal, variant, or spastic angina)
  - Diagnosed by severe chest pain, usually at rest, with concurrent ST segment elevation on ECG
  - Characterized by spasm of normal coronary arteries on arteriography
- Other forms of CAS
  - Without chest pain silent angina, diagnosed with Holter monitoring
  - CAS can be associated with ischemic heart disease and myocardial infarction
  - Effort angina, unstable angina, microvascular angina (female prevalence)
  - ECG changes may incl either ST segment elevation, ST depression or T wave abnormalities
  - Coronary arteriography can demonstrate normal or diseased coronary arteries

ICD9-CM: 414.0 (Coronary atherosclerosis)

Etiology

- The exact mechanism of coronary artery spasm is unknown. Several contributing factors thought to play a role:
  - Change in sympathetic activity
  - Vagal withdrawal
  - Coronary thrombosis
  - Endothelial dysfunction
  - Increased Ca^{2+} sensitivity
  - Reduced endothelial NO activity
  - *eNOS* gene polymorphism
  - Signs of chronic low grade inflammation
  - Oxidative stress

Usual treatment

- Cessation of smoking
- Calcium-channel blockers (primary)
- Long-acting nitrates (short when symptomatic)
- β-blockers (when associated with fixed lesions)
- Magnesium supplementation (may have a preventive effect)
- Statin therapy (improving endothelial function)
- Coronary angioplasty (medically intractable)
- Coronary artery bypass surgery (medically intractable)
- Automatic defibrillator implantation (life-threatening arrhythmias)

ASSESSMENT POINTS

System	Effect	Assessment by Hx	PE	Test
GENERAL		Risk factor search: Smoking, illicit drug use, esp cocaine		High sensitive C-reactive protein level
CV	Chest pain, myocardial ischemia, cardiogenic shock, ischemic sudden death, arrhythmias	Chest pain at rest or exertion, Hx of rapid heart rate, Hx of syncope	Palpitations, cold sweat, nausea, vomiting, syncope, hypotension	ECG, ST segment analysis, Holter, exercise testing Coronary arteriography, TEE or TTE—wall motion abnormalities, cardiac biomarkers

Key Reference: Yasue H, Nakagawa H, Itoh T, Harada E, Mizuno Y. Coronary artery spasm - clinical features, diagnosis, pathogenesis, and treatment. *J Cardiol.* 2008;51(1):2–17.

Perioperative Implications

Preoperative Preparation
- Continue treatment medication until the morning of surgery
- IV nitroglycerin, nicardipine, β-blockers available
- Have a plan for postop pain control
- Consider regional or neuroaxial techniques

Monitoring
- 2 lead (II. and V5) ECG & ST segment analysis
- Consider arterial line

Airway
- Blunt intubation reflexes, avoid sympathetic surcharge on intubation

Preinduction/Induction
- Cardio-stable induction
- Avoidance of hypotension and tachycardia

Maintenance
- Heart rate and BP control (maintain adequate diastolic BP)
- Avoid hypothermia
- Maintain Hct
- Optimize supply/demand

Extubation
- Smooth opioid wake up and extubation
- Heart rate and BP control
- Avoidance of hypercapnia and hypoxemia

Postoperative Period
- Adequate pain control
- Heart rate and BP control
- Treatment of shivering

Adjuvants
- Careful ST segment monitoring throughout periop period

- Immediate recognition and treatment of coronary ischemia by optimizing supply and demand, special attention to adequate diastolic blood pressure

Anticipated Problems/Concerns

- Anticipate potentially life-threatening arrhythmias
- Myocardial ischemia or infarction, LV and RV dysfunction
- Place defibrillator pads for high-risk pts

Craniosynostosis

Ryan Ball
Franklyn Cladis

Risk

- May be simple (non-syndromic) or associated with a syndrome
- 1/3–5000 live births for simple craniosynostosis
- 80% nonsyndromic, 20% syndromic
- Sutural involvement (decreasing incidence): Sagittal, coronal, metopic, lambdoid
- Prenatal or perinatal in onset, rarely later
- Majority of mutations found in fibroblast growth factor receptor genes

Perioperative Risk

- Difficult airway
- Blood loss (>1/2 blood volume)
- Venous air embolism (micro emboli common)
- Increased intracranial pressure (ICP), (all pts should have eye exam for papilledema)
- Associated cardiac anomalies

Worry About

- Difficult mask ventilation and intubation
- Management of intraop blood loss
- Monitoring for venous air embolism
- Management of increased ICP

Overview

- Premature closure of one or more cranial sutures
- Nonsyndromic type usually affects one suture and is not associated with other abnormalities
- Syndromic type typically affects >1 suture and has associated abnormalities
- May also be designated primary (abnormal cranial suture) or secondary (acquired from abnormal brain growth, example post-VP shunt)
- Most commonly associated syndromes are Apert, Crouzon, and Pfeiffer
- Degree of deformity depends on affected suture and time of closure
- Impaired brain growth, cognitive development, visual disturbances, and dysmorphic features can occur if left untreated

ICD9-CM: 756.0

Etiology

- Can be involved in more than 150 different syndromes
- Most often occurs by sporadic gene mutation (fibroblast growth factor receptor, TWIST), however can be inherited in autosomal recessive or dominant pattern

Usual Treatment

- Surgery is typically indicated for cosmetic reasons or increased ICP
- Results are best when surgery performed prior to 12 mo of age
- Important to consider associated syndromes prior to surgery
- Team usually incl plastic surgeon, neurosurgeon, and anesthesiologist

ASSESSMENT POINTS

System	Effect	Assessment by Hx	PE	Test
Airway	Diff mask vent and/or intubation	Hx or previous mask ventilation or intubation	Facial symmetry Size of mandible Neck range of motion	Neck films may be indicated (Apert may have cervical fusion)
RESP	OSA	Apnea during sleep, snoring	Noisy breathing from upper airway	Polysomnogram (apnea-hypopnea index) Overnight pulse oximetry Room air O_2 saturation
CARDIAC	CHD (ASD, VSD, tetralogy of Fallot)	Bottle feeds > 30 min Diaphoresis with feeds Failure to thrive	Murmur	ECHO
MS	Diff IV access Diff a-line access		Syndactyly (Apert) Fused elbows (Pfeiffer)	
CNS	Increased ICP	Irritable, vomiting, somnolence	Papilledema	Ophthalmology exam
HEME	Anemia (nadir at 3 mo of age)			Preop Hct, type and cross

Key Reference: Haas T, Fries D, Velik-Salchner C, Oswald E, Innerhofer P. Fibrinogen in craniosynostosis surgery. *Anesth Analg*. 2008;106(3):725–731.

Perioperative implications

Preoperative implications

- Determine whether surgery for cosmetic reasons related to isolated defect or for elevated ICP
- Determine if there is an associated syndrome
- Prepare for possible difficult airway if syndromic
- Prepared for significant blood loss with IV access, type and cross, and preparation of blood products accordingly

Monitoring

- At least two large (20–22G) peripheral IVs should be placed. *Endoscopic* surgery for single suture may have less blood loss, but it can still be significant.
- Multiple suture repairs require an open approach. Expect significant (>½–1 blood volume) blood loss. Will need 2–3 large bore IVs, arterial line for pressure monitoring and frequent lab draws. Central venous access may be needed for IV access and for CVP monitoring. Precordial Doppler monitoring should be considered in all pts.

Airway

- Have multiple airway devices (primarily LMA) available for multimodal airway management. May need to perform an asleep fiberoptic intubation.
- Consider awake fiberoptic as a possible choice for intubation.
- Depending on airway concerns and Hx, have surgeon available for possible tracheostomy.

Positioning

- May be supine or prone depending on suture involved
- If prone, be careful to avoid eye pressure (esp if proptosis is present).

Induction

- Standard inhalational induction is appropriate for most pts.
- An inhalation induction is often appropriate in the syndromic pt with potentially difficult airway because of lack of cooperation
- If increased ICP with symptoms, may need to do IV induction and avoid ketamine.

Maintenance

- General inhalational or IV maintenance with muscle relaxant
- Large fluid shifts can occur due to blood loss and massive transfusion.
- Need for frequent monitoring of blood gases, electrolytes, coagulation, and positioning
- Forced air warmer required due to length of case. IVF warmer should be used.
- Mannitol may be required prior to calvarial removal if increased ICP.
- Isotonic IVF should be used during the intraop period.

Extubation

- The majority of pts can be extubated at the end of the surgery.
- Place nasal pharyngeal airway prior to extubation.
- Have airway equipment available during extubation.
- Consider delaying extubation if tongue is edematous or if significant clinical or hemodynamic instability.

Adjuvants

- Preop Epogen may be used to increase the hematocrit.
- Cell saver for reclamation of blood loss during procedure
- Blood products in room prior to start of surgery
- Equipment available for transfer postop

Postoperative Period

- May require transfusion of red blood cells, factors, and platelets
- Hyponatremia common postop. Use isotonic IVF during the intra and postop period.

Surgical Stages

- Bicoronal incision, scalp and face are dissected to expose the calvarium.
- Calvarial removal. May be partial or complete calvarial removal (neurosurgery).
- Supraorbital osteotomies performed to mobilize superior orbital rim, nasion, and lateral temporal bones
- Calvarial vault remodeling and reconstruction with craniofacial plating system

Anticipated Problems/Concerns

- Difficult airway
- Massive blood loss and transfusion
- Extended length of surgery
- Possible postop intubation

CREST Syndrome

Risk

- Pts with Hx of exposure to silica dust or PVC
- Usual age group is of 30 to 50 y
- 4- to 9-fold higher in women than men, seen in all races
- In USA, systemic sclerosis has an estimated incidence of 19 cases per million and prevalence of 240 cases per million population (range 138 to 286)

Perioperative Risk

- Pts more likely to have compromised renal function at baseline
- Hypoxia from pulm Htn and/or restrictive lung disease
- Difficult intubation from narrow mouth opening

Worry About

- Reflux and thereby aspiration, renal crises, restrictive lung disease, CHF, pulm Htn, difficult intubation due to small mouth opening, keeping pt warm to avoid Raynaud's

Overview

- **C**alcinosis, **R**aynaud's phenomenon, **E**sophageal dysmotility, **S**clerodactyly and **T**elangiectasia (CREST)
- Symptoms involved in CREST or limited cutaneous systemic sclerosis are associated with the generalized form of systemic sclerosis

ICD-9-CM Code 710.1 (Scleroderma)

Etiology

- Exact etiology of systemic sclerosis is unknown; following pathogenic factors are always present: endothelial cell injury, fibroblast activation, cellular and humoral immunologic derangement

- Environmental factors like silica, industrial solvents and radiation exposure are all triggers or accelerators
- CMV, HHV5 and parvovirus are possible viral accelerators

Usual Treatment

- Glucocorticosteroid, immunosuppressive, chelating agents, endothelin receptor antagonist, PDE5 inhibitor and peripheral vasodilators
- Skin thickening with D-penicillamine, γ-interferon (not FDA approved)
- Pruritus with moisturizers, H1 and H2 blockers, tricyclic antidepressants, and trazadone
- Raynaud's with CCB, prazosin, PGE1, dipyridamole, aspirin, and topical nitrates
- GI symptoms with antacids, H2 blockers, PPIs, prokinetic agents and octreotide

ASSESSMENT POINTS

System	Effect	Assessment by Hx	PE	Test
SKIN and HEENT	Sclerodactly, few wrinkles or joint creases, decreased range of motion, hair loss, pruritus telangiectases	Observation	Tightness, indurations, hyper or hypopigmentation	Airway examination
CVS	Pericardial effusion, CHF, myocardial fibrosis, misconduction Cor pulmonale	Dyspnea, palpitation, irregular heart rate, chest pain from vasospasm	Rales and murmurs on auscultation	EKG, Holter monitoring, ECHO
RESP	Pulm Htn, aspiration pneumonia, dyspnea	SOB, cough, tachypnea, dec exercise tolerance	Dry rales	PFT, ABG, CXR, DLCO, HRCT
CNS	Carpal tunnel syndrome, trigeminal neuralgia (rare), entrapment neuropathies	Pain over wrist, other typical signs depending on nerve involved	Limited ROM	Conduction studies, CT
RENAL	Htn, oliguria	Headache, SOB, edema	Swelling of hands and feet	Check BP, UO & monitor serum creatinine
MS	Raynaud's phenomenon, arthralgias, myalgias, morning stiffness	Acroosteolysis, muscle weakness	Palpable tendon friction rubs, muscle wasting, flexion contractures	Increased serum CK and aldolase
GASTRO	GE reflux, esophagitis, esophageal strictures, watermelon stomach, primary biliary cirrhosis, colonic diverticula, anal sphincter incompetence	Bitter taste, dysphagia, retrosternal and abdominal pain, diarrhea, self-soiling	Abdominal tenderness, decreased rectal sphincter tone	Barium swallow CT or MRI, endoscopy Abdominal ultrasound, anti-mitochondrial antibodies for PBC

Key Reference: Highland KB, Garin MC, Brown KK. The spectrum of scleroderma lung disease. *Semin Respir Crit Care Med.* 2007;28(4):418–429.

Perioperative Implications

Preoperative Preparation
- Continue PPI, consider FOI, evaluate for regional anesthetic techniques for pulm issues

Monitoring
- If co-morbidities dictate A-line, (try to avoid due to Raynaud's, but difficult to get cuff pressure due to reduced flow, may need ABG)
- CVP ± PA catheter if pulm Htn, along with standard monitoring

Airway
- Airway may be a challenge due to small oral opening

Preinduction/Induction
- Worry about hypotension and hypoxemia at induction

Maintenance
- Choose drugs based on hemodynamic status
- Keep warm

Extubation
- May have to be delayed if significant pulm compromise

Adjuvants
- In the presence of compromised renal, cardiac, or pulm function modify anesthetic drugs accordingly

Anticipated Problems/Concerns

- Challenging airway, hypoxemia, CHF, renal function, and positioning challenges with contractures

Cri Du Chat Syndrome (5p Syndrome)

Mary Rabb

Risk

- 1:15,000 to 1: 50,000 births

Perioperative Risks

- Difficult airway management
- CHD—30%
- Aspiration risk

Worry About

- Difficult mask ventilation—airway obstruction secondary to hypotonia
- Difficult intubation
- Temp regulation
- Mental retardation

Overview

- Microcephaly with profound mental retardation and hypotonia
- Characteristic facies with micrognathia, low-set ears, facial asymmetry
- Characteristic high shrill cry may be due to laryngeal abnorm (narrow diamond-shaped larynx, long, floppy epiglottis) or neurogenic defect
- CHD, 30% ASD, VSD, PDA, or pulmonic stenosis

ICD-9-CM Code: 758.31

Etiology

- Partial or total deletion of the short arm of chromosome no. 5
- Loss of the critical 5p15.2 region is responsible for most of the features.
- Most cases occur by spontaneous gene mutation (90%).
- 10% arise by unbalanced translocations.

ASSESSMENT POINTS

System	Effect	Assessment by Hx	PE	Test
HEENT	Micrognathia	Resp distress in neonatal period; inspiratory stridor	Receding mandible	
CV	ASD, VSD, PDA, PS	SOB, cyanosis	Murmur, gallop	ECHO
RESP/GI	Pneumonia, chronic aspiration		Dyspnea, rales, rhonchi, wheezing	CXR
ORTHO	Scoliosis			
CNS	Mental retardation, seizures		Hypotonia in infancy, hypertonia later	

Key Reference: Cat cry syndrome. In Bissonnette B, ed. *Syndromes: Rapid recognition and perioperative implications.* McGraw-Hill; 2006: 140–141.

Perioperative Implications

Preoperative Preparation
- Difficult airway management

Monitoring
- Routine
- Pay particular attention to temp and neuromuscular blockade

Airway
- Laryngeal mask airway available
- Fiberoptic bronchoscope

- Wide assortment of laryngoscope blades and ETT available

Preinduction/Induction
- Presence of primary care giver for uncooperative pts
- Sedation in monitored setting
- Warm OR for temp regulation

Maintenance
- Measures to actively warm the pt (radiant heat lamp, forced air warming blankets, warm IV fluids)
- Monitor neuromuscular blockade

Extubation
- Extubate awake

Anticipated Problems/Concerns

- CHD
- Airway management may be difficult
- Extubation may be difficult; may have airway obstruction postop

Crohn's Disease

Mark C. Phillips

Risk

- Incidence of 4 cases per 100,000/y, prevalence of 80–150 per 100,000
- Race: Caucasians > African-Americans > Hispanics and Asians
- Three to four times more common in ethnic Jews than non-Jewish whites
- Peak occurrence between ages 15 and 25 y, with a second smaller peak between ages 60-80 y

Perioperative Risks

- Aspiration
- Arrhythmias due to electrolyte disorders

Worry About

- Intravascular fluid volume and electrolyte imbalances
- Chronic steroid use and need for periop supplementation
- Nutritional status, chronic weight loss, and malnutrition
- Difficult IV access due to chronic illness and frequent venipunctures
- Psychological mindset of the pt due to chronicity of the disease and relatively young age of the pts

Overview

- Chronic inflammatory disease of the GI tract that can give rise to strictures, inflammatory masses, fistulas, abcesses, and hemmorhage.
- Pt may develop bowel obstruction and perforation.
- Pt may develop rectocutaneous fistulas, rectal fissures, and perirectal abcesses.
- Pt may have anemia from several causes, chronic disease, chronic blood loss, folate and vitamin B$_{12}$ deficiency
- Chronic malnutrition and weight loss
- Extraintestinal manifestations occur in a minority of pts. These manifestations incl uveitis and episcleritis, erythema nodosum and pyoderma gangrenosum, ankylosing spondylitis, and primary sclerosing cholangitis. When present, their symptoms can be more serious than the primary intestinal disease.

ICD-9-CM Code: 555.9 (Regional enteritis of unspecified site)

Etiology

- Unknown
- Theories incl response to an infectious agent, defective mucosal barrier allowing exposure to antigens
- Smoking is a risk factor

Usual Treatment

- Pharmacologic: Aminosalicylates, steroids, immunomodulating agents such as azathioprine and cyclosporine, infliximab— a monoclonal anti-tumor necrosis factor-α antibody given in an effort to decrease inflammation
- Surgical: Indications for surgery are intractability, intestinal obstruction, intra-abdominal abscess, fistulas, fulminant colitis, toxic megacolon, massive hemmorage, cancer and growth, retardation
- Both medical and surgical management of Crohn's disease are aimed at providing long lasting symptomatic relief while avoiding excessive morbidity

ASSESSMENT POINTS

System	Effect	Assessment by Hx	PE	Test
CV	Hypovolemia	Bowel prep, wt loss, diarrhea	Hypotension, tachycardia	Electrolytes, Hct
GI	Bowel perforation	Abdominal pain	Abdominal tenderness, fever	WBC
	Malabsorption	Diarrhea, wt loss	Cachexia	Albumin
MS	Ankylosing arthritis	Joint mobility	Decreased ROM of joints	

Key Reference: Picco MF, Cangemi JR. Inflammatory bowel disease in the elderly. *Gastroenterol Clin North Am.* 2009;38(3):447–462.

Perioperative Implications

Preoperative Preparation

- Ensure volume status and electrolytes are normalized
- If pt is on hyperalimentation preop, continue it during the case; monitor glucose
- Assess current or recent steroid use and need for periop supplementation
- Discontinue methotrexate at least 2 wk before surgery as it has been shown to decrease wound healing
- Pts with significant anemia should be transfused preop

Monitoring

- Routine
- Consider CVL if pt has difficult IV access
- Consider arterial line if significant co-morbidities

Airway

- Aspiration risk if bowel obstruction present

Induction

- Rapid sequence induction in pts with gastric outlet or bowel obstruction
- Consider preinduction placement of NG tube to suction gastric contents

Maintenance

- Avoid nitrous oxide if bowel obstruction present
- Abdominal relaxation with non-depolarizing muscle relaxants usually needed. If liver disease present avoid muscle relaxants dependent on hepatic metabolism
- Check glucose regularly if on hyperalimentation

Extubation

- Awake extubation

Postoperative Period

- Consider epidural analgesia or IV PCA for pain control
- Monitor fluid status carefully in the postop period

Anticipated Problems/Concerns

- May need aggressive fluid replacement due to hypovolemia and anemia worsened by third space losses
- May have severe nutritional deficiency, esp with short bowel syndrome from extensive resection

Croup (Laryngotracheobronchitis)

Maurice S. Zwass

Risk

- Children between 6 mo and 6 y are at risk, (6 mo—3 y at greatest risk)
- Children with underlying airway abnormalities (e.g., subglottic stenosis) or difficult intubations (e.g., micrognathia) and symptoms are at increased risk and require particular planning

Perioperative Risks

- Difficulty with intubation because of very narrowed subglottic region
- Obstruction of the small tracheal tube because of airway secretions

Worry About

- Risk of rebound tracheal edema several hours after racemic epinephrine treatment
- Cardiorespiratory crisis in progressive or severe Sx, agitation, younger pts, difficulties with oxygenation or ventilation, failure to oxygenate
- Bacterial superinfection of airway

Overview

- Common childhood ailment with prodromal illness accompanied by a characteristic cough (often sounds like seal barking)
- Sx and resp compromise from progressive swelling of subglottic region tracheal mucosa
- Frequently present when inspiratory stridor and resp distress develop
- Radiographs of neck often demonstrate gradual progressive tracheal narrowing, most narrow just below level of vocal cords (referred to as steeple sign); upper glottis on lateral neck radiograph is normal
- When obtained, evaluation of CBC is consistent with viral illness

ICD-9-CM Codes: 464.4 (Croup); 464.2 (Laryngotracheitis)

Etiology

- Viral agents are usual etiologies and incl parainfluenza viruses (most common); adenoviruses, influenza virus, resp syncytial virus (RSV), and measles virus also associated

Usual Treatment

- Cool mist often greatly improves Sx; supplemental O_2
- If symptoms more severe, aerosolized racemic epinephrine can dramatically reduce airway swelling (rebound tracheal edema risk several hours after administration necessitates observation in hospital)
- Steroid administration controversial; may decrease severity of disease and decrease need for tracheal intubation or hasten improvement in first 24 hr of illness
- Small percentage with this disease needs tracheal intubation
- Parenteral steroids (dexamethasone) and inhaled (budesonide) have been used
- Breathing helium-oxygen mixtures has been reported as helpful in some cases (lower density and viscosity)

ASSESSMENT POINTS

Differential points between croup (laryngotracheobronchitis) and epiglottitis

	CROUP	EPIGLOTTITIS
AGE	3 mo–3 y	1–7 y
ONSET	Gradual	More rapid (usually <24 hr)
FEVER	Low grade	High
COUGH	Characteristic barking	None
SORE THROAT	Occasional	Frequently severe
POSTURE	Any	Frequently sitting forward, mouth open, drooling
AIRWAY SOUND	Inspiratory stridor	Inspiratory stridor
VOICE	Normal	Muffled
APPEARANCE	Nontoxic	Toxic
SEASONALITY	Peak winter, epidemic	Year-round

Key Reference: Jenkins I, Saunders M. Infections of the airway. *Paediatr Anaesth*. 2009;19(suppl 1):118–130.

Perioperative Implications

Airway

- Airway support with good mask fit and positive pressure ventilation can generally overcome obstruction from swelling of airway
- Identification of larynx generally routine, but tracheal tube 0.5–1.0 mm diameter smaller than usual may necessitate having available extra-long or microlaryngeal tracheal tubes
- Tracheotomy rarely needed as therapy for these pts with current management and reserved only for unusual cases

Induction

- Induction common with IV access already obtained

Anticipated Problems/Concerns

- Symptomatic pts who require intubation of trachea need tube 0.5–1.0 mm smaller in diameter than equivalent in children without croup.
- Pt who requires tracheal intubation usually requires sedative management to tolerate ventilation; often followed for development of leak around tracheal tube as a sign of improvement of edema; most pts improve within 2–4 d; when leak is present at 20–25 cm H_2O of pressure, extubation can be considered; complicated cases and pts with prolonged courses may benefit from examination of airway in operating room at time of extubation.
- Although a viral illness, some pts may acquire bacterial superinfection of airway and require antibiotic therapy.

Cryptococcus Infection

Pierre Moine

Risk

- 0.4–1.3 cases per 100,000 in general population. AIDS pts, 2–7 cases per 1000.
- Underlying immunocompromised conditions and other risk factors: Acquired immunodeficiency syndrome (AIDS), systemic lupus erythematous, prolonged treatment with corticosteroids, organ transplantation, advanced malignancy, diabetes, sarcoidosis, cirrhosis, idiopathic CD4 lymphocytopenia or use of immune-modifying monoclonal antibodies (alemtuzumab, infliximab, etanercept, or adalimumab).
- Only 20% of pts who have cryptococcosis without HIV infection have no apparent underlying disease or risk factor.

Perioperative Risks

- Resp insufficiency, severe ARDS
- Elevated intracranial pressure

Worry About

- Underlying immunocompromised conditions

Overview

- *C. neoformans* typically infects immunocompromised persons. 80–90% of infections occur in HIV pts in the USA

- Wide range of clinical presentations from asymptomatic resp colonization to dissemination of infection into any organ. In severely immunosuppressed pts, involvement of multiple body sites. Common sites for infection are the lungs and CNS.
- Pulm cryptococcosis: Multiple clinical presentations—asymptomatic nodules, lobar infiltrates, interstitial infiltrates, cavities, endobronchial colonization or masses, mediastinal adenopathy, hilar adenopathy, miliary pattern, or pleural effusions/empyema, pneumothorax, and life-threatening pneumonia with ARDS.
- Cryptococcal meningitis: Primary life-threatening infection. Mortality rate about 12%. Other CNS clinical manifestations: Cryptococcomas (abscesses) of brain, spinal cord granuloma, chronic dementia (from hydrocephalus).

ICD9-CM: 117.5 (Cryptococcosis)

Etiology

- *Cryptococcus neoformans* is an encapsulated heterobasidiomycetous fungus
- Enters the host primarily through the lungs but special predilection for invading the CNS

- No human-to-human transmission, except in cases of contaminated transplant tissue

Usual Treatment

- Cryptococcal meningitis or CNS infection: IV amphotericin B deoxycholate 0.7–1 mg/kg/d (or liposomal amphotericin B (AmBisome) 3–6 mg/kg/d with less nephrotoxicity) in combination with IV flucytosine 100 mg/kg/d for 2 wk. Adding flucytosine to amphotericin B reduces the rates of failure and relapse compared with amphotericin B monotherapy. Then fluconazole 400–800 mg/d for 10 wk. In HIV pts, maintenance fluconazole 200–400 mg/d po therapy lifelong.
- Corticosteroids not recommended for the treatment of cryptococcal meningitis.
- Control of increased intracranial pressures (external drainage or CSF shunt, or surgical drainage of abscesses).
- Antiretroviral therapy in HIV pts.
- Pulm disease in HIV-negative pts: fluconazole 200–400 mg/d for 6–12 mo.
- Pulm disease in HIV pts: Fluconazole 200–400 mg/d, lifelong.
- For more severe disease and immunocompromised hosts, treat like CNS disease.

ASSESSMENT POINTS

System	Effect	Assessment by Hx	PE	Test
RESP	Pneumonia	Fever, chest pain, cough, wt loss, dyspnea, sputum production	Signs of infection	ABGs, CXR, sputum culture, bronchoscopy, lung biopsy
CV	Endocarditis, myocarditis	Rare vascular instability		EKG, ECHO
HEME / IMMUNO	Cryptococcemia		Signs of infection	Blood cultures, serum cryptococcal antigen
GU	Prostatitis, renal cortical abscess		Signs of infection	UA, urine cultures
CNS	Meningitis, abscesses, dementia	Headache, fever, N/V, cranial nerve palsies, lethargy, coma, seizures, or memory loss	Mental status, focal signs	CSF India ink stain, CSF cultures and cryptococcal antigen, CT and MRI

Key Reference: Ritter M, Goldman DL. Pharmacotherapy of cryptococcosis. *Expert Opin Pharmacother*. 2009;10(15):2433–2443. Review.

Perioperative Implications

Preoperative Preparation

- Disposable anesthetic delivery circuits with bacterial filters
- Protect and maintain airways for altered mental status, seizures, focal neurologic signs, cranial nerve palsies
- Organ system effects of HIV infection or underlying immunocompromised conditions

Monitoring

- ARDS network low tidal volume protocol in severe ARDS pts
- Consider to monitor increased intracranial pressures

Airway

- None

Induction/Maintenance

- Anesthetic drugs associated with lower ICP and having neuroprotective qualities

- Possible interaction of antiretroviral drugs with the anesthetics and/or toxicity

Extubation

- Consider if it adequately protects airway

Adjuvants

- None

Postoperative Period

- Careful observation for resp and neurologic compromises

Cushing's Syndrome

Kathleen Smith
Justin L. Rountree

Risk

- Onset generally occurs in the third and fourth decades
- Cushing's disease is roughly three times more common in women than men
- 5-y mortality rate from adrenal carcinomas has been estimated to be >70%

Perioperative Risks

- Electrolyte abnormalities
- Consequences of untreated Htn
- Hyperglycemia

Worry About

- Challenges related to obesity, incl airway management and IV access
- Significant osteopenia secondary to impaired calcium absorption, making positioning difficult
- Htn due to fluid retention
- Increased risk of infection as a result of corticosteroid's immunosuppressive qualities
- Hypokalemic alkalosis, commonly seen in ectopic ACTH production

Overview

- The most common cause of Cushing's syndrome is iatrogenic administration of exogenous glucocorticoids.

- Spontaneous Cushing's syndrome can result from adrenal gland hyperplasia secondary to increased ACTH production from a pituitary tumor, or an ectopic non-endocrine ACTH tumor.
- Other causes incl primary gland disorders such as adrenal adenoma or carcinoma.
- Symptoms incl Htn, hyperglycemia, increased intravascular volume, hypokalemia, abdominal striae, truncal obesity, telangiectasias, muscle weakness and/or wasting leading to thin extremities, osteoporosis due to impaired calcium absorption, depression and insomnia.
- A 24-hr urine cortisol test can demonstrate elevated cortisol levels.
- Dexamethasone suppression test is used to aid in differentiating pituitary adenomas from adrenal tumors. Dexamethasone causes depression of cortisol and 17-hydroxycorticosteriod levels due to a negative feedback response, which is absent with ectopic ACTH or primary gland disease.
- ACTH plasma levels can also be tested directly.
- Radiologic evaluation incl: Abdominal CT scan to evaluate the adrenal glands, pituitary MRI scan with gadolinium contrast to evaluate the pituitary gland, and a chest CT scan when ectopic ACTH is the etiology.

ICD-9-CM Code: 255.0

Etiology

- ACTH dependent (excessive ACTH secretion, stimulating adrenal production of cortisol)
  - Pituitary microadenoma (70% of cases)
  - ACTH production from a non-endocrine tumor (e.g., tumors of the lungs, pancreas, or thymus)
- ACTH independent (excessive cortisol production by adrenals and suppression of ACTH production)
  - Adrenocortical adenoma or carcinoma
- Exogenous administration of glucocorticoids (e.g., treatment of asthma)
  - These pts will likely need periop stress dose steroids.

Usual Treatment

- ACTH dependent Cushing's disease
  - Transsphenoidal resection of a pituitary microadenoma
  - Radiation therapy
- ACTH independent Cushing's disease
  - Unilateral/bilateral adrenalectomy
  - Medical adrenalectomy

ASSESSMENT POINTS

System	Effect	Assessment by Hx	PE	Test
CV	Hypertension	HA, visual disturbances		Noninvasive BP
FEN	Hypokalemia	Weakness, constipation, nausea	Decreased strength	Basic metabolic panel, flat T waves on EKG
RENAL	Fluid retention	Leg swelling	Peripheral edema	Serum/urine osmolarity
ENDO	Hyperglycemia	Thirst, frequency		Fasting blood glucose
MS	Muscle wasting Impaired calcium absorption	Weakness	Thin extremeties	Difficulty rising from chair/ climbing stairs
		Osteoporosis	Easy fracture	Bone density scan

Key Reference: Nemergut EC, Zuo Z. Airway management in patients with pituitary disease: A review of 746 patients. *J Neurosurg Anesthesiol.* 2006;18(1):73–77.

Perioperative Implications

Preinduction/Induction/Maintenance

- Prior to induction, normalize volume status, electrolytes, BP, and blood glucose levels. Spironolactone can be used to mobilize fluid and normalize potassium levels.
- Anxiety can cause increased secretion of cortisol. This response may be blunted by premedication.
- Make preparations to deal with a potentially difficult airway.
- Cortisol secretion is unlikely to be affected by the type of anesthesia used.
- Choice of anesthetic agents used for induction and maintenance of anesthesia are not affected by the presence of Cushing's syndrome.
- Etomidate can be used at induction for its temporary suppression of the adrenal gland. However, this effect is likely overcome by the significant cortisol release with surgical stimulation.

Monitoring

- Intraop monitoring should be based on the pt's current clinical state.
- An arterial catheter may be indicated in cases of poorly controlled systemic Htn.

- CVP monitoring is often used to aid in fluid administration, particularly in transsphenoidal tumor resections.

General Anesthesia

- General anesthesia is often the anesthetic of choice in pts with significant skeletal muscle weakness/wasting due to the need for mechanical ventilation.
- Dose of muscle relaxant may need to be reduced in pts with skeletal muscle weakness.

Regional Anesthesia

- Regional anesthesia offers no significant advantage over general anesthesia in pts with Cushing's syndrome.

Postoperative Period

- Bilateral and unilateral adrenal resections require glucocorticoid and mineralocorticoid supplementation for life or until the remaining adrenal gland is able to compensate.
- Treatment doses start with 100 mg of IV hydrocortisone every 24 hr starting the day of surgery with titration over a week until a maintenance dose (20–30 mg/day) is reached. Hydrocortisone given in these quantities usually provides adequate mineralocorticoid activity.

- Bilateral adrenalectomy often requires the addition of fludrocortisone for mineralocorticoid supplementation.
- Close observation for pneumothorax when open adrenal resection is performed.
- Meningitis and transient DI are possible postop complications following a transsphenoidal microadenomectomy.
- Glucocorticoids decrease the tensile strength of healing wounds. Topical administration of vitamin A may improve wound healing in the face of increased glucocorticoids.

Anticipated Problems/Concerns

- Meningitis following microadenomectomy
- Obesity leading to a possible difficult airway
- Increased susceptibility to infection
- Hyperglycemia
- Increased risk of periop thromboembolic events.
- Increased risk for intraop pneumothorax with open adrenal resection when compared to laparoscopic approach

Cyanide Poisoning

Peter H. Breen

Risk

- Potent and rapid-onset toxin, esp inhalation of hydrogen cyanide (HCN, volatile liquid)
- CN ingestion results in slower onset
- Diffuses rapidly through body with high intracellular fixation to cytochrome aa_3 in cellular mitochondria to paralyze aerobic metabolism

Perioperative Risks

- Main target organs: CNS and heart
- Animal experiments: Apnea precedes cardiac collapse

Worry About

- If CN toxicity resulted from fire or smoke exposure, consider also carbon monoxide (CO) and other toxins
- ⅓ of pts from domestic fires with CO toxicity also have increased CN
- Be alert for CN poisoning in donor for organ transplantation

Overview

- Major route of CN detoxification: Conversion to thiocyanate, which requires sulfane sulfur donor (e.g., thiosulfate) and enzyme (e.g., rhodanase); without renal excretion, ↑ thiocyanate can cause CNS abnormalities
- Minor route: Hydroxocobalamin (one form of vitamin B_{12}) chelates CN to form cyanocobalamin
- Methemoglobin (metHb) ferric ion has high affinity for CN

ICD-9-CM Code: 989.0

Etiology

- Combustion product of natural and synthetic polymers
- Industrial chemistry (e.g., metals and plastics preparation)
- Plants: May contain cyanogenic glycosides
- Na nitroprusside: Overtreatment (>0.5 mg/kg/hr within 24 hr)
- Abuse (e.g., suicide, Chicago CN-laced-Tylenol murders [1982], terrorism, chemical warfare)

Usual Treatment

- Rescue victim from exposure
- Intubation and ventilation with 100% O_2 (hyperbaric O_2, effective experimentally, is not practical)
- Gastric decontamination (if necessary)
- Weigh risks and/or benefits of drug therapy since T½ of CN- is short (about 1 hr)
- Na thiosulfate (25%) 150 mg/kg IV (minimal side effects but thiocyanate requires renal excretion or hemodialysis)
- Hydroxocobalamin, 5–10 g IV, safe and rapid
- Methemoglobinemia induction (metHb, 30%) with 10% sodium nitrite (4 mg/kg IV) slow and unpredictable; can be hazardous in presence of carboxyhemoglobin (from CO toxicity) because neither metHb nor COHb carries O_2; can be fatal in G6PD deficiency
- Dicobalt EDTA (ethylenediaminetetraacetate), 300 mg IV, followed by glucose infusion; potent and rapid but unsafe (esp arrhythmias, hypotension, and allergic reactions)

ASSESSMENT POINTS

System	Effect	Assessment by Hx	PE	Test
HEENT	↓ CNS →↓ Airway maintenance/protection	Concomitant smoke inhalation injury	Perioral burns, airway edema	Laryngoscopy/bronchoscopy
CV	Stimulation at low CN conc Depression at high CN conc	Htn, tachycardia Hypotension, bradycardia	↑ Cardiac output ↓ cardiac output, arrhythmias	ECG: Arrhythmias, esp ↓ conduction, VTach, VFib
RESP	Aerobic cellular respiration paralyzed Thermal/toxic airway and parenchymal injury	Concomitant smoke inhalation injury	Bronchoconstriction and pulm edema	↑ Blood PvO_2 and ↑SvO_2 ↓ VO_2, ↓ VCO_2, ↓ $PETCO_2$ Chest x-ray Bronchoscopy
METAB	Cellular aerobic metabolism disabled	Combination of ↑ SvO_2 and lactic acidosis suggests CN		Lactic metabolic acidosis Whole blood CN levels (not available in all labs)
CNS	Stimulation at low CN conc	↑ Inhalatory CN intake Anxiety, dyspnea, headache Auditory/visual disturbances	↑ Resp rate Confusion	
	Depression at high CN conc		Apnea, convulsions, coma	Funduscopy: Red retinal veins (↑ SvO_2)

Key Reference: Breen PH, Isserles SA, Tabac E, Roizen MF, Taitelman UZ: Protective effect of stroma-free metHb during cyanide poisoning in dogs. *Anesthesiology.* 1996; 85:558–564.

Perioperative Implications

Preoperative Preparation
- Continuous 100% O_2

Monitoring
- SpO_2 unreliable in presence of metHb (or COHb if co-existant CO poisoning)
- Mixed venous continuous SO_2 (SvO2) or blood PO_2 (PvO_2)
- $PETCO_2$
- Measure of VO_2 and VCO_2 helpful

Airway
- Protect and maintain airway

Induction
- Avoid CV depressant agents

Maintenance
- 100% O_2 (no N_2O)

Extubation
- Ensure CNS status permits natural airway maintenance and protection

Adjuvants
- Consider treatment for concomitant CO poisoning (see Carbon Monoxide Poisoning in Diseases section)

Postoperative Period
- Maintain 100% O_2 breathing

Anticipated Problems/Concerns

- Heart and brain are target organs
- Prompt CPR (ventilation with O_2) determines outcome
- Follow CNS function
- Seek concomitant smoke inhalation injury and CO toxicity

Cystic Fibrosis

Daniel M. Roke
John T. Algren

Risk

- Prevalence ranges from 1:2500 births in Caucasians to 1:17,000 in African Americans
- Incidence ranges from 1:569 in Amish to 1:90,000 in Hawaiian Asians
- 2–5% of Caucasians are carriers

Perioperative Risks

- Pulmonary
  - Hypoxia and hypercarbia
  - Ventilation/perfusion (V/Q) mismatching
  - Pneumothorax
  - Airway obstruction with distal air trapping
- Pancreatic
  - Glucose intolerance
- Upper airway
  - Nasal polyps occlude nasal airways

Worry About

- Pneumothorax
- Atelectasis and air trapping
- Hemoptysis
- Copious, inspissated secretions
- Hypoxemia and hypercarbia
- Cor pulmonale

Overview

- A disease of the exocrine glands which affects the lungs, pancreas, GI and hepatobiliary tracts
- Pulm exacerbations are caused by airway obstruction with thickened mucus.
- Pulm infections are common, esp *P. Aeruginosa*
- Pancreatic insufficiency can develop leading to malabsorption, incl vitamins A, D, E, and K, as well as glucose intolerance.

ICD-9-CM Code: 277.0

Etiology

- Autosomal recessive trait due to mutation of gene on long arm chromosome 7
- Cystic fibrosis transmembrane regulator (CFTR) gene controls the transmembrane transport of chloride among other ions
- Thickened mucus is produced with obstruction of exocrine glands and subsequent infection

Usual Treatment

- Goals: Control infection, promote mucous clearance, improve nutrition
- Pulm: Chest physiotherapy, mucolytics (short term), bronchodilators, humidification, antibiotics for infections
- Pancreatic: Pancreatic enzyme replacement

ASSESSMENT POINTS

System	Effects	Assessment by Hx	PE	Test
HEENT	Frequent nasal polyps	Nasal obstruction Difficulty sleeping	Nasal polyps	Nasal endoscopy
	Sinusitis	Fever, headaches	Sinus drainage	Sinus x-ray, culture
CARDIO	Cor pulmonale	Dyspnea Orthopnea	Tachypnea Rales, rhonchi, wheezing Clubbing of fingers	ECG CXR
		Cyanosis	Cyanosis	
RESP	Bronchiectasis, atelectasis, pneumonitis, bronchospasm	Cough Dyspnea Poor exercise tolerance Orthopnea	Hyperinflation of lungs Poor ventilation, cyanosis Clubbing Cough, rales, rhonchi, wheezing	CXR PFTs A-a gradient
GI	Cholelithiasis, gallbladder dysfunction Pancreatic insufficiency Focal biliary cirrhosis Intestinal obstruction	Abd pain (may be asymptomatic) Poor fat absorption, glucose intolerance Abd pain	Jaundice Abd rigidity	US Cholangiography Glucose Liver function Abd x-rays
MS	Poor muscle development	Hx poor nutrition, muscle weakness	Cachexia	

Key Reference: Huffmyer JF, Littlewood KE, Nemergut EC. Perioperative management of the adult with cystic fibrosis. *Anesth Analg.* 2009;109(6):1949–1961.

Perioperative Implications

Preoperative Preparation
- Hx and evaluation of baseline pulm status, exercise tolerance
- CXR: Hyperexpansion indicated by flattened diaphragm
- PFTs: Obstruction indicated by increased RV to TLC ratio and decreased FEF 25–75%
- ABG, electrolytes, blood glucose, LFTs
- Medications: Bronchodilators, antibiotics
- Chest physiotherapy

Monitoring
- Routine plus arterial pressure and/or CVP as pt's cardiopulmonary status and procedure dictates
- Blood glucose should be checked frequently.

Airway
- Oropharyngeal airway for upper airway obstruction due to possibility of nasal polyps

Induction
- IV induction faster than inhalation due to larger FRC, smaller tidal volumes, and V/Q mismatching

Maintenance
- Volatile anesthetics useful as bronchodilators
- PPV may be necessary but should be used cautiously in light of pneumothorax risk.
- Warm and humidify gases
- Suctioning of airway mucus and bronchiolar lavage may help maintain oxygenation and ventilation.
- Muscle tone is important in maintaining patency of airways so muscle relaxants should be used only when needed.
- Opioids may be used as well, but pain control must be balanced with the risk of resp depression.

- Regional anesthetics may be particularly beneficial in minimizing instrumentation of the airways while providing postop pain control.

Extubation
- Carried out as soon as preop resp function resumes and after lung recruitment maneuvers

Adjuvants
- Bronchodilators, NSAIDs

Postoperative Period
- Pain control key in encouraging coughing/deep breathing
- Chest physiotherapy and early activity

Anticipated Problems/Concerns

- Pneumothorax
- Postop resp insufficiency
- Cor pulmonale
- Electrolyte disturbances (Na^+, Cl^-)

Cytomegalovirus Infection

Andrew D. Badley
Stacey A. Rizza

Risk

- Incidence in USA: <10 y: 25%; 10–25 y : 35%; 25–50 y :50%; >50 y : 50+%
- Disease from CMV rare in immunocompetent individuals; can cause mononucleosis like disease
- Disease from CMV in transplant recipients 10–40%
- Disease from CMV in HIV-positive pts 20–30% (increased risk with low CD4 count)
- Approx 1 in 150 children is born with congenital CMV

Perioperative Risks

- Related to degree of CMV-induced organ dysfunction: Pulm, CNS, hepatic, GI, cardiac, bone marrow, adrenal
- Risk of acquiring CMV from tissue or blood products from a CMV-seropositive donor

Worry About

- Giving CMV-seropositive blood products to a CMV-seronegative immunocompromised host. Alternatively, the use of filters that remove leukocytes from the blood can be used to prevent transmission of CMV if CMV-seropositive blood donors are used

- Abnormal hepatic metabolism if CMV hepatitis
- Elevated ICP if CMV encephalitis and/or meningitis
- Abnormal oxygenation if CMV pneumonitis
- Myocardial dysfunction or arrhythmias if CMV myocarditis
- Perforated viscus 2° to colonic and/or gastric CMV
- Abnormal bleeding from thrombocytopenia
- Adrenal insufficiency due to CMV adrenalitis

Overview

- Double-stranded DNA virus; member of herpes family of viruses. Vast majority of North American adults have had prior exposures and are CMV seropositive.
- CMV disease if:
  - Perinatal infection
  - Intrauterine infection leading to congenital CMV disease
  - Infection of normal host is asymptomatic; rarely may cause a heterophile antibody–negative mononucleosis-like syndrome.
- Infection in immunosuppressed individuals leading to symptomatic or asymptomatic viremia with or without organ involvement: retinitis, encephalitis, meningitis, myelitis, polyneuropathy, pneumonitis, esophagitis, gastritis, colitis, hepatitis, cholangitis, myocarditis, adrenalitis, vasculitis, bone marrow suppression.

ICD-9-CM Code: 078.5

Etiology

- Double-stranded DNA virus
- Transmission through blood/blood products, sexually, perinatally, other contact (day care, medical facilities)

Usual Treatment

- Medical treatment: Ganciclovir (IV or oral maintenance), valgancyclovir (oral), foscarnet (IV), occasionally IV immune globulin. Reduced immunosuppression.
- Surgical treatment: None

ASSESSMENT POINTS

System	Effect	Assessment by Hx	PE	Test
HEENT	Destruction of retina	Decreased visual acuity, blind stops	Funduscopy; white and red lesion	Ophthalmology evaluation
CV	Myocarditis; LV dysfunction	CHF symptoms, palpitations	Irregular rhythm, displaced PMI S$_3$	ECG, ECHO, heart biopsy
RESP	Pneumonitis; impaired gas exchange	Dyspnea, nonproductive cough	Wheezes, crackles	CXR, ABGs, bronchoscopy ± biopsy
GI	Viral infection of organ	Hepatitis/cholangitis –Right upper quadrant pain –Jaundice, itching, acholic stools –Esophagitis: dysphagia, odynophagia –Colitis: diarrhea, abdominal pain –Gastritis: pyrosis, anorexia	Signs of hepatic failure, fetor hepaticus, asterixis, jaundice, bruising, painful liver, nonspecific abdominal pain	Liver function tests, ERCP, US, viral blood cultures ± biopsy
HEME	Bone marrow suppression	Rash, fatigue	Petechiae, pallor, tachycardia	CBC
CNS	Encephalitis	Motor or sensory abnormalities, altered mental status	Motor weakness, sensory abnormality, cerebellar ataxia, abnormal tests of cortical function	CT MRI, lumbar puncture

Key Reference: Barber L, Egan JJ, Lomax J, et al. A prospective study of a quantitative PCR ELISA assay for the diagnosis of CMV pneumonia in lung and heart-transplant recipients. *J Heart Lung Transplant.* 2000;19:771–780.

Perioperative Implications

Perioperative Preparation
- Evaluate for signs of pulm, cardiac, hepatic, CNS, bone marrow, or adrenal dysfunction

Monitoring
- Routine

Airway
- May require high FIO$_2$ and PEEP

Preinduction/Induction
- Avoid tachycardia/hypotension

Maintenance
- Follow CO, PCWP, SaO$_2$, BP

Extubation
- No special concerns

Postoperative Period
- Monitor for clinical signs of disease progression

Adjuvants
- No special concerns

Deep Vein Thrombosis

Todd Dorman

Risk

- Incidence in USA: 170,000–200,000 diagnosed new cases/y 90,000–100,000 recurrent cases/y.
- True incidence (underdiagnosis) closer to 1 million cases/y. Could be as high as 2 million.
- Race with highest prevalence: Unclear. African-Americans have a higher rate of PE being diagnosed than DVT compared to Caucasians. Asians seem to have the lowest rates of either.
- Smoking, obesity, being bedridden, and decreasing LVEF are predisposing factors for developing DVT
- Risk factors incl age >40, previous DVT or family Hx of DVT, paraplegia, spinal cord trauma, major orthopedic surgery, malignancy, hypercoagulable states.
- Decreased risk with regional anesthesia vs. general, esp in LE orthopedic surgery.

Perioperative Risks

- Without prophylaxis, DVT develops in close to 30% of general surgery cases
- Incidence of fatal pulm emboli: 0.1% (general)—5% (total knee replacement)

Worry About

- Pulm embolism
- Cardiac arrest, electromechanical dissociation
- Hypoxemia and increased dead space potentially leading to resp acidosis in pt with controlled ventilation

Overview

- Clinical findings (e.g., Homans sign) helpful less than 50% of the time.
- Ascending phlebography (venography) is standard for comparison, but has 2–3% incidence of inducing peripheral thrombosis.
- Impedance plethysmography (IP), which detects proximal veins, reasonable in symptomatic pts, but lacks sensitivity and specificity in asymptomatic pts.
- Compression ultrasonography with Doppler flow imaging better than IP (proximal veins), yet sensitivity falls off in asymptomatic pts. If IP or Doppler-supplemented ultrasonography negative, pt needs serial exams to detect potential progression of distal disease.
- CT and MRI are reliable, yet are cumbersome, costly, and not routinely available.

- D-Dimer has a high negative predictive value.

ICD-9-CM Code: 453.9 (Thrombosis, vein unspecified)

Etiology

- Stasis
- Activation of coagulation cascade by tissue trauma
- Hypercoagulability related to congenital or acquired antithrombin III, protein C, or protein S deficiency, antiphospholid syndromes
- Hypercoagulability related to malignancy, smoking, sedentary lifestyle, increasing physiologic age, decreasing LVEF
- Hyperviscosity states such as polycythemia vera

Usual Treatment

- Heparin administration prior to warfarin to avoid acute decreases in endogenous anticoagulant protein C
- LMW heparin may be used
- Thrombolytics
- Thrombectomy, catheter or open surgical

ASSESSMENT POINTS

System	Effect	Assessment by Hx	PE	Test
CV			SVT RV strain	ECG
RESP	Pulm embolism	Chest pain Hemoptysis	Tachypnea, wheezing possible	ABGs, ETCO$_2$
HEME				PT, APTT Plt count Hgb, d-dimer
MS			Calf pain	Venography, US

Key Reference: Hirsh J, Guyatt G, Albers GW, Harrington R, Schünemann HJ, American College of Chest Physicians. *Executive summary: American College of Chest Physicians Evidence-Based Clinical Practice Guidelines.* 8th ed. *Chest.* vol. 133. 2008:71S–109S.

Perioperative Implications

Preoperative Preparation
- Sequential compression devices may decrease incidence by activating fibrinolytic system.
- Anticoagulation needed for 6 mo after diagnosis and up to the time of procedure.
- Consider preop placement of an IVC filter in high-risk pts
  - If pt on anticoagulants or antiplatelets drugs preop ensure adequate products available in blood bank
  - When possible, administer SQ heparin preop

Monitoring
- Bleeding from residual anticoagulation or drug-induced thrombocytopenia

- Screening US for ICU pts done on a weekly basis has started to become the vogue. Cost-effective data supporting this approach are pending.

Airway
- None

Preinduction/Induction
- Regional anesthesia may reduce risk in some orthopedic and genitourinary procedures

Adjuvants
- Depends on etiology: Examine specific etiology (e.g., Dilated Cardiomyopathy) in Diseases section
- Heparin, LMWH, warfarin tissue plasminogen activator, streptokinase/urokinase, anisoylated plasminogen-streptokinase activator complex all

increase periop bleeding diathesis. Some effect of these agents on other drugs (verify specific drug effects in Drugs section).

Postoperative Period
- In high-risk pts consider full anticoagulation postop as prophylaxis
- If using SQ heparin, it should be administered every 8 hr if possible
- Continue sequential use of elastic stockings until pt is ambulatory, but do not start in pts suspected of having DVT

Anticipated Problems/Concerns
- Pulm embolism represents life-threatening complication of DVT
- Post-thrombotic syndrome with chronic venous stasis with skin and wound effects

Degenerative Disk Disease

John E. Tetzlaff

Risk

Risk factors determined by spinal level
- Cervical spine: C3 and C4 most common, 10% of degenerative disk disease
- Thoracic: Uncommon, can be related to trauma, tumor, 0.2–1.8% of disk disease
- Lumbar: Very common, 85–90% of disk disease, third most-common cause of chronic pain in USA

Perioperative Risks

- Difficult airway
- Spinal cord injury from airway manipulation or positioning
- Positioning injury from prone position
- Ischemic optic neuropathy

Worry About

- Cervical spine instability or chronic subluxation
- Difficulty with intubation
- Injury to the spinal cord, nerve roots

- Pressure injuries or ventilatory difficulty with the prone position
- Optimum perfusion to the head. Ischemia, neck position, or venous congestion may contribute to ischemic optic neuropathy.
- Airway edema at the conclusion of surgery

Overview

- Pain from herniation of an intervertebral disk with nerve root compression is the third most-common chronic disease in the USA and the most common indication for elective spine surgery
- Incidence varies among spinal segments, being absent in sacral area, most common in lumbar area, next in cervical region, and uncommon in thoracic region

ICD-9-CM Codes: 722.40 (Cervical); 722.51 (Thoracic); 722.52 (Lumbar)

Etiology

- Osteoarthritis
- Trauma
- Connective tissue diseases such as rheumatoid arthritis or ankylosing spondylitis

Usual Treatment

- Conservative measures, incl rest, exercise, physical therapy, heat, and traction
- Symptoms are treated with analgesics and non-steroidal anti-inflammatory drugs
- In acute phase, disk herniation can be treated with epidural steroid injection
- Nonsurgical intervention, such as intra-discal electrothermy (IDET)
- Surgery is performed to relieve compression on the spinal cord or specific nerve roots, and to expand the space for nerve root exit from the spinal column

ASSESSMENT POINTS

System	Effect	Assessment by Hx	PE	Test
HEENT	Difficult airway	Neck pain	Decreased ROM	Flexion/extension x-ray to detect instability
	Visual acuity	Pt report	Pt report	Eye examination
RESP	Lung tumor can mimic symptoms of thoracic disk disease	Chest pain with chest excursion	Abnormal pulmonary auscultation	CXR, MRI
GI	GI malignancy can mimic symptoms of thoracic or lumbar disk disease	Truncal pain, abdominal pain	Abdominal mass	CT, MRI
RENAL	Pyelonephritis, cancer of prostate can mimic symptoms of lumbar disk disease	Lumbar pain, muscle spasm, fever/chills	Costovertebral angle tenderness to percussion	Urinalysis, prostate-specific antigen, lumbar spine x-ray, MRI
CNS	Myelopathy, anterior spinal cord syndrome	Radiating pain, incontinence, sexual dysfunction, paraplegia	Long tract signs, abnormal reflexes, pathologic, Babinski reflex	X-ray, MRI
PNS	Radiculopathy, absent deep tendon reflexes, peripheral nerve deficits	Sciatica, numbness, weakness of the extremities	Sciatic pain with ROM, motor deficits, patchy sensory deficits	EMG
MS	Pain, decreased ROM, calcification	Pain, night pain, disability from work	Decreased ROM in spine	Spine x-ray, MRI

Key Reference: Rothman RA, Simeone FA. *The Spine*. 4th ed. Philadelphia: Saunders; 1999 [Chapters 19–30].

Perioperative Implications

Preoperative Assessment
- Evaluate coagulation if heavy aspirin or NSAID use or symptoms of bleeding
- Airway assessment. If signs of cervical instability or other indicators of difficult airway management, flexion-extension x-ray of cervical spine.
- Antisialagogue if awake intubation
- If spinal or epidural anesthesia planned, lumbar x-rays may be needed
- Planned regional anesthesia may reduce minor complications, such as pain and nausea; intraop bleeding may be reduced

Monitoring
- Potential for air embolism, greater with sitting position for posterior approach to cervical spine
- Consider multilumen right atrial catheter, precordial Doppler if sitting position for cervical spine procedure
- If large blood loss estimated, arterial line becomes indicated.

Airway
- If cervical spine not involved, then routine

- If abnormal, choices incl awake intubation, inhalation induction, and intubation with induction drugs and muscle relaxants with the head maintained in a neutral position, possibly with traction
- Increasing role for videolaryngoscopy

Induction
- If airway secured, induction dictated by other aspects of pt's health
- If regional anesthesia, technical difficulty with placement due to anatomic abnormality of the spine
- Consider paramedian dural puncture. Higher levels for dural puncture may result in a better block with spinal stenosis.

Maintenance
- Movement while prone with spinal cord exposed is dangerous. Avoid muscle relaxants after induction if spinal stimulation is used.
- If regional anesthesia, be prepared to re-inject block if duration of surgery exceeds duration of action of local anesthetic injected.

Extubation
- Awake and supine are ideal
- Rapid-emergence agents (propofol, sevoflurane) may facilitate neuro exam in OR.

Adjuvants
- Injury in the prone position to eyes, lips, teeth, tongue, chin, brachial plexus, ulnar nerves, genitalia, peroneal nerves, skin of the patella, and ankles
- Identify full neurologic function prior to extubation, because re-exploration for compressive hematoma could be indicated for major deficit.

Postoperative Period
- Neurologic checks to identify deficits, pain control
- H_2-blocker therapy to prevent GI hemorrhage if large-dose steroid Rx chosen for nerve root swelling
- Evaluate visual acuity

Anticipated Problems/Concerns

- Difficult airway if cervical involvement
- Air embolism: Withdraw N_2O if any symptoms
- Transport bed availability and knowledge of how to remove frame, in case sudden transfer to supine position is necessary.
- Airway edema from prone position or anterior cervical dissection may present issues for immediate extubation. Consider leak test, and if in doubt, prolonged postoperative intubation with sedation may be indicated.

DISEASES

113

Delirium (Postanesthetic)

Nabil M. Elkassabany

Risk

• Risk factors for development of postop delirium (POD) are either pt or procedure related. Pt related factors can increase the pt's inherent risk for development of POD. Most important factors are:
  • Old age
  • Pre-existing cognitive dysfunction
  • Hx of stroke, depression, alcohol abuse, psychiatric diagnosis, diabetes, peripheral vascular disease, atrial fibrillation, and heart failure
• Procedure related factors that may trigger the development of delirium are:
  • Type of surgery: Cardiac, orthopedic, and vascular procedures are associated with the highest incidence of the syndrome
  • Emergent or urgent procedures
  • Anticholinergic medications
  • Poorly controlled postop pain
  • Benzodiazepines, polypharmacy, and meperidine
• Factors with no effects on the pt's risk for development of POD are length of surgery, type of anesthetic (general versus regional), and type of postop analgesia (regional techniques versus systemic opioids).

Perioperative Risks:

• Independent predictor of postop morbidity and mortality

• Increased length of hospital stay and ICU days after development of POD
• **Increased risk for falls, longer intubation/re-intubation, need for urinary catheters, urinary infections, pressure ulcers, aspiration pneumonia, periop myocardial ischemia, and wound infections**
• **Increased risk of subsequent functional loss and institutionalization**
• Added cost to the health care system

Worry About

• Other causes of change in mental status (i.e., rule out any metabolic causes for the syndrome).
• Pt can present with a violent behavior or symptoms of withdrawal. The first category can be harmful to themselves and others.
• Drug drug interaction in the periop period may result in the change in mental status.

Overview

• Acute confusional state that is characterized by disorientation, disturbed sleep-wake cycle, memory impairment, perceptual disturbance, and altered psychomotor activity.
• Reported incidence ranges from 5.1% to 52.2%. The wide range is due to the disparate and subjective symptoms and the different tests used to establish the diagnosis.

ICD-9-CM Code: 292.81 (Drug induced)

Etiology

• The pathophysiology of POD is not clearly understood. Some of the causes cited are:
  • Disturbed neurotransmitter systems esp cholinergic deficiency
  • Stress response to surgery and anesthesia
  • Global cerebral hypoperfusion
  • Drug–drug interaction
  • Alcohol and drug withdrawal in the periop period

Usual Treatment

• Supportive measures
  • Team approach is the best; physicians, nurses, and family members should be involved.
  • Anticholinergics, H_2-blockers, benzodiazepines, opioids, and antipsychotic medications should be replaced with drugs that have no central effects whenever possible.
  • Maintain adequate ventilation, oxygenation, cerebral perfusion, and normal electrolytes and acid-base balance.
  • Maximize awareness of the pt with his environment and surroundings.
  • Consider one-to-one companion rather than applying physical restrains unless the pt is posing a threat to themselves and others.
• Symptoms control
  • Low-dose haloperidol for symptoms control
  • Physostigmine for anticholinergic induced delirium

ASSESSMENT POINTS

System	Effect	Assessment by Hx	PE	Test
CNS	POD	*Preoperative:* Mental status, assess baseline risk, drug therapy *Intraoperative:* Anesthetic drugs, reversal drugs *Postoperative:* Pain state, assessment of mental state	Anxiety, agitation, violent behavior, impaired cognition, emotional lability, agitation, hallucinations, fluctuating states of consciousness	O_2 saturation, arterial blood gases, electrolytes, and blood glucose levels

Key Reference: Bagri AS, Rico A, Ruiz JG. Evaluation and management of the elderly patient at risk for postoperative delirium. *Clin Geriatr Med.* 2008;24(4):667–686.

Perioperative Implications

Preoperative Preparation

• The team effort should start by identifying pts at risk for POD when they present for the pre-admission screening process. The second step should focus on modifying the risk factors that are modifiable. Drugs are the most common reversible causes of delirium.
• Correct pre-existing electrolytes abnormalities
• Sensory impairments, visual and auditory, should be addressed preop.
• Pro-active geriatric consultation and involvement of anesthesia team with an expertise in dealing with geriatric population can prove to be very effective in prophylaxis against POD.

Monitoring

• Standard monitors. Monitor blood glucose level, electrolytes, and volume status.

Airway

• Maintain a patent airway, maintain adequate oxygenation and ventilation.

Preinduction/Induction

• Avoid centrally acting anticholinergics as premedications.

Maintenance

• As dictated by the type of surgery.
• Incl an effective plan for postop analgesia in your anesthetic regimen.

Extubation

• Standard criteria for extubation. Avoid hypoxia and hypercarbia.

Adjuvants

• Low-dose haloperidol 1–5 mg for symptoms control.
• If anticholinergic-induced delirium is suspected, use physostigmine 0.5–2 mg IV.

• Small doses of midazolam can help control pt agitation. Recommended dose is 0.5–1 mg IV.

Anticipated Problems/Concerns

• POD is a risk factor for increased functional loss and institutionalization. Confusion can be transient or can remain up to 6 mo after discharge. Quality of life measures are affected during and after an episode of delirium. Psychological stress to family members and caregivers should not be underestimated.
• Side effects of haloperidol incl extrapyramidal symptoms and neuropeptic malignant syndrome.

Dementia

Robert A. Whittington

Risk

- Worldwide, approx 24.3 million individuals have dementia, and it is estimated that this number will increase to 81 million people by 2040. Incidence in the USA: More than 5 million.
- Affects approx 10% of adults 65 y or older and up to 50% of community-dwelling individuals age 85 or older.
- Age and genetic susceptibility are risk factors. Increasing evidence suggests that vascular risk factors (Htn, obesity, DM, atherosclerotic cardiovascular disease (ASCVD), cerebrovascular disease, hyperlipidemia, tobacco use, and diets high in saturated fat) as well as psychosocial factors (degree of education, social disengagement, and physical activity) may also play a role in disease development.

Perioperative Risks

- Risks related to cognitive impairment (e.g., impaired ability to cooperate with anesthetic care, aspiration risk, trauma risk from falls).
- Risks associated with concomitant neuropsychiatric symptoms (e.g., agitation, hallucinations, aggressive behavior, delusions), the medications used to control these symptoms, and the potential interactions between these medications and drugs commonly utilized during anesthesia.

Worry About

- Central neurotransmitters levels may be reduced (particularly acetylcholine), and drugs administered during anesthesia may further attenuate these levels, potentially contributing to further cognitive deterioration.
- The immediate potential for anesthetics to further impair cognitive function periop as well as to exacerbate any accompanying neuropsychiatric symptomatology.
- Inability of the pt to fully comprehend and cooperate with the anesthetic plan.

- Baseline impairment of cognitive function and its impact on potential anesthesia-related injuries (e.g., increased aspiration risk, positioning injuries, inadvertent removal of indwelling catheters or ETT).
- Potential side effects of neuropsychiatric medications used in the treatment of dementia
- Consequences related to prolonged immobilization (e.g., limited exercise tolerance, risk of hyperkalemia with succinylcholine, presence of decubitus ulcers, development of DVT, and positioning injury risk).
- Obstacles to adequate postop pain relief incl the pt's limited ability to communicate as well as the potential for centrally acting analgesics to exacerbate cognitive impairment and neuropsychiatric symptoms.

Overview

- Dementia is a clinical syndrome characterized by memory impairment as well as one or more of the following disturbances: Language impairment (aphasia), perturbations in performing executive functions (e.g., organizing, planning, initiating, and abstract reasoning), the inability to recognize familiar objects or persons (agnosia), and the impaired ability to perform motor activities despite having intact motor function (apraxia).
- Although not part of the diagnostic criteria, dementia is commonly associated with neuropsychiatric symptoms incl agitation, personality changes, depression, delusions, hallucinations, aggressive behavior, repetitive vocalizations, and sleep disturbances.
- Alzheimer's disease (50–70%), and vascular dementia (15–20%) account for the majority of the cases; however, mixed pathologies (i.e., AD and VaD) are quite common (10–20%).
- All other dementias account for <10% of the total number of cases.

- Recent data suggest that the average survival time from the onset of dementia is 4.5 y.

ICD-9-CM Codes: 290.10 (Alzheimer's type); 290.40 (Multi-infarct dementia)

Etiology

- In Alzheimer's disease (AD), the two histopathological hallmarks incl senile neuritic plaques (comprised primarily of β-amyloid protein) and neurofibrillary tangles containing aggregated hyperphosphorylated tau protein. These pathological changes have been associated with a loss of cholinergic neurons and tracts, which are felt to correspond with the clinical cognitive impairment. Precise mechanisms of AD are still unknown.
- Extensive atrophy of cortical convolutions, esp in hippocampus and temporal lobes are commonly observed (much greater than normal aging).
- 10–30% of dementia cases can be potentially reversible if they are secondary to an underlying treatable cause incl structural or traumatic brain injury, medication toxicity, infectious causes, vitamin deficiencies, inflammatory diseases, as well as endocrine and metabolic disorders.

Usual Treatment

- Symptomatic treatment has incl the use of cholinesterase inhibitors: Donepezil, galantamine, rivastigmine, and tacrine.
- Neuropsychiatric symptoms are common in dementia and are often treated with the following classes of psychotherapeutic agents: Typical antipsychotics (haloperidol, perphenazine), atypical antipsychotics (risperidone, olanzipine), antidepressants (sertraline, citalopram, trazodone), mood stabilizers (carbamazepine, sodium valproate), cholinesterase inhibitors (donepezil, rivastigmine, galantamine), and NMDA antagonists (memantine).

ASSESSMENT POINTS

System	Effect	PE	Test
CV	~10% of those with dementia have CVD and generalized ASCVD, ischemic heart disease	Htn Chest pain or anginal equivalent	ECG ECG, ECHO, stress test, possibly angiography
GI	Hepatic injury due to cholinesterase inhibitor use (e.g., tacrine) or other drugs used to treat neuropsychiatric symptoms Hepatic injury possible with alcohol abuse etiology	Jaundice, tender hepatomegaly, splenomegaly	Liver enzymes
ENDO	Hypothyroidism can mimic or exacerbate dementia Type II diabetes mellitus		T_3, T_4 Serum glucose, HbA1C level
CNS	Baseline cognitive performance impairment, subdural hematoma and hydrocephalus possible causes, carotid artery disease	Neurologic exam Mini-mental state exam	EEG, MRI, CT Carotid Doppler studies
PNS	Poor motor skills	Neurologic exam	
MS	Generalized stiffness and slowness; psychiatric disorders	Neurologic exam	

Key Reference: Verbough C. Anesthesia in patients with dementia. *Curr Opin Anaesthesiol.* 2004;17:277–283.

Perioperative Implications

Preoperative Preparation

- Pt most likely cannot give consent or a reliable Hx; determine if guardian or surrogate is identified. Pre-existing medical records, nursing home medical documents, and the pt's relatives may be of critical importance.
- If possible, establish a general preanesthetic baseline of cognitive performance and behavior incl degree of orientation.
- Agitation and anxiety may be pronounced during this period. Sedatives best avoided, particularly in severe cases with low Mini Mental State Examination

scores. Benzodiazepines have been used to treat agitation in pts with mild cognitive decline, and should be performed in a monitored setting.
- Centrally acting anticholinergics (atropine, scopolamine) are best avoided; glycopyrrolate is acceptable, as it does not cross the blood brain barrier.

Monitoring

- Routine
- More invasive monitoring (e.g., A-line, CVP, PA catheter) may be necessary given that elderly pts with dementia may also demonstrate significant cardiac, pulm, or renal impairment.

Airway

- Cervical range of motion may be limited by arthritis.
- Check whether the pt has removable prosthetic dental appliances.

Preinduction/Induction

- Regional anesthesia (RA) may provide advantages incl reducing the cognitive and neurobehavioral side effects associated with the use of sedation. Furthermore, the need to manipulate the airway and to provide mechanical ventilatory support may be avoided. A reduction in the periop

development of DVT, particularly in pts with limited mobility, has also been observed.

• Monitored anesthetic care (MAC) with minimal sedation may also limit perturbations in cerebral functioning. However, the greater risk of aspiration in this pt population should be appreciated when considering this technique.

• Despite the theoretical advantages of RA and MAC, general anesthesia may still be necessary due to lack of pt cooperation.

• Propofol may offer most rapid recovery. Succinylcholine may present a risk of hyperkalemia in pts with a Hx of prolonged immobilization or prior stroke.

• DVT prophylaxis may be indicated (SQ heparin, intermittent pneumatic compression).

Maintenance

• No one technique or agent best.

• Avoid sedatives and narcotics with long half-lives.

• Consider using short-acting anesthetic agents (e.g., desflurane, sevoflurane, propofol, remifentanil).

• Consider the impact of potential renal or hepatic impairment on the metabolism of drugs administered during general anesthesia.

• The duration of action of succinylcholine may be prolonged by donepezil.

• The cholinesterase inhibitors used to treat dementia may antagonize non-depolarizing neuromuscular blockade.

• Bradycardia can be observed in pts treated with cholinesterase inhibitors; therefore, caution should be taken when using agents with known bradycardic effects.

• If bradycardia requires treatment with an anticholinergic medication, glycopyrrolate is preferred, as it does not cross the blood-brain barrier.

• The maintenance of normothermia as hypothermia may further depress pt's mental status and may increase myocardial O_2 demand.

Extubation

• Extubate when awake; orientation postop may be further impaired by anesthetics.

• Impaired cognitive performance and co-morbid diseases may increase the need for postop ventilatory support and critical care resources.

Adjuvants

• Can see prolonged effects on mental status with sedatives, hypnotics, and narcotics.

Anticipated Problems/Concerns

• Disorientation and delirium are common postop—provide familiar person and written orientation material.

• Close observation incl 1:1 nursing care may be necessary.

• Temporary restraints may still be necessary and requires familiarization with hospital and TJC policy on their use in the PACU.

• May be poor candidates for catheter-based postop regional analgesia (e.g., epidural or brachial plexus catheters) or for PCA in the postop period. Whenever possible, regional analgesia using single-dose peripheral nerve blocks should be considered, as this reduces the need for opioid analgesia.

• Consider the physiologic and pharmacologic effects of pre-existing decreases in renal and hepatic function whenever the use of parenterally or orally administered analgesics and sedatives is indicated in elderly pts.

Depression, Unipolar

Ashish C. Sinha

Risk
- Affects 2–4% of population
- Approx 15% of pts with major depression commit suicide.

Perioperative Risks
- Most periop issues arise from interactions between antidepressant medications and anesthetic agents. Withdrawal of antidepression medications can increase risk of suicide.

Overview
- Depression is the most common psychiatric disorder.
- Dx is clinical and based on persistent presence of 2 wk of symptoms.
- Distinguished from normal sadness and grief by severity and duration of disease

ICD9-CM: 296.2 (Major depressive disorder, single episode)

Etiology
- Unknown pathophysiology, but suspect abnormalities of amine neurotransmitter (serotonin, dopamine, and norepinephrine) pathway.
- Multifactorial. Familial pattern thought to exist.

Usual Treatment
- Selective serotonin reuptake inhibitor (SSRI): Works by blocking reuptake of serotonin at presynaptic membranes with little effect on adrenergic, cholinergic, histaminergic, or other neurochemical system. Associated with fewer side effects.

- Tricyclics: Inhibits synaptic reuptake of norepinephrine and serotonin. Also affects other neurochemical systems incl histaminergic and cholinergic systems resulting in side effects such as postural hypotension, prolonged QRS intervals (>0.1), cardiac dysrhythmias, and urinary retention.
- Monoamine oxidase inhibitor (MAOI): Prevents breakdown of catecholamine and serotonin. Orthostatic hypotension is most common side effect observed. Significant systemic Htn associated with ingesting food containing tyramine or sympathomimetic drugs.
- Electroconvulsive therapy (ECT) for pts who are resistant to antidepressant medications or with medical contraindication to antidepressants.

ASSESSMENT POINTS

System	Effect	Assessment by Hx	PE	Test
HEENT	Dehydration	Dry mouth, blurred vision	Glaucoma, retinal detachment decreased visual acuity	Fundoscopic exam
CV	AV conduction delays, bradycardia, tachyarrhythmia, hypertensive crisis, hypotension	Angina, symptoms of CHF, need for cardiac pacemaker, thrombophlebitis	Volume status, BP, S_3 gallop	12 lead ECG (± stress test), echocardiography
RESP	Resp depression	CHF, severe pulmonary disease	S_3, rales, wheezing	CXR, ABGs
GI	Delayed gastric emptying	Reflux		Gastroendoscopy
ENDO	Variable catecholamine levels	Symptoms suggestive of pheochromocytoma	Unexplained severe Htn	VMA levels
RENAL	Urinary retention	Difficulty urinating		
CNS	MS, neuroleptic malignant syndrome, seizures, coma, ALS, C-JD Alzheimer's disease	Recent CVA, intracranial surgery, intracranial mass lesion	Neurologic deficits, symptoms of increase ICP	CT, MRI, neurologic exam, toxicology screen
MS & COLLAGEN DISORDERS		Severe osteoporosis, major fractures, RA, SLE	Fractures, joint pain, and limited mobility	Skeletal x-rays, MRI

Key Reference: Hines RL, Marschall KE, ed. *Stoelting's Anesthesia and Co-existing disease.* 5th ed. 2008.

Perioperative Implications
- Serotonin syndrome
  - Potentially life-threatening drug reaction from interactions between SSRIs, atypical and cyclic antidepressants, MAOIs, opiates, and antibiotics, (e.g., phenylzine and meperidine, phenylzine and SSRIs, linezolide and citalopram).
  - Symptoms incl agitation, delirium, autonomic hyperactivity, hyperreflexia, clonus, and hyperthermia.
  - Treatment involves discontinuing the suspected agent(s), supportive measures, and control of autonomic instability, excess muscle activity, and hyperthermia.
  - In mild cases, lorazepam, propranol, or cyproheptadine (a 5-HT antagonist only available in PO form that binds to serotonin receptors) can be administered.
- Fluoxetine
  - Potent hepatic cytochrome P-450 inhibitor, which increases plasma concentration of drugs that depends on P-450 for clearance
  - Fluoxetine may increase the concentration of tricyclic antidepressants by two-to-five-fold.

- Some cardiac antidysrhythmic and beta-blockers may also be potentiated as a result.
- Tricyclics
  - Anticholinergic effect causes CV abnormalities such as orthostatic hypotension and cardiac dysrhythmias.
  - Due to increased availability of neurotransmitters in the CNS, anesthetic requirement may be increased. Likewise, increased availability of norepinephrine may cause exaggerated BP response in reaction to indirect-acting vasopressor such as ephedrine.
  - Acute treatment with tricyclics (first 2–3 wk) is associated with potential significant Htn, whereas long-term treatment is associated with down-regulation of receptors.
  - Tachydysrhythmias have been observed following administration of pancuronium, ketamine, meperidine, or local anesthetics containing epinephrine to pts who are also on imipramine.
- MAOIs
  - Anesthetic requirement may be increased due to increased concentration of norepinephrine in the CNS.

- Serotonin syndrome from combining MAOI and meperidine has been noted.
- Current belief is to continue MAOIs during the periop period despite previous thought of discontinuing MAOIs 14 d prior to elective surgery.
- Benzodiazepene (midazolam) may be used to treat preop anxiety.
- Ketamine, a sympathetic stimulant should be avoided.
- Serum cholinesterase activity may be decreased in pts on phenelzine, so the dose of succinylcholine may need to be reduced.
- The addition of epinephrine to local anesthetic solutions should probably be avoided.
- If hypotension develops direct-acting drugs such as phenylephrine are preferred. The dose should also be decreased to minimize the likelihood of an exaggerated hypertensive response.
- Anticipated concerns
  - In periop period, general rule is to try to continue antidepressant therapy.
  - Be aware of potential interactions between anesthetic agents and antidepressants.
  - Pts should be monitored for signs of serotonin syndrome.

Diabetes, Type I (Insulin-Dependent)

Michael F. Roizen

Risk

- Incidence in USA: 1.2 million
- Races with highest prevalence: Hispanics and Native Americans

Perioperative Risks

- Increased risk of CABG 5–10× if end-stage renal, CHF, or autonomic neuropathy; without renal, CHF, or autonomic dysfunction, risk is 1–1.5 × normal

Worry About

- Autonomic neuropathy, gastroparesis, and sudden postop death
- Painless myocardial ischemia
- Atlanto-occipital joint immobility
- Tight glucose control might be indicated if pregnant, difficult weaning from bypass (ECC), or predictable global or focal CNS ischemia.

Overview

- Endocrinopathy assoc with end-stage renal, ophthalmic, myocardial, and neuropathic disease

- Blood sugar control per se not assoc with increased periop risk in absence of
  - Hypoglycemia
  - Hyperosmolar coma
  - Ketoacidosis
  - CNS ischemia
  - Pregnancy
  - Extracorporeal circulation
- Causes deranged autoregulation to CNS (blood sugar, 250 mg/dL), renal (blood sugar, 225 mg/dL), and cardiac (blood sugar, 100 mg/dL) vessels
- Need to control BP or blood sugar to decrease damage to these vessels and organs
- Check pt glucose log for degree of control
- Variable control may predict periop hypoglycemic episodes

ICD-9-CM Code: 850.09

- See also Diabetic Ketoacidosis (DKA) in Diseases section

Etiology

- Genetic predisposition to autoimmune destruction of glucose transporter on islet cells leads to increased blood glucose, which affects proteins via nonenzymatic glycosylations
  - Swells cells (sorbitol is oncotically active)
  - Increased viscous proteins (macroglobins), which impede blood flow
  - Increased substrate for anaerobic metabolism
  - Deranges autoregulation of blood flow

Usual Treatment

- Insulin injections, lifestyle changes incl stress management, diet, and exercise
- Pancreas and islet transplant is option if renal disease is end-stage
- Control of BP

ASSESSMENT POINTS

System	Effect	Assessment by Hx	PE	Test
HEENT	Possible atlanto-occipital dislocation 2° to abn collagen glycosylation	Pain	Neck ROM, prayer sign	Usually not needed, neck x-rays in extension
CARDIO	Angiopathy LV dysfunction (4–10× with Htn) Ischemic PVD	Poor exercise tolerance Angina CHF symptoms	2-flight walk Chest exam for signs of CHF BP lying and standing	ECG, CXR
RESP	↓ Lung elastance; ↓ FEV; ↓ FVC	Poor exercise tolerance		Generally not needed
GI	Gastroparesis	Early satiety		
RENAL	Nephropathy, esp if hypertensive	N/V; impotence; orthostatic Sx Nonprotein foods		BUN/Cr
ENDO	↓ Insulin from islets			FBS, electrolytes
CNS	Autonomic dysfunction 2° to neuropathy	Early satiety, impotence, N/V, orthostatic symptoms		RR interval variation on ECG BP change on standing
PNS	Stocking-glove neuropathy → infections		PNS exam, esp. if regional planned	
MS	Impaired joint mobility 2° to non-enzymatic glycosylation of collagen	Joint mobility	↓ ROM of joints	

Key Reference: Daneman D. Type 1 diabetes. *Lancet*. 2006;367(9513):847–858.

Perioperative Implications

Preoperative Preparation
- Metoclopramide (10 mg/70 kg) in pts with gastroparesis
- Assess myocardial and volume status.

Monitoring
- Myocardial ischemia. Can have CHF if volume overload and LV dysfunction present.
- Blood sugar

Airway
- Atlanto-occipital dislocation possible—see HEENT. Do prayer sign test; may have gastroparesis.

Induction
- Osmotic diuresis can make hypovolemic; ANS and CV dysfunction make BP and HR fluctuate.

Maintenance
- CV instability; volume status key to avoid renal and myocardial dysfunction with operation; checking RR variation (HRV) to determine autonomic insufficiency likelihood still not widespread

Extubation
- CV and pulm drive insufficiencies common with neuropathies

Adjuvants
- Rx for tight control
- Regional: Diabetic nerves may be more prone to edema esp if epinephrine used. Reduce dose (e.g., lidocaine from 2.0% to 1.5%) for same effect.

Postoperative Period
- Sliding scale of insulin Rx based on q 1–3 hr blood glucose determinations

Anticipated Problems/Concerns

- Gastroparesis with presence of solid food 24 hr after last meal if ANS dysfunction present. Consider Rx with metoclopramide 10 mg IM 1½ hr prior to induction.
- ANS dysfunction assoc with sudden death postop; can keep in ICU/PACU overnight; vested adult who can measure blood glucose and call 911 if sent home postop

Diabetes, Type II (Noninsulin-Dependent)

Michael F. Roizen
Stanley H. Rosenbaum

Risk

- Incidence in USA: more than 25 million
- Highest prevalence: Hispanics and Native Americans
- Gender predominance: None

Perioperative Risks

- Increased risk 5–10× if end-stage renal, CV, CHF, or autonomic neuropathy; without renal, CV, or autonomic dysfunction, risk is 1–1.5× normal
- Metabolic abnormalities increased with periop insulin Rx
- Unclear if same risks as for type I diabetes

Worry About

- Autonomic neuropathy, gastroparesis, and sudden postop death
- Myocardial ischemia; CV instability
- Tight glucose control might be indicated in pregnancy (see under Diabetes, Type III), difficult weaning from bypass (ECC), predictable global or focal CNS ischemia
- Disordered autoregulation makes hypertensive BP fluctuations more dangerous
- Fluid and electrolyte imbalance

Overview

- Endocrinopathy that can cause same organ dysfunction as in diabetes type I: End-stage renal, myocardial, and neuropathic disease
- Associated with deranged blood flow autoregulation to CNS (at blood sugar 250 mg/dL), renal (at blood sugar 200 mg/dL), and cardiac (at blood sugar 100 mg/dL) vessels
- Ketosis is rare, since some endogenous insulin
- Primarily controlled by diet and/or oral agents, although insulin more frequently used
- Usually has high insulin levels for glucose level, but peripheral resistance to insulin effect. Can develop hyperosmolar nonketotic coma.
- Blood sugar control per se not associated with increased periop morbidity in absence of:
  - Hypoglycemia
  - Hyperosmolar coma
  - CNS ischemia
  - Pregnancy
  - Extracorporeal circulation
- Preoperative hemoglobin A1c levels (ideally <7%) indicate quality of recent blood sugar control. High levels correlate with chronic microvascular complications.

ICD-9-CM Codes: 250.00; 250.02 (Uncontrolled)

(See also Diabetes, Type I, in Diseases section)

Etiology

- Familial predisposition with very high concordance in identical twins
- Autosomal dominant with variable expression accentuated by conditions that increase peripheral insulin resistance (obesity, inactivity, certain changes, hormones), increase glucose production or metabolic demands (glucocorticoids, pregnancy), or decrease insulin secretion (certain β-adrenergic drugs)
- Increases nonenzymatic glycosylations
- Causes cell swelling
- Deranges autoregulation
- Increases viscous protein production
- Increases substrate for anaerobic metabolism

Usual Treatment

- Hypoglycemic agents (see oral hypoglycemic agents), diet, exercise, insulin
- BP control

ASSESSMENT POINTS

System	Effect	Assessment by Hx	PE	Test
HEENT	Possible atlanto-occipital dislocation	Pain	Neck ROM, prayer sign	
CV	Premature CAD Htn Peripheral vascular disease	Angina Claudication Symptoms of CHF	Peripheral pulses	ECG CAD-related tests as indicated
RESP	↓ Pulm elastance	Exercise tolerance		
GI	Gastroparesis	Early satiety		
ENDO	Hyperglycemia Osmotic diuretic–caused hypokalemia	Polyuria		Blood glucose, K+
HEME	Infection from ↓ WBC phagocytic function		Site of infections	
RENAL	Nephropathy	Asymptomatic although often associated with neuropathy		BUN/Cr, UA for protein
CNS	Cerebrovascular disease Medication-induced hypoglycemia	TIAs, CVAs, long-acting oral hypoglycemic agents	CNS exam	
PNS	Distal neuropathy Postural hypotension	Impotence Foot infections	PNS exam, esp prior to regional anesthetic	
MS	Impaired joint mobility		ROM of joints	

Key Reference: Roizen MF, Fleisher LA. *Miller's anesthesia*. 7th ed. Philadelphia: Churchill Livingstone; 2010:1069–1076.

Perioperative Implications

Preoperative Preparation

- Metoclopramide (10 mg/70 kg) if gastroparesis
- Assess myocardial and autonomic function and volume status, half-life of hypoglycemic agent(s) taken chronically

Monitoring

- Blood sugar (questionable need for very tight control in type II diabetes) and metabolic abnormalities
- Painless myocardial ischemia can cause CHF if volume overload and LV dysfunction
- Peripheral vasculature and nerves vulnerable to pressure ischemia

Airway

- Atlanto-occipital dislocation possible: See HEENT, do prayer sign test

Induction

- Osmotic diuresis, autonomic nervous system, and CV dysfunction can make BP/HR fluctuate.

Maintenance

- CV instability: Volume status and avoidance of Htn key to avoiding renal and myocardial dysfunction periop

Extubation

- CV and pulm drive insufficiencies common with neuropathies

Adjuvants

- Regional: Diabetic nerves may be more prone to edema, esp if epinephrine used. Reduce dose (e.g., lidocaine from 2.0% to 1.5%) for same effect.
- Oral hypoglycemics may ablate preconditioning.

Postoperative Period

- Debate as to whether control to tighter than 60–250 mg/dL is of value in absence of Htn

Anticipated Problems/Concerns

- Autonomic nervous system dysfunction associated with sudden death postop; can monitor for resp function in ICU/PACU overnight; presence of adult at home who can measure blood glucose and call 911
- Infections and end-organ risk substantially increased with blood sugar >250 mg/dL. Hypoglycemic symptoms hidden by autonomic nervous system dysfunction, effects of regional, sedative-narcotic, and β-adrenergic blocking agents.

Diabetes, Type III (Gestational Diabetes Mellitus)

Richard B. Clark
Danny Wilkerson

Risk

- Incidence of gestational diabetes mellitus (GDM) is about 7% of all pregnancies
- Increased in African-American, Hispanic, Asian, Native American, or Pacific Islander women
- Risk factors are:
  - Maternal age >25 y
  - Previous delivery of macrosomic infant
  - Glucosuria
  - History of polycystic ovarian syndrome
  - Previous unexplained fetal demise
  - Previous pregnancy with GDM
  - Strong immediate family history of NIDDM or GDM
    - Obesity
    - Fasting glucose >126 mg/dL or a glucose >140mg/dL after a 50g oral glucose tolerance test

Perioperative Risks

- Unlikely renal, ocular, cardiac, neurologic, or orthopedic complications in GDM
- Hypoglycemia if insulin is used

- Fetal risk (if not controlled: polyhydramnios or macrosomia [6× normal])
- RDS (2–3× normal); preeclampsia, neonatal hypoglycemia, prematurity

Worry About

- Hyperglycemia and hypoglycemia

Overview

- GDM is defined as a carbohydrate intolerance that occurs (or is first recognized) during pregnancy.
- A glucose tolerance test is used to identify GDM. For details of the test, see the Key Reference.
- Maternal complications with GDM are few, but the fetus is at risk.
- Complications, such as fetal polyhydramnios, macrosomia (6×), prematurity, birth trauma, RDS (2–3× normal rate), neonatal hypoglycemia, or morbidity, are as common with type III diabetes (GDM) as with type I diabetes (insulin-dependent)

ICD-9-CM Code: 648.0#

Etiology

- Occurs in genetically susceptible individuals
- Pregnancy, through secretion of substances from uterus, exerts diabetogenic effects

Usual Treatment

- Use of insulin in GDM is now more common as tighter control seems beneficial.
- Diet and exercise have been used in management.
- Insulin can be started if fasting glucose exceeds 105 mg/dL despite diet control.
- Oral hypoglycemic agents have been used, and there has been some success with glyburide.
- Many clinicians obtain a single HbA_{1c} level at 6–12 wk gestation. In pts with mildly elevated plasma glucose levels and normal concentration of HbA_{1c}, dietary modification alone and a modest increase in exercise are often sufficient to normalize plasma glucose levels.

ASSESSMENT POINTS

System	Effect	Assessment by Hx	PE	Test
HEENT	Possible facial/pharyngeal edema	Snoring	Neck ROM Mallampati exam	
CV	CV changes of pregnancy—possible worse hypovolemia from osmotic diuresis		BP/HR with orthostatic maneuvers	
RESP	Resp changes of pregnancy, ↓ FRC, etc.			
GI	Gastroparesis of pregnancy	Early satiety		
ENDO	Neonatal hypoglycemia if maternal hyperglycemia, obesity			Blood sugar, glucose levels, acid-base status of fetus, HbA_{1c} in mother
HEME	No change, unless type I diabetes			
RENAL	↓ Renal function			BUN/Cr
CNS	ANS dysfunction	Gastroparesis, early satiety	Orthostatic BP	Tilt table test
PNS	Neuropathy not present unless type I diabetes			

Key Reference: Serlin DC, Lash RW. Diagnosis and management of gestational diabetes mellitus. *Am Fam Physician*. 2009;80:57–62.

Perioperative Implications

Preoperative Preparation
- Full-stomach precautions: Nonparticulate antacid administration usual

Monitoring
- Blood sugar in maternal and umbilical vein blood

Airway
- Examine for edema

Induction
- Regional anesthesia preferred to general anesthetic due to risks of aspiration and failed airway attainment if C-section is performed

- Osmotic diuresis can cause hypovolemia and increase BP and HR fluctuations

Maintenance
- CV instability: Volume status is key to maintenance of uterine and other organ perfusion

Extubation
- Ensure pt is awake before extubation

Adjuvants
- Regional: Diabetic nerves may be more prone to edema esp if epinephrine used. Reduced dose (e.g., lidocaine reduced from 1.5% to 1%) for same effect.

Postoperative Period
- Usually GDM cured by delivery
- Women with GDM need a follow up GTT at 6–12 wk after delivery

Anticipated Problems/Concerns

- Fetal dysfunction, esp hypoglycemia and acidosis, if maternal hypoglycemia present
- Rapid changes in maternal blood glucose can accompany the pain and/or exertion of vaginal delivery of fetus and accompany the endocrine changes of uterine delivery.

Diabetes Insipidus

Natalie F. Holt

DISEASES

Risk

- Hereditary/familial (rare)
- Nephrogenic diabetes insipidus (DI) usually X-linked recessive transmission, but autosomal recessive and autosomal dominant forms exist; males>females
- Neurogenic DI due to mutations of the vasopressin (antidiuretic hormone, ADH) gene; usually manifests in childhood; males=females
- May also be part of developmental syndromes (Wolfram syndrome, Lawrence-Moon-Beidel syndrome)
- Acquired
- Trauma and/or surgery; infarction; inflammatory, infectious, infiltrative, and/or neoplastic process affecting the hypothalamic-neurohypophyseal region
- Renal disease (chronic renal failure, polycystic kidney disease, obstructive uropathy, renal transplantation)
- Systemic conditions (multiple myeloma, sickle cell disease)
- Electrolyte imbalances (hypokalemia, hypercalcemia)
- Medications (amphotericin B, colchicine, loop diuretics, demeclocycline, lithium) or toxins (methoxyflurane/fluoride)
- Gestational due to pregnancy-induced acceleration of vasopressin metabolism

Perioperative Risks

- Dehydration, hyperosmolarity, hypernatremia
- Altered mental status/seizures
- Hemodynamic instability
- Bladder distention, hydroureter

Worry About

- Fluid and electrolyte imbalance
- Contributing drugs and/or toxins (methoxyflurane/fluoride, lithium)
- Postop onset esp following pituitary surgery (1–6 d postop)

Overview

- Polyuria due either to insufficient production of vasopressin or inadequate renal tubular response to vasopressin
- Polyuria, excessive thirst, polydipsia; dehydration rarely present in competent pts with access to water
- Inadequate fluid replacement leads to hypernatremia, hyperosmolarity, and dehydration causing fatigue, weakness, altered sensorium, hemodynamic instability, seizures, and possible death

ICD-9-CM Codes: 253.5, 588.1

ICD-10 Codes: E23.2, N25.1

Etiology

- Neurogenic (central or hypothalamic)
- Inadequate release of vasopressin from posterior pituitary
- Primary genetic or secondary acquired condition due to trauma or surgery, inflammation or infiltration, infarction, neoplasm
- Nephrogenic
- Inadequate renal tubular response to vasopressin
- Primary genetic or secondary acquired due to medications/intoxications (lithium, amphotericin B, osmotic diuretics, fluoride toxicity), chronic renal disease, systemic diseases (multiple myeloma, sickle cell disease), electrolyte imbalances (hypokalemia, hypercalcemia)

Usual Treatment

- Central DI: Synthetic vasopressin or vasopressin analogue (desmopressin) supplementation; older treatments (chlorpropamide, carbamazepine, clofibrate) that increase ADH sensitivity or stimulate ADH release not commonly used due to systemic side effects
- Nephrogenic DI: Diuretics (e.g., hydrochlorothiazide, amiloride), salt restriction, non-steroidal anti-inflammatories

---

ASSESSMENT POINTS

System	Effect	Assessment by Hx	PE	Test
CV	Hypotension Tachycardia Myocardial ischemia	Fatigue Weakness Reduced exercise tolerance	Orthostatic hypotension	ECG
ENDO	Anterior pituitary dysfunction	Pituitary surgery, neoplastic or infiltrative disease	Multisystem effects due to hormone deficiencies	Tests of anterior pituitary function, hormone levels
RENAL	Polyuria	Copious production of dilute urine	Urine volume and specific gravity	24-hr urine collection; simultaneous measurements of plasma and urine osmolality; exclude hyperglycemia, hypercalcemia, hypokalemia
CNS	Altered sensorium Visual disturbance	Excessive thirst Polydipsia	Neurologic function	MRI

Key Reference: Fauci AS, Kasper DL, Longo DL, et al, eds. *Harrison's principles of internal medicine*. 17th ed. New York: McGraw-Hill Companies, Inc; 2008:2218–2222.

Perioperative Implications

Preoperative Preparation

- Recognition and appropriate treatment: Water deprivation test; desmopressin trial
- Assess electrolytes, serum osmolality, and volume status
- Rule out additional hormonal deficiencies, e.g., cortisol
- Discontinue provocative medications, e.g., lithium, mannitol

Monitoring

- Urine output
- Serum electrolytes
- Intravascular volume

Airway

- Not affected

Induction

- Pts may have exaggerated hypotensive response due to hypovolemia
- Arrhythmias may occur as a result of electrolyte abnormalities

Maintenance

- Fluid and electrolyte monitoring and replacement
- CV instability
- Variable sensitivity to neuromuscular relaxants depending on concomitant electrolyte imbalances (e.g., hypercalcemia, hypokalemia)

Extubation

- Altered sensorium may impair ability to protect airway

Adjuvants

- Early consideration for initiating vasopressin replacement therapy

- Administration of hypotonic IV fluids if oral intake inadequate to maintain normal plasma osmolality
- Supplemental corticosteroid therapy if anterior pituitary deficiency present
- Chlorpropamide treatment for DI may cause hypoglycemia

Anticipated Problems/Concerns

- High-dose vasopressin therapy may cause vasoconstriction and precipitate myocardial ischemia in at-risk pts
- Postop DI following pituitary surgery/traumatic brain injury usually manifests within 24–48 hr but may be delayed
- Vasopressin therapy will not increase urine osmolality in pts with DI of nephrogenic origin

Diabetic Ketoacidosis (DKA)

Shamsuddin Akhtar

Risk

- Typically seen in pts with type I diabetes mellitus; can occur in pts with type II diabetes (see Diabetes, Type I in Diseases section)
- Physiological (acute infection, trauma, myocardial infarction, stroke) or emotional trauma can precipitate DKA in diabetic pts.
- Poor compliance with insulin therapy or inadequate outpatient insulin regimen

Perioperative Risks

- CV collapse secondary to severe dehydration (diuresis, fluid deprivation, fever) and/or myocardial depression due to severe metabolic acidosis
- Cerebral edema and injury with rapid correction of DKA, esp in children
- Acute resp distress syndrome and bronchial mucus plugging
- Worsening of pre-existing end-organ dysfunction, (e.g., acute tubular necrosis) in the setting of baseline renal dysfunction or, periop MI in pts with pre-existing CAD

Worry About

- Fluid deficit of 5–10 L in established DKA (100 mL/kg)
- Cardiac arrest, severe shock or arrhythmias with onset of general anesthesia or regional anesthesia due to hypovolemia, acidosis, and electrolyte disturbances
- Severe electrolyte derangements and significant total body deficits of potassium (3–5mEq/kg), sodium (7–10 mEq/kg), phosphate (5–7 mmol/kg), calcium (1–2 mEq/kg), magnesium (1–2 mEq/kg)
- Necessity of surgical therapy to treat etiology of DKA (abscess, gangrene)

Overview

- DKA is the most common acute metabolic emergency with significant mortality (5%)
- Two primary hormonal abnormalities: Absolute or relative deficiency of insulin; and glucagon excess, causing severe hyperglycemia (> 250 mg/dL)
- Characterized by hyperglycemia (> 250 mg/dL), ketosis (positive ketones in serum and urine), anion-gap metabolic acidosis (anion gap >10)

- Intensive periop hemodynamic and metabolic management essential for favorable outcome

ICD-9-CM Code: 250.1

Etiology

- Type I diabetes with insulin deficiency caused by cessation, or inadequate dosing of insulin therapy, with or without significant pathological (infection, surgery) or emotional stress
- Elevation of counter-regulatory hormones (glucagon, epinephrine, cortisol and growth hormone) drive the catabolic and ketogenic state
- Osmotic diuresis 2° to sustained hyperglycemia leads to volume and electrolyte depletion
- Metabolic acidosis is a product of unrestrained free fatty acid release from adipose tissue and subsequent hepatic oxidation of fatty acids to ketone bodies (due to lack of insulin and glucagon excess)

Usual Treatment

- Search and treat initiating cause
- Insulin, aggressive rehydration, correction of electrolyte derangements, hemodynamic support

ASSESSMENT POINTS

System	Effect	Assessment by Hx	PE	Test
CV	Hypovolemia	Duration of initiating event, postural symptoms	BP, HR, JVD, skin turgor, mucous membranes, tilt table test, orthostatic hypotension	CVP ABGs
RESP	Hyperventilation (Kussmaul's respiration)		Ventilatory rate and depth, fruity odor of acetone	ABGs
GI	Anorexia, N/V	Appetite, N/V, abdominal pain	Abdominal distension, ileus, tenderness without rebound	
RENAL	Diuresis	Urinary frequency, thirst (polyuria, polydipsia)		UO, BUN/Cr, electrolytes (esp potassium), serum osmolality
ENDO	Insulin deficiency, glucagon excess during severe catabolic stress	Type I diabetes		Blood glucose ABGs (anion gap) Ketones (urine, blood)
CNS	Depression from lethargy to coma; late cerebral edema in children		Assess LOC Signs of ↑ ICP	

Key Reference: Vavilala MS, Souter MJ, Lam AM. Hyperemia and impaired cerebral autoregulation in a surgical patient with diabetic ketoacidosis. *Can J Anaesth.* 2005;52:323–326.

Perioperative Implications

Perioperative Preparation

- Vigorous 0.9N saline infusion (1–2.5 L) to restore hemodynamic stability, then use 0.5N saline if serum osmolality is >310 mOsm/L)
- Insulin Rx usually begins with 0.1 U of regular insulin/kg IV bolus (in adults) followed by infusion of 0.1 U/kg/hr. Adjust insulin infusion to decrease glucose by 10% or 50 mg/dL per hr.
- Sodium bicarbonate not generally indicated, administer if pH <6.9, hyperkalemia, or pt hemodynamically unstable with pH <7.1

Monitoring

- Check glucose, electrolytes hourly; check pH frequently: Foley catheter to determine urine output reliably during periop period; CVP catheter for fluid management, possibly PA catheter if pt

has pre-existing myocardial dysfunction or CAD; consider TEE in hemodynamically unstable pt

Airway

- Potential stiff joint syndrome with difficult intubation; at risk for aspiration

Induction

- Hemodynamic instability likely if intravascular volume depletion not corrected; pts frequently have pre-existing autonomic neuropathy and CV dysfunction

Maintenance

- Protect end-organs, esp heart, renal, and CNS as they are often compromised by DM

Extubation

- Awake. May require mechanical ventilation and ICU admission if pH <7.2, compromised mental status and /or high risk of aspiration.

Adjuvants

- See under Diabetes in Diseases section

Postoperative Period

- Potential for hypoglycemic injury from rapid increase in insulin sensitivity when surgical cause of DKA corrected
- Subsequent medical management should be continued by physician with expertise in diabetes

Anticipated Problems/Concerns

- Hemodynamic instability from combined volume deficiency, acidosis, and pre-existing CV disease
- CNS dysfunction from metabolic and electrolyte abnormalities, both early and late

Diaphragmatic Hernia (Congenital)

N. James Halliday
Jibin Samuel

Risk

- Occurs in ~1/2500–5000 births; 12–25% have associated anomalies in particular cardiac (20%), chromosomal (5–16%), and neurologic
- Parents who have one child with isolated defect have 2% chance with next child
- Usually left sided (90%) due to defect in foramen of Bochdalek and are more common in boys. Morgagni hernias (2–5%) located anterior are more common in girls. Remainder through esophageal hiatus.

Perioperative Risks

- 30–60% mortality despite improved diagnosis and management
- Degree of pulm hypoplasia and associated CNS and CV malformations affect mortality
- Timing of diagnosis associated with the prognosis

Worry About

- Hypoxemia and acidosis
- Pulm Htn and CHD
- Shock
- Tension pneumothorax

Overview

- Classified by site of herniation
  - Posterolateral defects (Bochdalek) are left-sided (largest and associated with greatest degree of pulm hypoplasia. Morgagni hernias rare; parasternal, less symptomatic, therefore, diagnosed at later age.
- Between 4–9 wk of age the pleuroperitoneal membrane forms with the left closing after the right. In Bochdalek and Morgagni normal development of the diaphragm and digestive tract does not occur.
- Degree of lung hypoplasia determined by time of defect during fetal development and amount of abdominal contents in chest. Though ipsilateral lung most affected, both lungs are abnormal and result in decreased numbers and function of alveoli; hypoplastic lung with smaller pulm artery and decreased arterial branching causes high vascular resistance.

ICD-9-CM Code: 756.6 (Congenital anomalies of diaphragm)

Indications/Usual Treatment

- Initial treatment involves determining the severity of associated congenital anomalies and degree of illness.
- Goal is semielective surgery when pt is medically stable.
- Posterolateral defects require surgical repair (does not resolve the pulmonary dysfunction).
- Small defects closed primarily; larger defects use artificial diaphragm, which contributes to postop resp failure.
- Most cases abdomen is closed primarily after correction but a silastic pouch may be used with increased intra-abdominal pressures.
- Fetal surgery has been accomplished in those severely affected with increased degree of pulm hypoplasia. Fetal Endoluminal Tracheal Occlusion (FETO) can be done to trigger lung growth. No maternal complications but preterm rupture of membranes is a drawback (20% <34 wk). Randomized control trials are ongoing to compare survival with controls.

ASSESSMENT POINTS

System	Effect	Assessment by Hx	PE	Test
CV	Mediastinal shift, associated ASD, VSD, coarctation, tetralogy of Fallot (23%)	Displaced cardiac impulse	CV exam	ECHO
RESP	Resp distress, pulm Htn	↓ Breath sounds on affected side Prominent ipsilateral chest	Pulmonary exam	CXR ABG
GI	Malrotation, atresia (20%)	Scaphoid abdomen	Abd exam	
GU	Hypospadias		Inspection	
CNS	Spina bifida, hydrocephalus, anencephaly (28%)		Inspection and neurologic exam	US, CT scan
METAB	Acidosis, hypoxemia, hypercarbia			ABGs

Key Reference: Suda K, Bigras JL, Bohn D, Hornberger LK, McCrindle BW. Echocardiographic predictors of outcome in newborns with congenital diaphragmatic hernia. *Pediatrics.* 2000;105:1106–1109.

Perioperative Implications

Perioperative Management

- ECMO provides temporary support until perinatal circulation matures and less sensitive to vasoconstrictive stimuli (1–2 wk)

Preoperative Preparation

- Avoid triggers for pulm vasoconstriction
- Goals incl a Pao_2 >80, $Paco_2$ 25–30, normal or elevated pH, and normothermia (hypothermia increases O_2 consumption)
- **For pulm Htn can also use nitric oxide 20–80 ppm, sildenefil**
- **Avoid gaseous distension of stomach with early placement of NG tube**
- **Compromised neonates, ET intubation, sedation, paralysis and ECMO may be required if conventional or high-frequency ventilation fails**
- **All neonates with resp distress require invasive monitoring using preductal Rt Radial**

a-line. Severe consider pre- and postductal a line and pulse oximetry
- **IV access best in upper extremities to avoid possible IVC obstruction from increased intra-abdominal pressure**
- Watch for pneumothorax (sudden deterioration in BP or oxygenation); consider prophylactic contralateral chest tube; equipment needed should be available.

Anesthetic Technique

- Opioids well tolerated; inhaled halogenated anesthetics may cause significant hypotension; avoid N_2O which distends gas-filled intestines
- Avoid peak pressures more then 25cm H_2O
- High frequency, low tidal volume preferred
- Continue nitric oxide if given preop
- Lung mechanics change during surgery; may require hand ventilation

Postoperative Considerations

- Continued muscle relaxation/opioids and ventilatory support
- Once stable, assess need for continued resp support
- If A—aDO_2 gradient >400 mmHg or if cardiopulmonary deterioration, continue resp assistance
- Persistent hypoxemia while on high FIO_2 suggests persistent pulm Htn with Rt to Lt shunting
- Minimize ET suctioning, correct metabolic acidosis
- Deliver adequate nutrition
- High degree of neurologic problems, whether or not infants placed on ECMO; seizures, developmental delay, and hearing loss in 20–30% but pulm outcomes are usually good

Diarrhea, Acute and Chronic

Michelle Braunfeld

Risk

- Incidence in the USA: 200–300 million new cases/y of acute, with >900,000 hospital admissions
- Chronic: 1–5% of population; increasing with age
- Acute: male = female
- Chronic: female > male

Perioperative Risks

- Hypovolemia with hemodynamic instability
- Electrolyte abnormalities, esp hypokalemia
- Acid-base abnormalities: May be non–anion gap acidosis or alkalosis, depending on underlying cause

Worry About

- Chronic
  - Underlying disease, especially iatrogenic (e.g., infection with antibiotic-induced diarrhea, end-stage liver disease with lactulose-induced diarrhea, or disaccharide [usually lactose] intolerance)
  - Hormone-producing tumors (e.g., carcinoid, VIPomas, gastrinomas)
  - Vitamin K malabsorption with coagulopathy
  - Extra-intestinal manifestations of inflammatory bowel disease (IBD) (e.g., deforming arthritis, cholangitis,)
  - Stress steroid therapy in IBD

- Psychological symptoms in up to 50% of patients with IBS; often alternates with constipation
- Postsurgical losses that may drain via ileostomy or fistula, or may be due to inadequate bowel absorption 2° to resection (short bowel syndrome)
- Acute
- Viral, bacterial, or protozoan disease

Overview

- Acute: Abrupt onset of loose stools in healthy individual: Viral—self-limited, 1–3 d causing changes in small intestinal cells with a shortened transit time; bacterial—tends to occur in groups of individuals (if within 12 h of a meal, usually due to preformed toxin); protozoan—prolonged watery diarrhea from contaminated water supply in endemic area
- Chronic: Too-frequent passage of stools that are too loose for too long; >200 g/day of stool for >4 wk
- Multifactorial medical problem that requires supportive therapy and attention to the underlying etiology
- Only one in a spectrum of medical problems associated with an underlying disease or with treatment of disease. Supportive therapy includes fluid and electrolyte repletion and attention to acid-base balance.

- Toxic megacolon—extreme manifestation of inflammatory or infectious bowel disease is a surgical emergency. Pts often septic.

ICD-9-CM Code: 558.9

Etiology

- Chronic:
  - Osmotic: Laxatives, indigestible carbohydrates
  - Secretory: Hormone-producing tumors
  - Exudative: Inflammatory bowel disease, pseudomembranous colitis
  - Decreased mucosal contact/mixing: short bowel syndrome, irritable bowel syndrome, hypermotility secondary to vagotomy, diabetic neuropathy
  - Malabsorption: Pancreatic exocrine insufficiency, celiac disease, Whipple's disease, small-bowel bacterial overgrowth
- Acute
  - Viral or bacterial (with or without toxin) or protozoan (see Overview)

Usual Treatment

- Volume and electrolyte replacement, including Na^+, K^+, $PO4^-$, Mg^{2+}
- Although acid-base correction often follows above, may occasionally need replacement
- Seek and treat underlying cause

ASSESSMENT POINTS

System	Effect	Assessment by Hx	PE	Test
CV	Hypovolemia	Postural symptoms, quantitation of bowel movements	Orthostatic changes Narrow pulse pressure Tachycardia Dry mucous membranes	
	Dysrhythmia 2° to electrolyte abnormalities			ECG
RESP	Compensatory hyperventilation			ABGs
METAB	Derangement dependent on underlying cause			Lab values include Ca^{2+}, Mg^{2+}, K^+, HCO_3^-; Na^+
RENAL	Prerenal azotemia	BUN/Cr		
CNS	Profound electrolyte abnormality		Range from drowsiness to obtundation	
	Anemia—can be acute or chronic from acute GI losses or chronic disease state	Melena or hematochezia	Stool guaiac	Hct

Key Reference: Cataldo R, Potash M. Atropine as a treatment of diarrhea after celiac plexus block. *Anesth Analg.* 1996;83:1131–1132.

Perioperative Implications

Preoperative Preparation

- Assess volume status, electrolytes, acid-base status
- Repletion

Monitoring

- Consider arterial and central venous catheter (or some other fluid status monitor such as TEE) if significant hypovolemia and CV compromise present

Airway

- May require full-stomach precautions

Induction

- Hemodynamic instability and decrease drug dosage if not repleted
- Sympatholytic drugs and sympathectomy with regional anesthesia can shorten transit time and increase diarrhea

Maintenance

- Tailor IV fluids to electrolyte and acidbase status (e.g., avoid normal saline if patient already has hyperchloremic acidosis)
- Continue electrolyte repletion if necessary

Extubation

- Routine, dependent on underlying condition

Adjustments

- Acid-base status and electrolytes may affect muscle relaxant duration and ability of antagonists to reverse block

Anticipated Problems/Concerns

- Most operations do not affect underlying condition, but narcotics can make diarrhea less problematic, but use with caution in severe IBD as they may promote toxic megacolon
- Regional anesthesia that causes sympathectomy leaves parasympathetic system unopposed, which can cause shortened transit time and increase diarrhea

Dilated Cardiomyopathy (DCM)

Frank W. Dupont

Risk

- Incidence: 5 to 8 cases per 100,000 per year
- Racial predominance: African-Americans > Caucasians
- Gender predominance: Male > female
- Marked limitation of exercise capacity is a reliable predictor of mortality

Perioperative Risks

- Increased periop morbidity and mortality, particularly in high-risk surgery cases
- CHF exacerbation
- Renal failure
- Systemic or pulm embolization from dislodged intracardiac thrombi

Worry About

- Autonomic instability
- Malignant tachydysrhythmias
- Worsening LV systolic and/or diastolic function, RV dysfunction

Overview

- Syndrome characterized by dilatation and impaired systolic function of left, right, or both ventricles
- LV systolic and diastolic dysfunction (noncompliant ventricle), RV dysfunction; possibly pulm Htn and AV valvular regurgitation
- High risk of sudden cardiac death

ICD-9-CM Code: 425.4 (Cardiomyopathy, idiopathic)

Etiology

- Cause of idiopathic dilated DCM remains unclear, but three possible basic mechanisms of damage: Familial and genetic factors; viral myocarditis and other cytotoxic insults; and immunological abnormalities

Usual Treatment

- Medical treatment primarily based on CHF treatment with diuretics, vasodilators, and β-adrenergic receptor–blocking agents; anticoagulants for thromboembolic prophylaxis; antiarrhythmics or ICD implantation for management of tachyarrhythmias
- Surgical treatment: Mitral valve annuloplasty, cardiomyoplasty, LVAD placement, heart transplant

ASSESSMENT POINTS

System	Effect	Assessment by Hx	PE	Test
CV	Arrhythmias	Palpitations	Narrow pulse pressure, pulsus alternans	ECG, EPS
	CHF	DOE	Displaced PMI	ECHO
		Orthopnea	Systolic murmur (MR), S_3, S_4	
		PND	JVD, ascites, pedal edema	
	Myocardial ischemia	Angina		Coronary angiography
RESP	Pulm edema	Dyspnea	Rales, wheezes	CXR
				ABGs
HEME	Coagulopathy	Bruising		PT/PTT
RENAL	Renal insufficiency	Oliguria		BUN/Crea
CNS	Cerebral infarcts	Stroke	Focal neurologic deficits	CT, MRI

Key Reference: Mohan SB. Idiopathic dilated cardiomyopathy: A common but mystifying cause of heart failure. *Cleve Clin J Med.* 2002;69:481–487.

Perioperative Implications

Preoperative Preparation

- Optimization of cardiac condition for anesthesia (consider cardiology consultation)

Monitoring

- ECG with ST-segment analysis
- Arterial line dependent on invasiveness of surgery
- Consider PA catheter if anticipation of large fluid shifts
- TEE is the monitor of choice for the assessment of biventricular function and AV valve regurgitation in invasive surgical cases

Airway

- None

Preinduction/Induction

- Anesthetic principles based on afterload reduction, preload conservation, and prevention of tachycardia and myocardial depression

Maintenance

- Higher doses of volatile anesthetic agents often poorly tolerated; thus a narcotic–based anesthetic with BZDP supplementation may be preferable
- Fluid management should be conservative to prevent fluid overload and acute CHF exacerbation
- Inotropic support may be necessary

Extubation

- Beware of tachycardia and Htn and treat proactively

Postoperative Period

- Consider ICU admission and mechanical ventilation if major intraop fluid shift has occurred

Adjuvants

- Regional anesthesia techniques are not contraindicated in the absence of coagulopathy and provided hypotension is prevented
- ICD management precautions should be taken if applicable
- DCM predisposes to decreased blood flow to liver and kidney, which prolongs action of many drugs; also increased volume of distribution requires drug dose adjustments

Anticipated Problems/Concerns

- CHF exacerbation, hemodynamic instability, tachydysrhythmias

Risk

• Incidence in USA: ~0.001 cases per 100,000 since 1980 (<5 cases a year)
• Endemic in developing countries
• Still common in countries where mass immunization programs are not enforced
• Risk factors for diphtheria outbreaks: Older age, lack of vaccination, alcoholism, low socioeconomic status, crowded living conditions, and Native American ancestry.

Perioperative Risks

• Early (days after exposure): Resp compromise; resp arrest; airway obstruction and hemorrhage; shock, coma, and death
• Late (2–6 wk): Myocarditis and neuritis

Worry About

• Resp diphtheria early toxic manifestations: Neck edema, pharyngitis, large pseudomembranes, massive swelling of the tonsils, bull-neck diphtheria (with massive edema of the submandibular and paratracheal region and foul breath, thick speech, and stridorous breathing), hoarseness and difficulty breathing are associated with severe advanced disease/poor prognosis, and with a significant early risk of airway obstruction
• Late toxic manifestations of diphtheria: Polyneuropathy (resembles Guillain-Barré syndrome) and myocarditis (cardiac arrhythmias or CHF)
• Other complications: Septic arthritis, pneumonia, renal failure, endocarditis, encephalitis, cerebral infarction, and pulm embolism
• Fatal pseudomembranous diphtheria typically occurs in pts with nonprotective antibody titers and in unimmunized pts. Death occurs in 5–10% of resp cases. Risk factors for death incl "bull-neck" diphtheria, myocarditis with ventricular tachycardia, atrial fibrillation or complete heart block, an age of >60 y or <6 mo, alcoholism, extensive pseudomembrane elongation, and laryngeal, tracheal, or bronchial involvement, and delayed antitoxin administration

Overview

• Prompt consideration of diphteria: Severe pharyngitis, difficulty swallowing, resp compromise, or signs of systemic disease incl myocarditis or generalized weakness, and presence of a pharyngeal pseudomembrane or an extensive exudate
• Resp diphtheria: A sore throat with low-grade fever and an adherent membrane of the tonsils, pharynx, or nose. Occasionally, weakness, dysphagia, headache, and voice change. The diphtheritic pseudomembrane is gray or whitish, sharply demarcated and tightly adherent to the underlying tissues. Attempts to dislodge the membrane may cause bleeding.
• Systemic manifestations of diphtheria: Neuritis and polyneuropathy (cranial nerve involvement, resp and abdominal muscle weakness, generalized sensorimotor polyneuropathy and autonomic manifestations), and myocarditis (dysrhythmia of the conduction tract and dilated cardiomyopathy).
• Cutaneous diphtheria: Infected skin lesions and nonhealing or enlarging skin ulcers which lack a characteristic appearance. Cutaneous diphtheria has a low mortality rate, rarely associated with myocarditis or peripheral neuropathy.

ICD9-CM: 032.#

Etiology

• *Corynebacterium diphtheria*, an aerobic non-encapsulated, nonmotile, nonsporulating gram-positive bacillus
• Two human isolate phenotypes: Nontoxigenic and toxigenic. Toxigenic strains express diphtheria toxin (mechanism of pathogenesis during human systemic infection). Toxin produced in the pseudomembranous lesion and distributed to all organ systems throught the blood. Toxigenic strains cause pharyngeal/resp diphtheria and systemic diseases, nontoxigenic strains cause cutaneous diseases.
• Direct person-to-person transmission via the aerosol route. Cutaneous lesions are also important in transmission. There are no significant reservoirs other than humans. The incubation period for resp diphtheria is usually 2–5 d.

Usual Treatment

• Prompt hospitalization in resp isolation with close monitoring of cardiac and resp function. Cardiac workup recommended.
• Start treatments as soon as possible even before confirmatory tests are completed due to the high potential for mortality and morbidity.
• Diphtheria antitoxin (DAT) available in USA only through CDC. DAT reduces the extent of local disease as well as the risk of complications of myocarditis and neuropathy. Rapid institution of DAT is associated with a significant reduction in mortality risk.
• Antimicrobial therapy: Procaine penicillin G 600,000 units (for children, 12,500–25,000 U/kg) IM 12 hr/ PO penicillin V 125–250 mg 6 hr daily to complete a 14-d course; or erythromycin 500 mg IV 6 hr (for children, 40–50 mg/kg/d IV in two or four divided doses) / PO erythromycin 500 mg Q 6 hr daily to complete a 14-d course alternative agents: Rifampin and clindamycin
• Sustained campaigns for vaccination of children and adequate boosting vaccination of adults.
• Resp diphtheria remains a notifiable disease in USA (National surveillance through the National Electronic Telecommunications System for Surveillance [NETSS]), whereas cutaneous diphtheria is not.

ASSESSMENT POINTS

System	Effect	Assessment by Hx	PE	Test
HEENT	"Membrane" spread and hemorrhage can cause airway obstruction	Altered speech, resp distress, croupy cough, hoarseness, chills, sore throat	Neck edema, fever, pharyngitis, large pseudomembranes, massive swelling of the tonsils, "bull-neck" diphtheria	Gram stain, culture of "membrane," indirect laryngoscopy
CV	Conduction abnormalities, dysrythmias, cardiogenic shock, CHF	Dyspnea with minimal exertion, symptoms of CHF, palpitations	Tachycardia, ectopic beats, atrial fibrillation, signs of CHF	ECG, CXR, serum troponin I, echocardiography
RESP	See HEENT	Tachypnea, dyspnea, presence of membrane	Progressive resp compromise	Indirect laryngoscopy
HEME/IMMUNO	Systems compromised dependent on amount of toxin			CBC, blood cultures, PCR assays
GU	Proteinuria			UA
CNS	Interference with phonation, swallowing, respiration, ressembles Guillain-Barré syndrome	Symptoms depend on involved nerves	Cranial nerves (most often III, VI, VII, X), peripheral nerves (motor > sensory)	

Key Reference: Jenkins IA, Saunders M. Infections of the airway. *Paediatr Anaesth.* 2009;19(suppl 1):118–130.

Perioperative Implications

Preoperative Preparation

• Initiate prompt treatments with diphtheria antitoxin and antimicrobial therapy
• Assessment of resp distress/airway compromise
• Assessment of cardiac involvement (for early detection of rhythm abnormalities. Initiate electrical pacing for clinically significant conduction disturbance and provide pharmacologic intervention for arrhythmias or for heart failure)
• Assessment of neurologic involvement
• Assessment of immunization status of exposed health care workers

Monitoring

• Maintain close monitoring of cardiac activity for early detection of rhythm abnormalities.

• Provide 2 large-bore IVs for pts with a toxic appearance; provide invasive monitoring and aggressive resuscitation for pts with septicemia.
• Initiate electrical pacing for clinically significant conduction disturbance and provide pharmacologic intervention for arrhythmias or for heart failure.

- Consider pulm artery catheter or transesophageal echocardiography to assess degree of myocardial involvement

Airway
- Secure definite airway for pts with impending resp compromise or the presence of laryngeal membrane (careful manipulation as membrane will bleed if manipulated)
- Early airway management allows access for mechanical removal of tracheobronchial membranes and prevents the risk of sudden asphyxia through aspiration.

Induction and Maintenance
- Compensate for problems of exotoxin shock and possible CHF, cardiac arrythmia

Extubation
- Early: May need prolonged ventilation
- Late: Cardiogenic shock/extensive polyneuritis may necessitate prolonged ventilatory support

Adjuvants
- Cardiac pacemaker for arrhythmia control and/or complete heart block
- Minimize use of sedative-hypnotics, as development of resp difficulties may be obscured

Postoperative Period
- Careful observation for resp, cardiac, and neurologic compromises

Anticipated Problems/Concerns
- Airway obstruction requiring tracheostomy/intubation
- Myocardial conduction problems that may necessitate electrical pacing
- Cardiogenic shock/CHF
- Neuritis that can present as a Guillain-Barré-like syndrome

Disseminated Intravascular Coagulation (DIC)

Adrian Hendrickse

Risk

- Most common coagulopathy in the ICU.
- Incidence of DIC in severe sepsis is nearly 35%.
- The most important initiators of DIC are sepsis; trauma (hypovolemic shock, extensive tissue damage, fat embolism, head injury); surgery (neurosurgery, CPB); obstetric emergencies (hemorrhage, pre-eclampsia, retained products, amniotic fluid embolism); malignancy (acute promyelocytic leukemia, disseminated metastases) and severe liver disease. Vascular abnormalities, immunological reactions, toxins, and drugs can also cause DIC.
- Gender and race predominance: None.
- Mortality: High and dependant on underlying condition.

Perioperative Risks

- Underlying disease process and nature of surgical intervention
- Existing coagulopathy
- Organ dysfunction

Worry About

- Uncontrollable bleeding from surgical and anesthetic access sites
- Further ischemic damage to end-organs
- Transfusion complications

Overview

- A syndrome characterized by the pathological imbalance of the thrombotic and fibrinolytic systems leading to systemic intravascular coagulation and the deposition of fibrin in the microcirculation.
- Ongoing activation of the coagulation system results in the consumption of platelets and the severe depletion of clotting factors, which can lead to generalized bleeding.
- Dx: There are no specific laboratory tests for DIC. DIC can be diagnosed clinically on the basis of the presence of a suitable risk factor along with a selection of laboratory findings: a rapidly falling platelet count or a count <100,000/mm³; prolongation of clotting times (APTT, PTT, INR); the presence of fibrin degradation products (FDPs); a reduction in plasma concentration of coagulation inhibitors (ATIII, Protein C).
- Serial testing showing temporal trends are valuable.

ICD9-CM:286.6 (Defibrination syndrome)

Etiology

- DIC is initiated in one of two ways:
  - A systemic inflammatory response resulting in the activation of the complement pathway and the release of cytokines leading to systemic coagulation
  - The activation of the extrinsic pathway of coagulation by the presence of increased concentrations of tissue factor
- An impairment of fibrinolysis, which normally keeps coagulation localized, also plays its part in the progression of the syndrome

Usual Treatment

- The primary goal is to remove the initiating stimulus and aggressive organ support.
- Mechanical ventilation, invasive monitoring and inotropic support are often required.
- Surgery intended to remove the cause of the DIC should be delayed no longer than is necessary to ensure hemodynamic stability.
- The early involvement of a hematologist
- Continuous monitoring of the coagulation tests will guide the use of blood products.
- Blood products:
  - PRBCs for significant hemorrhage
  - FFP for clotting factor deficiencies
  - Cryoprecipitate infusions to maintain fibrinogen >100 mg/dL
  - Platelet infusions to keep level >20,000/mm³ (without hemorrhage) or >50,000/mm³ (with hemorrhage)
- Pharmacological agents (controversial):
  - Heparin inhibits the activation of the coagulation process. Clinical trials have not shown improved outcomes but may have a role in the management of chronic (thrombotic) DIC.
  - Antithrombin III concentrates are also used to dampen down the process of thrombosis. Trials have shown improvements in the DIC, which haven't translated into improved mortality.
  - Activated Protein C helps to restore the anticoagulation pathway and has been shown to improve mortality in the severest of DIC cases.
  - ε-Aminocaproic acid is an antifibrinolytic agent and can be used in pts who continue to bleed.

ASSESSMENT POINTS

System	Effect	Assessment by HX	PE	Test
HEENT	Bleeding		Bleeding from minor sites of trauma	
CV	Sepsis Hypovolemic shock Microthrombi		Hypotension Signs of ↓ organ perfusion	ECG PAC ECHO
RESP	Bleeding Microthrombi	Dyspnea Hemoptysis	Tachypnea	CXR ABGs
GI	Bleeding Microthrombi	Hematemesis		NG suctioning Stool sample, LFTs, clotting studies
GU	Bleeding microthrombi	Hematuria PU/PV bleeding		Urine output, BUN, creatinine
HEME	Bleeding Consumption of factors and platelets	Hemorrhage		Hb, Plt count, clotting studies, TEG, fibrinogen, D-dimer, ATIII, protein C
CNS	Bleeding Microthrombi		Neurologic deficits	CT
MS	Bleeding Microthrombi		Extremity infarcts	

Key Reference: Levi M. Disseminated intravascular coagulation. *Crit Care Med.* 2007;35:2191–2195.

Perioperative Implications

Preoperative Preparation

- Treat underling cause
- Guided antibiotic therapy
- Correct coagulation where indicated
- Ensure blood product availability

Monitoring

- Routine
- Invasive where indicated by condition
- Serial CBC, coagulation studies and TEG

Airway

- Careful intubation to avoid trauma

Induction

- Consider full stomach
- Consider CV instability in shocked pts

Maintenance

- Resuscitation using invasive monitoring and laboratory tests to guide interventions

Extubation

- Organ dysfunction and/or failure may necessitate a protracted period of mechanical ventilation in an ICU

Adjuvants

- Hepatic and/or renal failure increases the duration of action of most muscle relaxants

Anticipated Problems/Concerns

- Postop management is best conducted in an ICU environment.
- Hemorrhage may continue into the postop period.
- End-organ damage from ischemia inducing microthrombi may indicate prolonged organ support.

Diverticulosis

Nancy C. Wilkes

Risk

- More prevalent in developed countries. Common in the United Kingdom and other parts of northern Europe, North America, Australia, and New Zealand, but uncommon in southern Africa, the Middle East, the Far East, and the Pacific Islands.
- **Prevalence in developing countries between 5–45% depending on age of population and method of diagnosis. African and Asian countries with prevalence around 0.2%.**
- Prevalence increases with age. In USA, seen in less than 5% of pts younger than 40. Approx 30% by age 60, 65% by age 85.
- Low-fiber diet is the highest risk factor. High fat and/or meat diets are high risk.
- Under age 50 y more common in men. Over 50 y more common in women.
- Colonic motility disorders contribute.

Perioperative Risks

- Pts who present with diffuse peritonitis or fail nonoperative management of acute diverticulitis may require emergency surgery.
- Risks may incl full stomach, obstruction, sepsis, and bleeding

Worry About

- 15–25% of pts with diverticulosis will develop diverticulitis.
- Acute diverticulitis may be complicated by abscess, fistula, obstruction, or perforation.
- 15% of individuals with diverticular disease will develop acute GI bleeding. Of those, one third will develop massive bleeding.
- Mortality rates of 22–39% reported for perforation and resultant fecal peritonitis.

Overview

- Multiple saclike herniations through weak points in the intestinal wall. Typically does not contain all layers of the wall but is a herniation of the mucosa and submucosa through the muscle layer.
- Vast majority (>90%) found in the sigmoid colon. Limited to the sigmoid in 65%, approx 25% involving sigmoid and other segments.
- Of pts with significant diverticulosis, 70% remain asymptomatic and without related complications.

ICD-9-CM Code: 562.1 (Colon)

Etiology

- Not completely understood but thought to be related to low-residue diet with long transit time, as opposed to diets with high-fiber content with shorter transit time
- Abnormalities of peristalsis and intestinal dyskinesis may contribute.
- With long transit times, intraluminal pressure increases, colon becomes distended, followed by acute and then chronic inflammation of diverticula

Usual Treatment

- Dietary modification, high-fiber emphasis long term for diverticulosis
- With the development of simple diverticulitis, 75% of cases are not associated with complications. Most are initially treated conservatively with medical therapy (low residue diet and antibiotics). 85% respond quickly, 15% will require surgery.
- Severe abdominal pain, fever, and clinical signs of peritonitis and/or pelvic abscess require initial resuscitation, parenteral antibiotics, and operative intervention.

ASSESSMENT POINTS

System	Effect	Assessment by Hx	PE	Test
CV	Hypotension Tachycardia Hemodynamic instability	Fatigue Weakness Angina	Auscultation	ECG BP Pulm artery catheter
RESP	Hypoxemia	Tachypnea Dyspnea	Auscultation	SpO_2 ABGs CXR
GI	Perforation Obstruction Abscess Fistula Hemorrhage	Abdominal pain N/V Fever Abdominal rigidity Rectal bleeding	Diffuse abdominal tenderness Rebound Absent bowel sounds Abdominal rigidity	Free air under diaphragm if perforation CT scan Ultrasonography
HEME	Anemia, leukocytosis, DIC with sepsis			CBC with differential PT/PTT, FSP, plt count, fibrinogen
RENAL	Colovesicular fistula	May pass air with urine if perforation into urinary bladder		Urinalysis Urine output
CNS	Disorientation with sepsis			

Key Reference: Young-Fadok TM, Sarr MJ. Diverticular disease of the colon. In: Yamada T, et al, ed. *Textbook of gastroenterology.* 4th ed. Lippincott; 2003 [Chapter 87].

Perioperative Implications

Monitoring
- Routine, incl urine output
- With sepsis, monitor arterial pressure; consider PAC monitoring

Maintenance
- Optimize intravascular volume and high O_2 content

Postoperative Period
- Maintain intravascular volume
- Continued monitoring of CV variables and urine volume

Adjuvants
- Antibiotics
- Volume expanders
- Component therapy if DIC develops
- Vasopressor support if required; no interactions

Anticipated Problems/Concerns

- Condition is chronic so flare-ups may occur. Diverticulosis may progress to uncomplicated diverticulitis and evolve to the complicated form (abscess, perforation, obstruction, bleeding, fistula)
- Any surgical intervention and bowel resection would therefore have the anticipated side effects and complications expected from that procedure.

Do Not Resuscitate (DNR) Orders

Alanna E. Goodman

Risk

- Violation of pt autonomy and self-determination if DNR orders aren't reconsidered and honored for the periop period
- Increasing numbers of pts have some form of advance directive
- Approx 15% of surgical pts have DNR orders

Perioperative Considerations

- Resuscitation preferences can change based on pt status and prognosis
- DNR orders do not become automatically suspended or continued when a pt goes to surgery
- Intraop arrests tend to have better outcomes because they are witnessed, acted upon quickly, and are often due to reversible causes
- Pts with DNR orders often undergo vascular access procedures, gastrostomy tube placement, tracheostomy, palliative procedures, repair of pathological fractures, and surgery for emergent conditions (bowel obstruction, appendicitis, etc.)

Worry About

- Ethical and legal obligation to honor and follow pt's wishes as well as provide optimal medical care
- Appropriateness of the DNR order
- Delineation of anesthesia care and resuscitation
- Iatrogenic events
- Intraop deaths
- Liability

Overview

- The Patient Self-Determination Act (1990) was established to allow pts to avoid undesired medical interventions. It requires federally funded healthcare institutions to ask pts about advance directives when admitted and provide information about their right to have one (Medicare and Medicaid are federally funded).

- The 1983 Report of the President's Commission for the Study of Ethical Problems in Medicine justified the "favoring of resuscitation of hospitalized pts with unexpected cardiac arrest"— which conveys implicit pt consent for CPR
- CPR is the only medical intervention that requires an M.D. order to be withheld.
- A DNR order is a limited advance directive which prevents resuscitative intervention in the event of a cardiopulmonary arrest.
- Many pts with DNR orders are terminally ill or have advanced disease.
- Policies should be set in place for re-evaluation of DNR orders for pts requiring surgery. These policies should be institutional, written, unambiguous, and flexible to individual pt needs.
- Anesthesiologists should be familiar with their institution's policies as well as state and federal laws.

ASSESSMENT POINTS

- What are the pts wishes?
- When was the DNR order written/last updated?
- Why was the DNR order initiated?
- Did the pt have a terminal condition?
- Did the pt have correct prognostic information?
- Who discussed/wrote the DNR order with the pt?
- Did the physician influence the decision to have the DNR order?

Key References: *Ethical guidelines for the anesthesia care of patients with Do Not Resuscitate Orders or other directives that limit care.* Park Ridge, IL: American Society of Anesthesiologists; 1993; amended 1998, Ewanchuk M, Brindley PG. Ethics review: Perioperative do-not-resuscitate orders-doing "nothing" when "something" can be done. *Crit Care.* 2006;(4):219–222. Ball A. Do-not-resuscitate orders in surgery: Decreasing the confusion by day. *AORN J.* 2009;89(1). Waisel D, Jackson S, Fine P. Should do-not-resuscitate orders be suspended for surgical cases? *Curr Opin Anesth.* 2003;16:209–214. Waisel D, Burns JP, Johnson J, et al. Guidelines for perioperative do-not-resuscitate policies. *J Clin Anesth.* 2002;14:467–473.

Perioperative Implications

- Review "required reconsideration" of the DNR orders
- All changes to DNR status must be communicated to all members of the periop team and documented in the pt's medical record.
- Best if discussion of DNR orders can be done preop to develop a better pt-doctor relationship, avoid production pressure influences, and to allow time to contact all appropriate parties (surrogate, surgeon, primary care physician).
- This discussion should incl what procedures are essential for the anesthetic and operation (i.e., intubation paralysis, etc.); iatrogenic arrest; and if the DNR order is modified when and if it should be reinstated.
- The document for *Informed Consent for Anesthesia Care in The Patients with An Existing Do-Not-Resuscitate Ord*er created by The American Society of Anesthesiologists Committee on Ethics provides three resuscitation options during the periop time period:
    - Full resuscitation
    - Limited resuscitation: Procedure-directed, documents specific procedures the pt refuses
    - Limited resuscitation: Goal-directed, allows resuscitation if the anesthesiologist and surgeon believe the adverse events are temporary and reversible. Allows resuscitation if the anesthesiologist and surgeon believe the resuscitation efforts support specified and documented goals of the pt
- Consider consultation with an ethics expert if there is disagreement or concern about DNR orders and the surgery isn't emergent.

Anticipated Problems/Concerns

- Anesthesiologists rarely have an established relationship with the DNR pt, but must discuss and clarify resuscitation wishes.
- Aspects of anesthesia care (intubation, vasopressors, IV fluid therapy, transfusion, etc.) are resuscitative therapies.
- Medications used for anesthesia may cause cardiac depression, resp and cardiac arrest
- Anesthesiologists may be morally conflicted with the pt's desire for limited intervention. For a nonemergent case, the anesthesiologist can decide not to perform the anesthetic as long as there is an another available physician and the change is not detrimental to the pt.

Double Aortic Arch

Anthony J. Clapcich

Risk

- Vascular rings account for <1% of CV malformations that require surgical correction; double aortic arch is the most common form of complete ring that encircles both the trachea and the esophagus.
- Race and gender predilection: None

Perioperative Risks

- Recurrent resp infections often aggravate chronic airway obstruction.
- Baseline dynamic tracheal compression can progress to complete airway obstruction upon induction and muscle relaxation.
- Persistent postop airway obstruction requiring prolonged mechanical ventilation and CPAP

Worry About

- Esophageal obstruction: Dysphagia, choking, emesis, aspiration, FTT
- Tracheal obstruction: Chronic cough, wheezing, barky-brassy cry, insp/expiratory stridor; acute episodes of severe resp distress, apnea, cyanosis, ALTE
- Associated cardiac anomalies (10–20%): VSD, ASD, interrupted aortic arch, transposition of the great arteries, tetralogy of Fallot, truncus arteriosis, complex univentricular lesions
- Chromosome 22q11 deletion syndrome (20%): Genetic defect associated with syndromes such as DiGeorge, velocardiofacial, CHARGE, VACTERL; features incl endocrine abnormalities (hypocalce-mia, thyroid/parathyroid dysfunction, short stature), palatal and laryngotracheal abnormalities, developmental delay/neurologic abnormalities, renal tract malformations, thrombocytopenia, T-cell deficiencies, and autoimmune disorders.

Overview

- Vascular rings can be classified as complete or incomplete; double aortic arch is the most common form of complete ring that encircles and compresses both the trachea and esophagus.
- Symptoms usually occur at birth or within the first 3 mo of life; the degree of tracheal and esophageal compression will dictate the severity of resp and GI perturbation.
- Initial work-up with CXR and UGI can reveal tracheal deviation and/or narrowing and proximal esophageal distention/indentation. Once diagnosis suspected, ECHO is used to examine arch anatomy and rule-out other intra-cardiac anomalies. Both MRI and CT are very useful in further delineating vascular, airway, and GI anatomy. Catheterization is now reserved for assessing complex cardiac defects that require additional hemodynamic information. Bronchoscopy is often performed at the time of repair to evaluate the location, degree, and extent of airway obstruction, which may help identify those pts at risk for postop resp compromise.

ICD-9-CM Code: 747.21

Etiology

- During normal human development, the branchial arches are penetrated by paired aortic arches that arise from the aortic sac and terminate in paired dorsal aortae (DA). By the 8th wk, the right DA largely involutes and forms the distal part of the right subclavian artery, leaving only the left DA to form the distal aortic arch and descending aorta. Failure of the right DA to involute results in a double aortic arch, whereby the ascending aortic arch divides into two arches, passes on each side of the trachea and esophagus, and joins posterior to form the descending aorta. The right carotid and subclavian arteries arise from the the usually dominant, posterior right arch, whereas the left carotid and subclavian arteries arise from the smaller, anterior left arch.

Usual Treatment

- Medical therapy: None
- Surgery: The goal is to relieve tracheal and esophageal compression by dividing the vascular ring and dissecting any fibrous bands. A thoracotomy is usually performed on the side ipsilateral to the minor arch: Right (posterior) arch is dominant >75% of cases, thus left posterolateral thoracotomy is commonly used to expose the left (anterior) arch. Video-assisted thoracoscopic repair is also an effective option. Median sternotomy with cardiopulmonary bypass is reserved for cases that require concomitant repair of associated cardiac anomalies.

ASSESSMENT POINTS

System	Effect	Assessment by Hx	PE	Test
HEENT	Chromosome 22q11 Deletion features:		Low set ears, short philtrum, hypertelorism, small mouth, small chin	
	Facial abnormalities	Previous difficulties w/anesthesia or intubation		
	Palatal abnormalities	FTT	Cleft palate	
	Velopharyneal incompetence	Nasal regurgitation of formula; delayed speech/poor articulation (childhood)	Hypernasal speech (childhood)	
	Congenital laryngeal web	Noisy breathing, abnormal cry	Insp/expiratory stridor; aphonia/weak high-pitched cry; hoarseness (childhood)	Flexible bronchoscopy Direct laryngoscopy/bronchoscopy
CV	Depends on presence of associated cardiac anomalies (10–20% cases) None if *only* double aortic arch present	Cyanotic spells, CHF, dyspnea, diaphoresis, FTT	Murmur, cyanosis, 4-limb NIBP discrepancy, grunting, rales/wheezes, hepatosplenomegaly	Pulse oximeter, EKG ECHO Cardiac MRI Cardiac catheterization
RESP	Airway obstruction Recurrent resp infection	Dyspnea, apnea, intermittent cyanosis, ALTE Coughing, wheezing	Insp/Expiratory stridor (+/- positional), hyperextended head, brassy-barky cry, intercostal retractions, nasal flaring	CXR Bronchoscopy MRI CT
GI	Esophageal obstruction	Dysphagia, FTT		UGI Esophagoscopy

Key Reference: Ruzmetov M, et al. Follow-up of surgical correction of aortic arch anomalies causing tracheoesophageal compression: A 38-year single institution experience. *J Pediatr Surg.* 2009;44:1328–1332.

Perioperative Implications

Preoperative Preparation

- O_2 therapy if decreased arterial O_2 saturation present
- Antibiotics for bronchopneumonia

Monitoring

- Bilateral upper extremity pulse oximetry and Doppler probe are useful for assessing subclavian, carotid and temporal pulses during temporary occlusion of the arch that is to be resected.
- Potential for hemodynamic and resp instability warrant placement of arterial catheter; presence of an aberrant subclavian artery may affect appropriate catheter site
- Large-bore IV access is essential; central venous line should be considered for pts with poor vascular access, and those that require extensive repair on CPB.

Airway

- Dynamic and static airway obstruction likely; significant tracheal compression may require smaller ETT size than predicted.

Induction

- Inhalation induction without neuromuscular blockade until airway maintenance is documented by mask and/or ETT is placed distal to area of obstruction.
- Bronchoscopy during spontaneous ventilation allows for direct assessment of tracheal pathology and degree of dynamic airway collapse, thus identifying pts at risk for postop resp compromise.

Maintenance
- Balanced technique of narcotics and volatile agent is usually well-tolerated

Extubation
- Extubation at end of case if tracheomalacia and stenosis absent

Postoperative Period
- Good pain control essential for stable hemodynamics and avoidance of resp complications; IV opioids, rectal acetaminophen, intercostal nerve blocks, one-shot caudal, and caudal epidural catheters have all been used with success.

Anticipated Problems/Concerns

- Despite surgical correction, persistent postop airway obstruction requiring prolonged mechanical ventilation and CPAP can occur secondary to edema, mucosal friability and/or reactivity, and long-segment tracheomalacia.

Down Syndrome

Stephanie Black

Risk

- Incidence in USA: >300,000
- 80% of children with this condition survive beyond 1 y
- Number >50 y will increase by 200% by the year 2010
- Male-female ratio 3:2
- No racial preponderance

Perioperative Risks

- Related to specific abnormalities in individual

Worry About

- Congenital heart disease: 50% born with congenital heart disease (CHD), 8% with cyanotic CHD (usually tetralogy of Fallot)
  - May become profoundly hypoxic with right to left shunting; accidentally injected air bubbles may exit into systemic circulation (coronary and cerebral air emboli)
  - Adults less likely to have CAD
- Upper airway obstruction
  - Soft tissue obstruction of upper airway common immediately on induction of GA due to large tongue, small mandible, short neck
- Subglottic stenosis is present in 20–25% and of particular concern in children
- Obstructive and central sleep apnea
- Cervical extension during intubation can cause neurologic symptoms (neck pain, arm pain, upper extremity weakness, torticollis)
- Generalized joint laxity; TMJ may sublux with jaw thrust
- Endocrine: hypothyroidism (4–6% in children; 15–20% in adults), hypothermia, obesity (difficult IV access)
- Mental retardation
  - May have overwhelming fears of unknown
  - Can become physically resistant to entering OR
  - Alzheimer's disease and other forms of mental illness (depression, psychosis) may co-exist

Overview

- Not a disease
- Incidence decreased by prenatal screening and elective termination of pregnancy

- Wide variation in abilities and disabilities; neurologic development enhanced by external stimulation
- Institutionalized individuals have high incidence of seropositivity for hepatitis B
- More people living in group homes in community and becoming more self-sufficient in ADL

ICD-9-CM Code: 758.00

Etiology

- Genetic: trisomy 21
- Risk of parenting a Down syndrome fetus greatest in older (>35 y) parents (well characterized in mothers)

Usual Treatment

- Depends on pathophysiology

ASSESSMENT POINTS

System	Effect	Assessment by Hx	PE	Test
HEENT	Large tongue Subglottic stenosis Hearing deficit in 66%	Hx of snoring Sleep apnea Intubation Hx		Audiology
CV	Tetralogy of Fallot in 4%	Sx of CHF "Tet spells"	Cyanosis Murmur	ECHO
ENDO	Hypothyroidism Obesity	Hypothermia	Obesity	
MS	Subluxation of C1/C2 Joint laxity			Cervical spine radiographs (controversy over whether these should be routine)

Key Reference: Mitchell V, Howard R, Facer E: Down's syndrome and anaesthesia. *Paediatr Anaesth.* 1995; 5:379–384.

Perioperative Implications

Monitoring
- Temperature (hypothermia)
- ECG (arrhythmias, ischemia); treat bradycardia from halothane or sevoflurane

Airway
- Have variety of alternative airway management devices available (e.g., oral and nasal airways, laryngeal mask, Bullard laryngoscope)
- Avoid neck extension during laryngoscopy if possible

- Smaller endotracheal tube may be necessary for narrowed subglottic space

Vascular Access
- Allow more time for IV placement
- Meticulously avoid injected air

Patient Management
- Soft, warm, kind, patient approach along with caregiver known to patient to help with initial management; warm, quiet OR

Anticipated Problems/Concerns

- Hypoxia if right to left shunting develops
- Resistance to separation from caregiver
- Life-threatening upper airway obstruction with difficult vascular access
- Spinal cord ischemia with neurologic damage

Drug Abuse, Lysergic Acid Diethylamide (LSD)

Eric Gewirtz

Risk

- True prevalence of LSD use impossible to determine.
- People began using it for recreational and spiritual purpose in 1960s. LSD is still illegally used as a major hallucinogen worldwide.
- LSD-related hospital visits remain low compared with those related to other major illicit drugs.

Perioperative Risks

- Acute intoxication has evidence of sympathetic nervous system stimulation incl mydriasis, increase body temp, systemic Htn, tachycardia, anxiety, agitation, vomiting, aspiration, apnea, and unrecognized injuries.
- May prolong succinylcholine neuromuscular blockade and delay metabolism of ester local anesthetics (speculated inhibition of plasma cholinesterase).
- May potentiate analgesics.

Worry About

- Systemic: Htn, tachycardia, hyperthermia, hyperglycemia, salivation, nausea, vomiting, seizures, and apnea
- Psychiatric: Hallucinations (visual, auditory, and tactile), labile mood, acute panic attacks, agitation, and hypertonia

Overview

- Lysergic acid diethylamide (LSD) is a semi-synthetic product of lysergic acid, a natural substance from the parasitic rye fungus *Claviceps purpurea*
- LSD is physiologically well tolerated, psychological complications result from overdose or uncontrolled use by layman
- There is high degree of psychological dependence but no evidence of physical dependence or withdrawal symptoms when acutely discontinued.
- Classified under Schedule I of the Controlled Substance Act

- Psychologic effects begin in 30–60 min and may last 8–12 hr

ICD-9-CM Code: 305.3

Etiology

- Mechanism of action is still unknown. Stimulation of sympathetic and parasympathetic system, central stimulation of sympathetic system, activation of higher cortical centers causes typical clinical effects.

Usual Treatment

- Supportive reassurance, transfer pt to calm, quiet area with minimum external stimuli
- Benzodiazepines seem to be the most effective agents for treating LSD psychosis and visual disturbances
- Rare cases require hemodynamic control, intubation, ventilatory and supportive care

ASSESSMENT POINTS

System	Effect	Assessment by Hx	PE
HEENT			Dilated, reactive pupils
CV	Sympathetic nervous system stimulation	Palpitations Sweating	Htn Tachycardia
RESP	No consistent changes	Diaphoresis	Tachypnea, apnea
ENDO	Hyperglycemia Mild hyperthermia		Elevated body temperature
CNS	Euphoria Anxiety, labile mood Tremors Visual hallucinations and illusions Synesthesia Distorted sense of time	Hx of drug ingestion	Altered mental status Hypertonia

Key Reference: Passie T, Halpern JH, Stichtenoth DO, Emrich HM, Hintzen A. The pharmacology of lysergic acid diethylamide: A review. *CNS Neurosci Ther.* 2008;14(4):295–314.

Perioperative Implications

Preoperative Preparation
- Rule out associated traumatic injury
- Hemodynamic control
- Aspiration prophylaxis
- Sedation if agitation is severe

Monitoring
- Temp
- Neuromuscular blockade

Airway
- Aspiration risk

Preinduction/Induction
- Salivation, N/V, which may warrant rapid sequence induction

- Ketamine should be avoided, which may have synergic effects with LSD
- Succinylcholine should be avoided
- Exaggerated response to endogenous and exogenous catecholamines

Maintenance
- Maintain normothermia

Extubation
- At risk for aspiration
- Continue supportive reassurance

Adjuvants
- May have exaggerated response to sympathomimetic agents

- Theoretical potential for ester local anesthetic toxicity due to inhibition of plasma cholinesterase activity
- Theoretical potential for prolongation of succinylcholine neuromuscular blockade due to inhibition of plasma cholinesterase activity

Anticipated Problems/Concerns

- Avoid injuries associated with agitation
- Possible concomitant drug and/or alcohol use by pt

Drug Overdose, Rat Poison (Warfarin Toxicity)

Michelle Braunfeld

Risk

- Major risk is hemorrhage, esp CNS or GI.
- Incidence: Risk of hemorrhage in 1.0%-7.4% of pts chronically anticoagulated. Risk is dose-related and proportional to PT prolongation. Risk of hemorrhage doubles as INR increases from 2.0-2.9 to 3.0-4.4. It further quadruples as INR increases from 3.0-4.4 to 4.5-6.9. (2) Age is associated with increased sensitivity to warfarin and increased incidence of bleeding complications.
- Rx for DVT, cerebral vessel atherosclerosis, prosthetic heart valves, mitral stenosis, paroxysmal atrial fibrillation.

Perioperative Risks

- Bleeding
- Drugs that potentiate anticoagulant effects: Antibiotics (esp metronidazole, sulfonamides, cephalosporins), NSAIDs, phenytoin, cimetidine, barbiturates, alcohol

Worry About

- Bleeding complications of invasive procedures
- Drug interactions

- Transient protein C deficiency preceding effect on procoagulant levels at initiation of warfarin therapy leading to thrombotic complications
- True poisoning with rodenticides (so-called super-warfarins) may result in prolonged clotting abnormality with abnormal PT values weeks to months post event because of the enormously long half-lives of these drugs

Overview/Pharmacology

- Vitamin K antagonist.
- Cleared by hepatic and renal transformation and excretion. $T_{1/2}$ is ~40 hr. Duration of action is 2–5 d.
- Onset of effect is delayed by 8–12 hr because of time required to clear already synthesized clotting factors. For similar reasons, peak effect of a dose occurs 48 hrs post-administration.

ICD-9-CM Code: 286.9 (Coagulation defect)

Drug Class, Mechanism of Action, Usual Dose

- Blocks vitamin K–mediated carboxylation of factors II, VII, IX, X (procoagulants); protein C, protein S (anticoagulants)

- Carboxylation of coagulation factors oxidizes vitamin K. The vitamin K epoxide must be reduced to become active again. Coumarin anticoagulants block reduction of the epoxide. Thus, large and/or repeat doses of vitamin K are needed for large overdoses or for long-acting forms
- Chronically taken for systemic anticoagulation for DVT, CVA, prosthetic valves, and atrial fibrillation either paroxysmal or associated with mitral stenosis
- Usual doses: Loading regimen varies, but maintenance dose is 2.5–10 mg/d
- Alternatives: None. An oral direct thrombin inhibitor investigated as a possible alternative to warfarin, ximelagatran, was withdrawn from distribution in 2006 because of hepatotoxicity. Heparin is drug of choice for acute anticoagulation, but must be given parenterally, usually as loading dose with an infusion

ASSESSMENT POINTS

System	Effect	Assessment by Hx	PE	Test
HEME	Abnormal levels of factor II, IV, IX, X, and protein C, protein S	Easy bruising, prolonged bleeding time	Ecchymoses	PT

Key Reference: Wiedermann CJ, Stockner I. Warfarin-induced bleeding complications—clinical presentation and therapeutic options. *Thromb Res.* 2008;122(suppl 2):S13–S18.

Possible Drug Interactions

Preoperative

- Increased effect: Antibiotics, NSAIDs, oral hypoglycemic, diazepam, cimetidine, diuretics, phenytoin
- Decreased effect: Methylxanthines, rifampin, antihistamines, corticosteroids, barbiturates
- Major surgical procedures warrant discontinuation of drug 1–3 d preop with a target PT within 20% of nl range. Alternatively, pt may be admitted 1–2 d prior to surgery. Warfarin is discontinued and heparin therapy instituted. Heparin is discontinued 6 hr prior to surgery
- For emergency surgery, pt may be given 10–20 mL/kg of FFP and 5–10 mg of vitamin K, with additional amounts of both given as needed

Adjuvants/Regional Anesthesia/Reversal

- Regional block: Relatively contraindicated without reversal of anticoagulation
- Peripheral block: Relatively contraindicated without reversal of anticoagulation

Anticipated Problems/Concerns

- Relatively minor surgical procedures may be performed without reversal of warfarin anticoagulation.
- The appropriate use of prothrombin concentrate complex (PCC) therapy for warfarin toxicity is controversial. PCC contains a combination of factors II, VII, IX, and X, and are given at a dose of 25–50 U/kg. Benefits incl smaller infusion volumes, no need for blood group testing, the fact that it is a virally inactivated product, and higher levels of factor IX compared to FFP. Evidence for significantly more rapid and more complete correction of INR with the use of PCC versus FFP in the setting of intracranial hemorrhage.
- Recommendation in the European Stroke Initiative guidelines to preferentially use PCC rather than FFP in the setting of warfarin-associated intracranial hemorrhage.

- Not all PCC formulations are identical. There may be relative factor VII deficiency, requiring concurrent VII administration. PCC also generally considered thrombogenic, although newer formulations may incl the coagulation inhibitors Protein C and Protein S.
- rFVIIa has also been reported to successfully correct INR in the setting of warfarin toxicity. The existing literature contains case reports and case series that describe administration of 20–135 ucg/kg of rFVIIa in various clinical settings, leading to correction of INR.
- Hypothermia will potentiate anticoagulant effect.

Duchenne Muscular Dystrophy (Pseudohypertrophic Muscular Dystrophy)

Stephanie Black
Richard I. Cook

Risk

- Males, 1/3500; few known cases in females
- Often undiagnosed until age 3–5 y
- Deterioration through puberty to death usually before age 25 y

Perioperative Risks

- Resp failure, prolonged mechanical ventilation
- Muscle weakness

Worry About

- Poor cardiac function, dilated cardiomyopathy, cardiac arrhythmias, MVP
- Poor resp function, pulm Htn from chronic sleep apnea, scoliosis
- Aspiration risk (gastroparesis)
- Hyperkalemic arrest with succinylcholine and some volatile agents
- Assoc with malignant hyperthermia-like syndrome
- Poor long-term prognosis

Overview

- Most boys die from pneumonia but CHF is also seen in the later stages
- Gradual onset of muscle wasting, eventually replaced by fat causing pseudohypertrophy
- Hyperkalemic response to depolarizing NMBs may develop years before the onset of DMD symptoms. The infant may appear entirely normal, with only mild gross motor delay.
- Increased sensitivity to nondepolarizing NM blockers
- Use of Ca^{2+}-channel blocker (e.g., verapamil) may prolong or even cause NMB.
- Up to a quarter of pts may have mitral valve prolapse.
- Resting tachycardia common; cardiac involvement in 70% of cases, cardiac debilitation usually late

ICD-9-CM Code: 359.1

Etiology

- X-linked recessive disease; the muscles (incl myocardium) are gradually replaced with fat and connective tissue. The defect is in the muscle cell membrane protein *dystrophin*.

Usual Treatment

- Corticosteroids have shown some promise by increasing strength and delaying progression.
- Spinal rodding and fusion, often with AP approach, for the scoliosis that begins at 10–12 y can prolong comfort and ease of wheelchair use. Pulm deterioration continues, and life may be only minimally prolonged.
- Tendon releases for contractures
- Exploratory laparotomy for ileus

ASSESSMENT POINTS

System	Effect	Assessment by Hx	PE	Test
CARDIO	Conduction Contractile force	Tachycardia Difficult (Hx CHF Sx: Orthopnea, DOE, PND)	Opening snap (MVP) CHF signs	ECG, 24-hr ambulatory ECG, ECHO, MUGA
RESP	↓ Volume and flows Sleep apnea/pulm Htn	SOB Snoring, apneic spells	Unreliable Unreliable	PFTs SaO$_2$ on RA, sleep study ECHO
GI	Dysmotility, gastric dilatation, paralytic ileus			
GU	Bladder paralysis, impotence			
CNS	↓ IQ		Mental status exam	
MS	Scoliosis, kyphosis Contractures Muscle destruction Macroglossia Poor IV access	Progressive weakness		Spine films Abn myogram Elevated CK levels

Key Reference: Birnkrant DJ, et al: American College of Chest Physicians consensus statement on the respiratory and related management of patient with Duchenne muscular dystrophy undergoing anesthesia or sedation. *Chest.* 2007;132:1977–1986.

Perioperative Implications

Preoperative Preparation

- Avoid or limit preprocedure sedation.

Monitoring

- Consider PA catheter and/or TEE based on EF and surgical procedure.
- Nerve stimulator

Induction

- Succinylcholine contraindicated because of hyperkalemia
- Avoid volatile anesthetics 2° to MH-like response.
- Avoid depressants of cardiac contractility.
- Consider long gastric emptying times, possible full stomach.

Maintenance

- Variable response to NM blockers; titrate to effect
- Consider a total IV anesthesia approach.
- Regional or neuraxial anesthesia when possible over GA
- Recommended to allow spontaneous recovery, as response to reversal agents varies
- Avoid hypoxemia, large fluid shifts, and anemia to prevent uncompensated cardiomyopathy

Emergence

- Potential for prolonged ventilator dependence greatest when vital capacity <30% of predicted
- For GA cases consider extubating directly to BIPAP and/or CPAP, weaning later

- Late resp depression reported (cause unclear); may make outpatient surgery inadvisable

Anticipated Problems/Concerns

- Resp failure
- CHF
- Supraventricular tachydysrhythmias
- Rhabdomyolysis, hyperkalemia, and cardiac arrest in response to succinylcholine and volatile agents have been described in boys years before clinical signs of DMD present.

Duodenal Atresia

Lynne G. Maxwell

Risk

- Incidence 1/10,000–40,000 live births
- M:F incidence is equal
- 20–30% have trisomy 21
- 45% are premature infants of pregnancy complicated by polyhydramnios
- Mortality 10%, due not to duodenal atresia but to associated CHD or prematurity

Perioperative Risks

- Hypoxemia associated with immature lungs
- Hypoxemia due to CHD, persistent fetal circulation

Worry About

- Ventilation problems associated with prematurity

- Other associated anomalies in 50% of cases: Esophageal atresia (7%), other intestinal atresias, renal anomalies (5%), malrotation of the gut (25%), volvulus, imperforate anus (3%), annular pancreas (25%)
- CHD associated with trisomy 21 (ASD, VSD, AV canal)
- Aspiration on induction of anesthesia 2° to bowel obstruction
- May be associated with cystic fibrosis
- Late presentation can be associated with dehydration, hypovolemia, and hypochloremic alkalosis

Overview

- Frequently premature infant of pregnancy complicated by polyhydramnios

- Vomiting after birth: May be copious and bile stained
- Flat abdomen
- Dx is made by "double bubble" on abdominal x-ray

ICD-9-CM Code: 751.1 (Atresia, small intestine)

Etiology

- Unknown in sporadic cases
- More common in trisomy 21

Usual Treatment

- Surgical repair is curative
- Surgical technique may be open laparotomy or laparascopic

ASSESSMENT POINTS

System	Effect	Assessment by Hx	PE	Test
CV	CHD—ASD, VSD, AV canal, Persistent fetal circulation	Trisomy 21	Murmur Cyanosis	ECHO CXR Pulse oximetry
RESP	Resp distress syndrome of prematurity	Polyhydramnios Gestational age <36 wk	Tachypnea Retractions Flaring Grunting	CXR Pulse oximetry
GI	Duodenal obstruction Associated esophageal atresia	Bilious vomiting No gas in abdomen	Scaphoid abdomen	Abdominal x-ray Unable to pass OG tube
RENAL	Structural anomalies		Palpation of kidneys	Abdominal US

Key Reference: Murshed R, Nicholls G, Spitz L. Intrinsic duodenal obstruction: Trends in management and outcome over 45 years (1951–1995) with relevance to prenatal counselling. *Br J Obstet Gynaecol.* 1999;106:1197–1199.

Perioperative Implications

Preoperative Preparation

- OG tube to decompress stomach, reduce gastric contents
- IV catheter placement with hydration (20 mL/kg NS) if diagnosis delayed beyond 24–48 hr; correct electrolyte abnormalities
- Surfactant for premature infants with significant lung disease
- Confirm intramuscular vitamin K given as part of normal newborn care

Monitoring

- Arterial monitoring for ABGs, electrolyte, and Hgb determination only in premature infants with significant lung disease, those with CHD, or those with extreme dehydration due to protracted vomiting; otherwise NIBP sufficient as minimal blood loss expected
- Temperature
- Urinary catheter (small feeding tube) may be helpful in assessing adequacy of fluid resuscitation
- Pulse oximetry, ECG, and end-tidal carbon dioxide and gas monitoring

Anesthetic Technique

- Suction OG tube with infant supine and in left and right decubitus positions prior to induction, intubation
- Awake intubation after preoxygenation only for actively vomiting, volume-depleted infants with abnormal airway anatomy
- Rapid-sequence induction after preoxygenation for normovolemic pts with normal airway anatomy
- Avoid N_2O to prevent intestinal distention

- Nondepolarizing muscle relaxant helpful for surgical exposure
- Second peripheral IV after induction

Airway

- Precautions to prevent aspiration
- Abnormal airway anatomy unlikely

Preinduction/Induction

- Pt may be hypovolemic due to vomiting, poor feeding
- Correct dehydration, hypochloremic alkalosis (failure to do so can shift oxyhemoglobin dissociation curve to left and reduce O_2 delivery to tissues)
- De-bubble IV lines to prevent paradoxical air embolism
- Type-specific blood available for transfusion—rarely needed

Maintenance

- Mechanical pressure ventilation with rate 15–20, PIP 20–25, PEEP 2-5 to achieve adequate ventilation (tidal volume 8–10 mL/kg)
- Air/O_2 mixture to achieve O_2 saturation 92–96%, although some use 100% O_2 to provide reserve; data on retinopathy of prematurity due to operative exposure to 100% O_2 is not conclusive, and surgical retraction may restrict ventilation and cause atelectasis, which can cause desaturation
- Surgical retraction/pressure on liver may decrease venous return and cause hypotension
- Hemorrhage and/or air or carbon dioxide embolus has been reported prior to or after trochar insertion when laparoscopic technique is used; this may result in CV collapse requiring CPR. Resuscitation drugs should be available.

- Cease insufflation of abdomen and evacuate gas from abdomen, left side down/Trendelenburg, 100% O_2, fluid administration, epinephrine bolus, cardiac compression if no cardiac output
- Fentanyl or remifentanil/pancuronium or vecuronium/isoflurane or sevoflurane for premature infants
- In full-term infants who may be immediately extubatable, consider caudal catheter threaded to low thoracic position. Dose with bupivacaine 0.25% (or ropivacaine 0.2%) with 1:200,000 epinephrine 0.5–0.75 mL/kg followed by continuous epidural infusion of 0.1% bupivacaine or ropivacaine at 0.2 mL/kg/hr for postop pain relief

Extubation

- May require postop ventilation if pt premature or has CHD
- Full-term infants with effective epidural anesthetic and no or low-dose opioid administration may be extubated if effective spontaneous ventilation

Anticipated Problems/Concerns

- Prematurity/resp distress syndrome/apnea
- CHD
- Hemorrhage, air, or gas embolus may occur at start of laparoscopic procedure
- Risk of aspiration may continue postop—leave OG or NG tube in place
- Later risk of GE reflux higher than normal (17%)
- Adequate fluid replacement
- Other associated anomalies

Echinococcosis

James M. Riopelle
Andrew Hemphill

Risk (Epidemiology)

- Men ≈ women
- *Echinococcus granulosus* causes *cystic* echinococcosis (*hydatid* disease) in people exposed to feces of dogs and other canids in endemic areas of nearly every continent.
- *E. multilocularis* causes *alveolar* echinococcus in people exposed to feces of infected foxes living in colder regions of the northern hemisphere.
- *E. vogeli* and *E. oligarthrus* cause *polycystic* echinococcocis in people exposed to feces of infected dogs and wild carnivores in rural Central- and South America.

Perioperative Risks

- Hydatid cyst rupture leads to anaphylaxis and spread of encapsulated organisms, which implant in exposed tissues (e.g., peritoneal cavity), later causing disseminated hydatidosis (bowel obstruction, cachexia, death)
- Failure to resect all echinococcal tissue due to microscopic or extensive disease extension
- Hemorrhage (if cyst attached to liver or major blood vessel)
- Systemic reactions to toxic agents instilled into cyst cavity; air embolism if cyst attached to a vein or hydrogen peroxide instilled into cyst cavity
- Postop jaundice, cholangitis, bacterial superinfection, vascular compression, hepatic failure

Overview and Etiology

- Parasitic disease caused by organism classified as flatworm (adult stage). Parasite cycles through 4 different stages (adult tapeworm, egg, oncosphere, metacestode) each adapted to maximize survival in the 2 host organisms:
    - *Definitive host:* Carnivore; intestines contain adult flatworms releasing eggs into feces.
    - *Intermediate host:* Herbivore/omnivore (sheep, small rodents, man); ingests minute amount of feces of definitive host, eggs hatch in stomach and release *oncospheres* (first larval stage), which penetrate gut blood vessels and distribute to potentially any organ, esp liver and lung. Develop into slowly expanding fluid-filled cysts (*metacestodes*). Inner (*germinal*) layer of metacestode buds off tiny encapsulated *protoscolices* [Gk: juvenile heads] which accumulate to form *hydatid sand*.
- A definitive host eats infected organs of intermediate host; protoscolices are released into intestinal lumen; these evaginate; anterior parts attach to intestinal epithelium and become adult tapeworms.

Adult *E. granulosus* (2–11 mm) inhabits small intestine of canid (dog, wolf, coyote, dingo, jackal); eggs distribute to grass eaten by sheep, goats, camels, yaks, cattle, pigs, horses, marsupials; man becomes infected via hand→oral contact with fecally-contaminated object. Cysts of volume up to 1000 mL form within intermediate host (or man—sometimes called *dead end host*), physically compromising organ function.

Adult *E. multilocularis* (1-5 mm) inhabits small intestine of fox (occasionally dog, bush dog, rarely cat); intermediate host usually a rodent. Cysts become multiple and invade target organs.

E. vogeli and *E. oligarthrus* rarely cause human disease (if present of polycystic type).

ICD-9-CM Codes: 122.0—122.9 (depending on parasite species and organ affected)

Usual Treatment

- *Echinococcus granulosus*
    - Medical: (cyst instillation with non-specific histotoxic solution—hypertonic NaCl, alcohol, silver nitrate, povidine-iodine, formaldehyde, hydrogen peroxide, chlorhexidine) in sequence of puncture, aspiration, injection, reaspiration (PAIR). Not appropriate if cysts multiple, cyst architecture subdivided into *daughter cysts*, or cysts balloon out via narrow passages to form *satellite cysts*. Increasing in popularity; complications incl biliocutaneous fistula, bacterial superinfection of residual cyst cavity. Technique variants incl percutaneous evacuation (sometimes using cutting-aspiration device), cyst catheterization/continuous irrigation
    - Laparoscopic: Cystotomy, toxin irrigation, partial cystectomy (± use of aspirator-grinder)
    - Open: Complete resection for concealed, extensive, or invasive disease; attempt to avoid spilling contents; histotoxic solutions often used in conjunction
- *Echinococcus multilocularis*
    - Radical open surgical resection if possible; liver transplantation considered if disease confined to liver. Prevent recurrence by treating infected family companion animals with oral anthelmintic, praziquantel.

ASSESSMENT POINTS

System	Effect	Assessment by Hx	PE	Test
GEN		Pt from endemic area, fever, itching, family Hx	Fever—if high, possible superinfection	US, CT, or MRI imaging of any part of body
GI	Liver mass (70%), biliary obstruction	Abdominal pain dyspepsia, vomiting fatigue; previous surgery for same disease	Jaundice; signs of cirrhosis	Abdominal US, CT or MRI; PT/ INR
RESP	Lung mass (20%) bronchial obstruction, pulm Htn	Chest pain, cough, SOB, hemoptysis	Fever (superinfection)	CXR; thoracic US, CT, or MRI; sputum microscopy for protoscolices
RENAL	Ureteral obstruction			Abdominal US, CT, MRI
HEME	Eosinophilia, antibodies	Duration of albendazole therapy (marrow toxicity)		CBC, eosinophil count; plt count; antibody-based tests (e.g., ELISA), newer DNA-based tests: problems with cross-reactivity, false negativity
CV	Obstruction, anaphylaxis			Echocardiography
GYN	Incidental occurrence	Last menstrual period	Signs of pregnancy	Blood or urine pregnancy test
CNS	Cyst (1.5%)	Seizure	Localizing neurologic findings, gait abnormality, hydrocephalus	Head CT, MRI

Key Reference: Junghanss T, da Silva AM, Horton J, et al. Clinical management of cystic Echinococcosis: State of the art, problems, and perspectives. *Am J Trop Med Hyg.* 2008;79:301–311.

Perioperative Implications

Preoperative Preparation

- Review all imaging studies.
- Ensure entire surgical team aware of nature of disease.
- If liver disease, OR table capable of intraop cholangiography; if cirrhosis, normalize coagulation status (vitamin K, ffp); ensure intraop availability of prbc (possibly ffp, platelets, cryoprecipitate).
- Know anatomic extent of disease, proposed surgical approach (position, laparoscopy/incision); know backup plan if disease more extensive than thought.
- Pt to take oral benzamidazole anthelminthic (albendazole)1 week preop, 3 mo postop.

Monitoring

- Based on planned/potential procedure
- Consider urinary catheter; if possibly extensive, consider invasive hemodynamic monitoring (art line, cent line), serial hct/coag/abg, precordial Doppler or TEE to diagnose embolism (air, CO_2, cyst contents), serial Na^+ if hypertonic NaCl used
- Observe for SQ emphysema if laparoscopic approach

Airway

- Tracheal intubation for laparoscopic or open procedure. Double-lumen tube to protect non-diseased lung if pulm echinococcosis

Induction

- Rx choice based on general health status and concurrent diseases

Maintenance

- Large-bore venous access and fluid warmer(s) if hemorrhage risk
- Consider gastric tube (whether laparoscopic or open)
- Immobile operative field essential, esp during portions of procedure where cyst spillage could occur
- Have on-hand in case of anaphylactic or hemorrhagic shock: Epinephrine, vasopressin, other inotrope/vasopressor, $CaCl_2$, and $NaHCO_3$, adequate crystalloid/colloid/blood products.
- If gas embolism suspected, aspirate central line; if none, consider subcostal insertion of spinal needle attached to large aspirating syringe directly into right ventricle.

Extubation

- Base on usual criteria, extent of operative procedure, pt age/physical condition, concurrent disease

Postoperative Period

- Base pain control plan on nature and extent of resection; regional anesthesia an option if coagulation status permits
- Base monitoring on extent of resection, blood loss, preop health status

- Watch for pneumothorax, subphrenic abscess, pneumonia, bronchobiliary fistula, jaundice, hepatic failure, septicemia

Anticipated Problems/Concerns

- If the pt is being treated in a non-endemic area, surgical team may be unfamiliar with disease; anthelmintic medications may require special order well in advance of procedure.

- Consider *Echinococcus* in any pt from endemic area presenting for surgical excision of cyst; search for others using US imaging; consider ID consult, serolologic testing
- Arrange US imaging in family/neighbors/farm animals capable of being intermediate hosts
- Examine stool of companion canids for eggs/segments.

Eclampsia

Emily Baird

Risk

- Incidence 0.01–0.1 % in developed countries
- 90% of women with eclampsia have accompanying manifestations of severe preeclampsia
- Risk factors incl age <20 y old, nulliparity, and multiple gestations

Perioperative Risks

- Eclampsia is a factor in up to 10% of all maternal deaths in developed countries.
- Maternal complications incl pulm aspiration, pulm edema, cerebral vascular accident, cerebral hemorrhage, acute renal failure, and cardiopulmonary arrest.
- Fetal complications incl placental abruption, severe prematurity, and intrauterine growth restriction.

Worry About

- Risk of pulm aspiration and hypoxemia with seizure.
- Fetal bradycardia may occur during or following seizure activity.

- Eclampsia often occurs with severe preeclampsia and its associated complications.

Overview

- Occurrence of seizure activity or unexplained coma during pregnancy or postpartum in a woman without a pre-existing neurologic disorder
- Eclamptic convulsions can occur antepartum, intrapartum, or postpartum.
- Onset of eclampsia is generally preceded by signs of severe pre-eclampsia but 10–15% present without Htn and/or proteinuria.

ICD-9-CM Code: 642.6

Etiology

- Etiology unknown: Two prevailing theories
- Forced dilation theory: The presence of blood pressures exceeding the upper limit of cerebral autoregulation leads to vasodilation and subsequent hyperperfusion and interstitial edema.

- Vasospasm theory: Severe acute Htn causes cerebral overregulation with resultant ischemia, infarction, and cytotoxic edema.

Usual Treatment

- Establish patent airway and ensure maternal oxygenation
- Prophylaxis against further seizure activity with magnesium sulfate (4–6 g bolus over 20 min followed by 1–2 g/hr infusion)
- BP management with labetalol (10 to 20 mg IV) and hydralazine (5 to 10 mg IV)
  - Severe Htn associated with an increased risk of cerebral hemorrhage
  - Maintain CPP (MAP – ICP) to avoid further neurologic injury
- Expeditious (preferably vaginal) delivery via induction or augmentation of labor
  - Immediately delivery indicated with persistent fetal bradycardia

ASSESSMENT POINTS

System	Effect	Assessment by Hx	PE	Test
CV	Htn LV dysfunction	Dyspnea, peripheral edema	Htn, peripheral edema	ECHO if suspect LV dysfunction
RESP	Airway edema Pulm edema	Snoring, stridor Dyspnea, orthopnea	Tachypnea, dyspnea, rales	CXR ABG
RENAL	Proteinuria Renal failure	Rapid wt gain, decreased urine output	Nondependent edema	24 hr urine protein, BUN, Cr, urine acid
HEME	Thrombocytopenia DIC	Mucosal bleeding, easy bruising	Petechiae, bleeding from puncture sites	Hgb, Hct, Plt, fibrinogen, and FSP
NEURO	Seizure Coma	Headache, visual disturbances	Hyperexcitability, hyperreflexia	CT/MRI if focal deficits or prolonged coma
FETUS	Fetal distress			Fetal heart monitor

Key Reference: Schneider MC, Landau R, Mörtl MG. New insights in hypertensive disorders of pregnancy. *Curr Opin Anaesthesiol.* 2001;14(3):291–297.

Perioperative Implications

Monitoring

- Standard maternal monitors incl non-invasive BP, pulse oximetry, and urine output
  - Invasive pressures indicated if (1) maternal BP poorly controlled; (2) need for frequent blood sampling; or (3) infusion of rapid-acting vasodilators (nitroprusside or nitroglycerin)
  - Pre-eclampsia/eclampsia is *not* an indication for invasive central monitoring
- Electronic fetal heart monitoring

Regional Anesthesia for Labor and Delivery

- Early epidural decreases likelihood of airway manipulation in the setting of emergency cesarean delivery and increases uteroplacental perfusion.
- Coagulation studies, as outlined above, should be checked prior to both placement *and* removal of epidural catheter.

- Because of increased risk of pulm edema, IV hydration prior to neuraxial anesthesia *not* recommended
- Pts may display greater sensitivity to vasopressors—systemic and neuraxial administration of vasopressors should be used with caution
- Neuraxial anesthesia preferable to general anesthesia for cesarean delivery

General Anesthesia for Cesarean Delivery

- Potential for difficult intubation secondary to airway edema
- Htn that may accompany laryngoscopy increases the risk of intracranial hemorrhage and pulm edema
- Induction with propofol or thiopental will terminate seizures and reduce $CMRO_2$ and CBF
- Magnesium increases the duration and potency of non-depolarizing muscle relaxants
- Avoid hypercarbia, which lowers seizure threshold

- Maintain CPP (MAP – ICP) and avoid hypoxia, hyperthermia, and hyperglycemia to prevent further neurologic injury

Postoperative Period

- Continue magnesium infusion for 24 hr after delivery and/or last convulsion
- Increased risk of pulm edema as extracellular fluid is mobilized leading to increased intravascular volume
- Most eclamptic pts have complete resolution of neurologic abnormalities

Anticipated Problems/Concerns

- 10% will have recurrent seizures in the absence of initial prophylaxis with initial seizure
- Eclamptic seizures can occur up to 4 wk postpartum
- Cerebral hemorrhage accounts for 15–20% of deaths from eclampsia

Eisenmenger's Syndrome

Inna Maranets

Risk

- 8% of all congenital heart disease (CHD) pts
- 11% of pts with intracardiac or aortopulmonary shunt allowing continuous exposure of pulm vasculature to systemic arterial pressure
- VSD is the most common lesion

Perioperative Risks

- High risk of CV complications when undergo non-cardiac surgery, mortality reaching 30%
- Severity of pulm Htn, cyanosis, tricuspid regurgitation and right ventricular dysfunction are important factors
- Additional acquired cardiac and systemic diseases, such as CAD and renal dysfunction
- Underlying pathology, urgency, duration of surgery and anesthetic choice contribute to the risk
- Bleeding due to platelet dysfunction
- Mortality rate of pts with ES carrying pregnancy to viability is 27–30%, most often at delivery or postpartum
- Fetal risks: ↑ Risk of preterm labor, intrauterine growth retardation; fetal demise of 75%
- C-section carries higher mortality: 70% versus 30% for vaginal delivery

Worry About

- R—L shunt, pulm Htn, right and left ventricular failure, hypoxemia, polycythemia
- Minor decrease in SBP can cause increase in R—L shunt, decrease pulm blood flow, hypoxia, and cardiovascular collapse
- Increased blood viscosity can lead to thromboembolic phenomena, paradoxical emboli, hemoptysis
- Arrhythmias, ventricular and supraventricular
- May not tolerate positive pressure ventilation
- Decreasing systemic vascular resistance of pregnancy worsens R—L shunt

- Inability to meet increasing demand for O_2 with gestation and labor
- Delivery produces autotransfusion with RV failure
- Excessive bleeding with previous heparinization
- Postpartum increase in PVR

Overview

- Eisenmenger's syndrome is defined as pulm Htn at systemic level due to high pulm vascular resistance with reversed or bidirectional shunt through communication between the two circulations
- Communication may be at aortic level (PDA, aortopulmonary window), intracardiac (ASD, VSD, AV canal, TAPVR) or single ventricle.
- Uncorrected L—R shunt leads to irreversible fixed pulm vascular obstructive disease
- Characterized by pulm Htn, R—L shunt, and right ventricular dysfunction
- Overall poor prognosis; mean age at death: 25 y
- Syncope, increasing right-sided filling pressures, and systemic arterial desaturation below 85% indicate poor prognosis
- 3%–70% of pregnant pts die in association with pregnancy
- Some pulm vascular reactivity may exist in the pulm vasculature of pregnant women; may be due to systemic hormonal changes of pregnancy

ICD-9-CM Code: 416.8 Pulmonary hypertension, secondary

Etiology

- Individuals with large unrestricted intracardiac or aortopulmonary communication have large L (systemic)—R (pulmonary) shunts
- Uncorrected L—R shunt overloads pulm vasculature and RV

- Continuous exposure to systemic pressure leads to pulm arteriolar medial hypertrophy, intimal proliferation and fibrosis
- Progressive pulm capillary and arteriolar occlusion leads to fixed increased PVR
- As pulm pressure exceeds systemic, shunt reverses to R—L

Usual Treatment

- Repair of intracardiac lesion is contraindicated
- Supplemental O_2 to decrease PVR
- Avoidance of medications that can cause hypotension, worsening cyanosis or hemorrhage (Ca channel blockers, antiplatelet agents, anticoagulants)
- Phlebotomy to treat hyperviscosity, extreme erythrocytosis (Hct >65%) and bleeding diathesis
- Single or bilateral lung transplantation with repair of the primary cardiac defect
- Combined heart-lung transplant in select pts
- With expected high maternal mortality, pregnant pts with ES should initially be counseled to terminate pregnancy
- For the pt who wishes to continue with pregnancy:
  - Hospital admission early in 3rd trimester
  - Anticoagulation with heparin: SQ heparin 5000–10,000 U bid
  - Pts with O_2 sat <80% on room air should be fully anticoagulated
  - O_2 Rx
  - Monitor for preterm labor
  - Medical Rx: Diuretics, antiarrhythmics, inotropes

ASSESSMENT POINTS

System	Effect	Assessment by Hx	PE	Test
CV	R⇒L shunt Right and left ventricular enlargement/failure	DOE, fatigue, syncope edema, orthopnea, anginal chest pain, arrhythmias	Elevated jugular venous pressure, increased intensity of S_2, split S_2 and S_3, decrescendo murmur of pulmonic regurgitation, holosystolic murmur of tricuspid regurgitation, rales. Right parasternal heave	ECG CXR ECHO MRI Cardiac catheterization
RESP	Pulm Htn	Dyspnea, hemoptysis	Palpable pulm artery Cyanosis, clubbing	Pulse oximetry ABGs, Hct (polycythemia)
NEURO	Neurologic abnormalities	Headache, dizziness, visual disturbances, CVAs	Neurologic exam	CT scan, MRI
HEME	Polycythemia, Hyperviscosity	Headache, weakness, blurred vision, pruritus	Splenomegaly, facial erythema, bleeding gums	CBC

Key Reference: Ammash NM, et al. Noncardiac surgery in Eisenmenger syndrome. *J Am Coll Cardiol.* 1999;33:222–227.

Perioperative Implications

Preoperative Preparation

- Continue antiarrhythmic medications, withhold diuretics
- Discontinuation of heparin; consider reversal with protamine
- Endocarditis prophylaxis depends on the type of operation (AHA Guidelines)
- In pregnant pts avoid aortocaval compression at all times
- IV lines must be carefully de-aired, consider placing air filters

Monitoring

- Pulse oximetry
- With uncorrected patent ductus arteriosus, use simultaneous right hand (preductal) and foot

(postductal) pulse oximetry to estimate changes in shunt fraction
- Arterial line for early recognition of sudden alteration of BP and repeated blood gas sampling
- CVP catheter
- PA catheter use must be balanced against potential complications:
  - Difficult to position in PA
  - High risk of arrhythmias, thrombi, paradoxical emboli, PA hemorrhage
  - Misleading data: Unreliable PCWP and measurement of CO with shunt

Airway

- Preop administration of Bicitra, metoclopramide, and ranitidine if needed
- NPO for 8 hr (if possible)

Preinduction/Induction

- No one best technique reported
- Goal of any technique is to maintain both cardiac output and SVR
- Combining short-acting IV narcotic (fentanyl), low-dose induction agent (sodium thiopental or ketamine) and inhalational agent (sevo- or isoflurane) with muscle relaxant devoid of CV effects (vecuronium or rocuronium)
- For labor:
  - Provision of effective analgesia prevents increased release of catecholamines, which increases PVR
  - Coaxial technique: Initial intrathecal dose of narcotic

- For C-section:
  - Regional: Slow induction of epidural anesthesia; counteract sympathectomy with vasopressor and maintenance of preload
- General anesthesia: Avoid rapid-sequence with risk of precipitating increase in PVR or inducing myocardial depression; maintain cricoid pressure through induction; avoid increase in PVR, decrease in SVR, hypoxia, hypercarbia, and myocardial depressants

Maintenance
- GA: Narcotic, low-dose inhalational agent, muscle relaxant
- Avoid hypotension (↓ SVR, acidosis, hypercarbia and hypoxia (↑ PVR)
- For labor:
  - Epidural infusion with low-dose local anesthetic/narcotic solution
  - Avoid Valsalva maneuver, pushing; delivery with vacuum or forceps

- For cesarean:
  - High-dose narcotic technique
  - Amnesia with benzodiazepine
  - Avoid halogenated agents: Myocardial depression, decreasing SVR
  - Avoid nitrous oxide: Increasing PVR, higher FIO_2

Extubation
- High-dose narcotic technique may necessitate postop ventilation

Adjuvants
- Avoid N_2O
- Maintain SVR with dilute solution of phenylephrine
- Inotrope, vasodilator for treatment of failure
- Cautious use of oxytocin (systemic vasodilation)
- Avoid prostaglandin F (increasing in PVR)
- Resume anticoagulation in postpartum period

Postoperative Period
- Pain management is critical
- In pregnant pts death most often occurs at delivery or postpartum
- Possible hemodynamic changes:
  - Excessive blood loss; replace volume
  - Autotransfusion; treat with vasodilator, inotrope, judicious use of diuretic
  - Arrhythmias: Sinus bradycardia, AV block, EMD
  - Pulm emboli
  - Postpartum increase in PVR; reason unknown

Anticipated Problems/Concerns
- Unresponsive, increase in PVR or decrease in SVR with loss of oxygenation
- CHF

Emphysema

William T. O'Byrne, III
William R. Furman

Risk

- Incidence in USA: 3.1 million
- Prevalence, incidence, mortality increase with age
- Higher in males than females
- Higher in whites than nonwhites

Perioperative Risks

- Intraop bronchospasm
- N_2O expansion of bullae
- Postop resp failure
- Postop pulm infection

Worry About

- Worsening of baseline pulm function, caused by
  - Bronchospasm
  - Acute bronchitis or pneumonia
  - Pulm embolism
- Worsening of baseline cardiac function caused by right heart failure

Overview

- Anatomic: Destruction of interalveolar septa and loss of pulm elastic recoil, leading to formation of bullae and development of irreversible expiratory airflow obstruction

- The "pink puffer" has dyspnea, hyperinflation, distant breath sounds, low diffusing capacity (decreasing D_LCO to <60% predicted)
- "Blue bloater" pts have chronic bronchitis, leading to hypoxemia, polycythemia, and CO_2 retention.
- Hypoxia, hypercarbia, cor pulmonale are late developments.
- Mucociliary clearance is often worsened after inhalational anesthetics.
- Diaphragmatic mechanics are impaired by anesthetics, sedatives, NMBs, interscalene blocks, supine positioning.

ICD-9-CM Code: 492.8 (Other Emphysema)

Etiology

- According to the elastase-antielastase hypothesis, the lung is normally protected from injury to its elastic tissues by antielastases, incl a_1 protease inhibitor (API), which is also called a_1-antitrypsin. According to this theory, emphysema may be acquired or genetic.
- Acquired: Related to inhaled oxidants (cigarette smoke or other occupational exposures), which are believed to inactivate API, thus compromising lung matrix repair after injury

- Genetic: Absent or abn API, also known as a_1-antitrypsin deficiency, which accounts for a small fraction of cases

Usual Treatment

- Smoking cessation (>6–8 wk may lessen anesthetic risk)
- Relief of symptoms by treatment of bronchospasm and infection
- In advanced cases, if hypoxia and cor pulmonale have developed: O_2 therapy may improve quality of life and survival.
- Lung volume reduction surgery may be considered for those with predominantly upper lobe disease and/or low exercise tolerance.

ASSESSMENT POINTS

System	Effect	Assessment by Hx	PE	Test
HEENT	Tumors 2° to smoking	Voice change	Hoarseness, stridor, inspiratory obstruction	Flow-volume loops
CARDIO	Cor pulmonale (late)	Edema, severe dyspnea	Signs of pulm Htn Hepatosplenomegaly Pedal edema, cyanosis, pleural effusions, usually without pulmonary edema	CXR ABGs
	Pulm emboli	Episodic SOB Arrhythmias Hard to differentiate from course of underlying illness	May reveal DVT in legs	CXR High resolution CT V/Q scan Pulm angiogram
RESP	Bronchospasm	Recent ↑ in dyspnea or ↓ in exercise tolerance	↑ Resp rate ↑ Expiratory time ↑ Accessory muscle use	Spirometry pre- and post-bronchodilators
	Pneumonia	Fever, dyspnea, ↑ sputum	Signs of pulm consolidation	CXR, WBC

Key Reference: Edrich T, Sadovnikoff N. Anesthesia for patients with severe chronic obstructive pulmonary disease. *Curr Opin Anaesthesiol.* Sep 21 2009.

Perioperative Implications

Preoperative Preparation
- Optimize bronchodilation
- Eradicate any underlying bacterial infection
- Encourage smoking cessation if this can occur >6 wk before surgery
- Consider regional anesthesia where appropriate

Monitoring
- Be cognizant of potential for increased gradient between $PETCO_2$ and $PaCO_2$

Airway
- None, unless tumor present in airway

Preinduction/Induction
- If patient has airway reactivity, consider issues related to asthma/chronic bronchitis
- Avoid N_2O when expansion of bullae is a risk
- May avoid high concentrations of desflurane if airway reactivity is of concern

Maintenance
- Recumbent positions impair chest wall muscle function, and abdominal muscle function usually needed for spontaneous ventilation
- Ventilator settings: Long expiratory times may be required; try to avoid high positive pressures (consider pressure control ventilation), esp. if bullae are present.

Extubation
- Residual anesthetics may compromise the ventilatory response to CO_2, increasing the risk of postop resp failure.
- Pre-extubation bronchodilators
- Unrelieved incisional pain, esp. after abdominal or thoracic surgery, will impair breathing—consider postop epidural analgesia.
- Consider regional block and/or NSAIDs to lessen risk of resp depression.
- Pts may be semiconscious and combative owing to hypoxia and hypercarbia on emergence.

- Evaluate whether postop ventilation may be the safest approach until the residual anesthetic effects have dissipated. Extubation to non-invasive positive pressure ventilation (NIPPV) may be useful in such cases.

Adjuvants
- β-Adrenergic agonists, anticholinergic agents for airway reactivity (may consider theophylline)
- Oral or inhaled steroids in selected pts

Anticipated Problems/Concerns

- Postop resp failure (consider NIPPV rather than reintubation in selected pts)
- Tension pneumothorax from ventilator-induced barotrauma
- Airway plugging from secretions

Encephalitis

Mary J. Njoku
David L. Schreibman

Risk

- Increased by exposure in endemic areas via human or zoonotic contacts. Transmission can be person-to-person, fecal-oral, via infected mosquito or animal bite, or infected saliva or secretions
- Increased during seasonal variation and epidemic outbreaks
- Assoc with 1° viral infection or reactivation, post-infectious/immune response, paraneoplastic syndromes or treatment-related immunosuppression

Perioperative Risks

- Assoc with mental status alteration, seizures, increased ICP, SIADH
- Assoc with increased sensitivity to sedative and amnestic effects of anesthetics and adjunct drugs
- Unrecognized, unexpected deterioration in mental status

Worry About

- Delayed awakening, postop delirium, clinical and subclinical seizures
- Hyperkalemic response to succinylcholine
- Transient myocardial dysfunction
- Electrolyte abn 2° to SIADH and CPM with rapid correction of Na+ abn

Overview

- Inflammation of brain parenchyma
- May be 1° manifestation of disease process or a component of another CNS or systemic illness
- Organisms enter CNS via bloodstream or peripheral nerves
- Symptoms incl altered mental status, altered consciousness, with or without focal neurologic abn, behavioral changes, in the presence of fever, headache, photophobia, nuchal rigidity, vomiting, disorientation, lethargy, confusion, hallucinations, memory loss, clinical or sub-clinical seizures, myoclonus, coma
- Dx is established by symptoms, epidemiologic Hx (exposure, season, geographic location), CSF culture, CSF bacterial and viral antigens, CSF viral PCR, virus specific DNA sequencing, MRI, EEG, CT scan. Brain biopsy is rarely performed.

ICD-9-CM Code: 064 (Viral encephalitis transmitted by other and unspecified arthropods), 054.3 (Herpetic meningoencephalitis), 052.0 (Postvaricella encephalitis)

Etiology

- Infectious
  - Viral: Herpes, varicella, CMV, EBV, influenza, RSV, enteroviruses, arboviruses, HIV, JC virus, rabies
  - Non-viral: Bacteria, protozoa, nematodes, fungi
- Noninfectious
  - Post-infectious/immune mediated
  - Autoimmune
  - Paraneoplastic

Usual Treatment

- Acyclovir effective for herpes simplex encephalitis
- Human rabies immunoglobin infiltration of inoculation site, immediately after bite
- Specific antimicrobial therapy, according to culture and sensitivity
- Supportive care
  - Intubate, ventilate, if dictated by mental status, airway reflexes
  - Hemodynamic support
  - Nutrition
  - DVT prophylaxis
  - GI prophylaxis
  - Physical therapy
  - Dx and treatment of extracranial infection
- Management of complications: Seizure, increasing ICP, SIADH, resp failure

ASSESSMENT POINTS

System	Effect	Assessment by Hx	PE	Test
HEENT	Virus access to CNS from nasal mucosa to olfactory bulb and olfactory tracts	Preceding URI		Nasopharyngeal swab Throat culture
CARDIO	Autonomic dysfunction Neurogenic stunned Myocardium	Transient myocardial dysfunction	Labile BP, HR	EKG, troponin, CK, echocardiography, LV angiography
HEME	↑ or normal WBC			CBC, WBC differential, serum antibody titers
RENAL	SIADH	Water intoxication Anorexia N/V Personality disorders Neurologic abn	No evidence of volume depletion Normal skin turgor Normal BP Mental status changes from lethargy to coma	Serum Na+ and osmolality Urine Na+ and osmolality BUN, Cr
CNS	Focal, global neurologic disturbances	Fever Headache Seizure Personality change Memory loss Confusion Weakness Sleep/awake abn	Focal neurologic deficits, altered mentation, papilledema, anisocoria; if spinal cord involvement: flaccid paraplegia, increased DTRs	CSF: Cell count (↑WBC, lymphocyte predominance), protein (↑), Gram stain, viral and bacterial culture, antibodies, antigens, viral polymerase chain reaction (PCR), viral DNA sequencing, MRI (temporal lobe involvement, hemorrhagic lesions, ± mass effect), EEG, CT

Key Reference: Rand KJ. Central nervous system infections. In: Layon AJ, ed. *Textbook of neurointensive care.* Philadelphia: Saunders; 2004.

Preoperative Implications

Preoperative Preparation
- Document neurologic exam
- Elicit Hx of increased ICP or seizure
- If SIADH present, correct electrolyte and free water abn
  - Sodium administration or fluid restriction depending on severity of hyponatremia
  - Beware of central pontine myelinolysis with rapid correction of hyponatremia

Monitoring
- Electrolytes
- Fluid I/O
- Consider ICP monitoring, EEG monitoring

Airway
- None

Induction
- Potential for hyperkalemic response to depolarizing NMBs if myopathy or paralysis, prefer use of nondepolarizing NMBs
- Autonomic instability and labile hemodynamics

Maintenance
- If pt is receiving seizure prophylaxis (e.g., phenytoin), be aware of potentiation of sedative effects and alteration of hepatic metabolism of anesthetics and muscle relaxants.

Extubation
- Delayed awakening
- Seizures on emergence

Postoperative Period
- Delirium
- Possible progressive deterioration

Anticipated Problems/Concerns

- Delayed awakening
- SIADH, careful selection of replacement fluid
- Hyperkalemic response to succinylcholine
- Universal precautions for contact with infected materials, sterilization of reuseable instruments

Encephalopathy, Hypertensive

Minda L. Patt
Christian Diez

Risks

- Most common clinical presentations of hypertensive emergencies are cerebral infarction (24.5%), pulm edema (22.5%), hypertensive encephalopathy (16.3%), and CHF (12%)
- Rapidly developing, fluctuating, or intermittent Htn carries a particular risk for hypertensive encephalopathy; pts with untreated or undertreated chronic Htn, renal failure, or preeclampsia-eclampsia are at increased risk
- Longstanding Htn disorders, coexisting renal disease, and immunosuppressive therapies are also risk factors.

Perioperative Risks

- Increased risk of myocardial ischemia, ventricular dysrhythmias, heart failure, cerebral hemorrhage, coma, long-term neurologic disability, aortic dissection, renal failure, or sudden death

Worry About

- Myocardial ischemia or infarction
- Cerebral infarction (ischemic or hemorrhagic)
- Aortic dissection
- CHF
- Acute renal failure
- Pulm edema
- Subarachnoid hemorrhage
- HELLP syndrome in eclamptic parturients
- Microangiopathic hemolytic anemia

Overview

- A relatively rapidly evolving syndrome of severe Htn in association with headache, N/V, visual disturbances, confusion, and—in advanced cases—stupor and coma that may be rapidly fatal
- More common with chronic hypertensive pts, renal failure, and eclampsia
- Occurs when the BP is elevated beyond autoregulatory thresholds of mean arterial pressures greater than 150–160 mmHg ('autoregulation breakthrough')
- Dx of exclusion; stroke and SAH also produce encephalopathy with acutely elevated BP; stroke is by far the most likely Dx; elevated BP, headache, papilledema, and altered consciousness are also seen with intracranial hemorrhage
- Pts with chronic Htn can tolerate higher mean arterial pressures before they have disruption of their autoregulation system; such pts, however, also have increased cerebrovascular resistance and are more prone to cerebral ischemia when flow decreases, esp if BP is decreased into normotensive ranges.
- BP >250/150 mmHg is usually required to precipitate the syndrome in pts with chronic Htn, while previously normotensive pts are affected at pressures as low as 160/100 mmHg (i.e., as with eclampsia or acute renal failure)
- Has been termed "hypertensive posterior reversible encephalopathy syndrome" or PRES

ICD-9-CM Code: 437.2

Etiology

- A sudden increase in BP, with or without preexisting chronic Htn, resulting in failure of cerebral autoregulation, leading to cerebrovascular endothelial dysfunction and vasogenic edema that renders the pt encephalopathic
- Most common in pts with untreated or undertreated chronic essential arterial Htn
- Renovascular disease or renal parencyhmal lesions
- Endocrine causes: Pheochromocytoma, rennin-secreting tumor, Cushing's disease, Conn's syndrome
- Preeclampsia and eclampsia

- Status post carotid endarterectomy (CEA hyperperfusion syndrome)
- Thrombocytopenic purpura
- Acute intermittent porphyria
- AIDS
- Autonomic hyperreactivity, as with spinal cord lesions
- Drug induced: D/C of antihypertensive drugs, erythropoietin, immunosuppressive therapy (cyclosporine, tacrolimus, cisplatin, interferon-alfa), MAOIs
- Ingestion of cocaine, amphetamine, or LSD
- Often multifactorial from the previous list

Usual Treatment

- Reduce mean arterial pressure by 20% within the first hour or to a target DBP of 100–110 mmHg, whichever value is greater
- Antihypertensive agents: Most commonly sodium nitroprusside, labetalol, fenoldopam, nicardipine, enalapril, or hydralazine; initiation of other therapy may be dictated by other end-organ damage (e.g., aortic dissection and β-blocker therapy)
- In general, vasodilators, like sodium nitroprusside, have a lesser effect on the cerebral circulation vs. other vascular beds, making them primary choices for pts with hypertensive encephalopathy (e.g., central agonists would be contraindicated)
- Clonidine should be avoided because of its CNS depressant effects.
- Anticonvulsant therapy: Phenytoin or fosphenytoin, benzodiazepines, barbituates, or a combination
- Withdrawal of exacerbating factors (immunosuppressive drugs, erythropoietin)
- In eclampsia, delivery of the baby and the placenta, as well as parenteral magnesium, are the mainstay of therapy.

ASSESSMENT POINTS

System	Effect	Assessment by Hx	PE	Test
CARDIO	Htn CHF Myocardial ischemia Aortic dissection	Hx of Htn Hx of preeclampsia Angina Hx of CHF Pain radiating to the back	S_3 S_4 gallop Rales	CXR EKG Arteriogram
RESP	Pulm edema ↓ Lung compliance ↓ FEV, FVC	SOB Frothy sputum Orthopnea	Rales	CXR O_2 sat
GI	Aortic dissection N/V	Abd pain Back pain	Abd mass	US or arteriogram (if indicated)
RENAL	Renal failure	Anuria		Measurement of UO, BUN/Cr May occur without presence of proteinuria
CNS	Cerebral hemorrhage Severe headache Visual disturbances Generalized or focal seizures Paralysis Stupor, coma	Mental status exam	Retinal arteriolar spasm on ophthalmoscopy Papilledema May have a normal fundoscopic exam	CT MRI

Key Reference: Vaughan CJ, Delanty N: Hypertensive emergencies. *Lancet.* 2000;356(9227):411–417.

Preoperative Implications

Preinduction

- Determine medications, compliance with antihypertensive regimens, and adequacy of BP control
- Evaluate for end-organ damage

Monitoring

- Arterial catheter
- Central venous catheter or pulm artery catheter may be used if extensive surgery is planned or there is evidence of other end-organ damage (LV dysfunction, renal failure)

General Anesthesia

- Volatile anesthetics are useful in attenuating sympathetic nervous system pressor responses; there is no evidence to suggest one volatile agent over another for control of intraop Htn
- Nitrous oxide–opioid technique can be used be used for maintenance of anesthesia in pts with labile pressure while under GA; a volatile agent

may be needed during periods of abrupt changes in surgical stimulation
- Antihypertensive agent by bolus or continuous infusion is an alternative to volatile agent BP control

Induction

- Induction of anesthesia may produce an exaggerated decrease in BP due, esp in the face of diastolic Htn (intravascular volume depletion)

- Direct larygoscopy and tracheal intubation can produce significant Htn; limit duration of DL and consider use of opioid, lidocaine, blocker, and vasodilator to blunt autonomic response

Maintenance
- Control BP and minimize wide fluctuations in BP, as aggressive treatment of Htn may worsen other end-organ function
- Monitor for myocardial ischemia

Regional Anesthesia
- Epinephrine-containing solutions may place the hypertensive pt at risk or worsen an existent hypertensive crisis (e.g., epidural in a pre-eclamptic parturient)

Postoperative Period
- Extubate with careful BP control
- Continue IV antihypertensive therapy and monitoring of BP and mental status

- Maintain monitoring for other end–organ morbidity such as myocardial ischemia, cardiac dysrhythmias, CHF, stroke, and bleeding

Anticipated Problems/Concers
- Particular caution is necessary with elderly pts and pts with preexisting Htn; over-aggressive reduction in BP may be accompanied by worsening neurologic status and stroke.

Encephalopathy, Metabolic

Charles Weissman

Risk

- 3.4–11% of medical ICU admissions
- 12–33% of multiple-organ dysfunction pts

Perioperative Risks

- With predisposing conditions, e.g., hepatic insufficiency, risk of developing or exacerbating metabolic encephalopathy
- Increasing severity of pre-existing encephalopathy

Worry About

- Worsening hepatic insufficiency causing hepatic encephalopathy
- Diabetics becoming hypoglycemic or with DKA/hyperosmolar coma
- Postop hyponatremia
- Deteriorating renal insufficiency leading to uremic encephalopathy
- Pre-existing encephalopathy may be exacerbated by anesthetics, e.g., benzodiazepines, in hepatic encephalopathy
- Undiagnosed sepsis, hypothermia, high fever, CNS-acting drugs, incl overdose
- CNS cause: Brainstem CVA, meningitis, occult head trauma, encephalitis, brain tumor

Overview

- Altered sensorium, stupor, or coma without any other explanation in the setting of a metabolic disturbance
- Process affects global cortical function by altering brain biochemistry
- Distinguished from structural lesions by a nonfocal neurologic exam
- EEG shows diffuse background slowing, triphasic waves in hepatic encephalopathy
- Increased spontaneous motor activity: restlessness, asterixis, myoclonus, tremors, rigidity

ICD-9-CM Code: 348.3 (Unspecified encephalopathy)

Etiology

- Hypoglycemic encephalopathy: Most commonly caused by accidental or deliberate overdosing with insulin or oral hypoglycemic agents or prolonged ethanol intoxication
- Hepatic encephalopathy: Acute or chronic hepatic insufficiency, Reye syndrome
- Uremic encephalopathy: Renal failure. After dialysis, disequilibrium syndrome caused by acute fluid and electrolyte shifts.
- Encephalopathy due to fluid and electrolyte abn: Hyperosmolar state, hyponatremia (acute decrease to <120 mEq/L), hypernatremia, hypercalcemia assoc with hypoparathyroidism (<4 mEq/L).
- Pulm encephalopathy: Combination of hypoxia and hypercarbia
- Drug overdose; sepsis; severe acute pancreatitis

Usual Treatment

- Uremic encephalopathy: Dialysis
- Hepatic encephalopathy: Lactulose (oral or rectal), neomycin
- Hypoglycemic encephalopathy: IV glucose
- Septic encephalopathy: Treatment of underlying infection
- Hyperosmolar/hyposmolar state: Slow and careful restoration of electrolyte balance
- Pulm encephalopathy: Quickly improve ventilation and oxygenation, mechanical ventilation

ASSESSMENT POINTS

System	Effect	Assessment by Hx	PE	Test
RESP	Sudden elevation Paco$_2$ (>65 mmHg)	COPD, drug overdose	Hypoventilation, periodic breathing, papilledema	Pulse oximetry and end-tidal capnography, or ABGs
GI	Hepatic insufficiency	Liver disease, cirrhosis, alcoholism, portosystemic shunt	Asterixis, jaundice, ascites	AST, ALT, bilirubin, ammonia PT (INR)
ENDO	Diabetes	Use of insulin or oral hypoglycemic agents		Blood glucose
	Apathy Thyrotoxicosis	Hyperthyroidism	Tachycardia Fever, sweating	T$_4$, T$_3$
	Hypothyroidism	Hypothyroidism	Hypothermia Pretibial edema	TSH
	Hypercalcemia	Hyperparathyroidism Malignancy		Serum Ca^{2+}, PTH
RENAL	Uremia Prerenal azotemia	Renal disease, ingestion of nephrotoxins, e.g., drugs	Asterixis	BUN/Cr, serum lytes Toxicology screen
CNS	Altered sensorium, stupor, coma, seizures	R/O Head trauma	Nonfocal neurologic exam, altered mental status	EEG, CT Lumbar puncture
MS	Multifocal myoclonus, rigidity		Myoclonus, asterixis, rigidity, tremors	

Key Reference: Ravin PD. Metabolic encephalopathy. In: Irwin RS, Rippe JM, eds. *Intensive care medicine*, 6th ed. Philadelphia: Wolters Kluwer/Lippincott Williams & Wilkins; 2008:1967–1975.

Perioperative Implications

Preoperative Preparation

- Assess and document preop mental status and neurologic function
- Uremic encephalopathy: Preop dialysis, if possible
- Hyperthyroidism, hypothyroidism: Initial treatment, if possible

Monitoring

- Routine
- In hyperosmolar states, uremia and liver failure with ascites may need central monitoring.

Preinduction/Induction

- Benzodiazepines should be avoided in hepatic encephalopathy.
- Increased potential for aspiration; consider rapid-sequence

Maintenance

- Carefully titrate anesthetics to avoid overdosing
- Careful attention should be paid to intravascular volume status, blood glucose, and lytes
- During and after TURP and hysteroscopy, sodium concentrations and volume status should be monitored.
- Correction of hypernatremia and hyponatremia should be gradual.
- In renal and hepatic failure, appropriate drugs and doses should be used. Long-acting drugs should be avoided. May be increased bleeding.
- Diabetics: Monitor intraoperative blood glucose to avoid hypoglycemia. Too rapid correction of hyperglycemia can lead to cerebral edema.

Extubation

- Extubate only if pt is able to protect airway and maintain adequate ventilation.

Anticipated Problems/Concerns

- Poor mental status at the conclusion of surgery may require continued intubation.
- Hyponatremia is a cause of postop metabolic encephalopathy.

Encephalopathy, Postanoxic

Risk

- After successful prehospital cardiac resuscitation: 59–65% of pts remain comatose
- 0–5% of successful resuscitations result in chronic vegetative state

Perioperative Risks

- Worsening of neurologic status; blindness most common residuum
- Postpone surgery in all but emergency situations
- Do what is necessary to treat precipitating cause and to decrease sequelae (e.g., treat elevated ICP)

Worry About

- Repeat of events that initially caused encephalopathy (e.g., arrhythmias leading to cardiac arrest)
- Hypotension, hypercapnia, hypoxia, and sepsis that can exacerbate encephalopathy.

Overview

- Definition: Brain injury resulting from prolonged period of insufficient cerebral oxygenation

- Clinical picture ranges from mild confusion to brain death
- Chances for acceptable neurologic recovery—1% with continued coma after 24 hr and lack of two of the following reflexes: pupillary, corneal, and oculovestibular
- Absence of brainstem function 72 hr after event associated with irreversible coma.
- Good prognosis seen in 50% of pts awakening within 24 hr of insult.
- Seizures occur in 25% of pts.
- Anoxic damage may have been sustained by other organs (e.g., MI, shock liver, acute renal failure, stress ulcers, ARDS)
- Diabetes insipidus poor prognostic sign

ICD-9-CM Code: 348.1 (Anoxic brain damage)

Etiology

- Caused by inadequate O_2 delivery to CNS due to inadequate cardiac output, resp dysfunction, severe anemia, and/or increased ICP

- Most often 2° to 1° cardiac (MI or arrhythmia) or pulm (asthma, pulm embolism) event
- May also be result of CO poisoning, suffocation, and cyanide poisoning

Usual Treatment

- Prevent recurrence of inciting event
- Ventilatory and hemodynamic support, as needed
- Stress ulcer prophylaxis
- Treatment of seizures (with anticonvulsants, e.g., phenytoin) and myoclonus
- Therapeutic hypothermia (esp. after cardiac arrest with initial VF or VT) to 32–34° C for 12–24 hr.
- BP should be maintained at normotensive or mildly elevated levels in normotensives and higher in hypertensives.
- Treat fever promptly with antipyretics.

ASSESSMENT POINTS

System	Effect	Assessment by Hx	PE	Test
CARDIO	MI	Assess if cardiac disease was cause of arrest		ECG, other cardiac assessment Troponins, CK
RESP	ARDS	Assess if resp disease was cause of arrest Resp failure	Wheezing, stigmata of COPD	Pre-arrest PFTs ABGs
GI	Shock liver Stress ulceration	Hx of GI bleeding	Jaundice	AST, ALT, bilirubin, alkaline phosphatase Hct NG output
RENAL	Renal failure	Assess if electrolyte abn or acidosis caused initial event	UO	BUN/Cr
CNS	Altered mental status, diffuse and focal neurologic abn	Changes in neurologic signs since hypoxic event	Neurologic and mental status exams, apnea test, brainstem reflexes	CT scan/CT angiography, MRI/MRA EEG SSEP, BAER
MS	Myoclonus, posturing	Hx of abnormal movements, posturing	Decerebrate or decorticate postures	
	Contractures	Prolonged immobility	Contractures	

Key Reference: Lippa CF, Moonis M. Generalized anoxia/ischemia of the nervous system. In: Irwin RS, Rippe JM, eds. *Intensive care medicine*. 6th ed. Philadelphia: Wolters Kluwer/Lippincott Williams & Wilkins; 2008:1976–1979.

Perioperative Implications

Preoperative Preparation

- Assess and document neurologic function and mental status
- Review cause of anoxic event
- Assess damage to other organs
- If pt hypothermic beware of possible increased blood loss

Monitoring

- If arrest was due to cardiac arrhythmias or MI/ischemia or if pt is hemodynamically unstable, may need specialized monitoring

Airway

- Assess potential for aspiration: Gag reflex, ability to cough and clear secretions

Induction

- Avoid succinylcholine

Maintenance

- Must consider that pts may have pain perception and will require analgesia
- Do what is appropriate to decrease sequelae (e.g., treat increased ICP); therapeutic hypothermia

Extubation

- If unable to maintain patent airway or sustain adequate minute ventilation, pt should remain intubated.

Adjuvants

- Avoid long-acting anesthetics so that neurologic status can be assessed soon after surgery.
- Avoid drugs that decrease seizure threshold.

Anticipated Problems/Concerns

- Repeat of events (e.g., arrhythmias) that initially led to anoxic encephalopathy
- Worsening of neurologic condition during periop period
- Postpone all but emergency surgery if fluctuating neurologic deficits or acute encephalopathic condition exists.

Endocardial Cushion Defect

Nathaen Weitzel

Risk

- 2% of CHD is endocardial cushion defect (ECD). No gender predilection.
- 30% of ECD assoc with Down syndrome

Perioperative Risks

- Shunt reversal caused by anesthetic drugs, airway stimulation during light anesthesia, or airway obstruction
- Paradoxical embolism, particularly with shunt reversal
- Subacute bacterial endocarditis; recommend antibiotic prophylaxis
- Pulm hypertensive crisis in pts with reactive pulm vasculature
- AV valve regurgitation, arrhythmias following surgical repair of ECD

Worry About

- Development of pulm vascular obstructive disease, reversal of shunt and RV failure

- Development of atrial arrhythmias due to significant atrial enlargement
- Extreme sensitivity to myocardial depressant effects of inhaled agents

Overview

- ECD causes various combinations of Ostium Primum atrial septal defects, ventricular septal defects in inlet septum, and clefts in anterior mitral and/or septal tricuspid valve leaflets
- Causes shunting at atrial or ventricular (or both) sites with or without assoc AV valvular regurgitation. Leads to heart failure (R > L), failure to thrive and repeated resp infections
- ECD can lead to shunt reversal, pulm vascular obstructive disease, and Eisenmenger's syndrome which can limit surgical therapy.
- Dx confirmed by TEE and cardiac catheterization

ICD-9-CM Code: 745.6

Etiology

- AV canal defects result from failure of the endocardial cushions to grow and fuse with portions of the interatrial and interventricular septa in the 5–6 mm embryo

Usual Treatment

- Medical: Typically unresponsive, but therapy with digitalis and diuretics for heart failure
- Surgical: Definitive therapy requires closure of the septal defects and repair of the clefts in the AV valves with reconstruction of tricuspid, and occasion mitral replacement

ASSESSMENT POINTS

System	Effect	Assessment by Hx	PE	Test
HEENT	Feeding difficulties	Failure to thrive	< Normal wt/ht for age	Comparison of wt/ht to published values
CARDIO	CHF	Diaphoresis, coughing	Wheezing, rales, hepatosplenomegaly Tachycardia, murmur	Cardiac cauterization, ECG with RVH, TEE
	Pulm Htn		Worsening CHF	TEE, cardiac catheterization
RESP	CHF	Dyspnea, tachypnea	Wheezing, rales	CXR
RENAL	Renal dysfunction due to heart failure			BUN, Cr
MS	Decreased exercise compared with peers			

Key Reference: Hudson J, Deshpande J. Septal and endocardial cushion defects. In: Lake CL, Booker PD, eds. *Pediatric Cardiac Anesthesia*. 4th ed. Philadelphia: Lippincott, Williams & Wilkins; 2005:329–343.

Perioperative Implications

Preoperative Preparation

- Prophylactic antibiotics for subacute bacterial endocarditis
- Premedication to minimize anxiety and possible shunt reversal
- Diuretic if prone to CHF

Monitoring

- Intra-arterial catheter and central venous catheter if required by surgical procedure
- TEE if available and appropriate to anesthetic and surgical procedure

Airway

- May be difficult if associated congenital anomalies such as Down syndrome are present

Preinduction/Induction

- Meticulous air removal to avoid paradoxical embolism
- IV or inhalation induction depending on pt preference/cooperation. Choice of IV induction agent depends on severity of CHF and pulm Htn.

Maintenance

- Volatile agents that decrease systemic vascular resistance may worsen R to L shunting. Combinations of narcotic with low concentrations of volatile agents may be appropriate in pts with moderate disease.

Extubation

- Possible in pts without CHF or pulm Htn. Proceed cautiously esp if reactive pulm vasculature, may develop pulm hypertensive crisis requiring hyperventilation, ↑ FIO_2, sedation, or even NO or ECMO, which is more easily accomplished during mechanical ventilation.

Adjuvants

- NO, nitroglycerin, prostaglandin to control pulm vascular tone. Inotropes for heart failure.

Postoperative Period

- Observe left and right atrial pressures, as LAP more than 6 mm > RAP suggests mitral valve incompetence and/or stenosis.

- Residual shunting at atrial or ventricular level should be excluded by TEE.
- Heart block or other conduction defects may result from surgical repair.
- Effective analgesia to minimize pulm hypertensive crisis, which may incl epidural or spinal analgesia in some centers

Anticipated Problems/Concerns

- Pts with partial or complete AV canal defects 2° to endocardial cushion defects who have CHF are likely to have moderate to severe AV valvular incompetence or pulm Htn following surgical repairs.
- Significantly increased pulm blood flow 2° to L to R cardiac shunting increases the risk of developing pulm vascular obstructive disease and postop pulm hypertensive crisis.

Epidermolysis Bullosa

Nancy B. Kenepp
Sumita Bhambhani

Risk

- 1/17,000, 50% dystrophic form
- Racial distribution equal

Perioperative Risks

- Difficult IV access, airway, intraop positioning, reflux, steroid dependence, intraop hemorrhage, sepsis, iatrogenic corneal abrasion, blister formation, airway obstruction

Worry About

- Problems similar to pts with severe skin burns. Pts are severely compromised.
- Difficult intubation (23%) 2° to microstomia
- Establishing monitoring, IV access
- Dehydration, malnutrition
- Anemia, hypoalbuminemia, electrolyte imbalance, thrombocytosis
- Septicemia
- Renal and adrenal dysfunction

Overview

- Characterized by epithelial blistering as a result of minor trauma by lateral shearing forces, not pressure
- 3 types: Simplex (SEB), junctional (JEB), dystrophic (DEB)

- Associated conditions: Growth retardation, pyloric stenosis, esophageal stricture, pseudosyndactyly, enamel hypoplasia, muscular dystrophy, squamous cell carcinoma, malignant melanoma
- SEB: Most common form. Blisters are intraepidermal and are on soles and palms only in Weber-Cockayne form, are generalized in Kobner form, are generalized herpetiform in Dowling-Meara form, and are generalized in association with muscular dystrophy in MD form.
- JEB: Blisters form in the intralamina lucida and are in intertriginous areas in inversa form, are generalized with growth retardation in Herlitz form, are generalized without growth retardation in non-Herlitz form, and are generalized with pyloric atresia.
- DEB: Blisters form in the sublamina densa and are in intertriginous areas in inversa form, are on ankles in pretibial form, are on arms and legs in pruriginous form. In the non–Hallopeau-Siemens form, the blisters are generalized. The blisters are also generalized with growth retardation and severe extracutaneous involvement in Hallopeau-Siemens form and very aggressive squamous cell carcinomas are common.

ICD-9-CM Code: 757.39

Etiology

- SEB: Inherited autosomal, usually dominant, mutation producing abnormal keratin intermediate filament proteins 5 or 14 which weaken the epidermal architecture. In MD form abn plectin (cytolinker protein) is the cause.
- JEB: Inherited autosomal recessive mutation producing abn laminin 5, abn type XVII collagen, and abn $\alpha_6\beta_4$ integrin
- DEB: Inherited autosomal dominant or recessive mutation producing abn type VII collagen

Usual Treatment

- Treatment is supportive similar to initial burn treatment with silver impregnated creams and collagen allografts.
- Use of retinoids and growth stimulator factors to induce wound repair keratin 6, 16, 17, which form a more normal epidermis.
- Emerging treatment: Isothiocyanate sulphoraphane which induces keratin 16 and 17 and occurs naturally in broccoli sprouts.
- Receive steroids and supportive treatment such as nutritional support, wound care, contracture release, esophageal dilation, oral surgery, and treatment of skin cancers.
- Future treatment: Gene therapy

ASSESSMENT POINTS

System	Effect	Assessment by Hx	PE	Test
HEENT	Enamel hypoplasia: Blisters, microstomia, ankyloglossia, supraglottic ulceration or narrowing	Delayed eruption, caries of teeth; painful peri- and intraoral lesions; hoarseness, resp obstruction; painful swallowing, spasm, food impaction	Poor oral hygiene, malocclusion; tongue atrophy; obliteration of vestibular sulci, stricture, webs, vocal cord lesions	Airway assessment, endoscopy
GI	Bullae Perianal blisters, poor absorption, diarrhea	Anal pain, tenesmus, constipation	Anal fissure or stricture	Endoscopy
GU	Blisters	Urinary diversion	Obstruction, sepsis	Renal function
MS	Contractures, growth retardation	Movement limitations, stature	Flexion contracture, pseudodactyly	
DERM	Blisters	Age at onset, Hx of remissions, infections	Scars, milia, nail dystrophy, cancer	Skin biopsy

Key Reference: Lin Y, Golinau B. Anesthesia and pain management for pediatric patients with dystrophic epidermolysis bullosa. *J Clin Anesth.* 2006;18(4):268–271.

Perioperative Implications

Preoperative Preparation

- Careful planning of monitoring, IV placement, positioning in the OR, prevention of reflux, and airway management

Monitoring

- No contraindication to pulse oximeter use
- Protect blisters on the face with foam adhesive inverted to pad mask
- Pad automated BP cuff heavily, limit intervals
- Cut off adhesive from ECG leads; hold in place with defibrillator jelly pads
- Suture invasive monitoring and IVs or wrap in place with petrolatum gauze
- Esophageal stethoscope may damage mucosa
- Avoid excessive heat or sweating, which increases risk of blisters

Induction

- Regional anesthesia encouraged; use spray antiseptics or pour prep solutions; no intradermal local anesthetics

- No GA or muscle relaxant specifically contraindicated

Airway

- All airway management techniques reported successful
- Mask (or nasal mask) lubricated and padded with petrolatum gauze; pad chin under fingers; bullae occurred in 1 in 50
- LMA one size too small, heavily lubricated, cuff soft with audible leak, extubated deep to prevent trauma; lingual bulla occurred in 1 in 57
- Intubation less frequent; blind nasal, fiberoptic, and oral techniques; heavily lubricated small tube; lubricate laryngoscope heavily; cricoid pressure without lateral movement permissible; 66% class I or II view of larynx, 7–23% difficult airway incidence; soft lubricated gauze to prevent tube movement in mouth, no lateral forces on mouth corners by tube, no tape; trachea lined with columnar epithelium, so less likely to blister

Emergence

- Aim for a quiet emergence
- No suction on intraoral mucosa

Anticipated Problems/Concerns

- Positioning: Pt performs if possible; lateral shear forces from lifting cause blisters
- Corneal abrasion: Poor eyelid retraction; use ointment generously, protect eyes in prone position
- Treat hemorrhage with epinephrine or thrombin-soaked sponge
- Avoid sweating; warming devices, if unavoidable, no warmer than skin temperature
- Extremity tourniquets, IM or rectal medications, EMLA can be used
- Common procedures: Release of syndactyly, dressing change, squamous cell carcinoma, esophageal dilatation, dental surgery

Epiglottitis

Maurice S. Zwass

Risk

- Children 1–7 y, although epiglottitis (sometimes called supraglottis) does occur in adults. (Decreasing incidence in children >3 y, related to vaccine against *Haemophilus influenzae* type B, but still found, particularly if not immunized.)
- Adult incidence remains constant with organisms group A *Streptococcus pneumoniae*, *Staphylococcus aureus*, *Klebsiella pneumoniae*

Perioperative Risks

- Acute deterioration of airway patency resulting in complete obstruction worse in children
- Difficulty in tracheal intubation due to severe edema of epiglottis and arytenoids

Worry About

- Airway compromise in children who appear toxic, with increasing distress, drooling, hypoxemia. The acute risks of airway compromise (of concern in small children) appear to be less critical in adults, most likely because of larger airway.
- Loss of airway control and aspiration

Overview

- An acute, potentially life-threatening cause of upper airway obstruction (etiologic agents may incl bacteria other than *H. influenzae* type B)
- Produces inflammatory edema of epiglottis and other supraglottic structures
- Onset usually rapid; progression to severe obstruction can occur in several hours
- High fever, sore throat, and dysphagia frequently so severe that swallowing is inhibited and drooling results
- Differential diagnosis also incl retropharyngeal abscess (a bacterial infection), which can have same presentation. It can be differentiated from epiglottitis by presence of torticollis and trismus and with radiographic studies (contrast CT). Treatment is with antibiotics and surgical drainage.

ICD-9-CM Codes: 464.30; 464.31 (With obstruction); 478.24 (Retropharyngeal abscess)

Etiology

- *H. influenzae* type B is most often traditional assoc pathogen, though can be caused by β-hemolytic streptococci, group A *Streptococcus pneumoniae*, *Staphylococcus aureus*, *Klebsiella pneumoniae*

Usual Treatment

- Antibiotic therapy against bacterium (usually *H. influenzae*) and airway support, which generally requires tracheal intubation
- Because of high incidence of ampicillin-resistant strains, ampicillin plus a β-lactamase inhibitor (such as sulbactam) and/or chloramphenicol, cefuroxime, ceftazidime, or another penicillinase-resistant antibiotic as indicated by blood and epiglottis culture results
- Tracheal intubation classically performed in OR in a controlled fashion with surgical support for possible tracheotomy or cricothyrotomy present and gowned

ASSESSMENT POINTS

Differentiation between epiglottitis and croup (laryngotracheobronchitis):

	Croup	Epiglottitis
AGE	3 mo–3 y	1–7 y
ONSET	Gradual	More rapid (usually <24 hr)
FEVER	Low-grade	High-grade
COUGH	Characteristic barking	None
SORE THROAT	Occasional	Frequently severe
POSTURE	Any	Frequently sitting forward, mouth open, drooling
AIRWAY SOUND	Inspir stridor	Inspiratory stridor
VOICE	Normal	Muffled
APPEARANCE	Nontoxic	Toxic
SEASONALITY	Peak winter, epidemic	Year-round

Radiographic studies may be helpful, because AP view of trachea appears normal but lateral neck view usually shows a markedly swollen, edematous epiglottis ("thumbprinting").

Key Reference: Jenkins I, Saunders M. Infections of the airway. *Paediatr Anaesth*. 2009;19(suppl 1):118–130.

Perioperative Implications

Preoperative Preparation

- With suspected epiglottitis, other personnel on pt care team can set up care (e.g., OR or ICU). Radiographs can be obtained, but a team member capable of monitoring and securing the airway should be present.
- Allow to remain in a position of comfort (often sitting with parent). Direct exam of oropharynx generally avoided, as are attempts to secure vascular access, because these may cause agitation leading to acute tracheal obstruction.
- Humidified O_2 should be delivered as tolerated.
- Aerosol therapy with racemic epinephrine may provide slight improvement of Sx, but not definitive. If Dx is confirmed, pt is taken to the location for intubation (most commonly OR).

Airway Management

- Anesthesia with sevoflurane or halothane and O_2, maintaining spontaneous ventilation
- IV catheter placed after induction of anesthesia, followed by direct laryngoscopy
- Large, swollen epiglottis can make identification of airway structures difficult, but once the epiglottis is identified, arytenoids and larynx are immediately below and tracheal tube can be inserted
- Because of upper airway swelling, a tracheal tube 0.5–1.0 mm smaller in diameter may be needed (tracheal tube of adequate length can be made available)
- Rarely is emergency tracheotomy necessary, but surgeons are "gloved" until airway secured
- Frequently orotracheal tube is changed to a nasotracheal tube for ease of securing and pt comfort

Post Airway Management Plans

- Once airway secured, cultures of blood and epiglottis are obtained, antibiotic therapy is initiated, and sedation plans are instituted.

Anticipated Problems/Concerns

- Resp support often for 24–72 hr until swollen epiglottis returns to normal
- Usually require sedative management to facilitate tolerating mechanical ventilation
- Many pts (~25%) have assoc pneumonia that requires treatment

Familial Dysautonomia (Riley-Day Syndrome)

Thomas J. Ebert
Darryl T. Tang

Risk

- Rare due to improved genetic screening measures. Incidence likely 1:10,000–20,000 in Jews originating from Eastern Europe (Ashkenazi)
- Carrier frequency in Ashkenazi Jews 1:27–32

Perioperative Risks

- Hemodynamic instability 2° to an erratic ANS
- Pulm insufficiency 2° to a relative insensitivity to hypoxemia and hypercarbia
- Altered response to hypoxia resulting in bradycardia and hypotension
- Impaired renal function in older pts due to renal hypoperfusion

Worry About

- Dysautonomic crisis: Triggered by physiologic and psychologic stressors and characterized by intractable vomiting, Htn, tachycardia, diaphoresis, and erythematous skin blotching
- QTc prolongation, dysrhythmias incl: Bradyarhythmias and asystole
- Heightened sensitivity to ACh and catecholamines

Overview

- Hereditary sensory autonomic neuropathy affecting primarily the sympathetic nervous system
- Primarily a disease of children; survival rates improving, with 50% of newborns expected to reach 40 y of age
- CV effects due to autonomic dysfunction resulting in episodic hyper/hypotension and arrhythmias
- Resp status compromised by dysfunctional swallowing leading to repeated aspiration pneumonias and impaired ventilatory response to hypoxia

ICD-9-CM Code: 742.8

Etiology

- Autosomal recessive mutation in *IKBKAP* gene of chromosome 8 leading to impaired neuronal development, differentiation, gene expression, and survival
- Symptoms due to denervation of chemoreceptors, baroreceptors, sympathetic and parasympathetic neurons

Usual Treatment

- Symptoms are managed by conventional direct-acting vasoactive therapies
- Dysautonomic crisis: First-line treatment with benzodiazepines

ASSESSMENT POINTS

System	Effect	Assessment by Hx	PE	Test
CARDIO	Orthostatic hypotension QTc prolongation Arrhythmias	Dizziness, syncope	Supine and standing BP, HR	Autonomic function, EKG
RESP	Pneumonia Bronchiectasis	Pleuritic chest pain Secretions	Wheezing, clubbing of digits	CXR
GI	Poor swallowing Aspiration pneumonia	Drooling, vomiting, Hx of "attacks"		Swallow study
GU	Dehydration Glomerulosclerosis	Emesis, nocturia, diaphoresis	Dry mucosa, skin turgor	Electrolytes, serum BUN, Cr
CNS	Seizure	Seizure		EEG

Key Reference: Ngai J, Kreynin I, Kim JT, Axelrod FB. Anesthesia management of familial dysautonomia. *Paediatr Anaesth.* 2006;16:611–620.

Perioperative Implications

Preoperative Preparation

- Consider regional anesthesia or adjunctive use of regional techniques combined with general anesthesia for improved intraoperative and postop pain control.
- Difficulty swallowing: Abundant secretions plus diminished laryngeal reflexes. Treat with antisialagogues
- Avoid medications that interact with the ANS
- Dysautonomic crisis: Prevent with anxiolytics. If symptoms develop, first-line treatment with midazolam, second-line treatment with clonidine for residual Htn or agitation
- H_2 blockers can decrease gastric volume and acidity.
- Phenothiazines are assoc with erratic hemodynamics at induction.
- Treat chronic dehydration 2° to dysphagia and emesis. Increased insensible losses 2° to increased sweating and drooling may require greater maintenance fluid volumes to maintain normovolemia.
- Insensitivity to hypoxia, hypercarbia: Minimize narcotics as premedication
- Insensitivity to superficial pain: Lines placed without discomfort. Poor thermal discrimination may affect assessment of regional blocks.

Monitoring

- Routine
- Consider arterial line

Induction

- Rapid sequence induction preferred. Titration of induction agents should be attempted to minimize risk of hypotension.
- Use of nondepolarizing agents must be balanced against the risk of postop hypotonia and unpredictable effect of reversal agents on ANS.
- Lubricate eyes to avoid corneal abrasions 2° to alacrima.

Maintenance

- Dysfunctional regulation can require fluids and vasoactive drug therapy.
- Titrate volatile anesthetic with processed EEG monitor to avoid overdose, supplement with short acting opioid.
- Aggressively treat blood loss, as hemodynamic instability exacerbated by decreasing intravascular volume
- Very sensitive to effects of exogenous catecholamines. Fluid boluses preferred over vasopressors. However, if vasopressors are required, use direct-acting agents.
- Consider controlled ventilation.

Emergence

- Titration of analgesics for pain control
- Spontaneous breathing may be delayed. $PaCO_2$ levels are a poor trigger for breathing 2° to chemoreceptor dysfunction.
- Aggressive pulm toilet: pts are at greater risk for atelectasis and bronchiectasis.

Postoperative Care

- Although peripheral pain sensation is diminished, visceral pain sensation is usually intact and presents as anxiety, Htn, or tachycardia and can precipitate dysautonomic crisis. Treat pain with careful titration of narcotics and/or consider NSAIDs.
- Maintain CV stability with fluids, plasma expanders, blood products, and mineralocorticoids as needed.
- Consider resp optimization with assisted ventilation, deep suctioning, inhalational therapies, and/or chest physiotherapy.

Anticipated Problems/Concerns

- Resp function often compromised by aspiration, hypotonic musculature, and scoliosis, and abn response to hypoxemia and hypercarbia; some authors advocate endotracheal intubation until pain Rx no longer needed
- Autonomic instability characterized by hypotension and/or Htn, arrhythmias, central sleep apnea, and temp dysregulation

Familial Periodic Paralysis (Hyperkalemic)

W. John Russell

Risk

- Rare, probably about 1/200,000
- Race appears to be exclusively Caucasian
- Presents usually in childhood

Perioperative Risks

- No reported increase in mortality with any procedure, but severe myotonia could create resp difficulty
- Succinylcholine may not give relaxation, and therefore an unexpected difficult intubation may result.
- Succinylcholine may also cause hyperkalemia and cardiac arrhythmia.

Worry About

- Cold can trigger an attack
- Hypoglycemia can trigger an attack; minimize fasting

Overview

- Intrinsic defect in muscle membrane allows depolarization of the muscle, but Na^+ channel does not close. Membrane thus remains inexcitable and a variable K^+ efflux continues.
- Pt may experience profound global stiffness and weakness after succinylcholine, exposure to cold, or spontaneously.
- Dx by family Hx

ICD-9-CM Code: 359.3

Etiology

- Na^+ channel in skeletal muscle membrane has a defective α subunit.
- Defect associated with chromosome 17 is substitution of a single base pair, usually methionine replacing threonine in fifth transmembrane segment of second domain.

- An autosomal dominant condition; allows a persistent Na^+ influx with activation threshold ~ 10 mV more negative than normal
- Persistence of a Na^+ influx is associated with K^+ leak from cell
- Episodes of weakness associated with elevated serum K^+ levels

Usual Treatment

- Avoid succinylcholine.
- Avoid cooling during anesthesia.
- Avoid hypoglycemia.
- Do not give K^+-containing solutions.
- Preop treatment with furosemide has been used.
- Severe postop weakness may be alleviated with Ca^{2+}.

ASSESSMENT POINTS

System	Effect	Assessment by Hx	PE	Test
MS	Weakness	Exercise, fatigue	Limb tone	Electromyography (discharges) K^+ load

Key Reference: Ashwood EM, Russell WJ, Burrows DD. Hyperkalaemic periodic paralysis and anesthesia. *Anaesthesia.* 1992;47:579–584.

Perioperative Implications

Preoperative Preparation
- 24 hr furosemide for K^+ depletion

Monitoring
- Temp (esophageal) (keep warm)
- ECG (detection of hyperkalemia)
- Neuromuscular (minimize relaxant dose)

Airway
- No special difficulty, but may need support

Preinduction/Induction
- Regional techniques are appropriate
- Avoid ketamine and succinylcholine
- Relaxation with nondepolarizing agents as indicated

Maintenance
- Keep warm
- Warm all IV fluid, use glucose 5% as maintenance

Extubation
- Normal reversal as indicated clinically
- Evidence of muscle weakness should be treated with IV calcium gluconate or chloride 10% 10 mL slowly over 5 min.

Adjuvants
- Some experimental evidence suggests that condition, e.g., postop weakness, may be helped by phenytoin or by salbutamol.
- Anticipate normal analgesic requirements for age and surgery.
- Regional techniques are appropriate.

Anticipated Problems/Concerns

- Severe myotonia may create resp difficulty.
- Succinylcholine may not give relaxation, and therefore intubation may be difficult.
- Cold or hypoglycemia can trigger hyperkalemic attack.
- Hyperkalemia can cause cardiac arrhythmia.

Familial Periodic Paralysis (Hypokalemic)

W. John Russell

Risk

- Rare, about 1 in 100,000
- Appears to occur in most races
- Presents usually in childhood or adolescence

Perioperative Risks

- Assoc with supraventricular or conduction defect–type cardiac arrhythmias
- Treatment with lidocaine is contraindicated.
- Weakness may be enhanced or precipitated by β-adrenergic blocking drugs
- Resp muscle weakness may occur postop.

Worry About

- Attacks after glucose intake or insulin administration
- Cold triggers attacks
- Serum K^+ levels should be maintained above 4.0 mEq/L.
- Cardiac dysrhythmias, esp bradycardias, during an attack

Overview

- Any severe hypokalemia may induce paralysis in susceptible persons even if they do not have familial disease. Limb weakness and paralysis have been reported after thyrotoxicosis, starvation, autoimmune and renal disease.
- Familial hypokalemic periodic paralysis is an autosomal dominant condition with reduced penetrance in females.
- Usually the pt will be aware of the onset of weakness
- Prompt treatment with K^+ will usually abort an attack, although as much as 40 mEq of K^+ may be required hourly
- Attacks are most likely with anything that increases muscle activity; can be precipitated by exercise and also cold, presumably because of the increased muscle activity in shivering. Usually there will be a CK increase during an attack.
- The symptoms in many pts can be controlled by regular K^+ supplements and acetazolamide.

ICD-9-CM Code: 359.3

Etiology

- The intrinsic defect in muscle membrane appears to be assoc with gene localized to 1q31–1q32 region near the dihydropyridine receptor gene.
- Unrelated to familial hyperkalemic disease
- Gene defect substitutes an arginine and impairs voltage-sensitive Ca^{2+} channel in about 70% of pts. Less commonly, in about 10% the Na^+ channel is affected. The change causes a compensatory increase in the $Na^+/K^+/Cl^-$ co-transport and a reduced overall efflux in K^+.

Usual Treatment

- Avoid cooling during anesthesia, hyperglycemia
- Give solutions containing K^+. Up to 30 mEq IV over 1 hr, aim for K^+ 4–5 mEq/L.
- Acetazolamide should be considered, if not already being given.
- Severe postop weakness may be aggravated by Ca^{2+}.
- Ventilation during anesthesia should be normocarbic to avoid K^+ shifts.
- Maintenance by IPPV if evidence of weakness in postop phase

ASSESSMENT POINTS

System	Effect	Assessment by Hx	PE	Test
RESP	Inadequate	Noticeable SOB	Resp rate high	ABGs
MS	Weakness	Exercise, fatigue	Limb tone	Serum K^+ elevation < Normal (normal = 0.8 ± 0.2 mEq/L) Glucose/insulin or ACTH infusion induces paralysis attack Plasma biochemistry after attack: Elevated myoglobin, creatine kinase Muscle fiber conduction velocity may be slower than normal.

Key Reference: Hecht ML, Valtysson B, Hogan K. Spinal anesthesia for a patient with a calcium channel mutation causing hypokalemic periodic paralysis. *Anesth Analg.* 1997;84(2):461–464.

Perioperative Implications

Preoperative Preparation

- 24-hr acetazolamide if not already given. Only glucose-free solutions IV. If Hx of frequent instability, prepare infusion with K^+.

Monitoring

- Temp (esophageal). Keep warm.
- ECG (detection of hypokalemia may not be seen until late)
- NM (minimize relaxant dose)

Airway

- No special difficulty, but may need support

Preinduction/Induction

- Regional techniques are appropriate.

Induction

- Successful relaxation with succinylcholine and with atracurium has been reported.

Maintenance

- Use warming blanket.
- Warm all IV fluid, use glucose-free solutions as maintenance.

Extubation

- Normal reversal as indicated clinically
- Evidence of muscle weakness should be treated with IV potassium chloride up to 40 mEq/hr

Adjuvants

- Ca^{2+}-channel blockers do not appear to be contraindicated in pts with concomitant CV disease.
- Anticipate usual analgesic requirements for age and surgery.

Anticipated Problems/Concerns

- May have assoc supraventricular or conduction defect arrhythmias
- Resp muscle weakness may occur postop.
- Cold triggers attack.
- Must maintain serum K^+ above 4.0 mEq/L

Fat Embolism

Brian J. McGrath

Risk

- Long bone fractures, pelvic fractures
  - 80–100% fat embolism
  - 0.2–19% fat embolism syndrome (FES)
- Male > female
- Adult >> pediatric
- Multiple fractures > single fractures
- Pathologic fractures > traumatic fractures
- Total hip, total knee replacement, intramedullary nailing:
  - 27–100% fat embolism
  - Unknown incidence FES
- Unusual causes: Liposuction, fat injection, bone marrow harvest and/or transplantation, vertebroplasty, cardiopulmonary bypass, CPR, burns, pancreatitis, sickle cell disease, osteomyelitis, fatty liver, soft tissue injury

Perioperative Risks

- FES: 7–20% mortality
- Pre-existing FES: Respiratory failure/ARDS, RV dysfunction, shock, coagulopathy, neurologic dysfunction
- Intraop fat embolism: Shock, hypoxemia

Worry About

- Pre-existing FES: Hypoxemia, reduced pulm compliance, hypotension, cardiac arrest, Pulm Htn, RV failure, abnormal CNS response to anesthetic, coagulopathy
- Intraop embolism: Hypotension, right ventricular failure, hypoxemia, paradoxical embolization, neurologic dysfunction

Overview

- Fat particles (globules of marrow fat) traveling into blood and lung
- Must distinguish fat embolism, which is common, from FES, a much less common consequence of fat embolism
- FES can produce mild pulm dysfunction to severe ARDS.
- Pulm Htn and acute right ventricular failure may occur in severe cases of FES.
- Typically, the onset of signs and symptoms of FES is delayed up to 72 hr following injury.
- Fat embolism occurs commonly during femoral reaming and cementing in hip arthroplasty.
- FES is confounded with cement reaction during arthroplasty.

ICD9-CM: 673.8 (Other pulmonary embolism)

Etiology

- Most frequently follows orthopedic trauma with release of marrow fat into venous circulation
- Pathology produced by mechanical obstruction by intravascular fat passing into the pulm and systemic arterial circulation and by production of endogenous inflammatory mediators

Usual Treatment

- Early fracture fixation to decrease embolization
- Use of noncemented prosthesis or venting of femoral shaft may reduce embolization during hip arthroplasty
- Unreamed nailing for fracture fixation to reduce embolization
- O_2 therapy to maintain SaO_2 >90%
- Low tidal volume ventilation strategy with PEEP for ARDS
- Aggressive hemodynamic support with fluid and/or inotropes for shock and/or RV failure
- Factor replacement for coagulopathy with bleeding
- Corticosteroids, heparin, ethanol, dextran, aspirin, prophylactic vena caval filter: Unproven benefit

ASSESSMENT POINTS

System	Effect	Assessment by Hx	PE	Test
CV	Intravascular fat	Fever		?Fat staining of blood ?Bronchoalveolar lavage, macrophage staining
	Hypoperfusion Pulm Htn RV failure	Syncope Dyspnea	Hypotension Tachycardia Oliguria Vasoconstriction Mental status changes	TEE, CVP, ?PA catheter Lactic acidosis
RESP	ARDS Hypoxemia	Dyspnea	Tachypnea Cyanosis Rales	CXR ABGs Pulm compliance
HEME	Thrombocytopenia DIC Anemia	Bleeding	Bleeding(rare)	CBC Platelets PT, PTT D-Dimer Fibrinogen
DERM	Capillary fat embolism		Petechiae (60%) Axilla, chest Base of neck Conjunctiva Oral mucous membranes	
CNS	Neurologic injury Cerebral edema	Mental status changes	Delirium Confusion Focal deficits (rare) Seizure (rare) Coma (rare)	? MRI

Key Reference: Bulger EM, Smith DG, Maier RV, Jurkovich GJ. Fat embolism syndrome, a 10 year review. *Arch Surg.* 1997;132:435–439.

Perioperative Implications

Preoperative Preparation

- Avoid sedatives and/or narcotics if hypoxemic and not mechanically ventilated or with obtundation

Monitoring

- Arterial catheter
- TEE, CVP, ?PA catheter to diagnose and manage right ventricular failure and/or pulm Htn

Airway

- May already be intubated and ventilated in severe cases
- Decreased FRC, O_2 reserve and tolerance of apnea with ARDS

Induction

- Minimize myocardial depression
- Avoid increases in PA pressures

Maintenance

- CV: Anticipate decrease in BP with femoral reaming/cementing: anesthetic reduction, fluid, vasopressors; pts with RV dysfunction may require longer-term inotropic support
- Resp: pts with ARDS may require increased FIO_2 and PEEP; utilize lung protective strategy with low tidal volume ventilation
- Heme: Factor replacement for coagulopathy with bleeding

Extubation

- Maintain intubation and mechanical ventilation in hemodynamically unstable pts and those requiring increased FIO_2, PEEP or with reduced compliance
- Pts with CNS involvement may have a prolonged or exaggerated response to anesthetics and narcotics and may require intubation postop for airway protection/patency

Anticipated Problems/Concerns

- Embolism during femoral reaming, prosthesis cementing
- FES may be delayed by up to 72 hr following fat embolism
- Pts with ARDS may be difficult to ventilate and oxygenate
- Hypotension is due to RV dysfunction and pulm Htn

Foreign Body Aspiration

Frederic Berry
Christopher Stemland

Risk

- Foreign body aspiration into the airway or esophagus is one of the most frequent and threatening pediatric surgical emergencies
- Morbidity and mortality ranges from 0–4.8%

Perioperative Risks

- Risk of aspiration is present but is very small. The danger period for vomiting or regurgitation with aspiration is primarily during the induction and recovery from anesthesia.

- Transfer to a specialized facility should be considered if a stable resp status.
- Urgent cases should go directly to the OR

Overview

- Acute presentation, with parent or caretaker witnessing the child swallowing or aspirating a foreign body and immediately developing cough, dyspnea, and stridor

- Delayed presentation with prolonged and often unexplained resp symptoms incl cough, wheezing, and recurrent resp tract infections

ICD-9-CM Code: 934.0 (Foreign body in trachea)

Usual Treatment

- Rigid bronchoscopy
- Foreign bodies found 70–90% of the time

ASSESSMENT POINTS

System	Effect	PE	Test
RESP	Main stem bronchus may have ball-valve effect	Involved lung cannot fully expire	Chest exam
	Pneumonia	Reactive airway with decreased breath sounds	CXR Hyperinflation or atelectasis

Key References: Litman R, Zur K. Pediatric foreign body retrieval: Surgical and anesthetic perspectives. *Paediatr Anaesth.* 2009;19(suppl 1):109–117. Woods AM. Pediatric endoscopy. In Berry FA (ed): Anesthetic Management of Difficult and Routine Pediatric Patients, 2nd ed. New York, Churchill Livingstone, 1990, pp 199–242. Higuchi O, Kazuteru Kawaski. Foreign body aspiration in children: A nationwide survey in Japan. *Inter J of Ped Otorhinolaryngology.* 2009; 73:659–661.

Perioperative Management

- Divided into three time periods: preop, intraop, and postop

Preoperative Concerns

- NPO period: The stomach will not empty, so proceed expeditiously.
- An IV should be started if possible and an anticholinergic agent administered. If the child has pneumonia, addition of antibiotics is indicated.
- Rapid sequence intubation for full stomach situations

Intraoperative Management

- Done in OR without presence of parents
- A technique of spontaneous ventilation usually with sevoflurane
- Controversy exists about whether to maintain spontaneous ventilation or administer a muscle relaxant.
- If child is struggling to breathe or cyanotic, induction is with sevoflurane and O_2.
- If only mild airway distress, nitrous oxide used for initial inhalation induction to facilitate administration of sevoflurane. Sevoflurane is the ideal induction agent. In addition, small doses of ketamine or a propofol infusion may be added to stabilize the maintenance anesthetic.

- Light anesthesia should be avoided.
- Small amounts of PEEP (3–5 cm H_2O) useful for any degree of obstruction
- Topical anesthesia of larynx and cords with 4% solution of lidocaine, 5 mg/kg (4% Lidocaine contains 40 mg lidocaine/mL) prior to laryngoscopy, so no response to introduction of ventilating bronchoscope
- If an IV is present, small doses of propofol (1 mg/kg) to make inhalation induction smoother

Monitoring

- $ETCO_2$ (also the wave form) may be elevated into the 80s or 90s. As long as O_2 saturation remains in 85–95 range, the CO_2 is usually not a problem.
- Using a ventilating bronchoscope with a sidearm attachment for anesthesia circuit, bronchoscope advanced through larynx into trachea and often into main stem bronchus. Desaturation may result from inadequate ventilation of contralateral lung. If this occurs consider administering PEEP until saturation can be returned to reasonable range.
- With pneumonia, saturations may not be able to be raised higher than the low 90s. Saturation of 85–90 is acceptable as long as it is stable. If rapidly falling O_2 saturation, bronchoscope must be

withdrawn from trachea and ventilation assisted with PEEP.
- The critical part of the surgery occurs when the surgeon extracts the foreign body from the airway. If the child starts to move or cough, management is either releasing foreign body and deepening the anesthetic; or administering either muscle relaxant such as succinylcholine, or 1 mg/kg of propofol, lidocaine, or ketamine (1 mg/kg) to deepen anesthesia.

Postoperative Management

- After trachea and bronchus are rechecked with ventilating bronchoscope, trachea is intubated and awake extubation performed. If pt is coughing but not sufficiently awake, lidocaine 1.5 mg/kg can be administered IV.

Anticipated Problems/Concerns

- Hypercarbia
- Hypoxia
- Atelectasis
- Bronchitis

Friedreich's Ataxia

Mark Helfaer

Risk

- Prevalence: 2/100,000; 80–90% have cardiac involvement

Worry About

- Cardiac involvement does not correlate with neurologic involvement
- Electrophysiologic disturbances
- Cardiac dysfunction and failure

Overview

- Progressive degeneration of posterior columns and corticospinal and posterior spinocerebellar tracts
- Muscle weakness
- Abnormal glucose homeostasis

- Usual onset in childhood
- Proprioceptive sensory loss, areflexia, ataxia of limbs, Babinski's sign
- Pes cavus and scoliosis
- Cardiomyopathy

ICD-9-CM Code: 334.0

Etiology

- Inherited: Usually autosomal recessive, but occasionally dominant
- Nucleotide has been mapped
- Fratoxin (mitochondrial iron content protein) deficiency

Usual Treatment

- Usually untreatable and progressive
- Medical management of cardiac abnormalities
- Scoliosis repair
- Can be mistaken for metabolic disorders (hexosaminidase A deficiency, adrenomyelo-neuropathy, vitamin E deficiency)
- Clinical trials of coenzyme Q10 (CoQ10)/vitamin E

ASSESSMENT POINTS

System	Effect	Assessment by Hx	Test
CV	LV hypokinesia Concentric and asymmetric hypertrophy Cardiomyopathy	Severities of heart and neurologic manifestations are not proportional	ECG ECHO Endomyocardial biopsy
RESP	Severe scoliosis Neuromuscular impairment	Noncardiac dyspnea	Lung functions
MS	Pes cavus Scoliosis Resp muscle weakness unpredictable and variable response to muscle relaxants	Ability to walk without assistance	

Key Reference: Pancaro C, Renz D. Anesthetic management in Friedreich's ataxia. *Paediatr Anaesth.* 2005;15(5):433–434.

Perioperative Implications

Preoperative Preparation
- Usual premedication

Monitoring
- Train of four to monitor effects of neuromuscular blocking agent with unpredictable response due to neuromuscular disease

Airway
- None

Preinduction/Induction
- Case report of sensitivity to curare (0.06 mg/kg caused 90 min apnea)
- Possibility of hyperkalemia and cardiac arrhythmias after succinylcholine

Maintenance
- Case reports of successful spinal and epidural anesthesia
- Case reports of spotty lumbar epidural block
- Case reports of successful GA with cautious use of nondepolarizing agents
- Case report of successful use of hypotensive anesthesia with isoflurane
- Case report of marked decrease in cardiac output and supraventricular tachycardia with nitroprusside for hypotensive anesthesia
- Case report of successful use of epidural narcotic

Extubation
- If adequate strength from neuromuscular blocker and adequate pulm function, extubation is appropriate

Adjuvants
- See under Maintenance

Gastrinoma

Christine Piefer

DISEASES

Risk

- Mean age of onset in the fourth decade
- Slight male predominance
- Less than 0.1% of all PUD caused by gastrinomas
- 60% of gastrinomas are malignant

Perioperative Risks

- Risks associated with PUD
- Assoc tumors (MEN type I)
- Risks assoc with metastatic disease (regional lymph nodes, liver, bone)

Worry About

- Large gastric fluid volume
- Esophageal reflux (common)
- Intravascular volume depletion

- Electrolyte imbalance 2° to watery diarrhea
- Coagulation abn due to liver metastases or poor fat absorption

Overview

- Gastrinoma is a gastrin-secreting neuroendocrine tumor (non-beta islet cell tumor) occurring most commonly in duodenum or pancreas
- Gastrin release stimulates gastric acid hypersecretion which causes symptoms of abdominal pain (due to refractory peptic ulcer disease), diarrhea and GERD known as Zollinger-Ellison syndrome
- Diagnosis often delayed several years from onset of symptoms because of difficulties distinguishing it from other cases of PUD

- Most cases are sporadic but 25% occur as part of the MEN I syndrome (parathyroid tumors, pituitary hyperplasia and pancreatic islet cell tumors)

ICD-9-CM Code: 235.5

See also Multiple Endocrine Neoplasia (MEN) Types I and II in Diseases section

Etiology

- May be inherited as autosomal dominant trait when associated with MEN I

Usual Treatment

- Control gastric acid hypersecretion with proton pump inhibitors and H_2 blockers
- Surgical exploration and resection

ASSESSMENT POINTS

System	Effect	Assessment by Hx	PE	Test
CARDIO	Hypovolemia	Weakness, dizziness	Vital signs	Orthostatics
GI	Gastric acid hypersecretion	Abdominal pain, esophageal reflux, diarrhea	Abd exam	Fasting gastrin levels Secretin stimulation test
FEN	Hypokalemia	Weakness, muscle cramps		Electrolytes, EKG
ENDO*	Hyperparathyroidism	Multiple systems involved		Serum parathyroid hormone
RENAL*	Nephrolithiasis	Flank pain, hematuria	Costovertebral angle tenderness	Urinalysis
CNS*	Pituitary adenoma	Headaches, visual changes	Visual fields	MRI; prolactin level
MS*	Weakness, arthralgias	Proximal muscle weakness	Motor strength Hyperreflexia	Ca^{2+} levels
HEME	Coagulation disorder	Bleeding abn		PT, PTT

* If gastrinoma presents as component of MEN I.
Key Reference: Jensen RT. Gastrinomas: Advances in diagnosis and management. *Neuroendocrinology*. 2004;80(suppl 1):23–27.

Perioperative Implications

Preoperative Preparation

- Assure adequate treatment of gastric hypersecretion
- Evaluate for other endocrinopathies of MEN I syndrome
- Assess volume status
- Check electrolytes and coagulation tests
- Consider preop NG tube placement

Monitoring

- May need central venous pressure monitoring and arterial line due to intravascular volume depletion causing hypotension and potential for fluid shifts. UO should be measured with a bladder catheter.

Induction

- Treat as full stomach due to increased gastric acid volumes and increased risk for aspiration
- Rapid-sequence induction with cricoid pressure

Extubation

- Assess adequate ventilatory function and recovery from neuromuscular blockade prior to extubation

Adjuvants

- May consider epidural catheter for postop pain control

Postoperative Period

- Decreased vital capacity and FRC due to pain and ileus
- Concern for continued symptoms if surgical resection not curative

Anticipated Problems/Concerns

- Lower cure rates after resection for pts with gastrinomas assoc with MEN I or in the presence of metastatic liver disease

Gastroesophageal Reflux in Children

Francine S. Yudkowitz

Risk

- Symptoms of gastroesophageal reflux (GER) persist past 6 wk of age in 1/500 infants
- 60% resolve by age 18 mo; 30% persist beyond age 4 y
- 5% develop esophageal stricture
- 5% die of complications of GER
- 10% of pyloric stenosis pts
- After diaphragmatic hernia, tracheoesophageal fistula, and esophageal atresia repairs
- Neurologically impaired or developmentally delayed children with spastic quadriplegia, hypoxic brain damage, or trisomy syndromes

Perioperative Risks

- Aspiration during induction of anesthesia
- Severe bronchospasm in pts with reactive airway disease (RAD)
- Decreased pulm reserve 2° to chronic aspiration and pneumonitis

Worry About

- Pulm complications from aspiration pneumonitis and RAD
- Anemia and malnutrition

Overview

- GER is defined as regurgitation without pathological consequences. GER disease (GERD) is defined as regurgitation resulting in esophagitis, nutritional compromise, and/or resp complications.
- Presence of a hiatal hernia does not necessarily mean pt will have GER
- Older children may complain of heartburn and chest pain
- Degree of reflux, duration of acid exposure in the esophagus, and ability of the esophagus to clear the reflux material determine extent of mucosal damage and degree of esophagitis
- Esophagitis may lead to bleeding, which may result in hematemesis, iron-deficiency anemia, and esophageal stricture. Also, predisposes to Barrett esophagus
- GER may be a cause of neonatal apnea.
- Diagnostic procedures incl upper GI series, esophagoscopy, and esophageal pH probe.

ICD-9-CM Code: 530.81

Etiology

- Immature maturation of the lower esophageal sphincter
- Dyscoordination of swallowing mechanism in neurologically impaired pts

Usual Treatment

- Medical
  - Thickening of feeds for infants. Avoidance of acidic foods and beverages in older children.
  - Maintaining the upright position after feeds in infants. Sitting position worsens reflux.
  - Antacids, H_2 blockers, or proton pump inhibitors to decrease gastric acidity
- Surgical
  - Indicated when medical therapy fails or in the presence of life-threatening disease.
  - Open or laparoscopic Nissen fundoplication. Success rate 95% in neurologically intact pts. Pts who are neurologically impaired have a greater morbidity and mortality with surgical repair.

ASSESSMENT POINTS

System	Effect	Assessment by Hx	PE	Test
RESP	Chronic aspiration	Cough, cyanotic episodes, apnea	Rales, rhonchi	CXR, ABGs (if indicated)
	RAD	Dyspnea, wheezing, cough	Wheezing ↓ BS, prolonged expiration	CXR, peak flow ABGs (if indicated)
HEME	Iron deficiency		Pallor	CBC
GENERAL	Malnutrition	Wt loss	↓ SQ tissue	Serum albumin

Key Reference: Cook-Sather SD, et al. Overweight/obesity and gastric fluid characteristics in pediatric day surgery: Implications for fasting guidelines and pulmonary aspiration risk. *Anesth Analg.* 2009;109:727–736.

Perioperative Implications

Preoperative Preparation

- Assess the severity of pulm compromise
- Optimize resp status: Treat pneumonia and control bronchospasm
- Correct anemia
- Improve nutritional status
- Confirm availability of blood
- Continue acid-suppressing therapy

Monitoring

- Consider arterial line

Induction

- At risk for aspiration. Rapid-sequence induction with cricoid pressure.
- For pts with RAD, ensure adequate depth of anesthesia prior to instrumenting the airway

Maintenance

- No one anesthetic preferred
- Avoid N_2O in laparoscopic procedure
- Esophageal bougie may be required
- Watch for possible pneumothorax, trauma to viscera, hemorrhage, and vena cava compression or laceration. Air embolism may occur during laparoscopic procedures.

- During laparoscopic procedures, intra-abdominal pressures of ≤12 mmHg should be maintained.

Extubation/Postoperative Period

- May be extubated after uncomplicated surgery
- Pts with severe resp compromise preop or with neurologic impairment may require a period of postop ventilation.
- Analgesic requirements will be less after laparoscopic procedures.

Surgical Procedure

- Fundus of the stomach is wrapped around the lower part of the esophagus. May be accomplished either open or laparoscopically.
- Pyloroplasty may be performed for associated delayed gastric emptying.
- Pneumoperitoneum created during laparoscopic surgery will result in increased SVR, increased CVP, increased CO, and increased BP. Intra-abdominal pressures >20 mmHg will decrease venous return and decrease CO, but the BP will remain unchanged due to increased SVR.
- Pneumoperitoneum will also elevate the diaphragms, which will decrease lung volumes, decrease FRC, decrease compliance, increased airway resistance, and increased V/Q mismatch.
- Pneumoperitoneum should not exceed 12 mmHg. Pts are placed in the reverse Trendelenburg position. This will help ameliorate both diaphragmatic elevation and the CVP elevation.
- Pneumoperitoneum is accomplished by the insufflation of CO_2, which may necessitate increased minute ventilation
- Laparoscopic procedures are associated with reduced rates of postop resp and wound complications and analgesic requirements, and shorter hospital stays.

Anticipated Problems/Concerns

- Resp compromise
- Unable to vomit postop and up to 3 mo after surgery. Therefore, intestinal obstruction in the postop period should be treated as a dire emergency.

Glaucoma, Closed-Angle

Risk

- Worldwide prevalence: 15.7 million pts with angle closure glaucoma (ACG) in 2009
- Second most common cause of irreversible blindness
- Risk factors: Eskimo, fhinese (87%), or Indian race, age (>60), female gender (69%), family Hx

Perioperative Risks

- Further damage to the optic nerve

Worry About

- Glaucoma pts may be at increased risk of sight-threatening complications from orbital injections because the optic nerve is already compromised and vulnerable to pressure/ischemic damage. Rather than a retrobulbar or peribulbar block, less invasive techniques of local anesthesia may be employed (anterior sub-Tenon, subconjunctival, topical, or intracameral placement.)

Overview

- ACG is a chronic (or sometimes acute) condition characterized by progressive pressure/ischemic damage to the optic nerve head, due to an obstruction to the outflow of aqueous humor and consequent rise in intraocular pressure. Acute ACG is an ophthalmologic emergency.

ICD – 9CM Codes: 365.20 (Primary ACG, unspecified), 365.21 (Intermittent ACG), 365.22 (Acute ACG), 365.23 (Chronic ACG), 365.24 (Residual Stage of ACG)

Etiology

- Multifactorial: Once thought to be primarily due to occluded drainage angles in the anterior chamber of the eye (leading to elevated IOP), optic nerve ischemia has been found to occur in pts with either elevated or normal IOP (which is 10–20 mmHg). Causative etiologies for the damage may also incl excitotoxicity, neurotrophin insufficiency, inflammatory cytokines, or immune abn.
- Precipitating factors: Dim/indoor light, anticholinergic agents (atropine, cyclopentolate, tropicamide, antihistamines, antipsychotics, antidepressants, antiparkinsonian, and GI spasmolytics), adrenergic agents (topical, e.g., epinephrine and phenylephrine), or systemic, (e.g., vasoconstrictors, central nervous system stimulants, bronchodilators, appetite depressants, and hallucinogenic agents), emotional stress

Usual Treatment for Acute ACG

- Topical β-blocker, α2-agonist, pilocarpine 2% or 4% (pilocarpine is effective in inducing miosis only when iris ischemia is relieved, i.e., when intraocular pressure falls to <50 mmHg)

- IV/oral acetazolamide 5–10 mg/kg (alternatives: hyperosmotic agents, e.g., IV 20% mannitol 1–2 g/kg, oral 50% glycerol 1–1.5 g/kg (contraindicated in diabetics), oral isosorbide 1.5–2.0 g/kg)
- Topical steroids
- Lie pt supine (to allow lens-iris diaphragm to move posteriorly)
- Analgesia and antiemetics
- After 1–2 hrs, if the attack is broken and corneal edema resolves (or if it is not broken but the cornea is clear), perform laser iridotomy.
- If attack is not broken and cornea is still hazy, pt should have laser iridoplasty first, followed by laser iridotomy later when cornea edema resolves.

Usual Treatment for Chronic ACG

- Reduction of IOP with prostaglandins (latanoprost, bimatoprost, travoprost)
- Other surgical options incl trabeculectomy, gonioplasty, or lens extraction.

ASSESSMENT POINTS

System	Effect	Hx	PE	Test
HEENT	Acute ACG	Sudden unilateral pain Blurred vision Photophobia Colored halos around lights Headache N/V	Ocular injection Hazy cornea Mid-dilated pupil	Penlight Gonioscope Slit-lamp US biomicroscopy
	Subacute ACG	Headaches (often mistaken for migraine) or asymptomatic		
	Chronic ACG	Generally asymptomatic		

Key Reference: SubakSharpe I, Low S, Nolan W, Foster PJ. Pharmacological and environmental factors in primary angle closure glaucoma. *Br Med Bull.* 2010;93:12543.

Perioperative Implications

Preoperative Preparation

- Avoid mydriasis, either due to stress, dim lighting, or drugs.
- Check electrolytes if pt is on a diuretic.
- Preop antisialogogues or scopolamine are generally ok.
- Many pts undergoing ophthalmic surgery take anticoagulants; the relative risks of a thrombotic complication must be weighed against possible bleeding. Glaucoma surgery is of intermediate risk for serious hemorrhagic complications. A consensus is developing that cataract surgery may be safely performed while maintaining pts on warfarin. For intermediate risk procedures, such as some glaucoma surgeries, stopping warfarin for 4 d preop is indicated. A pt may continue their clopidogrel.
- Echothiophate should be D/C 4 to 6 wk prior to surgery. Systemic absorption can inhibit plasma cholinesterase (causing prolonged muscle paralysis after succinylcholine) as well as inhibit metabolism of ester local anesthetics (LA), predisposing a pt to LA toxicity.

Induction

- Frequently, these cases may be done under very light sedation and topical anesthesia and possibly a block performed by the surgeon. Anesthetic goals center around minimizing interventions that may increase IOP or cause further damage to the optic nerve.
- General anesthesia may be required by the surgeon or due to individual pt factors. Succinylcholine increases IOP by 6–12 mmHg for 5 to 10 min, and may be used. Endotracheal intubation causes a similar increase in IOP. Bucking, coughing, and vomiting increase IOP by 30–40 and should be avoided. ET intubation causes a similar increase in IOP. An LMA may be preferred.

Maintenance

- Avoid hypercapnia, which will cause choroidal vascular congestion.
- Be prepared for bradycardia and/or arrhythmia due to elevated IOP and surgical pressure

Extubation

- Minimize coughing and bucking.

Anticipated Problems/Concerns

- 50–75% of pts will have ACG in the contralateral eye within 1 y; prophylactic iridotomy greatly reduces this risk.
- There is a phenomenon of severe visual loss after surgery, with no obvious cause, known as wipe out, or snuff syndrome. Local anesthetic injections are a putative cause, perhaps due to unnoticed direct trauma to the optic nerve from the needle, or to a hematoma in the nerve sheath, or simply due to the volume of the LA itself. High pressure around the nerve could potentially occur even with a low volume of LA if it were to be trapped between fascial layers and cause a compartment syndrome. Epinephrine in the LA mixture may contribute to ischemia due to a marked reduction in blood flow to the anterior optic nerve. This effect is not seen with anterior (e.g., subconjunctival) placement of LA.
- Topical β-blockers (esp. Timolol) may have systemic effects, and have been shown to exacerbate asthma and CHF, and produce bradycardia.

Glaucoma, Open-Angle

James W. Ibinson
Laura H. Ferguson

Risk

• Open-angle glaucoma is the leading cause of blindness among African Americans and the second leading cause overall in the USA.
• African American race, advanced age, elevated intraocular pressure (IOP), myopia, low diastolic perfusion pressures, and family Hx of open-angle glaucoma increase the risk for primary open-angle glaucoma.
• Incidence in USA: Estimates suggest over 2.25 million Americans over age 40 have open-angle glaucoma.

Perioperative Risks

• Vision loss secondary to optic nerve damage from pressure or ischemia.

Worry About

• Interactions between ophthalmologic drugs and anesthetics
• Increases in IOP
• Periop derangements in electrolytes secondary to ophthalmologic drugs

Overview

• Glaucoma is a degenerative optic neuropathy characterized by optic-nerve cupping that results in progressive vision loss and possibly blindness if not treated. Treatment does not reverse the blindness.
• Elevated IOP is often found in glaucoma but is not required for the diagnosis. Nonetheless, treatment for all forms is aimed at maintaining a low-normal IOP.
• Onset is gradual, bilateral, and often unnoticed. While juvenile forms exist, it is much more common in those above 40 y of age.

ICD-9-CM Code: 365.10

Etiology

• Likely caused by sclerosis of the trabecular meshwork near the canal of Schlemm which decreases aqueous humor outflow and elevates IOP
• Normal pressure, open-angle glaucoma is thought to be caused by insufficient blood flow leading to optic nerve damage, but treatment is the same as with primary open-angle glaucoma.

Usual Treatment

• Treatment goal is to maintain a low-normal IOP. Treatment is most successful if disease is detected early.
• Medical treatment incl topical timolol, betaxolol, epinephrine, echothiophate, or dipivefrin and oral acetazolamide.
• Surgical treatment incl laser trabeculoplasty, trabeculectomy, Baerveldt and Ahmed device implantation, and cycloablation.

ASSESSMENT POINTS

System	Effect	Assessment by Hx	PE	Test
HEENT	Optic nerve damage, increased IOP	Visual changes, family Hx of glaucoma, myopia	Decreased visual acuity, increased optic cup-to-disk ratio, visual field losses	Slit lamp exam Tonometry Visual fields Visual acuity
CV	Excessive beta blockade	Fatigue, syncope or near-syncope, SOB, chest pain	Hypotension, bradycardia	

Key Reference: Kwon YH, Fingert JH, Kuehn MH, Alward WL. Primary open-angle glaucoma. *N Engl J Med*. 2009;360(11):1113–1124.

Perioperative Implications

Preinduction

• Maintain miosis by continuing topical and systemic treatment medications except for echothiophate, which should be stopped four weeks prior to elective surgery.
• Pts taking acetazolamide, a carbonic anhydrase inhibitor, should have electrolytes checked preop with specific attention to Na⁺, K⁺, and bicarbonate levels.
• Antisialogogue premedication with glycopyrrolate or atropine is not contraindicated; however, several texts suggest scopolamine should be avoided due to its greater mydriatic effect.

Induction

• Blunt increases in IOP during laryngoscopy and intubation with the use of IV agents, which tend to decrease IOP. Controversy surrounds ketamine's effect.
• Succinylcholine is safe for induction and intubation, provided echothiophate has been discontinued.
• Hypotension should be avoided due to optic nerve perfusion concerns.

• Use of a laryngeal mask airway may not increase IOP as much as direct laryngoscopy and intubation.

General Anesthesia

• All inhalational agents decrease IOP. This should be taken into account when providing anesthesia for eye exams.
• Hypercarbia should be avoided since it increases IOP. Hypothermia, on the other hand, lowers IOP.
• Timolol is systemically absorbed and can cause asthmatic crises and severe sinus bradycardia, esp when other beta blockers are administered. Betaxolol is more oculospecific, but additional beta blockade during anesthesia should be done with extreme caution. Effects of calcium channel blockers like verapamil are addictive and should be administered with care.
• Pneumoperitoneum and head-down positioning can increase IOP, but maintaining adequate anesthetic depth likely eliminates any measurable pressure increase.

Regional Anesthesia

• Ester local anesthetics should be avoided in pts taking echothiophate due to reduced plasma cholinesterase activity and altered metabolism.

Extubation

• Avoid coughing and bucking, which can cause acute increases in IOP.
• Neuromuscular blockade reversal agents and antimuscarinics in usual dosages are considered safe.

Postoperative Period

• If emergency surgery is required in pts currently taking echothiophate, expect the need for prolonged postop ventilation.

Anticipated Problems/Concerns

• Avoid increases in IOP.
• Echothiophate therapy produces decreased plasma cholinesterase activity and should be stopped 4 wk prior to surgery to avoid a prolonged paralysis with the use of succinylcholine.
• Be aware that topical beta-blockers are systemically absorbed and can have systemic effects.

Glomus Jugulare Tumors

Ghaleb A. Ghani

Risk

- 0.6% of head and neck tumors
- M:F ratio: 1:2.5
- Slow-growing
- Can co-exist with other paragangliomas
- Histologically benign but can be malignant with metastases

Perioperative Risks

- Hypothermia
- Massive blood loss
- Venous air embolism
- Htn
- Bradycardia
- Hypotension
- Bronchospasm
- Tumor-parts embolization

Worry About

- Multiple locations, persistence of symptoms after resection of the tumor

Overview

- Tumors of neural crest at base of skull in jugular bulb area
- Highly vascular
- May extend into the posterior fossa
- May cause hydrocepehalus
- May damage the lower cranial nerves (IX–XII)
- May involve internal carotid artery
- May grow into lumen of the jugular vein, as far as the right atrium
- May secrete catecholamines: 5%
- May secrete serotonin, histamine

ICD-9-CM Codes: 194.6 (Malignant); 237.3 (Paraganglia)

Etiology

- Congenital (usually benign) hypertrophied arteriovenous anastomosis
- Epithelial cells with abundant capillary network

Usual Treatment

- Resection
- Embolization, alone or pre-resection
- Radiation
- Gamma knife

ASSESSMENT POINTS

System	Effect	Assessment by Hx	PE	Test
HEENT	Cranial nerve injury	Hoarseness Dysphagia Tinnitus Vertigo	Tongue movement Soft palate motion Gag reflex Hearing test	Video laryngoscopy
CV	Htn Intravascular growth	Headache Palpitations	BP	Catecholamines level MRI/CT scans Angio (if indicated)
RESP	Aspiration	Cough Fever SOB	Rhonchi, wheezing	CXR
GI	Delayed gastric emptying	Heartburn Regurgitation		
GU		No different from normal		
CNS	Intracranial extension	Hearing loss Headache Dizziness		CT scan MRI (if indicated) Paragangliomas in other locations

Key Reference: Jensen NF. Glomus tumors of the head and neck: anesthetic considerations. *Anesth Analg.* 1994;78:112–119.

Perioperative Implications

Preoperative Preparation
- Control Htn (in catecholamine-secreting tumors). Preparation is similar to pheochromocytoma (see under Pheochromocytoma in Diseases section)
- Treat pneumonia
- Metoclopramide for delayed gastric emptying
- Adequate venous access for rapid fluid infusion

Monitoring
- Consider A-line, CVP
- Monitor for venous air embolism (frequent ABG, $ETCO_2$, N_2; precordial Doppler)
- Cerebral oximetry
- Facial nerve

Maintenance
- Watch out for massive blood loss, Htn, hypotension, bradycardia, bronchospasm, venous air embolism, tumor-parts embolization
- Provide controlled hypotension if needed
- Measure to decrease the ICP for intracranial extension:
  - Mannitol
  - Hyperventilation
  - Optimize venous return from brain
  - CSF drainage

Extubation
- Evaluate for cranial nerves (IX–XII) injury

Adjuvants
- Controlled ventilation
- Muscle relaxants to prevent spontaneous ventilation intraop
- Controlled hypotension

Anticipated Problems/Concerns

- Loss of upper airway reflexes
- Airway obstruction
- Aspiration
- Delayed gastric emptying
- Ileus
- CNS insult
- CSF leak

Glossopharyngeal Neuralgia

R. David Todd

DISEASES

Risk

- Age of onset peaks between 40 and 60 y
- Pts with MS
- Increased prevalence with extracranial neoplasms, trauma/infection/inflammation to tonsils and pharynx, arachnoiditis
- No difference in frequency between men and women

Perioperative Risks

- Attacks of pain can trigger bradycardia/asystole, arterial hypotension, syncope, ECG changes (arrhymthmias)
- Convulsive limb and facial movements that resemble seizure activity can accompany attack of pain

Worry About

- Bradycardia, asystole, arterial hypotension, syncope, arrhythmias during pain attacks
- Drug interations with anticonvulsants-carbamazepine, phenytoin
- Chronic narcotic use

Overview

- Rare: Constitutes <1% of cases of facial pain
- Sudden and unilateral pain involving the pharynx, tonsils, base of tongue, with radiation to the throat and/or ear structures (cranial nerve IX and X distribution).
- Attacks may be triggered by chewing, swallowing (cold fluids), talking, coughing, or sneezing.
- Sudden paroxysms usually are <1 min and average 5 per hr but can be longer lasting and more frequent.
- Clusters of attacks can last weeks to months.
- Dx made when application of topical anesthetic solution to oropharynx relieves pain.
- Left side symptoms are more common, esp in women.
- Attacks can precipitate bradycardia, syncope, tachycardia, arterial hypotension.
- Easily misdiagnosed as trigeminal neuralgia, cluster headache, or sick sinus syndrome.

ICD-9-CM Code: 352.1

Etiology

- Usually idiopathic
- Secondary causes incl:
  - Vascular compression of the glossopharyngeal nerve
  - Neoplasms: Cerebellopontine tumors, laryngeal and tongue carcinomas
  - Infection and/or inflammation: Tonsillitis, pharyngeal abscess, arachnoiditis
  - Trauma: Tonsillectomy, dental extraction, impacted wisdom tooth

Usual Treatment

- Conservative treatment: Anticonvulsants-carbamazepine, gabapentin, phenytoin
- Microvascular decompression is the preferred surgical method with high success in pts with typical symptoms
- Surgical alternative incl sectioning of the glossopharyngeal (IX) nerve

ASSESSMENT POINTS

System	Effect	Assessment by Hx	PE	Test
CV	Bradycardia, tachycardia, syncope, hypotension	Syncope, palpitations	BP HR	EKG or biotelemetry to capture pain attacks
CNS	Pain in IX/X distribution	Paroxysmal pain attacks in IX/X distribution with various triggers	Attempt to trigger pain and find distribution	MRI/MRA to ID etiology and vascular compression

Key Reference: Patel A, Kassam A, Horowitz M, Chang Y. Microvascular decompression in the management of glossopharyngeal neuralgia: Analysis of 217 cases. *Neurosurgery.* 2002;50:705–711.

Perioperative Implications

Preoperative Evaluation

- Assessment of triggers and subsequent pain with emphasis on Hx of bradycardia, palpitations, syncope, seizures

Monitoring

- Preinduction arterial line in pts with significant CV symptoms and central venous catheter when temporary pacemaker might be indicated

Airway

- Direct laryngoscopy can trigger an attack.
- Topical anesthesia to oropharynx prior to laryngoscopy can blunt CV symptoms.
- Glossopharyngeal nerve block is an alternative to topical anesthesia for prophylaxis.

Maintenance

- Vigilance and promptness to treat cardiac symptoms and labile blood pressure
- Watch for sudden arterial hypotension, bradycardia, cardiac arrhythmias

Extubation

- Look for possible IX/X nerve palsy and subsequent vocal cord paralysis following microvascular decompression surgery.

Anticipated Problems/Concerns

- Direct laryngoscopy triggering a pain attack with hypotension, bradycardia, and cardiac arrhythmias
- Periop pain attack with severe uncontrolled pain
- Some pts have long Hx of narcotic use

163

Gonorrhea

Seth Eisdorfer
Edgar J. Pierre

Risk

- Decreasing; 120 per 100,000 as of 2006
- Most common in people ages 20–24 y, large urban areas, people with low socioeconomic status and/or low levels of education
- Incidence higher in men, prevalence higher in women

Overview

- Sexually transmitted disease
- High incidence of co-existing chlamydial infection

Clinical Features

- Local infection: Purulent, profuse urethral discharge; possible epididymitis, prostatitis, or proctitis in men. Often asymptomatic in women, may have cervical discharge, vaginitis, salpingitis, or proctitis. Ascending infection may lead to pelvic inflammatory disease (PID).
- Disseminated infection: Fever/rash, tenosynovitis/arthritis (common), conjunctivitis (usually from autoinoculation), possible myopericarditis, toxic hepatitis or perihepatitis (Fitz-Hugh–Curtis syndrome), rarely endocarditis or meningitis

ICD-9-CM Code: 098

Etiology

- *Neisseria gonorrhoeae*: Gram-negative intracellular diplococcus, usually found inside polymorphonucleocytes
- Humans only natural hosts for *N. gonorrhoeae*

Usual Treatment

- Diagnosis gold standard: Isolation of organism by culture, testing for antimicrobial resistance
- Test for other STDs: Syphilis, HIV; test partners as well
- Penicillins and tetracyclines not recommended as first line agents due to resistance
- Fluoroquinolones no longer recommended as first-line therapy due to increasing resistance, esp. in men who have sex with men

- Uncomplicated cervicitis/urethritis: Ceftriaxone is drug of choice; other 3rd generation cephalosporins (cefixime, cefpodoxime) also commonly used. Spectinomycin can be used in penicillin allergic pts.
- Add doxycycline or azithromycin for co-existing chlamydial infections
- Symptoms may subside without treatment, leaving chronic asymptomatic carrier state.
- Pharyngeal infection frequently asymptomatic; may clear spontaneously over several weeks, even without therapy. Ceftriaxone and trimethoprim-sulfamethoxazole can be used for treatment.
- Complicated infections: Penicillin G IV × 5 d or ceftriaxone × 5 d. Oral fluoroquinolones may be used provided susceptibility.
- PID requires second generation cephalosporin such as cefotetan or cefoxitin, or combination of clindamycin and gentamicin. Treat for chlamydial co-infection.
- Resolution of symptoms after treatment suggests cure; follow-up cultures are recommended.

ASSESSMENT POINTS

System	Effect	Assessment by Hx	PE	Test
HEENT	Conjunctivitis, ophthalmia neonatorum, adult gonococcal conjunctivitis			
	Pharyngeal infection		Exudative tonsillitis	Cultures
GI	Anorectal infections	Pain, pruritus	Purulent discharge, bloody diarrhea	Cultures
	Proctitis			
GU	*Women*			
	Urogenital tract disease	Abn vaginal discharge, dysuria, urinary frequency, lower abd pain, labial pain, abn menstruation	Mucopurulent cervicitis	Cultures from urethra and vagina
	Men			
	Acute epididymitis	Pain		
	Prostatitis			
CARDIO	Gonococcal endocarditis		Possible murmur	Echocardiography
GI	Perihepatitis (Fitz-Hugh–Curtis syndrome)		RUQ tenderness	Liver enzyme elevation
GU	*Women*			
	PID	Lower abdominal pain, vaginal discharge, fever, palpable adnexal mass	Severe pain to palpation	Endocervix cultures
	Men			
	Urethritis	Dysuria	Purulent urethral discharge	Cultures from urethra
CNS	Gonococcal meningitis		Meningeal signs	
MS	Septic arthritis	Most common cause of septic arthritis in young adults, tends to involve single joints	Warmth, tenderness of affected joint(s)	
SKIN	Disseminated lesions			Ranging from maculopapular to pustular or hemorrhagic, usually peripheral

Key Reference: Tapsall JW. *Neisseria gonorrhoeae* and emerging resistance to extended spectrum cephalosporins. *Curr Opin Infect Dis.* 2009;22(1):87–91.

Perioperative Implications

- Universal blood and body fluid precautions and/or barrier precautions

Monitoring
- Awareness: Foley catheter/temp probe placement

Airway
- Awareness if pharyngitis exists

Positioning
- Awareness of joint involvement

Maintenance
- Awareness of extent of disease

Adjuvants
- Vary with hepatic involvement

Anticipated Problems/Concerns

- No vaccine available
- Follow-up cultures
- Effective antibiotics
- Testing isolates for antibiotic susceptibility
- Routine culturing of high-risk populations
- Diligent contact tracing and prompt referral; treatment of sexual partners
- Education targeted at high-risk groups
- Use of condoms or other barrier methods

Guillain-Barré Syndrome

Gordon N. Finlayson
Jay B. Brodsky

Risk

- Prevalence: Both sexes, all races, all ages but mostly affects young and middle-aged adults.
- Worldwide illness, occurs all times of year.
- Mortality rate 5–20%. Most pts eventually fully recover, 20% have significant residual weakness.

Perioperative Risks

- Resp failure 2° to polyneuropathy
- Autonomic dysfunction with profound CV instability

Worry About

- Rapidity of symptoms—resp paralysis may occur within 24 hr of onset
- Pulm complications

Overview

- Polyneuropathy often encountered in critical care practice
  - Pts present initially with lower limb weakness that spreads
- Widespread, patchy, inflammatory demyelination of peripheral and autonomic nervous systems
- Dysautonomia from chromatolysis of antero-mediolateral cell column and autonomic ganglia: Fluctuating BP, Htn, hypotension, postural hypotension, tachycardia, arrhythmias
- CSF protein usually normal during first few days of illness, steadily rises and remains elevated for several months, even after recovery

ICD-9-CM Code: 357.0

Etiology

- Evidence points to infection induced aberrant immune response
- Typically antecedent illness within 4 wk of onset (resp or GI infection in 60–70% of cases)
- Other predisposing factors incl surgery, pregnancy, malignancy, acute seroconversion to HIV
- Epidural or spinal anesthesia may be antecedent event or associated with recurrence

Usual Treatment

- Basis of treatment is symptomatic care and plasma exchange or IVIG
- Daily bedside evaluation of vital capacity and resp muscle strength; pts with ↓ resp reserve should be moved to ICU
- Elective tracheal intubation and mechanical ventilatory support when signs of resp distress are present *even before* Paco$_2$ rises or vital capacity falls
- Anticipating requirement for ventilatory support
  - Vital capacity <20mL/Kg or reduction of 30% from baseline
  - Maximum inspiratory pressure <30cmH$_2$O
  - Maximum expiratory pressure <40cmH$_2$O
  - Facial and/or bulbar weakness, autonomic dysfunction, rapid disease progression
- Plasmapheresis or IVIG reduces hospital stay and time spent on ventilator if given to pts who do not improve or who worsen within first 2 wk of symptom onset

ASSESSMENT POINTS

System	Effect	Assessment by Hx	PE	Test
HEENT	Inability to close eyes	Dry eyes	Dry eyes	
CV	Fluctuating hypo- and Htn, postural hypotension, sinus tachycardia, arrhythmias	Orthostatic Sx Palpitations	BP/pulse	ECG
	DVT risk	Asymmetric limb swelling	Asymmetric limb swelling	Doppler US
RESP	Resp failure 2° to weakness	Stamina—for breathing	↓ Strength on repeated ventilation	VC Maximum inspiratory pressure
	Aspiration risk with bulbar dysfunction		Inability to sustain head lift	Maximum expiratory pressure
GI	Bowel obstruction	Constipation	Abdominal exam	Abdominal x-ray
CNS	Autonomic dysfunction	Early satiety Orthostatic hypotension Lack of sweating	BP lying and standing	ECG with R-R interval on deep breathing
	Pain: Acute nociceptive and chronic neuropathic	Pain		
MS	Weakness, joint fixation	Lack of stamina		

Key Reference: Asbury AK. New concepts of Guillain-Barré syndrome. *J Child Neurol.* 2000;15:183–191.

Perioperative Implications

Preoperative Preparation

- Avoid rapid turning of pt: Autonomic instability and postural hypotension may result.
- Avoid head-up (reverse Trendelenburg) position: Inability of pt to maintain CV stability with tilt.
- Increased gastric acidity: Treat with antacid and metoclopramide, 10 mg/70 kg.
- Maintain appropriate environmental temp.
- Coagulopathy and hypocalcemia may complicate plasma exchange therapy.

Monitoring

- Arterial line for continuous pressure monitoring started prior to anesthetic induction
- CVP or PA line to monitor for potential fluid shifts that result from positional changes and cardiac dysrhythmias
- Temperature: Pts may become poikilothermic
- Neuromuscular monitoring: Sensitive to relaxants

Airway

- Most pts have early tracheostomy; airway access should not be a problem; previous pts may have tracheal stenosis.
- Endotracheal suction may provoke bradydysrhythmias and asystole.

Induction

- Avoid barbiturates and phenothiazines, which may produce profound CV depression.

Maintenance

- Local anesthesia preferred
- GA: Non-sympatholytic technique
- Sensitive to positive pressure ventilation: May result in autonomic instability

Extubation

- Continue to ventilate postop if pt required ventilatory support preop
- Residual weakness from anesthetic agents and muscle relaxants may necessitate postop ventilation in pts not ventilated preop

Adjuvants

- Muscle relaxants
  - Avoid succinylcholine; can cause hyperkalemia with cardiac arrest
  - Pts have increased sensitivity to nondepolarizing muscle relaxants
  - May have residual muscle weakness after apparent full recovery from GA
- Volume
- Maintain blood volume
- CVP >5 cm H$_2$O

Anticipated Problems/Concerns

- Autonomic instability
- Resp failure
- Parturient: Third trimester and postpartum, risk of exacerbation; for labor a regional anesthetic indicated to avoid exaggerated hemodynamic response to pain from autonomic dysfunction. Aspiration pneumonitis and resp failure may result in premature labor and maternal mortality. For C-section a regional anesthetic relatively contraindicated even for pt with mild resp involvement. Case reported of newborn with GBS features following delivery by affected mother.
- Fecal impaction
- Stress ulcers

Hashimoto's Thyroiditis

Sanyo Tsai
Michael Williams

Risk

- Hashimoto's thyroiditis is the most common cause of hypothyroidism in iodine-sufficient countries and primary hypothyroidism in adults
- Incidence in USA: Approx 100,000–400,000 new diagnosis each year
- Causes thyroid failure in 10% of pts
- Prevalence increases with age, but also the most common cause of hypothyroidism in children as early as 1-to 2-y of age
- No documented ethnic predominance
- Gender predominance: F:M ratio: 7:1; age 30–50 y

Perioperative Risks

- Increased risk of thyroid storm even if euthyroid preop as the inflammatory process in the disease progression may involve enough apoptosis of thyroid follicles and cause thyroid hormone release. Clinical diagnosis of life-threatening illness if hyperthyroidism severely exacerbated by the stress of operation, typically manifested by hyperpyrexia, tachycardia, and alterations in consciousness
- Risk of resp failure or insufficiency and increased bleeding periop
- Chronic hyperthyroidism with its concomitants
- Co-existing autoimmune disease with adrenal failure

Overview

- Hashimoto's thyroiditis or chronic autoimmune thyroiditis is an autoimmune disease involving progressive thyroid dysfunction due to autoimmune-mediated destruction of the thyroid gland through apoptosis of thyroid epithelial cells. Typical manifestations of the disease may encompass high serum concentrations of antibodies against one or more thyroid antigens, diffuse lymphocytic infiltration of the thyroid, and destruction of thyroid gland resulting in thyroid failure.
- Chronic inflammation of thyroid (painful or painless) with lymphocytic infiltration due to autoimmune factors
- Acute inflammation results in increased release of preformed hormone with hyperthyroidism
- Chronic inflammation results in decreased thyroid gland function with resistant hypothyroidism.

ICD-9-CM Code: 423.9

Etiology

- Autoantibodies against thyroid peroxidase, thyroglobulin, or TSH receptors causing immune-mediated destruction of thyroid epithelial cells, though a small percentage of pts do not have the presence of such antibodies.
- Assoc with other autoimmune diseases: Sjögren's syndrome, SLE, RA, pernicious anemia, autoimmune endocrinopathies, Addison's disease, hypoparathyroidism, diabetes mellitus, gonadal failure
- Increased incidence in pts with a family Hx and with chromosomal disorders such as Turner's, Down, or Klinefelter's syndromes
- Also has been linked to several polymorphisms in genes for HLA and T-cell antigen receptors
- Precipitating causes: Thyroid injury (infection, radiation, and drugs), stress, steroids, pregnancy, and excessive iodine intake

Standard Treatment

- Thyroid hormone replacement chronically in hypothyroidism
- NSAIDs in acute thyroiditis for pain and propranolol to control symptoms of hyperthyroidism

ASSESSMENT POINTS

System	Effect	Assessment by Hx	PE	Test
HEENT	Swollen, tender neck Enlarged tongue Tracheal compression	Neck pain, hoarseness	Examine airway and neck	Lateral neck x-rays or CT of neck
CARDIO	Dehydration, tachy- or bradydysrhythmias	Orthostatic symptoms		Tilt table test ECG
RESP	Decreased resp muscle strength	SOB Dyspnea on exertion		
GI	Ileus Constipation			
ENDO	Acutely hyperthyroid Chronically hypothyroid	Shaking, anxiety, emotional lability	Reflex speed, HR Tremor, nervousness Mental status	Free T_4 estimate
HEME	Anemia			Hgb, Hct
CNS	Cold intolerance Slow or fast movement, depending on stage	Cold intolerance	Reflexes, mental status exam	
SKIN		Rough, pale skin Coarse, dry hair	Careful inspection of hair and skin	
MS		Arthralgias and myalgias		
GEN	Other autoimmune dysfunction	Weakness	Inability to arise from chair without using hands	Serum K^+/Na^+

Key Reference: Bennett-Guerrero E, Kramer DC, Schwinn DA. Effect of chronic and acute thyroid hormone reduction on perioperative outcome. *Anesth Analg*. 1997;85:30–36.

Perioperative Implications

Preoperative Preparation

- Assess NPO status (may have poor gastric emptying)
- Cautious use of preop drugs (increased sensitivity of central nervous and resp system to depressants)
- Ensure that pt is euthyroid to avoid thyroid storm.
- Assess fluid status.
- Assess for co-morbidities (autoimmune/adrenal/pancreatic dysfunction).

Monitoring

- Temp (consider placing cooling blanket on OR table as treatment for thyroid storm)
- Consider invasive monitoring if CV or resp compromise

Airway

- If normal preop, consider routine management
- If displaced or distorted, consider awake fiberoptic and armored tube intubation

Induction/Maintenance

- No data indicate one technique preferred over another

Extubation

- Consider extubation in optimal situation for reintubation

Postoperative Concerns

- Routine monitor and treatment of co-morbidities if co-existing autoimmune disease

Adjuvants

- Esmolol for acute hyperthyroidism
- Steroids sometimes necessary for adrenal dysfunction
- Oral hypoglycemics (chronic use) can cause hypoglycemia for longer duration and of greater severity in periop pt.

Headache, Migraine

Alan Kaye
Harry J. Gould, III

Risk

- Incidence in USA: >28 million; maximum prevalence 25–55 y of age
- Can start as early as 1 y of age, 10–20% of children by 20 y of age, male = female
- In adults: More frequent in women after age 11 y; approx 3:1: female: male; prevalence declines after age 40 y
- Familial aggregation; *CACNA1A* (P/Q voltage-gated calcium channel), *ATP1A2* (Na⁺-K⁺ ATPase), and *SCN1A* (Na$_v$ 1.1 voltage-gated sodium channel) genes implicated in genetic predisposition for variations of familial hemiplegic migraine
- Can be assoc with sinusitis; AVM; stroke; patent foramen ovale; epilepsy; ischemic myocardial infarction; depression; anxiety disorder; sensitivity to foods rich in tyramine, phenylethylamine, or octopamine (chocolate, wine, dairy products); electroencephalographic abn
- Socioeconomic status: Inversely related to household income and education

Perioperative Risks

- ↑ Incidence of hypertension, stroke, CAD
- Gastric stasis
- Drug toxicity and side effects

Worry About

- Toxic and side effects of antimigrainous preparations, adverse interaction with anesthetic drugs
- Assoc intracranial disorders

- ↑ Aggregation of plts with ↑ risk of stroke and CAD

Overview

- Recurrent, frequently unilateral, throbbing head pain with strong family Hx
- Often associated with increased sensitivity to touch, N/V, phonophobia and/or photophobia
- May be preceded by a visual, sensory or motor aura; headache and aura may present independently
- Dx is Hx dependent in the absence of 2° causes
- Migrainous infarction with permanent neurologic damage is rare.

ICD-9-CM Codes: 346.0 (Classic migraine); 346.1 (Common migraine. 5th digit subclassification: 0 without mention of intractable migraine, 1 with intractable migraine, so stated.)

Etiology

- Central or peripheral mechanisms incited by internal or external stimuli
- Lowering Mg²⁺ levels ↑ the affinity and release of serotonin at cerebrovascular and neuronal sites as well as NO production and activation of NMDA receptors
- Precipitated by trigger factors
- Cerebral and extracerebral arteries are most likely sources of pain.
- Pain results from exaggerated pulsations in association with trigeminal release of substance P (sP), calcitonin gene-related peptide (CGRP), and vasoactive intestinal polypeptide (VIP) and sensitization of nociceptors around blood vessels.

Usual Treatment

- No permanent cure
- Elimination of trigger factors when possible; chronobiologic regulation
- Abortive therapy: NSAIDs, barbiturates, ergotamines, triptans, phenothiazines, dihydroergotamine, sphenopalatine ganglion block, nonopioid and opioid analgesics
- Prophylactic therapy: Effective—β-blocking agents (metoprolol, tropranolol, timolol), TCA (amitriptyline), anti-epileptic drugs (AED; topiramate, divalproex sodium), serotonin agonists (frovatriptan; short-term prevention in menstrual migraine), petasites (butterbur); probably effective—ACE inhibitors (lisinopril, candesartan), AED (gabapentin), β-blocking agents (atenolol, nadolol), antidepressants (fluoxetine, venlafaxine), serotonin agonists (naratriptan, zolmitriptan; short term prevention in menstrual migraine), histamine, cyproheptadine, MIG-99 (feverfew), vitamins (riboflavin, CO-Q10, Mg²⁺); possibly effective—α-agonists (clonidine, guanfacine), Ca²⁺-channel blockers (verapamil, nicardipine, nifedipine, nimodipine), AED (carbamazepine); conflicting evidence for efficacy of MAOIs; botulinum toxin probably not effective
- Behavioral treatment with biofeedback, self-hypnosis, relief by dark surroundings, sleep

ASSESSMENT POINTS (Mainly side effects and toxicity of antimigrainous therapy.)

System	Effect	Assessment by Hx	PE	Test
CARDIO	Ergotamine, sumatriptan • Worsening of Htn, ischemic heart disease, PVD,serotonin syndrome β-adrenergic receptor blocking agents and Ca²⁺-channel blockers • Excessive depression of myocardial function Methysergide (no longer available) • Pericardial fibrosis, cardiac valvular fibrosis TCAs and Ca²⁺-channel blockers • Cardiac conduction abnormalities	Symptoms of angina and peripheral vascular insufficiency Symptoms of CHF Syncope	S₃ Rales ↓ Heart sounds Q-T prolongation	ECG Stress ECG CXR CXR, ECHO ECG
RESP	β-blockers • Worsening of COPD Methysergide (no longer available) • Pleuropulmonary fibrosis	Dyspnea Dyspnea	Expir wheezing Rapid shallow breathing	CXR ABGs PFTs
GI	Gastroparesis	Early satiety		
CNS	Intracranial disorders TCAs Anticonvulsants MAOIs • Anticholinergic and CNS stimulation	Tachycardia, dry mouth Blurred vision, urinary Somnolence, diplopia, ataxia, cognitive impairment Retention, delayed gastric emptying	Focal deficit	Neuroimaging ECG

Key Reference: Silberstein SD, Lipton RB, Dodick DW, eds. *Wolff's headache and other head pain.* 8th ed. New York: Oxford University Press; 2008.

Perioperative Implications

Preoperative Preparation

- Detailed pharmacotherapy Hx
- D/C MAOIs 14–21 d in advance, if possible (see Monoamine Oxidase Inhibitors in Drugs section)
- Gastroparesis: Metoclopramide (10 mg/70 kg pt)

Monitoring

- Routine, unless signs of ischemic heart disease

Airway

- None

Preinduction/Induction

- Pts receiving β-blockers and Ca²⁺-channel blockers may develop reduced CO and hypotension

Maintenance

- Exaggerated response to indirect-acting vasopressors may occur with pts on ergotamine, sumatriptan, TCAs, and MAOIs
- Hyperpyrexic coma reported after administration of narcotic to pts receiving MAOIs

Extubation

- Increased risk of CNS stimulation with sumatriptan, ergotamine, TCAs, and MAOIs

Postoperative Period

- Pain management may be critical
- Avoid withdrawal syndromes

Anticipated Problems/Concerns

- Possible adverse interactions of anesthetic drugs and antimigrainous preparations
- No unique hazards of anesthesia administered to pts with migraine

HELLP Syndrome

David J. Birnbach

Risk

- If severe preeclampsia, 20% may exhibit HELLP syndrome
- Preeclampsia occurs in 2–10% of pregnancies

Perioperative Risks

- High maternal and fetal morbidity and mortality
- Increased C-section rate (up to 94%)
- Urgent delivery after diagnosis to prevent maternal and fetal death

Worry About

- Confused with hepatitis, thrombotic thrombocytopenic purpura, gallbladder disease, and acute fatty liver of pregnancy. Malaria may also be mistaken for HELLP syndrome.
- Thrombocytopenia and coagulopathy increase risk of hematoma after regional anesthetic. Report of spinal hematoma associated with a HELLP pt who was not coagulopathic but had a platelet count of 91 X 10^9/L.
- High risk of hemorrhagic complications
- Upper airway and laryngeal edema leading to airway obstruction and difficult or failed intubation. Fluid management difficult; pulm edema may ensue.

Overview

- HELLP is an acronym for the findings that suggest hepatic involvement in preeclampsia pt: Hemolysis, Elevated Liver enzymes, Low Platelets.
- Diagnostic criteria incl hemolysis, defined by abnormal peripheral smear and increased bilirubin levels, elevated liver enzymes (SGOT >70 U/L, LDH >600 U/L), and thrombocytopenia (<100,000/mm^3).
- Failure to treat may lead to eclampsia or death due to hepatic hematoma or rupture.
- Not always associated with Htn

ICD-9-CM Code: 642.5 (Severe preeclampsia)

Etiology

- Poorly understood
- May be severe form of preeclampsia resulting from abnormal prostaglandin control, intravascular plt activation, and microvascular endothelial damage. Microangiopathic hemolytic anemia usual.

Usual Treatment

- Definitive treatment is delivery as quickly as possible.
- After delivery, many experience uneventful recovery, with plt counts returning to normal within 1 wk.
- Glucocorticoids may accelerate fetal lung maturity and may also improve mother's plt count and reduce liver enzyme abnormalities
- Plts, FFP, and cryoprecipitate administered as needed
- Magnesium sulfate for CNS irritability and antihypertensives for Htn

ASSESSMENT POINTS

System	Effect	Assessment by Hx	PE	Test
HEENT	Upper airway edema	Dyspnea, voice change	Poor visualization on airway exam	Mallampati assessment
CV	LV failure	Dyspnea, desaturation	Adventitious sounds	CVP and/or LVEDP
RESP	Resp depression	Magnesium administration	↓ Reflexes	MgSO$_4$ level
GI	Liver swelling Subcapsular hematoma	Epigastric pain N/V		Elevated SGOT, SGPT
HEME	Thrombocytopenia Hemolytic anemia	Bruising Pallor, jaundice	Bleeding (IV site oozing)	Plt count LDH, bilirubin Peripheral smear
RENAL	Acute renal failure	Oliguria		Elevated uric acid, BUN, serum Cr
CNS	Eclampsia, cerebral edema	Seizures		

Key Reference: Kulungowski AM, Kashuk JL, Moore EE, et al. Hemolysis, elevated liver enzymes and low platelets syndrome: When is surgical help needed? *Am J Surg.* 2009;198:916–920.

Perioperative Implications

Preoperative Testing
- Obtain CBC, PT, PTT, fibrinogen, SGPT, SGOT, LDH, BUN, Cr

Monitoring
- Consider arterial line
- Consider CVP or PA catheter if oliguria despite fluid administration or CHF

Airway
- Assess airway early and repeat airway exam periodically.

- Laryngeal edema may preclude normal tracheal intubation in the event of emergency C-section.
- Difficult intubation equipment should be readily available.
- Consider pre-emptive epidural or continuous spinal catheter.

Induction
- Controlled neuraxial anesthesia with incremental dosing of catheter, if not contraindicated due to coagulation abnormalities. Recent reports suggest that spinal techniques can be safely used in severe preeclampsia.

- If general anesthesia is required, the hypertensive surge associated with ET intubation can often be avoided by pretreatment with magnesium, antihypertensives, or opioids.

Adjuvants
- If significant Htn, antihypertensive therapy prior to laryngeal intubation
- If receiving magnesium sulfate and needs GA, small doses of neuromuscular blocking agents with close monitoring

Hemophilia

Vincent S. Cowell

Risk

- Incidence: Hemophilia A, factor VIII (FVIII) deficiency: 1/10,000 male births. Hemophilia B, factor IX (FIX, Christmas disease) deficiency: 1/30,000 male births
- Prevalence: Hemophilia A is 20.6/100,000 male individuals with 60% having severe disease. Hemophilia B is 5.3/100.000 male individuals with 44% having severe disease.
- Hemophilia A, FVIII deficiency, affects 80–85% of hemophiliacs; remainder has hemophilia B due to factor IX deficiency.
- Hemophilia A and B are X-linked recessive hereditary disorders.
- Females may be asymptomatic carriers of the hemophilia gene and may have partial deficiency of FVIII of FIX.
- Hemophilia is without ethnic or geographic predilection.

Perioperative Risks

- Prolonged and potentially fatal hemorrhage both during and after surgery
- Closed-space bleeding can lead to nerve injury, vascular or airway obstruction.

- Surgery should not proceed without adequate supply of factor concentrate to support the procedure and postop course.

Worry About

- Spontaneous bleeding
- Intra- and postop hemorrhage despite optimal replacement therapy of deficient coagulation factor
- Development of FVIII and FIX inhibitor antibodies (approx 20% for FVIII, 3% for FIX)
- Viral transmission from plasma derived factor replacement therapy

Overview

- Hemophiliacs can have severe deficiency (<1% nml levels), moderate deficiency (1–5% of nml levels), or mild deficiency (5–30% of nml levels)
- Congenital disorder, inherited as an X-linked recessive trait, affecting males almost exclusively
- Acute and chronic complications often due to recurrent spontaneous bleeding, the hallmark of which is bleeding into the joints (e.g., cycle of joint hemorrhage, inflammation, synovial proliferation, and erosion of cartilage, causing pain and disability)
- Pts with hemophilia generally have nml prothrombin time (PT), normal bleeding times, and a prolonged partial thromboplastin time, (aPTT). Specific laboratory factor assays make the distinction and plasma concentrations of FVIII or FIX determine the severity.
- Treatment generally follows bleeding episodes. New approaches to treatment involve the prophylactic use of clotting factors.

ICD-9-CM Code: 286.0.

Etiology

- Hereditary disorder, X-linked recessive
- Acquired hemophilia is the development of FVIII inhibitors (autoantibodies) in persons without a Hx of FVIII deficiency

Usual Treatment

- Desmopressin (DDAVP injection of Stimate nasal spray) whenever possible for mild hemophilia A
- Recombinant FVIII and FIX products
- Plasma concentrations of deficient factors maintained at minimum of 40–70% throughout the periop period (7–10 d postop) for adequate hemostasis
- Cryoprecipitate is no longer recommended as a treatment alternative except in life-threatening emergencies
- Recombinant factor VIIa (NovoSeven) for use in pts with inhibitors to FVIII of FIX
- Gene insertion therapy shows promising future

ASSESSMENT POINTS

System	Effect	Assessment by Hx	PE	Test
HEENT	Pharyngeal bleeding	Often seen in children	Tongue and mouth lacerations	Exam
GI	GI bleeding not common	When it occurs, bleeding can be excessive	Stool exam, endoscopy	Hemoccult, angio
HEME	Anemia, hematoma formation, bruising	Lethargy, SOB, skin discoloration	Hematomas	PT/PTT, plt count, bleeding FVIII and FIX assay, gene analysis
GU	Hematuria	Blood in urine		Urinalysis, cysto, IVP
CNS	Intracranial hemorrhage	Head trauma, headache, change in mental status	Any sign or symptom of head injury or trauma	Head CT
MS	Joint hemorrhage Joint deformities Muscle hemorrhage Compartment syndrome Chronic pain	Painful distention of the joint Bruising Restricted movement Narcotic dependence	Hemarthroses Limited ROM Tenderness	Physical exam X-ray

Key Reference: Agaliotic DP, Zaiden R, Ozturk S. *Hemophilia, overview*. Retrieved from: emedicine.medscape.com; Updated: Jan 2, 2008, National Hemophilia Foundation. www.hemophilia.org.

Hepatic Encephalopathy (HE)

Philip McArdle

Risk

• Incidence in pts with hepatic cirrhosis (about 0.1% of the population) is 50–70% of pts. Frequently subclinical, but can be exacerbated in the postop period by the surgical stress response, dehydration and postop infection.

• HE is acutely worsened, in about 20% of pts, following surgical portocaval shunts, minimally invasive transjugular intrahepatic portosystemic shunt (TIPS) and hepatic resections.

Perioperative Risks

• Precipitation of encephalopathy from benzodiazepines, surgical procedure (portocaval shunt), postop infection, GI hemorrhage, or erosive gastritis.

• In pts with severe underlying liver disease, Childs Class B and C, or high MELD score.

Worry About

• Preop resp depression from benzodiazepine premedication

• Hemorrhage from underlying hepatic dysfunction

• Underlying precipitating factor (infection, bleed) may create hemodynamic instability. HE in absence of precipitating factor, or when accompanied by seizure or focal nerologic deficit, should prompt brain imaging to rule out intracerebral bleed.

• Undiagnosed cerebral edema with risk of cerebral ischemia in fulminant hepatic failure presenting for liver transplantation

Overview

• A syndrome of alteration in mental status, from impaired concentration to coma, caused by portosystemic shunting, usually in the presence of liver failure. Hyperammonemia from protein breakdown is almost always present and the degree of hyperammonemia generally correlates with the degree of encephalopathy.

• Multifactorial in origin but altered neurotransmission and elevated levels of endogenous benzodiazepines and opioids appear important contributors. Although not effective in improving outcome, administration of flumazenil and naloxone temporarily improves mental status in about 50% subjects with HE.

• Underlying hepatocellular injury may arise from multiple etiologies but the most common are chronic alcohol abuse, chronic viral hepatitis, non-alcoholic steatohepatitis (NASH).

• HE usually reflects advanced hepatic dysfunction and is frequently seen in pts awaiting liver transplantation.

ICD9-CM: 572.2 (Hepatic coma)

Etiology

• Underlying liver disease with identifiable hyperammonemic precipitating cause in over 90% of cases: GI hemorrhage, infection, azotemia, diuresis, constipation, sedatives esp benzodiazepines

• Elevated levels of endogenous benzodiazepines, γ-aminobutyric acid agonists and opioids

• Direct ammonia neurotoxicity

Usual treatment

• Identify and treat precipitating cause.

• Reduce plasma ammonia with lactulose: 20g q6-12 hr orally or by NG tube until softening of stool; reduce dose if diarrhea. Alternately, 300 mL lactulose mixed with 700 mL tap water given as retention enema in pts with severe HE that cannot protect their airway.

• Consider combining lactulose with oral antibiotic such as metronidazole or neomycin.

ASSESSMENT POINTS

System	Effect	Assessment by Hx	PE	Test
CNS	Impaired concentration, drowsiness, coma	Amnesia	Transition of reflexes from hyperactive to hypoactive, and disappearance of asterixis, signify onset of severe HE	Plasma ammonia, CT scan
CV	Hypotension	Liver failure	Systolic BP 90 may be acceptable in liver failure	BP
RESP	Hyperventilation, hypoxemia	Dyspnea	Ascites, pleural effusions	CXR, ABG
METAB	Hyponatremia, hypokalemia	Correction of hyponatremia or worsening of hypokalemia can further impair mental status	Free water excess exacerbates ascites and anasarca	BMP
HEME	Anemia, coagulopathy	GI bleeding	Pallor, splenomegaly	Hemoglobin, plt count, prothrombin time

Key Reference: Zafirova Z, O'Connor M. Hepatic encephalopathy: Current management strategies and treatment, including management and monitoring of cerebral edema and intracranial hypertension in fulminant hepatic failure. *Curr Opin Anaesthesiol.* 2010;23(2):121–127.

Perioperative Implications for Liver Transplantation

• Recurrent or persistent HE predicts poor survival in cirrhosis and indicates decompensated liver disease which is best treated by liver transplantation.

• When severe, particularly in association with fulminant hepatic failure, HE is frequently associated with cerebral edema. The resulting intracranial Htn may be underestimated by CT scan and intracranial pressure monitoring is indicated to ensure adequate cerebral perfusion pressure periop.

Perioperative Implications for Other Surgeries

• Mental capacity may be impaired to degree that consent is problematic.

• Pt may be hypovolemic from impaired ability to maintain PO intake, lactulose therapy causing diarrhea, diuretic therapy for associated ascites, or recent GI bleed. Maintenance of hydration is important to prevent acute tubular necrosis the incidence of which is increased in liver failure.

• Placement of TIPS or surgically fashioned portosystemic shunt are performed for refractory esophagogastric variceal bleeding. HE may be precipitated or exacerbated postop, particularly if a significant degree of encephalopathy is present preop, or if the pt is elderly.

Hepatitis, Alcoholic

Alan Kaye
Amir Baluch

Risk

- Incidence in the USA: 8.5% of adults met DSM-IV criteria for current alcohol use disorder. 30.3% of adults met DSM-IV criteria for lifetime alcohol use disorder. Roughly 10–15% of alcoholics will develop alcoholic hepatitis and cirrhosis

Perioperative Risks

- Mortality rate of 60–100% of pts undergoing surgery during active alcoholic hepatitis
- Poorer prognosis when accompanied by increased bilirubin, increased Cr, PT >1.5× control, ascites, or encephalopathy
- >10% develop delirium tremens (DTs) without prophylaxis

Worry About

- Anemia and coagulopathy
- Pulm shunting leading to arterial hypoxemia
- Altered mental status and/or hepatic encephalopathy
- Hemodynamic instability secondary to DTs
- Insulin resistance

Overview

- Most common form of liver disease in USA
- Usually preceded by period of heavy alcohol consumption
- An intermediate stage between fatty liver and alcoholic cirrhosis
- Can vary from mild (with only elevated liver function tests) to severe liver inflammation (prolonged prothrombin time, and liver failure).
- Characteristic clinical features: Fever, hepatomegaly, jaundice, anorexia, abdominal bruit over liver (heard in > 50% pts)
- Mortality is 50% within 30 d of onset with pts having hepatic encephalopathy, derangement in renal function, hyperbilirubinemia, and prolonged PT

ICD9-CM: 571.1 (Acute alcoholic hepatitis)

Etiology

- A daily intake of more than 40 g of alcohol in men and 20 g in women significantly increases the risk of alcoholic hepatitis.
- Inflammatory process via leukocytic infiltration which leads to hepatocellular necrosis with intracellular deposition of alcoholic hyaline in the cytoplasm of liver cells (Mallory Bodies).
- Repeated episodes precursor to cirrhosis after healing and scar tissue formation

Treatment

- Abstinence with counseling
- Nutritional support: Diet, multivitamin and mineral supplementation
- Medications: Pentoxifyline, steroids (may reduce mortality in pts with severe alcoholic hepatitis or encephalopathy)
- Supportive care incl diet adjustment, multivitamin supplementation, lactulose, and neomycin if needed

ASSESSMENT POINTS

System	Effect	Assessment by Hx	PE	Test
CV	High CO Low SVR Low CO (in advanced disease)	Exercise tolerance	Hyperdynamic cardiac exam	ECG ECHO
RESP	Pulm shunts Restrictive disease Pulm effusions Central hyperventilation	Orthodeoxia Ascites	Effusions on CXR; ascites on abdominal exams	Resp alkalosis on ABG
GI/HEPATIC	Disrupted synthetic and metabolic function	Anorexia, N/V, malaise, wt loss, fever	Jaundice, ascites, tender hepatomegaly, splenomegaly	Elevated transaminases (AST/ALT>2), PT, alk phos, bilirubin Decreased albumin
RENAL	Mg^{2+} and PO_4^{2-} wasting Free water retention		Ascites	Serum Mg^{2+} and PO_4^{2-} Hyponatremia
ENDO	Insulin resistance			Glucose
HEME	Anemia and thrombocytopenia GI blood loss Hypersplenism	Bruising/bleeding	Splenomegaly	Hgb/Hct, platelets
CNS	Decreased clearance of amines	Altered mental status	Neurologic exam	NH_3 levels

Key Reference: Muilenburg DJ, Singh A, Torzilli G, et al. Surgery in the patient with liver disease. *Anesthesiol Clin.* 2009;27(4):721–737.

Perioperative Implications

Preoperative Preparation

- Pt should be assessed via Child-Pugh or MELD score. Elective procedures should be postponed for Child-Pugh score >7 or MELD > 8
- Increased sensitivity to sedative medications (increased cerebral uptake of benzodiazepines)
- Ascites may be treated by diuretics (spironolactone) or percutaneous drainage
- Hypokalemia and hyponatremia should be corrected slowly (over 24–36 hr)
- Correct coagulopathy with vitamin K, FFP, and platelets (if needed).

Monitoring

- Consider CVP or PA catheter: Following the removal of large amounts of ascitic fluid, IV colloid fluid replacement is often necessary to prevent profound hypotension and renal shutdown.
- Monitor blood glucose closely due to deranged insulin production secondary to liver pathology
- Arterial catheter for hemodynamic lability, frequent blood gas sampling, large fluid shifts.

Airway

- Rapid sequence intubation: Some pts at risk for aspiration due to ascites (increased abdominal pressure).

- Inadvertent esophageal intubation can cause enough trauma to damage the esophageal varices and cause significant bleeding.

Induction

- Hypoalbuminemia may decrease V_d and therefore increase pharmacologic response to standard drug dosages
- Water soluble drugs may have increased V_d owing to ascites
- Regional anesthesia well tolerated (if coagulation status permits)

Maintenance

- Impaired drug metabolism, detoxification, and excretion by the liver can prolong drug half-lives (volatile agents, muscle relaxants, analgesics, and sedatives may be affected).
  - Remifentail organ independent metabolism, fentanyl common choice
  - Cis/Atracurium are neuromuscular blockers of choice due to organ independent metabolism
- Decrease dose 50% for morphine, meperidine, barbiturates, and benzodiazepines.
- Desflurane most minimally metabolized inhalational agent; however, sevoflurane and isoflurane also shown to be safe in pts with impaired liver function. Factors known to reduce hepatic blood flow, such as hypotension, excessive sympathetic activation, and high mean airway pressures during controlled ventilation should be avoided

Extubation

- Extubate when pt fully awake to ensure highest degree of airway protection.

Adjuvants

- Multivitamins, minerals, and vitamin K 10 mg SQ or IM.

Postoperative Period

- Regional pain control ideal so as to avoid pharmacokinetic disturbances of systemic agents
- Maintain low threshold for transfer of pt to ICU environment.
- Vigilant observation for signs of acute hepatic decompensation (jaundice, encephalopathy, and ascites), delerium tremens, and sepsis (with secondary DIC).

Anticipated Problems/Concerns

- Increased risk of postop complications: Acute hepatic failure, sepsis, bleeding, renal dysfunction
- Need for prolonged airway protection because of altered mental status and pulm dysfunction
- Acute withdrawal from alcohol
  Multiple coagulation abnormalities due to synthetic dysfunction and hypersplenism

Hepatitis, Halothane

Mark G. Mandabach
A.J. Wright

Risk

- Multiple exposures to halothane is the most important risk factor
- Prior Hx of jaundice or fever after anesthesia
- Female sex
- Obesity
- Age:
  - Rare in pts <0 years old (3% of all cases)
  - Pts <30 years of age make up about 10% of all cases
  - Most cases occur in pts >40
  - In older pts the disease is more devastating
- Genetics: There is a strong family linkage associated with halothane hepatitis

Perioperative Risks

- Type or duration or extent of surgery not a risk factor
- Hx of non-halothane related liver disease also not a risk factor

Worry About

- Induction of cytochrome P450 2E1 enzyme by alcohol, barbiturates, or isoniazid

Overview

- Estimated incidence
  - First exposure: 0.3 to 1.5 per 10,000
  - With multiple exposures: 10 to 15 per 10,000
  - F:M ratio: 2:1
  - Latency period before clinical symptoms
  - After first exposure ~6 d, with overt jaundice in ~11 d
  - After multiple exposures ~3 d, with overt jaundice in ~6 d

- Presenting symptoms
  - Fever — 75%
  - Leukocytosis, eosinophilia — 20–60%
  - Myalgias — 20%
  - Rash — 10%
  - Jaundice — 25%
  - Ascites, coagulaopathy, GI hemorrhage — 20% to 30%
- Liver enzyme markers
  - Alanine aminotransferase — 25–250× upper limit of normal
  - Aspartate aminotransferase — 25–250× upper limit of normal
  - Alkaline phosphatase — 1–3× upper limit of normal
- Histological liver findings
  - Zone 3 necrosis (massive in 30% of cases, submassive in 70% of cases)
  - Inflammation, granulomas, eosonophilic infiltrates
- Clinical course
  - Mortality rate in preliver transplant era as high as 80% if encephalopathy present
  - Recovery becomes evident as symptoms resolve over 5–14 d, with full recovery taking weeks to months.

ICD-9-CM Code: 997.4 (Postoperative acute)

Etiology/Pathophysiology

- Two distinct types of hepatitis are associated with halothane exposure

- **Type I**
  - Subclinical disease with mild elevation of liver enzymes, no jaundice
  - Caused by the anaerobic, reductive metabolism of halothane
  - May occur in up to 30% of pts receiving halothane
- **Type II**
  - Fulminant liver failure with massive zone 3 liver necrosis
  - Caused by oxidative metabolism of halothane
  - Trifluroacetyl intermediates conjugate liver proteins
  - In susceptible individuals, antibodies to the metabolite-liver protein complex are formed causing an immune response
  - Incidence is 10 times higher in second exposure cases and severity of illness greater if second exposure follows soon after first exposure

Drug Class/Metabolism

- Halothane: A nonvolatile anesthetic— a halogenated hydrocarbon
  - Molecular formula $C_2HBrClF_3$
  - Systematic (IUPAC) name: 1-bromo-1-chloro-1,1,1-trifluoroethane
  - Metabolized in the liver through both oxidative and reductive pathways
- Comparison of oxidative metabolism of volatile anesthetics:
  - Halothane — 20%
  - Enflurane — 2%
  - Isoflurane — 0.2%
  - Desflurane — 0.02%
- There are a few case reports of Type II hepatitis associated with isoflurane and desflurane in the world literature.

ASSESSMENT POINTS

System	Assessment by Hx	PE	Test
	N/V, malaise	Jaundice (about 6 days after second exposure, longer if 1st exposure)	Eosinophilia, leukocytosis Elevated liver enzymes: 1) Aspartate aminotransferase 2) Alanine aminotransferase (25 to 250×upper limit of normal) 3) Alkaline phosphatase (1–3×upper limit of normal) Liver biopsy: Zone 3 Centrilobular necrosis

Key Reference: Lewis JH. Liver disease caused by anesthetics, toxins, and herbal preparations. In Feldman, ed. *Sleisenger & Fordtran's gastrointestinal and liver disease.* 8th ed. Saunders, An Imprint of Elsevier; 2006:1853–1855.

Preoperative Implications

- Prior records should be reviewed and prior exposure documented
- Avoid volatile anesthetics in a pt with a confirmed Hx of postop liver dysfunction from halogenated agents
- Total IV anesthesia is one approach if general anesthesia is planned
- Regional anesthesia not contraindicated

Anticipated Problems/Concerns

- How to evaluate postop liver dysfunction
  - Incidence: 25-75% of surgical pts may have some form of hepatic dysfunction, from mild elevation in liver enzymes to global liver failure
  - Up to 50% of pts with cirrhosis may have postop jaundice

Categories of postop liver dysfunction

- Hepatocellular injury (elevated alanine aminotransferase, +/– hyperbilirubinemia)

  - Etiologies: Inhalational anesthetics and other drugs, hypotensive shock, transfusion reactions, unrecognized preop liver dysfunction
- Cholestatic jaundice (elevated alkaline phosphatase, +/– elevated ALT; direct hyperbilirubinemia)
  - Etiologies: Benign postop cholestasis, prolonged cardiac bypass, sepsis, prolonged administration of total parenteral nutrition, cholecystitis, cholangitis, microlithiasis, drugs (esp antibiotics)
- Indirect hyperbilirubinemia (other liver enzyme markers often normal)
  - Etiologies: Multiple transfusions, hemolysis, glucose-6-phosphate dehydrogenase deficiency, Gilbert's syndrome

Differential Diagnosis for Inhalational Anesthetic Induced Hepatitis [AIH]

- First rule: AIH is a diagnosis of exclusion
- Preexisting liver disease
  - Viral hepatitis

  - Steatohepatisis: Alcoholic or nonalcoholic (NASH)
  - Autoimmune hepatitis
  - Wilson's disease
- Periop disorders
  - Drug reactions
  - Hypotensive shock, other causes of liver ischemia
- Second rule: In pts with drug-induced liver injury, jaundice may herald impending global liver failure and should be considered life threatening.
- Third rule: Treatment is supportive in nature and orthotopic liver transplant may be life saving
- Fourth rule: In a pt with documented or suspected AIH, avoiding all volatile anesthetics is the safest course for future anesthetics, due to immune cross reactivity, the possibility of trace amounts of volatile anesthetics in the anesthesia circuit, as well as the many unanswered issues regarding this disorder.

Hepatitis A

Arnold J. Berry

Risk

- Most common form of acute viral hepatitis in many parts of the world and about one third of the USA population has antibody to HAV.
- With more widespread use of the HAV vaccine, the rate has decreased from 150,000 in 1999 to 25,000 in 2007.
- Very common infection in economically developing countries of Africa, Asia, and Latin America; children are frequently sources for outbreaks in crowded households, day care centers, and institutions; increased risk of disease is associated with travel to developing countries, men who have sex with men, users of injecting and non-injecting drugs, persons with clotting-factor disorders.
- Health care workers do not appear to be at increased risk for occupationally acquired infection.
- Although pts with chronic liver disease are not at increased risk for HAV infection, they are at risk for fulminant hepatitis A.

Perioperative Risks

- Elective surgery should not be performed on pts with acute HAV infection.
- Worsening liver function

Worry About

- With fulminant hepatitis A and acute liver failure, there may be coagulopathy, encephalopathy, cerebral edema, and multiple organ failure; mortality rate of greater than 40%
- Maintanence of liver blood flow and O_2 delivery; metabolism of drugs with hepatic clearance; hypoglycemia; prolonged effect of sedatives

- In addition to use of universal precautions by anesthesia personnel, use of sharp devices for invasive procedures should be minimized and/or safety devices should replace standard sharps.

Overview

- HAV replicates in the liver and is shed in the stool; the concentration in the stool is highest during the 2-wk period before to 1 wk after the onset of clinical symptoms; the risk of transmission of infection via the fecal-oral route is greatest during this time.
- Symptoms do not occur until the viral load in the stool begins to decrease and most pts with hepatitis A do not require hospitalization for treatment.
- In children less than 6 y of age, most HAV infections are asymptomatic while among older children and adults, most infections are symptomatic with jaundice occurring in over 80%.
- The two most common physical findings are jaundice and hepatomegaly. In symptomatic pts, the most common laboratory findings are elevated levels of serum alanine aminotransferase and bilirubin.
- Chronic HAV infection does not occur; most acute infections resolve within 2 mo; 10–15% of symptomatic pts may have a relapse of illness for up to 6 mo.
- Fulminant hepatitis with acute liver failure occurs in about 0.5% of all pts with HAV infection; the rate is 1.8% among adults greater than 50 y of age; pts with chronic liver disease are at increased risk for fulminant hepatitis when infected with HAV.

Etiology

- HAV is a 27 nm RNA, non-enveloped virus transmitted by the fecal-oral route by either person-to-person contact or ingestion of contaminated food or water; rarely, HAV has been transmitted by tranfusion of blood or blood products collected from donors during the viremic phase of infection
- Transmission by saliva has not been demonstrated
- HAV infection diagnosed by IgM anti-HAV in the acute phase and IgG anti-HAV occurs later; IgG anti-HAV persists and confers lifelong immunity

Usual Treatment

Immune globulin (IG) provides protection through passive transfer of antibodies to exposed individuals; a single dose of IG should be administered as soon as possible after exposure.

- Hepatitis A vaccine provides pre-exposure protection from HAV infection and is recommended by the CDC Advisory Committee on Immunization Practices for all children at age 1 y and adults in high-risk categories (men who have sex with men, users of illicit drugs, travelers to areas of the world where HAV is endemic, people with chronic liver disease or who receive clotting factor concentrates)
- Most pts are treated at home unless there is dehydration from vomiting or anorexia; physical activity is curtailed; complete recovery usually occurs within 3 to 6 mo
- Pts with acute liver failure require intensive support and may require liver transplantation.

ASSESSMENT POINTS

For patients with acute hepatitis A or fulminant hepatitis A

System	Effect	Assessment by Hx	PE	Test
CV	Hypovolemia	N/V, GI bleed	Tachycardia, hypotension	Orthostatic BP changes; measure CO, SVR
RESP	Hypoxemia		Tachypnea	O_2 saturation, ABG
GI	Bleeding	Hx of bleeding	Hemoccult + material	Hct, endoscopy
	Jaundice	Dark urine	Icteric sclera	Bilirubin
	N/V	N/V	Edema, ascites	Serum albumin
	Hypoalbuminemia		Abdominal pain	ALT, AST
	Hepatitis			
ENDO	Hypoglycemia	Altered consciousness		Blood glucose
HEME	Anemia	Tachycardia	Bruises	Hct
	Thrombocytopenia	Easy bruising	Bleeding in wounds	Plt count
	Immunosuppression	Infections		PT (low factor V, VII, IX, X, fibrinogen)
	Coagulopathy	Abnormal bleeding		
RENAL	Hepatorenal syndrome	Oliguria		Urinary Na^+ low
	Hyponatremia	Altered consciousness, seizures		Serum Na^+
CNS	Encephalopathy	Mental status exam	Level of consciousness	Serum ammonia level
	Cerebral edema		Level of consciousness	Measure intracranial pressure

Key Reference: Centers for Disease Control and Prevention. Prevention of hepatitis A through active or passive immunization: Recommendations of the Advisory Committee on Immunization Practices (ACIP). *MMWR.* 2006;55(RR-7):1–18.

Perioperative Implications for Patients with Acute Hepatitis A or Fulminant Hepatitis A

Preoperative Preparation

- Elective surgery should be postponed in pts with acute hepatitis A
- Correction of clotting abnormalities with FFP, Plt, cryoprecipitate as needed
- Administration of vitamin K to facilitate production of coagulation factors (prolonged PT), if time permits

- Premedicant depressive or sedative drugs should be avoided.

Monitoring

- Arterial line for ABG, electrolytes, glucose, and BP
- Consider central venous or pulm artery catheter

Airway

- Consider rapid sequence induction if N/V, or upper GI bleeding exist

Preinduction/ Induction

- Consider ketamine or etomidate in hypovolemic pts
- Acute liver failure is not likely to reduce plasma cholinesterase levels so succinylcholine may be used if indicated
- Increased bioavailability of IV drugs if serum albumin concentration is decreased
- Limit sedative drugs

Maintenance

- Inhalation agent with high inspired O_2 concentration useful for maintaining hepatic blood flow and O_2 supply; should probably avoid halothane
- The effect of muscle relaxants with hepatic clearance may be prolonged
- Increased blood loss with coagulopathy

Extubation

- May need postop mechanical ventilation to ensure time for adequate metabolism of depressant drugs

Adjuvants

- Hypocalcemia may occur with citrate administration

Anticipated Problems/Concerns

- Worsening of hepatic or renal function
- Delayed awakening from prolonged drug metabolism or encephalopathy
- Need to protect airway with reduced consciousness
- Hypoglycemia

ANESTHETIC CONSIDERATION

Pt c̄ flu-like illness (i.e. fevers, chills, muscle aches, nausea, etc.) CXL SX!! (elective stuff) →

WHY?

B/c it "could" be hepatitis and you wouldn't want to miss that. Can be very dangerous c̄ an anesthetic

Hepatitis B

Arnold J. Berry

Risk

- Incidence in USA: 3–5% have had the disease and 0.3–1.0% are carriers of hepatitis B virus (HBV)
- High-risk groups incl immigrants from endemic areas, IV drug users, homosexual men, household contacts of HBV carriers, pts on hemodialysis, clients in mental institutions
- Before introduction of hepatitis B vaccine, about 20% of susceptible anesthesiologists had serologic evidence of prior hepatitis B infection

Perioperative Risks

- Depends on activity and stage of infection
- Worsening liver function, hepatic encephalopathy, coagulopathy

Worry About

- With acute hepatic failure or end-stage liver disease: Coagulation abn, decreased hepatic metabolism of drugs, decreased levels of plasma cholinesterase, hypoxemia from pulm shunting and edema, ascites and Na+ overload, hypokalemia, hepatic encephalopathy and cerebral edema, impaired glucose metabolism and hypoglycemia, portal Htn and GI bleeding, acute renal failure and hepatorenal syndrome, infection and sepsis, malnutrition
- Maintenance of liver and cerebral BF and O_2 delivery

- Hepatitis B vaccine is the primary strategy for disease prevention.
- Risk of disease transmission to susceptible anesthesia personnel assoc with a hepatitis B surface antigen positive needlestick injury may be as great as 30%.
- In addition to use of universal precautions by anesthesia personnel, use of sharp devices for invasive procedures should be minimized, and/or safety devices should replace standard sharp devices.

Overview

- Hepatotropic viral infection: 90% have self-limiting acute hepatitis; 10% become chronic HBV carriers with about half of those progressing to chronic active hepatitis, cirrhosis, or hepatocellular carcinoma; 0.5% of pts with acute infection develop fulminant hepatitic failure.
- 70% with acute hepatitis have subclinical hepatitis; symptomatic infection may produce jaundice, malaise, nausea, abd pain.
- HBV carriers are diagnosed by persistent positive serology for hepatitis B surface antigen (HBsAg).
- Hepatitis B surface antibody (anti-HBs) confers immunity (after resolution of infection or with immunization).

ICD-9-CM Code: 070.3 (Viral hepatitis B without mention of hepatic coma)

Etiology

- HBV (42-nm DNA virus, eight genotypes) carried in and spread by blood and body fluid contact
- Transmitted to non-immune individuals via parenteral or mucocutaneous exposure to HBV-infected blood or body fluids

Usual Treatment

- Prevention with hepatitis B vaccine
- Protocols should be in place for heath care personnel to report and have follow-up of percutaneous or permucosal exposures to blood or bloody body fluids.
- Hepatitis B immune globulin (HBIG) for passive immunization after susceptible individual is exposed
- Supportive treatment for most cases of acute hepatitis B; antiviral treatment may be used for pts with prolonged symptomatic acute hepatitis.
- Chronic hepatitis B is treated with interferon for pts without cirrhosis or oral antivirals such as tenofovir or entecavir (second-line antivirals incl adefovir)
- Orthotopic liver transplantation for liver failure; HBIG and antivirals (entecavir, tenofovir, lamivudine, telbivudine or adefovir) should be used to prevent HBV reinfection.

ASSESSMENT POINTS

The following are for patients with fulminant hepatitis or cirrhosis from chronic hepatitis.

System	Effect	Assessment by Hx	PE	Test
CARDIO	Hyperdynamic circulation		Tachycardia Skin spiders	Measure CO, SVR
RESP	Hypoxemia		Tachypnea	SpO_2
GI	Bleeding Ascites	Hx of bleeding Increasing abd girth	Ascites, pedal edema Abd pain	Hct, endoscopy
	Jaundice	Dark urine		Bilirubin
	Hypoalbuminemia Hepatitis			Serum albumin SGPT, SGOT
ENDO	Hypoglycemia	Altered consciousness		Blood glucose
HEME	Anemia			Hct
	Thrombocytopenia	Easy bruisability	Bruises	Plt count
	Immunosuppression Coagulopathy	Infections Abn bleeding		PT (low factors V, VII, IX, X, fibrinogen)
RENAL	Hepatorenal syndrome Hyponatremia Hypokalemia	Altered consciousness, seizures Taking diuretics	Oliguria	Urinary Na+ Serum Na+ Serum K+
CNS	Encephalopathy	Mental status exam	Level of consciousness Asterixis	Intracranial pressure Cerebral perfusion pressure

Key Reference: Stravitz RT. Critical management decisions in patients with acute liver failure. *Chest.* 2008;134:1092–1102.

Perioperative Implications

- For pts with end-stage liver disease from hepatitis B—emergency surgery only with acute infection

Preoperative Preparation

- Correction of clotting abn with FFP, plt, cryoprecipitate, rFVIIa as needed
- Administration of vitamin K to facilitate production of coagulation factors (prolonged PT), if time permits
- Paracentesis if resp compromise from massive ascites

Monitoring

- Arterial line for ABG and BP
- Consider need for central venous or pulm artery catheter
- Monitor intracranial pressure when cerebral edema present

Airway

- Consider rapid-sequence induction if pt has ascites or upper GI bleeding

Preinduction/Induction

- Ketamine or etomidate in hypovolemic pts
- Duration of action of succinylcholine may be prolonged
- Increased bioavailability of IV drugs with low serum albumin
- Limit sedative drugs

Maintenance

- Inhalation agent with high FIO_2 useful for maintaining hepatic blood flow; should probably avoid halothane
- Choose muscle relaxants not dependent on liver metabolism
- Increased blood loss with coagulopathy

Extubation

- May need postop ventilation to ensure time for adequate metabolism of depressant drugs

Adjuvants

- Hypocalcemia may occur with citrate administration

Anticipated Problems/Concerns

- Worsening of hepatic or renal function
- Fluid overload
- Delayed awakening from prolonged drug metabolism or encephalopathy
- Need to protect airway with reduced consciousness, esp with upper GI bleeding
- Hypoglycemia

Hepatitis C

Arnold J. Berry

Risk

- HCV accounts for about 20% of cases of acute viral hepatitis in the USA.
- HCV is the most common cause of chronic liver disease in the USA and is the most frequent indication for liver transplantation.
- HCV is transmitted through percutaneous exposure to infected blood (IV drug use); occupational and sexual transmission of HCV can occur; pts on hemodialysis are at increased risk for infection.
- About 2–3% of cases occur in health care workers.

Perioperative Risks

- Worsening liver function, hepatic encephalopathy, coagulopathy
- Risk of transmission of HCV from carrier to anesthesia personnel is ~2% after percutaneous exposure.

Worry About

- With end-stage liver disease: Coagulation abn, decreased hepatic metabolism of drugs, decreased levels of plasma cholinesterase, hypoxemia from pulm shunting, ascites and Na^+ overload, hepatic encephalopathy, glucose metabolism, portal Htn and GI bleeding, hepatorenal syndrome

- Maintenance of liver blood flow and O_2 delivery
- In addition to use of universal precautions by anesthesia personnel, use of sharp devices for invasive procedures should be minimized, and/or safety devices should replace standard sharp devices.

Overview

- Hepatotropic insidious viral infection; fulminant acute hepatitis C rare
- 60–70% of individuals with acute HCV infection are asymptomatic or have only a mild clinical illness.
- Over 80% of pts remain HCV-RNA positive with the majority having persistent elevation of liver enzymes.
- 70–85% of HCV infected pts develop chronic infection; cirrhosis develops in up to 50% of individuals with chronic hepatitis C and hepatocellular carcinoma in 1–5%.
- Pts over age 50 may have a more rapid progression of liver injury; alcohol use increases the risk of liver injury.
- Serologic testing for HCV infection incl testing for HCV RNA or immunoassay for anti-HCV; HCV RNA can be detected in serum within days after infection and HCV RNA quantification is useful in the management of treatment; ELISA tests for anti-HCV become positive about 8 wk after exposure, but anti-HCV is not associated

with resolution of infection and does not confer immunity

ICD-9-CM: 070 (Viral hepatitis)

Etiology

- HCV (30–60-nm RNA virus with at least 6 genotypes) carried in and transmitted by exposure to blood and body fluids

Usual Treatment

- For pts with acute HCV infection in which HCV RNA has not cleared after 3 mo, treatment with standard interferon or pegylated interferon alfa-2b, with or without ribavirin, should be considered.
- Some pts with chronic HCV infection may benefit from treatment with standard interferon or pegylated interferon, with or without ribavirin, but current guidelines should be consulted for specific details.
- Protocols should be in place for health care workers to report on and have follow-up of percutaneous or permucosal exposures to blood or bloody body fluids; immune globulin and antiviral agents are not recommended for postexposure prophylaxis after occupational HCV exposure.
- Currently there is no vaccine for prevention of HCV infection.
- Orthotopic liver transplantation for end-stage liver disease

ASSESSMENT POINTS

The following are for patients with end-stage liver disease from cirrhosis or chronic hepatitis.

System	Effect	Assessment by Hx	PE	Test
CARDIO	Hyperdynamic circulation		Tachycardia	Measure CO, SVR
	Pulm Htn		Telangiectases	Pulm artery pressure
RESP	Hypoxemia		Tachypnea	ABGs, SpO_2
	Hepato-pulm syndrome			
GI	Bleeding	Hx of bleeding	Hemoccult + material	Hct, endoscopy
	Ascites	Increasing abdominal girth	Fluid wave on abdominal exam	
	Jaundice	Dark urine	Icteric sclerae	Bilirubin
	Hypoalbuminemia		Ascites, pedal edema	Serum albumin
	Hepatitis		Abdominal pain	ALT, AST
ENDO	Hypoglycemia	Altered consciousness		Blood sugar
HEME	Anemia			Hct
	Thrombocytopenia	Easily bruised	Bruises	Plt count
	Immunosuppression	Infections		PT (low factors V, VII, IX, X, fibrinogen)
	Coagulopathy	Abn bleeding		
RENAL	Hepatorenal syndrome		Oliguria	Urinary Na^+ low
	Hyponatremia	Altered consciousness, seizures		Serum Na^+
	Hypokalemia	Taking diuretics		Serum K^+
CNS	Encephalopathy	Mental status exam	Level of consciousness Asterixis	Serum ammonia
	Cerebral edema			Intracranial pressure; cerebral perfusion pressure

Key Reference: Stravitz RT. Critical management decisions in patients with acute liver failure. *Chest.* 2008;134:1092–1102.

Perioperative Implications for Patients with End-Stage Liver Disease from Hepatitis C

Preoperative Preparation

- Correction of clotting abn with FFP, plt, cryoprecipitate, rFVIIa as needed
- Administration of vitamin K to facilitate production of coagulation factors (prolonged PT), if time permits
- Paracentesis if resp compromise from massive ascites

Monitoring

- Arterial line for ABGs and BP
- Consider central venous or pulm artery catheter (useful for diagnosis of pulm Htn)

Airway

- Consider rapid-sequence induction with ascites or upper GI bleeding

Preinduction/Induction

- Ketamine or etomidate in hypovolemic pts
- Duration of action of succinylcholine may be prolonged

- Increased bioavailability of IV drugs with low serum albumin
- Limit sedative drugs

Maintenance

- Inhalation agent with high FIO_2 useful for maintaining hepatic blood flow; should probably avoid halothane
- Choose muscle relaxants not dependent on liver metabolism
- Increased blood loss with coagulopathy

Extubation
• May need postop ventilation to ensure time for adequate metabolism of depressant drugs

Adjuvants
• Hypocalcemia may occur with citrate administration

Anticipated Problems/Concerns
• Worsening of hepatic or renal function
• Fluid overload
• Delayed awakening from prolonged drug metabolism or encephalopathy
• Need to protect airway with reduced consciousness, esp. with upper GI bleeding
• Hypoglycemia

Hereditary Hemorrhagic Telangiectasia (Osler-Weber-Rendu Disease)

Marina Shindell

Risk

- Affects varied in racial and ethnic groups, wide geographic distribution
- Men and women affected equally
- In Vermont, frequency 1:16,500
- Europe and Japan: 1:5,000–8,000

Perioperative Risk

- Excessive bleeding
- Paradoxical air, bland, or septic embolism to brain

Worry About

- Chronic anemia due to hemorrhage, esp. recurrent epistaxis
- Due to danger of intrapartum or postpartum pulm hemorrhage, a pregnant woman with HHT who has not had a recent pulm evaluation should be evaluated as soon as pregnancy is recognized.

Overview

- Mucocut and visceral vascular dysplasia
- Result from the combination of defective perivascular connective tissue, insufficient smooth muscle contractile element, endothelial cell junction defects, and increased endothelial tissue plasminogen activator impairing thrombus formation in case of vascular damage
- International consensus diagnostic criteria (Curacao criteria): HHT diagnosis classified as definite if 3 criteria present, possible or suspected if 2 criteria present and unlikely if, one criterion present. The criteria are
- Epistaxis: Spontaneous recurrent nosebleeds
- Mucocut telangiectasia
- Visceral involvement (i.e.; GI telangiectasia, pulm AVM, hepatic AVM, cerebral AVM, spinal AVM
- Affected 1° relative
- Manifestations of HHT are not present generally at birth, but develop with increasing age, with epistaxis usually being the earliest sign that may lead to chronic anemia. 90% of pts have signs and symptoms by age 40.

ICD9-CM: 448.0

Etiology

- Autosomal dominant trait with varying penetrance and expressivity

Usual Treatment

- Epistaxis is medically treated with Fe supplementation, estrogen therapy, and humidification. With intractable epistaxis ablative therapy with ND: YAG laser is effective, although multiple treatments required
- Multiple transfusions
- Pulm AVMs with feeding artery diameter greater than or equal to 3 mm require treatment with transcatheter embolotherapy with coils.

ASSESMENT POINTS

System	Effect	Assessment by Hx	PE	Test
HEENT	Telangiectasia of nasal mucosa, conjunctival telangiectasias, retinal vascular malformations	Recurrent frequent epistaxis		
CV	High-output heart failure, thromboembolism	Fatigue, SOB	Rales, neurologic deficits	CXR
PULM	AVMs with R to L shunt leading to hypoxemia, absence of filtering capillary bed allowing particulate matter to reach systemic circulation, fragile vessels may hemorrhage into bronchus or pleural cavity	Fatigue, dyspnea on exertion, hemoptysis, embolic cerebral events	Cyanosis, clubbing, neurologic deficits	CXR, CT, detection of R to L shunt via radionucleide perfusion scans or contrast ECHO
HEME	Anemia, coagulopathy, associated with von Willebrand disease	Recurrent epistaxis	Pallor	CBC, PT/INR, PTT
CNS	Cerebral AVM, aneurysms, cavernous angiomas paradoxical embolism, spinal AVM, migraines	CVA, brain abscess	Headache, seizure, hemorrhage, ischemia of the surrounding tissues due to a steal effect	MRI
HEPATIC	Hepatomegaly, high output heart failure, portal Htn, encephalopathy, biliary disease	Hemorrhage, sepsis	Jaundice	LFTs, PT/INR, PTT

Key Reference: Lomax S, Edgcombe H. Anesthetic implications for the parturient with hereditary hemorrhagic telengiectasia. *Can J Anaesth*. 2009;56:374–384.

Perioperative Implications

Preoperative Preparation

- Preop cardiac and pulm evaluation to exclude high-output cardiac failure and pulm AV malformations
- CBC for anemia from bleeding or polycythemia from pulm shunt
- Check liver and renal function
- Perform neurologic assessment to exclude previous paradoxical emboli and severe brain AVM
- Debubble IV lines to prevent paradoxical air emboli
- Use meticulous aseptic technique
- For regional technique, assess any possibility of AVMs in the neuraxial region prior to performing the technique

Monitoring

- Avoid or use with great caution TEE, gastric suctioning or esophageal stethoscope if esophageal varices or AVMs are present

Airway

- If oropharengeal AVMs are present, there is a high risk of airway bleeding
- Nasal intubation contraindicated if nasal telengiectasias are present
- Well-lubricated smaller size ETT to prevent any tissue trauma

Maintenance

- Risk of high-output heart failure, liver failure, modify anesthetic management
- Pulm AVMs could be large enough to lead to heart failure and polycythemia.
- Key aspects of anesthetic management are interventions to maintain nml hemodynamic parameters and to prevent bleeding and the formation of emboli.

Postoperative Period

- Avoid immobilization for prolonged periods of time to avoid thromboembolism to CNS.

Adjuvants

- Watch for incompatible drugs in IVs or peripheral veins to avoid particulate matter precipitation and embolization to the brain
- Broad spectrum antibiotic prophylaxis to decrease risk of CNS infections
- NSAIDs may precipitate GI or mucosal bleeding and impair renal function

Anticipated Problems/Concerns

- Anemia due to recurrent bleeding
- Transfusion is complicated: Low Hct may increase the risk of high-output CHF by increasing extent of arteriovenous shunting (decreasing viscosity effect), but a high Hct may increase risk of thromboembolism
- Coagulopathy: Multiple hemostatic defects, incl low-grade DIC, reduced plt aggregation, and factor XI deficiency, may aggravate bleeding caused by local vessel wall pathology
- Paradoxical embolism: Owing to pulm AVMs, peripheral microemboli (air, bland, or septic) bypass nml pulm capillary filtering and embolize, causing transient or permanent neurologic defects or brain abscess
- Special attention should be paid to pregnant women with the diagnosis of HHT. In the rare instances, deterioration of pre-conception AVMs and the development of new AVMs will present with clinically silent but potentially life threatening complications of the disorder. These are most commonly located in the pulm vasculature, followed in frequency by the cerebral, GI, and spinal circulation. With CV and hormonally induced enlargement of certain AVMs there is concurrent risk of rupture, as well as shunt-induced high cardiac output failure and systemic embolism.

Herniated Nucleus Pulposus

Christine Peeters-Asdourian

Risk

- Incidence of symptomatic disc herniation is 1–2% in the general population
- Most common age is during third and fourth decades of life
- Smoking (leads to a decrease in O_2 tension 2° to vasoconstriction with decreased nutrient supply to the nucleus pulposus)
- Chronic increases in disc strain (i.e., chronic coughing, sitting without lumbar support, heavy lifting)
- Poor posture combined with poor body mechanics stresses the lumbar spine and affects the distribution of the body's weight.
- Obesity and sedentary behavior

Overview

- Located between vertebral bodies
- The intervertebral disc is the largest avascular structure in the body.
- The nucleus pulposus is composed of H_2O, collagen, and proteoglycans (PGs). PG molecules are important because they attract and retain H_2O, making a hydrated gel–like matter that resists compression. The amount of H_2O in the nucleus varies throughout the day depending on activity. It decreases with age, leading to degenerative disc disease.
- The annulus fibrosus is an annular structure composed of concentric sheets of collagen fibers connected to the vertebral endplates. The sheets are oriented at various angles and enclose the nucleus pulposus.
- Disc herniation occurs when the annulus fibrosus breaks open or cracks, allowing the nucleus pulposus to escape. This is called a herniated nucleus pulposus (HNP) or herniated disc. The herniated disc material initiates an inflammatory reaction.
- Disc herniation typically gives rise to radicular pain, which is pain in the distribution of the nerve root affected by the herniation with a strong inflammatory and neuropathic component, with or without neurologic change. If radicular changes take place, the presentation is that of a radiculopathy.
- Lumbar region: L4–5 most common site (59%), followed by L5–S1 (30%), L3–4 (9%)

- Natural history of disease is favorable
- Majority of pts have substantial improvement of symptoms within a few mo

ICD-9-CM Code

Etiology

- The H_2O-retaining ability of the nucleus pulposus progressively declines with age.
- Nuclear material that is displaced into the spinal canal is associated with a significant inflammatory response (proinflammatory molecules interleukin-1 (IL-1), IL-8, and TNF α)
- Macrophages respond, which results in scar production, and an increase in substance P
- Symptoms do not always correlate with herniation size (asymptomatic herniations frequent)

Disease Presentation

- Frequently present with a combination of back pain along with radicular symptoms; neurologic signs such as weakness or sensory deficits are possible (isolated low back pain may also be the sole presentation)
- Pts often describe popping sensation prior to radicular symptom.
- Neural impingement is responsible for dysfunction (compression of a motor nerve results in weakness, and compression of a sensory nerve results in numbness).
- Radicular pain is caused by inflammation of the nerve (which can explain the lack of correlation between herniation size and pain symptoms).
- Ideal imaging modality is MRI, although CT may also be helpful, EMG/NCS aid in identifying nerve root (there is not always correlation between findings on imaging studies and clinical presentation).
- Maneuvers which increase intrathecal pressure (coughing, sneezing, prolonged sitting) aggravate pain.

Usual Treatment

- Conservative therapies
  - NSAIDs are literature supported
  - Systemic corticosteroids, opioids, muscle relaxants, neuropathic agents (empirical data, limited EBM data)
    - Contrary to prior beliefs, activity is now preferred over bed rest

- Physical therapy
- Several other modalities poorly supported by literature include bracing, traction, acupuncture, chiropractic manipulation, behavioral therapy, and biofeedback
- Favorable outcomes with higher education levels, self-motivated pts, return of nml neurologic examination within 12 wk, nml psychological profile, and absence of a workers compensation claim or litigation
- Injection therapy
  - Interlaminar epidural steroid injections are commonly performed
  - Transforaminal epidural steroid injections target area more precisely (commonly performed in lumbar region/controversial in cervical region).
  - Fluoroscopy improves accuracy of injectate and is preferred by most practitioners.
  - Randomized controlled studies have demonstrated superior efficacy of injections over conservative management (at least in short term).
  - Although used in other countries Chymopapain no longer used in USA 2° to severe allergic reactions
- Percutaneous discectomy
  - None directly remove herniated portion, rather removes nucleus pulposus with hope of herniation regressing (limited studies showed success rates around 30%)
  - Nucleoplasty
  - Laser disc decompression
  - Endoscopic discectomy
  - These techniques may be performed in ambulatory surgery settings or even office settings with moderate sedation or monitored anesthesia care.
- Surgical intervention
  - Most common procedure for a herniated or ruptured intervertebral disc is a microdiscectomy
  - 200,000 lumbar discectomies performed annually
  - Cauda equina syndrome or a high degree of motor dysfunction are surgical emergencies.
- Most recently a large study showed short-term benefit from surgery; however at long-term follow-up showed no benefit over conservative therapy.

ASSESSMENT POINTS

System	Effect	Assessment by Hx	PE	Test
MS	↓ ROM, pain	Lumbar sprain: Stiffness, ↓ ROM	Muscle tenderness	MRI MRI/CT
		Annular tear: Axial pain, difficulties sitting	↓ ROM referred dermatomal pain	MRI/CT EMG/NCS
		HNP: numbness, weakness or simply pain	↓ Reflexes, sensory loss	Surgical emergency
		Cauda Equina	"Saddle anesthesia"	
NEURO	↓ Reflexes or ↑ reflexes with severe spinal stenosis			
PSYCHOSOCIAL	Anxiety, chronic opioid intake, litigation issues	Medications preop	If opioid abruptly stopped, may present with withdrawal	Need for multimodal analgesia

Key Reference: Rathmell JP. A 50 year old man with Chronic Low Back Pain. *JAMA*. 2008;299:(17): 2066–2077.

Perioperative Considerations

- Pts on high doses of opioids may present a challenge intraop and postop.

- Multimodal analgesia is the best option incl the continuation of the preop dose of opioids as a baseline, gabapentin, NSAIDs (as allowed per surgical team), acetaminophen, clonidine (as allowed by CV status), and ketamine IV for its NMDA antagonist properties.

Herpes, Type I

Manuel C. Vallejo
Joel M. Pomerantz

Risk

- 500,000 new cases each year in USA; 58% of people worldwide are seropositive
- Symptoms are typically minor or absent except in immunocompromised pts

Perioperative Risks

- Theoretical risk that spinal anesthesia can spread HSV-1 infection to new dermatomes

Worry About

- Transmission of infection to health care workers or other pts
- Reactivation after organ transplantation and initiation of immunosuppression
- 2° infection of herpetic lesions with bacteria or fungi

Overview

- Transmission occurs after contact with secretions or mucus.
- Primary infection associated with fever/malaise; mean duration 19 d. Recurrences are milder, with a mean duration of 10 d.
- Lesions recur about 1/y (contrast with 4/y HSV-2) in immunocompetent pts
- 18–35% of populations are seropositive by age 5
- Oral symptoms incl gingivostomatitis/oral ulcers. Genital and ocular infection also exists
- Symptoms may last 1–4 wk
- Dx: Viral culture (titer 1000 times nml while active lesions exist) or HSV antibodies

ICD-9-CM Codes: 054.7 (Infection with specified complications); 054.8 (Infection with unspecified complications)

Etiology

- Transmission occurs after contact with lesions or body fluids such as saliva or genital secretions. 58% of world population is seropositive. Transmission can be vertical (transmission to infant via vaginal tract), which is a TORCH pathogen associated with greater risk of infant death or blindness. Other human herpesviruses (*Herpesviridae*) are varicella-zoster (HHV-3), Epstein-Barr virus (HHV-4), cytomegalovirus (HHV-5), and human herpesvirus 6 (HHV-6)
- No animal/insect reservoir or vectors exist for HSV-1.
- Infection is usually mild in pts with an intact immune system.
- Dx is by viral culture, PCR, fluorescent antibody testing, or serology.

Usual Treatment

- Acyclovir, valacyclovir, and famcyclovir are effective as episodic therapy when initiated within 72 hr of appearance of symptoms. Reduce viral shedding, lesion healing time, and symptoms.
- Suppressive therapy (lower dose initiated while asymptomatic) is effective in reducing frequency and severity of recurrences, as well as transmission to an uninfected partner.
- Foscarnet or vidarabine may be used in acyclovir-resistant herpes infections.

ASSESSMENT POINTS

System	Effect	Assessment by Hx	PE	Test
RESP	Pneumonitis	Aspiration of oral secretions; previous HSV esophagitis	Bilateral crackles	CXR—bilateral interstitial infiltrates
GI	Esophagitis	Odynophagia, dysphagia, substernal pain	Multiple shallow mucosal ulcers	
GU	Cystitis			
CNS	Encephalitis, meningitis	Headache, confusion, lethargy	Anosmia, memory loss, expressive aphasia, focal seizures	Brain biopsy
DERM	Cutaneous ulcers	Recurrent painful skin or mucosal ulcers	Multiple vesicular lesions on an erythematous base with subsequent ulceration	
	Stevens-Johnson syndrome	Extensive painful skin lesions	Deep bullous erosive lesions	

Key Reference: Chayavichitsilp P, Buckwalter JV, Krakowski AC, Friedlander SF, Herpes simplex, *Pediatr Rev*. 2009:30(4):119–129.

Perioperative Implications

Preoperative Preparation
- Cover exposed herpetic lesions
- Strict adherence to universal precautions

Monitoring
- Avoid disturbing active lesions

Regional Anesthesia
- Needle should not be inserted through lesion. Theoretical risk of spreading herpes from one infected ganglion to another, but regional anesthesia is not contraindicated

Postoperative Period
- Thorough disinfection of any surface area that might have been in contact with oral secretions or herpetic lesions. Most disinfectants are effective, incl chlorine and alcohol.

Anticipated Problems/Concerns

- No effective pre- or postexposure prophylaxis
- Acyclovir may reduce effectiveness of phenytoin.
- C-section should be offered for pregnant women with active HSV.
- Vaginal delivery is acceptable for women in remission; acyclovir is often used.

Herpes, Type II

Jay Shepherd
Santiago Gomez

Risk

- Incidence within USA: Estimated 40–60 million (20% of sexually active adults)
- Highest prevalence in women, African-Americans, and lower socioeconomic groups
- Frequency and severity of infection increased in immunocompromised pts, incl HSV encephalitis
- Incidence of neonatal HSV infection estimated at 1/2000–1/5000 deliveries

Perioperative Risks

- Vertical transmission from infected mother to fetus during vaginal birth
- Intrauterine fetal infection after rupture of membranes

Worry About

- Transmission of infection to health care personnel resulting in herpetic whitlow via inoculation of virus into fingers
- Neonatal herpetic infection during vaginal births
- Viremia 2° to needle placement within infected area during regional anesthesia
- Extension of genital infection to adjacent areas during exam and instrumentation
- 2° bacterial or fungal infection of herpetic lesions

Overview

- Causative primarily of infections below waist transmitted by sexual contact
- Maternal primary HSV-2 infection associated with spontaneous abortion
- Newborns infected with HSV-2 during vaginal delivery from the mother's genital infection (high neonatal mortality)
- Primary genital HSV-2 infection with highest incidence of systemic symptoms (malaise, fever, headache, myalgias)
- Latent infection remains dormant in sensory ganglia innervating infected area until reactivation
- Recurrent infection involves vesicular, ulcerative lesions in genital tract, labia, vulva, perineum, cervix, urethra
- No increased risk of reactivation of HSV-2 associated with neuraxial anesthesia
- Chronic recurrent HSV-2 infection associated with development of cervical and vulvar cancer
- Dx by viral culture (gold standard) most sensitive and specific (rapid Dx by Tzanck smear)

ICD-9-CM Codes: 054.9 (Infection); 771.2 (Congenital)

Etiology

- Double-stranded DNA virus in family of Herpesviridae
- Acquired genital infection primarily by sexual transmission of HSV-2
- Immunosuppression and increased number of sexual partners are risk factors for acquisition
- Diagnosed by multinucleated giant epithelial cells (polykaryocytes) with intranuclear (Cowdry type A) inclusion bodies on Giemsa stain smears (Tzanck preparation) taken from vesicle or tissue biopsy

Usual Treatment

- IV acyclovir for neonatal HSV-2 infection
- Oral acyclovir and topical cream shorten duration of lesions for recurrent infections
- Most recommend that full-term parturients with visible genital lesions (esp. primary infection) undergo abdominal delivery to decrease incidence of neonatal HSV infection. Neonates exposed to asymptomatic shedding of HSV during parturition (4-fold increase in HIV seropositive women) may also rarely acquire neonatal HSV.

ASSESSMENT POINTS (Primary and Recurrent)

System	Effect	Assessment by Hx	PE	Test
HEENT	Pharyngitis (primary)		Cervical adenopathy Mucosal ulceration	
GU (mucous membranes)	Cystitis (primary) Genital ulcers (recurrent)	Dysuria	Vaginal or urethral discharge Ulcerated lesions of penis or labia or cervix	Viral culture (gold standard) Tzanck smear; direct immunofluorescent assay Biopsy; intranuclear inclusion bodies
LYMPHATICS		Lymphadenopathy	Tender inguinal nodes	
SKIN	Herpetic whitlow (recurrent)	Painful vesicular or papular lesion	Pain	Tzanck smear
CNS	Aseptic meningitis (primary)	Headache	Cauda equina syndrome	
RECTAL	Herpes proctitis (primary)	Constipation Tenesmus Discharge		Proctosigmoidoscopy

Key References: Armitage and Salata. *Sexually Transmitted Diseases. Cecil's Essentials of Medicine*. 7th ed. [Ch. 106]. Augenbraun M, et al. Increased genital shedding of HSV-2 in HIV seropositive women. *Ann Intern Med*. 1995;123:845–847.

Perioperative Implications

Preoperative Preparation
- Universal precautions

Monitoring
- Routine

Regional Anesthesia
- Needle placement in infected area contraindicated 2° to risk of viremia and local extension into deep tissues
- Preferred in pregnant women with recurrent infection, no systemic symptoms, and no infection in area of block placement

Postoperative Period
- Universal precautions

Anticipated Problems/Concerns
- Difficulty identifying asymptomatic carriers of HSV-2 with viral shedding
- No effective prophylaxis for newborns

Hirschsprung's Disease

Sobia Mansoor

Franklyn Cladis

Risk

- Incidence: 1:5000 live births
- Male predominance of 4:1
- Most cases are sporadic but ~10% are familial
- Associated with neurologic, CV, urologic, and GI abn
- Trisomy 21 is seen in 10%, other associated anomalies incl Waardenburg syndrome, congenital hypoventilation syndrome ("Ondine's curse"), congenital deafness, MEN 2a and neuroblastoma

Perioperative Risks

- Intestinal obstruction with full stomach
- Septic shock
- Hypovolemia
- Electrolyte abn

Worry About

- Intestinal obstruction leading to regurgitation and aspiration
- Vomiting and diarrhea (enterocolitis related) may result in electrolyte and fluid abn
- Enterocolitis characterized by dehydration and septic shock
- Intestinal ischemia, perforation, and peritonitis leading to increases in third space losses

Overview

- 90% of pts have delayed (>48 hrs) passage of meconium
- 80% of pts present in the first few mo of life with constipation, poor feeding, and progressive abdominal distention
- Presentations vary from mild symptoms to severe disease with toxic megacolon, enterocolitis, peritonitis, or perforation.
- Dx may be made by radiographic imaging (transition zone seen with contrast enema), anorectal manometry, or histologic findings (definitive diagnosis) on rectal suction or full thickness biopsies

ICD-9-CM Code: 751.3

Etiology

- Disease is caused by the failure of neural crest cells to migrate cephalocaudally causing an absence of ganglion cells in all or part of the colon.
- Several genes incl *RET* and *EDNRB* have been linked to the disorder.
- Varying lengths of the distal colon are unable to relax, causing functional colonic obstruction over time.
- Aganglionic segment extends proximally from the anus and is limited to the rectosigmoid region in 75% of cases; however 10% of pts may have total colonic aganglionosis.

Usual Treatment

- Nasogastric decompression, antibiotics, volume resuscitation and correction of electrolyte abn
- Rectal irrigation to decompress bowel and prevent enterocolitis
- Healthy newborns with non-distended colons and short-segment disease can undergo a primary ileoanal pull-through procedure.
- If child has enterocolitis or a significantly dilated colon, a colostomy can be placed; with pull-through procedure being performed 4–6 mo later.
- Swenson's was the original pull-through procedure; newer techniques (Duhamel, Soave, and Boley) help preserve the nerve supply to the rectum and bladder.
- Recent advances incl laparoscopic-assisted endorectal pull-through and primary single-stage transanal pull-through without colostomy or intra-abdominal dissection. The colon and rectum are mobilized laparoscopically while the endorectal dissection is done through the anus. The laparoscopic approach minimizes postop analgesia requirements and hospital stay. Intraop pathologic evaluation of the bowel is essential for single-stage repair to ensure complete resection of aganglionic bowel.

ASSESSMENT POINTS

System	Effect	Assessment by Hx	PE	Test
RESP	Congenital hypoventilation "Ondine's curse"	Apnea		
CARDIAC	Hypovolemia, septic shock, tetralogy of Fallot	IV replacement Extent of vomiting	Mucous membranes Vital signs/UO Murmur, cyanosis	BUN and Cr BUN/Cr ratio ECHO
GI	Intestinal obstruction	No meconium Constipation Diarrhea Vomiting	No feces in rectum, abdominal distention, malnutrition	Electrolyte panel Abdominal films Barium enema

Key Reference: Kapur RP. Practical pathology and genetics of Hirschsprung's disease. *Semin Pediatr Surg*. 2009;18(4):212–223. Review.

Perioperative Implications

Preoperative Implications

- Assessment of volume status due to bowel preparation, vomiting, and diarrhea
- Other congenital anomalies: Cardiac malformations (2–5%) and trisomy 21 (5–15%) are associated with congenital aganglionosis, consider cardiac evaluation and genetic testing

Monitoring

- Routine

Airway

- No significant issues other than those related to newborns or associated syndromes

Induction

- Rapid-sequence induction required if bowel obstruction present
- Monitor BP
- Some IV and inhalational anesthetics may be poorly tolerated if hypovolemic

Maintenance

- Prevent heat loss with forced warm air device and heating lamps. Pts may be uncovered from mid chest down and procedures may be lengthy (4–6 hr)
- Need for muscle relaxation
- Use isotonic IVFs. Consider checking an intraop blood glucose
- Avoid N_2O
- Consider combined general and regional anesthesia for profound relaxation of anal sphincter muscles and reduction of need for IV narcotics or muscle relaxation

Extubation

- Can routinely be performed at the end of surgery. Pts should be awake.

Postoperative Period

- Apnea may occur in newborns receiving narcotics postop
- Association with congenital hypoventilation syndrome

- Consider postop pain management with continuous epidural/caudal anesthesia. The back may be prepped into the surgical field. Placement of regional technique may need to occur at the end of surgery.

Anticipated Problems/Concerns

- Aspiration pneumonitis
- Early postop surgical complications incl anastomotic leak (1–10%), pelvic abcess (5%) and wound dehiscence (3%).
- Late complications incl enterocolitis, constipation, incontinence, and stricture formation.
- Postop enterocolitis is the most serious and potentially life-threatening complication. Overall postop mortality is low at 2%.
- Definitive treatment of complications may require operative management involving a redo pull-through procedure, fecal diversion, or anorectal myomectomy.

Histiocytosis

Jeremy L. Gibson

Risk

- Langerhans cell histiocytosis (LCH)
- Incidence: 1 in 250,000
- M:F ratio: 1.5:1
- Seen in all ages, but peak incidence at 1–3 y of age
- Pulm LCH common in young adults

Perioperative Risks

- Dependent on organ systems involved and extent of dysfunction

Worry About

- Specific organ dysfunction caused by infiltration with histiocytes incl: Liver, lungs, hematopoietic system, pituitary, spleen, and bone
- Can involve single or multiple sites and organs
- Treated with steroids and chemotherapy; at risk for adrenal insufficiency and may require stress steroids
- Diabetes insipidus due to posterior pituitary involvement
- Cervical instability if lesions present in cervical vertebrae

- Severe pulm dysfunction possible; Pulm Htn without overt right heart failure

Overview

- Broad group of disorders involving infiltration of affected organs with monocytes, macrophages, and dendritic cells
- The most commonly discussed disorder is LCH, previously known separately as eosinophilic granuloma, Hand-Schüller-Christian disease, and Letterer-Siwe disease
- Severity of clinical symptoms varies markedly and can involve primarily skin and/or bone or liver, lung, or brain.
- Limited or progressive and fatal. Younger children with multiple or severe organ involvement of "risk organs" (liver, lungs, spleen, hematopoietic system) have a high mortality.
- Usual clinical presentation is in first decade of life
- Pathophysiology unclear and treatment is nonspecific

ICD-9-CM Codes: 277.89 (Acute chronic, subacute); 202.3 (Malignant); 202.5 (Acute, progressive)

Etiology

- Unknown; suggested factors incl immune dysfunction, viral infections, and genetic predisposition
- Smoking associated with pulm LCH

Usual Treatment

- 10–20% spontaneous regression rate
- Chemotherapy with steroids for multisystem disease with local or constitutional symptoms (vinblastine, etoposide, mercaptopurine, doxorubicin, cyclophosphamide, methotrexate, others)
- Immunomodulatory agents (cyclosporine A, antithymocyte globulin, FK-506, others)
- Surgery required for biopsy and Dx, isolated bone lesions, and occasionally splenectomy
- Orthotopic liver or lung transplantation has been performed for end-stage disease
- Radiation therapy (bone lesions, pituitary disease)
- Bone marrow or stem cell transplant

ASSESSMENT POINTS

System	Effect	Assessment by Hx	PE	Test
HEENT	Soft tissue distortion of airway, loose teeth, mucosal ulceration		Airway and dental evaluation	
RESP	Spontaneous pneumothorax, reactive airways, infiltrates, fibrosis, pulm Htn	Tachypnea, dyspnea		CXR, ABGs, PFTs, CT with cysts or nodular infiltrate
GI	Ulceration, obstruction, hepatic dysfunction		Jaundice Hepatomegaly	Bilirubin, albumin AST, ALT INR
CNS	Diabetes insipidus, neuropathy, exophthalmos	Polyuria, polydipsia	Neuro exam	Urine and serum Osm, electrolytes
HEME	Thrombocytopenia, anemia, leukopenia	Bruising or bleeding	Splenomegaly	CBC

Key Reference: Broscheit J, Eichelbroenner O, Greim C, Bussen S. Anesthetic management of a patient with histiocytosis X and pulmonary complications during Caesarean section. *Eur J Anaesthesiol.* 2004;21(11):919–921.

Perioperative Implications

Monitoring
- Routine

Preinduction/Induction
- Airway soft tissue or mandibular involvement may distort anatomy.
- Cervical vertebrae lesions may cause cervical instability.
- Ensure adequate preoxygenation, esp. if there is significant pulm involvement.
- Usual precautions depending on severity of organ involvement

Maintenance
- For pts with DI consider aqueous ADH infusion, frequent sodium monitoring, and isotonic crystalloid fluids.
- Stress dose steroids if patient has had steroid therapy.
- Usual precautions depending on severity of organ involvement

Extubation
- Consider awake extubation if anatomy distorted and airway difficult
- Severe pulm involvement may delay extubation

Regional Anesthesia
- Follow ASRA precautions if thrombocytopenic or elevated INR

Postoperative Period
- May need continued stress dose steroid coverage for several days postop.
- Closely monitor oxygenation and ventilation when pulm disease present

Anticipated Problems/Concerns
- Organ dysfunction (hepatic, pulm, hematologic, hypothalamic, or bone)
- DI
- Adrenal suppression due to chronic steroid therapy. May have intraop hypotension without stress steroids.
- Severe pulm involvement may increase risk of pneumothorax and complicate extubation.

Hydrocephalus

Joseph R. Tobin
Timothy E. Smith

Risk

- Newborns and children with anatomic CNS abnormalities (incl myelomeningocele)
- Head trauma and intracranial hemorrhage (prematurity, SAH, other causes)
- CNS tumors
- Meningitis
- Recurrent VP shunt malfunction

Perioperative Risks

- Cerebral ischemia and neurologic sequelae
- Impaired airway reflexes, level of consciousness, gastric emptying
- Cardiorespiratory arrest

Worry About

- Intracranial Htn
- Persistent N/V
- Bradycardia
- Decreased level of consciousness

Overview

- Excess accumulation of CSF due to obstruction in normal CSF flow pattern from ventricular system to cortical surface (obstructive hydrocephalus); or from impaired reabsorption of CSF at arachnoid villi (communicating hydrocephalus)
- Slow progressive hydrocephalus well tolerated for weeks with slowly worsening symptoms (headache, nausea, papilledema)
- Acute hydrocephalus results in acute symptoms and may be life-threatening owing to herniation of brain with catastrophic ischemic injury; bradycardia, Htn, depressed level of consciousness, depressed airway reflexes and resp drive, and gastric atony

ICD-9-CM Codes: 331.4 (Obstructive); 331.3 (Communicating)

Etiology

- *Congenital:* Anatomic abnormalities: Aque-ductal stenosis, Arnold-Chiari malformation, Dandy-Walker syndrome

- *Posthemorrhagic/Post-traumatic:* Intraventricular hemorrhage (newborns or adults) with blood clot in ventricular system
- *Neoplastic:* Brain tumor obstructing nml CSF flow
- *Postinflammatory:* Meningitis, abscess, meningoencephalitis, intracranial hemorrhage

Usual Treatment

- Surgical correction of underlying cause or CSF diversion procedures (ventriculoperitoneal, ventriculoatrial, or lumboperitoneal shunts)
- Glucocorticoids are used acutely to diminish edema associated with neoplasm or abscess and may diminish associated intracranial Htn.
- Acetazolamide to diminish CSF production
- Furosemide to acutely decrease cerebrovascular volume
- Mannitol to decrease ICP

ASSESSMENT POINTS

System	Effect	Assessment by Hx	PE	Test
CARDIO	Bradycardia, Htn	Late signs	Pulse, BP	
RESP	Impaired resp drive and airway reflexes		Cranial nerve exam, stridor, swallowing abn	Pulse oximetry
GI	N/V, aspiration, abnormal feeding	Hx of progression of N/V		
CNS	Depressed level of consciousness, increased ICP, headache	Timing of onset	Arousability and neurologic exam tense fontanel, inferior eye deviation	CT scan

Key Reference: Hamid RK, Newfield P. Pediatric neuroanesthesia. Hydrocephalus. *Anesthesiol Clin North America.* 2001;19(2):207–218.

Perioperative Implications

Preoperative Preparation
- Assessment of urgency of presentation. Catastrophic increased ICP requires emergent intubation and hyperventilation. In young infants, direct neurosurgical needle puncture of a proximal lateral ventricle or previously inserted shunt may diminish ICP sufficiently to avoid a catastrophe.
- Secure IV access if possible

Monitoring
- Level of consciousness
- Routine

Airway
- Head up 10–20° and midline may diminish ICP
- Aspiration risk due to gastric atony

Preinduction/Induction
- Sedatives usually not indicated so that resp compromise or sedation does not increase ICP. Minimal sedation or use of local anesthetic to secure IV access without causing increased ICP due to pain, crying, or struggling.
- Rapid-sequence IV induction preferred (because of aspiration risk) unless in doubt of airway anatomy

- Debate over use of succinylcholine versus rapid-onset nondepolarizing muscle relaxant (rocuronium); thiopental, propofol; or etomidate IV agents preferred; avoid ketamine
- Mask induction may increase ICP by increasing cerebral blood volume. Once fontanelles are closed, the brain is limited to a closed space within the cranium; prior to that time (<18 mo) the brain has some room to expand. Sevoflurane may be the preferable agent for inhalation induction (well tolerated and minimal effects on cerebrovascular tone). Isoflurane and desflurane are associated with coughing and are not recommended for induction.
- Lidocaine 1–1.5 mg/kg IV may be useful adjunct to minimize increase in ICP due to laryngoscopy and endotracheal intubation.

Maintenance
- Volatile anesthetic (most commonly sevoflurane or isoflurane) <1 MAC, N_2O 0–70% (debatable), and opioid (i.e., fentanyl 2–5 µg/kg or equivalent)
- Maintain normothermia, cardiac output. Hyperventilation may be acutely helpful until CSF is diverted and ICP reduced.

- Normal saline at restricted or maintenance rate. Glucose support only for infants, and avoid hyperglycemia.

Extubation
- Ensure return of airway reflexes, level of consciousness, and resp drive.
- Failure of achieving above criteria may require CT scan and/or ICU monitoring.

Postoperative Period
- Usually unremarkable; depressed level of consciousness is concern for periop ischemic insult or hemorrhage.
- EBL: Minimal

Adjuvants
- Lidocaine, mannitol, furosemide, spontaneous hyperventilation by pt

Anticipated Problems/Concerns

- Immediate postop neurologic exam should demonstrate improvement. If not im-proved, urgent CT scan and secure airway must be maintained. Postop ICU admission not required unless impaired neurologic status continues.

Hyperaldosteronism (Secondary)

James Duke

Risk

- Cause of Htn in as many as 20% of hypertensive pts, however, the numerical risk of 2° Htn cannot be estimated.
- These are high renin states and the greater risks may be associated with the primary problem leading to hyperreninemia.
- May have severe Htn refractory to therapy.

Perioperative Risks

- Htn, possibly refractory to treatment
- The volume status of these pts is uncertain. Some have edematous states with decreased plasma volume and some may be frankly hypovolemic.

Worry About

- The primary problem that leads to increased renin (and hence, aldosterone) secretion
- Hypokalemia and associated muscle weakness
- Metabolic alkalosis
- Renal insufficiency
- Pts with CHF can have 2° aldosteronism, so impaired myocardial function may be a concern.

Overview

- As opposed to primary hyperaldosteronism, where increased aldosterone is 2° to (usually) adrenal adenoma or adrenal cortical hyperplasia, increased aldosterone is a result of increased renin secretion.

- In some situations, such as pregnancy and chronic renal disease, increased aldosterone is an adaptive response and is not necessarily deleterious.
- Renin is released from the juxtaglomerular apparatus (JGA) as a response to decreased arterial pressure. Osmoreceptors in the macula densa will also stimulate renin release in the presence of decreased sodium. Renin enzymatically alters angiotensinogen (renin substrate), forming angiotensin I. Actions of angiotensin converting enzyme produce angiotensin II (a potent vasoconstrictor) in the lung. Angiotensin stimulates release of aldosterone from the zona glomerulosa of the adrenal medulla.
- Aldosterone stimulates distal tubular resorption of Na^+ and H^+ and K^+ secretion.
- Dx is suggested by increases in both plasma renin (>2 ng/mL) and aldosterone but the ratio of serum aldosterone concentration to renin activity is <10 (ratio >20 suggests primary hyperaldosteronism). This may not apply if the pt is already on a mineralocorticoid receptor antagonist.

ICD-9-CM Code: 255.14

Etiology

- Renovascular (hyper-reninemic) hypertension: Related to atherosclerosis (renal artery stenosis) or fibromuscular dysplasia

- Malignant Htn
- Renin-secreting tumors (e.g., JGA tumors or renal cell carcinoma)
- Heart failure, cirrhosis, nephrotic syndrome (edema plus relative intravascular depletion)
- Pheochromocytoma
- Aortic coarctation
- Noted with the traid of resistant Htn, obesity, and sleep apnea but the cause of increased aldosterone may be related to substances released from fat cells as renin is not increased. Loss of wt results in improvement in BP.
- Pregnancy
- Estrogen administration

Usual Treatment

- Treatment of the primary cause though this may not totally correct hypertension
- Htn may be drug-resistant
- Assess volume status
- Spironolactone, a K^+-sparing diuretic, due to its mineralocorticoid antagonistic effects
- Eplerenone is a more selective though weaker mineralocorticoid receptor antagonist when compared with spironolactone, but with fewer anti-androgen and progesterone effects.
- Amiloride, a diuretic

ASSESSMENT POINTS

System	Effect	Assessment by Hx	PE	Test
CARDIO	Htn, often resistant to therapy; increased sympathetic activity, cardiac output often increased except where heart failure is an etiology. May have unexplained congestive failure.	Exercise tolerance, dyspnea, hypertension- headache	BP (compare R to L or arms with legs with coarctation) Third heart sound, rales	BP, ABG, CXR, ECG
HEME	Hypovolemia (or decreased plasma volume in edematous states) may result in hypotension, hypokalemia, metabolic acidosis	Postural hypotension, tachycardia, weakness	Orthostatic BP	Serum electrolytes, biocarbonate, ABGs
RENAL	Increased renal tubular sodium absorption Azotemia may be caused by decreased renal perfusion or ineffective plasma volume. In setting of renal artery stenosis, ACE inhibitors may also result in renal failure; Hypokalemia	Htn, chronic renal disease, weakness	Abdominal bruit suggests renal artery stenosis Edema	BUN, creatinine, electrolytes, ABG
LIVER	Cirrhosis is an edematous state and pt may have decreased effective blood volume, altered metabolism of medications, hypoalbuminemia, coagulation abn	Alcoholism, hepatitis, other liver disease	Ascites, liver may be small, spider angiomas	Liver functions, coagulation tests, serum albumin

Key Reference: Goodfriend TL, Calhoun DA. Resistant hypertension, obesity, sleep apnea and aldosterone: Theory and therapy. *Hypertension*. 2004;43:518–524.

Perioperative Implications

Preinduction/Induction/Maintenance

- Correct severe hypokalemia; this may require larger than usual supplementation. Assess and treat other electrolytes disturbances.
- Correction of Htn with mineralocorticoid antagonists, ACE inhibitors, angiotensin receptor blockers
- Assess volume status and cardiac function and determine choice of induction agents on this assessment.
- Largely dependent on primary medical problems that led to increased renin secretion

Monitoring

- Consider intra-arterial monitoring
- Central venous or pulm arterial monitoring should be predicated on assessments of intravascular volume and cardiac function.

- Urine output
- Neuromuscualar blockade

General Anesthesia

- Consider co-morbidities and their impact on the pt.
- Hypokalemia may potentiate muscle relaxants.

Regional Anesthesia

- Consider volume status.
- Direct acting sympathomimetics may exacerbate pre-existing Htn; titrate carefully to effect.

Postoperative Period

- Appropriate care predicated on surgical procedure, co-morbidities, hemodynamic stability
- Evaluate volume status, electrolytes, BP, myocardial function.
- If decreased liver function or renal function is the cause of 2° hyperaldosteronism, pt may have

altered metabolism and excretion of medications and prolonged effects.
- Consider appropriate postop monitoring if sleep apnea is a concern.

Anticipated Problems/Concerns

- Labile blood pressure
- Pts with severe, longstanding Htn are at increased risk for left ventricular hypertrophy, myocardial infarction and stroke.
- Where CHF is an etiology, decreasing cardiac output under general anesthesia may exacerbate failure.
- Increased sympathetic activity leads to activation of the renin-angiotensin system.
- Decreased renal perfusion is a concern, esp. with renovascualar Htn

Hypercalcemia

Karene Ricketts
M. Concetta Lupa

Risk

- Pts with hyperparathyroidism
- Pts with cancer: Breast cancer accounts for 25–50% of malignancy-related hypercalcemia. Other cancers associated with hypercalcemia incl lung cancer, squamous cell carcinomas of the head, neck, and esophagus, gynecological tumors, renal cell carcinoma, and multiple myeloma.

Perioperative Risks

- Pts with nml renal and CV function who have moderate hypercalcemia (11.5–13 mg/dL) have no special preop problems but may exhibit lethargy, anorexia, nausea, and polyuria.
- Severe hypercalcemia (>13 mg/dL) carries risk for:
  - Hypovolemia and acid-base abn; therefore, normal intravascular volume and electrolyte status should be restored prior to surgery
  - Neuromuscular symptoms with muscle weak-ness
  - Neurologic disturbances ranging from poor concentration to coma
  - CV effects incl Htn, dysrhythmias, heart block, cardiac arrest, and digitalis sensitivity
- Total serum Ca^{2+} >14 mg/dL is a medical emergency and requires immediate treatment and delay of elective surgical procedures.

Worry About

- Volume status (hypovolemia 2° to polyuria, fluid overload 2° to treatment)
- Electrolyte disturbances
- Dysrhythmias and/or ECG changes
- Organ system manifestations of hypercalcemia (see table) and underlying disease

- Longstanding hypercalcemia can lead to calcification in the myocardium, blood vessels, brain, and kidneys. Beware of seizures from cerebral calcifications. Polyuria that is unresponsive to vasopressin may result from renal calcifications.

Overview

- Total body Ca^{2+} is stored in bone (99%) and in the serum (1%)
- Total serum Ca^{2+} exists in 3 fractions: 50% protein-bound (mainly to albumin), 40–50% free or ionized (the physiologically active fraction), and 5–10% anion-bound (to phosphate or citrate).
- The normal range for total serum calcium is 8.6 to 10.4 mg/dL; the normal range for ionized calcium is 4.7 to 5.3 mg/dL. Hypercalcemia is defined as total serum Ca^{2+} >10.4 mg/dL.
- The total serum Ca^{2+} level should be corrected for serum albumin level: for every 1 mg/dL decrease in serum albumin, there is a 0.8 mg/dL increase in Ca^{2+}.
- Normal serum Ca^{2+} is regulated by several hormones:
  - Parathyroid hormone, which increases bone resorption and renal tubular resorption of
  - Calcium
  - Calcitonin which inhibits bone resorption
  - Vitamin D, which augments intestinal absorption of Ca^{2+}

ICD-9-CM Code: 275.4

Etiology

- Disorders with increased bone resorption of Ca^{2+}: 1° or 2° hyperparathyroidism (common cause), malignancy (common cause – solid tumors elicit a PTH-like hormone that stimulates osteoclastic activity), hyperthyroidism, and immobilization
- Disorders with increased Ca^{2+} absorption from the GI tract: Milk-alkali syndrome, vitamin D and A toxicity, and granulomatous diseases such as sarcoidosis
- Disorders with decreased renal Ca^{2+} excretion: Thiazide diuretics, lithium therapy, familial hypocalciuric hypercalcemia, and renal failure

Usual Treatment

- Initiated in pts with total serum Ca^{2+} >14 mg/dL or symptomatic pt with total serum Ca^{2+} <14 mg/dL
- Volume expansion with saline to correct fluid deficit (from polyuria) and to increase urinary excretion of Ca^{2+}
- Loop diuretics to increase urinary excretion of sodium and Ca^{2+}
- Discontinuation of offending drugs, dietary Ca^{2+} restriction, and increased physical activity
- Calcitonin, bisphosphonates, or mithramycin may be required in disorders associated with osteoclastic bone resorption
- Hydrocortisone may be used to reduce GI absorption of Ca^{2+} in granulomatous disease, vitamin D intoxication, lymphoma, and myeloma. Hydrocortisone is not helpful in pts with hypercalcemia due to hyperparathyroidism or other malignancies.
- Dialysis may be required for life-threatening hypercalcemia.
- Surgical removal of the parathyroid glands to treat 1° or 2° hyperparathyroidism
- Treat underlying cause

ASSESSMENT POINTS

System	Effect	Assessment by Hx	PE	Test
CARDIO	Hypovolemia Shortening of the Q-T interval, prolonged P-R intervals, wide QRS complexes, bradycardia Htn	Postural symptoms Palpitations, fatigue, poor exercise tolerance, dizziness, syncope Headache	Orthostatic vital signs, narrowed pulse pressure, tachycardia Auscultation, variable or slow heart rate Elevated BP	ECG
NEURO	Decreased concentration, confusion, fatigue, stupor and/or coma, seizure (rare)	Confusion Obtundation and/or coma	Mini-mental exam	EEG
RENAL	Polyuria; polydipsia; renal tubular acidosis; nephrogenic diabetes insipidus Nephrolithiasis; nephrocalcinosis Acute and chronic renal insufficiency	Increased frequency of urination, excessive thirst, lithium use, abdominal pain Low urine output	Signs of dehydration (dry mucous membranes, poor capillary refill, decreased skin turgor) Flank pain	Electrolytes, BUN, creatinine, urinalysis Abdominal X-ray or CT scan Electrolytes, BUN, creatinine
MS	Muscle weakness Lytic bone lesions Osteopenia and/or osteoporosis	Muscle weakness Bone pain	Decreased muscle strength and tone, depressed deep tendon reflexes Pain on palpation or limited ROM	X-ray (lytic lesions or pathologic Fx) Densitometry (DXA)
ENDO	Excess PTH or production of PTH-related hormone			Radioimmunoassay of PTH or PTH-related peptides
GI	Anorexia, nausea and/or vomiting, bowel hypomotility and constipation, pancreatitis PUD	Poor appetite, nausea and/or vomiting, constipation, abdominal pain GI bleeding	Abdominal pain	Abdominal X-ray or CT scan, colonoscopy, LFTs (amylase and lipase) EGD

Key Reference: Prough DS, et al. Acid-base, Fluids, and Electrolytes. In: Barash PG, Cullen BF, Stoelting RK, eds. *Clinical anesthesia.* 5th ed. Lippincott, 2006:200–201.

Perioperative Implications

Preinduction
- Acquire knowledge of and treat the underlying cause.
- Determine if the hypercalcemia is acute or chronic.
- Assess volume status: Hydrate to attain normal intravascular volume and to promote renal excretion of Ca^{2+}.
- Administer diuretics to increase urinary Ca^{2+} excretion if serum Ca^{2+} >14 mg/dL.
- Correct other electrolyte imbalances: Hypophosphatemia, hypokalemia, and hypomagnesemia

Induction
- No specific anesthetic drug or technique has advantages in a pt with hypercalcemia however hemodynamic instability may occur if standard dosing is used in a hypovolemic pt.

Monitoring
- Standard ASA monitors
- Volume status (urine output and fluid administration); depending on the severity of hypercalcemia, underlying cause, the pt's CV status, and type of surgery, additional monitors of volume status (CVP or TEE) should be considered.
- Electrolytes (whether sampled via venous or arterial access)
- ECG to monitor for shortened Q-T interval, S-T changes, decreased T wave amplitude or T wave inversion
- BP to monitor for Htn (approx one third of hypercalcemic pts have Htn that usually resolves with treatment of the 1° disease)

General Anesthesia/Maintenance
- Routine maintenance tailored to the co-morbidities of the pt and the surgical needs
- Continued hydration and electrolyte replenishment to attain normal intravascular and acid-base status
- Hypercalcemia may be associated with decreased sensitivity to muscle relaxants and thus a shortened time course of neuromuscular blockade; however, associated electrolyte disturbances or renal insufficiency may prolong neuromuscular blockade.
- Careful positioning of the anesthetized pt is important because osteopenia/lytic bone lesions predispose these pts to pathologic bone fractures
- If the pt is mechanically ventilated, avoid resp alkalosis because alkalosis lowers plasma K^+, which would leave hypercalcemia unopposed.

Regional Anesthesia
- General anesthesia is most commonly used for parathyroid surgery; however, a cervical plexus block or local anesthesia with hypnosis has also been used.

Postoperative Period
- Continue to monitor the same intraop parameters
- After parathyroid surgery, monitor for bleeding, recurrent laryngeal nerve injury or hypocalcemia (2° to profound decrease in PTH).

Anticipated Problems/Concerns
- Fluid and electrolyte disturbances: Beware that Mg^{2+}, phosphate, and K^+ levels may be altered with treatment of hypercalcemia.
- ECG changes
- Neurologic impairment: Altered mental status may impair ability to protect airway
- When hypercalcemia is severe, do not hesitate to consult a specialist (endocrinologist, nephrologist, or cardiologist) and postpone surgery if possible.

Hypercholesterolemia

Dilipkumar K. Patel
Swapnil Khoche

Risk

- Incidence in USA: 102.2 million Americans age 20 and older have total cholesterol levels of 200 mg/dL or higher
- Risk factors: Male age >45 y, women age >55 y, family Hx of premature CAD, current cigarette smoking, DM, obesity, Htn, CAD, HDL level <40 mg/dL
- The LDL-C level of 130 to 159 mg/dL is considered borderline high, level of 160 to 189 mg/dL is classified as high, and level of ≥190 mg/dL is considered very high risk
- An HDL (good) cholesterol level below 40 mg/dL in adult is considered low and is a risk factor for CHD and stroke.
- A triglyceride level >150 mg/dL in adults is considered elevated and is a risk factor for CHD and stroke.
- Familial hypercholesterolemia, an autosomal dominant trait (LDL >260 mg/dL), risk for premature CHD
- Familial combined hyperlipoproteinemia elevated LDL and/or VLDL, increase risk of coronary disease.

Perioperative Risks

- Risk of acute coronary syndrome, myocardial ischemia and infarction
- Cardiac events, worsened CHF
- Stroke or death

Worry About

- New-onset angina or increasing frequency or severity of angina
- Worsening or new-onset CHF
- TIAs or stroke of the CNS
- Peripheral atherosclerosis, acute pancreatitis

Overview

- The mean level of LDL (bad) cholesterol for American adults ≥20 y is 115.0 mg/dL
- Normal total cholesterol < 200 mg/dL, borderline high 200–239 mg/dL, high ≥ 40 mg/dL
- Suggested treatment goals in high-risk pts with CHD or CHD risk equivalents is an LDL level <100 mg/dL, 2 or more risk factor LDL level <130 mg/dL, 0-1 risk factor LDL level <160 mg/dL along with triglyceride <120 mg/dL and HDL >45 mg/dL
- Intensive reduction of LDL-C to <70 mg/dL and ApoB <80 mg/dL is reasonable in highest risk pts.
- HDL ≥60 mg/dL is high and is considered protective
- Periop statins use is not assoc with rhabdomyolysis or myopathy
- Preop treatment with statins is assoc with improvement in early clinical outcome in pts undergoing cardiac surgery.

ICD-9-CM Code: 272.0

Etiology

- Can be 1° or 2° to systemic illness such as diabetes, nephrotic syndrome, chronic renal failure, hypothyroidism, or drugs that increase LDL such as anabolic steroids

Usual Treatment

- Life style modification: Dietary, physical exercise, and wt control
- Cholesterol and lipid statistics checked every year in high-risk pts
- HMG CoA reductase inhibitors (rosuvastatin, lovastatin, pravastatin, simvastatin, atorvastatin) are the drug of choice in most of the pts with hypercholesterolemia as they reduce LDL level effectively
- High-risk pts with high triglyceride or low HDL level— consideration can be given to combine a fibrate or nicotinic acid with an LDL lowering drug.
- Gemfibrozil or nicotinic acid may be better choice in pts with significant hypertriglyceridemia
- The combination treatment with reductase inhibitor and cholesterol absorption inhibitor (ezetimibe) highly synergistic in treating 1° hypercholesterolemia

ASSESSMENT POINTS

System	Effect	Assessment by Hx	PE	Test
CARDIO	Myocardial ischemia and infarction LV dysfunction	Angina or its equivalents Dyspnea, edema, exercise intolerance	Displaced PMI S_3	ECG, CXR, stress testing, ECHO, coronary angio
RESP	CHF	Dyspnea, orthopnea, cough	Rales and rhonchi	CXR
DERM	Lipid deposits		Xanthelasma, xanthoma, arcus juvenilis	
RENAL	Impaired renal perfusion	Nighttime urinary frequency		Cr
CNS	Cerebrovascular atherosclerosis	TIAs	Carotid bruit	Carotid US and angio

Key Reference: Brunzell JD. Lipoprotein management in patients with cardiometabolic risk: *J Am Coll Cardiol.* 2008;51(15):1512.

Perioperative Implications

Preoperative Preparation
- Assess for CAD, DM, and PVD
- Pts currently on statins and undergoing noncardiac surgery, statins should be continued
- Pts undergoing vascular surgery with or without clinical risk factors, initiation of statins should be considered
- Assessment for statin related myopathy and liver damage
- Assess and screen for obesity, related OSA and metabolic syndrome

Monitoring
- Consider appropriate invasive monitoring in presence of large fluid shifts, ischemic Hx, and high-risk surgery

- ST–T measurement or mapping in pts with CHD or risk factor for CHD

Airway
- May be overweight and difficult to intubate or ventilate

Induction
- Hypovolemia may lead to hypotension
- Aggressive treatment for tachycardia, Htn, or hypotension during induction

Maintenance
- Maintain hemodynamic stability without hypothermia or anemia (ideal Hct may be >27%)
- No anesthetic agent or technique proven superior
- Monitor for ischemia and CHF

Extubation
- For noncardiac surgery, this is the period of greatest risk for ischemia

Postoperative Period
- High incidence of tachycardia, ischemia, and MI for several days after noncardiac surgery
- Treat pain, unstable hemodynamic and biochemical abn aggressively

Adjuvants
- Depends on end-organ disease

Anticipated Problems/Concerns
- Problems are related to atherosclerosis in multiple organs incl heart, kidneys, and brain

Hyperglycemia

William L. Lanier

Risk

- Incidence in USA: Can occur in virtually any anesthetized or critically ill pt
- Race with the highest prevalence: None

Perioperative Risks

- Increased likelihood of neurologic injury following brain ischemia, and perhaps traumatic brain injury and spinal cord injury
- Dehydration resulting from osmotic diuresis
- Increased infection rate
- Diminished wound healing

Worry About

- Electrolyte abn, particularly hypo-kalemia, while treating hyperglycemia
- Hypoglycemia following insulin, resulting in insult to the CV system and CNS

- Polyuria complicates assessment of fluid balance

Overview

- Is not a disease
- Typically produces adverse effects by three mechanisms: Increases in plasma osmolality, increases in postischemic tissue lactic acidosis, and inhibition of white blood cell function
- Dx made by measuring blood glucose concentrations
- In acute setting, blood glucose concentrations can be estimated using indicator-impregnated strips or other point-of-care methods; confirmation can be made by mechanized techniques in a reference laboratory.

ICD-9-CM Code: 790.6

Etiology

- Results from DM (both insulin-requiring and non-insulin–requiring), other endocrinopathies (Cushing's syndrome, acromegaly, obesity, pheochromocytoma), physiologic stress, drug administration (particularly corticosteroids), and glucose-containing fluid infusions

Usual Treatment

- Insulin
- Isotonic IV crystalloid solutions to treat hypovolemia and dilute existing blood glucose
- If possible, treat underlying cause (e.g., D/C infusion of glucose-containing solutions, D/C corticosteroids, reduce physiologic stress to pt)

ASSESSMENT POINTS

System	Effect	Assessment by Hx	PE	Test
HEENT	Dehydration in extreme cases		Dry mucosa in extreme cases	
CARDIO	Mild positive inotropic effect with mild hyperglycemia Dehydration		Tachycardia, orthostatic hypotension	
GI		Polydipsia in extreme cases		
RENAL	Osmotically induced diuresis	Polyuria, urinary frequency		Elevated urine glucose
ENDO		See under Etiology		Elevated blood glucose
HEME	Diminished WBC activity; changes in serum sodium concentrations			Serum sodium concentration decreases 1.6 mEq/L for each 100 mg/dL increase in glucose concentration
CNS			Altered consciousness, neurologic deficits	Plasma osmolality

Key Reference: Pasternak JJ, McGregor DG, Schoreder DR, et al. IHAST Investigators. Hyperglycemia in patients undergoing cerebral aneurysm surgery: Its association with long term gross neurologic and neuropsychological function. *Mayo Clin Proc.* 2008; 83(4), 406–417.

Perioperative Implications

Preoperative Preparation
- Glucose reduction with insulin
- Hydration
- Normalization of lytes

Monitoring
- Blood glucose concentrations in all cases
- In severe cases, blood lytes, blood osmolality, UO

Airway
- Abn typically related to DM (reduced range of motion and abn atlanto-occipital contractions), acromegaly (distorted anatomy), or chronic corticosteroid use or Cushing's syndrome (cushingoid Sx, friable tissues)

Maintenance
- Maintain hydration
- Insulin therapy
- K+ replacement

Extubation
- No special considerations, other than those related to underlying disease

Adjuvants
- Limit attempted reduction of blood glucose concentration to ~75 mg/dL/hr to avoid problems with osmotic injury to brain and lyte disturbances.
- Monitor ECG during correction of profound hyperglycemia.

Postoperative Period
- Variations in physiologic stress, fluid administration, and drug usage make postop blood glucose concentrations difficult to predict and control.

Anticipated Problems/Concerns
- Increases in blood glucose concentrations by a mere 40 mg/dL may worsen outcome following cerebral ischemic insult. Hyperglycemia may also harm wound healing, increase infection rates, and worsen outcomes after myocardial infarction. In contrast, hypoglycemia resulting from excessive use of insulin may result in pt morbidity and mortality from neurologic and other causes, independent of ischemic events.

Hyperkalemia

Suzanne Strom

Risk

- Any pt with plasma K⁺ concentration >5.5 mEq/L

Perioperative Risks

- Muscle weakness and paralysis
- Cardiac conduction system abn
- CV collapse
  a) Peaked T waves (6 to 7 mEq/L)
  b) ST depression
  c) Prolonged P-R interval and widened QRS (10 to 12 mEq/L)
  d) Ventricular fibrillation or asystole

Worry About

- Adverse effects are likely to accompany acute increases in K⁺; chronic increases are better tolerated
- Depolarizing muscle relaxants, esp. if given to pts with burns, spinal cord transection, catatonia with immobility, or muscle trauma
- Digitalis toxicity
- Acidosis

Overview

- Condition that can be due to ↑ total body K⁺ content or alterations in distribution between intracellular and extracellular sites

ICD-9-CM Code: 276.7

Etiology

- Diminished renal excretion
- Acute oliguric renal failure
- Chronic renal failure
- Addison disease
- Hyporeninemic hypoaldosteronism
- Drugs: Potassium-sparing diuretics, nonsteroidal anti-inflammatory drugs, heparin, ACE inhibitors, angiotensin-receptor antagonists, K⁺-containing antibiotics
- Ingestion of K⁺-rich foods, salt substitutes in pt with renal insufficiency
- Transcellular shifts
- Acidosis—resp or metabolic
- Cell destruction—trauma, burns, rhabdomyolysis, hemolysis, tumor lysis, reperfusion of ischemic limb or organ
- Hyperkalemic periodic paralysis
- Diabetic hyperglycemia

- Depolarizing muscle relaxant causing K⁺ release esp. in pts with burns, spinal cord transection, catatonia with immobility, muscle trauma, or denervating muscle
- Massive transfusion, particularly with irradiated blood
- Factitious hyperkalemia
- Tourniquet method of drawing blood
- Hemolysis of drawn blood due to delay in chemical determination

Usual Treatment

- Promote transfer of K⁺ from ECF to ICF
- Glucose and insulin: 25–50 gm glucose with 10–20 units regular insulin/70 kg
- Sodium bicarbonate: 50–100 mEq/70 kg
- Hyperventilation: With each pH change of 0.1, there is an inverse change in K⁺ of 0.5 mEq/L (goal $PaCO_2$ 25–30 mmHg)
- Enhance K⁺ elimination: Diuretics, exchange resins (Kayexalate), dialysis
- Antagonism of cardiac effects: Ca^{2+} gluconate—10–30 mL of a 10% solution over 10–20 min/70 kg counteracts cardiac effects

ASSESSMENT POINTS

System	Effect	Assessment by Hx	PE	Test
CARDIO	Tall peak T waves ↓ Amplitude R wave Widened QRS complex Decreased and eventual disappearance of P wave QRS blends into T wave—"sine wave of hyperkalemia"			ECG
	Ventricular arrhythmia	Possible hemodynamic instability		ECG
	Cardiac arrest	CV collapse		ECG
NM	Weakness Paralysis			
ENDO	↑ Aldosterone Insulin release ↑ Glucagon Epinephrine release	↑ BP, HR		K⁺, renin, aldosterone, glucose

Key Reference: Cooper RC, Baumann PL, McDonald WM. An unexpected hyperkalemic response to succinylcholine during electroconvulsive therapy for catatonic schizophrenia. *Anesthesiology.* 1999;91:574–575.

Perioperative Implications

Preoperative Preparation
- Normal K⁺ levels before elective surgery
- Avoid sedatives (↓ ventilation) prior to K⁺ normalization

Monitoring
- ECG
- Plasma K⁺ levels
- ABG concentration
- Peripheral nerve stimulator

Maintenance
- Adequate ventilation to avoid respiratory acidosis
- Avoid metabolic acidosis: Arterial hypoxemia or excessive depths of anesthesia
- IV fluids: Avoid lactated Ringer's or others containing K⁺

Adjuvants
- Muscle relaxants: Avoid depolarizing agents; increase K⁺ 0.3–0.5 mEq/L with succinylcholine
- Dose of nondepolarizing relaxants required is unclear—may need diminished dose

Anticipated Problems/Concerns

- Acute increases in K⁺ leading to acute ECG changes or adverse cardiac effects. Rx: see Usual Treatment.
- Avoid use of depolarizing muscle relaxants in pts with burns, neuropathies, para- or quadriplegia, muscle trauma, or catatonia with immobility

Hypermagnesemia

David R. Gambling

Risk

- Pts with renal insufficiency, esp. those receiving Mg^{2+}-containing cathartics or antacids
- Parturients on $MgSO_4$ therapy
- "Runaway" infusion of Mg^{2+} during transportation to the OR can cause acute, life-threatening hypermagnesemia. Risk of developing very high serum Mg^{2+} levels in such cases can be reduced by always using a small volume Buretrol device in pts receiving IV Mg^{2+} therapy.

Therapeutic Uses

- Treatment of pre-eclampsia, eclampsia, and preterm labor
- Recent evidence indicates that Mg^{2+} therapy reduces the risk of cerebral palsy in women at risk of preterm delivery
- Treatment of ventricular dysrhythmias
- Treatment of severe asthma in pts who have not responded to initial therapy
- Treatment of migraine
- Lowers risk of metabolic syndrome

Perioperative Risks

- Potentiates nondepolarizing neuromuscular blocking agents
- May increase risk of modest hypotension during administration of regional anesthesia
- Potentiates hypotension associated with use of volatile anesthetics, Ca^{2+}-channel blockers, and butyrophenones
- Can exacerbate local anesthetic toxicity

- Hypermagnesemia may be associated with increased in bleeding time and TEG changes, although no clinically significant coagulopathies have been attributed to Mg^{2+}.

Worry About

- Intraoperative hypotension
- Muscle weakness (esp. resp)
- Excessive sedation
- Myocardial depression and cardiorespiratory arrest with very high levels

Overview

- Defined as an elevated Mg^{2+} concentration in plasma, in excess of 1.1 mmol/L
- Equivalent Mg^{2+} concentrations in the three unit systems in common use: mg/dL, mEq/L, mmol/L
  - Normal serum level 1.8–2.4 mg/dL, 1.5–2.0 mEq/L, 0.75–1.0 mmol/L
  - Therapeutic level 4.8–8.4 mg/dL, 4–7 mEq/L, 2–3.5 mmol/L
  - Neuromuscular toxic level >12 mg/dL, >10 mEq/L, >5 mmol/L
- Mg^{2+} elimination is dependent on GFR; with GFR <30 mL/min, pts are at significant risk
- Sx vary with plasma concentration and become more serious as the plasma concentration increases >4 mmol/L
- CV, resp, MS systems are predominantly affected
  - Pts with chronic renal failure frequently have Mg^{2+} levels up to 3 mmol/L but are seldom symptomatic.

- Acidemia will decrease serum level at which side effects occur; e.g., in presence of acidemia, cardiac arrest can occur at a serum level of 8–10 mmol/L.

ICD-9-CM Code: 275.2

Etiology

- Pts with chronic renal failure who are receiving Mg^{2+}-containing antacids or laxatives
- Often iatrogenic, e.g., excessive administration of $MgSO_4$ infusion to parturient pt with preterm labor or pregnancy-induced Htn
- Rarely Addison disease, myxedema, or lithium therapy

Usual Treatment

- D/C Mg^{2+} therapy and delay nonessential surgery
- Fluid load and diuretic therapy
- Adults: IV calcium gluconate 1 gm (temporary but effective).
- Neonates: IV calcium gluconate 100–200 mg/kg over 5 min and continuous infusion 100–300 mg/kg/d
- Peritoneal dialysis or hemodialysis for persistent or life-threatening hypermagnesemia
- Assist ventilation/protect airway if necessary

ASSESSMENT POINTS

The side effects of hypermagnesemia are more serious as the serum level of magnesium increases.

System	Signs and Symptoms	Serum Mg^{2+} Concentration
GENERAL	Normal	0.7–1.1 mmol/L (normal range)
CARDIO	Warmth, flushing, headache, nausea, dizziness	2–3 mmol/L (range during parenteral treatment)
	Decreased AV and intraventricular conduction	>2.5 mmol/L
	ECG—prolonged PQ and widening of QRS	
	Possible hypotension	
	Cardiac arrest in diastole*	>12.5 mmol/L
CNS	Sedation	2–3 mmol/L
MS	Absent deep tendon reflexes	4–5 mmol/L
	Progressive muscle weakness and resp arrest	6–7.5 mmol/L

*The ability of this degree of hypermagnesemia to cause cardiac arrest is uncertain if ventilatory support and normal acid-base balance are maintained.
Key Reference: Guerrera MP, Volpe SL, Mao JJ. Therapeutic uses of magnesium. *Am Fam Physician*. 2009;80:157–162.

Perioperative Implications

Preoperative Preparation
- D/C $MgSO_4$ unless being used to treat seizures or ventricular dysrhythmias
- Check serum level
- ECG, creatinine, electrolytes

Monitoring
- Routine

Airway
- Use full dose of succinylcholine for intubation
- Reduce dose of non-depolarizing NMBs by one third to one half

Preinduction/Induction
- Avoid sedative premedications
- Ensure full denitrogenation of lungs
- Avoid pre-curarization or priming dose of NMB

Maintenance
- May decrease requirement for anesthetics owing to decreased neurotransmitter release

Extubation
- Ensure full return of train-of-four, ability to sustain head lift and vital capacity >10 mL/kg
- Ensure pt responsiveness

Adjuvants
- Hypermagnesemia may exacerbate hypotension associated with hypovolemia, Ca^{2+}-channel blockers, volatile inhalation anesthetics, butyrophenones, lumbar epidural, or subarachnoid anesthesia
- Treat with IV calcium gluconate 1 gm and fluid load and diuretics

Postoperative Period
- Beware of excessive sedation, weakness, hypoventilation, cardiac arrest

- May cause or aggravate neonatal hypotonia and hypotension
- May reduce postop analgesic requirements by antagonism of N-methyl-D-aspartate

Anticipated Problems/Concerns
- Hypermagnesemia potentiates action of nondepolarizing NMBs by inhibiting release of acetylcholine from motor nerve terminal, decreasing sensitivity of postjunctional membrane, and reducing excitability of muscle fibers
- Many common anesthetic drugs exacerbate weakness and sedation associated with hypermagnesemia
- Potentiates local anesthetic toxicity
- Excessively high plasma Mg^{2+} concentrations can cause cardiorespiratory arrest

Hypernatremia

Samir Patel
James M. Hunter, Jr.

Risk

• Older age, infants, prior brain injury, DM, surgery, diuretic therapy, altered mental status; insufficient water intake, DI, hypertonic sodium solution (incl sodium bicarbonate), hyperalimentation, hyperaldosteronism, Cushing syndrome, hypothalamic injury

Perioperative Risks

• Increased incidence of morbidity and mortality, seizures, coma, cerebral bleeding, subarachnoid hemorrhage

Worry About

• Increased risk of hospital death, residual and/or permanent neurologic disability
• If Na^+ corrected too rapidly, cerebral edema, seizures, and death

Overview

• Hypernatremia is a relative deficit of body H_2O in relation to body sodium content
• Serum Na^+ is preserved within a fine physiologic range (138–142 mEq/L).
• Sodium metabolism is regulated by the kidney through the interaction of the renin-angiotensin-aldosterone system, sympathetic nervous system, atrial natriuretic peptide, brain natriuretic peptide, effective circulating volume, and serum H_2O content. H_2O metabolism is tightly regulated by arginine vasopressin.
• Most commonly found in pts with impaired sense of thirst (brain injury, altered mental status), lack of access to H_2O, diuretic therapy, and severe GI losses of H_2O.

Etiology

• Lack of access to H_2O
• Impaired thirst mechanism
• DI (central and nephrogenic)
• Osmotic diuresis (mannitol, glucose); diuretics (furosemide, thiazides)
• Insensible losses from the dermal or resp systems
• GI losses from diarrhea or osmotic cathartics (lactulose, sorbitol), vomiting, or nasogastric suctioning
• Seizures or severe exercise (transient intracellular shift of H_2O)
• Excess sodium administration; hyperalimentation
• Hyperaldosteronism and Cushing syndrome

Usual Treatment

• H_2O replacement (see below); central DI can be treated with desmopressin (5–20 mcg intranasal once or twice per day), nephrogenic DI can be treated with thiazide diuretics.
• Free H_2O deficit = total body water X [(serum Na^+/140)-1]
• Total body water is approx 0.6 and 0.5 × the lean body weight for men and women, respectively. Replace ½ of the free H_2O deficit over the first 24 hr as an initial starting point. Note that the free H_2O deficit does not take into account ongoing losses, so ultimately the rate of H_2O replacement must be guided by serial measurements of serum Na^+
• Rate of correction of Na^+ to level of 145 mmol/L.
• If hypernatremia developed acutely, Na^+ can be corrected rapidly (1 mmol/L per hr, with a limit of 12 mmol/L per 24 hrs)
• If hypernatremia developed slowly, Na^+ can be corrected at a maximum rate of 0.5 mmol/L per hr (or in the case of life-threatening complications, at 1 mmol/L/hr with a limit of 12 mmol/L per 24 hrs)
• Measurement of Na^+ at least every 4–6 hr and adjustment of the rate of H_2O replacement is important to ensure safe and expeditious correction of Na^+.

ASSESSMENT POINTS

System	Effect	Assessment by Hx	PE	Test
HEENT	Dry mouth/mucous membranes		Mouth exam	
CARDIO	Tachycardia/hypotension	Orthostatic changes	HR/BP	ECG
CNS	Restlessness, irritability, lethargy, seizures, coma		CNS exam	EEG
GI	NVD			
Renal	Polyuria	Urinary frequency/color		Serum and urine Na^+, K^+, osmolarity

Key Reference: Bagshaw SM, Townsend DR, McDermid RC. Disorders of sodium and water balance in hospitalized patients. *Can J Anaesth*. 2009;56:151–167.

Perioperative Implications

Preoperative Preparation
• Correct electrolytes, replace H_2O deficit, assess neurologic status.
• Consider delaying elective surgery until serum Na^+ is normal. If surgery cannot be delayed, care must be taken to avoid rapid correction of Na^+.

Monitoring
• Electrolytes

Airway
• None

Maintenance
• Restore circulatory volume
• Maintain uo
• Correct electrolytes

Extubation
• Assess neurologic status to determine whether the pt is a candidate for extubation.
• Possible muscular weakness

Adjuvants
• In central DI, vasopressin 5 units IVP will dramatically reduce UOP for 1–2 hr, making it possible to catch up on IV fluids.

• Caution must be used to avoid too-rapid correction of Na^+.

Postoperative period
• Assess for lethargy, irritability, muscular weakness, confusion.
• Monitor serum Na^+.

Anticipated Problems/Concerns

• Too rapid correction and resultant neurologic effects

Hyperglycemic Hyperosmolar State (HHS)

Jesse M. Raiten

Risk

- Elderly pts with DM, usually type II
- Debilitated pts who cannot care for themselves
- Chronically ill diabetic pts who experience exacerbation of an underlying co-morbidity
- Incidence increased in African Americans, Hispanics, Native Americans

Perioperative Risks

- Severe hypovolemia and hemodynamic instability
- Presence of diffuse organ system damage from poor glycemic control
- Altered mental status and increased risk of pulmon aspiration
- Periop stress causing further elevations in serum glucose

Worry About

- Cause of hyperglycemic hyperosmolar state
- Volume status and potential hemodynamic instability
- Electrolyte and acid-base abn increase the risk of cardiac arrhythmias

Overview

- Serious metabolic condition characterized by hyperglycemia, hyperosmolarity, and dehydration
- Is one of several potentially fatal states associated with poorly controlled DM
- Requires aggressive treatment and close electrolyte and hemodynamic monitoring

ICD9-CM: 250.2 (Hyperosmolar [nonketotic] coma)

Etiology

- Inadequate insulin production and increased counter-regulatory hormone production (catecholamines, glucagon, cortisol) in the setting of an acute insult leads to severe hyperglycemia, dehydration and electrolyte abn
- Triggering event may be infection, dehydration, CVA, inadequate dosing of insulin, silent myocardial infarction, pancreatitis, or drug ingestion (drugs that affect carbohydrate metabolism)

Usual Treatment

- Aggressive volume resuscitation with isotonic fluids to re-establish end-organ perfusion
- Insulin replacement and correction of electrolyte abn (start dextrose-containing fluids when serum glucose approaches 250 mg/dL to help prevent hypoglycemia and cerebral edema)
- Identify and treat underlying cause of hyperglycemic state
- Frequent evaluation of volume resuscitation and metabolic status in an ICU setting

ASSESSMENT POINTS

System	Effect	Assessment by Hx	PE	Test
NEURO	Altered mental status, obtundation, coma, seizures	Progression of mental status changes over days	Mental status exam, airway reflexes	Head CT, CSF culture
CARDIAC	Hypovolemia and shock	Polyuria progressing to anuria, sense of thirst, headaches, dry mouth	Orthostatic hypotension, tachycardia, dry mucous membranes	CVP, PAP, ECHO
PULM	Hyperventilation if severe metabolic acidosis, hypoventilation if brainstem malperfusion		Resp rate and pattern of ventilation	ABG
ENDO	Insulinopenia, hyperglycemia, hyperosmolarity	DM, recent infection or stress		Serum glucose and osmolarity
RENAL	Polyuria progressing to anuria, metabolic acidosis, electrolyte abnormalities			BUN and creatinine, FENa, UO, ABG, electrolytes

Key Reference: Kitabchi AE, Nyenwe EA. Hyperglycemic crises in diabetes mellitus: Diabetic ketoacidosis and hyperglycemic hyperosmolar state. *Endocrinol Metab Clin N Am.* 2006;35:725–751.

Perioperative Implications

Monitoring and Intravenous Access

- Large bore IV access for volume resuscitation, particularly before induction
- Invasive monitoring incl arterial line and CVP may be useful to guide volume replacement and allow for frequent glucose and electrolyte sampling.

Induction

- Aggressive volume resuscitation before induction
- Rapid sequence induction if altered mental status and concern for aspiration
- Limited use of succinylcholine if metabolic acidosis and hyperkalemia are present

- Be prepared for exaggerated hemodynamic changes with induction despite adequate volume resuscitation.
- Smaller doses than usual of induction agent if pt is obtunded

Maintenance

- Closely follow serum glucose, electrolytes, acid-base status.
- Continue volume resuscitation until UO is adequate and hemodynamics have stabilized.

Emergence

- Assessment of airway reflexes and ability to protect airway before tracheal extubation

- Ensure metabolic and electrolyte status is corrected, and pt meets the usual criteria for extubation.

Postoperative Period

- Continued insulin therapy and observation for worsening hyperglycemia due to surgical stress response

Anticipated Problems/Concerns

- Co-morbidities and diffuse end-organ damage increase morbidity and mortality of pts with HHS, particularly periop

Hyperparathyroidism

Michael L. Nahrwold
Daniel A. Nahrwold

Risk

- Incidence in USA: 100,000 pts per year
- Race with highest prevalence: None
- M:F: ratio: 1:2
- Prevalence: 50–100/100,000 (increases with age)
- 0.8% in pregnancy

Perioperative Risks

- Hypovolemia and lyte abn
- Increased risk of cardiac dysrhythmias 2° to hypercalcemia
- Aspiration from full stomach
- Postop hypocalcemia

Worry About

- Signs of hypercalcemia and other lyte irregularities
- Intravascular volume changes
- Fluid overload and Na^+ retention in CV fragile pts
- Renal, cardiac, skeletal, and CNS abnormalities
- Pancreatitis 2° to hypercalcemia

Overview

- Endocrinopathy assoc with elevation in PTH levels
- Primary problem is hypercalcemia
- Dx supported by increased PTH level assoc with hypercalcemia
- Most pts with primary hyperparathyroidism are hypercalcemic but asymptomatic
- Hyperparathyroidism in pregnancy is assoc with high (50%) maternal and fetal morbidity and can lead to neonatal hypocalcemia and tetany

ICD-9-CM Code: 252.0

Etiology

- Primary hyperparathyroidism usually due to benign parathyroid adenoma (80–90%), hyperplasia (15%), or parathyroid carcinoma (uncommon)
- May be manifestation of multiple endocrine neoplasia Type 1 or 2a
- 2° hyperparathyroidism may be seen in pts with chronic renal disease

Usual Treatment

- Surgically with parathyroidectomy
- Recent advances such as nuclear imaging for correct localization of parathyroid tumors, quick hormone assays, and radiologically-guided or video-assisted surgical techniques are allowing minimally invasive parathyroidectomy under local/regional anesthesia
- Medically with saline hydration, furosemide, and phosphate repletion in emergency situations to restore serum Ca^{2+} to a safe level (<14 mg/dL)
- Other Ca^{2+} lowering modalities such as calcitonin, cinacalcet, bisphosphonates (inhibit bone resorption), mithramycin (for more resistant hypercalcemia; toxic effects limit use), glucocorticoids, or hemodialysis
- Pregnant women with primary hyperparathyroidism should be treated with parathyroidectomy ideally in the second trimester

ASSESSMENT POINTS

System	Effect	Assessment by Hx	PE	Test
CARDIO	Htn, dysrhythmias	Palpitation, headache	Abn pulse rate and/or rhythm, ↑ BP	ECG, lytes, total and ionized Ca^{2+}, QT_c * interval
RESP	↓ Bronchial clearance of secretions	Cough	Adventitious sounds	
GI	Peptic ulcers, pancreatitis	Constipation, anorexia, N/V, epigastric pain		
RENAL	Nephrocalcinosis, nephrolithiasis → renal dysfunction	Polyuria, polydipsia, hematuria		BUN, Cr
CNS	EEG abn, seizures	Depression, personality change, psychomotor retardation, memory impairment	Psychosis, disorientation, obtundation, coma	
MS	Hyporeflexia, osteopenia, osteitis fibrosa cystica	Weakness, bone pain	Muscular atrophy, arthritis, pathologic fractures	

* $QT_c = \dfrac{QT}{\sqrt{R-R}}$; R-R = R-R interval.

Key Reference: Fraser WD. Hyperparathyroidism. *Lancet.* 2009;374:145–158.

Perioperative Implications

Preoperative Preparation

- Assess total and ionized Ca^{2+} levels.
- Reduce serum total calcium to <14 mg/dL.
- No intervention for Ca^{2+} level ≤12 mg/dL
- For higher Ca^{2+} levels use saline hydration, furosemide (rapid action), phosphate repletion, and consider calcitonin (acts in 1–2 hr), mithramycin (acts in 6–12 hr), cinacalcet, bisphosphonates, glucocorticoids, or hemodialysis
- Consider H_2-receptor antagonists, nonparticulate antacids, and metoclopramide

Monitoring

- Routine; pay attention to changes in QT_c interval (QT_c by itself poorly correlated with ionized Ca^{2+}, but changes correlate)

Airway

Possibility of pathologic fractures requires careful positioning for laryngoscopy

Preinduction/Induction

- No preferred agents or techniques
- Avoid ketamine in pts with psychosis due to hypercalcemia.
- Hypovolemia can lead to hemodynamic instability if usual dose of induction agents is given.
- Minimally invasive procedures can be performed using local/regional anesthesia.

Maintenance

- No preferred agents or techniques. Possibility of pathologic fractures requires careful positioning and padding of pressure points.

Extubation

- Airway edema, surgical site hematoma, or recurrent laryngeal nerve injury may cause airway compromise.

Adjuvants

- Response to NM blockers may be unpredictable if Ca^{2+} level elevated

Anticipated Problems/Concerns

- Cardiac arrhythmias due to hypercalcemia
- Postop airway compromise 2° to bleeding or recurrent laryngeal nerve injury
- Pneumothorax 2° to surgical procedure
- Fluid overload and lyte abn from too aggressive hydration

Hypertension

Simon J Howell
Karim Abdel Hakim

Risk

- Incidence in USA: Affects approx 50 million people
- The incidence of Htn increases with advancing age. Half of people aged 60–69 y and ¾ of people aged over 70 y are affected.
- There is a continuous relationship between BP and the risk of CV diseases incl MI, heart failure, stroke, and kidney disease. For people aged 40–70 y a 20-mm Hg increase in systolic pressure or a 10 mm Hg increase in diastolic pressure doubles the risk of CV disease across the entire range of BPs.

Perioperative Risks

- BPs of up to 180/100 mmHg are not independently associated with an increased risk of periop complications. There are limited data that suggest BPs greater than this may be associated with an increased risk of such complications.
- Intraop CV lability, esp. hypotension, which may precipitate myocardial ischemia or predispose to stroke.

Worry About

- Markedly elevated BP (>180/110 mmHg).
- Possible 2° Htn.

Overview

- Approx 95% of people with raised BP have essential Htn whilst in 5% of people an underlying cause for Htn can be identified.
- The aim of the long-term medical management of Htn is to reduce the burden of CV morbidity and mortality associated with chronically raised BP.

- The 1° concern of the anesthetist when managing a hypertensive pt through the periop period is to prevent or curtail the periop myocardial ischemia and BP lability that has been demonstrated to occur in Htn pts undergoing anesthesia and surgery.
- Target organ damage associated with Htn may of itself increase periop risk
  - Ischemic heart disease
  - Heart failure
  - Cerebrovascular disease
  - Renal impairment
  - Peripheral vascular and aortic disease

ICD-9-CM Code: 401

Etiology

- Essential Htn appears to be a complex mulit-factorial condiation for a single cause has not been identified. Factors that have a role in the development of essential Htn incl genetic factors, race (increased prevalence and severity in African Americans), age, sedentary lifestyle, obesity (in particular visceral obesity), sodium intake, alcohol intake, childhood influences (birth wt, BP tracking). Htn is part of the constellation of disorders that constitute the metabolic syndrome.
- 2° Htn is found in approx 5% of people with raised BP. Identifiable causes of Htn incl sleep apnea, drug-induced Htn, chronic renal disease, renovascular disease, primary aldosteronism, Cushing syndrome, chronic steroid treatmemt, pheochromocytoma, thyroid and parathyroid disease.
- Many pts who are found to have raised BP at presentation for surgery will be found to not to be hypertensive when the BP is rechecked in a less stressful setting.

Usual Treatment

- Lifestyle modification should be encouraged in all pts with elevated BP.
- Goals for long-term BP treatment are <140/90 for general CV disease prevention, <130/80 for pts with high CV risk, a Hx of ischemic heart disease, diabetes or chronic renal disease and <120/80 for pts with left ventricular dysfunction.
- BP reduction is more important than the choice of drug in the 1° prevention of CV complications. There is evidence to support ACEIs, angiotensin receptor blocking drugs (ARB), calcium channel blockers, or thiazide diuretics as first-line therapy. Combination therapy is frequently required to achieve and sustain long-term BP control.
- Specific classes of antihypertensive drugs may provide better 2° prevention in pts with compelling indications for BP control. In pts with a Hx of previous MI a beta-blocker (if the pt is hemodynamically stable) and an ACEI or ARB is indicated.

ASSESSMENT POINTS

System	Effect	Assessment by Hx	PE	Test
CARDIO	CAD	MI, angina, previous CABG or PCI		ECG
	LVH/LVF	Dysponea, orthopnea	Displaced apex beat S_3, basal crepitations	CXR, ECHO
	Peripheral vascular/aortic disease	Claudication/rest pain	Rales Pulses Ankle brachial pressure index	Doppler Angiography/CT angiography/MR angiography
METAB	Metabolic syndrome		Central obesity	Fasting blood glucose Triglycerides HDL-cholesterol
RENAL	Renal impairment			Creatinine Estimated creatinine clearance Microalbumin urine test
CNS	TIA/CVA	Hx of TIA/CVA	Neurologic signs Carotid bruit	Doppler CT/MRI Angiography/CT angiography/MR angiography

Key Reference: Fleisher LA, Beckman JA, Brown KA, et al. ACC/AHA 2007 Guidelines on perioperative cardiovascular evaluation and care for noncardiac surgery: A report of the American College of Cardiology/American Heart Association Task Force on Practice Guidelines. *J Am Coll Cardiol.* 2007;50:159–241.

Perioperative Implications

Preinduction/Induction/Maintenance

- There is no clear evidence to support deferring surgery or for acute management of BP in pts presenting with moderate Htn.
- Severe Htn (>180/110 mmHg) confirmed on multiple readings should be controlled prior to surgery if the delay necessary to achieve this will not compromise the pt (esp. if the pt has evidence of target organ damage).
- Consider withholding ACEI and ARBs for 12 hr before surgery as they may be associated with an increased incidence of intraop Htn.
- Maintain treatment with other antihypertensive medications (in particular beta-blockers) unless

the pt is hypotensive or has evidence of postural hypotension.
- If beta-blockers are started de novo in the periop period begin with a low dose and titrate this up gradually ensuring that the pt does not become hypotensive relative to their usual resing BP.
- Maintain euvolemia, esp. in pts taking vasodilating drugs such as ACEI or ARB.

Monitoring

- Standard monitoring
- Frequent BP readings should be taken at times of potential CV instability such as induction in order to detect sudden changes in BP.

- Consider direct arterial pressure monitoring if surgery is proceeding in the face of severe Htn.
- Consider dynamic (e.g., pulse pressure variation) or static (CVP) volume monitoring if significant hypovolemia is suspected.

General Anesthesia

- Pts may develop profound hypotension at induction and Htn at intubation.
- Consider a fluid preload prior to induction if relative hypovolemia is suspected.
- Prepare a short acting vasopressor prior to induction.
- Consider the use of opiates or short-acting vasoactive drugs to control the response to intubation in pts with significant CV disease.

- Aim to keep intraop BP within 20% of best estimate of preop BP with appropriate use of fluids and vasoactive drugs.
- No anesthetic maintenance technique has been demonstrated to be superior in this setting.

Regional Anesthesia

- Risk of hypotension with neuroaxial blockade
- Consider a fluid preload prior to neuroaxial blockade.

- Take BP readings every 1–2 min immediately after neuroaxial blockade if using non-invasive monitoring.
- As with general anesthesia, aim to keep intraop BP within 20% of best estimate of preop BP.

Postoperative Period

- Resume normal antihypertensive treatment as soon as possible.
- If the pt is not on appropriate CV prevention make appropriate medical referrals to rectify this if possible.

- In some cases parenteral treatment of BP may be required if the pt cannot take oral medications.
- Consider parenteral beta-blockade if a pt who is chronically treated with a beta-blocker is unable to resume this treatment.

Anticipated Problems/Concerns

- In pts with pre-existing CV disease poorly controlled BP in the postop period may precipitate myocardial ischemia and cardiac complications.

Hypertension, Uncontrolled with Cardiomyopathy

Valeriy V. Kozmenko
Lien B. Tran
Alan Kaye

Risk

- 1.5 billion worldwide in 2005
- USA highest prevalence: African American
- Male=female

Perioperative Risks

- Increased risk of MI and/or ischemia
- Increased risk of stroke
- Increased risk of CHF
- Increased risk of renal failure
- Increased blood loss
- Increased risk of cerebral hypoperfusion due to the shift to the right of the curve for the autoregulation of cerebral blood flow
- Prolonged hospitalization

Overview

- Possibility of masked hypovolemia

- Silent myocardial ischemia may occur from supply-demand mismatches, even in absence of CAD
- May be forerunner of renal failure and/or stroke
- CHF may be presenting sign
- May develop left ventricular hypertrophy (LVH) ± strain pattern on ECG
- May require >6 wk of treatment for regression of LVH

ICD-9-CM: 402 (Hypertensive heart disease)

Etiology

- Idiopathic with genetic predisposition (>90%)
- 2° due to thyroid, renal, and adrenal abn
- Substance abuse (alcohol, cocaine, amphetamines)
- Valvular heart pathology (e.g., aortic insufficiency)

- High peripheral resistance is accelerated with time

Usual Treatment

- Preload optimization (diuretics, venodilators)
- Afterload optimization (ACE inhibitors, angiotensin receptor blockers, calcium channel blockers, alpha$_1$-blockers, beta-blockers with alpha$_1$ activity, alpha$_2$ adrenomimetics, direct vasodilators, and sodium nitroprusside for emergencies)
- Drugs with negative inotropic effect (beta-blockers, calcium channel blockers)
- Atherosclerosis prophylaxis (statins)
- Surgical correction of 2° forms of Htn

ASSESSMENT POINTS

System	Effect	Assessment by Hx	PE	Test
CARDIO	LV function LVH	Exercise tolerance	2-flight walk	ECG, CXR ECHO, MUGA Stress thallium
RESP	Pulm edema	Orthopnea Dyspnea	Rales	CXR
CNS	Stroke	Blackouts	Carotid bruit	Carotid study
RENAL	Nephropathy		Edema	BUN/Cr

Key Reference: Howell SJ, Sear JW, Foëx P. Hypertension, hypertensive heart disease and perioperative cardiac risk. *Br J Anaesth.* 2004;92(4):570–583.

Perioperative Implications

Preoperative Risks

- Continue and/or increase antihypertensive medicine
- Short-acting vasodilators prepared, incl nitroglycerin
- Assess myocardial and volume status
- Anxiolytics on the day before surgery
- Correct electrolyte imbalance if present

Monitoring

- Arterial monitoring
- Foley catheter to monitor urine output for traumatic or long procedures or for the procedures with expected significant blood loss
- Volume status monitoring depending on LV function (e.g., CVP, possibly PA catheter, or TEE)
- Consider brainwave monitoring to ensure adequate depth of anesthesia and optimal anesthetic dosing

Induction

- Pre-intubation opiates to blunt hypertensive response to laryngoscopy and ETT placement
- Consider administration of the high end of the dose range of the IV induction agent with uncontrolled Htn, with significant cardiomyopathy, consider etomidate to maintain cardiac hemodynamics
- Use of defasciculating dose of non-depolarizing NMB to prevent mesenteric blood mobilization during abdominal muscle contractions during acetylcholine-induced muscular fasciculations

- Avoiding significant BP fluctuations during induction by using esmolol
- Consider administration of short-acting beta-blockers prior to induction (e.g., esmolol)
- Rapid correction of arterial hypotension induced by propofol or thiopental administration by increasing infusion rate and/or administering ephedrine or propofol
- If severe uncontrolled Htn, consider starting prior to induction, vasodilators, incl either nitroglycerin or nitroprusside

Maintenance

- Careful monitoring of the depth of anesthesia to avoid light anesthesia masking intravascular volume deficit
- Maintaining euvolemic status
- Pre-emptive analgesia to prevent 1° sensitization phenomenon
- Consider high-dose opioids if high hemodynamic stability is needed and prolonged postop ventilation is not an issue.

Extubation

- Adequate pain relief prior to termination of anesthesia
- Short-acting vasodilator and/or β-blockers to prevent Htn and tachycardia

Adjuvants

- Regional: May prevent severe increases in BP, since intubation not needed. Severe dehydration may be present, resulting in profound hypotension.

- Continuous infusions of nitroglycerin, nitroprusside, or esmolol
- Severe hypotension may not respond to usual doses of vasoconstrictor due to prior drug treatment.
- Consider use of alpha$_2$ adrenomimetics
- Inhalational agents, in particular, above 1 MAC can cause dose-dependent increase in heart rate and have different hemodynamic effects

Postoperative Period

- Restart antihypertensive medication as soon as possible in postop period
- Patch therapy for some drugs must be started 12 hr prior to anticipated need due to slow absorption from skin., e.g., clonidine and fentanyl
- Effective pain control using opioids and/or NSAIDs or continuous blockade

Anticipated Problems/Concerns

- Watch for symptoms of CNS, renal, or myocardial dysfunction
- Preop period affords opportunity to educate pt about importance of complying with antihypertensive therapy
- Hypotension if therapy is continued, esp. angiotensin-receptor blocking drugs and receptor inhibitors; or if pt is untreated and volume depleted
- Rebound Htn if certain medications are discontinued (e.g., clonidine)

Hyperthyroidism

Michael F. Roizen

DISEASES

Risk

- Incidence in USA: 440,000/y develop hyperthyroidism plus 5–15% of pregnant females (highest prevalence in 2nd trimester); 1/1000 females; 1/3000 males
- Race with highest prevalence: Unknown

Perioperative Risks

- Risk related to occurrence of thyroid storm; increased risk of storm, even if made euthyroid prior to surgery
- Some increased risk of resp insufficiency
- Progressive increased risk of hypothyroidism after surgery on thyroid, radioactive Rx of hyperthyroidism, and thyroiditis

Worry About

- Assessing that pt is euthyroid
- Securing airway in pt with large goiter or displaced trachea
- Postop risks of nerve injury (immediate stridor requires immediate reintubation), surreptitious bleeding (examine wound—can drain externally—prior to PACU discharge), and thyroid storm (uncommon without another acute illness or after 3 d postop)

Overview

- Endocrinopathy with CV disease—tachycardia (commonly idiopathic if no prior Dx of hyperthyroidism has been made), CHF, dysrhythmias (AFIB) as major manifestation
- Other target: Resp and CNS (decreases drive to breathe; worsens anxiety, psychoses) and metabolic (hypermetabolism and increased protein turnover resulting in weakened muscles and malnourishment); can present as unintentional wt loss
- If euthyroid prior to operation, risk of storm and of periop CV problems diminished by >90%
- If not euthyroid, try to delay operation until euthyroid
- If emergency (life-threatening trauma, ruptured viscus), use β-blocking agents and iodides to decrease periop effects and decrease further synthesis and release of thyroid hormones; keep in ICU until risk of storm has passed

ICD-9-CM Codes: 242.9 (Hyperthyroidism [thyrotoxicosis]); 242.0 (Graves' disease); 245 (Thyroiditis); 193 (Malignant thyroid disease); 198.89 (Metastatic malignant thyroid disease)

Etiology

- Multinodular diffuse enlargement (Graves' disease); almost never malignant, soft large gland, thought autoimmune (thyroid-stimulating IgGs that bind to TSH receptors on thyroid associated with goiter and ophthalmopathy)
- Pregnancy (ectopic TSH-like substance)
- Thyroiditis (autoimmune) in acute phase—often with sore neck, and hoarseness
- Thyroid adenoma—toxic multinodular goiter (firm gland) later in life and rarely (almost never) malignant; unilateral solitary nodule with autonomous function earlier in life, also almost always benign
- Choriocarcinoma
- TSH-secreting pituitary adenoma
- Surreptitious ingestion of T_4 or T_3

Usual Treatment

- Antithyroid drugs for 2–6 mo; if recurs, retreat; if recurs again, consider surgery or radioiodine Rx

ASSESSMENT POINTS

System	Effect	Assessment by Hx	PE	Test
HEENT	Weakened tracheal rings, distorted/displaced trachea Ophthalmopathy	Snoring, hoarseness, neck pain	Ask to vocalize "e"; examine airway and neck; look at eyes; test for diplopia; change over time in measure of eye protrusion	Check CXR (PA and lateral) lat neck films; CT scan or US of neck
CARDIO	Dysrhythmias, AFIB, sinus tachycardia, mitral valve prolapse CHF, cardiomyopathies	Palpitations; ↑ HR during sleep DOE, orthostatic SOB	Standard exam	Rhythm strip or full ECG CV system is involved in either Hx or PE
GI	Wt loss, diarrhea, dehydration	Dizziness on arising; Hx of diarrhea, constipation	Skin turgor; other measures of volume status such as orthostatic vital signs	Increased serum alkaline phosphatase
HEME	Mild anemia, thrombocytopenia; agranulocytosis 2° to propylthiouracil or methimazole		Skin/mucous membranes for infection/petechiae	CBC with plt count and differential
CNS		Shaking, anxiety, emotional lability	Reflex speed, tremor, nervousness, mental status	
METAB	Need to assess if euthyroid; malnourished	Refer to all other systems, esp. reflex speed, tremor, heat intolerance; fatigue; weakness; wt loss; anorexia, increased appetite	Reflex speed; HR	Free T_4

Key Reference: Roizen MF, Fleisher L. Anesthetic implications of concurrent diseases. In: Miller RD, ed. *Anesthesia*. 7th ed. New York: Churchill Livingstone/Elsevier; 2010:1077–1080.

Perioperative Implications

- See also under thyroidectomy, subtotal

Preoperative Preparation

- Assess if euthyroid
- Assess for associated autoimmune diseases

Preinduction/Induction

- Prehydrate liberally if CV status will tolerate
- Check and protect eyes

Anesthetic Technique

- No one technique has proved superior
- Hyperthyroidism is associated risk factor for halothane hepatitis

Monitoring

- Temp (also place cooling blanket on OR table to treat thyroid storm if it occurs)
- Consider invasive monitoring if pt has dilated cardiomyopathy/thyroid storm/severe dysrhythmia

- If head-up position is utilized, consider air embolus monitoring and therapy

Airway

- Consider awake fiberoptic intubation if questions about adequacy of airway or distortion/involvement of trachea present.
- Consider armored tube or equivalent if tracheal rings are affected.

Induction/Maintenance

- Routine

Adjuvants

- Usually no requirement for muscle relaxants

Anticipated Problems/Concerns

- Thyroid storm is life-threatening illness if hyperthyroidism has been severely exacerbated by illness or operation. Manifested by hyperpyrexia, tachycardia, striking alterations in consciousness. Early signs incl delirium, confusion, mania, excitement. Differential Dx: malignant hyperthermia, pheochromocytoma crisis, NMS.
- Rx incl supportive care, methimazole or propylthiouracil followed in 1 hr by iodides and propranolol, decrease conversion of the less active T_3 to the more active T_4
- Surreptitious bleeding behind neck bandages, or into chest if minimally invasive technique is used from axilla, can suddenly compromise airway function or result in CV collapse
- Recurrent laryngeal nerve injuries post thyroidectomy usually result in damage to abductor fibers, which results in hoarseness
- Bullous glottic edema can require immediate reintubation
- Occasionally late tetany (usually 2–3 d post thyroidectomy) can occur from accidental removal of or damage to parathyroid glands

Hypertriglyceridemia

Tim Pawelek
Richard M. Layman

Risk

- Elevated triglyceride levels are an independent risk factor for CAD after adjustment for other risk factors. The risk increases proportionally with increasing triglyceride levels.
- 30% of the population have elevated levels at age 20 and 43% have elevated levels by age 50.
- Component of the metabolic syndrome (increased waist circumference, low HDL, Htn, impaired glucose metabolism) each of which are risk factors for CAD.

Perioperative Risks

- Atherosclerosis with coronary and peripheral vascular sequelae.
- Pancreatitis sequelae incl hemorrhage, dysregulation of glucose, electrolye imbalance, dehydration, pseudocysts, and pancreatic exocrine insufficiency. Levels needed to trigger acute pancreatitis varies but is usually above 1000 mg/dL.

Worry About

- Myocardial ischemia and infarction.
- Alteration of medication 2° to fatty acid sequestration of albumin.
- Pseudohyponatremia.

Overview

- Triglycerides are glycerol molecules with three free fatty acid side chains of variable length and saturation. They are the major form of stored and circulating energy.
- The two main sources of plasma triglycerides are exogenous (dietary) and endogenous (liver). The exogenous form is carried in chylomicrons while the endogenous form is carried in very-low-density lipoprotein (VLDL) particles.
- Normal level is below 150 mg/dL, Borderline high is 150–199 mg/dL, high is 200–499 mg/dL and above 500 is very high.
- The autonomic nervous system regulates lipolysis of adipose cells. Increases in sympathetic stimulation can increase levels.

ICD-9-CM Code: 272.1-3

Etiology

- Primary hypertriglyceridemia incl: familial chylomicronemia, primary mixed hyperlipidemia (both having pathologically increased chylomicron levels), familial hypertriglyceridemia (elevated VLDL), familial combined hyperlipoproteinemia (elevated VLDL and LDL), familial dysbetalipoproteinemia (elevated triglyceride remnants, Beta-VLDL).
- 2° hypertriglyceridemia is caused by obesity (esp. visceral), DM type 2, hyperinsulinemia, metabolic syndrome, alcohol consumption, renal disease, pregnancy, hypothyroidism, autoimmune disorders and medications incl: thiazide diuretics, beta-blockers, oral estrogen compounds, retinoids, protease inhibitors, antipsychotics, corticosteroids.

Usual Treatment

- Lifestyle modification such as increasing exercise, wt reduction and dietary changes such as decreasing intake of fat and refined carbohydrates as well as elimination of alcohol.
- Fibrates: Gemfibrozil, bezafibrate and fenofibrate reduce triglyceride levels by 50%.
- Niacin: 45% reduction but can cause flushing, pruritis, and light-headedness.
- Fish oil (Omega-3 fatty acids): Can reduce triglyceride levels by 20%

ASSESSMENT POINTS

System	Effect	Assessment by Hx	PE	Test
CARDIO	Atherosclorosis, ventricular changes	Hx of MI, angina, CHF, exercise tolerance	JVD, peripheral edema, S3, S4	EKG, CXR, ECHO, stress test, coronary angiography
ENDO	Associated with altered glucose metabolism	Hx of diabetes, ketoacidosis; hypothyroidism		Blood glucose, hemoglobin A1C; thyroid function tests when applicable
RENAL	Caused by nephrotic syndrome, renal failure	Urinary frequency		BUN, Cr, electrolytes; can falsely affect serum electrolyte tests
CNS	Worsens hard macular exudates of diabetes; can resemble dementia	Visual changes; irritability	Ophthamologic exam, presence of lipemia retinalis	
GI	Fat accumulation in liver and spleen; acute pancreatitis	Abdominal discomfort/pain	Hepatosplenomegaly, obesity	Amylase, lipase; can falsely affect serum LFTs
DERM			Cutaneous palmar xanthoma; eruptive xanthoma on back, gluteal, extensor surface of arm	

Key Reference: Yuan G, Al-Shali KZ, Hegele RA. Hypertriglyceridemia: Its etiology, effects and treatment. *CMAJ.* 2007;176:1113–1120.

Perioperative Implications

Preinduction/Induction/Maintenance

- Electrolyte levels (pseudohyponatremia) and liver function test may be falsely affected.
- Binding of fatty acid to albumin may compete with induction agents that bind albumin, hence altering kinetics.
- No apparent differences in agent choice for maintenance.
- Concerns for associated co-morbidities should be addressed.

Monitoring

- Standard ASA monitors unless co-morbid conditions dictate otherwise.

General Anesthesia

- Increasing serum triglyceride levels will increase blood-gas partition coefficient and increase volatile solubility.
- Renal function may be diminished, therefore, uo should be closely observed.

Regional Anesthesia

- Neuraxial anesthetic poses theoretical benefit as sympatholysis will result in decreased lipolysis of adipocytes.

- Associated co-morbidities such as obesity and cardiac sequelae may affect choice.

Postoperative Period

- Possibility of cardiac event requires vigilance.
- Consider familial hyperchylomicronemia syndrome if changes in mental status.

Anticipated Problems/Concerns

- Known complications of CAD.
- Complications regarding comorbidities.

Hypokalemia

Daniel Cormican
Shawn T. Beaman

Risk

- Defined as plasma K⁺ <3.5 mEq/L
- Common conditions and/or treatments place pts at increased risk, incl:
  - Those on diuretics (esp. loop and thiazide diuretics) to treat Htn, CHF, etc
  - Those experiencing significant GI fluid loss (e.g., vomiting, diarrhea, or gastric suction)
  - Those with increased serum pH (metabolic or resp alkalosis)

Perioperative Risks

- Increased risk of cardiac dysrhythmias (with greater concern in those with pre-existing heart disease and in setting of acute onset hypokalemia)
- Increased risk of muscle weakness (which incl possible resp muscle weakness and prolonged neuromuscular blockade)
- Increased risk of GI hypomotility

Worry About

- Cardiac dysrhythmias are the most worrisome complication of hypokalemia.
- Many medications regularly used in periop treatment can cause or worsen hypokalemia (e.g., diuretics, antibiotics, β_2 agonists, epinephrine).
- Pts requiring significant/urgent K⁺ replacement may require central line placement.
- Over-replacement: Any pt requiring K⁺ replacement may be at risk for hyperkalemia and thus the malignant dysrhythmias associated with hyperkalemia.

Overview

- K⁺ ions have essential role in maintaining cellular resting membrane potentials and in generating functional activity in muscle cells, neurons, and cardiac tissue.
- Overall, intracellular K⁺ concentration is ~30 times greater than extracellular K⁺ concentration; this ratio is maintained by cell membrane Na⁺/ K⁺ ATPase.
- Decreases in extracellular K⁺ impairs nml gradients required for membrane potential/action potential transmission.
- Acute/rapid decreases in serum K⁺ concentration create more concerning derangements in cellular membrane potential physiology than chronic or slowly developing decreases in K⁺.

ICD-9-CM Code: 276.8

Etiology

- Inadequate K⁺ intake: Seen in eating disorders, inability to eat, "tea & toast" diet, alcoholism, and those receiving K⁺-poor TPN.
- Increased K⁺ excretion
  - Renal losses: Mineralocorticoid excess (1° or 2° hyperaldosteronism, Cushing disease, congenital adrenal hyperplasia), hyperreninism, congenital renal disorders (Bartter/Gitelman/Liddle syndromes), medication-induced (loop and thiazide diuretics, carbonic anhydrase inhibitors, amphotericin B, some penicillins, gentamicin)
  - GI losses: Vomiting, diarrhea, NGT/OGT suction, villous adenoma, ureterosigmoidostomy
- Intracellular K⁺ shifts: Alkalosis (metabolic or resp), medication induced (insulin administration, β_2 agonists, epinephrine, terbutaline, ritodrine), refeeding syndrome, periodic paralysis, barium toxicity

Usual Treatment

- Identify and attempt to correct the underlying/precipitating factors causing the hypokalemia (e.g., adjust diet intake, review/reconsider medications, lower pH of pts with alkalosis by treating 1° disorder)
- K⁺ repletion: It is reported that each 10 mEq of K⁺ given will raise serum K⁺ by 0.1 mEq/L.
  - Oral K⁺: Can use K⁺ paired with gluconate, phosphate, chloride, or citrate, with delivery via tablet or solution
  - IV K⁺: Most commonly as K⁺ chloride. Careful repletion required via programmable infusion pump to avoid hyperkalemic complications — pts receiving >10–20 mEq/hr should have cardiac monitoring in place. Peripheral IV administration can cause burning sensation and vascular epithelium damage; consider placement of central line.

ASSESSMENT POINTS

System	Effect	Assessment by Hx	PE	Test
NERVOUS	Muscle weakness Cramping/myalgia	↓ Mobility, falls, ↓ ADL c/o muscle pain	↓ Muscle strength	TOF intraop
RESPIR	Respir muscle failure	SOB, hypoventilation, ventilator dependence	Poor insp effort, low TV	ABG, NIF
CV	Dysrhythmias	c/o palpitations, syncope, cardiac arrest		EKG
	Vasomotor instability	Syncope, falls, disorientation	Refractory shock, hypotension	
GI	↓ GI motility	Constipation, abd pain	Loss of bowel sounds, abd tenderness and distention	KUB
RENAL	Polyuria Polydipsia ↑ Renal ammonia Edema and sodium retention	Frequent urination Frequent drinking		Urine ammonia Urine sodium

Key Reference: Gennari FJ. Hypokalemia. *N Engl J Med.* 1998;339:451–458.

Perioperative Implications

Preoperative Preparation

- Obtain serum K⁺ concentration preop if pt presents with risk factors for hypokalemia
- Attempt to identify and/or address the etiology of hypokalemia
- For elective cases, replete serum K⁺ concentration to >2.6 before going to OR. Discuss concerns/implications with pt/family/surgical team.
- Have ACLS meds on hand, and transport with cardiac monitoring.

Monitoring

- EKG/continuous cardiac monitoring (watch for T wave flattening, U waves, PVC, VT/VF)
- BP cuff or arterial line (watch for hypotension related to vasomotor insufficiency)
- Periodic ABG and electrolyte panels as needed (watch for pH and K⁺ trend)
- Twitch monitor (watch for prolonged neuromuscular blockade)

Maintenance

- Judicious use of medications associated with causing or exacerbating hypokalemia
- Control glucose and fluid volume
- Control ventilation to avoid hyperventilation and resp alkalosis

Anticipated Problems/Concerns

- Pts with symptomatic hypokalemia (esp. with cardiac symptoms) that are not well controlled after initial treatments may need elective surgical procedures delayed
- Cardiac dysrhythmias are greatest concern in hypokalemia, as these can be lethal. Risk is greatest when hypokalemia is acute and serum K⁺ <3.0.
- Preop problems: EKG changes and volume status (related to diuretics or polydipsia)
- Intraop problems: Persistent hypotension after induction (related to refractory vasomotor response to catecholamines), prolonged neuromuscular blockade, resp muscle weakness

Hypomagnesemia

Mehmet S. Ozcan
James M. Feld

Risk

- General population (up to 25%) may be deficient because of poor eating habits.
- 12% of all hospitalized pts as well as 44–60% of all pts admitted to medical/surgical and pediatric ICUs were hypomagnesemic.

Associated With

- Poor nutrition
- Gastrointestinal losses
  - Diarrhea
  - Malabsorption (steatorrhea, bowel resection, intestinal fistulas)
  - Acute pancreatitis
- Renal losses
  - Diuretics (esp. loop diuretics)
  - Antimicrobials (e.g., aminoglycosides, amphotericin B)
  - Chemotherapeutics (e.g., cisplatin, foscarnet, cyclosporine)
  - Phosphorus depletion
  - Metabolic acidosis
  - Alcohol abuse
- Miscellaneous
  - Diabetes mellitus
  - Prolonged IV therapy
  - Massive blood transfusions
  - Digitalis

Perioperative Risks

- Arrhythmias (atrial and ventricular, esp. torsades)
- Worsening cardiac ischemia and CHF
- Increased susceptibility to seizures, bronchoconstriction, and vasospasm
- Inability to correct low K+ and Ca2+ levels
- Resistance to vasodilators
- Insulin resistance in the diabetic pt

Worry About

- Weakness, lethargy, paresthesias, muscle spasms
- Seizures (esp. in preeclampsia)

- Arrhythmias (esp. torsades)
- Hypokalemia and hypocalcemia (may be difficult to treat if hypomagnesemia is the underlying cause)
- Coronary artery spasm and CHF
- During treatment of hypomagnesemia: Burning at IV site, overall sense of warmth and flushing, transient and mild hypotension may occur if $MgSO_4$ is given too fast

Overview

- Hypomagnesemia is defined as plasma Mg^{2+} <1.7 mg/dL. Most symptomatic pts have levels <1 mg/dL
- Mg^{2+} levels are not routinely checked in screening tests. Hypomagnesemia should be suspected esp. in chronic diarrhea, alcoholism, malnutrition, long-term hospitalization, and hypoalbuminemia.
- Mg^{2+} is primarily an intracellular ion. Plasma levels may not reflect the true magnitude of deficit. Intracellular shift may occur with the administration of insulin and thyroid hormone.
- Normomagnesemic Mg^{2+} depletion has been described; if clinical suspicion of hypomagnesemia present, Mg^{2+} should be administered, even with normal plasma levels.
- Differentiation of renal from non-renal causes is helpful to investigate etiology. In a 24-hr urine sample, Mg^{2+} loss of >3-4 mEq/d supports renal etiology.
- Alternatively, a fractional excretion of Mg^{2+} can be calculated in a spot-urine sample.
- $FE_{Mg} = [(U_{Mg} \times P_{Cr})/(0.7 \times P_{Mg}) \times U_{Cr}] \times 100$, where U_{Mg}/U_{Cr} and P_{Mg}/U_{Cr} denotes urinary and plasma concentrations of Mg^{2+} and creatinine.
- Usually, FE_{Mg} greater than 2% indicates renal etiology. In a study of 74 hypomagnesemic pts, ranges of FE_{Mg} in non-renal and renal causes were 0.5–2.7% and 4–48%, respectively.

ICD9-CM: 275.2 (Disorders of magnesium metabolism)

Usual Treatment

- Acute administration of 2 gm $MgSO_4$ over 20–30 min
- 1 gram $MgSO_4$ with every 20-40 mEq of KCl
- Give at the beginning of an anesthetic, as $MgSO_4$ may interfere with neuromuscular blockade reversal
- Usual doses for preeclampsia are 4–6 gm bolus followed by 1–2 gm/hr, targeting a plasma level around 6 mg/dL (normal up to 2.5 mg/dL)
- Each gram of $MgSO_4$ has 98 mg of elemental Mg^{2+} (equivalent to 4 mmol or 8 mEq)
- As long as renal function is intact, excessive Mg^{2+} levels will be cleared over several hours.

Therapeutic Uses

- Besides correction of hypomagnesemia, Mg^{2+} replacement can be used.
- CV: Myocardial protection, decreases CHF, improves contractility, diastolic relaxation, attenuates or prevents tachycardic arrhythmias, minimizes changes in heart rate and BP during intubation
- Neurological: May improve memory, decrease cerebral vasospasm, limit any neuro insult to brain or spinal cord
- Endocrine: Attenuates insulin resistance, helps in hemodynamic control in pheochromocytomas, may increase HDL levels
- OB: Widespread use in treatment of preeclampsia, decreases risk of cerebral palsy in preterm infants
- Pulm: Bronchodilation esp. in severe asthmatic
- Anesthesia: Decrease need for inhalation agent to maintain same BIS level
- Pain: Decreases need for postop opiates through its blockade of NMDA receptors
- MS: Relaxes muscle rigidity and decreases autonomic dysfunction in tetanus
- Intoxication/recreational drugs: Helpful to treat CV problems associated with cocaine and methamphetamines

ASSESSMENT POINTS

System	Effect	Assessment by Hx	PE	Test
CNS	Seizures, cerebral vasospasm (after SAH)	Lethargy, SAH (vasospasm)	Altered mental status	Plasma Mg^{2+}, TCD, cerebral angiogram
CARDIO	Arrhythmias (torsades), wide QRS, tall T waves (flattens in severe depletion), CHF (impaired diastolic relaxation)	Tachyarrhythmia, Htn, dyspnea		EKG, plasma Mg^{2+}, BNP, ECHO
MS	Hypocalcemia (decreased secretion and resistance to PTH)	Weakness, tetany	Chvostek and Trousseau signs	Plasma Ca^{+2}, Mg^{2+}
ENDO	Insulin resistance, may affect lipid profile	Diabetes (type 1 and 2) Hyperlipidemia		Glucose, plasma Mg^{2+}, HDL, triglycerides
RESP	Bronchospasm	Asthma	Wheezing	Plasma Mg^{2+}
RENAL	Hypokalemia (K+ loss from loop of Henle)	Alcohol abuse, nephrotoxins (antibiotics, chemo), diuretics		Creatinine, BUN, Plasma K+, Mg^{2+}

Key Reference: James MFM. Magnesium: An emerging drug in anaesthesia. *Br J Anaesth.* 2009;103(4):465–467.

Perioperative Implications

Preoperative Preparation

- Check serum Mg^{2+} level (<1.7 mg/dL is hypomagnesemia)
- Obtain 12-lead EKG
- Start replacing Mg^{2+} (e.g., 2 gm over 20 min; faster replacement safe but may cause burning at the IV site)

Monitoring

- EKG
- Plasma Mg^{2+} levels (normal range 1.7–2.5 mg/dL)
- TOF monitoring (replacing Mg^{+2} potentiates NMB agents)
- Consider BIS (or other depth of anesthesia) monitoring, since replacing Mg^{2+} may alter anesthesia requirement

Induction

- Mg^{2+} IV bolus during induction is safe (e.g., 2–4 gm IV bolus)
- May cause mild and transient drop in BP
- Replacing Mg^{2+} minimizes changes in heart rate and BP during intubation
- Hypomagnesemia may cause or exacerbate bronchospasm

Maintenance

- Replacing Mg^{2+} decreases anesthetic requirement (i.e., maintain same BIS level with less anesthetic)
- Hypomagnesemia may decrease cardiac contractility and impair diastolic relaxation in pts with CHF; improved by replacing Mg^{2+}.
- Replacing Mg^{2+} attenuates or prevents tachyarrhythmias.
- Insulin resistance may occur in the hypomagnesemic pt.

Emergence

- Replacing Mg^{2+} attenuates shivering.

- Replacing Mg^{2+} maintains hemodynamic stability.
- Titrate NMB agents and reverse residual NMB, esp. if Mg^{2+} was replaced intraop.

Postoperative Period

- Hypomagnesemia may increase analgesic (i.e., opioid) requirement; Mg^{2+} replacement leads to decreased opioid consumption.
- Hypomagnesemia may worsen bronchospasm in asthmatic pts.
- Increased catecholamine levels may exacerbate tachyarrhythmias in the hypomagnesemic pt.

Anticipated Problems/Concerns

- Although Mg^{2+} replacement is usually well tolerated, potential problems with overdose include the following:
  - Levels above 8–10 mg/dL may cause diaphragmatic weakness and above 10–12 mg/dL may cause widening of QRS and conduction blocks. These levels are rarely reached with the above-recommended doses and in the absence of decreased GFR.
  - Potentiation of neuromuscular blockade

Hyponatremia

Charles Fox
Paul J. Primeaux
Alan Kaye

Risk

- Premenopausal women, esp. those undergoing procedures associated with rapid irrigant absorption, at particularly high risk.
- Conditions associated with syndrome of inappropriate antidiuretic hormone (SIADH), or adrenocortical insufficiency (Addison disease).
- Pts with liver, heart, or renal failure
- Hyponatremia esp. common in elderly pts and associated with increased morbidity and mortality
- Up to 25% of men undergoing TURP
- Infants and/or children receiving multiple tap H_2O enemas

Perioperative Risks

- Risk of CV collapse with adrenocortical insufficiency and inability to cope with stress of surgery
- Iatrogenic dilution in TURP and endoscopic gyn procedures associated with CNS, cardiopulmonary, and skeletal muscle abn
- Increased ADH secretion extremely common periop and may cause further decrease serum NA^+
- Isotonic saline (0.9%) will result in free H_2O gain and decrease in serum NA^+ in presence of SIADH.

Worry About

- Acute iatrogenic hyponatremia associated with TURP syndrome
- Development of cerebral and/or pulm edema
- Cardiac dysrhythmia
- Visual or motor disturbances attributed to ammonia intoxication with glycine irrigation

- Consider Dx in surgical pts exhibiting headache, lethargy, obtundation periop
- Seizures, coma, pulm edema, and resp arrest can be seen with NA^+ concentration below 115 to 120 mEq/L

Overview

- Hyponatremia defined as serum Na^+ <135 mEq/L; most common cause is an excess of total body H_2O.
- Hyponatremia can be associated with low, nml, or high tonicity (tonicity defined as the contribution to osmolality of solutes that cannot freely cross cell membranes)
- Change in tonicity causes free H_2O shift leading most importantly to cerebral intracellular volume changes (edema in hypotonic hyponatremia)
- Extracellular volume may be decreased, nml, or increased

ICD-9-CM: 276.1 (Hyposmolality and/or hyponatremia)

Etiology

- Most common causes of severe hyponatremia in adults: Postop state, thiazide diuretics, clinical scenarios associated with SIADH, polydipsia in psychiatric pts, TURP
- Mutiple tap H_2O enemas most common cause in infants and children
- Hypervolemic hyponatremia
  - Cirrhosis
  - CHF
  - Renal failure
  - TURP
- Normovolemic hyponatremia
  - SIADH (associated with CNS, pulm diseases/malignancy, pain, stress)

- Hypothyroidism
- Pseudohyponatremia syndrome e.g., factitious hyponatremia (normotonic hyponatremia): hyperlipidemia states (e.g., chylomicronemia) or hyperproteinemia
- Hypovolemic hyponatremia
  - Trauma
  - Thiazide diuretics
  - Mineralcorticoid difficiency

Usual Treatment

- Free H_2O restriction
- IV or oral sodium chloride (incl hypertonic saline with caution in symptomatic pts)
- Loop diuretics (limits extracellular volume expansion with 3% saline)
- Vasopressin antagonists
- Risk of osmotic demyelination syndrome with overly aggressive correction of plasma Na^+ concentration
- Goal: Raise plasma sodium <10 mEq/L in first 24 hr; <18 mEq/L in first 48 hr
- If needed, dose of sodium required to correct a deficit may be calculated using the following formula: Dose (mEq) = (Weight [kg] × (140 – [Na]) [mEq/L]) × 0.6
- The optimal rate of correction appears to be 0.6 to 1 mmol/L/hr until the Na^+ concentration is 125 mEq/L, and then correction proceeds at a slower rate. One half the deficit can be administered over the first 8 hr and the next half over 1 to 3 d if symptoms remit.
- Targeted therapy for end-organ dysfunction (diuresis, vasodilation in CHF, airway protection with mental status changes)
- Hypovolemic pts require careful isotonic fluid resuscitation to maintain hemodynamic stability

ASSESSMENT POINTS

System	Effect	Assessment by Hx	PE	Test
CARDIO	Dysrhythmias	Palpitations		Oscillation, ECG (wide QRS, ↑ ST, VT/VF)
	CHF, hypervolemia	DOE, orthopnea	S3, rales	CXR
	Hypovolemia	Lightheadedness, weakness	Orthostatic hypotension, ↓ CVP, tachycardia	BP, CVP
RESP	Pulm edema	DOE	S3, rales	CXR
CNS	Confusion, restlessness, gait disturbance, lethargy, seizures, visual disturbances, obtundation, coma			Serum Na^+ <115-120 mEq/L associated with profound symptoms
MS	Weakness, cramps	Weakness, cramps	Weakness, hyporeflexia	Reflexes
RENAL	Free H_2O retention Salt wasting			Urine Na^+, serum and urine osmolality

Key Reference: Yeates KE, Singer M, Morton AR. Salt and water: A simple approach to hyponatremia. *CMAJ.* 2004;170:365.

Perioperative Implications

Preinduction

- Ensure medical optimization of co-morbid diseases (hyponatremia greater risk with increasing severity of disease: ASA III and IV)
- Caution with sedatives
- Preop lytes in high risk procedures
- Consider regional in TURP to facilitate monitoring of mental status
- Increased ADH and volume changes associated with surgical trauma likely to decrease Na^+ further
- Identify irrigating solution and prepare for irrigant-specific side effects

Monitoring

- TURP
  - Metal status with regional technique

- Consider EEG with GA
- Consider invasive monitoring (CVP/PA cath/TEE) with development of TURP syndrome and CHF in elderly pts
  - Visual acuity with glycine irrigation
- Hyponatremic pts undergoing therapy to correct serum Na^+
  - Serum Na^+
  - Mental status
  - ECG

General Anesthesia

- Isotonic fluids for volume resuscitation
- Ensure adequate depth of anesthesia as pain and/or stress associated with ADH release

Regional Anesthesia

- Neuraxial blockade technique of choice for TURP

- Prepare for emergency airway protection if resp distress, seizures, obtundation

Postoperative Period

- Ensure adequate pain control
- Monitor serum Na^+
- Initiate appropriate therapy in symptomatic or severely hyponatremic pts
- Avoid too rapid correction and associated demyelination syndrome
- Restore blood and/or volume loss if necessary

Anticipated Problems/Concerns

- TURP procedures of long duration and with significant bleeding or increased hydrostatic pressure of irrigant predictive for large amounts of irrigation fluid absorption. (Increased vigilance required)

- Attempt to optimize pts with cardiopulmonary disease preop
- Isotonic saline in SIADH will result in increased free H_2O and worsening hyponatremia (close monitoring of serum Na^+ required with 0.9% saline administration necessary if unclear diagnosis)
- Premenstrual women at greater risk of both symptomatic hyponatremia and osmotic demyelination with Na^+ correction
- Chronic hyponatremia tolerated better than acute hyponatremia

Hypophosphatemia

William H. Daily

Risk

- Incidence: 1% of population, 5–20% of hospitalized pts

Perioperative Risks

- Acute resp or cardiac failure, generalized weakness, confusion, or seizures

Worry About

- Periop resp or cardiac failure
- Too rapid correction can cause hypocalcemia or Ca^{2+} deposition in tissues

Overview

- Total body phosphorus is distributed 90% in bone, 10% intracellular and < 1% in the extracellular fluid.
- Normal ionized phosphorus (Pi) is 2.7–4.5 mg/dL. May fall by 30% after administration of carbohydrates/insulin. Higher in childhood and postmenopausal women. Lower in AM than PM.
- Serum concentration does not correlate closely to body stores.

- Normal requirements 1 mmol/kg/d
- 1° absorption of Pi is in the duodenum and the jejunum, stimulated by vitamin D
- Kidney: Primary filtration in the kidney with 1° reabsorption in the proximal tubules with only 10% reabsorption in the distal tubules. Regulated by PTH, cortisol, high dietary intake, and calcitonin. Increased Pi excretion with volume expansion.
- Functions: Phosphates provide the 1° energy bond in ATP, creatine phosphate. Severe Pi depletion can cause cellular energy depletion, lack of cAMP, also important for cellular structures as phospholipids, nucleic acids, and cellular membranes. As part of 2,3 diphosphoglycerate, phosphates promote O_2 release from hemoglobin.

ICD-9-CM Code: 275.3

Etiology

- Decreased intake, increased loss, redistribution, occasionally genetic

- Decreased absorption and/or intake: Malnutrition, malabsorption syndromes, Crohn's disease, celiac disease, inadequate replacement in TPN, hemodialysis, Mg^{2+} and aluminum antacids, sucralfate, Vitamin E deficiency
- Increased losses: Rapid volume resuscitation, steroids, pancreatitis, burns, alcoholism, dialysis, hyperparathyroidism, diuretics
- Redistribution: Shift from serum into cells-hyperglycemia, glucose infusion, hormonal effects-catecholamines, insulin, glucagon, calcitonin
- Resp alkalosis, leukemic blast cell crisis

Usual Treatment

- Prefer oral over parenteral because of risk of resultant hypocalcemia or calcification of tissues. Suggested dose of KPHOS 2–5 mg/kg/d.
- If parenteral therapy is required, administration of 10–45 mmol of IV Na^+ or K^+ phosphate over 6–12 hr. Important to monitor Ca^{2+}, K^+, and Mg^{2+} levels.

ASSESSMENT POINTS

System	Effect	Result
CARDIO	Depressed ATP, impaired response to Norepinephrine/angiotensin	Heart failure
Blood WBC	Impaired phagocytic, migration and bacteriocidal activity	Sepsis
Platelets		Thrombocytopenia, impaired clot retraction
RBC	Reduced RBC 2,3 DPG	Increased Hgb O_2 affinity
CNS	Neurologic dysfunction	Seizures, coma, hyperreflexia, paresthesia, dysarthria
MS	Resp failure, motor weakness	Proximal > distal, rhabdomyolysis, myoglobinuria

Key Reference: Bugg NC, Jones JA. Hypophosphatemia. Pathophysiology, effects and management on the intensive care unit. *Anaesthesia*. 1998;53:895–902.

Perioperative Implications

- Correction of severe hypophosphatemia should be done slowly over several hours to days to prevent severe hypocalcemia and vascular and interstitial Ca^{2+} precipitation.

- Consider hypophosphatemia in the pt who is difficult to wean off the ventilator as this might be the cause.

Hypopituitarism

Amir Baluch
Alan Kaye

Risk

- Most frequent cause: Pituitary tumor (61%). The incidence is 45.5 people out of 100,000.
- 30% of pituitary macroadenomas (>10 mm) cause one or more hormone deficiencies
- 50% of pts after pituitary radiation therapy by 4.2 y have hypopituitarism.

Perioperative Risks

- If adequate hormone replacement, surgery presents no increased risk
- If due to secreting tumor, then there is an increased risk of Cushing disease, acromegaly, SIADH, or hyperthyroidism

Worry About

- Concerns with manifestations of disease process (Cushing disease (hypercortisolism 2° to an adrenocorticotropic hormone-secreting adenoma), acromegaly (2° to a growth hormone-secreting adenoma), hyperthyroidism in the setting of thyrotropic adenomas.

- Operative risks, incl bleeding, DI, the syndrome of inappropriate antidiuretic hormone secretion)
- GH-secreting adenoma predisposing to airway abn and OSA
- Hypoglycemia
- Altered volume status due to ↑ urinary losses
- Adequacy of adrenal function
- Increased risk of CV disease
- Possible increase in ICP

Overview

- Partial or complete disruption of pituitary gland secretion. Symptoms result from end-organ hypofunction or dysfunction. Organs affected incl adrenals, thyroid, reproductive system, liver (glucose production), and kidneys.
- May manifest cortisol deficiency, hypothyroidism, amenorrhea, infertility, insulin-induced hypoglycemia, DI
- Pituitary apoplexy is sudden loss of pituitary function with hypotension, eye pain, blindness, ophthalmoplegia

ICD-9-CM Codes: 253.2 or 253.7 (if due to radiotherapy, post ablative, post hypophysectomy, or secondary to hormone therapy)

Etiology

- 61% 2° to tumors of the pituitary gland
- 9% due to other types of lesions
- 19% due to other causes (radiation, hemorrhage, infarct, head trauma, infiltrative diseases)
- 11% no cause could be identified

Usual Treatment

- Surgical resection of adenoma with appropriate hormonal replacement therapy for ACTH: Prednisone or cortisone PO; for TSH: Thyroxine PO; for LH and FSH: Women: estrogen and progesterone PO; Men: testosterone esters IM; for ADH: Desmopressin intranasal

ASSESSMENT POINTS

System	Effect	Assessment by Hx	PE	Test
HEENT	Mandibular and oral soft tissue hyperplasia in acromegalics		Airway exam Check ring size	
CARDIO	Hypovolemia Catecholamine resistance		Orthostatic hypotension	Give steroid replacement and observe effect on BP
GI	Hypoaldosteronism	Anorexia, N/V, wt loss, abdominal pain		Hyperkalemia, hyponatremia, hypocalcemia, hypovolemia
ENDO	Decreased ACTH	Fatigue, fever, stress-induced hypotension, and hyponatremia	Fever, hypotension, wt loss, mental status	AM cortisol level, rapid ACTH stimulation test, insulin tolerance test
	Decreased LH, FSH	Decreased libido and sexual function, amenorrhea	Regression of 2° sexual characteristics	FSH, LH serum levels, serum estradiol and testosterone
	Decreased GH	Fatigue		Insulin-induced hypoglycemia, serum IGF-I
	Decreased TSH	Wt gain, cold intolerance, depression, constipation, hair loss	Myxedema, hyporeflexia	TSH, T$_4$
	Increased prolactin	Lactation, amenorrhea	Galactorrhea	Serum prolactin
MS	Increased GH in acromegalics		Large hands, feet, mandible, tongue	
RENAL	↑ Vasopressin	Excessive thirst		Hyponatremia
	↓ Vasopressin	Increased UO and thirst	Hypovolemia Hypotension	Hypernatremia Dilute urine

Key Reference: Nemergut EC, Dumont AS, Barry UT, et al. Perioperative management of patients undergoing transsphenoidal pituitary surgery. *Anesth Analg.* 2005;101(4):1170–1181.

Perioperative Implications

Preoperative Preparation

- Ensure adequacy of hormone replacement therapy
- Check serum Na⁺, Ca⁺⁺, and K⁺ and correct if necessary
- Determine volume status and adequacy of fluid replacement
- In acromegalics: Careful airway assessment and cardiac workup
- Steroid supplementation considerations (hydrocortisone 100 mg/70 kg tid)
- Clinically assess for signs of increased ICP (N/V, papilledema, headache, blurry vision)

Monitoring

- Consider arterial line if severe CV compromise, central venous pressures if indicated by inadequate preop correction of fluid status
- Frequent monitoring of electrolytes if hypo or hypernatremia is not corrected preop
- Consider glucose monitoring

Airway

- Acromegalics with normal airway exam may be difficult to intubate. Have LMA, fiberoptic, or glidescope available.

Induction

- Little risk of increased ICP with pituitary adenomas

- No special technique if hormone replacement and volume status are adequate

Maintenance

- Maintain normocarbia for pituitary surgery
- Careful titration of narcotics and benzodiazepines in pts with OSA 2° to GH-secreting tumors

Extubation

- Routine (for nonpituitary surgery). May need CPAP postop if pt requires use at home for possible OSA

Adjuvants

- Intraop DI treated with vasopressin 5–10 IU SQ or IM q 4–6 hr

Postoperative Period
• Polyuria and polydipsia with dilute urine may indicate development of DI
• Postop hypopituitarism may require steroid replacement therapy

Anticipated Problems/Concerns
• Acromegalic should be treated as a difficult airway
• Pt with GH deficiency may manifest hypoglycemia
• Electrolyte abn (K^+, Na^+, Ca^{++}) and possible hypovolemia resulting predisposing to arrhythmias and CV instability

Hypothermia, Mild

Daniel I. Sessler

Risk

- Greater in infants and children
- Greater in longer, larger operations
- Similar in regional and GA

Perioperative Risks

- Myocardial ischemia
- Surgical wound infections
- Coagulopathy
- Reduced drug metabolism
- Prolonged recovery and hospitalization
- Shivering and thermal discomfort

Benefits

- Improved neurologic recovery after cardiac arrest
- Improved neurologic recovery in asphyxiated neonates
- Decreases triggering and severity of malignant hyperthermia

Overview

- Core temp normally protected by responses incl sweating, vasoconstriction, shivering
- Typical doses of general anesthetics have little effect on the sweating threshold, but decrease vasoconstriction and shivering thresholds 2–4°C, thus increasing the range of temp *not* triggering protective responses 10-fold from ~0.4°C to ~4°C
- Regional anesthesia inhibits thermoregulatory control by preventing peripheral responses (such as vasoconstriction) and centrally by reducing afferent input

ICD-9-CM Code: 991.6 (Accidental)

Etiology

- Initial 0.5–1.5°C decrease in core temp from core-to-peripheral *redistribution* of body heat
- Subsequently, slow, linear decrease in core temp from *heat loss exceeding heat production*

- Finally, a core-temp plateau results when thermoregulatory *vasoconstriction decreases cutaneous heat loss and constrains metabolic heat* to core thermal compartment

Usual Treatment

- Forced-air is the most effective generally available warming method, typically increasing mean body temp 1°C/hr.
- 1 L of crystalloid at 20°C or 1 U of blood at 4°C decreases mean body temp ~0.25°C in adults. Fluid warming should be restricted to pts given large volumes of fluid (i.e., ≥2 L/hr).
- Passive insulation (e.g., surgical drapes, cotton blankets) decreases heat loss only 30% which is usually insufficient to maintain periop normothermia.
- Circulating-H_2O mattresses less effective and may cause burns. Airway heating and humidification is ineffective.

ASSESSMENT POINTS

System	Effect	Dx	Treatment
CNS	Ischemia protection Thermal discomfort	None Visual analogue scale	Induce and maintain hypothermia Active cutaneous warming
CARDIAC	Myocardial ischemia (usually postop)	ST-segment depression Troponin	Active cutaneous warming
VASC	Precapillary dilation; reduced SVR Arteriovenous shunt constriction; ↑ BP, ↓ HR	Associated with sweating Fingers feel cold, ≈10 mmHg increase in mean arterial pressure	Active or passive cooling Active cutaneous warming
MS (shivering)	2–3-fold ↑ metabolic rate Pt discomfort Interference with monitoring	Visual inspection O_2 consumption	Prevent hypothermia Meperidine 10–25 mg IV Clonidine 75 µg IV Active cutaneous warming
IMMUNO	Incidence of infections increases 2–3-fold	Clinical infections	Prevent hypothermia
HEME	10% ↑ /°C in blood loss	Bleeding time PT/PTT *falsely* normal	Prevent hypothermia Defect probably *not* reversed by FFP and platelet transfusions
METAB (increased drug action)	MAC decreases ~5%/°C ↓ Drug metabolism	Monitor drug action (rather than dose)	Titrate drug administration to desired endpoint Monitor twitch depression

Key Reference: Sessler DI. Temperature monitoring and perioperative thermoregulation. *Anesthesiology*. 2008;109:318–338.

Perioperative Implications

Preoperative Preparation

- Active prewarming for 30–60 min helps prevent redistribution hypothermia

Monitoring

- Four core temp sites are accurate: Pulm artery, distal esophagus, tympanic membrane, nasopharynx
- Four additional sites suitable except during cardiopulmonary bypass: Mouth, axilla, rectum, bladder
- The best site for postop temp monitoring is the mouth

Intraoperative

- Maintain normothermia (core temp >36°C) unless otherwise indicated
- Sufficient passive or active reduction of heat loss will prevent hypothermia, however, active warming is usually required
- Once triggered, thermoregulatory vasoconstriction effective in preventing further core hypothermia
- Current standards (Surgical Care Improvement Project and Physicians Quality Reporting Initiative) require that nearly all surgical pts have regional or general anesthesia lasting ≥1 hr be normothermic near the end of anesthesia *and/or* that active over-body warming be used

Postoperative

- Hypothermic pts should be rewarmed with forced-air
- Shivering and thermal discomfort can be specifically treated
- Postop warming not a routine substitute for maintaining intraop normothermia

Anticipated Problems/Concerns

- Thermal discomfort has been proven to cause numerous life-threatening complications and should be actively prevented unless therapeutic hypothermia is specifically indicated

Hypothyroidism

John Butterworth

Risk

- Subclinical hypothyroidism may be present in as many as 8–10% of adult women and 1–2% of adult men; about 3% of adults receive chronic thyroid replacement.

Perioperative Risks

- Potential increased risk for hypothermia, hypotension, cardiac failure, and GI dysfunction
- Periop mortality rate not increased unless overtly hypothyroid
- During pregnancy maternal hypothyroidism associates with adverse obstetric outcomes and developmental delays in the offspring

Worry About

- Predisposition to hypothermia
- Neuromuscular weakness may impair weaning from mechanical ventilation

Overview

- A common condition, particularly in adult women
- Elevated thyrotropin (TSH) concentration in blood is hallmark laboratory finding and may be present months to years before decreased T_4 concentration.
- Adequacy of T_4 replacement defined by TSH concentrations in the low-normal range
- Total and free thyroxine (T_4) (and usually triiodothyronine [T_3]) concentrations usually reduced

- Symptomatic pts with TSH >10 mU/L should receive maintenance thyroid replacement. (levothyroxine 1.6 µg/kg daily).
- Pts presenting with severe, untreated hypothyroidism or myxedema coma may also demonstrate hypothermia, hypoventilation, hyponatremia, hypotension, heart failure, bowel obstruction, and hypoglycemia

ICD-9-CM Code: 244.9

Etiology

- Hypothyroidism (decreased thyroid hormone secretion) most often results from primary disease of thyroid gland (most commonly autoimmune thyroiditis). Less frequently it results from disorders of the pituitary gland or hypothalamus.
- Previous treatment for hyperthyroidism and previous total thyroidectomy are also relatively common causes of hypothyroidism.
- Pts with critical illness may have reduced total T_4 and reduced total and free T_3 despite normal TSH concentrations (euthyroid sick syndrome) but usually do not require thyroid hormone replacement.
- Primary TSH deficiency may result from pituitary tumors and cysts or their treatment (either surgery or radiation), pituitary infiltration, necrosis, or infarction; 2° TSH deficiency may result from congenital deficiency of thyrotropin-releasing hormone (TRH), radiation

therapy, infections, or tumors or cysts impinging on the hypothalamic-pituitary portal circulation.

Usual Treatment

- Maintenance outpatient therapy for adults consists of oral thyroxine 0.1–0.2 mg (1–3 µg/kg) daily.
- There may be a delay of up to 4 wk for TSH to stabilize after T_4 dosage adjustment.
- Long $T_{1/2}$ of T_4 (about a week) permits oral T_4 to be withheld safely for several NPO days.
- Chronic rifampin, carbamazepine, phenobarbital, and phenytoin, and increase T_4 dosage requirements by increasing metabolism or clearance of T_4.
- Pts with known or occult CAD may have increased symptoms unless T_4 replacement is initiated at a reduced dose and only cautiously increased.
- Myxedema coma may require use of IV T_3 (liothyronine) 0.15–0.3 µg/kg every 6 hr and IV hydrocortisone 0.5–1 mg/kg every 8 hr to cover for possible hypothyroid-impaired adrenal response to stress.
- IV liothyronine may also be indicated in other circumstances when peripheral conversion of T_4 to T_3 is impaired (e.g., hypothermic cardiopulmonary bypass).

ASSESSMENT POINTS

System	Effect	Assessment by Hx	PE	Test
HEENT	Puffiness below eyes, enlarged tongue	Snoring	Enlarged tongue	TSH, T_4 (or T_3) concentrations
CARDIO	Bradycardia, ↓ BP, heart failure	Palpitations, myocardial ischemia, arrhythmias, peripheral edema	Bradycardia, tachycardia	TSH, T_4 (or T_3) concentrations, ECG
RESP	Hypoventilation			TSH, T_4 (or T_3) concentrations; arterial Pco_2; or venous HCO_3^-
GI	Ileus, wt gain	Constipation, ascites	↓ Bowel sounds	TSH, T_4 (or T_3) concentrations
RENAL	Decreased free water clearance	Fluid retention, edema	Edema	TSH, T_4 (or T_3) concentrations; serum Na^+ concentration
CNS	Obtundation, depression, muscular weakness, cold intolerance	Lethargy, weakness, mental slowness	Decreased deep tendon reflexes, impaired mental status examination	TSH, T_4 (or T_3) concentrations

Key Reference: Vaidya B, Pearce SHS. Management of hypothyroidism in adults. *BMJ*. 2008;337:a801.

Perioperative Implications

Preoperative Preparation

- Chronic thyroid replacement to maintain euthyroid state

Monitoring

- Temp
- Other monitors as indicated by surgery

Airway

- Rarely incidence of macroglossia

Maintenance

- No effect of hypothyroidism on MAC for inhaled anesthetics

- Keep the pt warm
- Potential increased periop risk of heart failure, hypotension, and GI dysfunction (controversial)

Extubation

- Weaning from mechanical ventilation may be impaired.

Adjuvants

- None needed (except in cases of myxedema coma, in which IV liothyronine and hydrocortisone may be indicated

Anticipated Problems/Concerns

- Only those pts who have been inadequately treated with T_4 carry risks; those who chronically receive an appropriate dose of T_4 probably have (at most) minimally increased risks compared with other pts.
- Inadequately treated hypothyroidism can lead to lethargy and fatigue, wt gain, dementia, heart failure, resp insufficiency, fluid retention and edema, hyponatremia, clotting abn, and generalized weakness.

Hypoxemia

Risk

- All pts undergoing anesthesia and surgery (7–35% in large series have Pao_2 <60 mmHg in OR or PACU)
- Pts with pre-existing pulm disease

Perioperative Risks

- Hypoxemia may lead to hypoxia and eventual severe neurologic/cardiac sequelae or death

Worry About

- Inadequate delivery of O_2 to blood—greatest concern to the anesthesiologist is inadequate delivery of O_2 to pt
- Concern that inadequate delivery of O_2 to blood will lead to inadequate delivery of O_2 to tissues
- Misinterpretation of clinical manifestations of hypoxemia

Overview

- Hypoxemia:—Denotes low PaO_2 in blood (versus hypoxia, which denotes inadequate delivery of O_2 to tissues)
- Hypoxemia defined as resting Po_2 >2 SD below normal for age and FIO_2, SaO_2 <90%, PaO_2 <60 mmHg on room air, and a fall in SaO_2 >5%
- Multiple clues in vital signs and pt symptoms that should be assumed to be due to hypoxemia

ICD-9-CM Code: 799.0 (Hypoxia)

Etiology

- Decreased FIO_2 failure to provide adequate inspired O_2 (e.g., O_2 supply failure, gas machine disconnect, airway disconnect, pts at higher altitude)
- Inadequate alveolar ventilation or alveolar hypoventilation: Venous admixture accounts for majority of causes

- V/Q mismatch: Asthma, COPD, pulm embolism, pulm vascular disease, passive atelectasis due to pneumonia. Resorption atelectasis is most common when O_2 is taken up from an obstructed area of tracheobronchial tree; adhesive atelectasis seen with decreased surfactant; alveoli filled with blood, vomitus; FRC > closing capacity
- R to L cardiac shunts: ASD, VSD (*Note*: will not respond to increased FIO_2)
- Diffusion problems: Very rare cause

Usual Treatment

- Determine cause of decreased O_2 delivery and treat
- Increase FIO_2: This will help in all situations of hypoxemia except those due to R to L shunts

ASSESSMENT POINTS

System	Effect	Assessment by Hx	PE	Test
CARDIO	Sympathetic stimulation Htn Arrhythmia Bradycardia (late sign)	Htn	Tachycardia BP	ECG
RESP	Cyanosis Atelectasis lung collapse evidence of aspiration		Tachypnea	SaO_2 ABG Decreased PaO_2 CXR
CNS	Altered mental status	Anxiety Confusion seizures		

Key Reference: Blum JM, Fetterman DM, Park PK, Morris M, Rosenberg AL. A description of intraoperative ventilator management and ventilation strategies in hypoxic patients. *Anesth Analg*. 2010;110(6):1616–1622.

Perioperative Implications

Monitoring
- Routine: Pulse oximetry is mandatory
- ABGs

Airway
- Must ensure patency and intact circuit at all times

Maintenance
- Adequate FIO_2 and alveolar ventilation

Anticipate Problems/Concerns

- Must have a high index of suspicion whenever SaO_2 decreases or any of the clinical subjective or objective signs and symptoms are present. Always assume the decreased SaO_2 does not reflect a problem with the pulse oximeter but signifies a real problem. Stable vital signs may not fully eliminate significant arterial hypoxemia.

IgA Deficiency

Jahan Porhomayon
Paul R. Knight III

Risk

- The most common immunodeficiency disorder
- Incidence has been estimated to be 1/100 to 1/1000
- More prevalent among European descendants
- Most pts are clinically normal
- Increased risk of allergies and anaphylaxis
- Increased risk of malignancies

Perioperative Risks

- Increased incidence of pulm complications, atopic disorders, and postop infections

Worry About

- Recurrent sinopulmonary infections leading to decreased pulm reserve
- Associated autoimmune disorders (e.g., lupus, DiGeorge syndrome)

- Associated GI disorders leading to volume depletion
- Anaphylactic reactions from transfusion of blood products containing IgA

Overview

- An immunodeficiency syndrome with increased susceptibility to nosocomial infection
- Cell-mediated immunity is usually nml
- Co-existing diseases may incl atopy, recurrent sinopulmonary infection, GI disease, and autoimmune disease
- Decreased synthesis or secretion of IgA

ICD-9-CM Code: 279.01

Etiology

- Absence of IgA on mucosal surface

- Decreased IgA blocking antibodies against environmental antigens
- Associated with histocompatibility groups HLA-A1, -B8, and -Dw3
- There have been several reported cases of acquired IgA deficiency
- Usually decreased rather than absent lymphocyte IgA secretion
- Overt clinical disease presentation may relate to changes in IgG subclass and/or compensatory IgM secretion

Usual Treatment

- Do not treat with gammaglobulin
- Increased suspicion of infections and aggressive antibiotic therapy
- Therapy directed toward specific co-existing disease(s)

ASSESSMENT POINTS

System	Effect	Assessment by Hx	PE	Test
CARDIO	Decreased reserve, hypovolemia	Dypnea or exertion	Tachycardia, orthostatic hypotension	ECG, ECHO
RESP	Recurrent sinopulmonary infection, hemosiderosis, asthma	↓ Exercise tolerance	Wheezing, rales	CXR, PFTs Sinus x-rays
GI	Chronic gastroenteritis, malnutrition, malabsorption	Chronic diarrhea	Cachexia	Electrolytes, BUN, serum albumin
HEME	Nonspecific	Depends on the extent of co-existing diseases		Serum IgA, anti-IgA antibody, Coombs' test
RENAL	Nonspecific	Varies in severity depending on the extent of co-existing diseases		BUN, Cr
CNS	Degenerative, demyelinating	Mental retardation associated with ataxia-telangiectasia		MRI

Key Reference: Knight PR. In: Lema MI, ed. *Problems in anesthesia*. Philadelphia: JB Lippincott; 1993:375–391.

Perioperative Implications

Preoperative Preparation
- Consider antibiotic therapy
- Work up any indication of infection
- Optimize any underlying organ dysfunction and volume status

Monitoring
- Consider invasive hemodynamic monitoring in debilitated pts

Airway
- Strict aseptic technique
- Universal precautions
- May encounter difficult intubation in pts with associated rheumatoid arthritis

Induction
- Hypotension 2° to hypovolemia and/or decreased cardiac reserve
- Wheezing allergies relatively resistant to conventional therapy

Maintenance
- May require high inspired O_2
- Regional anesthesia and careful titration of anesthetic agents due to potential underlying CV and pulm diseases
- Use only thoroughly washed RBC transfusions

Extubation
- Careful assessment of neuromuscular function due to potential drug-drug interaction

Adjuvants
- Depend on organ dysfunction

Postoperative Period
- May require intensive pulm therapy
- Maintain strict antiseptic precaution
- Increased suspicion of bacterial infection

Anticipated Problems/Concerns

- Anaphylactic reaction from transfusions of blood or blood products containing IgA to individual with IgA antibodies
- Asthmatic pt with IgA deficiency is relatively resistant to treatment
- Increased risk of nosocomial infection

Immune Suppression

Padmavathi R. Perela
Paul R. Knight III

DISEASES

Risk

- Incidence in USA: 0.25 to 1.5% of population has HIV or other cause of immune suppression
- 20–25% of HIV infected pts will require surgery
- Major risk factors: Neutropenia, yeast overgrowth, and/or nosocomial colonization of skin and mucosa

Perioperative Risks

- 22.2% 30-d mortality in one study of AIDS pts undergoing intra-abdominal surgery
- Mortality greatest at the extremes of age
- Greatest source of morbidity and mortality is 2° to infection
- Pneumonia accounts for ~40% of all deaths
- Increased incidence of postop pneumonia, wound infection, postop sepsis, resp insufficiency, SIRS, and hypotension due to CV instability
- Increased healing time

Worry About

- Nosocomial transmission of infection
- Interactions with other drugs (IV street drugs, antiviral agents)
- Transmission of pathogenic drug-resistant strains of microbial agents to medical personnel (e.g., new strains of TB)
- Decreased pulm reserve due to repeated infections
- Decreased myocardial reserve 2° to underlying disease and generalized poor health
- Translocation of intestinal bacteria due to severe mucositis

Overview

- Immune suppression can arise from multiple causes both primary and acquired
- Intraop, surgical trauma, anesthetic agents, blood transfusion with/without severe hemorrhage decreases the immune response

ICD-9-CM Code: 279.3 (Immune deficiency)

Etiology

- Primary immune deficiency (most are familial)
- The very young have immature immune systems
- Aging alters some cellular immune responses
- Acquired
  - Malnutrition, drugs (glucocorticoids, chemotherapy, antiviral), massive burns, or trauma
  - Cancers (leukemia, lymphoma, and multiple myeloma)
  - Infections (HIV stages 2-4, influenza, sepsis),
  - Smoking decreases resp defense mechanisms

Usual Treatment

- Selective use of antibiotic prophylaxis, antivirals (e.g., acyclovir), antifungal agents (e.g., fluconazole), or immune enhancement (e.g., immune globulin)
- Strict sterile procedures and universal precautions
- Fastidious personal hygiene

ASSESSMENT POINTS

System	Effect	Assessment by Hx	PE	Test
HEME	Anemia, neutropenia, lymphocytopenia, hypoglobulinemia, recurrent bacteremia, coagulation abn, thrombocytopenia	Easy fatigue, recurrent fever, sweats, and chills	Pale, petechiae	Hct/Hgb, WBC, platelets, plasma proteins, coagulation studies, special lymphocyte counts (e.g., CD4+ cells)
CARDIO	SBE, decreased CV reserve, hypovolemia, drug-induced injury (e.g., arabinomycin), mycotic aneurysms, pericardial effusion, vasculitis, pulm Htn	Decreased exercise tolerance	Murmurs, orthostatic hypotension, abn HR	ECG, ECHO
RESP	Recurrent acute pulm infections, pulm fibrosis, pulm obstruction, chronic TB and/or fungal infections	Decreased exercise tolerance	Airway lesions	CXR, spirometry
GI	Chronic gastroenteritis, chronic malnutrition, severe mucositis	Severe "cramping", dysphagia, odynophagia diarrhea	Cachexia, leukoplakia	Electrolytes, albumin Blood cultures
RENAL	Chronic pyelonephritis, bladder infections, chronic cystitis, drug-induced nephropathy (e.g., cyclosporine), end-stage renal pathology	Recurrent UTIs, frequency		BUN, Cr, pyelogram
CNS	Mycotic infarcts, AIDS, dementia and encephalopathy	Minor strokes	Focal deficits, decreased mental function	Brain scan
MS	Osteomyelitis	Deep pain located over involved area	Point tenderness	X-ray

Key Reference: Knight PR. In: Lema MJ, ed. *Problems in anesthesia*. Philadelphia: JB Lippincott; 1993:375–391.

Perioperative Implications

Preoperative Preparation
- Continue or initiate antibiotic therapy and immune therapy
- Assess and optimize underlying organ system dysfunction (HIV-associated cardiomyopathy).
- Assess volume status and electrolytes due to chronic diarrhea
- Involved assessment may be required (pulm function tests, ECHO cardiography).
- Identify timing of administration of immune suppressive drug(s)

Monitoring
- Consider arterial line, PA line, or other invasive hemodynamic monitors in severely debilitated pts

Airway
- Strict aseptic technique and universal precautions when handling the airway
- Examination of upper airway for potentially obstructive lesions (i.e., Kaposi's sarcoma)

Induction
- Chronic resp injury due to repeated lung infections may cause rapid desaturation.
- Hypotension due to decreased myocardial reserve and/or relative hypovolemia
- Decreased drug requirements 2° to decreased plasma proteins

Maintenance
- Increased inspired O₂ may be required due to chronic lung infections.
- Decreased myocardial reserve may require careful selection and titration of anesthetic agents or local or regional anesthesia for peripheral procedures.
- Pre-emptive pain management may protect against additional immune suppression

Extubation
- Due to weakness and drug-drug interactions, return of strength should be carefully evaluated.

Adjuvants
- Transplantation and anticancer drug interactions need to be considered (e.g., cyclosporine

and barbiturates, narcotics, and muscle relaxants); bleomycin and O₂ administration

Postoperative Period
- Resp adequacy should be carefully followed and may require intensive care monitoring.
- Maintain careful antisepsis procedures for extended periods.

Anticipated Problems/Concerns

- The greatest intraop risk to these pts is infection; therefore, strict hygienic practices are required.
- The general state of nutrition, recurrent infections, and the underlying cause of the immune suppression all tend to generally decrease resp reserve and CV stability.
- Risk of transmission of drug-resistant pathogenic microbial agents to medical personnel (needle stick or resp, e.g., drug resistant TB). Follow CDC recommendations if exposed.

Implantable Cardioverter-Defibrillators (ICDs)

Marc A. Rozner

Epidemiology

- 450,000 pts/y in USA suffer sudden cardiac arrest (SCA); 550,000 new cases /y of CHF
- Incidence in USA: Approx 300,000 have implantable cardioverter-defibrillator (ICD)
- Incidence worldwide: Approx 500,000 have an ICD
- ICD therapy for SCA, VT, VF and primary prevention remains substantially better than drug therapy.
- Associated diseases incl cardiomyopathy, CAD, long QT syndrome, arrhythmogenic right ventricular dysplasia, Brugada syndrome, and LV noncompaction. Some pts will also have sinus node and/or AV nodal disease.
- New implants (based on registry data) currently exceed 10,000 per mo in USA
- ICD implant is indicated for any cause cardiomyopathy with EF ≤35% and without evidence of dysrhythmia; thus some pts undergo ICD implantation for primary prevention.
- At current implant and survival rates, nearly 700,000 pts in USA with ICD in 2020
- ALL ICDs can provide pacing for bradycardia; some pts might be pacing dependent.
- Some ICDs also have atrial, RV, and LV pacing capability for cardiac resynchronization therapy (CRT).
- Premature ICD failure rate might approach 2%. For the ICD pt without evidence of pacing, determining battery function is difficult.*

Perioperative Risks

- No proven increase in risk due to ICD itself, although an inappropriate high voltage therapy (HVT) might induce tachydysrhythmia, injure the myocardium releasing troponin, or both.
- These pts might be at increased risk owing to associated disease(s).
- Risk related to incorrect interpretation of events (pseudomalfunction), which is similar to the issues with pacing
- Risk related to incorrect interpretation of device type, i.e., confusing an ICD for a pacemaker, because ICD pts tend to have more medical issues and ICDs are more complicated

Worry About

- EMI entering the ICD on the ventricular channel, which might result in an ICD discharge. For the pacing dependent pt, EMI-induced ventricular oversensing with pacing inhibition can also result in asystole.
- Intraop increase in ventricular pacing owing to EMI entering a dual chamber DDD ICD on the atrial channel with resultant tracking
- Intraop increases in pacing rates with misinterpretation as inadequate anesthesia owing to activation of the exercise sensor, whether due to direct mechanical stimulation (such as preparation of the chest) or pressure on the device (personnel leaning)
- Failure to capture (i.e., pacing output without depolarization) due to inadequate preop output (i.e., inadequate safety margin) or increase in pacing threshold, which can result from myocardial ischemia/infarction, drug administration, or electrolyte shifts. Note that any or all chambers can undergo failure to capture, with possible hemodynamic derangement but not apparent outright pacing failure.
- Magnet† placement will change pacing rates only in ICDs from ELA (Sorin, Milan, Italy). Only Boston Scientific (BOS)‡ ICDs emit tones confirming appropriate magnet placement. NO confirmation of magnet placement is available in Medtronic, St Jude Medical (SJM), or Biotronik ICD. ICDs from BOS and SJM can have the magnet switch disabled by programming. In fact, some older ICDs from BOS (with the "GDT" or "CPI" x-ray code) can undergo permanent disabling of tachy therapy by magnet placement.
- Careful attention to sterility (gown, gloves, hat, mask, body drape) if central access is placed. ICDs should have HVT disabled during central access procedures in the chest to prevent inappropriate discharge due to guidewire contact with the RV lead. Central line placement in the chest is relatively contraindicated for the first 6 wk of implant for any new lead.

Overview

- Indications for initial ICD placement: SCA (incl spontaneous or induced VT or VF), cardiomyopathy from any cause with LV EF ≤35%, long QT syndrome, arrhythmogenic RV dysplasia, Brugada syndrome.
- Despite considerable "intelligence", inappropriate shocks are delivered to 10–15% of pts.

- Tachydysrhythmia therapy in most devices incl antitachycardia pacing (ATP), which uses less battery energy and is better tolerated (sometimes not even noticed) by pts. Some ICDs will deliver ATP while charging.
- Codes: The NASPE / BPEG generic defibrillator code has 4 positions. The 1st position refers to the chamber(s) shocked (A=atrium, V=ventricle, D=both, O=none). The 2nd position refers to the chamber(s) where ATP is programmed (A,V, D, O). The 3rd identifies the detection method: either heart rate (E=electrogram) or hemodynamic (H), although no hemodynamic sensors are currently in clinical use. The 4th position identifies chambers (A, V, D, O) where pacing for bradycardia has been programmed. The most robust form of this code uses only the first 3 positions and adds the 5-position generic pacemaker code. Thus a current model ICD with anti-afib therapy and CRT might be DDE-DDDRV.

ICD-9-CM Code: V53.32 (Implanted cardioverter-defibrillator)

Indications and Usual Treatment

- Primary prevention in a pt with LVEF ≤35% (and more than 40 d from an ischemic event or 3 mo from vascular intervention) who is receiving optimal medical therapy and has a reasonable expectation of survival with good functional capacity for >1 y
- Survivors of cardiac arrest presumably due to VT/VF, not associated with reversible factors, such as acute coronary syndrome
- Pts with inducible VT/VF by EP study and no reversible cause
- Treatment for LV cardiomyopathy should incl (unless a contraindication is noted on the chart): beta blocker and ACE inhibitor and/or angiotensin receptor blocker therapy (see ACC/AHA Heart Failure Guidelines). Many pts will also have antiarrhythmic, diuretic, nitrate, or digoxin therapy.

ASSESSMENT POINTS

System	Effect	Assessment by Hx	PE	Test
CARDIO	Myocardial ischemia LV dysfunction Heart rate (guidelines suggest <80 bpm) Frequency of ICD therapy Need for pacing	Angina symptoms Exercise tolerance, DOE	ECG, pulse S_3, rales	Nuclear imaging Echocardiography B-type natriuretic peptide ICD interrogation
RESP	Amiodarone toxicity	Exercise tolerance, DOE		SpO_2, CXR, PFTs, ABGs
ENDO	Amiodarone toxicity			TSH, T_4
RENAL	Renal insufficiency		Edema	BUN, Cr
NEURO	CV disease	Stroke, TIAs	Bruits	Carotid duplex
LYTES	Reversible VT/VF	Diuretic Chemotherapy (platins)		Serum K^+ and Mg^{2+}

Key Reference: Rozner MA. Pacemakers and implanted cardioverter-defibrillators. In: Miller RD, Eriksson LI, Fleisher LA, Wiener-Kronish JP, Young WL, eds. *Miller's anesthesia*. 7th ed. Philadelphia: Churchill Livingstone / Elsevier; 2009:1387–1409 [Chapter 43].

Perioperative Implications

Preoperative Preparation

• Comprehensive ICD evaluation and/or interrogation should be performed in a timely manner (<3 mo) prior to surgery. An EP pacing and/or ICD service consult might be needed. The remaining battery life, tachy zones and therapies, pacing behavior, and prior dysrhythmia treatment should be documented. Many ICDs have ventricular-only (VVI) pacing capability; for the pt with intact atria and AV node, periop care must be directed to prevent the sinus rate from falling below the VVI pacing rate, since ventricular-only pacing will likely compromise hemodynamics. For the pt with hemodynamically advantageous pacing capability who is chronotropically incompetent or pacing dependent, consideration should be given to increasing the pacing rate for a significant procedure.

• For ventricular multisite pacing (called cardiac resynchronization therapy), assurance that the LV pacing lead is functioning. If central access is planned in a CRT pt, a recent CXR might be prudent to document the position of the LV lead.

• Alternate defibrillation (and pacing modality [e.g., transvenous, transcutaneous] for the pacing-dependent pt) should be available. While transesophageal pacing might work as backup, it is contraindicated in atrial fibrillation, AV nodal block, and any pt with a permanently implanted pacing device.

• IV chronotropes (epinephrine, ephedrine)

• Discuss monopolar electrosurgery (ESU) precautions with surgeon and nursing staff. If monopolar ESU will be needed, then the ICD should have the HVT disabled for the procedure. If magnet use is planned for this function, the interrogation should ensure that a magnet mode is present and enabled.

• Regional technique offers CNS perfusion monitoring.

• Placement of defibrillation pads should be considered, esp. if a pt has been receiving HVT from the ICD.

Monitoring

• Mechanical pulse wave monitoring is required. It can be accomplished with the pulse oximeter plethysmogram, any invasive hemodynamic monitoring modality, or Doppler technique.

• Electrocardiographic (ECG) monitoring is required by ASA standards, but EMI perturbs the signal, and monitors frequently report incorrect heart rates (both too high and too low).

• For high risk cases with large potential fluid shifts, TEE might be indicated.

Induction

• Succinylcholine or etomidate might lead to inappropriate muscle activity, resulting in pacing inhibition, increased rates, or false VT/VF detection, but this has not been reported for ICDs. Succinylcholine-induced K⁺ fluxes theoretically can change pacing thresholds, but this has not been reported.

Maintenance

• Vigilant ECG/pulse monitoring

• Monopolar electrosurgical (ESU) cautery (i.e., the Bovie), which emits radiofrequency energy, has potential to cause inappropriate VT/VF detection (and HVT) as well as transient or permanent changes in ICD function. The most common problem is inhibition of pacing. Prevention includes: use of bipolar-only ESU, use of pure unblended monopolar ESU, and placement of the ESU current return pad so that the presumed current path of the ESU does not cross the chest. For all head and neck or contralateral breast surgery, the pad can be placed on the shoulder contralateral to the CIED. For ipsilateral breast surgery, the pad can be placed on the ipsilateral arm and the wire prepped into the field if needed.

• Magnet: Assuming that the magnet is appropriately placed and that the magnet mode is enabled, placement might be useful to suspend HVT. NO ICD provides asynchronous pacing upon application of a magnet, and, except for ELA (Sorin) ICDs, no ICD will change its pacing rate in response to appropriate magnet placement. If interference from the ESU creates hemodynamically challenging issues, the current return pad should be relocated to the extent possible (for abdominal or pelvic surgery the pad could be moved to the other leg) or the ICD will require reprogramming.

Postoperative Period

• Monitoring of mechanical pulse in the postoperative care unit

• ICD interrogation/reprogramming required if ICD was reprogrammed preop; advisable if monopolar ESU employed, any problems noted, or cardioversion/defibrillation has taken place.

• Some pts will require pacing changes to incl increased pacing rate, disabling of battery saving features, and adjustments to AV delays to optimize postop hemodynamics

• Other risks related to associated medical problems

Anticipated Problems/Concerns

• Inappropriate delivery of HVT, which will occur without warning if due to EMI and will likely be missed by the intraop personnel

• Intraop failure to pace, most likely related to monopolar electrosurgery

• Periop pacing and sensing threshold changes

• Risks related to associated medical problems

• Iatrogenic misadventures resulting from misunderstanding of pacing system behavior

---

* Some ICDs allow demonstration of battery function without interrogation:
-Boston Scientific‡ ICDs will emit beeps if the magnet switch is enabled and the magnet is appropriately placed. A constant tone indicates that the ICD is disabled. No tone indicates magnet switch deactivation or a dead battery
-ELA (Sorin) ICDs will change pacing rate to 90 bpm if battery ok, 80 if elective replacement. But the patient rate must be less than 90 (80) to observe this function. No change indicates battery or other failure
-Medtronic ICDs will emit a tone for at least 15 seconds when the magnet switch (nonprogrammable) is activated, even briefly, by a magnet. A warbling tone indicates a problem with the ICD, and no tone indicates a nonfunctioning device.

†MAGNET CAUTION: NO ICD provides asynchronous pacing to appropriate magnet placement. Only ICDs from ELA (Sorin) will change pacing rate (to 90 bpm if battery is ok) upon appropriate magnet placement. For many ICDs (Boston Scientific§ and St Jude Medical§), the magnet switch can be programmed "OFF." Only ICDs from Boston Scientific and its previous companies emit tones that identify correct placement of a magnet. Some older ICDs from Boston Scientific (with the "GDT" or "CPI" xray code) can undergo permanent disabling of tachy therapy by magnet placement.

‡Boston Scientific owns the Guidant and CPI brands, and St Jude Medical owns the Pacesetter brand.

Infratentorial Tumors

Tod B. Sloan

Risk

- Highest incidence: Age 3–12 and 55–65 y
- 2/3 of children: ~1.6–2.2/100,000 children – 1,300–2,000 new tumors in USA
- 1/3 of adult tumors: ~14,600 adults in the USA had new tumors in 2005

Perioperative Risks

- Very confined space, brain tolerates tumor poorly leading to symptoms and less forgiving with surgery than supratentorial
- CSF obstruction with hydrocephalus common, ICP tolerated poorly

Worry About

- Increasing ICP, hydrocephalus
- Impaired protective airway reflexes, aspiration
- Irregular resp due to brainstem compression, swelling
- Impaired level of consciousness

Overview

- Survival 60% in children
- Prognosis is poor with glioblastoma, infiltrating brainstem glioma.
- Benign lesions such as meningioma, acoustic neuroma have low morbidity, mortality, but may recur if resection is incomplete.
- Degree of head elevation influences incidence, severity of air embolism (sitting > prone > park bench/lateral position).

ICD-9-CM Codes: 191.6; 191.7; 225.1; 225.2

Etiology

- Primary intra-axial lesions are generally malignant; extra-axial lesions are typically benign.
- Children primary most common: Astrocytoma, medulloblastoma, brainstem glioma are the most common posterior fossa tumors in children. Most common tumors in child age 3–12 y
- <1 y, astrocytoma, cerebellar PNET medulloblastoma common, epidymoma, brainstem glioma
- <2 y, 70% are medulloblastoma and low-grade glioma
- Pediatric cystic cerebellar astrocytoma is associated with 80% survival at 20 y
- Adult, most are metastases or acoustic tumors (most >60 y are acoustic)
- Acoustic neuroma (assoc neurofibromatosis NF II), metastases, meningioma are the most common posterior fossa tumors in adults. Metastases (lung and breast most common and vasogenic so inc ICP common). Metastases to cerebellum forms mass lesion.
- Differentiate from AVM and aneurysms
- Neurofibromatosis with some acoustic neuromas

Usual Treatment

- Surgical removal or debulking
- CSF diversion (ventriculostomy or shunt)
- Dexamethasone to decreased peritumor vasogenic edema
- Primary or adjuvant radiotherapy

ASSESSMENT POINTS

System	Effect	Assessment by Hx	PE	Test
HEENT	Tonsillar herniation, cranial nerve VII compression	Dysphagia, change in voice tinnitus, vertigo	Gag dysfunction, hyperthermia, ipsilateral hearing impairment	Indirect laryngoscopy, hearing exam
CARDIO, HEME	Progressive brainstem compression, ischemic cardiomyopathy		Cushing response: Htn, bradycardia, raised ICP, S_3 gallop, CHF	ECG, HCT, T&C
RESP	Progressive tonsillar herniation		Hyperventilation, irregular resp, apnea	CT exam, MRI
RENAL, GI	↑ ICP	N/V (esp. near 4th ventricle)		CT scan, MRI, glucose
CNS	↑ ICP	Listlessness, headache, nausea, drowsiness, diplopia	Papilledema, classic triad (headache, vomiting, ataxia)	CT scan, MRI
MS	Lesion in cerebellar hemisphere or midline	Truncal ataxia	Nystagmus hypotonia, limb ataxia intention tremor	Extraocular movement abnormalities

Key Reference: Irefin SA, Schubert A, Bloomfield EL, DeBoer GE, Mascha EJ, Ebrahim ZY. The effect of craniotomy location on postoperative pain and nausea. *J Anesth.* 2003;17(4):227–231.

Perioperative Implications

Preoperative Preparation

- Neuro exam: Cranial nerve deficits
- Presence and status of VP shunt
- Patent foramen ovale if sitting position
- Assess volume status from decreased intake, vomiting, diuresis (will increase risk of hypotension if sitting).
- Avoid narcotic premedication or any resp depressants if risk of ↑ ICP.

Monitoring

- Goals are maintenance of adequate CNS perfusion and cardiorespiratory stability, detection/treatment of air embolism, and surgical brainstem compression.
- Monitor CPP (MAP-ICP) measure BP at ear level; watch for hypotension when sitting.
- Capnography, precordial Doppler US, right atrial catheter for air embolism detection/retrieval (TEE if available),
- Brainstem auditory evoked responses and cranial nerve VII stimulation may reduce morbidity from surgical manipulation. SSEP, MEP, and multiple cranial nerves often monitored.
- Watch for deep breath from brainstem compression resp center, watch for BP decreases and arrhythmias from brainstem compression.
- ECG, pulse oximetry to watch for arrhythmias (bradycardia common) from manipulation of brainstem cranial nuclei and dura (innervated by vagus n.) Avoid treating with anticholinergic as eliminate heart rate as monitor of brainstem
- If sitting position: Precordial Doppler and CVP with tip at right atrium needed.
- Watch eyes if prone for pressure and prep solutions

Airway

- Verify appropriate ETT position after final positioning; avoid large bite blocks and oral airways to minimize tongue and soft tissue compression, postop airway swelling.
- Watch for ETT kinking with neck flexion (armored tube if indicated).

Induction

- Hypotension on induction can be offset by pre-induction IV hydration.

Maintenance

- Positioning: Protect eyes, kink vertebral artery when truning head
- Preserve autonomic reflexes; avoid long-acting vasodilators.
- Monitor for changes in electrolyte balance due to loop and osmotic diuretics, replace diuresis if needed.
- Maintain normothermia, normovolemia, normotension, normnatremic fluids.
- Avoid hyperglycemia and hyperthermia.
- Controlled PPV, adequate hydration decreases risk of air embolism
- Avoid NMB with cranial nerve and MEP monitoring.
- Limited inhalational agents with SSEP and TIVA if MEP monitored.
- Dose, redose antibiotics
- Avoid anticholinergics and beta blockers to mask CV changes with brainstem compression

Extubation

- Pt should be awake, following commands, and showing return of protective airway reflexes (swallow)

Adjuvants

- Short-acting vasopressors or vasodilators for maintenance of CV stability
- Antiemetics

Postoperative Period

- Suspect brainstem compression or hematoma if postop Htn or profound bradycardia persists in previously normotensive pt.
- Suspect brainstem injury if persistent hypotension or apnea.
- Avoid potent narcotic analgesic drugs that may produce hypercarbia, decreased intracranial compliance.

Anticipated Problems/Concerns

- Intraop air embolism: Notify surgeon who should flood field, turn off N_2O if on, acute CPAP may help find source, lay down supine if needed.
- Pts with higher-grade malignancy have greater likelihood of postop brain swelling.
- Postop inability to protect airway (loss of lower cranial nerves) watch for swallowing prior to extubation, use NG if question
- Loss resp drive in brainstem injury resp center
- Delayed awakening from pneumocephalus if sitting position (tension possible requiring relief), also supratentorial hemorrhage when sitting
- Massive tongue swelling, cervical spinal cord ischemia if sitting position
- Loss facial nerve (corneal ulceration from failed eye closing)
- Aseptic mengitis (blood irritating meninges)

Insulinoma

Jesse J. Muir
Molly Solorzano

DISEASES

Risk

- Most common functional islet cell tumor of pancreas
- Incidence 1–4/100,000 person-years
- Mean age of onset: 47 y
- Presentation earlier (mean age 25 y) if part of multiple endocrine neoplasia syndrome type 1 (MEN-1)
- More common in females

Perioperative Risks

- Hypoglycemia

Worry About

- Preop and intraop hypoglycemia
- Post-excision rebound hyperglycemia (not always present and not reliable to validate completeness of resection)
- Possibility of MEN-1 or multiple islet cell tumors

Overview

- 80–90% are <2cm, solitary, and benign
- Malignant lesions typically invade locally into surrounding soft tissue or structures, to the lymph nodes, or to the liver
- Insulinomas are found equally distributed throughout the pancreas (i.e., head, body, and tail)
- 5–10% occur in the setting of MEN-1; increased risk of recurrence if associated with MEN-1
- Presentation: Post-absorptive hypoglycemia (fasting hypoglycemia), hypoglycemia after exercise, awakening at night to eat, wt gain due to frequent meals to avoid hypoglycemic symptoms
- Differential diagnosis: Factitious hypoglycemia, liver or metabolic disease, noninsulinoma pancreatogenous hypoglycemia syndrome (NIPHS)
- NIPHS is associated with diffuse islet cell hyperplasia and presents with postprandial symptomatology rather than postabsorptive
- Dx strongly suggested by Whipple's triad: (1) symptoms of hypoglycemia provoked by fasting; (2) blood glucose levels <50 mg/dL; and (3) relief of symptoms with glucose administration
- Typically, blood glucose <45 mg/dL, insulin level >6uU/mL, and C-peptide elevated to >200pmol/L
- Gold standard for Dx: Measurement of plasma glucose, insulin, C-peptide, and pro-insulin during a 72 hr fast with or without betahydroxybutyrate and absence of plasma levels of sulfonylurea
- Preop localization techniques incl: CT, MRI, PET, endoscopic US, octretotide scintigraphy, selective mesenteric angiography with intra-arterial calcium stimulation, and hepatic venous sampling for plasma insulin. Extensive preop imaging may not be helpful.

- 20–60% of insulinomas remain undetected at the time of surgery, likely due to small size and/or decreased density of somatostatin receptor subtypes compared to other neuroendocrine tumors.
- Recent data suggests intraop US along with surgical exposure and palpation is the most cost-effective approach.
- Gold standard is firm biochemical Dx and selected preop imaging along with thorough pancreatic exploration and intraop US
- In absence of preop localization and intraop detection, blind pancreatic resection is not recommended.
- **Neurogenic symptoms are 2° to autonomic system discharge in response to hypoglycemia. Neuroglycopenic symptoms are 2° to CNS glucose deprivation.**

ICD-9-CM: 211.7 (Benign neoplasm of islets of Langerhans)

Etiology

- Unknown: Most are solitary adenomas
- 5–10% of insulinomas assoc with the autosomal dominant MEN-1 syndrome

Usual Treatment

- Operative management only curative option
- Laparoscopic (14% conversion rate) versus open
- Most studies conclude laparoscopic approach feasible and safe, esp. for benign and distal pancreatic tumors (role for pancreatic stump and malignant lesions remains more controversial)
- Enucleation may be performed for lesions that are clearly localized preop, near or at the pancreatic surface, and easily defined intraop
- Resection recommended for lesions that are multiple, near the pancreatic duct or major vessels, MEN-1 cases, and suspected malignancy (infiltrating tumor, puckering of surrounding soft tissue, distal dilation of pancreatic duct, or lymph node involvement)
- Medical management reserved for unresectable malignant disease, high-risk surgical candidates, or unsuccessful operation with persistent symptoms
- Medical treatment of unresectable disease consists of small frequent meals, diazoxide, verapamil, and octreotide
- Octreotide is a somatostatin analogue that relieved symptoms in 50% of pts.
- Octreotide should be used with caution because many insulinomas lack octreotide receptors. Treatment may fail to suppress insulin production and blunt compensatory growth hormone and glucagon response leading to worsening hypoglycemia.
- Molecular targets are being investigated.

Perioperative Implications

Preoperative Preparation

- Maintain/optimize physiologic condition
- Evaluate for MEN-1
- Avoid severe hypoglycemia with frequent meals, avoidance of prolonged exercise
- Diazoxide, octreotide, and verapamil to control hypoglycemia if necessary
- Admit the night before and maintain on 10% dextrose infusion while NPO
- Remove dextrose from IV solution just prior to entering the operative room
- Monitor plasma glucose every 10–15 min

Monitoring

- Measure plasma glucose every 10–15 min
- Maintain plasma glucose >60 mg/dL
- Consider arterial line and/or CVP to facilitate sampling ease

Airway

- Nothing specific, although these pts may have significant wt gain

Induction

- Propofol has not been shown to significantly affect the release of insulin or glucose regulation

Maintenance

- Length of procedure highly variable
- Careful attention to fluid status
- Have dextrose solutions available to treat hypoglycemia

Extubation

- Nothing specific

Anticipated Problems/Concerns

- It has been proposed that glucose solutions be avoided intraop so that hyperglycemic rebound can be used to confirm tumor removal.
- More recent studies show that less than half of pts will have this rebound in the first 30 min following tumor removal, and therefore, hyperglycemic rebound cannot be used as proof of complete tumor removal.
- Intraop insulin assays may be an alterative.
- Pts who have hyperglycemic rebound and/or successful tumor removal can still have hypoglycemic episodes, so pts must be monitored for hypoglycemia in the postop period
- Most pts are discharged home with nml fasting glucose levels
- Postop complications incl pancreatic duct leak causing pseudocyst, abscess, and/or fistula (octreotide can be used to decrease fistula output)

ASSESSMENT POINTS

System	Effect	Assessment by Hx	PE	Test
RENAL	Renal stones if MEN-1	Renal colic	Flank pain	Serum Ca^{2+}
ENDO	MEN-1	Renal colic	Flank pain	Parathyroid hormone, serum Ca^{2+}
	Pituitary tumors	Vision changes	Signs of pituitary dysfunction	Skull x-rays and appropriate endocrine tests
	Insulinoma	Neurogenic symptoms: Hunger, sweating, and paresthesias (cholinergic) and anxiety, tremor, and palpitations (adrenergic) Neuroglycopenic symptoms: Behavioral changes, death, confusion, vision changes, fatigue, seizure, loss of consciousness	Mental status exam	Fasting glucose, insulin levels, C-peptide
CNS	Symptoms of hypoglycemia	Neuroglycopenic symptoms	Mental status exam	Blood glucose

Key Reference: Abood GJ, Go A, Malhotra D, Shoup M. The surgical and systemic management of neuroendocrine tumors of the pancreas. *Surg Clin North Am.* 2009;89(1):249–266.

Intracranial Hypertension (ICH)

Kevin J. Gingrich

Risk

- Incidence in USA: >50% of pts presenting with head trauma or other intracranial pathology (>600,000/y)
- Gender predominance: Depends on etiology

Perioperative Risks

- Increased risk of brain ischemia and herniation leading to brain infarction, disability, coma, and death
- Increased risk of permanent CNS dysfunction

Worry About

- Controlling intracranial pressure and preventing brain ischemia/herniation
- CV and resp instability
- Co-existing injuries in trauma pts (occult cervical spine and intra-abdominal injuries)

Overview

- Intracranial compartment has fixed volume with three components (brain = 85%, CSF = 10%, cerebral blood volume [CBV] = 5%)
- Increased volume of one component (e.g., tumor, hydrocephalus, or hemorrhage) elevates ICP, leading to ICH (ICP >20 mmHg, >40 mmHg = severe life-threatening)
- ICH reduces CPP = MAP – ICP, causing brain ischemia and/or infarction
- ICH causes intracranial pressure gradients that may extrude brain parenchyma through dural or bony passages, resulting in herniation
- Some anesthetic agents, Htn, hypercapnia, and hypoxemia increase CBF, increasing CBV and ICP

ICD-9-CM Code: 348.2 (Benign)

Etiology

- Usually a 2° process accompanying other pathology (e.g., head injuries, hemorrhage, hydrocephalus, abscess, 1° and metastatic brain tumors, cerebral infarcts, hypertensive and metabolic encephalopathies, venous thrombosis, infection, burns, near-drowning, and status epilepticus) that increases brain, CSF, or cerebral blood volumes

Usual Treatment

- Treatment of 1° disease (e.g., removal of tumor, hematoma, or abscess)
- Control ventilation, avoid hypoxemia (PaO_2 >90 torr), hyper- and hypocapnia
- Establish stable hemodynamics (normotension but estimated CPP > 60 mmHg)
- Head elevation (head above heart) and neutral neck position to promote cerebral venous return
- Osmotic therapy (mannitol or hypertonic saline) to decrease brain size
- Corticosteroids (neoplasm or abscess)
- CSF drainage
- Sedation and NMB in responsive pts

ASSESSMENT POINTS

System	Effect	Assessment by Hx	PE	Test
CV	Dysrhythmias, unstable vital signs Inferior wall myocardial ischemia		BP Pulse S_3 gallop	Tachycardia, bradycardia, prolonged QT interval, ECG, ECHO
RESP	Irregular breathing		Resp rate and pattern	
GI	Reduced gut motility	Vomiting		
RENAL	SIADH Central DI		Oliguria Polyuria	Urinalysis, serum electrolytes
CNS	Altered function	Headache, vomiting, unconsciousness	Neurologic deficits, papilledema	Direct ICP measurement (ventriculostomy, intracranial bolt, etc.)

Key Reference: Kofke WA, Stiefel M. Monitoring and intraoperative management of elevated intracranial pressure and decompressive craniectomy. *Anesthesiol Clin.* 2007;25:579–603.

Perioperative Implications

Preoperative Preparation

- Judicious or no preop sedation due to risk of depressed ventilatory drive/hypoventilation/hypercapnia
- Assess volume status

Monitoring

- Consider arterial catheter for BP monitoring and for serial ABGs to properly manage mechanical ventilation
- Consider ICP monitor and CVP line
- Glucose

Airway

- Neutral cervical spine position for tracheal intubation if possible traumatic injury
- Possible aspiration risk (emergency procedure or severe ICH)

Preinduction/Induction

- Neutral neck position and head elevation
- If pt cooperative, establish voluntary hyperventilation; otherwise hyperventilate as soon as possible
- Induction technique should maintain CV stability and not ↑ CBF (e.g., fentanyl, thiopental, nondepolarizing NM blocker; avoid succinylcholine unless airway concerns override)

Maintenance

- O_2, N_2O (controversial) or hypnotic (thiopental or propofol) infusion, and narcotic infusion with 0.25% isoflurane or equivalent sevoflurane, up to 1.2% isoflurane without narcotic infusion, avoid halothane and enflurane
- Normoventilation ($PaCO_2$ to 35–40 torr) and avoid PEEP
- Maintain MAP such that estimated CPP >60 mmHg

Extubation

- Maintain tracheal intubation if concerns about postop resp function or persistent ICH; otherwise, prompt extubation for early neurologic evaluation

Adjuvants

- Benzodiazepines, β-blockers, antihypertensives

Postoperative Period

- If ICH persists, adequate ventilation and/or oxygenation, pain control, sedation essential

Anticipated Problems/Concerns

- Use isotonic crystalloid or colloid IV solutions to minimize brain H_2O and cerebral edema. Avoid dextrose since it may exacerbate effects of brain ischemia.
- Renal dysfunction and severe hypovolemia are possible from preop osmotic therapy.

Intraoperative Recall

G. Richard Benzinger

DISEASES

Risk

- Incidence in USA: 20 million anesthetics annually

Perioperative Risks

- Incidence is approx 0.1% in general surgical population and increases to about 1% in high risk populations.
- Procedure risk factors incl OB surgery, cardiac surgery, trauma, and rigid bronchoscopy.
- Pt risk factors incl prior awareness, significant CV disease, COPD, substance abuse, chronic opioid use, and chronic benzodiazepine use.
- Anesthetic risk factors incl absent/low benzodiazepine premedication, absent/low halogenated agent, and dense NM blockade.

Worry About

- PTSD is a common sequela (up to 50% incidence).

- Awareness caused 1.9% of closed claims against anesthesia personnel.
- Many cases are preventable, and identified as attributable to lapses in technique.

Overview

- Explicit recall: Conscious, articulable recollection of events when intended to be unaware.
- Implicit recall: Change in behavior attributable to perception of intraop events, but no explicit awareness. Much harder to study.
- Hemodynamic changes are neither sensitive nor specific signs of awareness.
- Processed EEG monitoring (such as the bispectral index, BIS) may decrease incidence of awareness.
- Maintenance of adequate end-tidal halogenated agent (≥ 0.7 MAC, age-adjusted) may decrease incidence of awareness.

Etiology

- Inadvertent awake paralysis is usually due to drug labeling or administration error.
- Other awareness is frequently associated with light anesthesia: Intentional, unintentional, or equipment malfunction.

Usual Treatment

- Discuss incident with pt postop.
- Offer psychiatric referral to all pts with recall as screening or treatment for PTSD.
- Preliminary work suggests that beta blockers may reduce development of PTSD when administered shortly after a traumatic event; consider administration in PACU if explicit recall is reported there.
- Benzodiazepines are not effective in producing retrograde amnesia; can't use for rescue of awareness.

ASSESSMENT POINTS

System	Effect	PE	Test
CV	Htn Tachycardia		BP EKG
RESP	Tachypnea Bronchospasm Decreased compliance	Observation Auscultation	Resp rate PIP
CNS	Increased sympathetic tone Spontaneous movement	Lacrimation Diaphoresis Observation	Processed EEG, bispectral index End-tidal agent monitoring

Key Reference: Ghoneim MM, Block RI, Harrarnan M, et al. Awareness during anesthesia: Risk factors, causes, and sequelae: a review of reported cases in the literature. *Anaesth Analg.* 2009;108:527–535.

Perioperative Implications

Preinduction/Induction/Maintenance

- Counsel all pts about risk of awareness as part of routine consent process.
- Consider benzodiazepine premedication in all pts without contraindication; titrate dose to clinical effect.
- Avoid muscle relaxant if not indicated. If needed, titrate to avoid dense paralysis.

Monitoring

- Consider use of bispectral index in high-risk pts.

- Keep inhaled agent ≥ 0.7 MAC with audible alarms in high-risk pts.
- Continue to monitor NM blockade.

General Anesthesia

- Consider redosing induction agent or using inhaled agents if time between induction and securing airway is prolonged.

Regional Anesthesia

- Counsel pts that awareness during regional anesthesia is expected, even with sedation.
- Limit incidental and alarming conversation during surgery with regional or any other anesthetic technique.

Postoperative Period

- Structured interview for recall
  - Last thing remembered before sleeping?
  - First thing remembered after awakening?
  - Anything in between?
  - Remember any dreams?
  - Worst thing about anesthetic?
- Many pts with awareness don't report in recovery room. Serial interviews are necessary for complete surveillance.

Anticipated Problems/Concerns

- High risk of serious psychiatric sequelae.

Jaundice

William T. Merritt

Risk

- Chronic liver disease consistently ninth most common cause of death in USA
- M:F ratio: 2:1
- African-American to Caucasian 2:1

Perioperative Risks

- Jaundice per se poses no special risks
- Risks associated with co-existing or underlying conditions
- Use of regional anesthesia limited by coagulopathy and ascitis

Worry About

- Chronic liver disease
  - Hepatopulmonary syndrome, hypoxemia
  - Portopulmonary hypertension
  - Hepatorenal syndrome
  - CV dysfunction (cirrhotic; alcohol)
  - Infection, protein-malnutrition
  - Encephalopathy (hepatic and alcoholic); cerebral edema
  - Esophageal varices (incompetent lower esophageal sphincter)
  - Ascites; renal dysfunction
  - Low systemic vascular resistance/hyperdynamic circulation
  - Bleeding
  - Inability to extubate at end of surgery
- Altered drug pharmacodynamics and pharmacokinetics
- Universal precautions
- Invasive monitoring

Overview

- Mostly unconjugated
  - Excess production
- Hemolytic anemias (e.g., sickle cell anemia; β-thalassemia major)
- Extravascular hemolysis (tissue infarction; hemorrhage into tissue, postop jaundice)
- Ineffective erythropoiesis
  - Decreased hepatic uptake
- Drugs (e.g., flavaspidic acid, novobiocin, some cholecystographic dyes)
- Severe, prolonged fasting
  - Decreased conjugation
- Neonate: Physiologic jaundice of the newborn; breast milk jaundice; hypothyroidism; galactosemia
- Sepsis
- Acquired transferase deficiency: Drug inhibition (e.g., pregnanediol, chloramphenicol); hepatocellular disease (cirrhosis, hepatitis)
- Gilbert's disease: Decreased glucuronyl transferase
- Crigler-Najjar I (absent) and II (partial decrease) in glucuronyl transferase
- Mostly conjugated
  - Decreased hepatic excretion
- Hereditary and/or familial: Dubin-Johnson, Rotor syndromes; recurrent intrahepatic cholestasis, benign; gestational cholestatic jaundice—(~1:13,000 deliveries; third trimester; preeclampsia, nulliparity; twin; decreased plt)
- Acquired: Sepsis; hepatocellular disease (drug- and viral-induced hepatitis); postop jaundice (pigment overload [transfusions, resorption of hematomas, hemolysis]; hepatocellular damage [drugs, incl halothane; shock]; benign postop jaundice); drug-induced cholestasis (e.g., oral contraceptives, methyltestosterone)
  - Extrahepatic biliary obstruction (e.g., mechanical, from stones, stricture, tumor)
- Pseudojaundice
  - Dietary carotenoids (primarily infants; excessive intake of vegetables, such as carrots, tomatoes); TPN-associated liver dysfunction
  - Poisoning (picric acid)

ICD-9-CM Code: 782.4 (Jaundice, unspecified, non-newborn)

Usual Treatment

- No specific treatment outside of newborn period
- For neonates: Fluids, phototherapy, exchange transfusion, albumin, tin mesoporphyrin and IV immunoglobulin Rx have been shown to decrease the level of unconjugated bilirubin below levels regarded to be toxic to the neonatal brain
- The smaller and sicker the premature infant, the more aggressive the therapy needed

ASSESSMENT POINTS

System	Effect	Assessment by Hx	PE	Test
HEENT		Duration	Yellow sclerae	
CV	Hyperdynamic Poss ↓ SVR	General Sx	↑ HR; ↓ BP	
RESP	Cirrhotics have 6× increase in pulm Htn	Severe dyspnea, hypoxia, clubbing	Clubbing Cyanosis	ECHO; right-sided heart catheterization if indicated
GI	Severe dysfunction Prolonged effects of most anesthesia drugs	General Sx, reflux, ascites, varices, edema	Signs of chronic liver disease	LFTs Coagulation time Hgb, plt
ENDO/METAB	↓ Synthetic function, ↑ enzymes, ↑ albumin, ↓ hepatic coag factors; ↓ clearance of toxins	General malaise Sx Easy bruising/bleeding	Jaundice Ecchymoses Hematoma Ascites	LFTs Coagulation time NH$_3$
HEME	↓ Plt	Easy bruising/bleeding	Ecchymoses, hematoma	
DERM		Duration; evidence of bleeding	Yellow color	
RENAL	↓ Function		Edema	BUN, Cr; Cr may be spuriously lower with high bilirubin
CNS	Recurrent encephalopathy in cirrhosis Cerebral edema in fulminant hepatic failure Autonomic dysfunction	Mental status Duration of illness Abn autonomic function	Normal to encephalopathy/comatose Orthostatic BP changes	Bilirubin interferes with cerebral near-infrared oximetry

Key Reference: Yang LQ, Song JC, Irwin MG, Song JG, Sun YM, Yu WF. A clinical prospective comparison of anesthetics sensitivity and hemodynamic effect among patients with or without obstructive jaundice. *Acta Anaesthesiol Scand.* 2010 Aug; 54:871-877.

Perioperative Implications

• Drug: Decreased protein production leads to decreased albumin binding, more active drug

• Cimetidine and/or ranitidine: Clearance reduced, esp. in pts with ascites, hypoproteinemia, encephalopathy

• Benzodiazepines: Clearance of oxidative pathway markedly decreased; glucuronidation path (e.g., lorazepam) not greatly altered. Excessive sedation in severe liver disease.

• Narcotics: Meperidine clearance is severely affected; succinylcholine activity may be prolonged somewhat because of decreased levels of pseudocholinesterase.

• Miscellaneous: Phenobarbital and lidocaine have reduced clearance; diuretics may have reduced natriuretic efficacy.

• Halogenated agents: Halothane should be avoided; association of enflurane with hepatic toxicity is less clear; isoflurane, seroflurane are preferred agents in setting of liver disease and best preserves liver hemodynamics.

• Pregnancy: Jaundice may signal HELLP syndrome and pregnancy-induced Htn.

• Cardiac surgery: Jaundice occurs in about 20% post-CPB pts; risk factor for mortality

Preoperative Preparation

• Hydration should be adequate; if chronic liver failure, may be total body fluid increased, but intravascularly decreased

Monitoring

• NMB: Dose muscle relaxants to effect and consider path of elimination

Airway

• May have bleeding disorder

Induction

• Avoid benzodiazepines
• Consider cricoid pressure if varices present

Maintenance

• Be mindful of metabolic clearance paths
• When practical, use drugs cleared chiefly by nonhepatic paths

Extubation

• May have delay in awakening

Anticipated Problems/Concerns

• Inability to extubate immediately postop due to prolonged action of NMB and sedative/hypnotic/narcotic medications

Jehovah's Witness Patient

Meg A. Rosenblatt
S. William Pinson

Risk

- Incidence in USA: Approx 1.9 million members, 7.1 million worldwide
- Headquartered in Brooklyn, New York

Perioperative Risk

- Morbidity and/or mortality from massive hemorrhage 2° to religious dogma banning members from accepting blood transfusions

Worry About

- Understanding the rights and desires of pt vs. duty of physician in regards to blood or blood product administration
- Trauma and emergency situations in which little time is available to discuss blood product transfusion
- Competent adults are those who know the nature and consequences of their actions; such adults have the right to refuse specific therapies
- *Parens patriae* ("parent of the nation"), refers to the public policy power of the state, represents the duty and interest of the state to preserve the health of minors. Medicolegally, when a child's right to live and parental religious beliefs collide, the courts have consistently ruled that the child's welfare is paramount.

Overview

- Began as Bible study group in 1869; adopted the name Jehovah's Witnesses (based on Isaiah 43:10–12) in 1931
- Strict interpretation and adherence to Biblical passages, which forbid eating of blood; interpreted as prohibition of acceptance of blood products to sustain life
- In 1942 the Watchtower Society, the governing body of Jehovah's Witnesses, introduced the blood ban which forbids members from accepting allogeneic blood products incl: whole blood, red blood cells, white blood cells, plts, and plasma
- There is variability among members to the interpretation of the prohibition regarding blood; Jehovah's Witnesses may consider the use of one's own blood in the course of a medical procedure or therapy provided there is no advanced storage. They may accept fractions of plasma such as albumin, recombinant human erythropoietin (rHuEPO), immunoglobulin, or factor concentrates

Usual Treatment

- Discuss and document preop the potential for life-threatening hemorrhage and therapies/interventions that would be acceptable to the pt.
- Seek evidence of advance directive, an affidavit that confirms the pt's refusal to accept a transfusion (which forces discussion and releases physicians/hospitals of responsibility for outcome of the pt's decision).
- Optimize Hct with rHuEPO prior to elective procedures in which risk for the need for a transfusion is high.
- Consider contacting a Jehovah's Witness Hospital Liaison Committee, which consists of a group of individuals trained to work as intermediaries in avoiding conflict between pts and physicians.
- Contact legal counsel if pt is a minor, unconscious, or is an incompetent adult.

ASSESSMENT POINTS

System	Assessment by Hx	Test
HEME	Evaluate for treatable forms of anemia	Hg/Hct, Folate, B12 Levels, Fe, Ferritin, Transferrin saturation

Key Reference: Bodnaruk ZM, Wong CJ, Thomas MJ. Meeting the clinical challenge of care for Jehovah's Witnesses. *Transfus Med Rev.* 2004;18:105–116.

Perioperative Implications

Preoperative Preparation

- Iron therapy, esp. if evidence of decreased iron stores; ferrous sulfate 325 mg PO 23 × daily or
- Iron dextran 100–200 mg IV × 45 daily doses if unresponsive to oral medication or evidence of malabsorption
- Consider rHuEPO; 75100 U/kg SQ or IV, 3 ×/wk × 34 wk
- Delay elective surgery until red cell mass is optimal

Monitoring

- Minimize phlebotomies; consider pediatric sampling tubes
- Consider oximetric pulm artery catheter if high possibility of hemorrhage

Intraoperative Therapeutic Options

Maintain Blood Volume

- Acceptable treatment
  - Nonblood volume expanders (saline, lactated Ringer's, hydroxyethyl starches, dextrans)
  - Synthetic oxygen therapeutics (recombinant human or bovine hemoglobin, perfluorocarbons)
- Personal decision
  - Hyper- or normovolemic hemodilution (maintain continuous circuit with pt) in the absence of CAD or Hg <7gm/dL
  - Blood salvage techniques (equipment must be arranged in continuous series with the pt's circulation)
  - Autotransfusion of shed mediastinal or wound blood
  - Plasma derived fractions (albumin, cryoprecipitate)

Maximize Oxygen Delivery

- Increase FIO_2
- Hyperbaric O_2
- Inotropic agents to augment cardiac index once volume resuscitated
- Synthetic O_2 carrying solutions

Prevention of Intraoperative Blood Loss

- Acceptable
  - Meticulous surgical technique, use of hemostatic surgical instruments
  - Laparoscopic, endovascular, or minimally invasive surgical techniques
  - Hypotensive anesthetic techniques
  - Preop angiographic embolization
  - Pharmacologic agents: Tranexamic acid, epsilon aminocaproic acid, desmopressin, recombinant factor VIIa. Careful consideration must given to the use of aprotinin.
- Personal decision
  - Hemostatic products containing blood fractions (fibrin glue/sealant, thrombin sealants)

Minimize O_2 Consumption and Demand

- Hypothermia 30° to 32° C (reduces O_2 consumption 50%)
- Sedation and/or analgesia
- Paralysis

Postoperative Considerations

- Consider postop ventilation with paralysis, sedation, and hypothermia for severe anemia.
- Consider PA catheter to measure and follow CO and SvO_2 to assess O_2 delivery/consumption without resorting to phlebotomy.
- Supplement with IV hyperalimentation, rHuEPO, and iron dextran.

Jeune Syndrome (Asphyxiating Thoracic Dystrophy)

Anne Marie Lynn
Stefan Budac

Risk

- Incidence in USA: 1:100,000–130,000 live births and prevalence of 2.6:100,000
- No race or sex predilection
- Skeletal survey by US after 14 wk gestation can detect defining deformities
- Four clinical forms: Lethal, severe, mild, latent

Perioperative Risks

- 70–80% mortality of homozygous carriers in infancy from restrictive lung disease
- Resp failure from small thoracic cage and hypoplastic lungs
- Progressive renal disease with cystic lesions and periglomerular fibrosis
- Liver and pancreatic involvement with fibrosis and cysts

Worry About

- Resp failure with hypoxia and hypercapnia
- Barotrauma with positive pressure ventilation

- Renal failure requires careful fluid and electrolyte management and selection of non-renally cleared muscle relaxants and opiates
- Liver involvement, and rarely cirrhosis, may affect drug handling

Overview

- Rare autosomal recessive disease with skeletal dysplasia and variable renal, hepatic, pancreatic and retinal abnormalities
- Poor survival beyond early infancy
- Narrow, rigid thoracic cage due to short horizontal ribs, short limbs, underdeveloped iliac wings and acetabula and occasional polydactyly
- Resp failure from restrictive thorax and hypoplastic lungs
- Changes in renal, hepatic, and pancreatic systems if survival past infancy
- Chronic renal failure can lead to transplantation
- Hepatic dysfunction can be controlled with ursodeoxycholic acid but those with severe portal Htn require liver transplantation

- Occasional pulm Htn and cor pulmonale
- Surgical enlargement of the thorax has been undertaken to increase pulm compliance

ICD-9-CM Code: 756.4

Etiology

- Autosomal recessive inheritance
- Postulated involvement of chromosome 15q13 or *IFT80* gene on chromosome 3

Usual Treatment

- Vertical expandable prosthetic titanium rib (VEPTR) thoracoplasty has been successful for Jeune syndrome but may require postop ventilation and has a high incidence of barotrauma
- Older children may require surgery related to renal failure (dialysis catheters, renal transplantation)

ASSESSMENT POINTS

System	Effect	Assessment by Hx	PE	Test
HEENT	Cleft lip or palate Small larynx		Airway exam	
CARDIO	Pulm Htn	Syncope	↑ 2nd heart sound	ECG (RVH) ECHO
RESP	Stiff, small rib cage Hypoplastic lungs	Pneumonia/resp failure Assisted ventilation Asynchronous ventilation with agitation/crying	Small chest Horizontal ribs Cyanosis with crying	ABGs CXR Oximetry
GI	Hepatic fibrosis/cysts Pancreatic fibrosis/cysts Foregut dysmotility/malrotation	Failure to gain wt	Hepatomegaly	Abdominal US Bilirubin/LFTs
RENAL	Cysts Nephritis	Polyuria, polydipsia		BUN, Cr, lytes, Ca²⁺, PO₄ abdominal US
CNS	Occasional hydrocephalus Retinal degeneration		Increased OFC (head circumference)	
MS	Short limbs and stature Polydactyly of hands and feet			X-ray of thorax, pelvis

Key Reference: Waldhausen JH, Redding GJ, Song KM. Vertical expandable prosthetic titanium rib for thoracic insufficiency syndrome: A new method to treat an old problem. *J Pediatr Surg*. 2007;42(1):76–80.

Perioperative Implications

Preoperative Preparation

- Assess ventilation
- Evaluate for possible pulm Htn
- Evaluate renal function and consider liver function testing

Monitoring

- Consider arterial catheter

Airway

- Small larynx requires smaller ETT size

Induction

- Agitation may make resp asynchronous (chest and/or abdomen), causing hypoxemia

Maintenance

- Lung hypoplasia makes barotrauma high risk; maintain low peak airway pressures

Extubation

- Document adequate ventilation before extubation; postop ventilation may be needed for a prolonged period, esp. after thoracoplasty

Adjuvants

- Renal function assessment guides selection of muscle relaxant and fluid management

Anticipated Problems/Concerns

- Asynchronous ventilation during crying with hypoxia
- Barotrauma during assisted mechanical ventilation
- Renal and/or liver disease and drug metabolism
- Postop resp failure requiring ventilatory support

Kartagener's Syndrome

Matthew L. Garvey
Nancy C. Wilkes

Risk

- Kartagener's syndrome (KS), first described in 1933, is part of a larger family of diseases classified as Primary Ciliary Dyskinesia (PCD)
- The triad of KS consists of bronchiectasis, chronic sinusitis, and situs inversus, and it has an incidence estimated at 1:15,000–40,000 births
- The disease is likely underdiagnosed, as a limited amount of centers have resources to provide an accurate diagnosis
- No predilection for race or gender
- Symptoms more prevalent in children in the first decade of life

Perioperative Risks

- Morbidity: Lung infection, pulm edema, atelectasis, sinusitis

Worry About

- Pulm function and anatomy
- Airway obstruction due to ineffective clearance of secretions
- Bronchiectasis, which can lead to cor pulmonale, amyloidosis, and pulm edema and is usually found in the middle or lower lobes in KS pts as opposed to the upper lobes in cystic fibrosis pts
- Chronic disease with variable onset
- Chemical injury from aspiration in left lung, which is the larger lung in pts with KS
- Unintended bronchial intubation with single-lumen ETT resulting in non-ventilation of right lung (in those with pulm inversion)
- Left-sided double-lumen tubes may occlude orifice of left upper lobe
- Nasal catheters relatively contraindicated because of risk of paranasal sinusitis and ear infections
- Increased susceptibility to overall infection due to impaired neutrophil chemotaxis

Overview

- Complete situs inversus (incl dextrocardia)
- PCD resulting in chronic respiratory tract infections, bronchiectasis and sinusitis
- Approximately half of pts with PCD have situs inversus and, thus, are classified as having KS

ICD-9-CM Code: 759.3

Etiology

- Congenital defect in synthesis of various parts of cilia (dynein arms, radial spokes, nexin links, microtubules) that results in abn/dyskinetic ciliary movement
- Ciliated epithelium covers most areas of the upper resp tract, incl the nasal mucosa, paranasal sinuses, middle ear, eustachian tube and pharynx The lower resp tract contains ciliated epithelium from the trachea to the resp bronchioles
- Autosomal recessive inheritance pattern; genetically heterogeneous with multiple chromosomes likely responsible for phenotype

Usual Treatment

- Aerosol administration to reduce secretion viscosity
- Antimicrobial therapy for chronic resp tract infections, sinusitis
- Surgical intervention for persistent bronchiectasis
- Conventional and assisted airway clearance techniques (chest physiotherapy, positive expiratory pressure [PEP] mask, forced oscillation techniques, exercise programs and physical activity)
- Nasal steroid sprays
- Inhaled bronchodilators and anti-inflammatory medications to treat bronchospasm

ASSESSMENT POINTS

System	Effect	Assessment by Hx	PE	Test
CARDIO	Dextrocardia		Right-sided heart tones	CXR, ECHO, ECG
RESP	Bronchiectasis	Dyspnea	Decreased breath sounds, rhonchi, crackles, wheezes	CXR, bronchoscopy, spirometry, bronchography
	Ciliary dyskinesia	Cough		
		Halitosis		
IMMUNO	Chronic sinusitis	Nasal drainage	Frontal and maxillary tenderness	CT sinuses
		Morning sore throat		
	Bronchitis	Cough	Rhonchi	Sputum and tracheal aspirate for culture and Gram stain
		Mucus production		
	Pneumonia	Cough	Rales	CXR
		Fever	Rhonchi	SpO_2
	Otitis media	Earache	Erythematous tympanic membrane	Audiometry Tympanotomy

Key Reference: Mathew PJ, Sadera GS, Sharafuddin S, Pandit B. Anaesthetic considerations in Kartagener's syndrome – a case report. *Acta Anaesthesiol Scand.* 2004;48(4):518–520.

Perioperative Considerations

Preinduction

- Consider omitting anticholinergics and cough suppressants from preanesthetic medication.
- Chest physiotherapy, bronchodilators, and incentive spirometry are often beneficial.
- Treat underlying pulm infections.
- Immunize against influenza A and pneumococcal organisms.

Monitoring

- In dextrocardia, position of ECG leads should be the mirror image of normal, as should that of paddles of external defibrillation, cardioversion, and pacing.
- Since the great vessels and thoracic duct are likely to be reversed, consider cannulation of the internal jugular vein from the left.
- Pulm artery catheters should be oriented in anticipation of a clockwise direction of migration.
- Pregnant pts with KS should be positioned in right uterine displacement rather than left.

Induction/General Anesthesia

- Emphasize aseptic technique 2° to abn neutrophil chemotaxis.
- Aim for non-traumatic airway manipulation to avoid possible infection.
- Humidify inspired gases.
- Inhalation injury usually occurs in left lung, which is also larger lung.
- Bronchial intubation with a single-lumen ETT usually involves left side.
- Right bronchial suctioning will be more difficult to perform with nonangulated suction catheters.
- Left-sided double-lumen tubes may occlude orifice of left upper lobe.
- When lung isolation is needed, consider tracheal intubation first with a bronchial blocker in the appropriate bronchus.
- If a double-lumen tube is required, consider inserting a left-sided tube with the bronchial tube on the right; the endobronchial stylet and the upper part of tube must be bent 180° from original orientation prior to insertion such that the normal curvature of the oropharynx is still followed. The same principles apply to use of a right-sided tube.
- Extubation of the trachea should occur as soon as possible after the pt meets common extubation criteria.

Regional Anesthesia

- Employ regional or local anesthetic techniques when possible to avoid airway manipulation/complications and to preserve resp muscle function intraop and postop.

Postoperative Period

- Consider nonnarcotic analgesia and/or epidural analgesia for postop pain.
- Avoid excessive sedation and encourage early ambulation to aid in clearance of airway secretions.
- Chest physiotherapy, bronchodilators, incentive spirometry may be beneficial.
- Oral airway preferred over nasal airway 2° to increased risk of sinusitis.

Anticipated Problems/Concerns

- Lung infection is common as result of ciliary dyskinesia.
- Fluid overload can precipitate cor pulmonale and pulm edema.
- Avoid nasal catheters and/or airways to minimize chances of paranasal sinusitis.

Klippel-Feil Syndrome

Ronald S. Litman

Risk

- Incidence estimated at 1:40,000 live births (probably underestimate, as milder cases go unrecognized)
- Slight female predilection (63%)

Perioperative Risks

- Cervical spine instability and cardiopulmonary complications
- Often occurs in association with other clinical syndromes (e.g., fetal alcohol, Goldenhars)

Worry About

- Exacerbation of cervical spine instability during airway maneuvers, endotracheal intubation, and subsequent positioning

Overview

- Congenital abnormality consisting of the following triad of Findings: Fusion of two or more cervical vertebrae; low posterior hairline; cervical immobility
- Severity ranges from mild (often not recognized until late in life) to severe (recognized at birth because of obvious deformity)

- Careful preop assessment of cervical spine anatomy and degree of instability
- Review of systems for other congenital abn (many reported; see below)

ICD-9-CM Code: 756.16

Etiology

- Unknown

Usual Treatment

- Symptomatic, depends on organ system involvement

ASSESSMENT POINTS

System	Effect	Assessment by Hx	PE	Test
HEENT	Head and neck immobility		Decreased ROM of cervical spine, low posterior hairline, webbed neck, facial asymmetry, cleft palate, torticollis, vocal cord dysfunction	Flexion/extension radiographs of cervical spine Consider MRI of cervical spine
CARDIO	Bradyarrhythmias and AV conduction pathway abn (due to CNS malformations) Cardiac defects (most commonly VSD)	Syncope	Murmurs	ECG ECHO
RESP	Central alveolar hypoventilation, pulmonary agenesis or hypoplasia, restrictive lung disease (due to severe scoliosis)	Sleep apnea, snoring, difficulty breathing		ABGs CXR (if symptomatic)
RENAL	Urinary tract abn, renal agenesis, ureteral duplication			BUN, Cr if indicated, renal US
CNS	Hindbrain abn (e.g., syringomyelia, Arnold-Chiari malformation) Mental retardation, deafness, strabismus	Peripheral neurologic dysfunction (e.g., weakness, paresthesias, paraplegia, quadriplegia)	Neurologic exam	
MS	Scoliosis, Sprengel's deformity (scapular elevation), hypermobility of C-spine, spondylosis/decreased mobility of C-spine		Exam of spine and shoulders	Radiographs if indicated

Key Reference: Stallmer ML, Vanaharam V, Mashour GA. Congenital cervical spine fusion and airway management: A case series of Klippel-Feil syndrome. *J Clin Anesth.* 2008;20(6):447–451.

Perioperative Implications

Preoperative Preparation
- Careful and complete evaluation of cervical spine anatomy and instability and of other major organ system abn

Monitoring
- Depends on pt's physical condition

Airway
- If indicated, awake intubation using maneuvers to stabilize cervical spine; complete immobility with use of fiberoptic intubating bronchoscope ideal

Preinduction/Induction
- Depends on pt's physical condition

Maintenance
- Careful positioning of head and neck with maintenance in neutral position

Extubation
- Depends on extent of cervical spine pathology and resp compromise

Adjuvants
- No special considerations

Anticipated Problems/Concerns
- Exacerbation of pre-existing cervical spine instability leading to neurologic deterioration

Latex Allergy

Robert H. Brown

Risk

- Myelomeningocele (25–50%)
- Congenital urologic anomalies (25–50%)
- Health care workers (3–17%)
- Atopic individuals (6–11%)
- General population (0–6%)

Perioperative Risks

- Anayphylactic reaction leading to hypotension, bronchospasm, CV collapse

Worry About

- A latex allergy is a Type I immediate hypersensitivity reaction. Life-threatening anaphylaxis can be the first manifestation of the reaction. Latex-containing medical products are common throughout most medical environments.

Overview

- Type I (immediate) hypersensitivity reaction: Immune mediated and involve IgE-specific latex proteins. Exposure can occur by either direct contact or through inhaled airborne particles. Symptoms can be localized or generalized, mild to life-threatening and incl pruritus, hives, angioedema, wheezing, hypotension, tachycardia, and CV collapse.

- Type IV (delayed or contact dermatitis) hypersensitivity reaction: Cell mediated, occurs 24–48 hr after exposure and is localized. Symptoms incl localized pruritus, swelling, and blisters.
- The increase in latex allergies coincided with the advent of universal precautions and the increased use of latex examination gloves, many with high allergen content.
- Exposure can occur both by contact and by inhalation of latex-containing powder.
- Considered to represent ~10% of all anaphylactic reactions reported for pts while under anesthesia.
- Increased risk with repeated exposures.
- Reaction caused by crosslinking latex specific IgE on mast cells leading to degranulation and release of both immediate and delayed inflammatory mediators.
- DX incl a Hx consistent with a latex reaction (e.g., time and exposure), nonspecific blood markers (e.g., serum mast cell tryptase), serology testing (radioallergosorbent [RAST] testing) and skin testing where available.

ICD-9-CM Code: V15.07

Etiology

- Exposure with subsequent sensitization in at-risk individuals is the usual etiology of a latex allergy. At-risk individuals commonly have identified risk factors such as atopy, food allergies, and or a Hx of multiple surgeries.

Usual Treatment

- Avoidance of exposure should be the 1° consideration.
- There is no evidence any premedications can prevent or attenuate a Type I hypersensitivity reaction.
- In cases of an anaphylaxis reaction, treatment includes stopping the exposure, intravascular volume expansion, epinephrine as needed to support BP, bronchodilators to treat bronchospasm. Antihistamines and corticosteroids are distant 2° therapies.
- A latex-safe environment, one with minimal latex allergen, insufficient to elicit a latex allergic reaction, should be considered for all health care locations.

ASSESSMENT POINTS

System	Assessment by Hx	PE	Test
CARDIO	Hypotension, tachycardia, CV collapse	Tachycardia, vasoconstriction	ECG, BP
PULM	SOB, stuffy nose, cough, elevated airway pressures	Wheezing, excessory muscle use	Spirometry, airway pressure
SKIN	Pruritus, edema	Hives, urticaria, erythema, swelling	Visual exam
EYES	Red, itching	Angioedema	Visual exam
GI	Cramps, N/V, diarrhea		

Key Reference: Mertes PM, et al. Periopertive anaphylaxis. *Immunol Allergy Clin North Am.* 2009;29:429–451.

Perioperative Implications

- Ask all pts about any Hx of an allergy or reactions to latex products.
- Do not attempt to prevent with premedications.
- Provide a latex-safe environment incl the pre-, intra- and postop environment.
- If latex allergic reaction suspected, make sure the postop environment is latex safe.

Anticipated Problems/Concerns

- Many latex-sensitized individuals are unaware of their allergic status.
- 10% of anaphylactic reactions under anesthesia are presumed due to a latex reaction.

- Maintain vigilance with regard to potential inadvertent latex exposures.
- Consider allergic reaction if hypotension is unresponsive to usual pressor agents.

Lesch-Nyhan Syndrome

Roberta Hines

Risk

- X-linked recessive disorder (deficiency on the enzyme hypoxanthine-guanine-phosphoribosyl-transferase (HGPRT), resulting in buildup of uric acid)
- Incidence ~5.2 per million male births (where symptoms appear)

Perioperative Risks

- Hyperuricemia and hyperuricosuria (gout)
- Airway problems 2° to scarification from self-mutilation (clip and finger bitting)
- Involuntary writhing
- Repetitive movement of arms and legs

- Impairment of renal function due to obstructive uropathy

Worry About

- Aspiration pneumonia (poor muscle control)
- May have associated megaloblastic anemia (poorly utilize Vitamin B_{12})
- Drug metabolism and prolonged drug effects 2° to metabolic defect and impaired renal function

Overview

- Pts usually mentally subnormal
- Pts exhibit characteristic pattern of compulsive self-mutilation, spasticity, and choreoathetosis
- Primary biochemical defect is almost complete absence of HGPRT

- Enzyme defect leads to excessive purine production and elevated uric acid concentrations

ICD-9-CM Code: 277.2

Etiology

- Genetic disease inherited as X-linked recessive trait (female carriers generally asymptomatic)

Usual Treatment

- No specific treatment of enzyme deficiency
- Benzodiazepines frequently used to control self-mutilation and spasticity (bacluten may be helpful)
- Gene therapy possibility
- Gabapentin
- Gout can be treated with allopurinol

ASSESSMENT POINTS

System	Effect	Assessment by Hx	PE	Test
HEENT	Distortion of airway structures due to self-mutilation		Examine airway	
CV	Htn, CAD Adrenergic pressor response to stress is absent	Angina, angina-equivalent symptoms, PND	Displaced PMI S_3	ECG Pharmacologic stress testing Coronary angiography and ECHO
RESP	Aspiration pneumonia	SOB following vomiting episode	Rales Wheezing	CXR
GI	Vomiting Athetoid dysphagia	Dysphagia		
RENAL	Decreased renal function due to obstructive uropathy			BUN Cr IVP
CNS	Retardation Seizure disorders Decreased MAO activity	Mental status questioning		EEG Mental function tests
MS	Spasticity, contractures		ROM	

Key Reference: Williams KS, Hankerson JG, Ernst M, Zametkin A. Use of propofol anesthesia during outpatient radiographic imaging studies in patients with Lesch-Nyhan syndrome. *J Clin Anesth*. 1997;9:61–65.

Perioperative Implications

Preoperative Preparations
- Antacids
- H_2 blockers
- Metoclopramide
- IV access may be difficult

Monitoring
- Routine
- ST-segment analysis if CAD present

Airway
- Rapid-sequence induction
- Avoid succinylcholine
- Awake fiberoptic intubation

Preinduction/Induction
- Premedication where appropriate to help with behavioral issues
- Avoid agents with renal metabolism (adjust dosing)

Maintenance
- Avoid agents with renal toxicity
- No one agent or technique shown superior
- Administer exogenous catecholamines with caution (due to assoc Htn)

Extubation
- Awake to avoid aspiration

Adjuvants/Postoperative Period
- Make some space accessible to avoid injury to child
- Benzodiazepines for spasticity

Anticipated Problems/Concerns
- Hx unavailable or inaccurate because of retardation

Leukemia

Dilipkumar K. Patel

Risk

- Incidence in USA: 245,225 people living with, or in remission from leukemia. AML and CLL are the most common type of leukemia in adults.
- Leukemia causes about one third of all cancer deaths in children younger than 15 y. ALL is most common type of leukemia in children.

Perioperative Risks

- Neutropenic fever, opportunistic infection, sepsis, interstitial pneumonitis, acute resp failure and encephalopathy
- Hematoma and/or bleeding, diffuse alveolar hemorrhage from thrombocytopenia and splenic sequestration of plts

Worry About

- Bone marrow suppression with NO, potential for malignant hyperthermia in ALL, neuropathy, upper airway edema, anterior medistinal mass, pleural effusion, and pulm fibrosis

Overview

- Hematologic malignancy with proliferation of cells may cause decrease in amino acids, causing fatigue and metabolic starvation
- Invasion possible in all organ systems
- Usually outpatient treatment, but may require several procedures incl bone marrow aspiration, central venous access placement, lumbar puncture, bronchoscopy, pericardiocentesis, external beam radiation

ICD-9-CM Codes: 208.0 (Undifferentiated, acute, blastic); 204.0 (Lymphoblastic); 205.0 Myeloid leukemia

Etiology

- Unknown
- Strong suspicion that leukemia and lymphoma are virus-induced
- Chronic exposure to benzene (primarily from tobacco smoke), extraordinary doses of radiation, and certain cancer therapies, can be causes of the leukemia

Treatment

- Supportive treatment: Antimicrobial, blood transfusion, nutrition and pain control
- Newer approaches: Monoclonal antibody, experimental cancer vaccines, donor lymphocyte infusion, gene therapy, autologous and allogeneic transplantation, stem cell transplantation
- Treatment varies with type of leukemia, phase, age
- AML
  - Ara-C
  - Anthracyclines: Daunorubicin, idarubicin
    - Gemtuzumab ozogamicin: ATRA (All Trans Retinoic Acid)
    - Arsenic trioxide: Vinca alkaloids: vincristine/vinblastine
    - Bone marrow transplant
- CML
    - Imatinib mesylate (initial treatment of choice)
  - Nilotinib
  - Dasatinib
  - Busulfan
  - Hydroxyurea
  - Interferon alfa, allopurinol
  - Splenectomy, radiation, bone marrow transplant
- CLL
  - Cyclophosphamide
  - Corticosteroid
  - Fludarabine
  - Cytarabine
  - Bendamustine, rituximab
  - Alemtuzumab
- ALL
    - Imatinib, clofarabine, L-asparaginase, daunorubicin, vincristine, dexamethasone, doxorubicin, cytarabine (ara-C)
    - Radiation therapy, intrathecal chemotherapy

ASSESSMENT POINTS

System	Effect	Assessment by Hx	PE	Test
HEENT	Ulceration, oral lesions	Dysphagia	Airway assessment	
CV	Rare: Pericardial effusion, conduction defects, murmurs, CHF Mediastinal mass	Dyspnea, fatigue	Narrow pulse pressure, pericardial friction rub, cardiomegaly	CXR, CT scan, ECG, ECHO
GI	Hepatosplenomegaly hypoalbuminemia	Loss of appetite wt loss	Hepatosplenomegaly	Albumin
HEME	Anemia Leukostasis Thrombocytopenia	Weakness, easy fatigue,	Pallor Ecchymoses Petechiae, easy bruising, nosebleeds	CBC Bone marrow aspirate results
RENAL	Renal failure from tumor lysis syndrome (acute loss of tumor)	↓ UO	↓ UO	BUN/Cr ↑ Phosphate, ↑ or ↓ Ca^{2+} ↑ K^+
CNS	Cranial nerve infiltration (very rare), meningeal leukemia (less common in adults), vincristine neuropathy	Cranial nerve palsies, clouding of mental status, peripheral neuropathy	Weakness	EMG
MS	Infiltration of bony cortex and periosteum, synovial membranes	Bone pain	Bone swelling	X-ray CT scan

Key Reference: Foon KA, Hallek MJ. Changing paradigms in the treatment of chronic lymphocytic leukemia. *Leukemia*. 2009;Dec 24. [Epub ahead of print].

Perioperative Implications

Preoperative Preparation
- Assess volume status, CBC, electrolytes, renal function, N/V, diarrhea, oral mucositis

Monitoring
- Routine

Airway
- Signs of dysphagia, ulcerations from chemotherapy and candidiasis
- Oral leukemia lesions can occur prior to or during therapy
- Mediastinal mass

Induction
- Brief heparinization and thrombocytopenia may influence choice of local, spinal, or epidural

Maintenance/Extubation
- Routine

Anticipated Problems/Concerns
- Risk of infection, aseptic technique with placement of all lines

Lipidemias

Alan Kaye

Amir Baluch

Arushi Kak*

Risk

- Incidence in USA: 18% of adult population (aged 20 and over)
- Race with highest prevalence: None
- Cigarette smoking
- Age ≥45 for men or ≥55 for women
- Htn
- Low HDL (<40mg/dL)
- Family Hx of premature CHD in first degree relative (male <55 y or female <65 y)

Perioperative Risks

- Pancreatitis with hypertriglyceridemia
- Stroke and transient ischemic attacks
- Myocardial ischemia, infarction, CHF

Worry About

- Angina of increasing frequency or severity and new-onset angina
- Peripheral atherosclerosis
- Worsening or new-onset CHF
- Transient ischemic attacks of CNS

Overview

- Hypertriglyceridemia, hypercholesterolemia lipodystrophy: Köbberling-Dunnigan syndrome (familial lipodystrophy of limbs and trunk, autosomal dominant, may lead to macrosomia); familial generalized lipodystrophy (Berardinelli-Seip syndrome: Autosomal recessive, leads to macrosomia)
- Hypolipidemia: LDL deficiency (autosomal recessive abetalipoproteinemia, autosomal dominant familial hypobetalipoproteinemia); normotriglyceridemic abetalipoproteinemia (LDL absent); autosomal recessive Tangier disease (severe deficiency of HDL); 2° to cancer, myeloproliferative disorders, liver failure familial hypoalphalipoproteinemia (HDL deficiency)

ICD-9-CM Codes: 272.0–9

Etiology

- Autosomal dominant or recessive inheritance

- 2° to systemic illness (i.e., primary hypothyroidism, nephrotic syndrome, and extrahepatic obstruction of bile)

Usual Treatment

- Cholestyramine and colestipol inhibit absorption of bile acids derived from cholesterol
- Neomycin blocks cholesterol absorption
- Diet and exercise
- Thyroid hormone clears LDL
- Fish oils (omega-3 fatty acids) reduce triglyceride levels
- Probucol reduces LDL but also HDL
- Nicotinic acid inhibits VLDL, LDL production, and is an HDL-raising drug*
- Fibric acids clofibrate and gemfibrozil cause catabolism of triglyceride-rich lipoproteins
- Niacin/statin combination therapy promotes optimal lipid values for several at-risk pt populations
- HMG CoA reductase inhibitors (lova-statin, pravastatin, simvastatin, rosuvastatin, atorvastatin) reduce cholesterol synthesis and are commonly used

ASSESSMENT POINTS

System	Effect	Assessment by Hx	PE	Test
HEENT	Tangier disease		Lobulated, bright orange-yellow tonsils Hepatosplenomegaly Peripheral neuropathy (in 50% of pts)	Lipoprotein profile
CV	Myocardial ischemia and infarction LV dysfunction	Angina or its equivalents Dyspnea, edema, exercise intolerance, MI	Displaced PMI S_3 S_4	ECG, CXR, stress testing, ECHO, coronary angiography
RESP	CHF	Dyspnea, orthopnea, cough	Rales and rhonchi	CXR
RENAL	Impaired renal perfusion	Nighttime urinary frequency		BUN, Cr
CNS	Cerebrovascular atherosclerosis	TIAs	Carotid bruit	Carotid US and angiography

Key Reference: Ballantyne CM. Hyperlipidemia: Diagnostic and therapeutic perspectives. *J Clin Endocrinol Metab.* 2000;85:2089–2112.

Perioperative Implications

Preoperative Preparation
- Assess for CAD and peripheral vascular disease
- β-blockers and nitrates periop (as tolerated)

Monitoring
- Consider pulm artery catheter, transesophageal echocardiogram in the presence of large fluid shifts, Hx of ischemia, and high-risk surgery

Airway
- Pts may have large head and neck and be overweight—making it difficult to intubate

Maintenance
- Avoid hypothermia and anemia
- Monitor for ischemia and cardiac failure
- Insulin increases activity of lipoprotein lipase and releases free fatty acids (FFAs)
- Sympathetic stimulation, stress, and catecholamines release FFAs
- Spinal or epidural anesthesia and β-blockers reduce FFA levels
- Heparin releases two triglyceride hydrolases: Lipoprotein lipase inhibited by protamine and hepatic lipase resistant to protamine

Extubation
- During noncardiac surgery, this may be period of greatest risk for ischemia

Adjuvants
- Depends on lipid-drug binding and end-organ disease

Postoperative Period
- High incidence of ischemia, tachycardia, and MI for several days after noncardiac surgery
- Treat pain, hemodynamic, and biochemical abn

Anticipated Problems/Concerns
- Concerns are related to issues associated with atherosclerosis

* Sophomore Medical Student, Howard University College of Medicine, Washington, D.C.

Ludwig's Angina

Risk

- Odontogenic infections esp. of second and third molars (account for 90% of all cases). Dental and gingival disorders, bacterial infection of floor of the mourh, peritonsillar abscess, IV drug abuse, mandible fracture, tongue piercing, sialdenitis, puncture wounds of floor of mouth. Predisposing factors: DM, alcoholism, acute glomerulonephritis, SLE, and aplastic anemia

Perioperative Risks

- Airway obstruction, aspiration pneumonia, sepsis, descending mediastinitis, subphrenic abscess, empyema, cervical or mandibular osteomyelitis

Worry About

- Airway obstruction, sepsis, jugular vein thrombosis, pneumothorax, pericardial/pleural effusion, infection of carotic sheath structures, descending, necrotizing mediastinitis occurring through the retropharyngeal space and carotid sheath

Overview

- Potentially lethal, rapidly spreading cellulitis of the sublingual and submandibular spaces. Five characteristics: Submandibular cellulitis; involvement of more than one space; progression of cellulites to gangrene; progression of cellulites to connective tissue, fascia, and muscles; and spread of cellulites by continuity and not via the lymphatics. Infection often starts as a periapical dental abscess of the third and fourth mandibular molars (the roots of these teeth penetrate the mylohyoid ridge such that any abscess or dental infection has direct access to the submaxillary space) usually with elevation and posterior displacement of the tongue.
- Presents with painful neck swelling, laryngeal edema, tooth pain, dysphagia, dyspnea, fever, and malaise. Neck swelling and protruding or elevated tongue are seen in the vast majority. Stridor, trismus, cyanosis, and tongue displacement suggest impending airway crisis.

ICD-9-CM Code: 641.2

Etiology

- Results from bacterial infection: Polymicrobial most common: Predominantly *Streptococcus viridans, Staph aureus*. Also: *Bacteroides, Fuso-bacterium, Actinomyces, Haemophilus influenza*

Usual Treatment

- Airway control: EARLY (incl IV dexamethasone and nebulized adrenaline which has been shown to aid in reducing airway obstruction)
- Antibiotics: Penicillin, clindamycin, flagyl
- Sugical decompression

ASSESSMENT POINTS

System	Effect	Assessment by Hx	PE	Test
HEENT	Airway edema, elevation and posterior displacement of tongue	Dysphagia Dyspnea	Stridor, drooling, cyanosis, tongue displacement, redness and swelling of neck and face, trismus	MRI/CT with IV contrast
PULM	Pneumonia, pneumothorax, empyema Pleural effusion Subphrenic abscess	Pleuritic pain, cough, dyspnea, generalized SOB	Unequal breath sounds, tachycardia, cyanosis, tactile fremitus	CXR Thoracentesis for pleural effusion and empyema
CARDIO	Pericardial effusion Hypovolemia	Poor PO intake Hypotension	Orthostatic hypotension Tachycardia Arrhythmia, decreased CO, JVD	ECHO Pericardocentesis

Key Reference: Rajeev S, Panda NB, Batra YK. Anaesthetic management of Ludwig's angina in pregnancy. *Int J Obstet Anesth*. 2009;18(1):96–97.

Perioperative Implications

Preinduction/Induction

- Fully developed Ludwig's: ET intubation is associated with high rate of failure with acute deterioration in resp status resulting in emergency slash tracheostomy.
- Elective, awake tracheostomy using local anesthesia is the preferred method of airway management in pts with fully developed Ludwig's.
- In cases not fully advanced, awake nasal fiberoptic is the logical choice.

- The use of 10 mg of dexamethasone initially and 4 mg every 6 hours helps to decrease edema and cellulites. Nebulized adrenaline (1 mL of 1:1000 diluted to 5 mL of 0.9% saline) is also believed to help relieve upper airway obstruction. Pt must be maintained in sitting position and surgeon should be immediately available for tracheostomy.
- The first airway should be the definitive airway and induction should occur after airway has been secured. For mild cases that have not progressed, one may elect to do an inhalational induction but the majority of cases require awake intubation and then induction.

Monitoring

- Large-bore access should be obtained. Central line is not be advised with involvement in the neck.

Maintenance

- Avoid NO in case of pneumothorax.

Anticipated Problems/Concerns

- Blind nasotracheal intubation should not be attempted in Ludwig's, given the potential for bleeding and abscess rupture.

Lyme Disease

Ahmed M. Darwish
Philip D. Lumb

Risk

• Accounts for >95% of all reported cases of vector-borne illness in USA; it is by far the most common arthropod-borne infection in USA
• During 1992–2006, 93% of cases were reported from 10 states (Connecticut, Delaware, Massachusetts, Maryland, Minnesota, New Jersey, New York, Pennsylvania, Rhode Island, and Wisconsin). Incidence was highest among children aged 5–14 y, a disproportionate increasing trend was observed in children and in young males compared with other demographic groups. The majority of pts had onset in June, July, or August.
• Gender predilection: Male (53.4%)
• Children <15 y; adults 30–59 y

Perioperative Risks

• Increased risk of dysrhythmias and CHF in pts with cardiac involvement

Worry About

• CV: Volume overload, CHF, and AV block
• Neuro: Hyperkalemia from muscular weakness or paralysis, facial muscle paralysis (Bell's palsy), peripheral neuropathy and muscle weakness, meningitis, and confusion

Overview

• Stage 1, Early localized infection: Chills, fever, headache, lethargy, muscle pain, erythema migrans (rash spreads centrifugally; lesion usually occurs at site of bite) in 68% of pts.
• Stage 2, Early disseminated infection: Arthritis, aseptic meningitis, cranial neuritis (Bell's palsy), and peripheral radiculoneuritis are neurologic manifestations.
• Carditis occurs in 4–8% of pts during this stage of disease.
• Second and third degree AV block and myocarditis may be documented by ECG and heart failure; symptoms resolve in days to weeks.
• Stage 3, Late persistent infection: Over years 60% of pts with untreated infection will begin to have intermittent bouts of arthritis, with severe joint pain and swelling. Large joints are most often affected, particularly the knees. In addition, up to 5% of untreated pts may develop chronic neurologic complaints months to years after infection.

These incl shooting pains, numbness or tingling in the hands or feet, and problems with concentration and short-term memory.

ICD-9-CM: 088.81

Etiology

• Lyme disease is caused by the spirochete *Borrelia burgdorferi*, which is transmitted by the tick *Ixodes dammini*.

Usual Treatment

• Early doxycycline prevents infection in high percentages, amoxicillin, cefuroxime, and ceftriaxone. Pts with certain neurologic or cardiac forms of illness may require IV treatment with drugs such as ceftriaxone. Antibiotic therapy for 10–21 up to 28 d generally aborts stages 2 and 3. Pts may benefit from a second 4-wk course of therapy.
• Vaccine available for adults

ASSESSMENT POINTS

System	Effect	Assessment by Hx	PE	Test
CV	AV node block	Palpitations	Bradycardia	ECG
	CHF	Fatigue	Tachycardia	ECHO
		Dyspnea		
		Dizziness with exercise		
RESP		SOB	Rales	CXR
DERM	Erythema chronicum migrans	Erythematous annular lesions	Erythematous circular rash	
CNS	Meningitis	Headache	Cranial nerve facial palsy	Serology
	Bell's palsy	Cognitive impairment	Numbness, tingling	Lumbar puncture
	Radiculoneuritis	Memory deficit	Muscular weakness	EMG
MS	Arthritis	Joint pain and swelling	Swelling of one or a few joints	
		Musculoskeletal pain	Erythema of joints	

Key Reference: Lelovas P, Dontas I, Bassiakou E, Xanthos T. Cardiac implications of Lyme disease: Diagnosis and therapeutic approach. *Int J Cardiol.* 2008 16;129(1):15–21.

Perioperative Implications

Preoperative Concerns
• Ensure antibiotic Rx and cure of carditis prior to all but life-or-death emergency operations.

Monitoring
• Consider invasive monitoring with an arterial line based on cardiac manifestations.

Airway
• Routine

Preinduction/Induction
• Avoid depolarizing muscle relaxants.

Maintenance
• Routine

Extubation
• Usually routine but might be delayed due to generalized muscle weakness

Adjuvants
• Avoid depolarizing muscle relaxants on induction, because of hyperkalemia.

Postoperative Period
• Depends on the cardiac and neurologic manifestations of the disease if present.

Anticipated Problems/Concerns

• Pts may develop arrhythmias or CHF.

Lymphomas

Alisa C. Thorne

Risk

- Hodgkin's disease (HD) and non-Hodgkin's lymphoma (NHL) are most common hematologic malignancies in the USA.
- HD and NHL represent 4–5% all new cancers
- Race with highest prevalence of HD and NHL: Caucasian
- In past 40 y, striking↑ in incidence of NHL partly due to lymphoma in AIDS pts

Perioperative Risks

- Morbidity and mortality related to compression of organs and chemotherapy
- Mediastinal mass
- Superior vena cava syndrome; anthracycline cardiac toxic effects
- Bleomycin pulm toxic effects
- Pericardial effusion
- Radiation pneumonitis

Worry About

- Tracheal or bronchial compression by large mediastinal mass

- Increased cardiac/pulm toxic effects with combination chemotherapy/radiation therapy (RT)

Overview

- Two major types of lymphoma: HD and NHL, many subtypes
- Seventh most common cause of cancer-related death in the USA
- Third most common childhood malignancy
- Average age at diagnosis: 42 y
- Often curable
- Accurate Dx and staging critical in determining Rx and prognosis

ICD-9-CM Codes: 200–202.8

Etiology

- HD: Pathogenesis remains obscure, genetic predisposition, increased risk with inherited immunodeficiency syndromes, EBV, increased educational level
- NHL: Pathogenesis involves clonal malignant expansion of B or T cells, increased risk with congenital and acquired immunodeficiency states, autoimmune disorders, infectious agents, phenoxyherbicides, organophosphates, ionizing radiation

Usual Treatment

- Diagnostic laparoscopy or laparotomy no longer routine, reserved for pts with limited disease, treated with RT alone.
- RT
- Chemotherapy with multiple agents
- Combination RT and chemotherapy
- Chemotherapy commonly incl: Bleomycin, doxorubicin, prednisone, etoposide, vincristine, cyclophosphamide
- RT commonly incl neck, chest
- Both chemotherapy and RT have cardiac and pulm toxic effects
- Advanced or recurrent HD: Treatment with biologics (e.g., radiolabeled immunoglobulin therapy)

ASSESSMENT POINTS

System	Effect	Assessment by Hx	PE	Test
HEENT	Bulky nodal disease Compression	SOB, DOE Tracheal deviation	Neck mass Wheeze, stridor	Indirect laryngoscopy CXR CT/MRI
CARDIO	Mediastinal mass	SOB, DOE	Facial swelling, wheeze, may be asymptomatic	CXR, CT/MRI ECHO
	SVC syndrome (SVC obstruction)	Cough, orthopnea Mental status change	Dilated veins upper half of body Edema of head, neck, and upper extremities, cyanosis	CT of airway
RESP	Pericardial effusion CHF due to anthracyclines	Frequently asymptomatic SOB, DOE	↑ HR, ↓ BP, neck vein distention Rales, pedal edema	CXR, ECHO
	Bronchial compression	Cough		
	Obstructive pneumonia	Wheeze		CT/MRI
	Pneumonitis due to bleomycin and/or RT	Sx worse in supine position Fever, cough		Flow-volume loop ABGs, PFTs, DLco
GI	Abdominal mass Upper/lower GI bleed Perforated viscus	Abdominal pain, GI bleeding	Palpable mass	CT/MRI
HEME	Bone marrow involvement			Alk phos, CBC, plts, bone marrow biopsy
CNS	Leptomeningeal disease or single or multiple mass lesions	Headache Cranial nerve abn	Abnormal neuro exam	Spinal tap CT/MRI
RENAL	Ureteral compression			IVP, BUN/Cr

Key Reference: DeVita Jr VT, Lawrence TS, Rosenberg SA, eds. *Cancer: Principles and practice of oncology*. 8th ed. Philadelphia: Lippincott Williams & Wilkins; 2008 [chapter 51].

Perioperative Implications

Preoperative Preparation
- Assess extant bulky nodal disease causing upper or lower airway and/or cardiac compression
- Assess LV function after anthracyclines
- Assess pulm function after bleomycin, RT
- If large mediastinal mass, use local anesthetic if possible

Monitoring
- Routine

Airway
- Routine, unless large anterior mediastinal mass calls for awake fiberoptic intubation
- Use armored ETT
- Rigid ventilating bronchoscope on hand

Induction
- If large mediastinal mass: Consider awake fiberoptic intubation, maintaining spontaneous ventilation, and semi-Fowler's position

Maintenance
- Spontaneous ventilation as above; avoid muscle relaxants
- Choose shortest acting agents for rapid wakeup
- After bleomycin use lowest FIO_2 possible

Extubation
- If mediastinal mass, extubate pt awake and breathing spontaneously and have rigid ventilation bronchoscope on hand

Adjuvants
- If asymptomatic with mediastinal mass, airway obstruction and/or cardiac compression may develop on induction

Postoperative Period
- Airway obstruction if mediastinal mass: Observe longer in intensive nursing setting
- Monitor fluid status if significant LV dysfunction

Anticipated Problems/Concerns
- If bulky nodal disease in neck and chest, at risk for SVC syndrome, difficult airway, and tracheobronchial compression on loss of spontaneous ventilation
- May have significant cardiac/pulm impairment due to combination chemotherapy and RT

Malignant Hyperthermia (MH) and Other Anesthetic-Induced Myodystrophies (AIM)

Henry Rosenberg

Risk

- Incidence of MH: 1/15,000–20,000 anesthetics in children; 1/50,000–100,000 in adults depending on use of trigger agents, gene pool
- Male > female
- Family Hx of MH or unexplained death may predict MH susceptibility.
- Improved outcome by avoiding trigger agnets in MH susceptibles, availability of dantrolene, and using succinylcholine on indication

Perioperative Risks

- Mortality with MH in North America <10%, when event in a hospital; ~20% when pt transferred into a hospital; untreated, mortality >80%
- Mortality with other AIMs unknown
- Masseter muscle rigidity (MMR)—10–20% of pts experiencing MMR develop clinical MH; generalized rigidity predicts clinical MH in >60%
- Central core myopathy—very high risk for MH
- Multiminicore is also associated with MH susceptibilty
- Hyperkalemia and cardiac arrest with Duchenne, Becker's dystrophy when succinylcholine used and sometimes with volatile agents only
- Certain forms of myotonia lead to risk for MH and/or hyperkalemia with succinylcholine
- Muscle rigidity common with all myotonias when succinylcholine used

Worry About

- Unexplained tachycardia, tachypnea elevated $ETCO_2$ during anesthesia
- Potent volatile anesthetics and succinylcholine contraindicated in MH and pts with AIM
- Availability of dantrolene
- Purge machine with 100% O_2 15–20 min prior to case. Newer anesthesia workstations (e.g., Drager Fabius) require longer period of purging—up to 60 min.

- Recrudescence of MH in 25% of cases despite treatment
- If working in ambulatory center, prearranged transfer protocol and blood gas analysis
- Counseling family regarding risk, muscle biopsy and genetic testing

Overview

- Malignant hyperthermia (MH)
- Autosomal dominant myopathy in humans
- No phenotypic signs predict MH other than previous Hx of MH or family Hx or unexplained elevated CK.
- Hypermetabolic disorder manifested by $\uparrow CO_2$ production/O_2 consumption, acidosis, hyperkalemia, myoglobinuria/emia, tachycardia, tachypnea, increased $ETCO_2$
- Dantrolene is the only specific treatment
- Dx by halothane/caffeine contracture test of biopsied muscle is most sensitive and specific.
- DNA testing available in two laboratories in the USA and in many centers in Europe. Pts must be selected. Sensitivity is ~30%, specificity close to 100%.
- Pts with MD/myotonia may develop hyperkalemic arrest with succinylcholine and occasionally with potent volatiles only
- Signs of dystrophy subtle or not apparent in young children
- Obtain muscle specimens for dystrophin analysis; genetic testing if cardiac arrest
- Test for CK elevation in suspicious cases
- Information for provider and pt available through MHAUS, the Malignant Hyperthermia Association of the US, Sherburne NY. www.mhaus.org, 607–674–7901
- MH hotline 1-800-MH –HYPER

ICD-9-CM Code: 995.86 (MH) Other AIMs

Etiology

MH

- Defect in intracellular calcium release/control in skeletal muscle leads to $\uparrow$ intracellular calcium
- Heterogenetic predisposition
- Ryanodine receptor of skeletal muscle is defective in 70% of cases. Dihydropyridine receptor (DHPR, the CACNA1S locus) in about 1% of cases. Unknown loci, the remainder.
- *RYR-1* gene on chromosome 19. Over 120 mutations of which 29 have been shown to be causal. The others are being clarified.

Other AIMs

- Muscular dystrophies: X-linked inheritance, several mutations
- Myotonia: Genetic abn of sodium, chloride channels, or protein kinase, linked to chromosomes 19, 17, others
- Central core disease: In most families, linked to ryanodine receptor
- Pts with CPT-2 deficiency may develop rhabdomyolysis with MH triggers.

Usual Treatment

MH

- D/C triggers
- Hyperventilate pt with 100% O_2
- Dantrolene 2.5 mg/kg IV; may use more to treat acute episode
- Treat metabolic acidosis; actively cool
- Increase fluids 1½ to 2 × maintenance
- No calcium-channel blockers
- Maintain UO 1–2 mL/kg, diuretics if necessary
- Assess for hyperkalemia and treat appropriately
- Coagulation profile, DIC a problem
- Continue treatment for at least 36 hr at 1–2 mg/kg /4–6 hr

Other AIMs

- Treat for hyperkalemia

ASSESSMENT POINTS

System	Effect	Assessment by Hx and PE	Test
HEENT	Masseter muscle rigidity	Difficult intubation	ABGs/acidosis Hypercarbia Myoglobinuria
CARDIO	MH: Tachycardia, arrhythmias AIM: Sudden bradycardia VFIB, asystole	Hyper/hypotension	Mixed venous and ABGs: $\uparrow ETCO_2$, myoglobinuria, hyperkalemia
RESP	Tachypnea	Tachypnea	$\uparrow ETCO_2$
MS	Generalized rigidity	Developmental delay Muscle weakness	CK Muscle biopsy contracture test and histology DNA testing
RENAL	Renal failure	Low UO Dark urine	Myoglobin in serum and urine, serum potassium
SKIN	Vasoconstriction Heat	Mottled appearance (late) Hot skin Sweating	Core temp

Note: The caffeine/halothane contracture test is used to assess MH susceptibility.

Key Reference: Rosenberg H, Dirksen RA, Sambuughin N. Malignant hyperthermia susceptibility. In Baskin P, Pagan R, eds. *Gene Reviews.* www.Genetests.org; 2003, revised 2006, 2009.

Perioperative Implications

Perioperative Preparation for Known MH
- Avoid triggers (succinylcholine, all potent volatile agents)
- Use local anesthesia (amides and ester OK)
  - Regional anesthesia (epidural, spinal, regional block)
  - General: All following drugs are *not* triggers: pentothal (barbiturates), etomidate, ketamine, propofol, NO, all nondepolarizing muscle relaxants, narcotics, benzodiazepines. Suggest TIVA
- Anesthesia machine
  - Change circuit and bag
  - Remove and/or drain vaporizers

- O_2 flow at 10 L/min for 15–20 min prior to use
  - Newer anesthesia workstations (e.g., Fabius) require up to 60 min of purging
- Dantrolene prophylaxis not necessary
- Dantrolene and calcium-channel blockers together produce hyperkalemia

Monitoring
- Routine incl $ETCO_2$, core temp (e.g., esophageal, axillary, bladder, pulm artery)

Perioperative Implications, Other AIMs
- Some, not all, pts with DMD and Becker's dystrophy will develop hyperkalemia with MH triggers

- Avoid succinylcholine in pts with myotonia and most other myopathies and neuromuscular disorders

Anticipated Problems/Concerns
- Sudden cardiac arrest in PACU
- Myoglobinuria, renal failure
- Postop rhabdomyolysis, follow CKs
- Hyperkalemia
- Postop muscle pain/weakness and persistently elevated CK
- Have pt enter the North American MH Registry of MHAUS. MHreg.org

Malnutrition

Joseph Rinehart

Risk

- Rate about 4% in general population, 10–20% in surgical pts, and rises to 40% or more in severely ill hospital admissions
- Risk increases with severity of underlying disease, presence of malignancy (esp. GI), and advancing age
- Hospitalized pts lose an average of 5% body wt during time of admission

Perioperative Risks

- **Postop complications are significantly higher in the malnourished.**
- Severe undernutrition may result in CHF, resp failure, and immunologic dysfunction.

Worry About

- Need for early postop nutritional supplementation, particularly enteral if possible.
- Infection risk: Care should be taken with invasive procedures and sterile technique.
- Intraop problems may incl low cardiac output and resp failure.

Overview

- Results from inadequate intake of macronutrients (carbohydrate, protein, fat); referred to as protein-calorie malnutrition (PCM)
- There are two types of PCM:
  - Marasmic form (MF-PCM), which results in uniform loss of fat and muscle mass in all tissues and a concomitant loss of H_2O in proportion to nonaqueous mass
  - Stress-induced hypoalbuminemic form of protein-calorie malnutrition (HAF-PCM), which results from neurohumoral modulation leading to depletion of visceral protein (in excess of muscle mass) and fat and is assoc with an expansion of extracellular fluid compartment. Stress may be surgery, infection, inflammation, trauma, neoplasia.
  - In hospitalized pts, marasmic-kwashiorkor type (i.e., wasting of muscle and fat with hypoalbuminemia) is most common.

ICD-9-CM Code: 263.9 (Unspecified protein-calorie malnutrition)

Etiology

- Decreased dietary intake: Advanced age, physical debilitation, GI-related illnesses, neck mass
- Increased metabolic demands and nutrient loss: Stress (physical and psychological), disease states (particularly GI and resp illness like emphysema), infections, burns, liver failure
- Conditions assoc with N/V
- Malignant conditions, esp. those involving the GI tract

Usual Treatment.

- Early PO intake postop is advantageous, esp. in GI malignancies; enteral intake reduces infections
- Enteral nutrition via g-tube or j-tube preferable to TPN if direct PO intake not possible but gut can still be utilized (e.g., esophageal surgery)
- TPN value is inconclusive, but probably indicated in severe malnutrition states. TPN reduces noninfectious complications but increases infectious complication rates in most studies.

ASSESSMENT POINTS

System	Effect	Assessment by Hx	Test
CARDIO	↓ Preload and stroke volume		ECHO
RESP	↓ FRC and diaphragmatic activity		CXR Expiratory spirogram
GI	↓ Gastric motility Gastric ulceration Gastric and intestinal atrophy	Anorexia, vomiting	Generally not needed
GENERAL	Malnutrition	Preadmission wt loss >10% of body wt in 6 mo or 5% in 1 mo, edema, anorexia, vomiting, diarrhea, ↓ food intake, chronic illness	BMI <20 kg/m² Voluntary hand-grip test Anthropometric measurements (midarm muscle circumference or triceps skinfold thickness: Both <15th percentile of reference data)
IMMUNO	Impaired cell-mediated immunity Surgical wound infection and sepsis		Abnormally low lymphocyte count (<1500/mm³) Anergy to a battery of 4 or 5 standard skin antigens
RENAL	↓ Body mass ↓ Cr clearance and impaired ability to concentrate urine	↓ UO	Serum Cr/BUN
HEPATIC	↓ Protein synthesis		↓ Serum albumin (<3.5 mg/dL) and ↓ serum transferrin (< 200 mg/dL)
PNS	↓ Peripheral nerve conduction and sensory abnormalities	Tingling and numbness in extremities	Generally not needed

Key Reference: Corish CA, Kennedy NP. Protein-energy undernutrition in hospital in-patients. *Br J Nutr.* 2000;83:575–591.

Perioperative Considerations

Preinduction

- Use of a malnutrition risk assay (e.g., Nutrition Risk Score) for screening will help identify at-risk pts
- Nutritional and caloric supplementation in the days before surgery may be beneficial if possible
- Consider prophylaxis for aspiration of gastric contents if GI process is responsible for malnutrition (malignancy, obstruction, etc.)

Monitoring

- Routine

Induction

- If resp muscle weakness/fatigue is suspected, avoidance of long-acting NMDBs may be prudent.

Maintenance

- Pts receiving TPN should continue to receive it in the OR as abrupt discontinuation may result in severe hypoglycemia. Many sources recommend a rate reduction of 50% intraop. Alternatively, TPN may be replaced with dextrose during surgery.
- Standard hydration and UOP monitoring

Extubation

- Resp muscle failure may preclude early extubation; careful attention to resp status warranted in PACU

Adjuvants

- Hepatic drug metabolism may be impaired
- Decrease binding (volume of distribution) of protein-bound drugs in hypo-albuminemic pts

Anticipated Problems/Concerns

- Because edema is prominent feature of HAF-PCM, interpretation of anthropometric measurements like arm circumference may be unreliable.
- Serum markers like albumin, transferring, and prealbumin can be unreliable in a wide array of disease states and do not correlate well with outcomes and complications.
- Pts with end-stage chronic obstructive lung disease usually have malnutrition, and sudden feeding periop may precipitate acute resp failure and re-feeding syndrome.

Marfan's Syndrome

William J. Greeley

Risk

- Prevalence is 2–3/10,000 population
- Inherited as autosomal dominant trait
- 25% of cases are sporadic due to de novo mutations

Perioperative Risks

- Aortic arch dissection, MVP, mitral or aortic valve regurgitation, coronary artery abn, cardiac arrhythmias, pneumothorax, restrictive lung disease

Worry About

- Symptoms referable to progressive dilatation or rupture of ascending thoracic aortic aneurysm (e.g., chest pain radiating to interscapular region)
- Symptoms of mitral (midsystolic click) or aortic valvular insufficiency
- Myocardial ischemia (angina) due to medial necrosis of coronary arterioles
- Arrhythmias and conduction disturbances (palpitations)
- SOB (dyspnea) due to restrictive lung disease

Overview

- Familial disorder of connective tissue (CT) underlying defect of collagen synthesis decreases tensile strength and elasticity of CT. Involves skeleton, eye, and CV system, skin, fascia, lungs, skeletal muscle, CNS, and adipose tissue.
- Common causes of death are CV: Aortic dilation, dissection, or rupture; aortic or mitral valvular regurgitation; coronary artery insufficiency
- Airway features: High-arched palate, facies dolichocephaly (long narrow skull), malar hypoplasia (an underdeveloped mid-face), retrognathia
- Skeletal features: Increased length of long bones, joint laxity, scoliosis, pectus excavatum and carinatum, possible laxity of cervical spine, hernia, lumbar sacral dural ectasia
- Pulm: Spontaneous pneumothorax, restrictive lung disease with thoracic deformity, and obstructive problems during sleep due to laxity of soft tissue
- Ocular: Lenticular subluxation or dislocation, flat cornea, increased globe axial length (myopia), hypoplastic iris or ciliary muscle, enophthalmos

ICD-9-CM Code: 759.82

Etiology

- Mutation in *FBNI*, the gene that encodes fibrillin-1, a major component of extracellular microfibrils (major components of elastic fibers, anchoring the dermis, epidermis, and ocular zonules). The new understanding is that many aspects of the disease are caused by altered regulation of transforming growth factor β (TGFβ), a family of cytokines that affects cellular performance.
- A rapid and efficient molecular diagnostic test does not currently exist for this disorder.

Usual Treatment

- No specific treatment exists however, pts can be considered for prophylactic beta blocker therapy or other antihypertensives to reduce hemodynamic stresses and the progression of aortic dilation.
- Life expectancy can be normal.

ASSESSMENT POINTS

System	Effect	Assessment by HX	PE	Test
HEENT	Lens dislocation	Myopia	Retinal detachment	Ophthalmoscopy
CV	Aortic dissection	Chest pain		MRI, ECHO
	Myocardial ischemia	Angina		ECG
				Radionuclide studies
				Stress testing
				Angiography
	Arrhythmias	Palpitations	Pulse	Holter monitor
				Electrophysiology
RESP	Restrictive lung disease	Dyspnea	Pectus scoliosis	PFTs
				CXR
MS	Tall stature			Arm span:height ratio >1.05
	Joint hypermobility			
	Recurrent dislocation			
	Hernias			

Key Reference: Judge DP, Dietz HC. Marfan's syndrome. *Lancet.* 2005;366:1965–1976.

Perioperative Implications

Preoperative Preparation

- Consider antibiotics for SBE prophylaxis.
- Consider preop β-blockade Rx to mitigate increases in myocardial contractility and aortic wall tension (dP/dT).

Monitoring

- ST-segment analysis; QT interval analysis, consider TEE
- Invasive monitoring as appropriate for planned surgery

Airway

- High-arched palate
- Potential cervical laxity/instability
- Potential for TMJ dislocation with direct laryngoscopy

Preinduction/Induction

- Avoid sudden increases in aortic wall tension
- Careful positioning to avoid dislocations

Maintenance

- No one technique has demonstrated superiority

Exubation

- Avoid sudden increases in CO, BP as this may increase dP/dT
- High risk for developing myocardial ischemia

Adjuvants

- Adequate pain management is important
- May require ↑ doses of local anesthetic due to ↑ size and enlargement of the neural canal

Anticipated Problems/Concerns

- CV: Aortic dissection, MVP, mitral or aortic regurgitation, myocardial ischemia, cardiac arrhythmias
- Resp: Pneumothorax, restrictive lung disease with thoracic deformity

Mastocytosis

Jeremy L. Gibson

Risk

- Cutaneous mastocytosis (CM) is primarily a disease of children and affects 1 in 1000 to 1 in 8000
- Systemic mastocytosis (SM) is more prevalent in adults and affects between 1 in 10,000 and 1 in 80,000
- Equal male and female prevalence

Perioperative Risks

- Increased risk of hypotension and bronchospasm as a consequence of paroxysmal release of mast cell mediators
- Anesthetic drugs and procedures may induce mast cell degranulation
- Mast cell degranulation may present as an anaphylactic shock with CV collapse. Fatal cases have been reported.

Worry About

- Increased risk of hypotensive shock and bronchospasm
- Clotting factors may be disturbed as result of vitamin malabsorption, hepatic fibrosis, and massive heparin release from mast cells (uncommon).
- Profound CV collapse and death without signs of flushing or bronchospasm

Overview

- Group of rare mast cell proliferative disorders
- CM is limited to the skin, SM may involve the bone marrow or other non-cutaneous organs, and may or may not affect the skin.
- CM usually presents in childhood and often resolves by adolescence.
- CM is classified as urticaria pigmentosa, diffuse cutaneous mastocytosis, or solitary mastocytoma
- SM is more common in adults and is identified as indolent systemic mastocytosis, smoldering systemic mastocytosis, systemic mastocytosis with another associated non–mast-cell hematologic lineage disorder, aggressive systemic mastocytosis, and mast cell leukemia.
- Mast cells release histamine, heparin, leukotrienes and various cytokines.
- Degranulation can be caused by certain medications, physical pressure, extreme temp, spicy food, ingestion of hot beverages, alcohol, and emotional upset.
- Medications to be avoided: Morphine, atracurium, mivacurium, rocuronium, NSAIDs, vancomycin
- Thorough pt trigger Hx is critical
- Lower risk medications incl fentanyl, sufentanil, remifentanil, acetaminophen, cisatracurium, midazolam.
- Avoid aspirin in those with no exposure Hx, but for those who can tolerate aspirin, its ability to block prostaglandin D_2 is a potential benefit in SM.
- Volatile anesthetics do not cause histamine release.
- For many the initial manifestation is a cutaneous eruption.
- Common symptoms incl episodic flushing, headaches, N/V, diarrhea, fatigue.
- May see vascular collapse with syncope and palpitations, abdominal pain, wheezing
- Serum tryptase levels correlate with total body mast cell burden.
- Pts with systemic disease at greater risk for CV collapse.
- Main concern: To avoid mast cell degranulation
- Rare: Mast cell lymphoma/leukemia; rule out carcinoid syndrome as cause of symptoms (elevated urinary 5-HIAA)

ICD-9-CM Codes 202.6 (Mastocytosis); 238.5 (Mastocytoma); 757.33 (Mastocytosis syndrome)

Etiology

- Pathogenesis incompletely understood but frequently involves mutations in the tyrosine kinase receptor c-kit. It is a mast cell proliferative disorder.

Usual Treatment

- H_1 blockers, e.g., diphenhydramine, chlorpheniramine maleate, hydroxyzine, terfenadine
- H_2 blockers, e.g., cimetidine, ranitidine
- Aspirin to control flushing (if pt has a past Hx of safe aspirin use) to block PGD_2 synthesis
- Proton pump inhibitors if H_2 blockers ineffective for abdominal symptoms
- Antileukotriene inhibitors, e.g., montelukast, zafirleukast
- Cromolyn sodium for GI symptoms
- Ketotifen mast cell stabilizing and H_1 antihistamine (Canada and Europe)
- Shock: IV epinephrine (Adults: 2–10 μg/min infusion; children: 0.1 to 1 mcg/kg/min infusion) and volume repletion
- EpiPen and epinephrine inhalers should be carried by pts with known or suspected disease.
- PUVA (psoralens plus ultraviolet A) for cutaneous manifestations
- Steroids: Topical and systemic
- Chemotherapy
- Splenectomy for hypersplenism with anemia and thrombocytopenia
- Protamine sulphate rarely necessary when endogenous heparin prolongs prothrombin time

ASSESSMENT POINTS

System	Effect	Assessment by Hx	PE	Test
HEENT	Rhinorrhea	Allergic rhinitis		
CV	Episodic CV collapse			Episodic elevations of plasma histamine levels, serum tryptase levels
RESP	Asthma	Wheezing		
GI	Malabsorption, GI bleeding Abdominal pain, N/V, diarrhea		Hepatosplenomegaly	
HEME	Anemia, thrombocytopenia, leukopenia, mast cell leukemia, excess bone marrow blasts			CBC clotting studies Bone marrow biopsy
DERM	Mastocytoma/urticaria pigmentosa; Telangiectasia macularis eruptive perstans (TMEP)	Pruritis, urticaria	Skin biopsy	(+ Giemsa)
PNS	Polyneuropathy		CNS exam	
MS	Bone pain			X-ray, ^{99m}Tc bone scan

Key Reference: Ahmad N, Evans P, Lloyd-Thomas A. Anesthesia in children with mastocytosis—a case based review. *Paediatr Anaesth.* 2009;19:97–107.

Perioperative Implications

Preoperative Preparation
- Refrain from ethanol, NSAIDs, aspirin (unless known tolerance for aspirin).
- Premedication with histamine-releasing drugs should be avoided.
- Diazepam, midazolam premedication—reported to be safe
- Start prophylactic H_1 and H_2 blockers
- May give diphenhydramine, 25–50 mg PO 1 hr prior, ranitidine 150 mg PO 1 hr prior, montelukast 10 mg PO 1 hr prior, prednisone 50 mg PO 24 hr and again 2 hr prior to procedure
- Prophylactic cromolyn sodium: Yet to be confirmed (100 mg q6h)

- Predictive prick tests for drugs such as muscle relaxants are inconclusive because metabolites not seen in skin tests may cause degranulation.
- Serum tryptase levels correlate with mast cell burden.

Monitoring
- Routine monitors
- Intra-arterial catheter (sudden BP changes)

Airway
- Intubation may be dangerous in the presence of mucosal lesions, as pressure can cause degranulation and bronchospasm or hypotension.

Preinduction/Induction
- Avoiding atropine, scopolamine, and sodium thiopental has been recommended.

- Midazolam and fentanyl both with good safety records
- Muscle relaxants: Cisatracurium recommended. Avoid atracurium, mivacurium, rocuronium, ditubocurarine
- Inhalational agents: Safe (may even increase mast cell stability)

Maintenance
- Maintain normothermia
- Hypotension due to histamine release: IV epinephrine, (Adults: 2–10 μg/min infusion; children: 0.1 to 1 mcg/kg/min infusion)
- Dopamine: Not helpful
- Avoid dextran as colloidal solution

Extubation
- Should be smooth
- Keep pt warm

Adjuvants
- Blood transfusion—should be warmed and given only when essential
- Regional: Has been advocated but hypotension and bronchospasm reported to be even more common as well as urticaria and pruritus

- Antibiotics: Avoid polymyxin B sulfate, vancomycin. Used safely: Amikacin, cefazolin, metronidazole
- Miscellaneous drugs: Avoid dipyridamole, papaverine, quinine, thiamine
- Radiologic contrast dyes can induce acute episode.

Postoperative Period
- Continue with analgesics, H_1 and H_2 blockers

Anticipated Problems/Concerns
- Hypotensive and bronchospastic crisis due to mast cell degranulation induced by anesthetic or surgical procedures
- Anaphylaxis

Mediastinal Masses

Frank Gencorelli

Ashish C. Sinha

Risk

- Usually a congenital lesion, occurring at 1:5000, no gender bias
- Benign or malignant; cysts or aneurysms that arise from the lung, pleura, or another structure of anterior mediastinum
- Lymphoma (Hodgkin's or NHL), thymoma, germ cell tumor, granuloma, bronchogenic cancer, thyroid tumors (retrosternal goiter), bronchogenic cysts and cystic hygroma

Perioperative Risks

- Periop mortality is rare
- Sudden CV collapse from inability to ventilate or oxygenate (collapse of great vessels)
- Hypotension or tamponade
- Increased dyspnea (orthopnea) or cough when supine (increased risk of airway complications)
- Syncopal symptoms or pericardial effusion (increased risk of CV complications)
- Major airway complications in these pts are now more likely to occur in the post-anesthetic care area rather than in the OR

Worry About

- Inability to get on cardiopulmonary bypass rapid enough to avoid permanent neurologic damage

- Superior vena cava syndrome with airway edema and increased bleeding
- Recurrent laryngeal nerve injury
- Pts at risk with cough and pain, dyspnea and dysphagia, superior vena cava syndrome, tracheal deviation, Horner's syndrome, cyanosis, mediastinal widening, and hoarseness

Overview

- Severity of symptoms does not predict intraop course.
- Airway obstruction or hemodynamic compromise has occurred with induction of GA, intubation, muscle relaxation, position change, and after extubation.
- Pts may present with Sx that incl chest pain or fullness, dyspnea, cough, sweats, superior vena cava obstruction, hoarseness, syncope, or dysphagia.
- Pts can be asymptomatic and have a mass diagnosed on a screening chest radiograph or CT scan.

ICD-9-CM Codes: 164.0 (Malignant thymoma) 201.9 (Hodgkin lymphoma); 202.8 (NHL)

Etiology

- Adults: 97% malignant, 80% metastatic bronchogenic carcinomas; 17% lymphomas (50% of lymphomas have mediastinal involvement); 20% thymomas (50% malignant, 35% assoc with myasthenia gravis)
- Pediatric: 8% malignant, 16–36% NHL and 54–81% Hodgkin lymphomas, bronchial cysts, and teratomas
- Superior vena cava syndrome in 6–7% of lung cancer
- Others incl parathyroid or thyroid tumors; lymphoid tumors; teratomas; aortic aneurysms; esophageal achalasia or diverticula, diaphragmatic hernia

Usual Treatment

- For tissue diagnosis: Biopsy under local
- If no tissue can be obtained or pt is uncooperative, approach is selective radiotherapy sparing some tumor for later diagnosis – if not diagnostic, then biopsy under GA.
- Surgical resection for some tumors
- Anesthesia complications are usually fewer after radiation.

ASSESSMENT POINTS

System	Effect	Assessment by Hx	PE	Test
HEENT	Possible tracheal compression by mass, bulky nodal disease	Dysphonia, dysphagia, coughing paroxysms when supine or orthopnea	Palpable neck mass, wheezing, stridor,	Indirect laryngoscopy, CXR, CT scan, MRI, pulm flow volume studies (not very helpful though)
CARDIO	SVC syndrome, compression of PA, cardiac failure	Dyspnea, fatigue, syncope, peripheral edema, crackles, headache, chest pain, SOB	Facial or neck swelling, upper body edema, cyanosis, increased JVP, hypotension	CXR, ECHO EKG, stress ECHO, CT/MRI
CNS	Recurrent laryngeal nerve compression, spinal cord compression	Stridor, dysphonia, focal symptoms based on point of compression	Anatomical distortion of neck or thorax	CXR, CT
RESP	Decreased lung volumes, bronchial compression, obstructive pneumonia	SOB, ↑ respiratory rate, dyspnea, cough	Wheezing, distant breath sounds, hypoxemia, pedal edema	PFT, ABG, CXR, DL_{CO}

Key Reference: Slinger P, Karsli C. Management of the patient with a large anterior mediastinal mass: recurring myths. *Curr Opin Anaesthesiol.* 2007;20:1–3.

Perioperative Implications

Preoperative Preparation
- Consider (incl pediatric pts) an IV prior to induction (lower extremity if SVC syndrome)
- All pts should have a CXR and a chest and neck CT scan prior to any surgical procedure to plan airway management.
- Those with PA or heart compression may need cardiopulmonary bypass (check availability prior to induction with cannulation sites prepped and draped)
- Studies of flow-volume loops have shown a poor correlation with the degree of clinical airway obstruction and have not demonstrated usefulness in managing these pts.
- Reserve use of premedication except for anticholinergic.

Monitoring
- Consider intra-arterial catheter, central venous, or pulm artery catheter.
- If SVC syndrome, insert central venous access or PA catheter via femoral vein.

Airway
- Tracheal or distal compression; may become obstructed with induction and muscle relaxation

- Maintain spontaneous ventilation throughout procedure unless ETT is below obstruction.
- Pts who are symptomatic in supine position are best induced sitting or semi-sitting.
- Awake fiberoptic intubation may be skipped if asymptomatic in supine position and CXR and/or CT scan do not reveal airway obstruction or compression.
- If in doubt, consider awake fiberoptic bronchoscopy to rule out obstruction or compression.
- If compression seen in thoracic trachea, consider a single lumen armored ETT with its tip distal to the compression.
- If compression is at level of carina or distal, endobronchial intubation or a double-lumen endobronchial tube is recommended.

Preinduction/Induction
- May develop airway obstruction with inability to ventilate
- May develop hypoxia from obstruction of pulm artery and blood flow to lungs
- If muscle relaxants are required, assisted ventilation should first be gradually taken over manually to assure that positive-pressure ventilation is possible and only then can a short-acting muscle relaxant be administered.
- Development of airway or vascular collapse at induction demands immediate awakening.

Maintenance
- Consider local anesthesia, otherwise consider keeping pt breathing spontaneously.
- If obstruction occurs, consider altering pt's position, attempt rigid bronchoscopy, median sternotomy, or femorofemoral cardiopulmonary bypass

Extubation
- Deep extubation during spontaneous breathing recommended; try to minimize straining, coughing, or bucking which would all increase intrathoracic pressure.
- Observe in a monitored bed for several hr after extubation to detect and treat delayed airway obstruction

Anticipated Problems/Concerns

- Airway obstruction with the inability to ventilate
- Vascular compression with hypotension, hypoxia, and arrest.
- Consider radiation and/or chemotherapy before surgery.
- If GA required, consider inspection of tracheobronchial tree with fiberoptic bronchoscopy.
- If GA required, maintaining spontaneous ventilation preferable.
- The most useful information for the anesthesiologist to guide management of these pts comes from the pt's Hx and the chest imaging.

• Special problems in pediatric populations: Anesthetic deaths have mainly been reported in children, possibly due to the more compressible cartilaginous structure of the airway or because of underestimation of the severity of the airway compression in children due to the difficulty in obtaining a clear Hx of positional symptoms. Even with proper management, children with tracheobronchial compression more than half cannot be safely given general anesthesia. Further increasing risk in pediatric pts, securing the distal airway with awake fiberoptic intubation and placement of an ETT distal to a tracheal obstruction, an option for some adults with masses compressing the mid-trachea, is not an option in most children.

Mesothelioma

Srinivasan Rajagopal
John R. Moyers

Risk

- Incidence in USA: ~2000–3000 new cases annually, and decreasing. Increasing incidence in developing countries due to poor regulation of asbestos in mining and industrial use.
- Attributable mortality: 14 deaths per million USA population
- M: F: ratio 3–6:1
- 0.16% of all malignancies

Perioperative Risks

- Usually discovered in geriatric male undergoing lung biopsy
- Pleural effusion
- General debilitation from malignancy

Worry About

- Previous needle biopsy of lung and thoracentesis make pneumothorax a concern

Overview

- Diffuse malignant mesothelioma arises from the mesothelial surface of the pleura, peritoneum, and pericardium, and the tunica vaginalis of the testis
- 80–90% originate from the pleura
- Peak incidence 20–40y after asbestos exposure
- Usual onset of symptoms at age 55–70y
- Median survival after onset of symptoms is approx 18mo

ICD-9-CM Codes: 162.9 (Lung neoplasm); 199.1 (Mesothelioma, malignant site unspecified); 162.9 (Malignant neoplasm of bronchus and lung unspecified)

Etiology

- Diffuse mesothelioma related to asbestos exposure in 12–93% of cases
- Also assoc with radiation therapy, erionite exposure, chronic inflammation and fibrosis, and other agents

Usual Treatment

- Treatment has been controversial and largely ineffective
- Therapy has consisted of combinations of radiation to hemithorax, chemotherapy, and sometimes surgery (parietal pleurectomy and decortication or extrapleural pneumonectomy)

ASSESSMENT POINTS

System	Effect	Assessment by Hx	PE	Test
HEENT	Tracheal displacement Superior vena cava syndrome			Lateral and AP CXR
CARDIO				ECG, echocardiography
RESP	Pneumothorax	Cough, chest pain, increased SOB		ABGs, PFTs (for lung resections) CXR (post biopsy; in expiration)
	Restrictive lung disease	Dyspnea with exercise	Percussion and auscultation of chest	
GI	Wt loss, debilitation, peritoneal tumors	Past body weights		CT scan of abdomen (not for periop care) Albumin (for degree of malnutrition) CBC (for malnutrition)
ENDO	Not associated with paraneoplastic syndromes			

Key Reference: Ng J, Hartigan PM. Anesthetic management of patients undergoing extrapleural pneumonectomy for mesothelioma. *Curr Opin Anaesthesiol.* 2008;21:21–27.

Perioperative Implications

Perioperative Preparation

- Usually come to surgery for lung biopsy via thoracoscopy or open-lung biopsy; some pts are scheduled for pleuropneumonectomy
- Assess pulm status; size of effusion, no pneumothorax
- Pt often had one or more recent needle biopsies of lung or thoracenteses
- Review radiographic studies for size and location of tumor

Monitoring

- Routine monitors
- Resp system via stethoscope, SpO_2, and $PETCO_2$
- Intra-arterial catheter for complex surgical procedures

Airway

- Look for tracheal and mediastinal displacement on radiographic studies

Induction

- Propensity for hypoxia, particularly from restrictive lung disease

Maintenance

- High FIO_2 may be necessary
- One-lung ventilation
- Lateral positioning

Extubation

- Ensure pt meets extubation criteria

Adjuvants

- Pain control after thoracoscopy or thoracotomy
- No special considerations for muscle relaxants, reversal agents, local anesthetics, or special drug interactions

Postoperative Period

- Monitor ventilation and oxygenation
- Pain relief; consider epidural or spinal analgesia after thoracotomies
- May have air leak postop

Anticipated Problems/Concerns

- Anesthesia with one-lung ventilation for a geriatric pt with incurable malignancy
- Recent lung biopsy and thoracentesis prior to surgery and potential for complications from those procedures, incl pneumothorax and dehydration
- With extrapleural pneumonectomy a possibility of massive blood loss, dysrhythmias, and hemodynamic instability during pericardial window and patch
- Effective pain relief and monitoring of resp function postop
- Consider ICU stay for those undergoing complex procedures

Methemoglobinemia

H. Michael Marsh

Risk

- Incidence within USA: Rare
- Gender prevalence: None
- Socioeconomic/ethnic prevalence: None

Perioperative Risks

- Inadequate O_2 carriage and delivery to tissues
- Hemolysis may be induced by methylene blue, esp in pts with G6PD deficiency.

Worry About

- Percent of methemoglobin or sulfhemoglobin. Acutely developing methemoglobinemia or sulfhemoglobinemia may become symptomatic at 1% with cyanosis; at 60%, acute CV collapse, coma, or death may occur.

Overview

- Present when >1% of circulating hemoglobin is oxidized to ferric form
- Two hereditary forms: Due to NADH-diaphorase (cytochrome b5 reductase) deficiency, inherited as an autosomal recessive trait; and due to abn globins, hemoglobin M, which are inherited as autosomal dominant traits
- Toxic methemoglobinemia occurs from exposure to agents that directly oxidize hemoglobin or facilitate its oxidation by molecular O_2: nitrates ingested, nitroglycerin, isobutyl nitrite, and some local anesthetics

ICD-9-CM Code: 289.7

Etiology/Pathogenesis

- Fe^{2+} in hemoglobin is constantly oxidized in vivo, by NO and reactivity with O_2, to Fe^{3+}, methemoglobin. NADPH-diaphorase utilizes NADH generated by glyceraldehyde dehydrogenase, in the Embden-Meyerhof pathway, to reduce cytochrome b5, which in turn reduces Fe^{3+} in methemoglobin to Fe^{2+} in hemoglobin.

Usual Treatment

- Medical therapy: Ascorbic acid 300–600 mg/d in divided doses. Methylene blue 1 mg/kg IV, repeated once provided that pt is not G6PD-deficient, since hemolysis will occur in this case.
- Methylene blue may also be taken orally as 60 mg tid.

ASSESSMENT POINTS

System	Effect	Assessment by Hx	PE	Test
RESP	SOB DOE	Hx of cyanosis if hereditary form	RR	Co-oximetry
HEME	Cyanosis if 1% methemoglobin is present or sulfhemoglobin seen	Cyanosed	Cyanosis	Spectrometry at 630 nm

Key Reference: Kern K, Langevin PB, Dunn BM. Methemoglobinemia after topical anesthesia with lidocaine and benzocaine for a difficult intubation. *J Clin Anesth*. 2000;12:167–172.

Perioperative Implications

Preoperative Preparation

- Consider treatment if methemoglobin level is >1%. If sulfhemoglobin is present, may mean exchange transfusion.

Monitoring

- Use co-oximeter (IL282), since presence of methemoglobin will render pulse oximetry unreliable.

Airway

- Routine

Induction

- Routine

Maintenance

- Routine

Extubation

- Routine

Adjuvants

- Avoid nitrates and local anesthetics that act as oxidizing agents.

Postoperative Period

- See Monitoring

Anticipated Problems/Concerns

- O_2 carriage is interfered with, proportional to concentration of altered hemoglobin present, and the interference with O_2 release and shift of tension-saturation curve from normal position.
- Pulse oximetry overestimates SaO_2 in presence of methemoglobin. Methylene blue will decrease the SaO_2 for about 30 min after injection.

Mitochondrial Myopathy

Jerry H. Kim
Jeremy M. Geiduschek

Risk

- More common than previously thought. Prevalence ranges from 1 in 7000 to 1 in 15,000
- Occurrence is usually sporadic or maternally inherited

Perioperative Risks

- Metabolic acidosis
- Resp and cardiac insufficiency/failure
- Delayed emergence

Worry About

- Resp failure following sedation
- Consider aspiration risk
- Metabolic acidosis
- Hypotension during induction

Overview

- Clinically heterogeneous collection of diseases with myopathy of mitochondrial origin as common trait
- Commonly assoc with encephalopathy

- Incl Kearns-Sayre syndrome (KSS); Pearson's syndrome (PS); maternally inherited Leigh syndrome (MILS); late-onset Leigh syndrome; mitochondrial encephalomyopathy, lactic acidosis, and stroke-like symptoms (MELAS); myoclonic epilepsy with ragged-red fibers (MERRF); Leber hereditary optic neuropathy (LHON); chronic progressive external ophthalmoplegia (CPEO); neuropathy, ataxia, and retinitis pigmentosa (NARP)
- Onset is variable. Most severe phenotypes present in infancy
- Most common symptom is muscle weakness, and most common sign is lactic acidosis, resulting from the inefficient metabolism of pyruvate and shift to anaerobic resp
- Muscle biopsy often used for suspected cases. Hallmark is appearance of ragged red fibers.
- Anesthetic sensitivity may manifest as decreased MAC of inhaled anesthetics (e.g., Complex I disorders), increased resp insufficiency from sedatives

and narcotics, and decreased hepatic clearance or renal excretion of IV agents.

ICD-9-CM Code: 359.8

Etiology

- Genetic variation in either mitochondrial DNA (mtDNA) or nuclear DNA (nDNA)
- Large-scale mtDNA deletions (e.g., KSS, PS, PEO) are most often acquired sporadically.
- Single-base mtDNA changes (e.g., MELAS, MERRF, MILS, LHON) are often inherited maternally, and usually affect mitochondrial protein synthesis (via mRNA, tRNA, or rRNA) or components of the electron-transport chain (i.e., Complex I, III, IV, V).
- Single-base nDNA changes (e.g., late-onset Leigh syndrome) are often inherited in Mendelian patterns (autosomal dominant or recessive).

Usual Treatment

- Supportive measures
- Dietary vitamins and supplements, coenzyme Q

ASSESSMENT POINTS

System	Effect	Assessment by Hx	PE	Test
HEENT	Dysphagia	Coughing, choking, aspiration with feeding	Sialorrhea	Swallow study
CARDIO	Cardiomyopathy Conduction defects (KSS)	Sx of CHF	Murmur, gallop, crackles	CXR, ECHO ECG, exercise testing (VO$_2$ max)
RESP	Disorganized resp muscle effort	Hypoventilation, hypoxia following sedative use	Rhonchi	CXR
GI	Chronic diarrhea Exocrine pancreatic failure (PS)	Dehydration Steatorrhea		Serum electrolytes
ENDO/METAB	Lactic acidosis Hepatic insufficiency	N/V Prolonged Rx effects	Hyperventilation	Serum lactate, CSF pyruvate/lactate ratio
GU	Renal tubular defects (PS), nephropathy	Urinary changes		Urinalysis Serum BUN, Cr, electrolytes
CNS	Encephalopathy (MILS) Ophthalmoplegia (CPEO, KSS) Stroke (MELAS) Seizure (MELAS, MERRF) Retinopathy, ataxia (NARP), blindness (LHON), deafness	Developmental delay Poor visual tracking Poor coordination Vision loss	↓ ROM of extraocular mm ↓ Visual acuity, ptosis Focal neurologic deficits Signs of seizures Pigmented retinas	Head CT or MRI Ophtho exam
PNS	Peripheral neuropathy	Weakness, clumsiness	↓ Strength	
MS	Hypotonia, weakness Myoclonus (MERRF)		↓ Strength	Muscle biopsy-ragged red fibers

Key Reference: Muravchick S, Levy RJ. Clinical implications of mitochondrial dysfunction. *Anesthesiology.* 2006;105:819–37. Clinical findings listed above may be characteristic of one or more mitochondrial myopathies. A specific disorder may follow in parentheses if the finding is a primary feature.

Perioperative Implications

Preoperative Preparation

- Assess cardiac involvement
- Preop anticholinergic for excessive oral secretions
- Avoid prolonged fasting and dehydration, which can worsen acidosis
- When possible, start IV fluid (IVF) at NPO time, allow for late (2 hr prior) clear fluid intake, and book as first case

Airway

- Possible aspiration risk

Monitoring

- Routine, assuming no severe cardiomyopathy or CHF
- Consider bispectral index (BIS) monitor prior to induction, for possible increased anesthetic sensitivity

Induction

- Avoid lactate-containing IVF (e.g., lactated Ringer's)

- Consider dextrose-containing IVF (e.g., 2–5% dextrose in normal saline)
- Avoid succinylcholine for uncharacterized myopathy or in face of neuropathy

Maintenance

- Many techniques have been used safely
- Avoid prolonged infusion of IV anesthetics, esp propofol, which is a known electron-transport chain de-coupler, due to worsened acidosis and reduced ATP production
- Hepatic and renal insufficiency may increase IV anesthetic half-life and prolong elimination
- If NMB agent is required, consider careful titration with shorter-acting agents
- Implement aggressive temp control; recommend active warming techniques
- Avoid tourniquets

Extubation

- Muscle weakness and anesthetic sensitivity may delay extubation

Regional Anesthesia

- Used successfully, but caution in those with underlying cardiac conduction block
- Local anesthetics have potential to de-couple electron transport chain

Postoperative Period

- Close monitoring of resp function
- For cases of longer duration, consider serum electrolytes or blood gas to assess acidosis
- Some have reported increased incidence of PONV

Anticipated Problems/Concerns

- Generally not associated with malignant hyperthermia (MH); however, scenario of critical ATP depletion may lead to muscular contraction mimicking MH
- Although succinylcholine is not contraindicated as in Duchenne or Becker MD, acidosis and neuropathy may predispose to accentuation of hyperkalemia.

Mitral Regurgitation

Raj K. Modak

Risk

- May include 5 million Americans
- Incidence of moderate/severe mitral regurgitation: Nearly 20% for age >55 y
- Most frequent diagnosed valve abnormality
- Females > males

Perioperative Risks

- Acute mitral regurgitation
- Atrial arrhythmias (tachycardia, atrial fibrillation, atrial flutter)
- Left ventricular dysfunction yielding reduced cardiac output, acute CHF, pulm edema, and acute RV failure
- Bacterial endocarditis

Worry About

- Worsening symptoms of fatigue, orthopnea, dyspnea on exertion
- Acute or chronic mitral regurgitation
- New-onset atrial fibrillation
- Hemodynamic instability in setting of poor LV function and acute myocardial infarction

Overview

- The mitral valve allows one-way blood flow through the left heart.
- During diastole, it acts as an open conduit for blood flow from the left atrium to the LV. During systole, it closes preventing back flow while the heart contracts.
- With mitral regurgitation, retrograde flow occurs from the LV to the LA during systole. This can occur as an acute or chronic process.
- The acute form results in sudden elevations in LA pressure. Elevated pressures in the pulm artery result in pulm edema and RV strain and possible failure.
- Chronic mitral regurgitation is tolerated well. LV hypertrophy is followed by dilation and failure. Similar changes in the RV and pulm circulation occur, as in the acute form, but are better tolerated over the longer time period.
- As a general rule, the more precipitous the onset, the more significant the sequelae.

ICD–9–CM Code: 424.0

Etiology

- Acute: Myocardial ischemia or infarction causing papillary muscle dysfunction, ruptured chordae causing a flail mitral valve from infarction or endocarditis, trauma, prosthetic valve dysfunction
- Chronic: Incl acute processes over longer time, mitral valve prolapse, dilated LV, rheumatic disease, lupus, congenital valvular disease, LA myxoma. All forms can be accelerated by systemic Htn.

Usual Treatment

- Medical therapy: Afterload reduction, CHF regimens, arrhythmia control, endocarditis prophylaxis
- Pharmacology incl: Angiotensin inhibitors, hydralazine, cardiac glycosides, diuretics, nitrates, antibiotics
- Surgical therapy: Mitral valvuloplasty (repair) or mitral valve replacement

ASSESSMENT POINTS

System	Effect	Assessment by Hx	PE	Test
CARDIO	Mitral regurgitation	Fatigue, exertional or nocturnal dyspnea	Pansystolic and late systolic murmur, rales	Doppler ECHO
	LA enlargement			2D-ECHO ECG
	AFib	Palpitations, defibrillation, anticoagulation	Irregular rhythm, bruises	ECG, PT/INR
	RV failure	Peripheral swelling, RUQ pain, tenderness	Ankle edema, hepatomegaly, hepatojugular reflux	Cardiac catheterization, 2D and Doppler ECHO
	Cardiomegaly		Displaced posterior MI	CXR, 2D-ECHO
RESP	CHF, pulm edema	Dyspnea, orthopnea	Gallop, rales	CXR
GI	Congestive hepatopathy	Bleeding with minor trauma	Bruises	PT, PTT, LFTs
RENAL	↓ Perfusion	Oliguria		↓ BUN, Cr
	Diuretic-induced	Palpitations	Muscle weakness	Serum K*, Mg
	↓ K+, Mg²⁺		↓ Reflexes	ECG
MS	Cachexia	Wt loss	Muscle wasting	↓ Wt

Key Reference: Stout KK, Verrier ED. Acute valvular regurgitation, *Circulation*. 2009;119:3232–3241.

Perioperative Implications

Preoperative Preparation

- Antibiotic prophylaxis
- Manage anticoagulation issues related to atrial fibrillation and the possible use of regional techniques
- Optimize HR issues related to atrial fibrillation
- Optimize symptoms related to CHF

Monitoring

- In procedures with expected wide variations in BP, direct arterial BP monitoring should be considered esp. with moderate or severe mitral regurgitation.
- In settings of LV failure, a pulm artery catheter or transesophageal echocardiogram may be useful in assessing changes and guiding pharmacologic therapy.

Airway

- Avoid hypoxemia and hypercarbia, which maintains the lowest pulm vascular resistance and reduces risk of RV failure

Preinduction/Induction

- "Faster, Fuller, Forward"
- Avoid bradycardia, maintain high-normal preload, reduce afterload
- Maintain stoke volume by avoiding myocardial depression and atrial fibrillation

Maintenance

- Cardiac and pulm goals, same as induction
- Avoid excessive PEEP, which reduces preload
- If possible, follow cardiac output, utilizing pharmacology as needed
- Regional anesthetic techniques may be considered as they help reduce afterload, however, caution is recommended in the setting of impaired LV function

Extubation

- Airway management to avoid hypoxia and hypercarbia inducing right ventricular strain and failure
- Requires vigilance on BP management to avoid Htn

Adjuvants

- No known drug interaction problems

Postoperative Period

- Pain management critical to avoid hypertensive episodes
- Both pt-controlled analgesia and postop epidural useful for pain control
- Fluid shifts and intraop volume management may alter LV function and antiarrhythmic blood concentrations
- New onset atrial fibrillation from fluid shifts and electrolyte abn
- Consideration for restarting anticoagulation for chronic atrial fibrillation

Anticipated Problems/Concerns

- High periop risk is best predicted by impaired LV function, symptoms of both LV and RV dysfunction
- Htn can acutely worsen mitral regurgitation causing CHF and pulm edema

Mitral Stenosis

Albert T. Cheung

Risk

- Bimodal age distribution: 20–39 y and 50–60 y
- Mitral stenosis is 2–3 times more common in women and is the most common valve disease affecting pregnant women.
- Most common among immigrants to the USA from regions where rheumatic fever is prevalent (e.g., Middle East, Asia, Latin America)

Perioperative Risks

- Increased risk of periop cardiac complications that incl infectious endocarditis, pulm edema, resp failure, heart failure, tachyarrhythmias, new-onset AFIB or atrial flutter, embolic stroke of cardiac origin

Worry About

- Fluid status
- Paroxysmal AFIB or flutter
- Pregnancy
- Limited ability to increase cardiac output in response to increased metabolic demands or intravascular volume expansion
- Cardiomyopathy, pulm Htn, RV failure, hepatic dysfunction, tricuspid regurgitation, and assoc aortic valve disease
- Pulm edema

Overview

- The normal mitral valve has an area of 4–6 cm^2. Symptoms start when the mitral valve area is reduced to 1.5 cm^2. Diastolic emptying of blood from the left atrium into the left ventricle is impaired critically when the mitral valve area is <1 cm^2.
- Transmitral pressure gradient varies directly with blood flow across the valve; acute increases in cardiac output or venous return to the heart increases the mitral valve gradient and increases LA and pulm venous pressures. Pulm edema occurs when the pulm venous pressure > pulmonary capillary oncotic pressure.
- Pulm venous Htn leads to left atrial dilation, left atrial thrombosis, AFIB, pulm Htn, RV failure, and tricuspid regurgitation.
- Symptoms of mitral stenosis can be elicited by conditions (fluid overload, exercise, pregnancy, sepsis, operation) that demand an ↑ in cardiac output or diastolic blood flow across the mitral valve (e.g., MR).
- Deformity of the mitral valve apparatus may cause mitral stenosis in combination with mitral regurgitation or left ventricular dysfunction.

ICD-9-CM Code: 394.0

Etiology

- Congenital heart disease (rare)
- Mitral valve repair with restrictive ring annuloplasty (rare)
- Acquired mitral stenosis is sequela of rheumatic carditis developing after group A streptococcal pharyngitis
- Rheumatic carditis produces exudative and inflammatory lesions that lead to fibrosis, calcification, thickening, and commissural fusion of the mitral valve apparatus

Usual Treatment

- Anticoagulation to decreased risk of thromboembolic events
- Digoxin, beta-blockers, or calcium channel blockers to control ventricular rate in pts with AFIB
- Diuretic therapy for symptomatic pulm edema, CHF, or RV failure
- Percutaneous balloon valvotomy in pts without extensive valve calcification, leaflet restriction, leaflet thickening, or involvement of the subvalvular apparatus
- Mitral valve replacement, repair, or open valvotomy

ASSESSMENT POINTS

System	Effect	Assessment by Hx	PE	Test
CARDIO	Mitral stenosis	DOE, NYHA class Chest pain or tightness	Diastolic murmur	ECHO Cardiac cath
	AFIB	Palpitations	Irregular pulse	ECG
	Pulm Htn	DOE	Sternal heave Prominent S$_2$	CXR
RESP	Pulm edema	DOE Orthopnea Paroxysmal nocturnal dyspnea Hemoptysis	Tachypnea Rales Wheezes	CXR
GI	Cardiac cirrhosis		Hepatomegaly	Liver function tests
RENAL	Fluid retention Diuretic therapy	Dependent edema	Pedal edema	Serum lytes
CNS	Embolic stroke	Neurologic deficits, TIAs	Focal neurologic deficits	Head CT scan, TEE
HEME	Bleeding	Anticoagulation therapy	Ecchymosis	INR, PT, PTT

Key Reference: Chandrashekhar Y, Westaby S, Narula. Mitral stenosis. *Lancet.* 2009;374:1271–1283.

Perioperative Implications

Preoperative Preparation

- Determine if pt is a candidate for percutaneous balloon valvotomy
- Optimize fluid status of pts in CHF
- Control ventricular rate in pts with AFIB
- Replete K$^+$ in pts with hypokalemia on digoxin therapy
- Antibiotic prophylaxis for infectious endocarditis according to guidelines
- Keep pt calm using reassurance, anxiolytics, and analgesics
- Assess the risk of bleeding in anticoagulated pts and correct the prolonged PT (INR) with FFP if necessary

Monitoring

- ECG to detect paroxysmal AFIB or flutter
- Consider arterial catheter for continuous BP monitoring and ABG sampling

- Consider CVP line, PA catheter, or TEE to measure pulm artery pressure, assess RV function, and guide intravascular volume management when large fluid shifts are anticipated.

Preinduction/Induction

- Cautious administration of drugs that decrease myocardial contractility, increase HR, or cause vasodilation.
- Hypoventilation and hypoxia may worsen pulm Htn and RV failure
- Positive inotropic drugs may precipitate pulm edema

Maintenance

- Control fluid administration

Extubation/Postoperative Period

- Provide adequate analgesia
- Increased risk of postop resp failure

Adjuvants

- Consider regional anesthesia or periop epidural anesthesia and analgesia, esp. for labor and delivery in the pregnant pt with mitral stenosis
- Inhaled NO or epoprostenol for RV failure assoc with pulm Htn

Anticipated Problems/Concerns

- Pts have a limited ability to increase their cardiac output
- Acute pulm edema is precipitated by increased cardiac output, increased HR, pregnancy, anxiety, fluid overload, exercise, and postop mobilization of sequestered (third space) interstitial and extracellular fluid
- Bleeding in anticoagulated pts

Mitral Valve Prolapse

Albert T. Cheung

Risk

- Believed to be most common form of valvular heart disease, with an incidence of 5% of the general population
- Based on strict ECHO criteria, the incidence of MVP is 2–3% with no predilection for gender or age
- The severity of disease varies widely in pts with the diagnosis of MVP depending on the severity of mitral regurgitation (MR), the degree of structural abn of the mitral valve apparatus, and LV function as a consequence of MR.

Perioperative Risks

- Infectious endocarditis
- HF as a consequence of acute or chronic MR
- Embolic stroke
- Sudden cardiac death

Worry About

- Severity of MR
- LV dysfunction, CHF, AFIB, sudden cardiac death, infective endocarditis, or embolic stroke as a consequence of MR
- Associated conditions: Marfan syndrome; Ehlers-Danlos syndrome, osteogenesis imperfecta, or pseudoxanthoma elasticum
- MVP syndrome: Atypical chest pain, palpitations, syncope, exertional dyspnea, or anxiety

Overview

- Severity of disease in pts with MVP varies widely based on the clinical and ECHO criteria used to establish the diagnosis.
- MVP is defined as isolated prolapse of the mitral valve leaflets ≥2 mm beyond the mitral valve annular plane into the left atrium during systole by ECHO. The severity of myxomatous degeneration of the mitral valve apparatus causing MVP is characterized by leaflet thickening, leaflet redundancy, chordal elongation, or chordal rupture by ECHO.
- Structural abn in MVP lead to weakness and deformity of the valve apparatus. Annular dilation, stretching of valve leaflets, and chordal elongation impair leaflet coaptation causing progression of MR.
- A flail leaflet is caused by acute rupture of weakened chordae and produces severe MR.
- Chronic MR causes progressive LA dilation, eccentric left ventricular hypertrophy, HF, and AFIB.
- MVP syndrome is used to describe MVP assoc with a spectrum of nonspecific symptoms incl atypical chest pain, palpitations, exertional dyspnea, exercise intolerance, syncope, anxiety, lean body habitus, and electrocardiographic repolarization abn. A pathophysiologic basis establishing a link between these nonspecific symptoms and MVP has not been defined.

- Risk factors for HF, sudden cardiac death, infective endocarditis, stroke, or need for mitral valve surgery in pts with MVP are LV dilation, depressed LV ejection fraction (<50%), severity of MR, AFIB, LA enlargement, flail leaflet (chordal rupture), leaflet thickening (>5 mm) and age >50 y.

ICD-9-CM Code: 424.0

Etiology

- Inherited connective tissue disorders
- Myxomatous degeneration caused by dysregulation of collagen and elastin matrix protein synthesis and degradation
- Inherited myxomatous mitral valve prolapse

Usual Treatment

- No treatment in asymptomatic pts or pts with MVP syndrome without significant MR by ECHO.
- ACE inhibitors, β-blockers, and diuretics in pts with significant MR or CHF (see mitral regurgitation)
- Antiarrhythmic agents and anticoagulation therapy in pts with AFIB (see atrial fibrillation)
- Mitral valve repair or replacement in patients with symptomatic MR or evidence of LV dilation, reduced LV ejection fraction, AFIB, pulm Htn, or severe MR by ECHO

ASSESSMENT POINTS

System	Effect	Assessment by Hx	PE	Test
CARDIO	Mitral valve prolapse	Atypical chest pain	Mid- and late-apical nonejection systolic clicks	ECHO
	Mitral regurgitation	DOE	Mid- to late-apical systolic murmur	ECHO
	AFIB	CHF	Irregular pulse	CXR
	Infectious endocarditis	NYHA class	Embolic phenomena	ECG
		Palpitations		TEE, blood culture
		Fever, chills		
CNS	Stroke	Neurologic deficits	Focal neurologic signs	Head CT scan
		TIAs		TEE
MS	Connective tissue disorders		Pectus excavatum	
			Scoliosis	
			Lean stature	

Key Reference: Hayek E, Gring CN, Griffin BP. Mitral valve prolapse. *Lancet.* 2005;365:507–518.

Perioperative Implications

Preoperative Preparation

- Assess existence and severity of MR
- Assess for signs and symptoms of HF
- Antibiotic prophylaxis for infectious endocarditis in pts with Hx of infectious endocarditis and procedure that may result in transient bacteremia

Monitoring

- Routine
- Consider invasive hemodynamic monitoring for major operations in symptomatic pts with severe MR and LV dysfunction.

Preinduction/Induction/Maintenance

- Avoid Htn and acute increases in sympathetic tone
- Consider regional anesthesia

Adjuvants

- Therapeutic interventions that increase BP, myocardial contractility, preload, or sympathetic tone may increase severity of MVP, MR, or the risk of chordal rupture.
- Antihypertensives, afterload reducing agents, and positive inotropic drugs are effective for increased cardiac output in pts with significant MR.

Extubation/Postoperative Period

- Avoid Htn and acute increases in sympathetic tone.

Anticipated Problems/Concerns

- Htn and intravascular volume expansion may increase severity of MVP, the regurgitant LV ejection fraction when MR is present, and the risk of CHF.

- Presence of severe MR, LV dysfunction, or assoc connective tissue disorders may alter routine managment of pts with isolated MVP (see Mitral Regurgitation and individual connective tissue disorders in Diseases section)
- MVP is assoc with a 3–8 fold higher risk of infective endocarditis. Traditionally, antibiotic prophylaxis was recommended for pts with MVP and significant MR undergoing procedures with a risk of transient bacteremia. The AHA revised recommendations for antibiotic prophylaxis in 2007 to incl only pts with Hx of infectious endocarditis or who have had mitral valve repair or replacement.

Mobitz I (Second-Degree Atrioventricular Block)

James R. Zaidan

Risk

- Occurs after inferior MI, or occasionally in trained athletes or in normal, sleeping people
- Incidence varies based on etiology.

Perioperative Risks

- Without assoc heart disease and without symptoms, should not present undue risk during anesthesia, for instance in trained athletes
- If occurs 2° to inferior myocardial infarction, the periop risk depends on extent of ischemic area

Worry About

- Advancing to a higher-degree block if ischemic zone extends to anterior wall
- Papillary muscle dysfunction may occur

Overview

- Found usually in presence of CAD
- Block generally occurs in AV node, resulting in normal QRS complexes
- ECG reveals progressive lengthening P-R intervals at decreasing increments and progressively shortening R-R intervals leading to a regular atrial rhythm and an irregular ventricular ryhythm
- Bradycardia usually responds to atropine

ICD-9-CM Code: 426.13 (Mobitz I)

Etiology

- Acquired, usually with MI
- Increased resting parasympathetic tone relative to resting sympathetic tone

Usual Treatment

- Specific therapy in absence of heart disease not necessary unless pt is symptomatic
- Treatment of an infarction-related Mobitz I block incl observation and medical therapy with atropine
- Temporary pacing is necessary only if a medically unresponsive pt is symptomatic
- Permanent pacing seldom required and considered only in persistently blocked, symptomatic pts

ASSESSMENT POINTS

System	Effect	Assessment by Hx	PE	Test
CARDIO	Commonly no Sx Bradycardia on occasion	Exercise tolerance Angina SOB	Signs of CHF and ↓ perfusion	ECG CXR
RENAL	Likely normal			Renal function testing?
CNS	No effect or ↓ perfusion of CNS	No Sx or only mild Sx: fainting, dizziness	Normal Bruits	PE Carotid US

Key Reference: Epstein AE, DiMarco JP, Ellenbogen KA, et al. ACC/AHA/HRS 2008 Guidelines for device-based therapy of cardiac rhythm abnormalities. *J Am Coll Cardiol.* 2008;51:2085–2105.

Perioperative Implications

Preoperative Preparation
- Consider availability of transcutaneous pacing

Monitoring
- Based on co-existing disease
- Observe for and prepare to treat 3° block when positioning PA catheter in pt with Mobitz I block.

Airway
- None

Induction/Maintenance
- Regional or general
- No contraindications to any standard anesthetic drugs
- Intraop processes and drugs that increase atrial rate could decrease ventricular rate.

Extubation
- None

Adjuvants
- Cautious use of drugs that slow AV conduction

Anticipated Problems/Concerns

- Extension of infarcted area with higher degree block and CHF

Mobitz II (Second-Degree Atrioventricular Block)

James R. Zaidan

Risk

- Occurs after anterior infarction and can quickly proceed to a 3° heart block

Perioperative Risks

- Risk of developing 3° block

Worry About

- Rapid development into a 3° block, which requires temporary transvenous pacing

Overview

- Unlike Mobitz I block, Mobitz II block is located in bundle of His or bundle branches, resulting in lengthening QRS duration
- P-P and R-R intervals are constant, and P-R intervals are constant prior to the dropped QRS complex

ICD-9-CM Code: Mobitz II: 426.12

Etiology

- Acquired, usually associated with MI

Usual Treatment

- Temporary pacemaker insertion should be considered soon after onset of this block, because 3° block commonly occurs.
- Pacing does not improve survival.
- Atropine usually does not improve conduction.

ASSESSMENT POINTS

System	Effect	Assessment by Hx	PE	Test
CARDIO	Bradycardia	Exercise tolerance Angina SOB	Signs of CHF and ↓ perfusion	ECG CXR Other tests as indicated
GU	Likely normal			Renal function testing?
CNS	↓ Perfusion of CNS	Fainting, dizziness	Normal? Bruits	PE Carotid US

Key Reference: Epstein AE, DiMarco JP, Ellenbogen KA, et al. ACC/AHA/HRS 2008 Guidelines for device-based therapy of cardiac rhythm abnormalities: A report of the American College of Cardiology/American Heart Association Task Force on Practice Guidelines (Writing Committee to Revise the ACC/AHA/NASPE 2002 Guidelines update for implantation of cardiac pacemakers and antiarrhythmia devices) developed in Collaboration with the American Association for Thoracic Surgery and Society of Thoracic Surgeons. *J Am Coll Cardiol.* 2008;51:2085–2105.

Perioperative Implications

Preoperative Preparation

- Evaluation of CAD important
- Likely a transvenous pacemaker will be in place
- Transcutaneous pacing should be available if temporary transvenous pacing was not established prior to induction of anesthesia.

Monitoring

- Based on severity of heart disease and extent of infarcted area

- Prepare to treat 3° block when positioning a PA catheter

Airway

- None

Induction/Maintenance

- No contraindications to any standard anesthetic drugs
- Any intraop process or drug increasing atrial rate could worsen block and decrease ventricular rate

Adjuvants

- Cautiously use drugs that slow conduction through AV node unless they also slow SA nodal rate and allow 1:1 AV conduction and increased ventricular rate.
- 1° AV block will persist if 1:1 conduction occurs.

Morbid Obesity

Ashish C. Sinha

Risk
- Incidence in USA: ~5% morbidly obese

Perioperative Risk
- Increased morbidity/mortality versus normal BMI, from resp and cardiac issues

Worry About
- Challenging procedures: IV start, intubation, ventilation, epidural catheter placement
- Restrictive pattern of resp disease, hypoxemia, larger O_2 demand, small FRC; obstructive sleep apnea (OSA) is common, with assoc cardiac issues
- Htn; systemic and pulm
- DM
- Nonalcoholic steatohepatitis (NASH)
- Reflux, hiatal hernia, and depression

Overview
- Defined by BMI, (wt in kg/ht in m²), >30 obese, >35 morbidly obese
- Cardiac and resp issues mainly due to size. Large body mass to be perfused and oxygenated; increased cardiac strain and resp effort of breathing. OSA common, increased sensitivity to narcotics.
- Depression common

ICD-9-CM Code: 278.0

Etiology
- Disputed role of genetics, mainly environmental and nutritional habits; essentially a form of severe malnourishment

Usual Treatment
- Medical treatment incl psychological counseling along with decreased calorie consumption with increased exercise, if physically able.
- Surgical treatment incl gastric banding, Roux-en-Y, sleeve gastrectomy, or intestinal bypass.

ASSESSMENT POINTS

System	Effect	Assessment by Hx	PE	Test
CARDIO	Htn Pulm	Fatigue, dyspnea	Auscultation, increased heart size, ± rales	BP, EKG, CXR
	Htn Cardiac failure Coronary disease	Dyspnea, fatigue, syncope inc JVP, peripheral edema, hepatomegaly, crackles Chest pain, SOB	Auscultation, palpation, auscultation	CXR, EKG, ECHO EKG, ECHO EKG, stress ECHO Cor angiogram
RESP	Restrictive disease OSA	SOB, inc resp rate, decreased exercise tolerance Hx of snorning, periods of apnea in sleep, non-restful sleep, daytime somnolence and tiredness	Rapid shallow breathing, hypoxemia, large neck, redundant soft tissue in neck Large neck, redundant soft tissue in neck	PFT, ABG, CXR, Hg, pulse ox for room air saturation Overnight sleep study for apnea hypopnea index
NEURO	Depression	Hx	Question and answers, survey instruments	By psychologist and/or psychiatrist
AIRWAY	Potentially difficult intubation	Mallampati, upper lip bite test	Evaluation	
GI	NASH NIDDM	Hepatomegaly, icterus, ascites Polyphagia, polyuria, polydispsia	Palpation	LFT, PT, PTT, BUN, Cr UA, BS, GTT, HgA1c

Key Reference: Sinha AC, Eckmann DM. Anesthesia for bariatric surgery. In: Miller RD, Eriksson LI, Fleisher LA, Wiener-Kronish JP, Young WL, eds. *Miller's textbook of anesthesia*. 7th ed. Philadelphia: Elsevier; 2009:2089–2104 [Chapter 64].

Perioperative Implications

Perioperative Preparation
- All medications except for DM
- Sedation titrated to effect preop
- Consider prophylactic preop IVC filter placement if risk of DVT is high

Monitoring
- Routine with ± arterial catheter if cardiac status dictates or ultra obese (BMI >70kg/m² or weight >200kg)
- If severe cardiac or resp disease, ABGs
- UO
- Central venous access if peripheral access difficult, or CVP or pulm pressures need to be monitored for cardiac disease

Airway
- Position at 30° head elevated to improve probability of intubation with direct laryngoscopy
- Minority of pts may need awake FOI
- Prepare for difficulty; with multiple airway option like laryngeal masks and video laryngoscopes

Induction
- Pre-oxygenate with pressure support if possible, complete denitrogenation
- Rapid sequence with cricoid pressure preferable

Maintenance
- Drug dosing lipophilic dosed to real body wt; lipophobic to IBW or LBM
- Desflurane preferable due to complete and rapid recovery

- Appropriate fluid infusion based on deficit, losses, and UO
- Ventilation: Start at TV 10–12 mL/kg IBW; RR 12–14/m; PEEP 8–10; adjust as needed

Extubation
- Wide awake, no residual volatile agent, normocapnic, responsive with appropriate resp effort and partially sitting up

Postoperatively
- Rapid placement on CPAP or BiPAP decreases atelectasis
- Good analgesia with IV PCA, NSAIDs and local infiltration with LA and rapid mobilization helps resp function and decreases DVT

Moyamoya

Francine S. Yudkowitz

Risk

- Occurs in both children and adults
- Occurs predominantly in children, highest incidence in first decade of life
- More frequent in females
- Highest incidence in Japanese and Asian population, familial occurrence 10%

Perioperative Risks

- Stroke

Worry About

- Hypocarbia and hypercarbia
- Adequate cerebral blood flow
- Hypotension
- Hypothermia

Overview

- Moyamoya means "puff of smoke," which describes the angiographic appearance
- Chronic progressive cerebrovascular disease consisting of concentric stenosis or occlusion in the distal internal carotid arteries and large vessels of the circle of Willis with prominent basal collateral vessels
- Adults present with intracerebral/intraventricular hemorrhages
- Children present with TIAs and strokes that lead to neurologic deficits. Symptoms may start from birth to age 5 y, with rapid deterioration in neurologic function over the next 2–3 y.
- Symptoms in children are precipitated by activities that involve hyperventilation, which results in hypocarbia. Changes in body temp may also precipitate attacks.
- Abn vessels have intimal thickening or deficiency of the internal elastic lamina.

ICD-9-CM Code: 437.5

Etiology

- Not clearly defined
- Moyamoya disease (congenital): Angiographic appearance with or without other risk factors, both cerebral and systemic vasculature involved
- Moyamoya syndrome: Present with other known associated conditions, e.g., meningitis, neurofibromatosis, connective tissue disease, sickle cell disease, SLE, trisomy 21, prior radiation therapy, brain tumors, and chronic inflammation in the neck region

Usual Treatment

- Medical
  - Aspirin in select pts such as asymptomatic, mild disease, increased risk for surgery. Not indicated in adult population with Hx of intracranial hemorrhage.
- Surgical
  - Direct: Superficial temporal artery or middle meningeal artery to middle cerebral artery bypass
  - Indirect: EDAS (encephalodural arteriosynangiosis). The scalp artery or temporal artery is placed onto the arachnoid surface of the brain. Collaterals to ischemic brain occur over time.

ASSESSMENT POINTS

System	Effect	Assessment by Hx	PE	Test
CNS	Decreased CBF Seizures	TIAs, strokes	Neuro deficits	CT/MRI/MRA EEG

Key Reference: Baykan N, Ozgen S, Ustalar ZS, Dagcinar A, Ozek MM. Moyamoya disease and anesthesia. *Pediatric Anesthesia*. 2005;15:1111–1115.

Perioperative Implications

Preoperative Preparation
- Assess for associated abn
- Avoid sedatives and narcotics that would result in hypercarbia

Monitoring
- Arterial line for BP monitoring and blood gas analysis

Induction/Maintenance
- Balanced anesthesia or total IV anesthesia
- Maintaining cerebral and systemic hemodynamics is paramount.
- Avoid cerebrovasodilators.
- Minimize increases in CMRO$_2$ with adequate levels of anesthesia during painful stimuli.
- Ensure adequate CBF by avoiding hypotension, hypocarbia, and hypercarbia.
- Maintain normothermia with warming blanket if needed.

Postoperative Period
- Monitor for hypoventilation to avoid hypercarbia-induced neurologic symptoms.
- Provide adequate analgesia.
- Maintain normotension, normocarbia, normovolemia, and normothermia.

Anticipated Problems/Concern

- Stroke
- Subdural hematoma
- Intracerebral hemorrhage

Mucopolysaccharidoses

Megan A. Brockel

James J. Fehr

Risk

- Mucopolysaccharidosis type I (MPS I), Hurler syndrome, is inherited as an autosomal recessive disorder.
- MPS II, Hunter syndrome, is X-linked (only males affected)
- Incidence in USA: Estimated at 1/30,000

Perioperative Risks

- Estimated periop mortality: 20%
- Difficult intubation (25%), failed intubation (8%)

Worry About

- Difficult airway, cardiac lesions, poor IV access, resp failure

Overview

- MPS is a group metabolic disorder caused by a lack of lysosomal enzymes required to break down glycosaminoglycans which, over time, build up in blood and connective tissue.
- The child may appear normal at birth but by age 1 y will often show signs of both growth and mental retardation. The Dx is made by characteristic physical findings and increased urinary mucopolysaccharides (MPs).

- Hurler syndrome, considered the prototypic and most severe sub-type of MPS I, is characterized by involvement of heart, liver, and bones. It is also assoc with corneal clouding, developmental delay, frequent resp infections, stiff joints and an abn airway.
- Scheie syndrome is a milder form of Hurler syndrome; pts have normal intelligence and life expectancy but may have stiff joints and aortic regurgitation.
- Hunter syndrome has diffuse joint limitations, short neck, short stature, and ischemic cardiomyopathy.
- Morquio syndrome (MPS IV) has severe kyphoscoliosis, possible cervical subluxation, and aortic regurgitation.
- Maroteaux-Lamy syndrome (MPS VI) has kyphoscoliosis, cardiac involvement, and mild joint stiffness.
- Recurrent hernias often occur in mucopolysaccharidoses.

ICD-9-CM Code: 277.5

Etiology

- Hereditary, progressive disorders of lysosomal enzymes responsible for metabolism of MPs resulting in intracellular accumulation of incompletely metabolized MPs in tissues throughout body. This leads to progressive alteration of cellular structure and function; death often results from cardiac or pulm failure.
- All forms are autosomal recessive except for Hunter syndrome, which is X-linked recessive.

Usual Treatment

- Hematopoietic stem cell transplantation can prevent and/or reverse many clinical features of MPS but must be performed early in the disease course (before developmental deterioration begins) and it carries significant risk of morbidity and death.
- Enzyme replacement therapy is lower risk but does not cross the BBB and therefore cannot preserve CNS function.

ASSESSMENT POINTS

System	Effect	Assessment by Hx	PE	Test
HEENT	Large tongue, small mouth, micrognathia; Difficult airway anticipated; Atlantoaxial subluxation possible; Corneal clouding; Chronic recurrent rhinitis and frequent ear infections		Neck ROM	X-ray
CARDIO	Frequent valvular lesions; Arrhythmias; Cardiomyopathy/CHF; Severe CAD (even at a young age); Difficult IV access	Exercise tolerance Angina Hx		ECG CXR ECHO
RESP	Restrictive lung disease; Propensity to develop pneumonia; Obstructive sleep apnea; Asthma; Bronchospasm			PFTs Sleep studies
GI	Frequent hepatomegaly; Hepatic function usually normal; Inguinal and umbilical hernias;			
CNS	Mental retardation, deafness, minimal language skills; Hydrocephalus in Hurler and Hunter syndromes; Cervical myelopathy in Morquio syndrome			CT/MRI
MS	Short neck, severe progressive skeletal and joint disease; Characteristic gibbus deformity of lumbar spine; Defective ossification (dysostosis multiplex); Anticipate difficulty in positioning			

Key Reference: Muenzer, et al. Mucopolysaccharidosis I: Management and treatment guidelines. *Pediatrics.* 2009;123:19–29.

Perioperative Implications

Preoperative Preparation

- May be resistant to sedative premedications
- Anticipate possible upper airway obstruction and/or cardiopulmonary difficulties
- Antisialagogue, such as glycopyrrolate
- Antibiotic prophylaxis for pts with Hx of endocarditis, prosthetic valves, or foreign material in the heart

Monitoring

- Routine

Airway

- Abn airway and short neck predispose to complicated airway management, incl difficulty in performing a tracheotomy.
- Limited jaw movement, enlarged tongue, and thick secretions compound airway challenges.

- ETT may need to be smaller than anticipated for the age and size of the pt.
- Consider fiberoptic bronchoscopy.
- LMA may be useful.

Preinduction/Induction

- IV placement before induction
- Padding and positioning

Maintenance

- Avoid myocardial ischemia.

Extubation

- Conscious with intact airway reflexes prior to extubation

Adjuvants

- Utilize local anesthetics and regional techniques when appropriate

Postoperative Period

- Delayed emergence
- Resp complications incl pneumonia, bronchospasm, and apnea

Anticipated Problems/Concerns

- Airway is likely to be difficult to manage
- Cardiac and pulm systems frequently affected

Multiple Endocrine Neoplasia (MEN) Type I and II

Mary A. Blanchette

Risk

• Neoplastic syndromes, inherited in an autosomal dominant pattern, variable penetrance, rare incidence. Syndromes involve more than one endocrine gland.

• MEN tumors and their effects may be underdiagnosed, unrecognized when pt presents for nonrelated surgery. (MEN2a and 2b assoc with pheochromocytoma)

• Medullary carcinoma of thyroid (MEN2a, 2b) is inherited with almost 100% penetrance, prophylactic thyroidectomy is recommended. Genetic screening tests are available.

Perioperative Risks

• See specific syndrome, risk related to functional components of tumors

Overview

• MEN I "Werner's syndrome" incl: Parathyroid hyperplasia (95%), anterior pituitary tumors (30%), pancreas (insulinoma, glucagonoma) (50%), gastrinoma ("Zollinger Ellison") (20–60%)

• MEN II has 3 distinct clinical subtypes: IIa, IIb, and familial medullary carcinoma (FMTC)

• MEN IIa: "Sipple's syndrome" incl: Medullary carcinoma of the thyroid (97%), parathyroid hyperplasia (20%), pheochromocytoma (50%)

• MEN IIb: Extremely rare subtype, (5% of all MEN II syndrome) incl: Medullary carcinoma of thyroid, pheochromocytoma, neuromas of oral mucosa, intestinal ganglioneuromas, marfanoid body habitus, rare parathyroid hyperplasia

ICD-9-CM Code: 258.0

Etiology

• MEN I/II: autosomal dominant, variable penetrance. MEN I caused by mutation in MEN-1 gene (tumor suppressor/regulatory), men and women equally affected. MEN II caused by oncogenic mutation in c-Ret gene (regulatory). Incidence of MEN2a > FMTC > MEN 2b

Usual Treatment

• MEN I: parathyroid hyperplasia: Treat hypercalcemia medically, surgical resection of hyperplastic tissue with parathyroid reimplantation.

Pituitary adenoma: Prolactinoma (58%) treated medically with dopamine agonist, growth hormone adenoma/acromegaly (23%), and nonsecreting adenoma (10%), treated surgically with transphenoidal resection. Pancreatic tumors treated surgically with glucose management (insulinomas), gastrinoma treated medically, then surgery.

• MEN IIa: Parathyroid hyperplasia, treat as in MEN-I. Medullary carcinoma is treated with total thyroidectomy and neck dissection. Pheochromocytoma pts must be medically optimized with alpha-adrenergic blockade first, then beta blockade, before surgical resection of tumor is attempted, otherwise high morbidity/mortality. Pts with Hx of pheo, and parathyroid hyperplasia should have prophylactic total thyroidectomy.

• MEN IIb: Treatment for medullary carcinoma is total thyroidectomy; pheochromocytoma, same treatment as in MEN2-a.

ASSESSMENT POINTS

System	Effect	Assessment by Hx	PE	Test
MEN I	Parathyroid hyperplasia (assoc nephrolithiasis) Pancreatic tumors (insulinoma, glucagonoma), gastrinoma Ant pituitary tumor (prolactinoma, growth hormone (GH) tumor, ACTH/Cushings)	Family Hx of endocrine tumors Fatigue, muscle weakness, flank pain/renal stones/ Hx pathological fractures Diaphoresis, palpitation, abdominal pain Diarrhea, reflux, dyspepsia Headache, visual changes	Htn Neck nodule Altered mental status Flank tenderness Tremor, mental status changes (hypoglycemia) Visual field defect Acromegaly (GH) Cushingoid habitus	NIBP and EKG Serum calcium Sestamibi scan, PTH level, neck CT, bone density, BUN/creatinine, pelvic x-ray Serum glucose, electrolytes, CT/MRI Endoscopic US Head CT/MRI metabolic panel, specific hormone level
MEN IIa & b	Pheochromocytoma	Family Hx, episodic sweating, palpitations, anxiety, tremor	Htn (paroxysmal), arrhythmia	CT/MRI, NIBP EKG/consider ECHO, 24 hr urine for catecholamines, metanephrines
	Medullary cancer of thyroid Parathyroid adenoma (see MEN I)	Can be asymptomatic Family Hx Hx urinary stones Symptoms of hypercalcemia	Thyroid mass Neck nodule	Calcitonin levels Serum calcium, serum PTH level, BUN/creatinine Pelvic x-rays

Key Reference: Grant, F. Anesthetic considerations in the multiple endocrine neoplasia syndromes. *Curr Opin Anaesthesiol.* 2005;18(3):345–354.

Perioperative Implications: Men I

Monitoring

• Parathyroid surgery: ECG signs of hypercalcemia (arrhythmias, prolonged PR, short Q-T), consider using EMG ETT tube for monitoring recurrent laryngeal nerve intraop. Unpredictable response to muscle relaxants with hypercalcemia, monitor TOF. PTH levels; significant decrease expected post successful resection, monitor calcium level postop.

• Pituitary adenomas: Tight BP control; acromegalics may have impaired ulnar circulation to hand which increases risk morbidity from radial a-line; monitor urine output (risk diabetes insipidus, SIADH)

• Insulinoma surgery: Requires tight, careful blood glucose control, increased risk hypoglycemia periop, arterial line

• Gastrinomas: Arterial line, pts at risk for labile BP

Airway

• Acromegaly: Increased risk of difficult mask airway and intubation, also increased incidence of sleep apnea; have difficult airway equipment ready.

• Parathyroidectomy: Risk of surgical damage to recurrent laryngeal nerve, and vocal cord paresis periop (risk of hoarseness to stridor to complete airway obstruction if bilateral)

Maintenance

• Parathyroidectomy: Draw post resection PTH levels, to confirm removal of tumor.

• Insulinomas, gastrinomas: Monitor volume status, glucose, BP control

• Pituitary adenomas: Usually transphenoidal approach, tight BP control, watch UO

Perioperative Implications: Men II

Monitoring

• Pheochromocytoma: Standard ASA monitors, arterial line, CVP, UO

• Total thyroidectomy: Standard ASA monitors. Consider use of EMG ETT to monitor recurrent laryngeal nerve intraop. Postop PTH levels to check for adequate parathyroid function

• Parathyroidectomy: See MEN-1 section

Airway

• Thyroidectomy and parathyroidectomy: Review ENT preop evaluation, incl ENT's fiberoptic exam of larynx, CT/MRI scans, sestamibi localization scans for potential mass effects of tumor on airway, also note baseline vocal cord function. Communicate with surgeon for plan.

Maintenance

• Pheochromocytoma: Tight BP control before and during resection (anesthetics, nipride, phentolamine, esmolol, Ca channel blockers, epidural infusions); after adrenal ligation, BP support with fluid boluses, prn pressors (NE, phenylephrine). Monitor glucose.

- Thyroidectomy: If using EMG ETT, avoid muscle relaxants.
- Parathyroidectomy: See MEN I

Adjuvants

- Pheochromocytomas: Require adequate preop treatment to control BP, HR, and restore blood volume (10–14 d alpha adrenergic blockers (ex. phenoxybenzamine, or prazosin), hydration, then initiate beta blockade)

- Hyperparathyroidism with symptomatic hypercalcemia: Preop hydration, diuresis with furosemide, consider biphosphonates, calcitonin or glucocorticoids

Anticipated Problems/Concerns

- MEN I: Parathyroidectomy: Postop hypocalcemia, recurrent laryngeal nerve damage/VC paresis, neck hematoma/airway compromise.

Transphenoidal pituitary adenoma resection: Hypopituitarism, SAIDH/DI. Acromegaly: Potential difficult airway. Pancreas tumors: Hyper/hypoglycemia. Gastrinoma/VIPoma: Labile BP
- MEN II: Pheochromocytoma; malignant Htn and labile BP, increased risk of CVA, MI.

Multiple Myeloma

Susheela Viswanathan
Alan Kaye
Alecia L. Sabartinelli

Risks

- Incidence: 4.3/100,000 white males; 3/100,000 white females; 9.6/100,000 black males; 6.7/100,000 black females
- Race: 1.1% of all malignancies in white population; 2.1% of all malignancies in black population
- M:F ratio: 3:2
- Age: Median age 68 y men, 70 y in females
- Survival: Median survival 3 y; 100% fatality rate

Overview

- MM is a part of a spectrum ranging from monoclonal gammapathy of unknown significance (MGUS) to plasma cell leukemia (malignancy of antibody forming cells)
- Also known as plasmacytosis or Kahler's disease; classified within non-Hodgkin's lymphomas
- Proliferation of plasma cells results in functioning peripheral blood cells and leads clinically to:
  - Impaired production of blood cells > pancytopenia (leucopenia anemia thrombocytopenia)
  - Formation of plasmacytoma (mass), leading to lytic lesions in bone
  - Impaired immunity (humoral) > infection

ICD-9-CM Code: 203.0

- Increased plasma cells (antibody forming cells) > amyloidosis (soft tissue, lungs, kidneys) and hyperviscosity
- Presenting signs: High sedimentation rates, anemia, signs of coagulopathy
- Renal failure from toxic immunoglobin deposition in renal tubuli most common cause of mortality; 10% of pts develop amyloidosis

Etiology

- Genetic instability: Translocation at 14q32 and/or deletion of chromosome 13 leading to either neoplastic plasmacytes producing either a monoclonal immunoglobulin (IgG, IgA, IgD) or isolated light chains (Bence Jones plasmacytoma)
- Environmental/occupational causes
- Radiation (increased incidence in survivors of the atomic bombing of Nagasaki)

Treatment

- Alkylating chemotherapeutic agent
- Thalidomide (delayed progression of disease)
- Stem cell transplantation
  - Autologous
  - Allogenic
- Glucocorticoids

- Interferon alpha-2b (maintenance therapy)
- Bortezomib (PS-341)
  - Inhibitor of 26S proteosome > inhibition of proteosome in myeloma

Treatment of Complications of Multiple Myeloma

- Bone disease: Narcotics (pain), radiation (refractory pain and cord compression), surgical intervention
- Anemia: Iron, B$_{12}$, folate, erythropoietin, transfusion
- Infection: Vaccination against strep pneumonia, *haemophilus influenzae*, H1N1, seasonal flu; antibiotics; IV immune globulin
- Hypercalcemia: IV fluid and corticoid steroid, bisphosphonates (if unresponsive to hydration), calcitonin, furosemide
- Renal failure: Treat dehydration, hypercalcemia, and hyperuricemia; chemotherapy (ex. vincristine, doxorubicin, etc.); alkaline diuresis; trial of plasma exchange in acute evolving renal failure; hyperviscosity syndrome; exchange of plasma (plasmapheresis)

ASSESSMENT POINTS

System	Clinical Manifestations	Signs and Symptoms	Anesthetic Implication
MS	Bone pain Pathological fracture	Usually lumbar 95% more than one side	Positioning to prevent fracture
HEME	Bleeding and bruising Coagulopathy Normochromic normocytic anemia Capillary fragility	2° Thrombocytopenia Absorption of clotting factor Weakness Purpura Dark circles (raccoon like) around eye, 2° prolonged valsalva	Availability of FFP and plts ↑ Transfusion requirements, ventilator management
METAB	Hypercalcemia Infection	Confusion, somnolence, constipation, nausea, thirst, bone pain 2° humoral immunity of normality	↑ Fluid requirements, maintenance of adequate UO Antibiotic coverage
	Hyperviscosity	Epistaxis Visual disturbance Carpal tunnel Headache Somnolence, bruisability	Preop: Plasmapheresis, ↑fluid requirement intraop Temp maintenance to prevent microvascular sludging
CNS and PNS	Spinal cord compression Meningitis Carpal tunnel Peripheral neuropathies Stroke (hyperviscosity)	Signs of weakness and numbness of extremities	Positioning of pt Diligent use of muscle relaxants Avoidance of depolarizing muscle relaxants
RENAL	Renal insufficient/failure	2° Direct tubular injury Amyloidosis Involvement by plasmacytoma	Adequate hydration
RESP	Pneumonia Resp insufficiency	2° rib fracture	Extubation problems Pneumothorax intraop
HEENT	Amyloidosis	Macroglossia Skin lesions of lips	Airway problems

Key Reference: Palumbo A, Gay F. How to treat elderly patients with multiple myeloma: combination of therapy or sequencing. *Hematology Am Soc Hematol Educ Program.* 2009;566–577.

Perioperative Implications

Preoperative

- Recombinant erythropoietin increased hemoglobin and decreased transfusion requirement
- Antibiotics and gammaglobulin prophylaxis

Airway

- May be difficult due to macroglossia

Maintenance

- Regional anesthesia is contraindicated due to bony lesions, coagulopathy, and neurologic deficit
- Unpredictable pharmacokinetic of protein-bound drugs

Post Operative

- Continue adequate hydration
- Aggressive pulm toilet
- Treat specific complication (refer to Treatment of Complication of Multiple Myeloma)

Anticipated Problems/Concerns

- Careful positioning to prevent fractures

Multiple Sclerosis

Armin Schubert
Logan Emory

Risk

- Prevalence: 10–90/100,000 in North America
- Occurs primarily in temperate climates, with a North to South gradient in the USA
- Female predominance up to 2:1
- Onset usually in third or fourth decade of life
- Racial predominance: Caucasian 6 × the incidence of all other races

Perioperative Risks

- Exacerbation of Sx with temp elevation, stress of surgery, infection, emotional trauma, postpartum state
- Risk of positioning injury (muscle wasting), hyperkalemia with succinylcholine, DVT
- Steroid therapy predisposes to adrenal suppression, gastric ulceration

Worry About

- Advisability of major conduction block; greater neurotoxicity of local anesthetics due to demyelination. Spinal anesthesia has been reported to exacerbate symptoms.

- Presence of transverse myelitis and other major motor neuron disease (risk of hyperkalemia with depolarizing NMB)
- Cranial nerve involvement with loss of airway integrity
- Temp increase: As little as 0.5° can aggravate symptoms
- Autonomic dysfunction

Overview

- Demyelinating disease of brain and spinal cord (peripheral nerves are not affected), with chronically remitting and relapsing or progressive course
- Assoc conditions incl seizures and uveitis; CNS components involved are cortex (cognitive dysfunction, memory loss, personality change, emotional lability) and spinal cord
- Chronic dysesthetic pain and spasticity contribute to disability
- Paroxysmal Sx may mimic cerebral ischemia, spinal cord compression, tic douloureux

ICD-9-CM Code: 340

Etiology

- Cause unknown
- Autoimmune, genetic, environmental factors thought to combine to attack CNS myelin

Usual Treatment

- No treatment curative
- Steroids, interferon, azathioprine, cyclophosphamide ameliorate relapses; methotrexate may also be used.
- Intrathecal baclofen pumps are sometimes seen for control of spasticity.
- Carbamazepine used for paroxysmal Sx (incl pain); baclofen, and, occasionally, surgery for spasticity (thalamotomy)
- Interferon-β now a first line treatment, shown to decrease rate and severity of relapses, may delay onset of disability

ASSESSMENT POINTS

System	Effect	Assessment by Hx	PE	Test
HEENT	Pseudobulbar palsy	Hx of swallowing difficulty	Cranial nerves IX, X	
RESP	May have aspirated from bulbar dysfunction, seizure	Review with family	Auscultation	CXR, oximetry
GI	GI effects of steroids	Hx of pain, bleeding		
CNS	Cognitive dysfunction, optic neuritis, seizures, dysesthesias, ophthalmoplegia, autonomic dysfunction, monoplegia, transverse myelitis, quadriplegia	Hx of memory loss, emotional lability, "dropping things", visual problems Lhermitte's sign (electric shock to legs); check with family for description of seizures	Mental status exam Neurologic exam (esp. motor and sensory) Orthostatic vital sign changes	CSF electrophoresis (elevated IgG and myelin basic protein); MRI (plaques); evoked potentials; EEG

Key Reference: Dorotta IR, Schubert A. Multiple sclerosis and anesthetic implications. *Curr Opin Anaesthesiol.* 2002;15(3):365–370.

Perioperative Implications

Preoperative Preparation

- Consider steroid supplementation; avoid anticholinergics
- May need benzodiazepine premedication to reduce risk of stress-induced exacerbation
- Carefully document preop neurologic status
- Adequate volume status
- Orthostatic intolerance and inappropriate heart-rate responses may be seen due to autonomic instability.

Monitoring
- Routine

Airway
- None

Preinduction/Induction

- Spinal anesthesia implicated in aggravating MS symptoms and considered contraindicated
- Caution with epidural anesthesia: Need clear indication, such as in obstetrics, pt informed of possible symptom exacerbation, use lower concentrations of local anesthetics, and epidural opioids are OK to use

- Peripheral nerve blocks OK
- Succinylcholine may precipitate hyperkalemia; both sensitivity AND resistance to NMDBs reported
- Avoid elevation of body temp
- Avoid proconvulsant anesthetics
- Sedation, confusion, and nausea are all possible from intrathecal baclofen infusions

Maintenance
- Careful maintenance of normothermia
- Continue steroid stress coverage
- Careful titration of nondepolarizing NMBs

Extubation
- Pts with brainstem involvement should be extubated awake
- Spasticity may diminish maximal insp effort

Adjuvants
- Duration of most NMBs shortened by phenytoin and carbamazepine

Postoperative Period

- Exacaerbations common in postop period regardless of anesthetic technique; perform neuro exam
- Continue supplemental steroid coverage
- Treat hyperthermia
- Spasticity may interfere with pulm toilet

Anticipated Problems/Concerns

- Unpredictable appearance of new neurologic deficits periop
- Exacerbation of MS symptoms with hyperthermia, stress, pain
- Hyperkalemia with succinylcholine, unpredictable blockade with NMDBs
- Emotional lability and need for sedative premedication

Multisystem Organ Failure, Lung Dysfunction In

Muhammad Fareedul Azam

Risk

- The incidences of adult respiratory distress syndrome (ARDS) and acute lung injury (ALI) are 8 and 50 cases per 100,000 person-years, respectively.
- ARDS/ALI are the manifestations of lung dysfunction in MODS.

Risk Factors

- Systemic sepsis, polytrauma, severe pancreatitis, multiple transfusions
- Pneumonia, lung contusion, near drowning, inhaled toxins, DIC
- ARDS affects 15% ICU pts and has a mortality rate of 40%.
- Refractory hypoxia is an uncommon cause of death in these pts.
- Majority of ARDS deaths due to MODS

Perioperative Risks

- Hypoxemia
- Systemic hypotension
- Pulm Htn, RV dysfunction/failure

Worry About

- High PEEP reducing preload causing hemodynamic instability
- Barotrauma and auto PEEP (esp in obstructive pulm diseases)

Overview

- Four overlapping disease states exist in a spectrum of severity, incl SIRS
- Descending order of severity; MODS > severe sepsis > sepsis > SIRS
- ALI is characterized by massive inflammation and leakage of protein rich fluid from pulm capillaries into the alveoli. This phase lasts a few days, inhibiting gas exchange ($\downarrow$ PaO$_2$ / $\uparrow$ PaCO$_2$) and decreasing pulm compliance
- ALI subsequently becomes a fibro-proliferative process, frequently permanent

- Definition: ARDS and ALI, American and European 1994 Consensus Conference
  - Acute onset hypoxemia and resp failure
  - Bilateral diffuse infiltrates on chest radiography
  - Pulm artery occlusion pressure <18 mm Hg (no left atrial Htn)
  - PaO$_2$ / FIO$_2$ ratio of ≤300 for ARDS, ≤200 for ALI

ICD-9-CM Code: 995.92 (Severe sepsis)

Etiology

- ALI in MODS may have pulm or extra pulm causes

Usual Treatment

- Aggressive Dx, treatment of underlying cause with timely antibiotics
- General supportive therapy using well established sepsis bundles
- Lung protective strategies (LPS) to minimize ventilator-induced lung injury
  - Plateau <30 cm H$_2$O, TV 6 mL/kg, permissive hypercapnia

Perioperative Implications

Preoperative Preparation

- Transport from ICU to the OR, consider RRT/RN/perfusionist/intensivist help
- If not intubated, ensure equipment, medications, personnel, monitors present
- Consider ICU ventilator for case (high PEEP +/- inhaled NO), oscillator

Monitoring

- Consider arterial line, central line, PA catheter, TEE

Airway

- Ensure airway is secure. Decompensation may be rapid and hard to recover from.

- Consider continuous suction catheter ETT (potentially reduces incidence of ventilator-assoc pneumonia)

Preinduction/Induction

- Hypoxemia and/or hypercarbia may exacerbate pulm Htn and RV dysfunction
- Reduced FRC exacerbates ventilation/perfusion (V/Q) mismatch, worsening PaO$_2$

Maintenance

- Adequate PEEP restores FRC, decreasing shunt, improving V/Q and oxygenation
- Appropriate fluids and blood products for optimum preload
- Vasopressors and inotropic support when indicated
- Surgical manipulation of septic focus may cause adverse hemodynamic effects
- Consider use of spectral edge EEG analysis to guide mixed balance anesthesia
- Consider cisatracurium for organ-independent elimination
- Maintain case-appropriate temp

Extubation

- Consider leaving pt intubated for continued postop ventilation
- Avoid shivering, which increases O$_2$ consumption dramatically

Adjuvants

- iNO, inhaled prostaglandins, surfactant, bronchoscopy

Postoperative Period

- Close monitoring and treatment of volume status, PEEP, hemodynamic support
- Reduce FIO$_2$ as soon as reasonably possible, maintaining SpO$_2$ > 90%

Anticipated Problems/Concerns

- Ventilator-assoc pneumonia
- Barotrauma (pneumothorax/mediastinum/pericardium)

ASSESSMENT POINTS

System	Effect	Hx	Exam	Test	Rx
CARDIO (septic shock)	Low CO RV dysfunction	$\downarrow$ MAP $\uparrow$ PAOP	Edema Gallop S$_3$	ECG, troponin ECHO PA catheter BNP	Euvolemia Conservative fluids if no hypoperfusion Vasopressors
RESP (ALI/ARDS)	Hypoxemia $\downarrow$ Compliance Pulm Htn and edema	Respiratory distress	Crackles $\uparrow$ P2	ABG CXR PA catheter	Protective strategies TV – 6 mL/kg High PEEP Prone position
GI, HEPATIC (shock liver)	Ileus Dysfunction Hemorrhage	Pain N/V Distension	Hypoactive Ascites Tense abdomen Guaiac stool	Lactate KUB CT scan Bladder pressures	NPO, NGT, IV fluid +/– TPN GI stress ulcer Rx
RENAL (ATN)	Acute kidney injury	RIFLE criteria	Urine volume Urinalysis	Chem 7, FeNa US	Renal replacement therapy
HEME	Anemia Coagulopathy DIC	$\downarrow$ Hgb	Pallor Bleeding	CBC Plts PT/PTT Fibrinogen	PRBC: Hgb 7–9 g/dL Plts: 5–30 k FFP: High risk/IR/OR Cryo: ≤80 fibrinogen
CNS ($\downarrow$ mental status)	Cerebral hypoxia	$\downarrow$ GCS	Deficits: CNS/PNS	CT brain, MRI ICP monitor Lumbar puncture	Maintain CPP Avoid hypotension
ENDO	Insulin resistance	$\uparrow$ BG	Goal <150 mg/dL	Frequent blood sugars	Insulin—sliding scale or infusion

Key Reference: Levy MM, Dellinger RP, Townsend SR, et al. The Surviving Sepsis Campaign: Results of an international guideline-based performance improvement program targeting severe sepsis. *Crit Care Med.* 2010;38(2):367–374.

Myasthenia Gravis

Cecil O. Borel

Risk

- Incidence in USA: 50–142 cases per million
- Affects all races
- M:F ratio: 2:1

Perioperative Risks

- Postop NM ventilatory failure
- Postop pneumonia due to poor cough and secretion clearance

Worry About

- Preop optimization of muscle strength
- Anticholinesterase medications, steroids, plasmapheresis

Overview

- Characterized by weakness and fatiguability of skeletal muscles
- Insp muscle weakness from residual paralysis from nondepolarizing NM blocking agents
- Exacerbation of underlying bulbar (airway) musculature weakness
- Increased sensitivity to hypoventilation with narcotic analgesics
- Muscle strength improves similarly in both myasthenia gravis and nondepolarizing blockade after administration of anticholinesterase drugs.

ICD-9-CM Code: 358.0

Etiology

- Autoimmune disease of NM junction mediated by reduction in number of acetylcholine receptors at NM junction

Usual Treatment

- Anticholinesterase medications (pyridostigmine, Mestinon)
- Immunosuppression: Steroids, azathioprine
- Plasmapheresis
- Intravenous immunoglobulin (IVIG)
- Thymectomy

ASSESSMENT POINTS

System	Effect	Assessment by Hx	PE	Test
NM	Peripheral muscle weakness	Easy fatiguability	Arm adduction times <1 min	Repetitive nerve stimulation
RESP				
Airway	Bulbar weakness	Difficulty swallowing	Head lift <5 sec	Formal swallowing evaluation
Ventilation	Insp muscle weakness	Orthopnea, breathlessness	Paradoxical insp motion	NIF <30 cm H_2O FVC <1000 mL
Ventilatory drive	CO_2 retention	Morning headache	↓ Ventilation of bases	ABGs
Secretion clearance	Weak cough	Recurrent pneumonia		CXR

Key Reference: Borel CO, Hanley DF. Muscular paralysis—myasthenia gravis and polyneuritis. In: Parrillo JE, Bone RC, eds. *Critical care medicine: Principles of diagnosis and management*. Philadelphia: Mosby–Year Book; 1994:1193–1215.

Perioperative Implications

Preoperative Preparation

- Anticholinesterase medications
  - Hold 2–4 hr preop
  - Postop: May use IV neostigmine to replace pyridostigmine PO, 1 mg IV/60 mg PO or start IV neostigmine 1 hr before emergence at 1/30–1/60 daily pyridostigmine dose, infuse over 24 hr
- Steroid maintenance

Monitoring

- Routine
- Train-of-4 twitch monitor if short-active nondepolarizers used

Induction/Intubation

- Consider inhalational anesthestic breathe-down techniques

Intubation Without Muscle Relaxation, Using Propofol/Remifentanil Maintenance

- Minimize or avoid use of muscle relaxants
- TIVA or inhalational anesthesia

Extubation

- Check NIF (>30 cm H_2O), head lift, cough, gag, ensure full return of twitch

Adjuvants

- Avoid or minimize use of nondepolarizing muscle relaxants

- Depolarizing relaxants may have ↑ or ↓ efficacy
- Consider epidural analgesic, particularly for thymectomy.

Anticipated Problems/Concerns

- Postop ventilatory failure, pneumonia, aspiration
- Cholinergic crisis if excess anticholinesterase medications given

Mycoplasma pneumoniae Infection

Carlos A. Puyo

Risks

• Endemic and/or pandemic worldwide every 3–5 y
  • Outbreaks likely during summer, early fall
  • Affects persons of all ages
  • Long incubation periods 1-3 wk
  • Transmitted person to person via aerosols
• Frequent in closed and semiclosed communities
• Common cause of upper and lower resp infections
  • Up to 40% of community-acquired pneumonias, walking pneumonia
  • Up to 5% of bronchiolitis in children
  • 3–10% of adults may develop bronchopneumonia
  • Clinical manifestations similar to *C. pneumonia*, *S. pneumonia* and resp viruses
• Fulminant pneumonia may occur in children with sickle cell disease (functional asplenism), Down syndrome, and immunosuppressive conditions.
  • Extrapulmonary complications in 25% of pts infected with *M. pneumoniae*.

Perioperative Risks

• No periop risk data; hemolytic anemia, DIC, cross-reacting cold agglutinins are of concern esp if CPB is required.
• Hyperreactive airway disease

Worry About

• Multisystem organ dysfunction

Overview

• Clinical manifestations of resp involvement are mediated by activity of cytadherence on the airway epithelium and incl:
  • Sore throat, hoarseness, fever, cough (pertussis-like), may play a role in asthma, COPD.
  • Conjunctivitis, headache, chills, coryza, myalgias, earache, and generalized malaise are common.
  • Extrapulmonary manifestations are the result of direct invasion or immune reactivity.

Diagnosis

• Hx and clinical manifestations: Nonspecific
• CXR: Diffuse reticular infiltrates in perihilar and lower lobe regions. Bilateral in 20% of cases

• Pathology: Ulceration, edema, ciliary loss, bronchoalveolar Inflammatory cell infiltration
• Culture: Incubation period of several weeks. Sensitivity around 60%. Not practical for routine Dx
• Serology: Current or recent infection likely if antibody titer increase ≥ 4-fold
• Cold agglutinins: IgM within 1–2 wk after initial infection. Titers ≥ 1:32 correlate with severity of lung involvement
• Polymerase chain reaction: RNA-amplification techniques are highly sensitive and indicate viable bacterium.

ICD-9-CM Code: 483.0

Etiology

• *Mycoplasma pneumoniae*, slow-growing bacterium.

Usual Treatment

• Antibiotic treatment will shorten resp symptoms.
• Macrolides, tetracyclines, and fluoroquinolones. Macrolide resistance has been reported.

ASSESSMENT POINTS

Organ	Effect	Assessment by Hx	PE	Test
HEENT	Otitis Retinitis conjunctivitis	Ear symptoms may affect 30%	Mucosal congestion	
RESP	Tracheobronchitis Pneumonia Asthma	Failure to respond to treatment with sulfonamide or penicillin	Persistent cough Expiratory wheezes	CXR Sputum
CARDIO	Pericarditis Pericardial effusion Cardiac tamponade Myocarditis	Incidence: 1–8.5% Almost 50% will develop cardiac symptoms within 16 mo of *M. Pneumoniae* infection	Distant heart sounds S_3, JVD Pericardial rub	ECG ECHO Tap effusion
CNS	Aseptic meningitis Meningoencephalitis Transverse myelitis Guillian-Barré Peripheral neuropathy Cerebellar syndrome	Incidence 7%, children more likely to die or have severe neurologic deficits	Focal or general neurologic symptoms, diplopia, coma	CSF Elevated cytokines IL-6, IL-8 MRI Serology
HEM	Hemolytic anemia Cold agglutinins DIC	More common in children Likely due to cross-reactive antibodies	Peripheral cyanosis	IgG-free Hgb D Coombs'
DERM	Maculopapular Vesicular rash Stevens-Johnson Syndrome	May affect up to 25%	Rash, but needs to rule out rash due to Abx	*M. Pneumoniae* has been detected in cutaneous lesions
RENAL	Glomerulonephritis Tubulointerstitial nephritis IgA nephropathy Paroxysmal cold Hemoglobinuria	Brisk hemolytic anemia		UA renal biopsy Ig G, M, A

Key Reference: Waites KB, Balish MF, Atkinson TP. New insights into the pathogenesis and detection of Mycoplasma pneumonia infections. *Future Microbiol.* 2008;3(6):635–648.

Perioperative Implications

Preoperative Evaluation
• Routine physical exam: Emphasis on, resp, CNS, CV, and HEME systems.
• Resp-increased minute ventilation, low sat, prolonged ventilation may be required.
• CNS-document preexistent neuropathy
• CV-JVD, rule out tamponade physiology
• HEM-hemolysis and anemia. If cold agglutinins are suspected, determine temp range and titers.
  • If surgery is non-urgent, consider postponing it until active issues resolved

Monitoring
• Invasive monitoring necessary if resp and CV concerns.

Airway
• Desaturation is possible due to decreased FRC
• High incidence of hyperreactive airway disease

Maintenance
• Normothermia is essential to avoid cold agglutinins. Warm all fluids, humidify airway.
• If hemolysis develops; optimized UO, alkalinized urine and use diuretics.

Extubation
• Clear mental status, good resp mechanics, able to clear secretions.

Anticipated Problems/Concerns

• Resp distress 2° to asthma, COPD, high O_2 requirements may result in prolonged intubation
• Neurologic deficit may delay extubation
• CPB and/or cold agglutinins may result in circuit obstruction and impair myocardial protection.

Myocardial Contusion (Blunt Cardiac Injury)

Andrew L. Rosenberg

Risk

- Incidence unknown, in part due to absence of clear diagnostic criteria/test
- Two million motor vehicle accidents/y with ~ 40% involving closed chest injury
- 20–70% incidence by clinical criteria
- 16–20% incidence by autopsy
- Motor vehicle > falls > crush injuries
- Males > females (5:1)
- Commotio cordis is a rare form of BCI
  - Due to low impact chest injury (sports) causing sudden death

Perioperative Risks

- Abn ECG
- Nonspecific ST-T wave changes (70%) in trauma pts
- Q wave and ST elevation
- 7–17% false negative
- 60% false positive
- Ventricular arrhythmias most common in contusion
  - Trifasicular conduction block
- Other cardiac conditions: Thrombosed, lacerated coronary arteries in spasm; ventricular hypofunction; pericardial effusion/tamponade; pericarditis; valvular insufficiency, left-sided > right-sided; ventricular wall rupture (incl septum)
- Possible increased risk of cardiac complications (arrhythmias, hypotension) with increased CK-MB troponins, and abn ECHO
- No evidence of increased mortality assoc with GA

Worry About

- Malignant ventricular arrhythmia (acute and delayed)
- Cardiac conduction blocks incl complete heart block
- Volume status
- Acute hypotension
- Delayed myocardial rupture
- Assoc injuries: Pulm contusion–hypoxemia, thoracic aorta injuries, flail chest

Overview

- Traumatic injury with hemorrhagic, well-circumscribed lesions of partial or full thickness from myocardial contusion
- Usually of RV but can be multichambered
- Frequently in severe blunt chest trauma and after CPR, precordial thumps, but difficult to definitively diagnose
- Incorporation of clinical suspicion, anginal chest pain unrelieved by nitrates, ECG—esp. ventricular dysrhythmia, CK-MB, troponin I and T levels, 2-D ECHO for Dx
- Amount of malignant arrhythmias may be proportional to severity of myocardial contusion
- See also under Trauma in the index

ICD-9-CM Code: 861.01

Etiology

- Mechanical contusion of myocardium from posterior sternum
- Ram effect from increased transdiaphragmatic pressure or sudden deceleration
- Automobile accident most common cause = 15%
- Falls ~10%
- Crash, sports-related assaults ~15%

Usual Treatment

- Supportive
- Adequate volume replacement

ASSESSMENT POINTS

System	Effect	Assessment by Hx	PE	Test
CARDIO	Ventricular contusion	Angina-like chest pain unrelieved by nitrates	Chest wall, sternal tenderness	ECG, serial
				↑ Troponin I and T within 6 hr
		Dyspnea	Hypotension with severe dysfunction	ECHO
				SPECT
			S$_3$	MRI
			Rales	
	Arrhythmia	Palpitations, dizziness, syncope	Pulse	ECG monitoring
	Valvular disruptions	Dyspnea	Auscultatory murmurs	ECG
	Coronary artery injury: thrombosis, laceration, spasm	Chest pain		Angio
	Effusion/tamponade	Chest pain	Pericardial friction	TTE
			Diminished heart sounds	2–D cardiography
			Distended neck veins	PA catheter
RESP	CHF	Dyspnea	S$_3$	
	Pulm contusion	Orthopnea	Rales	
		Chest tightness	Wheezing	CXR
			Tachypnea	O$_2$ saturation

Key Reference: Lindstaedt M, Germing A, Lawo T, et al. Acute and long-term clinical significance of myocardial contusion following blunt thoracic trauma: Results of a prospective study. *J Trauma.* 2002;52:479.

Perioperative Implications

Preoperative Preparation
- 2-D ECHO or TEE abn predict periop hypotension
- Assess and ensure adequate volume replacement
- Assess and treat assoc concurrent injuries
- No evidence for benefit of prophylactic antiarrhythmic agents

Monitoring
- Continuous ECG for arrhythmias
- PA catheter for large fluid shift operations or pts with signs of LV dysfunction
- Increased risk of periop arrhythmias without increased mortality

Airway
- Evaluation for assoc airway injury

Preinduction/Induction
- Adequate volume replacement
- Hypotension more likely with large contusions
- Extra attention to avoid hypoxia, hypovolemia

Maintenance
- No one agent or technique shown superior
- Avoid known pulm vasoconstrictors: catecholamine, hypoxia, acidosis, histamine-releasing agents (MgSO$_4$, mivacurium)
- Consider high inspired O$_2$ if contusion
- NO can aggravate pulm Htn
- Elevations in PVR may unmask RV failure
- Increased LV filling pressures and decreased cardiac output often reflect hypovolemia or are 2° to RV failure, not LV failure

Extubation
- May leave intubated if concerns for resp failure and hypoxia present

Adjuvants
- Combination of appropriate intravascular volume replenishment and vasodilators (nitroglycerin) for pulm Htn

Postoperative Period
- Delayed hypoxia from pulm injury common and can cause pulm Htn leading to hypotension if RV severely contused

Anticipated Problems/Concerns
- Variable diagnostic criteria, total CK-MB >50 U/L and ≥5% total CK
- Possible higher risk of cardiac complications with ↑ CK-MB
- Almost any arrhythmia reported, esp. conduction delays; more severe contusion assoc with ↑ malignant ventricular arrhythmia
- Watch for RV failure leading to increase LV pressure but decrease LV diastolic filling.

Myocardial Ischemia (MIsch)

Dennis T. Mangano

Michael F. Roizen

Risk

- Incidence in USA: 1.5 million/y develop acute myocardial infarction (MI); decreased rate of death in USA balanced by increased population has kept MI numbers constant since 1970 despite increased population; 7 million worldwide had MI/year
- 10 million in USA have ≥70% narrowing of 1 or more coronary arteries
- European, Indian, and African-American heritage > Japanese, but environment of North America equalizes risks
- Highest in pts with known other atherosclerotic disease (incl prior MI): smokers (3.5-fold increase); hypertensives (3-fold increase); diabetics (4-fold increase); hypercoagulable or chronic inflammatory diseases (3-fold increase); stressed, divorced, or unstable marriage (2.5-fold increase); with wt gain since age 20 y (1.5-fold increase for each 5 kg increase); increase LDL cholesterol in those who do not exercise (0.5% increase for each 1% increase than 100 mg/dL); who do not drink or take vitamin D or aspirin; whose parent died of CAD at < age 40 y (1.4 to 2.5-fold increase); age (3–fold increase per decade over 50), family Hx (1.1 to 2.4-fold increase)

Perioperative Risks

- Increases risk 9-fold of periop CV complication (MI, CHF, Rt HF, arrhythmia requiring Rx)

- 2-y survival: Rate in high-risk pt with periop MIsch is 25%, vs. 85% for those without periop MIsch
- Inadequate coronary perfusion (1.5 to 6% reinfarction rate with general surgery; higher with vascular/thoracic/upper abd surgery); lower with cataract/prostate/peripheral surgery with 1-limb anesthesia only
- Can lead to increase LV or RV compliance and CHF and dysrhythmias
- Can lead to inadequate perfusion of other organs and their insufficient function (brain, kidney, liver, gut)

Worry About

- Postop period if stressed by perturbations that increase demand (pain, sepsis, fever, hyper- and hypovolemia, and tachycardia), or limit supply (thrombosis, hyperviscosity states, diseases limiting pulm function and gas exchange [restrictive, obstructive, parenchymal], Hct <28%)

Overview

- Condition of inadequate supply of O_2 and nutrients to myocardial cells relative to need assoc with the increased stress of perioperative period
- Treatment and prophylaxis of this and related disorders consume 10–20% of total health expenditures. Periop CV complications increased 1-fold with MIsch, with 3-fold reduction in 2–y survival and 3-fold increase in periop costs for major surgery.

- Major focus of clinical and basic studies to decrease incidence of and risks from concern over risk-benefit ratio and cost-effectiveness, identifying high-risk pts prior to surgery and segregating them for prior therapy (smoking cessation, control of Htn, hypercholesterol states, hypercoagulable states, PTCA, CABG) or increased periop vigilance and care (PA lines, TEE, ICU care, prophylactic pain therapy)

ICD-9-CM Code: 410.09

Etiology

- Known atherosclerotic risks (genetic predisposition, smoking, Htn, diabetes, divorced or unstable marriage, inflammation, hypercoagulable states, increase LDL or decrease HDL cholesterol, weight gain)
- Known conditions that increase periop demands on heart (tachycardia, 2-fold greater for HR >90; 11-fold greater for HR >110); or limit supply (vasospastic states; $Paco_2$ <25; Hct <28%; hyperviscosity and hypercoagulable states; inadequate O_2 exchange)

Usual Treatment

- Decrease atherogenic risk factors
- Decrease periop demands on heart
- Consider preop segregation for statin or aspirin or β-blocker and nitrate therapies, antispasm and sympatholytic therapies, PTCA or CABG considerations, or stepped-up postop care of increased monitoring, intensive normalization of hemodynamics, greater prophylactic pain therapies

ASSESSMENT POINTS

System	Effect	Assessment by Hx	PE	Test
HEENT	Plaques in other areas	Risk factor search: Smoking stain; hypercholesterolemic lesions	McArdle's earlobe	
CARDIO	↓ LV or RV compliance ↓ Pump function arrhythmias Autonomic pain	SOB, DOE Angina ↓ Exercise tolerance Palpitations PND	HR/BP prior to and after 2-stair climb; S_3; rales; JVD; use character and rhythm	ECG, CXR, stress ECHO or dipyridamole thallium or ambulatory Holter, troponins, and myeloperodiase tests
RESP		Nocturnal cough, orthopnea		
RENAL	Perfusion insufficiency	Nocturia Erectile dysfunction (male) Loss of ability to acheive orgasm (female)		BUN/Cr
CNS	Autonomic pain syndromes Other atherosclerotic syndromes	Pain in neck or left arm Stroke/TIA Hx	CNS and cranial nerve exam	Carotid Doppler ANS testing

Key Reference: Jeremias A, Kaul S, Rosengart TK, Gruberg L, Brown DL. The impact of revascularization on mortality in patients with nonacute coronary artery disease. *Am J Med.* 2009;122:152–161.

Perioperative Implications

Preoperative Preparation
- Consider segregation procedures and prophylactic regimens (see under Usual Treatment)

Monitoring
- ST-T waves of area of myocardium identified as at risk (or II and V_5) (II esp. for CNS surgery); ST-segment trend analysis
- Consider TEE and arterial line and approaches to intensively normalize hemodynamics
- Management of arrhythmia management devices (see Practice Advisory for the Perioperative Management of Patients with Cardiac Rhythm Management Devices: Pacemakers and Implantable Cardioverter–Defibrillators, *Anesthesiology* 2005; 103:186–198)

Airway
- Routine

Induction
- Without hemodynamic disturbance and esp. with HR control

Maintenance
- Tachycardia or hypovolemia and Hct <28 can precipitate ischemia.
- No agent with demonstrated outcome superiority.
- Intensively normalize hemodynamics and HR

Extubation
- In nonstressful fashion for pt without compromising supply of O_2 to myocardium
- Aggressive stepped pain therapy recommended; alpha-2 adrenergic agonist recommended by some

Adjuvants
- CHF decreases liver blood flow and clearance of drugs requiring hepatic metabolism (such as lidocaine)

- β-adrenergic receptor antagonists and nitrates can be assoc with profound hemodynamic disturbances if drug interactions or sudden preload, afterload, or contractility perturbations (such as rapid onset of spinal anesthesia) occur.

Anticipated Problems/Concerns

- Pre- and postop periods at least as great a cause of morbidity as intraop period
- Restart anti-anginal and antiplaque therapies, i.e., statins, CO Q10, aspirin, DHA, etc., and physical activity rehab program as soon as possible postop if D/C preop
- Consider compassionate anxiety-relieving yet aggressive preop consultation and intensive stepped pain prophylaxis consultations postop.

Myotonia Dystrophica (Myotonic Dystrophy, Steinert's Disease)

Saroj Mukesh Shah
Adam J. Broussard
Alan Kaye

Incidence

- Myotonic dystrophy is a rare disease with an incidence of about 1 in 8000. The incidence of the congenital form is higher with an incidence of 1/100,000

Perioperative Risks

- Operative/anesthetic and postop morbidity/mortality are increased and not proportional to severity of disease
- High incidence of cardiopulmonary complications, incl sudden death, cardiac failure, cardiomyopathy

Worry About

- Increasing frequency of symptoms
- Signs of resp or cardiac decompensation

Overview

- Degenerative disease of skeletal muscles. Progressive distal muscle wasting. Triad of characteristic features described as frontal baldness, cataracts, and mental retardation.

- Extremely variable in presentation: Asymptomatic cases to congenital with mental retardation and resp insufficiency.
- Typically onset of symptoms in 2nd and 3rd decades of life with progressive muscular weakness and wasting most common in the cranial and distal limb muscles—temporalis and masseter muscle, atrophy known as hatchet face and limb muscles; initial affected result in footdrop and weak handshake. Deep tendon reflexes reduced and muscles of the vocal cord apparatus result in nasal speech. Proximal muscle variant recently recognized; death frequently in 5th or 6th decade of life, usually due to cardiopulmonary complications incl sudden death from conduction abn, cardiomyophy, and CHF.
- Persistent contracture after cessation of stimulation or voluntary contraction of the muscle. This inability of the skeletal muscle to relax is diagnostic. EMG is corroborative and pathognomonic, showing continuous low-voltage activity with high-voltage, fibrillation-like potential bursts.

- Intrinsic disorder of skeletal muscle linked to myotonin-protein kinase gene on chromosome 19q13.2. Defect in Na^+ and Cl^- channel function produces electrical instability of the muscle membrane and self-sustaining runs of depolarization. May also have abn Ca^{2+} metabolism.

ICD-9-CM Code: 359.2

Etiology

- Inherited autosomal dominant trait; abn expansion of the nucleotide CTG on chromosome 19, which codes for a serine-threonine protein kinase. Variable gene expressivity as within same family can have minimally affected and severely affected individuals.

Usual Treatment

- Quinine, procainamide, phenytoin, tocainide, mexiletine (depress Na^+ influx)

ASSESSMENT POINTS

System	Effect	Assessment by Hx	PE/Clinical Sequelae	Test
HEENT	Visual disturbance		Presenile cataract, ptosis, strabismus, retinal pigmentation	Exam by ophthalmologist
	Speech/swallowing impaired		Generalized weakness of pharyngeal, mandibular (and thoracic) musculature	
			Dysarthria, facial weakness	
			Expressionless facies	
CARDIO	Dysrhythmias	CHF uncommon but may occur with pregnancy	Delayed intraventricular conduction	ECG
	Cardiomyopathy		Heart block, hypotension	ECHO, Holter
			Up to 20% with mitral valve prolapse, sudden death	Cardiology consult
RESP	Restrictive lung disease	Weak cough	Wasting of sternocleidomastoid muscles; resp muscle weakness	PFTs
	Chronic aspiration	Dyspnea		ABGs
	Central hypoventilation	Hx of pneumonia	Lungs intrinsically normal; $\downarrow$ VC, $\downarrow$ ERV, $\uparrow CO_2$	
GI	High aspiration potential	Weak swallowing ability		
	Delayed esophageal and gastric emptying			
	Gastric dilation/atony			
	$\uparrow$ Incidence of cholelithiasis			
ENDO/ IMMUNE	Testicular atrophy		Thyroid nodules	Blood/urine glucose tests
	DM		$\downarrow$Immunoglobulins	Thyroid function tests
	$\downarrow$ Thyroid function			
	Adrenal insufficiency			
	Frontal balding			
	?Malignant hyperthermia			
CNS	Mental retardation		Myotonic handgrip (delayed, incomplete release), $\uparrow$ CK in serum	EMG
	Assoc with central sleep apnea and hypersomnolence		Myotonia can be initiated or worsened by exercise or cold temp; $\downarrow$DTR	CK
	Emotional abn			
GYN	Pregnant pt is a challenge. Resp function threatened by $\downarrow$ FRC and myotonic weakness, which may be exacerbated by pregnancy. Seems to be added risk for uterine hemorrhage at delivery due to uterine atony and retained placenta. C-section may be safer.			

Key Reference: Aldredge LM. Anaesthetic problems in myotonic dystrophy. A case report and review of the Aberdeen experience comprising 48 general anesthetics in a further 16 patients. *Br J Anaesth.* 1985;57:1119–1130.

Perioperative Implications

Preoperative Preparation

- Ensuring NPO status (increased aspiration) and recent ECG
- No preop analgesics or sedatives and caution with benzodiazepines
- Warm ambient room air in OR may $\downarrow$ incidence and severity of myotonia

- Routine monitoring

Airway

- Propensity for frequent jaw dislocation
- Potential inability to secure airway because of jaw muscle spasm

Preinduction/Induction

- Risk for aspiration of gastric contents

- Induction: Gaseous; avoid slow metabolizing hypnotics; use lower doses on propofol
- Relaxation: Avoid succinylcholine (link to malignant hyperthermia, severe extended contractures); use short-acting non-depolarizing agents at lower doses; recovery may be prolonged.
- May be hard to differentiate from onset of MH.

Maintenance
- Myotonia may be precipitated by drugs (propofol, succinylcholine, anticholinesterases, halothane, neuroleptics, liquid paraffin, etc.), physical factors (cold, shivering), surgical manipulation, or electrocautery.
- Avoid K^+ containing fluids
- Regional or local anesthesia acceptable, but will not block myotonic response
- Regional +/– TIVA may be preferable when suitable

Extubation
- Beware of airway obstruction because of jaw muscle weakness.
- Delayed recovery from anesthetic common

Adjuvants
- Increased sensitivity to ventilatory depressant effects of all premedicants, sedatives, opioids
- Reversal agents can theoretically precipitate skeletal muscle contraction by facilitating depolarization of NMJ, but adverse responses do not predictably occur.

Postoperative Period
- Increased sensitivity to resp depressant effects of opioids or sedatives, incl epidural opioids; explore analgesic methods (e.g., regional or NSAIDs)
- Pulm complications due to poor cough possible
- Cardiac and resp monitoring and early chest physiotherapy

Anticipated Problems/Concerns
- If myotonia develops intraop, neither general or regional anesthesia, nor NMBs will attenuate it. Local infiltration of involved muscles may help. Even asymptomatic pts may have some degree of cardiomyopathy. Beware of premature extubation, consider postop ventilation.
- 57% of these of pts have conduction defects with one third have 1° block unresponsive to atropine, it is advisable to have antiarrhythmics and transthoracic pacing readily available as many anesthetic agents can increase vagal tone.
- For numerous reasons, it is advisable to avoid general anesthetics (myocardial depressants, conduction effects, link to malignant hyperthermia).

Myxoma

Solomon Aronson

Risk

- Although primary cardiac tumors are rare (<0.01%) this is the most common (50%)
- 75% develop in LA
- Rarely develop in ventricle
- More common in females (70%)

Perioperative Risks

- May be friable and embolize
- Risk of LV or RV inflow obstruction
- May simulate pulm Htn and/or constrictive pericarditis

Worry About

- Hypotension due to obstruction of ventricular inflow and/or incompetence of tricuspid (right) or mitral (left) valve

- Tumor flips on stalk across valves, causing stenotic or incompetent symptoms
- RV hypertrophy due to longstanding left inflow obstruction
- Rare pulm or systemic embolization

Overview

- Is a true neoplasm and distinct from a thrombus
- Usually polypoid with 1–2 cm stalk projecting into cavity; round with smooth margins
- Typically grows very slowly before symptomatic (10–20 y)

ICD-9-CM Code: D21.3 (Thorax myxoma)

Etiology

- Polyhedral cells with small nuclei are separated by an afibrillar, eosinophilic myxomatous stroma that is predominantly a mucopolysaccharide
- Rarely extends deeper than endocardium
- Although benign, this tumor can undergo malignant degeneration

Usual Treatment

- Surgical
- Cardiopulmonary bypass required
- Atriotomy with transseptal approach through fossa ovalis

ASSESSMENT POINTS

System	Effect	Assessment by Hx	PE	Test
CARDIO	Mitral stenosis or insufficiency syndromes	Edema, CHF	Left atrial enlargement Systolic murmur (MI) Diastolic murmur (mitral stenosis)	ECHO ECG CXR
RESP	Pulm emboli (right)	DOE, cough	Rales, wheezing, $\uparrow P_2$	ECHO, CXR, ECG
GI		CHF	Hepatic enlargement	Hepatic enzymes (if Sx of CHF)
RENAL	Emboli (left)			Urinalysis Cr clearance
CNS	Stroke (left)	CNS dysfunction	CNS dysfunction	ECHO
GENERAL	Constitutional symptoms	Fever, malaise	Weight loss	

Key Reference: Tagawa T, Okuda M, Sakuraba S. Anesthetic management of a patient with giant right atrial myxoma. *J Cardiothorac Vasc Anesth*. 2009; Jul 28.

Perioperative Implications

Preoperative Preparation

- Differential Dx incl mitral stenosis/insufficiency (left), tricuspid stenosis/insufficiency (right), constrictive pericarditis, pulm Htn, subacute bacterial endocarditis.
- Mitral stenosis: Hemodynamic aim is to keep in normal sinus rhythm with adequate preload and high normal afterload (see Mitral Stenosis in Diseases section).
- Mitral insufficiency (regurgitation): Hemodynamic aim is to keep HR normal or fast and vasodilate.
- Hemodynamics can mimic any or all of above depending on load-dependent variables prevailing in the cardiac cycle at the time (e.g., preload, afterload, HR).

Monitoring

- Routine monitors otherwise needed for cardiopulmonary bypass (e.g., temp, ECG, coagulation, Foley)
- Intra-arterial catheters

- Beware of central line with right-sided atrial myxoma (may cause dislodgment of friable debris as pulm emboli)
- TEE most sensitive way to guide hemodynamic management and assess therapeutic approach

Airway

- Routine

Preinduction/Induction

- May develop hypotension if preload is decreased or HR increased
- Avoid insertion of central venous or PA monitoring catheters or cannula with right-sided tumor
- Intraop TTE helpful diagnostic (prior to induction): Concern about right inflow obstruction exacerbated by PPV

Maintenance

- May dislodge pieces during CPB venous cannulation; direct assessment of anatomy, physiology; and even placement of cannula should be guided by TEE.

- If pedunculated, tumor may obstruct inflow track and hemodynamics may present as low BP, low CO; increased CVP (right) or increased PCWP (left)

Extubation

- Expect excellent recovery from primary myxomatous lesion and ventricular function.
- Criteria should be based on myocardial protection techniques and post-CPB bleeding risk.
- Early extubation consideration is reasonable.

Postoperative Period

- Beware residual ASD (as tumors typically originate in atrial septum in region of fossa ovalis)
- Beware conduction, dysrhythmia disturbance (esp. in pediatric population)
- Symptoms of pulm Htn usually regress quickly

Anticipated Problems/Concerns

- Hypotension with inadequate preload when lesion obstructs inflow dynamics

Narcolepsy

Douglas Martz

Risk

- Prevalance: 1/2000, more common in males
- Race with highest prevalence: None

Perioperative Risks

- Risks related to treatment medications
- Possible increased sensitivity to anesthetic agents
- Possible increased incidence of delayed emergence and postop hypersomnia after GA

Worry About

- Tricyclic drugs increase incidence of periop hypotension
- Tricyclic drugs blunt pressor response to indirect-acting sympathomimetic agents (e.g., ephedrine) and exaggerate pressor response to direct-acting sympathomimetic agents (e.g., phenylephrine)
- Possible increased incidence of postop apneic episodes
- Possible increased sensitivity to anesthetic agents

Overview

- Lifelong disease. Peak age of onset 15–30 yr

- Initial symptom is excessive daytime sleepiness with irresistible sleep attacks
- 2° symptoms of cataplexy, hypnagogic hallucinations, disrupted nocturnal sleep, and automatic behavior have variable incidence and can occur later in the disease.
- Sleep attacks appear as clinically normal sleep lasting from seconds to minutes. Can be easily awakened by auditory or tactile stimulation.
- 80% incidence of cataplexy (sudden brief loss of voluntary muscle control). Usually precipitated by strong emotional response (e.g., laughter, anger, surprise). Pt remains conscious. Majority of pts develop a flat affect to suppress the emotional trigger.
- Diagnostic work-up incl nocturnal polysomnogram (documents adequacy of sleep and rules out obstructive sleep apnea) followed by a Multiple Sleep Latency Test (MSLT) to document hypersomnolence and REM onset sleep. Pts with narcolepsy fall asleep quickly (usually <5 min) and have early onset of sleep.

- Often confused with obstructive sleep apnea syndrome

ICD-9-CM Code: 347

Etiology

- Assoc with HLA-DR15 and DQ6 antigens and low CSF levels of hypocretin-1

Usual Treatment

- Psychosocial support, therapeutic naps, medications
- Sleep attacks most commonly treated with modafinil (provigil) and/or indirect sympathomimetic drugs such as pemoline, methylphenidate, and dextroamphetamine
- Cataplexy and other 2° symptoms treated with gamma hydroxybuturate (xyrem), tricyclic antidepressants and/or SRIs

ASSESSMENT POINTS

System	Effect	Assessment by Hx	PE	Test
HEENT			Obstructive symptoms (rare)	
CARDIO	Conduction abn due to tricyclics			ECG
CNS	Flat affect Fatigue		Daytime sleep attacks	

Key Reference: Burrow B, Burkle C, Warner D. Postoperative outcome of patients with narcolepsy. *J Clin Anesth.* 2005;17:21–25.

Perioperative Implications

Preoperative Preparation

- Avoid sedative premedication
- Continue all medical therapy related to narcolepsy on day of surgery.
- If antisialagogue needed use non–central acting agent

Monitoring

- May have conduction abn on ECG
- Pts with a Hx of chronic amphetamine therapy may benefit from direct arterial pressure monitoring.

Induction

- May have exaggerated hypotension if taking tricyclics
- Hydrate prior to induction

Maintenance

- Increased sensitivity to anesthetic agents. Consider use of propofol, desflurane, sevoflurane, and N₂O instead of longer acting intravenous/inhalation agents.
- Exaggerated pressor response to direct-acting sympathomimetics (e.g., phenylephrine) if taking tricyclics. Use small doses if clinically indicated.
- Blunted and/or unpredictable pressor response to indirect-acting sympathomimetics if taking tricyclics. Probably best to avoid.

Adjuvants

- Muscle relaxants: Life-threatening arrhythmias have been reported with the use of pancuronium in pts on tricyclics.
- Anesthetic agents: Life-threatening arrhythmias have been reported with the use of halothane in pts on tricyclics.

Postoperative Period

- May be prone to postop apneic episodes esp. with use of IV and/or neuraxial narcotics for postop analgesia.

Anticipated Problems/Concerns

- Pts often on tricyclic therapy and CNS stimulant therapy. Will often be sensitive to anesthetic agents. If on tricyclics need to be concerned about exaggerated pressor responses with direct-acting sympathomimetics. Indirect-acting sympathomimetics have a blunted pressor response and probably should be avoided. Postop apnea is of theoretical concern. Postop obstruction symptoms are extremely rare. Small retrospective study showed no increase in postop complications in pts receiving GA.

Necrotizing Enterocolitis

Robert M. Insoft

Risk

- Most common life-threatening intestinal surgical emergency in the newborn
- Occurs predominantly in premature infants, with 75% in infants <1500 g
- Increasing incidence in term and near-term neonates as well

Perioperative Risks

- CV instability, acidosis, shock, bowel ischemia, bacteremia, patent ductus arteriosus, polycythemia

Worry About

- Persistent metabolic acidosis and intestinal perforation are ominous signs

Overview

- Presents commonly with generalized signs of sepsis, incl glucose instability, hypothermia, apnea, feeding intolerance, and metabolic acidosis
- Terminal ileum most commonly involved, followed by the distal small bowel and ascending colon. Bowel ischemia may lead to gangrene of bowel with perforation as well as peritonitis, CV and resp collapse, shock, and death.
- Multisystem failure is commonly assoc involving the resp, CV, renal, and hepatic systems. Abn elevated inflammatory mediators, such as TNF, IL-6, and PAF, are assoc.
- In severe cases, abd wall may be erythematous, signifying intestinal perforation and peritonitis
- Pneumatosis intestinalis is evident as a linear collection of air and hydrogen gas in the wall of dilated loop of bowel; may extend into portal venous circulation

ICD-9-CM Code: 777.5

Etiology

- Assoc with bowel ischemia, enteral feeds, infection, and prematurity. Clearest link is with prematurity, leading to the theory that an underlying developmental immaturity of bowel is potentially the initiating problem leading to this life-threatening condition.

ASSESSMENT POINTS

System	Effect	Assessment by Hx	PE	Test
CARDIO	Shock PDA	Pulm edema, RDS, shock	Murmur BP/HR	ABGs, BP UO
RESP	RDS	Apnea or tachypnea		ABGs CXR
ID	Sepsis	Bacteremia Peritonitis	Abd wall cellulitis, peritonitis	Blood and peritoneal fluid cultures
GI	Peritonitis, bloody stools, malabsorption	Large feeding residuals, bilious emesis	Residuals, guaiac stools	Lytes, bowel sounds, KUB Temp instability
RENAL	Prerenal failure		UO, BP	BUN, Cr
HEME	DIC Polycythemia	Bleeding		Hct, plt count, fibrinogen PT/PTT

Key Reference: Henry MW, Moss RL. Necrotizing enterocolitis. *Annu Rev Med.* 2009;60:111–124.

Perioperative Implications

Preoperative Preparation

- Most neonates may be treated medically with fluid resuscitation, antibiotics, ventilatory support, and hyperalimentation.
- Surgery indicated for pneumoperitoneum from intestinal wall perforation, intestinal gangrene (detected by abd paracentesis), and presence of portal vein gas. Other indications incl clinical deterioration, abd wall erythema, and an unresolved ileus.
- D/C enteral feeds and insert NG tube connected to suction for intestinal decompression.
- Therapeutic goals incl normalization of vital signs, ensuring adequate oxygenation and ventilation (e.g., tracheal intubation, mechanical ventilation, adequate perfusion)
- Vigorous fluid resuscitation to keep up with third space losses from peritonitis and sepsis
- Correct metabolic acidosis—achieved through fluid resuscitation
- Inotropic agents such as dopamine and dobutamine may be required to optimize cardiac output
- Correct coagulopathy with FFP, plts, and packed RBCs
- Administer broad-spectrum antibiotics, with anaerobic coverage highly considered as well

Monitoring

- Routine plus glucose and electrolytes

Induction/Maintenance

- Potent anesthetic agents are poorly tolerated.
- Carefully titrated narcotic and muscle relaxant technique is satisfactory.
- N_2O is usually avoided because of its potential for causing bowel distention.
- Fluid resuscitation (lactated Ringer's, 5% albumin, and sometimes packed RBCs) is actively carried out during surgical procedure.

Postoperative Period

- Closely monitor in NICU for ongoing fluid requirements as third space loss continues.
- Prolonged TPN is often required.
- Stricture formation leading to partial or total bowel obstruction is a common complication in both medically and surgically treated neonates.
- Short-bowel syndrome can occur, leading to long-term complications.

Anticipated Problems/Concerns

- Hypovolemia and bowel ischemia
- Acidosis, shock, and death

Necrotizing Fasciitis

Hernando Gomez
A. Murat Kaynar

Risk

- Incidence in USA: Approx 9 to 11.5 cases of invasive streptococcal infections/y, from which 1–1.8 die each year.
- Streptococcal toxic shock syndrome (STSS) and necrotizing fasciitis (NF) each comprise an average of 6–7% of these invasive cases, with an assoc mortality of 35–50% for the former and 29% for the latter.
- Predisposing risk factors: Diabetes, peripheral vascular disease, alcoholism, IV drug abuse, immunosuppression, obesity, or malnourishment

Perioperative Risks

- Shock, hypoperfusion, and organ dysfunction
- Multiple organ dysfunction syndrome (MODS) and death

Worry About

- Making an early Dx and beginning treatment accordingly. This is the single most important factor to decrease morbidity and mortality and always includes surgery.
- STSS and septic shock.

- Multiple organ dysfunction incl pulm (ARDS), renal, hepatic failure, and hematologic (disseminated intravascular coagulation).
- Postop ICU often required

Overview

- Necrotizing fasciitis constitutes one of the two severe manifestations of Group A streptococci, along with STSS, and often is assoc with it during its initial presentation.
- NF is a common cause of CV collapse, shock, and hypoperfusion which could be aggravated by the anesthetics. High suspicion is important to ensure early detection and treatment of hypovolemia and hypoperfusion. A suitable anesthetic procedure should be planned. Aggressive and continuous assessment of the CV status is required to have a stable hemodynamic condition during the septic process.
- Despite the low incidence of the disease, prompt recognition is important given its devastating consequences, not only as a major cause of mortality but also morbidity, incl:
  - Organ failure with long-term requirement of support therapy (i.e., dialysis, home O$_2$).

- Physical disfiguration and amputations causing physical and psychological disability.
- Acute and chronic pain syndromes, difficult to control.

ICD-9-CM Code: 728.86

Etiology

- Polymicrobial (incl *S. aureus*, *E. coli*, enterobacteria, *Clostridium spp.*, *Peptostreptococcus*, *Fusobacterium*, *Bacteroides spp.*) in 70% of cases and Group A streptococci (GAS) in 30% of cases
- Majority (80%) are due to skin and soft tissue infections, whereas 20% are due to contaminations from distant sources (bacteremia)

Usual Treatment

- Early Dx and repeated surgical excision of necrotic tissues are often required.
- Adequate antibiotic coverage is based on cultures and sensitivities.
- Support of organ systems, metabolism, and nutrition are necessary.
- Hyperbaric O$_2$ therapy is still under study.

ASSESSMENT POINTS

System	Effect	Assessment by Hx	PE	Test
CARDIO	Vasodilation, hypovolemia early after local symptoms (i.e., 24–48 hr)	Dizziness, alteration in mental status	Signs of dehydration, orthostatism, tachycardia, hypotension	Hemodynamic monitoring
HEME	DIC, hemorrhage, leukocytosis	Petechiae, skin discoloration	Bleeding, poor coagulation, fever, chills, myalgias	Hemoglobin and Hct, clotting evaluation with platelets, PT/PTT, fibrinogen, fibrin split products, CBC
RENAL	Prerenal and acute renal failure	UO	Signs of hypovolemia	Urinalysis with specific gravity, Na excretion, serum creatinine and BUN
PULM	ALI/ARDS	None	Hypoxia, increased work of breathing	Arterial blood gas with low P/F ratios <300
SKIN AND SOFT TISSUES	Inflammation, necrosis, blistering	Hx of skin/soft tissue injury (i.e., insect bite, contusion, ingrown nail)	Pain, erythema, edema, cellulitis with rapid progression to bluish discoloration, blisters, subcutaneous crepitus	Congelation biopsy, with fascia involvement.

Key Reference: Edlich RF, Cross CL, Dahlstrom JJ, Long 3rd WB. Modern Concepts of the diagnosis and treatment of necrotizing fasciitis. *J Emerg Med.* 2008;Dec 10.

Perioperative Implications

Preinduction/Induction/Maintenance

- Establish large bore venous access promptly and optimize CV status and perfusion. Anticipate additional fluid loss from exposed debrided areas and large fluid shifts.
- Type and cross.
- Consider ketamine 1–2 mg/kg vs. etomidate 0.2 mg/kg as induction agent. Watch for CV depression during induction. Anticipate the potential for adrenal insufficiency with etomidate.
- Provide adequate pain control.
- Consider procedure contaminated and use all recommended infection control guidelines.

Monitoring

- Establish invasive CV monitoring (CVC/PAC, A-line and UO), pulse-pressure wave form analysis (PPWF), ECHO, and temp monitor.
- H&H, clotting studies and CBC as above.
- Pulm pressures, tidal volumes, ABGs.
- Perfusion to end organs: ScvO$_2$/SvO$_2$, lactate, base excess.
- General anesthesia

Preinduction/Induction:

- Hydrate aggressively with crystalloids/colloids.
- Establish invasive CV monitoring (CVC/PAC/A-line). Pre-oxygenate adequately.
- Aspiration prophylaxis
- Do not delay antibiotics if required at the time of surgery.

Maintenance

- Monitor volume status (CVP/SVV/PPWF/UO) and perfusion adequacy as above to optimize accordingly, incl volume responsiveness and consider requirement of vasopressors (such as norepinephrine).
- Monitor blood loss, coagulopathy, and electrolyte imbalance and replace accordingly.
- Avoid hypothermia, monitor for fever.
- Watch for the presentation of bacteremia during/after debridement (hypotension, tachycardia, fever).
- Extubation: Consider delaying extubation according to CV/pulm status.
- Regional anesthesia
- Do not use in the acute setting. Only use in the absence of shock, occult shock, hemorrhage, and

significant coagulopathy. Usually adequate in later stages of the disease, while still requiring surgical management.
- Spinal versus epidural: Use dependent on affected region and length of the procedure.
- Anticipate important loss of sympathetic tone in the setting of potential hypovolemia.
- Do not use if anesthetic application implies puncture through potentially contaminated site.

Postoperative Period

- Potential requirement for continued intubation to maintain adequate oxygenation and to be admitted to ICU.
- Must be directed at obtaining adequate end-organ perfusion. Same strategies of monitoring.
- Optimize support according to requirement (i.e., CVVH, HD, mechanical ventilation, etc.).

Anticipated Problems/Concerns

- Pts often in septic shock, hypovolemic and hypoperfused to begin with. Optimize CV and perfusion status in pre-induction and be cautious during induction. Always consider assoc co-morbidities.

- Surgical debridement and combined with antibiotic therapy is the only strategy to decrease poor outcome. Do not delay surgical intervention. Surgical procedures may incl amputation of limbs, which if delayed may cause uncontrolled systemic involvement and response.

- Complications such as organ failure (renal failure 80%, ARDS 50%), bacteremia (60%) are the rule, not the exception. Be prepared to support failing organs and troubleshoot acute destabilizations.

- Pts may require additional surgical interventions such as diverting colostomies or urinary diversions to avoid further contamination.
- Specific complications may arise depending on the location of NF.

Neurofibromatosis (NF)

Jane C. Ahn
Zeev N. Kain

Risk

- NF-1 birth incidence: 1/3000
- NF-2 birth incidence: 1/33,000–1/40,000

Perioperative Risks

- Risk depends on tumor and location

Worry About

- Difficult intubation
- Intraop Htn and tachycardia

Overview

- NF-1, also known as von Recklinghausen disease, is a genetic disorder with variable clinical presentation in which multiple organs, such as skin and peripheral nervous system, are site of tumors and hamartomas.

- Hallmarks incl café-au-lait spots (more than 6 that are >1.5 cm in diameter), Lisch nodules (benign iris hamartomas), axillary and groin freckling, and multiple neurofibromas
- Laryngeal and tracheal compression may occur 2° to assoc tumors
- Surgery may be indicated for pts with NF-1, esp. for removal of tumors (e.g., neurofibromas, pheochromocytoma), skeletal dysplasia (e.g., tibial pseudoarthrosis), scoliosis, and renovascular Htn
- NF-2, also known as central neurofibromatosis, is a genetic disorder characterized by bilateral vestibular schwannomas, hearing loss, and CNS tumors.

ICD-9-CM Codes: 237.71 (NF-1); 237.72 (NF-2)

Etiology

- NF-1 and NF-2 are both autosomal dominant, although about 50% of cases represent new mutations.
- The gene for NF-1 resides on the long arm of chromosome 17.
- The gene for NF-2 resides on chromosone 22.

Usual Treatment

- Radiation and surgical treatment for various tumors involved

ASSESSMENT POINTS

System	Effect	Assessment by Hx	PE	Test
HEENT*	Pharyngeal compression Laryngeal compression Vocal cord and arytenoid involvement Airway obstruction	Dyspnea, dysphonia, stridor, and voice changes	Evaluation of airway	X-ray CT of neck
CARDIO	Renovascular Htn Pheochromocytoma Autonomic dysfunction	Headache, perspiration		BP/HR Urinary catecholamines
RESP*	Restrictive lung disease Cor pulmonale Interstitial lung disease Hypoxemia	Exercise tolerance	Cyanosis Clubbing	CXR ECG ABGs PFTs (rare)
GI	Carcinoid tumor			
GU*	Obstruction and uremia			
CNS	Mental retardation Seizures Intracranial tumors and increased ICP Paraspinal tumors			MRI of brain and spine for neuraxial technique
MS*	Kyphoscoliosis Macrocephaly Craniofacial dysplasia Cervical dislocation Pectus excavatum			X-ray of neck

* In severe cases

Key Reference: Hirsch NP, Murphy A, Radcliffe JJ. Neurofibromatosis: Clinical presentations and anaesthetic implications. *Br J Anaesth.* 2001;86:555–564.

Perioperative Implications

Preoperative Preparation
- Evaluation of airway for possible laryngeal and pharyngeal tumors

Monitoring
- Routine
- Consider arterial line depending on resp status and presence of pheochromocytoma.

Airway
- Consider awake fiberoptic intubation or awake tracheotomy if laryngeal and pharyngeal involvement.

Preinduction/Induction
- No particular anesthetic drug or technique recommended
- Consider potential for increased ICP.

- Consider potential of pheochromocytoma (see Pheochromocytoma in Diseases section)
- Although there are case reports of abn response to NMBs, recent evidence suggests no or minimal effect.

Maintenance
- CV instability if pheochromocytoma present

Extubation
- Routine considerations

Postoperative Period
- Pain management may be critical

Regional Anesthesia
- Asymptomatic paraspinal neurofibromas can make identification and entry into epidural and subarachnoid spaces very difficult. A careful exam of the back is indicated before any regional technique is considered.

- Paraspinal and intracranial tumors are exacerbated during pregnancy.
- Consider potential for epidural hematoma, tumor trauma, brainstem herniation.
- Recommend MRI of brain and spine for tumor assessment prior to neuraxial technique.

Anticipated Problems/Concerns

- Difficult airway
- Presence of pheochromocytoma
- Potential for increased ICP with expanding intracranial tumor
- Difficult epidural or spinal placement. Potential for complications due to tumor involvement.

Occlusive Cerebrovascular Disease

Ian A. Herrick

Risk

- Prevalance: Approx 1 in 59, or 1.69%
- Annual incidence of stroke: 600,000 annually incl 500,000 new cases and 100,000 recurrences
- Incidence in the USA: Approx 1 in 453, or 0.22%
- Races with highest prevalence: Japanese and Eastern European (incidence 0.3%/y)

Perioperative Risks

- Stroke
  - Major general surgery at age >50 y = 0.4%; at age >80 y = 2.5%
  - Major peripheral vascular reconstruction = 1%
  - CABG = 1–5%, carotid endarterectomy (CEA) = 3% or less

Worry About

- Cerebral ischemia
- Myocardial ischemia (CAD, leading cause of morbidity following CEA)
- Control of co-existing CAD, DM, Htn

Overview

- Two main clinical presentations
  - Pts with known occlusive CVD undergoing CEA or carotid angioplasty. Risk factors incl CAD/CHF; stroke in evolution, frequent TIAs; severe Htn; carotid siphon stenosis; COPD; poor cerebral collateral flow; age >70 y; intraluminal thrombus. Criteria for pt selection and acceptable periop morbidity and mortality rates are now well established for CEA.
  - Pts with known or possible CVD presenting for other surgery. Risk factors are poorly defined. Most periop strokes occur postop and do not correlate with presence of CVD. Highest risk with CABG.
- Asymptomatic carotid bruits are inconsistent predictors of CVD but predict poor CVD survival

ICD-9-CM Code: 434.9

Etiology

- Vasculopathy 2° to advanced atherosclerosis
- Risk factors incl age, Htn, DM, smoking
- High incidence of concomitant CAD and PVD

Usual Treatment

- Antiplatelet drugs (esp. ASA, clopidogrel)
- CEA
- Carotid angioplasty with or without stent placement

ASSESSMENT POINTS

System	Effect	Assessment by Hx	PE	Test
HEENT	Possible positional cerebral ischemia	Sx of cerebral ischemia with head movements	Neck ROM	
CARDIO	Htn Vasculopathy LV dysfunction, CHF	Exercise tolerance Angina, MI, CHF Claudication	Arterial BP S_3 Peripheral pulses	ECG, CXR ECHO Stress test
RESP	COPD due to smoking Irritable airway	Dyspnea Chronic cough Smoker	Wheezing Accessory muscles	CXR ?ABGs ?PFTs
ENDO	Possible diabetes			Glucose
RENAL	Possible nephropathy	Diabetes, Htn		Cr, urea
CNS	Cerebral ischemia	TIA, stroke	Neurologic deficits	Cerebral angio prior to CEA

Key Reference: O'Kelly CJ, Butcher KS, Marchak BE, Findlay JM. Carotid revascularization: an update. *Can J Neurol Sci.* 2010;37(3):320–335. Review.

Perioperative Implications

Preoperative Preparation
- Neurologic assessment
- Optimize control of co-existing Htn, CAD, diabetes, COPD
- Evaluate normal BP range

Monitoring
- Arterial catheter and ST-segment monitoring
- For CEA, consider neurologic monitor: EEG or regional anesthetic with awake pt (if practical)
- Carotid angioplasty usually performed with the pt awake

Induction/Maintenance
- Have surgeon block carotid sinus nerve if bradycardic

- Maintain hemodynamic stability based on preop BP range
- Maintain normocapnia based on preop pH and $Paco_2$
- Light IV sedation often administered during angioplasty
- Embolic stroke or severe, vagal-mediated, bradycardia can accompany carotid dilation during angioplasty

Extubation
- Be prepared to manage hemodynamic instability following CEA
- Avoid straining on ETT with fresh arteriotomy following CEA

Postoperative Period
- Hemodynamic instability due to baroreceptor dysfunction following CEA

- Adequate analgesia, supplemental O_2
- Awake pt allows early and frequent neurologic evaluation

Anticipated Problems/Concerns

- Most pts with CVD also at high risk for CAD. Consistent approach to management of both problems incl hemodynamic stability, adequate oxygenation, normocapnia, adequate analgesia, normoglycemia.
- Caution regarding use of succinylcholine in pts with previous paretic CVA
- Angioplasty is not assoc with substantial discomfort. Only minimal sedation is typically needed for comfort.

Opitz-Frias Syndrome (The G Syndrome)

Roberta Hines

Risk

- Overall incidence not reported
- Very rare congenital disorder

Preoperative Risks

- Very high risk of recurrent pulm aspiration; hypoplasia of both pulm and vascular components of one lung (pulm hypoplasia)
- High mortality rate in infancy

Worry About

- NM dysfunction of laryngoesophageal apparatus
- Laryngotracheoesophageal cleft or fistula
- Difficult tracheal intubation due to assoc craniofacial deformity(s)
- Assoc congenital anomalies (Htn, hypospadius, wide eyes, cleft lip, cleft palate, cryptorchidism, imperforate anus, cardiac deficits)

Overview

- Also known as the hypospadias-dysphagia syndrome
- Emergency presentations are for cardiopulmonary resuscitation, upper resp obstruction, severe resp stridor, regurgitation, aspiration
- Presence of one hypoplastic lung
- Laryngeal hypoplasia
- Laryngotracheoesophageal cleft or fistula
- Anticipate very difficult tracheal intubation
- Thorough preop cardiac evaluation need to access for cardiac abn (? ECHO)
- Any male infant presenting for TEF with genital defect should be suspected.
- Classically—weak, hoarse cry

ICD-9-CM Code: 759.9 (Congenital Anomaly, unspecified)

Etiology

- X-linked recessive inheritance
- Autosomal dominant inheritance or new mutation
- Partial male sex limitation
- Autosomal recessive inheritance, high parenteral consanguinity
- Females can be equally or nearly as severely affected as males

Usual Treatment

- Prophylactic gastrostomy
- Feeding jejunostomy
- Cervical esophagostomy if unable to swallow
- Prophylactic antibodies (pulm infection)

ASSESSMENT POINTS

System	Effect	Assessment by Hx	PE	Tests
HEENT	Cleft lip–palate (35%) Ankyloglossia Micrognathia	Feeding difficulties, speech anomalies	Short lingual frenulum	
CNS	Dolichocephaly (20%) Large metopic sagittal suture and anterior fontanel	Mental dysfunction, prominent forehead	"Cone-head" Palpation	CT (if indicated)
FACIES	Hypertelorism/telecanthus (90%) Mongoloid palpebral fissures Strabismus	Mother-related disease	Large nasal bridge downslanting	Face X-ray
CARDIO	Congenital heart defects (40%) (ASD, VSD, PDA, coarctation of aorta)	Failure to thrive	Auscultation	ECG TEE, ABGs
RESP	Agenesis, hypoplasia of one lung Tracheoesophageal cleft, fissure Hypoplasia of vocal cord Tracheomalacia Short trachea, high carina	Polyhydramnios on delivery Coughing, choking, cyanosis Hoarse, weak cry Stridorous resp	Auscultation Tracheal stenosis	CXR Bronchogram Esophagogram
GI	Achalasia of the cardia (70%) NM dysfunction of esophagus	Dysphagia		Esophagogram (if indicated) Cinefluoroscopy of swallowing (if indicated)
GU	Hypospadias with descended testis Ureteral stenosis or duplication		Perineal or penoscrotal	Nephrogram

Key Reference: National Library of Medicines: OS. www.nih.gov/mesh/jablonski/syndromes/syndroms 498.html.

Perioperative Implications

Preoperative Preparation

- Evacuation of the stomach with NG tube (if pt has gastrectomy open to air)
- Feeding: Clear water or apple juice (standard NPO guidelines)
- Consider H_2 blocker
- No atropine IM or metoclopramide preop
- Give sodium citrate through NG tube
- Complete cardiac evaluation
- Assessment of renal function
- Not appropriate for outpatient or same day process
- IV access 24 hr before surgery to reduce stomach content

Monitoring

- All standard monitors
- Invasive arterial pressure if indicated due to procedure or unstable hemodynamics

Airway

- Tubes smaller than normal 2° (as assessed by age) to laryngeal hypoplasia

Preinduction

- Warm OR
- Decompress stomach with suction
- Atropine and succinylcholine backup

Induction

- Maintain spontaneous respiration
- Danger of regurgitation and aspiration requires careful inhalation induction
- Cricoid pressure should be applied
- Atropine 20 μg/kg of induction to prevent bradycardia during intubation

Maintenance

- Hand ventilation (low PPV)
- Avoid hypothermia

Extubation

- Based on pts lung condition and preop assessment and/or lung function

Adjuvants

- All medications can be used (no contraindication to IV or inhaled anesthesia)

Anticipated Problems

- Regurgitation and pulm aspiration. Difficult tracheal intubation. Increased incidence of pneumothorax. High mortality rate in infancy.
- Unanticipated cardiac issues
- Difficult to access recovery from anesthesia due to assoc mental conditions

Osteoarthritis

Denise Wedel

Risk

- Osteoarthritis (OA) most common cause of impairment in the elderly
  - Incidence in USA: 63–85% >65 y have radiographic signs
  - 35–50% have pain, stiffness, or limitation of movement
  - 9–12% are significantly disabled
  - 46 million doctor visits and 68 million work d lost per year
- Risk factors differ across joints: Knee, obesity, injury; hand, repetitive use; hip, congenital or developmental abn, male preponderance

Perioperative Risks

- Often assoc with obesity
- Common analgesics incl NSAIDs and intra-articular steroid injections
- Rarely affects neck or jaw
- Reported assoc with diabetes, hypothyroidism, hyperparathyroidism, gout

Worry About

- Anesthetic problems with assoc obesity
- Positioning may be difficult owing to joint pain and stiffness
- Possible assoc metabolic conditions
- Effect of medications on plt function and frequent steroid injections

Overview

- OA is age-related but not caused by aging
- Early radiographic findings incl joint space narrowing, osteophytes, subchondral stenosis
- With progression, osteophytes, subchondral cysts, intra-articular osseous bodies seen
- Subchondral bone collapse is a late finding
- Knees most common joint affected (41%), followed by hands (30%) and hips (19%)
- Risk factors for symptoms are obesity (knees) and severe radiographic findings

ICD-9-CM Code: 715.0 (Generalized)

Etiology

- Cartilage shows increase in water with softened cartilage and depletion of keratin sulfate
- Age-related decreases in blood supply, followed by changes in distribution of forces causing damage to cartilage nutrition
- Repetitive use or previous injury may cause subchondral microfractures over time with strain on overlying cartilage
- Autosomal dominant in some with co-segregation of OA with a mutation in type II procollagen gene

Usual Treatment

- Conservative therapy: Wt loss, PT to maintain function and mobility, analgesics (aspirin, acetaminophen, NSAIDs), steroid injections
- Surgical replacement
- Acupuncture

ASSESSMENT POINTS

System	Effect	Assessment by Hx	PE	Test
HEENT	Rare C-spine involvement	Pain	Neck ROM	Usually not needed C-spine x-rays
CARDIO	Age-related changes	Exercise tolerance may be limited by joint changes	HR and tolerance to 2-flight stair climb	ECG CXR
RESP	Nonspecific	Exercise tolerance		CXR
GI	Sensitivity to NSAIDs	Gastric upset		
ENDO	Associated diabetes			Fasting blood sugar
CNS	Age-related changes	TIAs or stroke		
MS	Multiple joint involvement	Joint pain	Joint ROM	
RENAL	Age-related changes			Cr

Key Reference: Wang SM, Kain ZN, White PF. Acupuncture analgesia: II. Clinical considerations. *Anesth Analg.* 2008;106(2):611–621.

Perioperative Implications

Preoperative Preparation

- Assess joint involvement and ROM
- Question pt regarding nonprescription analgesics
- Consider regional anesthetic techniques
- Evaluate for steroid need

Monitoring

- Routine

Airway

- Assess neck ROM

Induction

- Age-related considerations: Elderly pts may have slow circulation times, CV disease, fluctuations in BP

Maintenance

- Position with consideration of other joint involvement

Extubation

- No special considerations

Adjuvants

- Elderly pts may be more sensitive to narcotics.

Postoperative Period

- Consider continuous regional technique with local anesthetic and/or narcotic for pain management

Anticipated Problems/Concerns

- Usually neck and airway normal
- Concomitant risk factors, esp. obesity
- Often several joints involved with pain and decreased ROM
- Regional anesthesia well suited

Osteoporosis

Risk

- Most common metabolic bone disease in USA
- All elderly pts of European descent considered at risk
- Non-Hispanic white women and Asian women at highest risk
- 10 million Americans have osteoporosis, 34 million have low bone mass and therefore at risk for osteoporosis
- Female > male: 3:1
- Postmenopausal female, small frame, low wt
- Risk factors for osteoporosis, such as advanced age and reduced bone density, have been established by virtue of their direct and strong relationship to the incidence of fractures; however, many other factors have been considered risk factors based on their relationship to bone density value as a surrogate indicator of osteoporosis. Risk factors incl the following:
  - Advanced age, female sex, white or Asian ethnicity, family Hx of osteoporosis, body wt less than 127 pounds, amenorrhea, late menarche, early menopause, nulliparity, physical inactivity, alcohol and tobacco use, androgen or estrogen deficiency, calcium deficiency
- 2° osteoporosis attributable to diseases (hyperparathyroidism, rheumatoid arthritis, sarcoidosis, thalassemia, idiopathic scoliosis, multiple myeloma, and thyrotoxicosis) and drugs (lithium, anticonvulsants, excessive alcohol use, excessive thyroxine, prolonged unfractionated heparin use [> 6 mo of >15,000 IU/day], glucocorticoids, and cytotoxic drugs).

Perioperative Risks

- Concomitant medical conditions in elderly
- Pneumonia
- Co-existing metabolic or endocrine disorders
- Fractures

Worry About

- Positioning because of increased risk of bone fractures
- Vertebral fractures: Vertebral compression fractures assoc with increased morbidity/mortality.
- Hip fractures: Significantly increased risk of morbidity/mortality in first year after fracture; men > female
- Pulm function/restrictive disease, esp. if kyphosis present

Overview

- Osteoporosis is a systemic skeletal disease characterized by low bone mass and microarchitectural deterioration of bone tissue, with a consequent increase in bone fragility.
- Imbalance between bone resorption and formation causes loss of bone substance, resulting in bone fractures.
- Most common fracture sites: Vertebral body, neck of femur, distal radius, proximal humerus, pelvis
- 1.5 million fractures due to osteoporosis occur each year: Spine (700,000), hip (300,000), wrist (200,000)
- Severe kyphosis common
- Type I (postmenopausal) osteoporosis: Women 15–20 y after menopause; vertebral and Colles' fractures most common

- Type II (age-related) osteoporosis: Men and women ≥70 y. Hip and vertebral fractures most common. Also pelvis, humerus, femur.
- Biphasic pattern of bone loss
  - Slow phase occurs in both sexes beginning at age 40 y; 0.6–1%/y, cortical and trabecular bone
  - Accelerated phase in women after menopause: 2–3%/y cortical bone; 4–6%/y trabecular bone

ICD-9-CM Code: 733.00

Etiology

- Insufficient accumulation of bone mass during skeletal growth
- Age-related factors: Decreased bone formation at cellular level begins in 4th decade and becomes more severe with age. Age-related ↑ in parathyroid function with age-related ↓ in calcium absorption.
- Menopause: Accelerated phase of bone loss is the result of estrogen deficiency
- Sporadic factors: Twofold increased risk with cigarettes and high alcohol consumption

Treatment

- Vitamin D and calcium
- Selective estrogen receptor modulators (SERMs): Raloxifene
- Bisphosphonates: Alendronate, risedronate
- Human recombinant PTH: Teriparatide
- Calcitonin
- D/C of glucocorticoid (if osteoporosis due to chronic use)
- Surgical stabilization of fractures: Kyphoplasty/vertebroplasty for spine fractures, ORIF (hip, wrist)

ASSESSMENT POINTS

System	Effect	Assessment by Hx	PE	Test
HEENT	Osteoporosis of skull Vertebral fractures	Pain		Skull x-ray Neck x-ray
RESP	Kyphosis	Dyspnea	Dowager's hump	Flow-volume loop ABGs
ENDO	Parathyroid function ↓ in Type I ↑ in Type II Calcium absorption ↓ Metabolic disorders of vitamin D			Ca^{2+}
MS	Back pain Loss of ht Spinal deformity Fractures	Acute back pain Remittance and recurrence until chronic	Dowager's hump ↓ Height Multiple fractures	X-ray Vertebral bone density

Key Reference: Canalis E. New Treatment Modalities in Osteoporosis. *Endocr Pract.* 2010;Mar 29:1–23.

Perioperative Implications

Preoperative Preparation
- Move and position carefully owing to risk of bone fractures
- Pulm function tests indicated in kyphoscoliosis present
- Preop cervical x-rays and thorough evaluation of cervical spine. Document range of motion. Document any preop neurologic deficits.

- Detailed Hx to determine co-existing metabolic/endocrine disorders

Monitoring
- Routine
- Consider arterial line and frequent ABGs if pulm disease or pneumonia present

Airway
- Cervical fractures may require neck stabilization and fiberoptic intubation.
- Acromegaly may occur with osteoporosis.

Musculoskeletal
- Vertebral collapse may make spinal/epidural anesthesia more difficult

Anticipated Problems/Concerns

- Susceptible to fracture with routine positioning and moving
- Restrictive lung disease if scoliosis present may impair oxygenation

Otitis Media

Vincent J. Kopp
Karene Ricketts

Risk

- Age: The highest incidence occurs between 6 and 24 mo of age. Incidence subsequently declines except for an increase at the time of school entry (between 5 and 6 y of age)
- Day care attendance
- Tobacco smoke and air pollution
- Other factors: Poor social and economic conditions, season (fall and winter), altered host defenses, and diseases with assoc craniofacial abn such as cleft palate and Down syndrome.

Perioperative Risks

- Active or concurrent disease, such as upper and lower resp infections, may increase risk of airway reactivity, laryngospasm, bronchospasm, periop O_2 requirement, and postop mechanical ventilation.
- Inherent risks of assoc craniofacial abn may predispose to airway obstruction and/or difficult airway.
- N/V related to the infection, antibiotic therapy, and vestibular imbalance

Worry About

- Chronic or recurrent otitis media can cause hearing loss (usually conductive) that may lead to problems in development of speech, language, and cognitive abilities in the child. This may impair communication in the periop period.
- Rare but important complications: Mastoiditis, petrositis, labyrinthitis, meningitis, epidural abscess, brain abscess, lateral sinus thrombosis, cavernous sinus thrombosis, subdural empyema, and carotid artery thrombosis
- Pts with fever ≥38 °C and/or concurrent disease, incl upper and lower resp infections with their potential risks
- Pts with assoc vestibular, balance, and motor dysfunctions

- Pts with adenotonsillar hypertrophy or craniofacial abn that may predispose to airway obstruction and/or difficult airway

Overview

- Acute otitis media (AOM) is a common infectious disease. It is defined by the presence of fluid in the middle air, accompanied by acute signs of illness, and signs or symptoms of middle ear inflammation.
- Otitis media with effusion (OME) is defined by the presence of middle ear fluid without acute signs of illness or inflammation of the middle ear mucosa. OME may be caused by allergies, but usually occurs after AOM. OME typically leads to a conductive hearing loss.
- Otitis media is most prevalent in infancy, but it can occur at all ages.

ICD-9-CM Code: 382.9

Etiology

- Pathogenesis: Dysfunction or obstruction of the eustachian tube (usually from nasal congestion assoc with an upper resp infection or allergic rhinitis) leads to negative pressure and accumulation of secretions in the middle ear. The middle ear secretions serve as a growth medium for viruses and bacteria that colonize the upper resp tract resulting in suppuration and clinical signs of otitis media.
- The most common bacterial causes of otitis media are *Streptococcus* pneumonia, *Haemophilus* influenza, and Moraxella catarrhalis.
- The most frequent viral pathogens assoc with otitis media are the resp syncytial virus, rhinoviruses, influenza viruses, and adenoviruses.

Usual Treatment

- Analgesics such as ibuprofen, acetaminophen, and auralgan (topical anesthetic) for symptomatic treatment of ear pain (otalgia)

- Antimicrobial therapy
  - First line therapy is amoxicillin (80 to 90 mg/kg orally per day divided into 2 doses). Other commonly used antibiotics incl cephalosporins (cefuroxime, ceftriaxone), macrolides (erythromycin, azithromycin), and trimethoprim sulfa sulfamethoxazole
  - Should be administered to any child younger than 6 mo
  - Should be administered to children 6 mo to 2 y in whom the Dx of acute otitis media is certain **or** if the Dx is uncertain but the illness is severe (moderate to severe otalgia or fever ≥39 °C). If the Dx is uncertain and illness is not severe, the child may be observed without treatment with antibiotics.
  - Should be administered to pts older than 2 y if the Dx is certain and illness is severe. When the Dx is certain but illness is not severe, observation alone is an option.
- Acute otitis media usually resolves in 24–72 hr with appropriate antimicrobial therapy, however fluid may persist for weeks to months despite treatment. Placement of tympanostomy tubes is performed for pts with persistent middle ear effusion or severe and recurrent episodes of otitis media. Adenoidectomy may be indicated in selected pts.
- Prevention is an important management strategy for otitis media: Minimize risk factors if possible (smaller day care groups and decrease smoke exposure), administer vaccines (influenza and pneumococcal), and encourage breastfeeding for at least 3 mo (diminishes colonization of the nasopharynx by bacterial pathogens and offers protective factors).

ASSESSMENT POINTS

System	Effect	Assessment by Hx	PE	Test
GENERAL	Patient age varies	Childhood vs. adult dz.	Find co-morbidities	As indicated
HEENT	Nasal secretions Middle ear fluid/drainage	Allergy vs. infection Acute vs. chronic OM, ear pain, ear tugging	Clear vs. green mucous Fever vs. afebrile, inflamed tympanic membrane (red, opacified, bulging, immotile) vs. fluid level	Eosinophil smear Tympanogram
	Hypertrophic T&A	OSA, mouth breathing, snoring	Inspection	
RESP	Cough Laryngo-tracheomalacia Pneumonia	Dry vs. wet OSA/feeding difficulty Fever, cough, dyspnea	Upper vs. lower tract Sx Retractions, stridor Fever, tachypnea, crackles	Pulse ox Bronchoscopy Pulse ox, CXR, CBC
GI	NPO status, reflux Hx	Clear vs. fatty liquid	Non-fussy child	None
CNS	Developmental status Hearing (usually conductive loss) Complications of untreated OM (such as meningitis)	Developmental Hx Delayed speech and cognition Fever, headache, mental status changes, photophobia	Congenital anomalies Fever, Brudzinski's and Kernig's signs, meningismus	Genetic testing Audiometry MRI, lumbar puncture, cultures
INTEG	Eczema	Allergy/steroid history	Allergic/non-allergic rash	Skin biopsy

Key Reference: Hoffmann KK, Thompson GK, Burke BL, Derkay CS. Anesthetic complications of tympanostomy tube placement in children. *Arch Otolaryngol Head Neck Surg.* 2002;128(9):1040–1043.

Perioperative Implications

Preoperative Preparation

- Lower resp tract pathology or pneumonia may warrant further evaluation and case rescheduling; runny nose (rhinorrhea) is usually not an indication for case cancellation

- Children: Avoid oral premed for myringotomy and pressure equalizing tubes (PETS) alone (short surgical time); consider parental presence for induction; allow comfort object in OR; developmentally appropriate review of procedures; consider preop oral acetaminophen to give analgesic regimen time to work

- Adult: IV midazolam or fentanyl before induction; topical local anesthetic drops in ear may be indicated

Monitoring

- Standard ASA monitors, skin temp probe
- Precordial stethoscope very helpful

Airway
- Children: Inhalation induction and mask airway maintenance for straightforward cases
- Adults: IV induction with mask airway or LMA maintenance
- Oral and/or nasal airways as indicated
- Be prepared to intubate if obstruction or as case direction changes
- Maintenance
- Volatile anesthetic in oxygen with NO usually sufficient
  - 70/30 N_2O/O_2 plus 8% Sevo for induction, followed by 50/50 N_2O/O_2 plus 4% Sevo for maintenance until first tube in place
  - Turn off anesthetics at second myringotomy to avoid prolonged anesthesia for short operation.
- Consider IV propofol infusion to maintain spontaneous ventilation if laryngoscopy/bronchoscopy also planned
- Otherwise as required for additional operative procedures after PETs placed

Extubation
- Routine precautions and criteria

Adjuvants
- Determined by course and complexity of operation(s) to be performed
- PETs are frequently placed before other procedures (cleft lip/palate repair, auditory evoked potentials)

Postoperative concerns
- Postop analgesia: Multimodal approach
  - Children: Belly analgesia first (bottle, cup, soda); consider nasal fentanyl and/or oral acetaminophen if rectal not given intraop
  - Adults: IV / oral analgesics as needed; antiemetic may be needed more so than in children
- Emergence delirium: Nasal or IV clonidine or dexmedetomidine an option for children
- Slow introduction of PO fluids; limit volume if possible
- Plan to reunite child with parent and/or proxy after pt settled in PACU

Anticipated Problem/Concerns

- Separation of child and parent and/or proxy: have guardian present for induction

- Separation from child's comfort object: Label with pt's name
- Charting vital signs and maintaining anesthesia record in a short case with a lot to do: assistant or electronic medical record is helpful
- Difficulty maintaining mask airway: Use LMA, ET intubation
- Laryngospasm: Hold positive pressure, IM/IV succinylcholine and/or atropine, propofol if IV present, possible ET intubation
- Antibiotics: Start PIV if required
- Ear drops applied by surgeon: Can sting if pH is basic
- Unanticipated pathology: Cerumen impaction, cholesteatoma, other tumors, ossicular dislocation
- Excessive bleeding (ear canal trauma): Topical epinephrine application
- Small external ear canals: Change type of PE tube used
- Unable to place PE tube because of prior scarring: Abandon case
- PE tube falls into middle ear space: Surgical retrieval required

Pacemakers

Marc A. Rozner

Epidemiology

- Incidence in USA: Exceeds 3 million; 6 million worldwide have conventional pacing (but not high voltage) cardiac implantable electrical device (P-CIED)
- >600,000 pacemakers implanted per year in USA
- Some pts with cardiomyopathy have atrial, RV, and LV pacing
- Since all implanted cardioverter defibrillators (ICDs) provide pacing, this section also applies to these pts as well*

Perioperative Risks

- No proven increase in risk due to CIED itself, although these pts might be at increased risk owing to assoc disease(s)
- Risk related to assoc medical problems
- Risk related to incorrect interpretation of events (pseudomalfunction)

Worry About

- Intraop decrease in pacing rate due to inhibition of pacing output from electromagnetic interference (EMI) entering the P-CIED on the ventricular channel, esp. in the pacing dependent pt, which will result in asystole
- Intraop increase in ventricular pacing owing to EMI entering a dual chamber DDD P-CIED on the atrial channel with resultant tracking
- Intraop increases in pacing rates with misinterpretation as inadequate anesthesia owing to activation of the exercise sensor, whether due to direct mechanical stimulation (such as preparation of the chest), pressure on the device (personnel leaning),

or EMI interaction with a minute ventilation sensor.
- Failure to capture (i.e., pacing output without depolarization) due to inadequate pacing output (i.e., inadequate safety margin) or increase in pacing threshold, which can result from myocardial ischemia/infarction, drug administration, or electrolyte shifts. Note that any or all chambers can undergo failure to capture, with possible hemodynamic derangement but not apparent outright pacing failure.
- Hemodynamics can be degraded by magnet* placement, which might produce asynchronous pacing 85-100 bpm (depending upon brand, model, and programming) with short (100 msec) AV delay.
- Careful attention to sterility if central access is placed. Central line placement in the chest is relatively contraindicated for the first 6 wk of implant for any new lead.

Overview

- Indications for permanent pacing: Symptomatic failure of impulse formation (sinoatrial disease), symptomatic failure of impulse conduction (AV block), hypertrophic or dilated cardiomyopathy, long QT syndrome
- Indications for temporary pacing (usually reversible issue): post-cardiac surgery, treatment of drug toxicity resulting in dysrhythmias, certain dysrhythmias complicating MI
- Codes: The NASPE/BPEG generic pacing code has 5 positions. The first position refers to the chamber(s) paced (A=atrium, V=ventricle, D=both, O=none). The second position refers to

the chamber(s) sensed (A,V,D,O). The third identifies the response to sensed events (I=inhibit, D=dual chamber pacing and tracking). The fourth position will be "R" if the P-CIED will increase its rate in response to "exercise;" it will be "O" if rate responsiveness is programmed off and a fifth position is present. The fifth position identifies a multisite (A=biatrial, V=biventricular, or D=both) P-CIED.

ICD-9-CM Code: V53.31 (Permanent pacemaker)

Etiology

- Congenital electrical disease
- Acquired: Mostly idiopathic or a result of necessary antiarrhythmic drug therapy. Some neurally mediated syncope. Other issues incl: AV ablations, CAD, MI, Htn, post-cardiac surgery, post-evoked potential study, dilated and infiltrative cardiomyopathy, inflammatory, infectious, neoplastic, radiation

Usual Treatment

- Pt should be undergoing regular in-office (yearly) and telephone (q 3 mo) pacemaker checks. As the pacemaker generator ages, checks become recommended q monthly.
- Pt should have recent (within 1–3 mo) in-office check to verify pacemaker integrity, sensing and pacing safety margins, and evaluate for the occurrence of arrhythmia. If the P-CIED will be in the surgical field, or if the pt is pacing dependent and monopolar electrosurgery will be needed, then a plan will have to be constructed to ensure pt safety.

ASSESSMENT POINTS

System	Effect	Assessment by Hx	PE	Test
CARDIO	Dysrhythmia Pacemaker	Pacemaker indication	ECG/pulse	Preop pacemaker check; CXR unnecessary to evaluate a properly working device except for multisite pacing device
	Palpitations	Exacerbating cause(s), such as arm movement, body position, or exercise	Pacemaker pocket manipulation while monitoring pacemaker; arm movement, flexion/extension of shoulder	Pacemaker telemetry
	Exercise intolerance	Exercise tolerance, angina, Sx CHF	2-flight walk	Walk test to ensure correct settings of rate response sensor
ENDO	Atrial tachydysrhythmias	Hypo-, hyperthyroidism		TSH, free T4
CNS	Other causes of syncope	TIA, CVA	Bruits	Carotid Doppler exam

Code	Indication	Function	Perioperative Management
VVI	Ventricular bradycardia without need for preserved AV conduction	Demand ventricular pacing	Magnet* utilization might be helpful to produce asynchronous (VOO) pacing 85-100 bpm. Magnet* effect can depend on programming.
VVIR	Ventricular bradycardia without need for preserved AV conduction, chronotropic incompetence	As above, but adjusts pacing rate to allow somewhat physiologic response to exercise	Pacemaker may sense periop changes (e.g., mechanical stimulus or resp rate) and increase pacing rate, misleading the anesthesia provider to treat "increased pain."
DDD	Bradycardia when AV synchrony can be preserved	Provides more physiologic response, maintains AV concordance	Magnet* utilization might be helpful to produce asynchronous (DOO) pacing 85-100 bpm. Magnet* effect can depend on programming.
DDDR	Pts requiring AV synchrony and have chronotropic incompetence	Allows somewhat physiologic response to exercise, maintains AV concordance	Pacemaker may sense periop changes (e.g., mechanical stimulus or resp rate) and increase pacing rate, misleading the anesthesia provider to treat "increased pain."

Key Reference: Rozner MA. Pacemakers and implanted cardioverter-defibrillators. In: Miller RD, Eriksson LI, Fleisher LA, Wiener-Kronish JP, Young WL, eds. *Miller's anesthesia* 7th ed. Philadelphia: Churchill Livingstone; 2009:1387–1409 [Chapter 43].

Perioperative Implications

Preoperative Preparation

- Comprehensive pacemaker evaluation and/or interrogation. A pacing consult might be needed. Consideration should be given to increasing the pacing rate for any pt undergoing a significant procedure who is chronotropically incompetent or pacing dependent in the atrium.

- For ventricular multisite pacing (called cardiac resynchronization therapy), assurance that the LV pacing lead is functioning. If central access is planned in a CRT pt, a recent chest x-ray might be prudent to document the position of the LV lead.
- Alternate pacing modality available (e.g., transvenous, transcutaneous). While transesoph-

ageal pacing might work as backup, it is contraindicated in atrial fibrillation, AV nodal block, and any pt with a permanently implanted pacing device.
- IV chronotropes (epinephrine, ephedrine)
- Discuss monopolar electrosurgery precautions with surgeon and nursing staff.

- Regional technique offers CNS perfusion monitoring

Monitoring

- Mechanical pulse wave monitoring is required. It can be accomplished with the pulse oximeter plethysmogram, any invasive hemodynamic monitoring modality, or Doppler technique.
- Electrocardiographic (ECG) monitoring is required by ASA standards, but EMI perturbs the signal, and monitors frequently report incorrect heart rates (both too high and too low).

Induction

- Succinylcholine or etomidate might lead to inappropriate muscle activity, resulting in pacing inhibition or increased rates. Succinylcholine-induced K^+ fluxes theoretically can change pacing thresholds, but this has not been reported.

Maintenance

- Vigilant ECG and/or pulse monitoring
- Monopolar electrosurgical (ESU) cautery (i.e., the "Bovie"), which emits radiofrequency energy, has potential to cause transient or permanent changes in pacemaker function. The most common problem is inhibition of pacing. Prevention includes use of bipolar only ESU, use of pure unblended monopolar ESU, and placement of the ESU current return pad so that the presumed current path of the ESU does not cross the chest. For all head and neck or contralateral breast surgery, the pad can be placed on the shoulder contralateral to the CIED. For ipsilateral breast surgery, the pad can be placed on the ipsilateral arm and the wire prepped into the field if needed.
- Magnet*: Assuming that the magnet converts the P-CIED to asynchronous pacing, it might be useful to prevent asystole from EMI-induced pacing inhibition. However, the asynchronous pacing rate must be greater than the pt's own rate, or competition will result. Atrial competition usually just lowers the BP, but ventricular competition can lead to R-on-T pacing with triggering of ventricular tachycardia. Not all ICDs have a programmable asynchronous pacing mode, a possible concern where a pt might require pacing from their ICD.

Adjuvants

- K^+ rapid fluctuations could affect capture.

Postoperative Period

- Monitoring of mechanical pulse in the postop care unit
- Pacemaker interrogation advisable if monopolar ESU employed, any problems noted, or cardioversion/defibrillation has taken place.
- Some pts will require pacing changes to incl increased pacing rate, disabling of battery saving features, and adjustments to AV delays to optimize postop hemodynamics
- Other risks related to assoc medical problems

Anticipated Problems/Concerns

- Intraop failure to pace, most likely related to monopolar electrosurgery
- Periop pacing and sensing threshold changes
- Risks related to assoc medical problems
- Iatrogenic misadventures resulting from misunderstanding of pacing system behavior

---

*CAUTION: If the pacing device is actually an implanted cardioverter defibrillator (ICD), then magnet application rarely affects brady pacing. For many ICDs (Boston Scientific [which owns Guidant and CPI brands] and St Jude [which owns Pacesetter]), the magnet switch can be programmed "OFF." Only ICDs from Boston Scientific and its previous companies emit tones that identify correct placement of a magnet. Some older ICDs from Boston Scientific (with the "GDT" or "CPI" x-ray code) can undergo permanent disabling of tachy therapy by magnet placement. Only ICDs from ELA (Sorin) will change pacing rate (to 90 bpm if battery is ok) upon appropriate magnet placement.

Pancreatitis, Acute

Jeffrey J. Schwartz

Risk

- Incidence of 100–200/1 million in larger cities
- No racial predilection; gallstone more common in women; alcohol more common in men

Perioperative Risks

- Most mortality occurs with surgery for complications of severe pancreatitis: 10–30%
- Risk of nonpancreatic surgery probably dependent on severity of attack

Worry About

- Severe hypovolemia 2° to sequestration of fluid in retroperitoneal space
- Electrolyte abn, incl hypocalcemia, hyperglycemia, acidosis
- Systemic complications such as alcohol withdrawal, ARDS, acute renal failure, DIC, multisystem organ failure, sepsis (see these topics in Diseases section)

Overview

- Intense inflammatory response caused by release of activated pancreatic enzymes with resultant tissue destruction, fluid and electrolyte loss
- Most commonly a mild self-limited disease diagnosed by abd pain radiating to the back, elevated serum amylase and lipase, CT imaging
- Occasionally severe with renal, pulm, coagulation, septic complications

ICD-9-CM Code: 577.0

Etiology

- Many diverse causes
- Most commonly gallstones, alcohol, trauma, CPB, medications, hypertriglyceridemia, infection
- 10% of cases idiopathic

Usual Treatment

- In most cases, nonspecific and supportive only
- Adequate volume replacement and correction of electrolyte abn
- Intensive care of organ system failures
- Parenteral opioid analgesia
- Thromboprophylaxis
- Early nutritional support; enteral better than parenteral
- Rarely, judiciously timed open or endoscopic surgery to drain abscesses or debride necrotic tissue

ASSESSMENT POINTS

System	Effect	Assessment by Hx	PE	Test
CARDIO	Hypovolemia	Orthostatic dizziness Cold	Lying and sitting BP and HR Hypotension Oliguria	BUN/Cr Hct (hemoconcentration)
RESP	ARDS	Dyspnea Tachypnea	Chest exam may be nonspecific	ABGs CXR
GI	Ileus GI bleed	N/V Hematemesis		
ENDO	Hyperglycemia			Serum glucose
HEME	DIC		Bleeding	PT/PTT, plt FSP, fibrinogen Hct
RENAL	Acute renal failure Hypocalcemia		Tetany	BUN/Cr Serum Ca^{2+}
CNS	Psychosis Encephalopathy		Mental status	

Key Reference: Tonsi AF, Bacchion M, Crippa S, Malleo G, Bassi C. Acute pancreatitis at the beginning of the 21st century: The state of the art. *World J Gastroenterol.* 2009;15(24):2945–2959.

Perioperative Implications

Preoperative Preparation

- Assess and correct volume status, hypocalcemia, hyperglycemia, acidosis

Monitoring

- Consider bladder catheter for monitoring of UO
- Consider arterial catheter if need for blood draws or hypovolemia
- Consider CVP or PA catheter for monitoring of volume status

Airway

- Routine

Induction

- Peritoneal irritation frequently leads to ileus and ↑ risk of aspiration
- Anticipate hypovolemia

Maintenance

- CV instability due to massive sequestration of fluid; depending on severity >10 L of isotonic fluid may be required over 24 hr

Extubation

- Will likely require postop mechanical ventilation

Adjuvants

- Multiple interaction of protein-bound drugs, esp. if pt malnourished or undergoing alcohol withdrawal (see Malnutrition in Diseases section and Alcohol Abuse in Diseases section)

Anticipated Problems/Concerns

- Pts with pancreatitis presenting for abd surgery are typically critically ill and require postop intensive care to manage hypovolemia, ARDS, DIC, acute renal failure, sepsis
- Hypoglycemia, hyperglycemia are life-threatening risks after pancreatectomy
- Alcohol withdrawal can be life-threatening.

Pancreatitis, Chronic

Jeffrey J. Schwartz

Risk
- Unknown

Perioperative Risks
- Periop mortality directly related to chronic pancreatitis (rare)
- Assoc malnutrition may lead to difficulty with wound healing and infection.
- Endocrine insufficiency leads to glucose intolerance, but ketosis, coma, and chronic diabetic complications are rare.

Worry About
- Management of pain and opioids if pt is tolerant owing to chronic administration

Overview
- A nonlethal condition characterized by fibrosis, inflammation, loss of exocrine pancreatic tissue
- Characterized by severe persistent or episodic abd pain
- Malabsorption and DM are consequences of loss of pancreatic tissue
- Endocrine insufficiency occurs later than exocrine insufficiency.

ICD-9-CM Code: 577.1

Etiology
- Most commonly chronic alcohol use leads to proteinaceous plugs in the ducts and atrophy of acinar tissue with fibrosis
- Other causes are pancreatic duct obstruction, cystic fibrosis, protein-calorie malnutrition
- Acute pancreatitis does not lead to chronic pancreatitis
- 30–40% of cases are idiopathic

Usual Treatment
- Strict avoidance of alcohol
- Pancreatic enzyme supplements for exocrine insufficiency
- Insulin for glucose intolerance
- Selected pts may occasionally achieve pain relief with surgery

ASSESSMENT POINTS

System	Effect	Assessment by Hx	PE	Test
GI	Malabsorption	Diarrhea	Orthostatic hypotension	BUN/Cr Albumin
ENDO	Glucose intolerance	Polyuria, polydipsia		Serum glucose

Key Reference: Nair RJ, Lawler L, Miller MR. Chronic pancreatitis. *Am Fam Physician.* 2007;76(11):1679–1688.

Perioperative Implications

Preoperative Preparation
- If pt is receiving chronic opioids, the usual dose should be given on the day of surgery.
- Glucose/insulin management

Monitoring
- Routine

Airway
- Routine

Induction
- Consider full stomach if abd pain

Maintenance
- Consideration of opioid tolerance must be incorporated in plan.

Extubation
- Routine

Adjuvants
- Multiple interventions and adjustments needed for protein-bound drugs if pt is malnourished (see Malnutrition in Diseases section)

Anticipated Problems/Concerns
- Difficulty managing pain and opioids in pts on large doses of opioids for chronic pain
- Pancreatic endocrine insufficiency may lead to impaired glucose intolerance without chronic sequelae of DM.

DISEASES

Parkinson's Disease (Paralysis Agitans)

Molly Fitzpatrick
Seema Deshpande

Risk

- Advancing age
- 3% of population >65 y
- Slight increased prevalence in males

Perioperative Risks

- Hemodynamic instability, hypotension, arrhythmias
- Aspiration and upper airway obstruction from poor coordination of upper airway muscles
- Laryngospasm; 90% of pts have vocal fold bowing/adduction
- Postop confusion and hallucinations

Worry About

- Acute dystonic reaction with alfentanil
- Neuroleptic malignant syndrome with dopamine agonists
- Worsening of Parkinsonism with dopamine antagonists (phenothiazines, metoclopramide, butyrophenones (droperidol, haloperidol))
- Serotonin toxicity syndrome (clonus, hyperreflexia, hyperthermia, and agitation) due to interaction between MAOIs and phenylpiperidine series of opioids-meperidine, methadone, dextromethrophan, tramadol, and propoxyphene (weak serotonin re-uptake inhibitors)

Overview

- Pathophysiology: Loss of dopaminergic fibers in substantia nigra in basal ganglia leads to dopamine deficiency.
- Dx based on clinical presentation: Resting tremor, muscle rigidity, bradykinesia, postural instability, facial immobility, with or without dementia or depression
- Aspiration pneumonia—most common cause of death

ICD-9-CM Code: 332.0

Etiology

- Etiology unknown
- Possible genetic link
- Exposure to environmental toxins (MPTP), pesticides may play a role.

Usual Treatment

- Pharmacologic
- Dopamine precursors -L-Dopa (prodrug converted to dopamine in brain) mainstay of therapy, usually in combination with a Dopa decarboxylase inhibitor (carbidopa) to prevent peripheral conversion to dopamine in bloodstream.
- Treatment with levodopa characterized by "on" periods of symptom amelioration and possible dyskinesias, followed by "off" periods with decreasing therapeutic levels of dopamine and return of Parkinsonism symptoms.
- Dopamine agonists: Ergot alkaloids (bromocriptine, carbegoline, lisurid) and non-ergot alkaloids (pramiprexole, ropinirole, rotigotone); A D-1/D-2 receptor agonist, apomorphine, is an effective treatment for "off" episodes. It is administered via subQ, intranasal, or sublingual route; high incidence of nausea and/or vomiting.
- Antivirals-amantadine, useful for treatment of L-dopa induced dyskinesias
- MAO-B inhibitors—selegiline, rasagiline
- Catechol-O-Methyl Transferase Inhibitors (COMT): Entacapone and tolcapone inhibit breakdown of dopamine
- Anticholinergics—trihexyphenidyl, benztropine
- Surgical
- Deep brain stimulation: Inhibits neuronal activity at site of stimulation and therefore mimics an ablative lesion; stimulation to either subthalamic nucleus (most promising; treats tremor, bradykinesia and rigidity), internal globus pallidus, or unilateral thalamus (treats tremor)
- Pallidotomy, thalamotomy: Rarely used today; replaced by DBS
- Continuous infusion of levodopa via implanted intraintestinal catheter
- Experimental use of fetal stem cell implantation

ASSESSMENT POINTS

System	Effect	Assessment by Hx and PE	Test
NEURO	Tremor, akinesia, depression, confusion, dementia, hallucination	Resting tremor that disappears with purposeful movement Muscle rigidity Akinesia Speech impairment Confusion Dementia	Mini-mental status exam
ENT	Pharyngeal muscle dysfunction, dysphagia, post extubation laryngospasm, sialorrhea, papillary abn, oculogyric crises	Dysphagia Sialorrhea Retained secretions	Swallowing evaluation
PULM	Atelectasis, resp infections, aspiration pneumonia, diaphragmatic spasm, uncoordination of resp muscles, postop resp failure	Resp impairment Atelectasis Aspiration pneumonia Post extubation laryngospasm	CXR PFTs ABG
CARDIO	Hypovolemia, orthostatic hypotension, arrhythmias, depletion of myocardial norepinephrine stores	Orthostatic hypotension Arrhythmias Htn Hypovolemia	ECG ECHO
GI	Wt loss, malnutrition, GERD	Wt loss Malnutrition	Swallow eval, serum albumin/transferrin
ENDO	Abnormal glucose metabolism (selegiline)		Blood glucose concentration
UROL	Bladder dysfunction from autonomic instability	Difficulty in urination	
DERM	Seborrhea		

Key Reference: Deiner S, Hagen J. Parkinson's disease and deep brain stimulator placement. *Anesthesiol Clin*. 2009;27:391–415.

Perioperative Implications for DBS Surgery

Preoperative Implications

- Hold Parkinson medications the morning of surgery
- Avoid benzodiazepines that could interfere with cooperation or resting tremor

Monitoring

- Routine

Airway

- Poor airway access due to stereotactic headframe, hence always have plan to access airway, should need rise, incl having a key to the frame.
- Nasal cannula generally used, facemask, LMA, cuffed opharyngeal airway and awake ET intubation with local anesthetic have also been used to secure the airway, when required.

Intraoperative

- DBS surgery requires the pts to be secured in a stereotactic headframe and be awake to allow identification of areas of brain, accurate electrophysiologic recording and for intraop neurologic assessment.
- Different techniques used are awake technique with local anesthesia, regional anesthesia using scalp nerve blocks or IV sedation, and general anesthesia.

- Dexmedetomidine ideal sedation agent as it does not interfere with Parkinsonian symptoms, generally used in doses of 0.3–0.6 mcg/kg/hr
- Propofol not ideal as may mask tremor but can be used during certain stages of procedure (CT and MRI studies) in a low dose infusion (up to 50 mcg/kg/min)
- Small doses of fentanyl or low dose remifentanil (less than 0.1 mcg/kg/min as a dose of 0.1 mcg/kg/min can cause rigidity) have been used.
- Ketamine may lead to exaggerated sympathetic response but recently has been reported to be used safely and successfully in a low dose for

preop sedation and dyskinesia attenuation during internal pulse generator placement
- Optimize pt comfort while positioning
- Minimize IV fluids (no Foley)
- Complications of DBS surgery incl intracranial hemorrhage, seizure, venous air embolism, infection

General Anesthesia
- Reserved for pts who cannot tolerate awake procedure
- Must decide on GA prior to procedure as difficult to access airway after headframe positioned
- Volatile anesthetics, IV anesthetics or combination used. Limit amount of anesthetic used. Using <1 MAC of volatile anesthetics, reportedly, does not drastically affect microelectrode mapping

Perioperative Implications for Non-DBS Surgery

Preoperative Implications
- Continue Parkinson medications the morning of surgery

- Administer L-dopa via OG/NG at regularly scheduled intervals during surgery to prevent Parkinson's exacerbation.

Monitoring
- Routine

Airway
- Aspiration risk
- Upper airway obstruction

Induction
- Propofol ideal induction agent
- Thiopental may cause parkinsonian episodes

Maintenance
- Exaggerated vasodilatation and cardiodepressant effects with volatile anesthetics
- Nondepolarizing NMB drugs well tolerated, but mask tremor
- Anecdotal reports of hyperkalemia with succinylcholine
- Enhanced opioid-induced muscle rigidity following fentanyl administration
- Increased risk of neostigmine-induced bronchoconstriction

General Anesthesia
- May see transient appearance of otherwise pathological neurologic reflexes (hyperreactive stretch reflexes, ankle clonus, Babinski reflex, decerebrate posturing) on emergence

Regional Anesthesia
- Advantageous
- Diphenhydramine useful for sedation

Postoperative Period
- Confusion, delirium, hallucinations common
- Shivering common

Anticipated Problems/Concerns

- Be aware of all Parkinson's medications and possible drug interactions, particularly with MAO inhibitors.
- Avoid drugs that exacerbate parkinsonism (phenothiazines, butyrophenones, and metoclopramide).
- Use caution with airway management, esp. keeping in mind postextubation laryngospasm and resp failure.

Paroxysmal Atrial Tachycardia

David Amar

Risk

- May be seen in ICU pts and indinstinguishable from paroxysmal SVT
- Digitalis toxicity, acute electrolyte or acid-base imbalance
- Incidence of 2% in the periop period (excl AF or atrial flutter)
- No racial prevalence and all age groups
- May be seen with mitral valve prolapse esp in females

Perioperative Risks

- Rapid heart rate impairs LV filling and may adversely affect LV function in pts with LV failure, hypertrophic cardiomyopathy, aortic or mitral stenosis
- Cerebrovascular disease

Worry About

- Syncope: ~15% on initiation or abrupt termination of rapid SVT
- Syncope may also indicate AF and rapid conduction over an accessory pathway
- Hypotension: In pts with systolic or diastolic dysfunction
- Chest pain: Pts with CAD
- ST-T segment changes: Common with rapid rates and reduced coronary filling even with normal coronaries
- VF: In Wolff-Parkinson-White (WPW) pts who develop AF
- Dig level, electrolyte and acid-base status

Overview

- Paroxysmal atrial tachycardia (PAT) is among a larger group of narrow (<120 ms) QRS-complex tachycardias defined by the ACC/AHA/ESC task force to incl: paroxysmal supraventricular tachycardia (PSVT), AF/flutter, permanent junctional tachycardia and focal atrial tachycardia and macro re-entrant tachycardia
- Rapid atrial arrhythmias occur after any major surgery in pts >60 y of age (3–4%) but with a greater incidence of cardiac (20–40%), thoracic

(4–27%) and peak 2–3 d after surgery. Acute postop events such as pneumonia or ARDS may increase the incidence.
- Causes poorly defined, probably multifactorial, and may incl catecholamine excess and pericardial inflammation
- Common mechanisms of narrow complex tachycardias in the periop period
- Re-entrant rhythms: AV nodal re-entrant tachycardia; AV reciprocating tachycardia through accessory pathway, AF/flutter (most common in over 90%)
- Unifocal or ectopic atrial tachycardia
- Multifocal atrial tachycardia in pts with chronic pulm disease

ICD-9-CM Code: 427.0

Etiology

- Re-entrant rhythms
  - AV nodal re-entry: Re-entrant pathway within AV node. Most common form of PAT; seldom assoc with organic heart disease.
  - Accessory pathway mediated: Re-entrant rhythm that involves an accessory pathway from atrium to ventricle. In sinus rhythm, the bypass tract may cause a pre-excitation pattern on ECG (WPW syndrome: Short P-R interval and *delta* wave on ECG) or may not be apparent.
- Unifocal atrial tachycardia arising from a single atrial muscle site other than SA node and assoc with catecholamine excess states (uncontrolled pain, light anesthesia) or digitalis toxicity (triggered activity with variable AV block).
- Multifocal atrial tachycardia arising from multiple atrial sites, usually seen in pts with pulm disease or CHF

Usual Treatment

- Initial therapy: Vagal maneuvers (i.e., valsalva, carotid massage (avoid in known carotid disease) or facial immersion in cold water) should be initiated to terminate the arrhythmia

- IV adenosine or Ca^{2+}-channel blockers (diltiazem or verapamil) are the drugs of choice but beta-blockers may also be used. Adenosine may provoke bronchospasm in pts with reactive airway disease, or excessive (prolonged) bradycardia in pts taking carbamazepine or in denervated heart transplant pts. Higher doses of adenosine may be needed in pts taking methylxanthines (i.e., theophylline). Adenosine may initiate AF in 1–15% which is usually transient.
- The goal of second-line therapy is to achieve ventricular rate control and possible conversion when PAT does not respond, or rapidly recurs, after adenosine. IV digoxin is not effective unless CHF is present.
- When AV nodal block is unsuccessful, electrical cardioversion is considered. If infeasible or unsuccessful, antiarrhythmic agents may also be used. When LV function is preserved, IV options incl procainamide and amiodarone. The proarrhythmic potential of these agents makes them less desirable than AV nodal blockade. In pts with poor LV function, IV amiodarone is preferred.
- Pts with accessory pathway re-entrant rhythms who develop AF are at risk for VFIB, and this scenario is exacerbated by agents that reduce the accessory bundle refractory period (digoxin, Ca^{2+}-channel blockers, β-blockers, and adenosine). Hence, WPW pts who experience AF should not receive AV nodal blockers, and IV procainamide and amiodarone are preferred agents for slowing the rate and to achieve conversion.
- Multifocal and unifocal PAT: Correct underlying hypoxia, electrolyte imbalance. Therapy: Electical cardioversion and procainamide are not effective. Effective IV agents available for use incl AV nodal blockers (Ca^{2+}-channel blockers, β-blockers) and amiodarone. While digoxin slows the ventricular rate, toxicity may provoke automatic atrial tachycardia.

ASSESSMENT POINTS

System	Effect	Assessment by Hx	PE	Test
CARDIO	WPW AV nodal re-entry Symptomatic unifocal atrial tachycardia	Palpitations, diaphoresis Hypotension, chest pain	Prominent jugular venous pulsations	ECG (150-250 bpm, abn P waves preceding QRS, rarely discernible) Electrophysiologic studies, ECHO
NEURO	Rapid arrhythmia	Fatigue, presyncope or syncope		
RESP	Rapid arrhythmia	Dyspnea	Rales, wheezes	CXR
RENAL	Atrial dilation	Polyuria		BNP, BUN/Cr

Key Reference: ACC/AHA/ESC. Guidelines for the management of patients with supraventricular arrhythmias-executive summary. *J Am J Cardiol*. 2003;42:1493–1531.

Perioperative Implications

Preoperative Preparation
- If possible, continue Ca^{2+}-channel blockers and β-blockers periop to avoid withdrawal-assoc arrhythmias.
- Correct hypoxemia and electrolyte imbalance
- Consider proven prophylactic regimens for high-risk pts undergoing cardiac or thoracic surgery.
- Pts with recurrent arrhythmias may be taking drugs such as flecainide, propafenone, amiodarone or dofetilide for prevention.

- Pts with refractory arrhythmias have usually had electrophysiologic studies and in some, catheter ablation procedure

Monitoring
- Continuous intraop ECG monitoring and postop ECG monitoring in high-risk pts

Induction/Maintenance/Extubation
- Aim for effective postop analgesia.
- Consider β-blockers in hyperadrenergic postop pts with adequate cardiac output.

Anticipated Problems/Concerns

- Transient side effects with adenosine incl flushing, dyspnea, and chest pain. Adenosine may provoke hypotension, esp in pts with borderline hemodynamic status.
- Wide-complex rhythms: Adenosine may be used if the rhythm is confirmed by other means to be supraventricular in origin. The use of adenosine to discriminate VT from SVT is now discouraged due to vasodilatory side effects (worsened hypotension) in pts with VT.

Patent Ductus Arteriosus

Aris Sophocles
Mark Twite

DISEASES

Risk

- Full term infants: 1 in 2000
- Preterm infants: 8 in 1000
- Highest in preterm and low-birth-weight infants
- F:M ratio: 2:1
- Assoc with congenital rubella infection and genetic defects incl trisomy 21, CHARGE, and a familial recurrence rate of 3%

Perioperative Risks

- Surgery: Hemorrhage; hemodynamic instability esp in premature and low-birth-weight neonates; single lung ventilation resulting in hypoxia, atelectasis, and pneumothorax; recurrent laryngeal nerve injury; chylothorax; ligation of the incorrect vessel (aorta or pulm artery); thoracic scoliosis long term
- Cardiac cath lab device closure: Obstruction of the pulm artery and/or aorta from the occlusion device, arrhythmias, incomplete closure, and embolization of the device

Worry About

- Premature infant: Lung disease and high mechanical ventilator settings, hemodynamic instability after duct closure due to poor cardiac reserve

- Term infant and young child: Preop dehydration, ability to tolerate single lung ventilation, post-extubation stridor due to recurrent laryngeal nerve injury, postop analgesia
- Older child and adult: pulm Htn

Overview

- Preterm and low-birth-weight infants: PDA may cause CHF and worsening of chronic lung disease which makes weaning from mechanical ventilation difficult.
- Term and older infants: PDA may be asymptomatic or assoc with failure to thrive, recurrent resp infections, and CHF
- Silent duct is a small PDA detected with echocardiography with no murmur heard
- PDA leads to an increased risk of endocarditis

ICD-9-CM Code: 747.0

Etiology

- Normal: The arterial duct is the connection between the pulm artery and the aorta that shunts blood away from the lungs during in-utero fetal development. The duct normally constricts shortly after birth due to the postnatal drop in circulating prostaglandin levels as well as the rise in systemic O_2 tension. Constriction is followed by permanent duct closure from endothelial and

smooth muscle cell hypertrophy and eventual formation of the ductal ligament
- PDA: In preterm infants the ductal muscle layer is thin and poorly contractile and has a poor constrictor response to changes in arterial oxygen tension

Usual Treatment

- Medical management: Neonates often receive a trial of ibuprofen or indomethacin. These act by inhibiting prostaglandin forming cycloxygenase (COX) enzymes. Adverse drug effects incl renal dysfunction and necrotizing enterocolitis.
- Surgical management
  - Bedside left lateral thoracotomy: Reserved for critically ill ventilated pts who have failed medical therapy
  - OR left-lateral muscle sparing thoracotomy or video-assisted thoracoscopic surgery (VATS): Stable child, technique is surgeon's preference with most children receiving a thoracotomy. Candidates are usually not suitable for device closure (less than 8 kg) or unusual duct anatomy
  - Cardiac cath lab: Reserved for children greater than 8 kg due to the size of the femoral sheaths through which the occluding device is introduced. Large PDAs are occluded with an Amplatzer device while small PDAs are occluded with coils.

ASSESSMENT POINTS

System	Effect	Assessment by Hx	PE	Test
CARDIO	CHF	FTT, difficulty feeding	'Machinery' murmur Wide pulse pressure Bounding pulses	ECHO
	Pulmonary Htn		Pulsus bisferiens Tachycardia Diaphoresis	
RESP	Pulm edema	Recurrent resp infections ↑ O_2 requirement	Worsening mechanical ventilation parameters Rales	CXR
GI	Necrotizing enterocolitis	Abd distention Poor feeding Blood in stool Free air in peritoneum	Distended tense abdomen Edema of abd wall Tender abdomen	Abdominal XR
RENAL	Oliguria	↓ UO due to ↓ renal blood flow		Serum chemistry
CNS	CNS hemorrhage	↑ Fontanel pressure ↓ Hct	↑ Fontanel size and tension	Head USS

Key Reference: Jacobs JP, Giroud JM. Evolution of strategies for management of the patent arterial duct. *Cardiol Young*. 2007;17:68–74.

Perioperative Implications

Preoperative Preparation
- Surgery
  - Bedside unstable neonate: Cross-matched blood at bedside, adequate IV access with extension tubing, familiar with ventilator function and settings, check current running infusions (TPN, vasopressors)
  - OR stable child: Cross-matched blood in the OR
- Cardiac cath lab: Routine setup for general ET anesthesia

Preinduction/Induction
- Unstable neonate: Induce with fentanyl (10–30 mcg/kg)
- Cath lab/OR stable child: Premedication and mask induction

Monitoring
- Standard ASA monitors
- Unstable neonates require an arterial line for continuous BP measurement and blood gas analysis and central venous access for inotrope drug delivery.

- Stable older children do not require invasive monitoring.

Airway
- Critically ill neonates are already intubated and ventilated. Check tube size for leak and confirm position on CXR.
- OR cases: Intubate for single lung ventilation (right main stem a single lumen ETT, bronchial blocker, or double lumen tube)
- Cath lab cases: Young children often require intubation, older cooperative children may be done with a natural airway.

Maintenance and extubation
- Bedside critically ill neonate: Fentanyl, paralytics, and remain intubated at the end of the procedure
- Stable child in the OR: Balanced anesthetic technique with the goal of early extubation and adequate analgesia (consider regional techniques)

- Cath lab: Balanced anesthetic technique and extubate at the end of the procedure. Analgesic requirements are minimal and related to the femoral vessel puncture sites

Adjuvants
- Antibiotic prophylaxis for all cases (usually cefazolin 30–50 mg/kg)

Postoperative Period
- Adequate analgesia

Anticipated Problems/Concerns

- Critically ill neonates: Often require a transient increase in BP and resp support.
- Stable children postop surgical ligation via a thoracotomy may have atelectasis from single lung ventilation and thoracotomy pain.

Pemphigus

James M. Sonner
Jeffrey A. Katz

Risk

- Incidence in USA: 0.1–0.5/100,000/y for pemphigus vulgaris (the most common form of pemphigus)
- Age: Most common from age 30–60 y; can occur in children or elderly
- Most common in people of Mediterranean descent

Perioperative Risks

- Infection
- Electrolyte abn with extensive lesions

Worry About

- Pharyngeal blisters, sloughing of mucosa, bleeding produced by airway manipulations
- Consequences of steroid treatment (e.g., Htn, hyperglycemia, gastric or duodenal ulceration, myopathy, infection, psychic disturbances, osteoporosis) or immunosuppressive therapy (bone marrow suppression)

Overview

- Autoimmune, intraepidermal blistering disease of skin and mucous membranes. Oral lesions most common. Blisters rupture easily, heal slowly, usually do not scar.
- Four types: Vulgaris (most common and severe form), vegetans, foliaceus, erythematosus
- 5 y mortality 5–15% for treated pemphigus vulgaris. Most common cause of death is infection, usually with *Staphylococcus aureus*.
- Occasionally co-exists with other autoimmune diseases, thymoma (with or without myasthenia gravis), or malignancies

ICD-9-CM Code: 694.4

Etiology

- Autoimmune disease in which autoantibodies are produced to cell adhesion molecules (desmosomal glycoproteins) on keratinocytes. More common in pts with certain HLA haplotypes. Immune response leads to acantholysis and blistering.

- Uncommonly, pemphigus is drug induced.
- Rarely, may occur in association with malignancy (paraneoplastic pemphigus)
- Endemic pemphigus foliaceus (South America) possibly caused by an infectious agent

Usual Treatment

- Corticosteroids
- Adjuvant therapy
  - Immunosuppressive agents (e.g., azathioprine, cyclophosphamide, methotrexate, cyclosporine)
  - Oral gold, dapsone, or mycophenolate mofetil occasionally used
  - Plasmapheresis or photopheresis occasionally used to decrease antibody titer in refractory disease
  - Rituxan is a biologic that may also be effective in treating pemphigus

ASSESSMENT POINTS

System	Effect	Assessment by Hx	PE	Test
HEENT	Oral and pharyngeal erosions and blisters	Painful oral lesions ↑ Salivation Painful swallowing	Oral lesions	
CARDIO	Htn (due to steroids)		BP	
RESP	At risk for pneumonia	Fever, cough, sputum	Diminished breath sounds, dullness to percussion	CXR
GI	Gastric or duodenal ulcer (due to steroids)	Epigastric pain Dark stools		
MS	Myopathy (due to steroids)	Fatiguability, weakness		
DERM	Blisters Denuded areas Lyte abn	Blisters	Blisters Denuded or crusted areas of skin	Electrolytes

Key Reference: Mahalingam TG, Kathirvel S, Sodhi P. Anaesthetic management of a patient with pemphigus vulgaris for emergency laparotomy. *Anaesthesia.* 2000;55(2):160–162.

Perioperative Implications

Preoperative Preparation

- Pts may require supplemental steroids.
- Avoid tape on skin because it can generate new lesions.
- Secure IV with loose cloth bandage or suture.

Monitoring

- Consider monitors that do not adhere to skin. Consider removing adhesive from ECG pads and oximeter probes and securing with loose bandage. Place soft padding (e.g., Webril) under BP cuff.

Airway

- Pts may have oral erosions or blisters; new blisters may form from airway management. Risk is of airway obstruction or bleeding. Consider lubricating mask and laryngoscope blade to decrease

friction, using small ETT; minimal cuff inflation; and suture or hold tube in place. Avoid LMA owing to unquantified risk of pharyngeal trauma.

Preinduction/Induction

- Lubricate eyes, do not tape
- Allow pt to position self on well-padded OR table, to decrease risk of blister formation with positioning. Ensure all pressure points are padded once pt is on table.

Maintenance

- Neither general nor regional anesthesia clearly superior
- Local infiltration probably contraindicated owing to risk of blister formation

Extubation

- Minimize coughing during extubation

Postoperative Period

- New lesions of skin or mucous membranes may appear

Adjuvants

- Depends on agents and effects of agents used for chronic treatment
- Consider need for steroid supplementation

Anticipated Problems/Concerns

- Minor frictional trauma to skin or mucosa may generate new lesions. Airway must be instrumented gently and tape avoided anywhere on the skin.
- Pts are at risk of infection and lyte abn from pemphigus and of side effects of steroid and immunosuppressive therapy.

Pericardial Effusion

Terence Wallace
Bruce D. Spiess

Risk

- Occurs rarely
- Postop open heart or PTCA: Blood and/or serous
- Infection: Viral, bacterial, fungal
- Neoplastic: Lymphoma, leukemia
- Post acute MI (esp transmural)
- Trauma
- Gender predominance: Male > female

Perioperative Risks

- If unknown, tamponade causing CV collapse possible with low probability of determining cause ante mortem
- If known, risk of CV collapse, esp with induction and institution of positive pressure ventilation

Worry About

- Hypovolemia
- Limited filling of cardiac chambers

Overview

- Found in sac surrounding heart; if severe can restrict filling of heart
- Ventricular filling is depressed in both RV and LV
- Fluid bolus and inotropes do little to improve cardiac output
- Cardiac output becomes more dependent on heart rate
- Must have surgical drainage for proper treatment

ICD-9-CM Code: 423.9

Etiology

- Postsurgical and catheterization procedures
- During or after viral, bacterial, or fungal infection
- Postinflammatory process: Acute transmural, SLE, rheumatoid arthritis
- Neoplastic
- Trauma

Usual Treatment

- Drainage either percutaneous or open
- Medical management is generally ineffective

ASSESSMENT POINTS

System	Effect	Assessment by Hx	PE	Test
CARDIO	Tamponade limiting CO Hypotension	Chest pain	Neck veins HR BP	Equalization of all pressures in heart (catheterization)
	Arrhythmias			ECG TEE
RESP	↓ CO on institution of IPPB (mechanical ventilation)	Dyspnea Change in BP on institution of mechanical ventilation		Pulm artery, RA, LA pressures
METAB	Metabolic acidosis			ABGs

Key Reference: Collins D. Aetiology and management of acute cardiac tamponade. *Crit Care Resusc.* 2004;6(1):54–58.

Perioperative Implications

Preoperative Preparation

- Appropriate monitoring before induction
- Preoxygenation is not always effective
- Support hemodynamics-catecholamines, keep acid-base balance full and fast
- Consider draining transthoracically if hemodynamic compromise severe
- Consider prep and drape prior to induction with surgeon ready
- Positive pressure ventilation may significantly worsen hypotension, resulting in shock and death
- Consider placing external defibrillator patches prior to anesthetic induction

Monitoring

- Arterial line indicated as BP may change suddenly; sampling of Hct for bleeding and acid-base status in low cardiac output state is useful
- Consider PA catheter, useful in making diagnosis and following surgical treatment. If pressures not relieved on surgical drainage, question original diagnosis.
- TEE, useful but less so than PA monitoring

Induction/Maintenance

- Do not decrease preload
- Slowly titrate small doses of barbiturates or propofol
- Monitor hemodynamics and use anesthetic, if tolerated, or etomidate
- Consider placing before induction invasive hemodynamic monitoring
- Ketamine and pancuronium have been advocated for new tamponade situations
- Initiation of positive pressure ventilation may cause severe CV compromise due to decreased filling of RV and LV

Treatment Approach

- Post open heart surgery hemorrhage—reopening sternum to explore for sites of hemorrhage—usually relieved by first few sutures released
- Infections and/or neoplasia: Subxyphoid pericardial window
- Small incision: Open pericardium under direct vision; chest tube placed behind heart
- Insertion of a pericardioscope provides the ability to visualize the pericardium and obtain biopsies

Adjuvants

- Depends on etiology

Extubation

- Consider awake extubation or postop mechanical ventilation, depending on etiology

Anticipated Problems/Concerns

- Many different causes, all with different sequelae
- Hypotension on induction of anesthesia or positive pressure ventilation

Pericarditis, Constrictive

Ribal Darwish

Risk

- CHF
- Cardiac tamponade
- Cardiac cirrhosis
- Arrhythmias

Perioperative Risks

- Heart failure
- Atrial arrhythmia
- Myocardial infarction
- Abn drug metabolism secondary to liver failure
- Intraop major hemorrhage
- Postop resp failure

Worry About

- Difference between CP and restrictive heart failure.
- When providing general anesthesia, be prepared for CPB.

Overview

- CP is an inflammation of the pericardium, leading to an impaired filling of the ventricles and reduced ventricular function.
- Restriction of the pericardium results in increased ventricular interdependence and a reciprocal relation between the left and right heart filling.
- During spontaneous ventilation, the transtricuspid blood flow is increased, resulting in increased filling of the RV. This will lead to the septum to shift to the left and the decrease in the LVEDV with subsequent hypotension, causing pulsus paradoxus.
- During expiration, the septum is shifted to the right. Opposite changes take place during mechanical ventilation.
- Pts present with dyspnea, fatigue, orthopnea, right heart failure with venous congestion and chest pain.

ICD-9-CM Code: 423.2

Etiology

- In developed countries, idiopathic or viral infections are the most common cause of CP followed by cardiac surgery and mediastinal irradiation.
- Bacterial infectious causes are more common in underdeveloped countries such as: Tuberculosis, staphylococci, group A and B streptococci and gram-negative rods.
- Less common causes are uremia, connective tissue disorders, and drug reactions.

Usual Treatment

- In advanced stages, the standard treatment is pericardiectomy. Both median sternotomy and left thoracotomy approaches are used.

ASSESSMENT POINTS

System	Effect	Assessment by Hx	PE	Test
HEENT	Lymphoadenopathy if the CP is caused by viral or bacterial infection, cyanosis	Hx of fever, chills, upper resp tract infections.	Enlarged cervical lymph nodes, jugular venous distention	Blood and sputum cultures, immunological assays for viral infections
RESP	Pulm edema if heart failure develops	Dyspnea, dry cough	Tachypnea, rales on auscultation	Chest x-ray, arterial blood gas analysis
CARDIO	Right and left heart failure, arrhythmia, hypotension	Dyspnea, orthopnea, chest pain, peripheral edema, fatigue, palpitations, and hepatomegaly	Tachycardia, muffled and distant heart sounds, friction rub, apical pulse is not palpable	MRI and CT scans EKG -low voltage and ectopic AT. increased CVP (W shape). Left heart catheterization shows "square root sign" Doppler echo—restrictive LV diastolic filling, characterized by TMF E/A ratio >>1, short deceleration time (DT) of TMF E velocity, and PVF S/D ratio <1
MS	Muscle atrophy, myositis if there is an underlying connective tissue disorder	Significant wt loss and muscle wasting	Clinical evidence of weakness	CPK to r/o myositis; specific tests if connective tissue disorder is suspected

Key Reference: Schwefer M, Aschenbach R, Heidemann J, Mey C, Lapp H. Constrictive pericarditis, still a diagnostic challenge: Comprehensive review of clinical management. *Eur J Cardiothorac Surg*. 2009;36(3):502–510. Epub 2009 Apr 25.

Perioperative Implications

Preoperative Preparation
- Cardiac medications incl antidysrhythmics should be continued.

Monitoring
- Have invasive monitoring incl arterial line and pulm artery catheter.
- Intraop TEE is of significant help

Maintenance
- Conducted under general anesthesia
- Narcotic-based technique is preferred
- The intraop hemodynamic goals are adequate preload, maintenance of sinus rhythm, and rate control if sinus rhythm cannot be maintained.

Adjuvants
- Inotropic support is indicated if there is evidence of ventricular dysfunction.
- Most pericardioectomies are done without the need for CPB, but CPB should be on stand by.

Anticipated Problems/Concerns

- Myocardial infarction, major intraop hemorrhage, atrial and ventricular arrhythmias, and worsening of the heart failure.

Peripheral Vascular Disease

Jacqueline M. Leung

Risk

- 10–15% of those >age 50 y
- Long-term mortality increased 2–3× in those with overt CAD, large vessel arterial disease, DM
- 5-y mortality rate: 30–40%

Perioperative Risks

- High prevalence of co-existing CAD and carotid artery disease
- Presence of CAD increases operative mortality
- Pulm and renal insufficiency can cause prolonged recovery or morbidity

Worry About

- Aortic clamping: May induce myocardial ischemia or ventricular failure; hypotension with declamping
- Increased risk of periop myocardial ischemia and cardiac complications
- Postop thrombosis in arterial grafts
- Postop delirium, esp if >70 y

Overview

- Vascular abn involving extremities increase in frequency with age
- Co-existing diseases common (DM, COPD resulting from smoking, Htn, CAD)

ICD-9-CM Code: 443.9

Etiology

- Chronic arterial occlusive disease
- Less common: Takayasu's syndrome and thromboangiitis obliterans

Usual Treatment

- Reconstitute pulsatile blood flow to distal vascular tree to allow healing of ulcerated or gangrenous tissue, relieve ischemic rest pain with the goal of salvaging a functional limb
- Most common surgical procedures are aortofemoral bypass, femoropopliteal bypass, femorotibial bypass or endovascular approach
- Angiogenesis gene therapy now being combined with percutaneous angioplasty techniques in experimental protocols

ASSESSMENT POINTS

System	Effect	Assessment by Hx	PE	Test
CARDIO	Htn Coronary artery stenoses MI	Usually asymptomatic Angina, may be asymptomatic	Normal if treated S_3 and/or S_4 cardiomegaly	Vital signs ECG Exercise ECG Treadmill Pharmacologic stress test Coronary angiography ECHO Radionuclide studies
	Ventricular dysfunction	Exercise intolerance Sx of heart failure		
PERIPHERAL VASC EXAM	Occlusive lesions Abd aortic aneurysm may co-exist	Claudication Abd pain, may be asymptomatic	↓ Pulses Pulsatile abd mass	Angio Aortogram MRI
RESP	COPD (many are smokers)	DOE	↓ Breath sounds Prolonged expiration Wheezes	ABGs PFTs
ENDO	DM and assoc effects such as angiopathy, peripheral and autonomic neuropathy, nephropathy	Attention to CV, PNS for ANS and other evaluation	Obesity (in DM type II) Cardiomegaly Foot ulcers	Fasting blood sugar
CNS	Ischemic CNS disease	Scotoma CNS and mental status evaluation Absence spells	CNS exam Search for carotid bruits	Doppler or angio (if indicated)

Key Reference: Swangard DM. Anesthesia for vascular surgery. In: Leung JM, ed. *Cardiovascular and vascular anesthesia: the requisites in anesthesiology*. St Louis, Mosby; 2004:186–210.

Perioperative Implications

Preoperative Preparation

- Attention to and stabilization of concomitant medical conditions such as CAD, COPD, DM
- High-risk pts scheduled for noncardiac surgery may not benefit from a better periop outcome from preop coronary revascularization.
- Consider periop β-blockade in vascular surgery pts with CAD to decrease myocardial ischemia, but caution about acute preop implementation and the potential in increasing periop stroke rate. Ideally, office evaluation should be scheduled several weeks in advance to allow dose titration. Pts already on β-blockade should be have their medication continued.

Monitoring

- ST trending if available
- In aortic surgery, consider placement of CVP or TEE for monitoring preload
- Use of transesophageal ECHO may elucidate the mechanism(s) of declamping hypotension (hypovolemia versus ventricular dysfunction) and regional ventricular function (myocardial ischemia)

Airway

- None

Preinduction/Induction

- Prevent tachycardia (use of short-acting β-blockers desirable) and treat BP changes aggressively.
- Epidural anesthesia combined with epidural analgesia shown to decrease incidence of reoperation and arterial thrombosis of graft as compared with GA

Maintenance

- See above

Extubation

- Same hemodynamic concerns as in induction
- Use of postop epidural analgesia decreases likelihood of arterial graft thrombosis

Adjuvants

- β-blockers and other antihypertensives useful in hyperdynamic situations
- Prophylactic nitroglycerin and Ca²⁺-channel blockers to treat myocardial ischemia not conclusively proven efficacious

Anticipated Problems/Concerns

- Periop myocardial ischemia and cardiac complications, thromboembolic events of grafts, CHF, renal failure

Pertussis (Whooping Cough)

Raj K. Modak

Risk

- Increased prevalence 1976 (lowest) vs. 2007:1010 vs. 10,454 cases
- Incidence highest for infants <1 y, 23% of all cases
- Adolescent group 10–19 y, 33% of all cases
- Incidence of death highest for infants <6 mo, 91% of all deaths
- Females > males (54%)
- Whites > minorities (90%)
- 90% susceptibility following exposure to index case, if unimmunized
- Only 2% of adult population protected against pertussis

Perioperative Risks

- Most common complications age <6 mo: Hospitalization (69%), pneumonia (13%), seizures (2%), encephalopathy (<2%)
- Common complications in adults: Cough-related incontinence (28%), syncope (6%), pneumonia (5%), rib fractures (4%), hospitalization (3%)

Worry About

- Infectivity and contagion
- Secretions, pneumonia, altered mucociliary function, apnea, and decreased pulm reserves causing hypoxemia
- Postop complications related to coughing

Overview

- Pertussis is an acute resp infection caused by *Bordetella pertussis*
- Transmission occurs by resp droplet with a 7–10 d incubation
- Organism releases multiple toxins that damages the epithelial cells of the resp tract
- Characterized by 3 phases: Catarrhal (cold symptoms), paroxysmal (cough symptoms), convalescent (persistent or episodic cough)
- Infectivity highest in catarrhal and early paroxysmal phases
- Adolescents and adults display milder symptoms that may be indistinguishable from less serious causes of URI/LRI.
- Immunization in childhood has decreased but not eliminated incidence.
- Vaccine estimated 80–85% effective after 3 exposures, usually given as combination tetanus, diphtheria, acellular pertussis (TDaP) vaccine
- Increased in incidence in adolescence (age 10–19) indicating a need for booster immunization

ICD–9–CM Code: 033.0

Etiology

- *Bordetella pertussis*, a fastidious, gram–negative, pleomorphic or rod bacillus

- A whooping cough syndrome also caused by *B. parapertussis*, *Chlamydia trachomatis*, and many adenoviruses

Treatment

- Infectivity and contagion control
- Most effective treatment occurs in catarrhal and early paroxysmal phases
- Macrolides (erythromycin, azithromycin, clarithromycin) and trimethoprim-sulfamethoxazole
- Cough suppression: Dextromethorphan and codeine; expectorant: guaifenesin
- Corticosteroids and β_2 agonists have an unclear role in paroxysmal stage.
- In some cases, hospitalization may be required to suppress cough, institute antibiotic treatment, monitor for apnea and hypoxemia, and general nutrition
- Intensive care treatment may be needed for severe sequelae of pneumonia, seizures, and encephalopathy
- Antibiotic therapy is not recommended in the convalescent phase.

ASSESSMENT POINTS

System	Effect	Assessment by Hx	PE	Test
HEENT	Upper airway obstruction	Difficulty feeding Difficulty breathing	Rhinorrhea Lacrimation Conjunctivitis	Nasal culture Direct fluorescent antibody (DFA)
CARDIO	High 0₂ consumption	Irritability	Tachycardia	ECG
RESP	Cough V/Q mismatch Hypoxemia Pneumonia	Apnea, SOB Tachypnea, rales As above	Inspiratory whoop Cyanosis Rales	Culture + DFA Pulse oximetry, ABGs CXR
GI	Poor oral intake Post–tussive emesis Fatty liver Cough–induced hernias	Dehydration Inability to retain food Inguinal hernias	Altered turgor Wt loss Hepatomegaly Reducible hernias	Weigh on scale LFTs
RENAL	Hypovolemia	Oliguria	Altered turgor	BUN, Cr, FeNa
CNS	Seizures Encephalopathy	Seizure type Altered neuro status	Seizure type Neuro exam	EEG, CT, MRI LP, glucose, ammonia, BUN
ID		Immunization Hx Physical contacts		Culture + DFA

Key Reference: Centers for Disease Control and Preventive. Pertussis — United States, 2001–2003. *MMWR*. 2005;54(50):1283–1286.

Perioperative Implications

Preoperative Preparation

- Postpone elective surgery until noninfectious and symptom-free; uncomplicated disease resolves in 6–10 wk
- Emergency surgery based on risks and benefits
- Infectivity and contagion control with isolation precautions
- Usage of disposable anesthesia circuit system
- If possible, optimize resp function and nutrition prior to surgery
- If in early phases, consider premedication with topical or oral decongestants (ephedrine, pseudoephedrine, xylometazoline) to reduce upper airway secretions, β_2 agonists (albuterol, metaproterenol) to minimize risk of bronchospasm
- Optimize preop volume status from dehydration.
- Premedication with resp depressants may increase risk of hypoxemia.

Monitoring

- Arterial catheterization may be useful in scenarios of impaired oxygenation for frequent blood gas sampling.

Airway

- Acute and chronic coughing increase the risk of upper and lower airway edema with possible obstruction.
- Nasal and tracheal secretions increase the risk of laryngospasm and bronchospasm.
- Inspissated secretions can cause hypoxemia by mucous plugging and atelectasis, barotrauma by airway obstruction, and an inability to ventilate by ET obstruction.

Preinduction/Induction

- In some scenarios, regional anesthesia may be favorable.
- Inhalational techniques with pungent agents should be avoided.
- Avoid agents assoc with coughing.

- Usage of IV or topical lidocaine may decrease tracheal irritation and coughing.

Maintenance

- Keep warm and hydrated.
- Airway humidity should be controlled with a passive device to minimize humidity loss or an active humidifier, which warms and humidifies the airway gases.
- Controlled ventilation allows optimal oxygenation and minimizes atelectasis.
- Consider PEEP for alveolar recruitment.
- Be prepared to contend with airway secretions, suction the ETT as needed, saline-moistened secretions are more readily removed.

Extubation

- Oral and tracheal suctioning should be performed with anticipation of copious secretions.
- Consider the use of pre-emergence bronchodilator treatment to minimize bronchospasm.

- Emergence techniques using NO may carry an increased risk of post-extubation hypoxemia.
- An H₂-blocker should be considered with postop N/V prophylaxis to minimize risk of aspiration of acidic gastric contents.

Postoperative Period

- Infectivity and contagion control with isolation precautions should be maintained.

- Supplemental O_2 therapy should incl the use of a humidifier.
- Aggressive pulm toilet
- Monitoring for apnea and hypoxia are needed.
- Regional techniques for pain management may be useful in avoiding serious resp complications related to IV analgesics

- Infection risk to all contacts, incl family, other pts, and hospital personnel
- High risk of resp insufficiency causing hypoxemia from tissue damage, edema, and secretions
- Infants at higher risk for sequelae and death compared to adults

Pheochromocytoma

Michael F. Roizen

Risk

- Incidence in USA: 0.03–0.04% (~80,000) by autopsy of nonselected individuals; 0.1–0.3% of individuals with sustained Htn have pheochromocytoma. At least 20% are now diagnosed when the tumor is incidentally found during abd MRI or CT for other reasons
- Race with highest prevalence: Caucasian

Perioperative Risks

- If emergency (life-threatening trauma, ruptured viscus), use α- and β-blockers and nitroprusside and keep in ICU until most painful time has passed or adrenergic control is attained.
- ↑ Risk of hypertensive crisis with bleeding into myocardium, brain, or kidney or ischemia
- Mortality rate of 0–3% even if appropriately prepared for tumor resection and in "good" hands for adrenalectomy—may be higher for undiscovered case undergoing nonadrenal surgery
- 25–50% of those who die in hospitals of pheochromocytoma crisis do so during induction of anesthesia, during stressful periop periods, or during labor and delivery.
- Assoc with cholelithiasis and renal stones

Worry About

- Pheochromocytoma (catecholamine excess) crisis with hemorrhage/infarcts in vital organs

- Major goal is to avoid pheochromocytoma crisis; pre- and intraop goals of management of extraadrenal surgery are same as for adrenal surgery. If adrenergic blockade not present prior to surgery, try to delay operation until pt has appropriate degree of α-blocker. Judge appropriate blockade by
  - No BP readings >165/90 mm Hg for 48 hr.
  - Presence of orthostatic hypotension, but BP on standing should not be <80/45 mm Hg
  - ECG free of ST-T changes
  - Absence of other signs of catecholamine excess, and presence of signs of α-blocker

Overview

- Tumor of catecholamine-producing tissue (90% in adrenals). Painful (stressful) events cause exaggerated stress response if less than perfectly anesthetized or in daily living. Even small stresses can lead to blood catecholamine levels of 2000–20,000 pg/mL. However, infarction of tumor, with release of products onto retroperitoneal surfaces or pressure causing release of products, can result in blood levels of 200,000–1 million pg/mL–a situation that should be anticipated during tumor resection.
- Endocrinopathy assoc with CV disease–tachycardia, CHF, dysrhythmias (AFIB)

- Need α-blocker prior to β-blocker unless vasoconstrictive effects of latter go unopposed, thereby increasing risk of dangerous Htn. β-blocker suggested if persistent arrhythmias or tachycardia not resolving with α-blocker or when aggravated by α-blocker.
- If α-blocker, appropriately, risk of crisis diminished by >90%

ICD-9-CM Code: 194.0

Indications and Usual Treatment

- 90% are spontaneously arising and 10% familial (autosomal dominant genetics involving chromosome 7 implicated)
- Assoc with MEA IIA (medullary thyroid carcinoma; primary hyperparathyroidism) and IIB (medullary thyroid carcinoma and mucosal neuromas) with mutation often at chromosome location 17q11.2
- Assoc with neurofibromatosis, von Hippel–Lindau disease (retinal and cerebellar hemangioblastoma), ataxia-telangiectasia syndrome, Sturge-Weber syndrome, with mutation often at VHL gene localized to chromosome 3p25–26

ASSESSMENT POINTS

System	Effect	Assessment by Hx	PE	Test
HEENT		Nasal stuffiness (from α-adrenergic blockade)		
CARDIO	Htn; dysrhythmias; AFIB, sinus tachycardia, mitral valve prolapse; CHF, myocardial fibril necrosis or myocarditis	SOB, poor exercise tolerance, palpitations, Htn (50% sustained, 40% paroxysmal)	Standard exam + BP q 1 min in stressful environment + orthostatic maneuvers with BP/HR q 1 min	ECG, ECHO (if cardiomyopathy is suspected)
GI	90% of tumors adrenal or abd	Wt loss, diarrhea Dehydration	Palpating abdomen can trigger pheo crisis	No different from normal
HEME		Mild polycythemia, thrombocytopenia (2° to ↓ intravascular fluid)		Hgb (↓ polycythemia way to judge volume expansion by α-blocker)
GU	Renal stones from dehydration			
CNS	↑ Catecholamine effects	Headache, tremor, anxiety, ↓ pain threshold, fatigue		
METAB	Associated with hyperparathyroidism	Glucose intolerance from α-adrenergically induced gluconeogenesis and ↓ insulin secretion		Insulin Rx often before Dx made; Ca²⁺

Key References: Witteles RM, Kaplan EL, Roizen MF. Safe and cost-effective preoperative preparation of patients with pheochromocytoma. *Anesth Analg.* 2000;91: 302–304; Amar L, Servais A, Gimenez-Roqueplo AP, Zinzindohoue F, Chatellier G, Plouin PF. Year of diagnosis, features at presentation, and risk of recurrence in patients with pheochromocytoma or secreting paraganglioma. *J Clin Endocrinol Metab.* 2005;90:2110–2116.

Perioperative Implications

Preoperative Preparation

- Prehydrate liberally over 6–60 d if CV status will tolerate; expand with high salt/fluid diet while increasing α-adrenergic blockade over 7–60 d (some use calcium channel blockers, but increased complications assoc with this process epidemiologically)

Monitoring

- Temp
- Art line placement prior to induction difficult and painful but desired because of variations in BP
- PA catheterization or TEE if CV system severely affected; CVP used in minority of cases

Anesthetic Technique

- No technique/group of agents assoc with better outcome; use of droperidol controversial; agents that block reuptake (ketamine) or cause catecholamine release might be avoided.

Induction/Maintenance

- Prehydrate liberally if CV status will tolerate
- Gentle induction with nitroprusside infusion plugged into IV line and running slowly
- Dopamine infusion in reserve for ready use
- Painful or stressful events often cause exaggerated response. Caused by release of catecholamines from nerve endings that are "loaded" by the reuptake process.

Postoperative Care

- See Adrenalectomy for Pheochromocytoma in Procedures section
- Postop: If catecholamine-producing tumor removed or if α-adrenergically blocked, do not chase or force high UO with large crystalloid infusions, as pts have tendency to CHF because they have been on endogenous inotrope for many years.

- Early mobilization and deep breathing a must but fraught with difficulty owing to disturbed psyche that removal of catecholamines present for a long time often causes

Adjuvants

- Drug interactions possible with chronic antiadrenergic agents such as between verapamil or diltiazem and β-blockers in depressing AV nodal conduction if pt chronically or acutely receiving a β-blocker or decreased clearance of phenytoin, barbiturates, rifampicin, chlorpromazine, and cimetidine

Anticipated Problems/Concerns

- Important to interview family members and perhaps advise them to inform their future anesthesiologists about potential for such familial disease

Physiologic Anemia and the Anemia of Prematurity

Jessica Miller

Risk

• Physiologic anemia is a normal process in term infants.
• Anemia of prematurity is a pathologic anemia occuring in preterm infants. Extent of prematurity and co-morbidities correlates with extent of anemia.

Perioperative Risk

• Term infants with physiologic anemia tolerate minor surgery well.
• Premature infants must be evaluated for symptoms due to anemia that may contribute to increased risk of preop events.

Worry About

• Major surgery occurring at the physiologic nadir of anemia may require blood transfusion.
• Preterm infants with anemia undergoing physiologic stress due to surgery are at risk for tachycardia, tachypnea, lactic acidosis, and periop apnea and bradycardia.

Overview

• Physiologic anemia is normal response to extrauterine life. Nadir at 9th–12th wk of life, Hbg level varies 9 to 11 g/dL.

• In preterm infant, nadir occurs at 4–8 wk of life and may decrease to 8 g/dL.
• Anemia of prematurity may be asymptomatic or have non-specific symptoms such as tachycardia, tachypnea, lethargy, pallor, apnea and bradycardiac, poor feeding, poor growth, and lactic acidosis.

ICD-9-CM Code: 776.6 (Anemia, prematurity neonatal)

Etiology

• Transition to extrauterine life incl increased O_2 available to bind to hemoglobin (HbO_2 saturation 50% in utero, 95% ex utero). Fetal hemoglobin with high O_2 affinity starts to be replaced with low O_2 affinity adult hemoglobin.
• Survival of neonatal erythrocytes is shorter than that of adult erythrocytes. Hemoglobin decreases until O_2 needs are greater than O_2 supply. Production of erythropoietin (EPO) is triggered and erythropoiesis increases.
• Rapid growth in infants causes a rapid increase in blood volume resulting in hemodilution. Growth is more rapid in preterm than term infants.

• Preterm infants have more severe anemia because the less sensitive hepatic O_2 sensor triggers EPO production until 40 wk PCA. After 40 wk PCA, an extremely sensitive renal O_2 sensor takes over triggering and production of EPO.
• Iron storage occurs in last trimester, thus premature infants are relatively iron deficient and have difficulty increasing stores by feeding.
• Extent of prematurity correlates with the amount of blood loss due to blood sampling.

Usual Treatment

• No treatment required in term infants
• Preterm infants benefit from prevention: Reduction of blood draws, appropriate dietary supplementation, and erythropoietin therapy.
• Treatment of anemia of prematurity with blood tranfusion occurs when symptoms of reduced O_2 supply are present. Symptoms incl continued need for mechanical ventilation, apnea and bradycardia, tachycardia (>180 bpm for 24 hr), inadequate wt gain, metabolic acidosis, or anticipation of major surgery.

ASSESSMENT POINTS (Apply to Preterm Infants Only)

System	Effect	Assessment by Hx	PE	Test
CARDIO	Tachycardia	Review of VS trends	Tachycardia	± ECG
RESP	Apnea/bradycardia	No. episodes, treatment required or spontaneous resolution		

Key Reference: Aher S, Malwatkar K, Kadam S. Neonatal anemia. *Semin Fetal Neonatal Med.* 2008;13(4):239–247.

Perioperative Implications

Preoperative Preparation
• Timing of elective blood-losing surgery depending on Hgb levels

Monitoring
• Routine

Airway
• None

Preinduction/Induction
• Routine

Extubation
• Recent Hx of apnea and bradycardia: Consider delaying extubation to allow metabolism of anesthetic agents and sedatives.

Adjuvants
• Spinal anesthesia, when appropriate, may be beneficial in preterm infant.

Postoperative Care
• Consider monitoring preterm infant for apnea and bradycardia for 24 hr.

Anticipated Problems/Concerns

• Anemia is significant risk factor for postop apnea in preterm infant undergoing surgery and anesthesia.

Pickwickian Syndrome

Ryan Rubin
Aaron M. Fields

Risk

- 5–10% of morbidly obese pts
- Usually assoc with long-standing obesity

Perioperative Risks

- Marked increased risk from normal body mass index (BMI) pts
- 40% serious morbidity in intra-abdominal or intrathoracic procedures of >2 hr duration

Worry About

- Hypoventilation
- Hypercarbia
- Hypoxemia
- Polycythemia, thrombophlebitis, and subsequent pulm embolism
- Pulm Htn
- Hypersomnolence
- Biventricular cardiac failure

Overview

- Obesity hypoventilation syndrome is defined as the combination of obesity (BMI above 30 kg/m^2), hypoxia during sleep, and hypercapnia.
- Morbidly obese pts who hypoventilate due to sleep apnea and severe restrictive ventilatory disorder and have permanent pulm Htn, acidosis, and polycythemia because of their chronic hypoxemia and CO_2 retention.

- Usually assoc with systemic Htn and compensatory increased circulating blood volume, leading to right and left ventricular failure.
- Two subtypes are recognized, depending on the nature of disordered breathing detected on further investigations. The first is OHS in the context of obstructive sleep apnea; this is confirmed by the occurrence of 5 or more episodes of apnea, hypopnea or resp-related arousals per hr (high apnea-hypopnea index) during sleep. The second is OHS primarily due to "sleep hypoventilation syndrome"; this requires a rise of CO_2 levels by 10 mmHg (1.3 kPa) after sleep compared to awake measurements and overnight drops in O_2 levels without simultaneous apnea or hypopnea. Overall, 90% of all people with OHS fall into the first category and 10% in the second.
- On physical examination, characteristic findings are the presence of a raised jugular venous pressure, a palpable parasternal heave, a heart murmur due to tricuspid regurgitation, hepatomegaly, ascites, and leg edema.

ICD-9-CM Code: 278 (Obesity)

Etiology

- Work of breathing is increased as adipose tissue restricts the normal movement of the chest muscles and makes the chest wall less compliant causing the diaphragm to move less effectively. Resp muscles are fatigued more easily, and airflow is impaired by excessive tissue in the head and neck area.
- Under normal circumstances, central chemoreceptors in the brainstem detect decreased pH, and respond by increasing the resp rate; in OHS, the ventilatory response is blunted.
- Episodes of nighttime acidosis due to sleep apnea lead to renal compensation with retention of bicarbonate.
- Nightime apnea leads to hypoxia causing hypoxic pulm vasoconstriction (HPV). HPV in turn leads to pulm Htn and right ventricular failure and remodeling.
- The chronically low O_2 levels in the blood also lead to increased release of erythropoietin causing polycythemia.

Usual Treatment

- Wt loss through diet and exercise, which is rarely successful, or bariatric surgery
- Continuous positive airway pressure (CPAP)
- Uvulopalatopharyngoplasty
- Tracheostomy

ASSESSMENT POINTS

System	Effect	Assessment by Hx	PE	Test
HEENT	Difficult airway access	Snoring	Poor visualization	X-ray of neck may be helpful
CARDIO	Biventricular failure	Dyspnea, poor exercise tolerance	Venous engorgement, S_3 and S_4, dyspnea	ECG, ECHO, CXR
	CAD	Angina, poor exercise tolerance		ECG, stress ECHO, angio
RESP	Hypoventilation	Dyspnea, sleeping upright Poor exercise tolerance	Rapid shallow breathing, cyanosis	ABGs, Hct, CXR

Key Reference: Littleton SW, Mokhlesi B. The pickwickian syndrome-obesity hypoventilation syndrome. *Clin Chest Med.* 2009;30(3):467–478.

Perioperative Implications

Preoperative Preparation

- Consider pulm function tests with bronchodilator to determine if reversible restrictive component exists.
- Assess for bronchitis/pneumonia that can be improved with pulm toilet and antibiotic therapy.
- Assess myocardial and volume status using a central venous catheter or pulm artery catheter (PAC).
- Consider maintaining semi-sitting position to avoid sudden shifts of volume to central circulation and pulm edema.

Monitoring

- Consider an arterial line to monitor frequent ABGs.
- Resp volumes and pressures
- Consider PAC or transesophageal ECHO to monitor filling volumes and wall motion.

Airway

- Awake intubation frequently required
- Shoulders and head elevated on bolster can sometimes facilitate laryngoscopy

Induction

- Do not expect to ventilate pt adequately by mask. Establish airway first.

Maintenance

- May have to remain in reverse Trendelenburg position to allow adequate ventilation.

Extubation

- Perform in sitting position without residual sedation.
- Ensure adequate tidal volume and consider preop levels of CO_2 retention when making decision to extubate as a normal CO_2 level may not be attainable in these pts.

Adjuvants

- Regional anesthesia only if pt is able to maintain ventilation
- Residual sedation or narcosis may preclude early extubation.

Postoperative Period

- Consider prophylaxis for thromboembolism—early ambulation may minimize pulm and thromboembolic complications.
- May be extremely sensitive to resp depressant effects of benzodiazepines and narcotics

Anticipated Problems/Concerns

- All those assoc with morbid obesity apply to Pickwickian pts.
- Early ambulation may minimize pulm and thromboembolic complications.
- Prepare the pt for a possible prolonged course of postop mechanical ventilation, esp. after upper abd procedures.

Pierre Robin Syndrome

Charles B. Cauldwell

Risk
- 1/8500 live births
- No known sex or race predilection

Perioperative Risks
- Assoc congenital anomalies, e.g., cardiac
- Pulm Htn, cor pulmonale, or pulm edema 2° to chronic airway obstruction
- Cachexia due to feeding difficulties

Worry About
- Airway obstruction
- Difficult intubation

Overview
- An anomaly consisting of micrognathia (or retrognathia), glossoptosis (posterior displacement of the tongue), and cleft palate, leading to varying degrees of airway obstruction and feeding difficulties. Some authors incl resp distress as necessary for diagnosis.
- Airway obstruction can lead to hypoxia, brain damage, or CHF.
- Feeding problems may cause malnutrition or aspiration.
- Obstruction often improves by several mo of age, 2° to mandibular growth, if hypoxia and malnutrition are avoided.

ICD-9-CM Code: 756.0

Etiology
- Congenital, found either as isolated syndrome or as part of multiple defect syndromes. In several series, about 50%–60% of cases are isolated, the rest are part of other syndromes, esp. Stickler and velo-cardio-facial.
- Also named Pierre Robin Sequence, reflecting the several disease processes that can lead to mandibular maldevelopment

Usual Treatment
- Prone positioning, lavage feeding
- Nasopharyngeal or oral airway, for short-term treatment
- Glossopexy or tracheotomy, if surgery necessary
- Mandibular distraction osterotmy for selected cases

ASSESSMENT POINTS

System	Effect	Assessment by Hx	PE	Test
HEENT	Airway obstruction	Sleep apnea Feeding difficulties	Micrognathia Cleft palate	Sleep study
CARDIO	Pulm Htn Cor pulmonale Congenital defects	Cyanotic episodes Tachypnea	Loud S_2 Murmur	EKG ECHO CXR SpO_2
RESP	Hypoxia Pulm edema Aspiration pneumonitis	Tachypnea	Labored inspiration or stridor	SpO_2 CXR
GI	Failure to thrive	Feeding problems	Wt	Wt gain
CNS	Hypoxia	Seizures Developmental delay		

Key Reference: Nargozian C. The airway in patients with craniofacial abnormalities. *Paediatr Anaesth.* 2004;14:53–59.

Perioperative Implications

Preoperative Preparation
- Avoid sedative premedication.
- Consider atropine as antisialogogue and to maintain heart rate.

Monitoring
- Oximeter and precordial stethoscope particularly important

Airway
- Intubation may be very difficult.
- Consider awake intubation in neonates.
- Airway management and intubation tends to get easier with age, esp. in isolated Pierre Robin.

Preinduction/Induction
- May obstruct in supine position while awake or early during inhalation induction
- Consider oral or nasopharyngeal airway.
- Have difficult airway cart available.
- Consider use of LMA with fiberoptic bronchoscope and exchange catheter, or light wand.
- Have surgeon in OR capable of performing tracheotomy when induction begins.

Extubation
- Pt should be awake for extubation, may need to recover in ICU.

Adjuvants
- Do not use muscle relaxants unless absolutely sure pt can be intubated.

Anticipated Problems/Concerns
- Airway obstruction during all phases of anesthesia very common

Pituitary Tumors

Ira J. Rampil

Risk

- Surgical incidence in USA: 7500/y
- Incidental small adenomas occur in 17% adults
- M:F ratio: 1:8 in some histologies, gender neutral in others

Perioperative Risks

- Risks due to 2° endocrine syndromes from secreting (functional) adenomas, e.g., acromegaly, Cushing's syndrome, DM, hyperthyroidism

Worry About

- Angina, cardiomyopathy with evidence of CHF, electrolyte imbalance
- Difficult airway in acromegaly

Overview

- Symptoms due to hormonal dysregulation or local mass effect
- Microadenomas (secreting)
  - Prolactinoma (increased PRL)
  - Cushing's disease (increased ACTH)
  - Acromegaly (increased GH)
- Macroadenoma (mass lesion)
  - Panhypopituitarism
  - Increased ICP
  - Bitemporal hemianopsia

ICD-9-CM Code: 253.8

Etiology

- Usually a nonmalignant clonal tumor derived from Rathke's pouch
- May occur as a component of MEN I, an autosomal dominant trait assoc with deletion at q13 locus of chromosome 11

Usual Treatment

- Incidental (asymptomatic) microadenoma: Conservative
- Prolactin-secreting microadenoma: Bromocriptine or cabergoline (dopaminergic agonists)
- Somatostatin analogs (e.g., octreotide) usually effective in acromegaly
- Transsphenoidal resection is viewed as safe, and curative in ~90%
- Endoscopic approach generally less traumatic than traditional approach

ASSESSMENT POINTS

System	Effect	Assessment by Hx	PE	Test
HEENT	Acromegaly: Prognathism, lingular and laryngeal hyperplasia, mandibular enlargement		Mallampati class	Indirect laryngoscopy
CARDIO	Cushing's disease: ↑ BP Acromegaly: ↑ BP, cardiomyopathy	Exercise tolerance	Volume status, BP	ECG (± stress test) ECHO
RESP		Sleep apnea		Usually not needed
ENDO	Acromegaly: DM Cushing's disease: Hyperglycemia Prolactinoma: Infertility, amenorrhea, galactorrhea, impotence (male) Macroadenoma (usually due to a glycoprotein-secreting adenoma leading to panhypopituitarism by compression/atrophy)		Truncal obesity, striae, moon facies	Serum cortisol; petrosal venous sampling of corticotropin; dexamethasone suppression test Serum GH and glucose suppression Serum prolactin, glycoprotein, TSH
CNS	Suprasellar compression of optic chiasm	Visual field cuts		Formal visual field testing
MS	Acromegaly: Hypertrophy of facial bones and airway tissue Cushing's disease: Osteoporosis, truncal obesity, skin fragility		Weakness	

Key Reference: Nemergut EC, Dumont AS, Barry UT, Laws ER. Perioperative management of patients undergoing transsphenoidal pituitary surgery. *Anesth Analg.* 2005; 101(4):1170–1181. Review.

Perioperative Implications

Preoperative Preparation
- Replacement therapy for panhypopituitarism

Monitoring
- Invasive arterial pressure monitoring usually required if intercurrent disease
- Continuous ETCO$_2$ and N$_2$ to detect venous air embolism when incision >10 cm above right atrium
- Consider CVP in severe acromegaly

Airway
- Have variety of laryngoscope blades and small ETT available
- Consider awake, oral fiberoptic intubation if macroglossia is present

Maintenance
- Htn frequently associated with epinephrine infiltration of nasal mucosa and hammering of nasal speculum in classic approach. Anticipate and pretreat.

Extubation
- Despite pharyngeal packing and suctioning, pharynx and stomach may contain blood and irrigant. Pt should be fully awake and capable of protecting airway to prevent aspiration following extubation.

Postoperative Period
- UO should be followed to detect onset of DI

Adjuvants
- Esmolol and possibly phentolamine (during epinephrine infiltration)

Anticipated Problems/Concerns

- Pts with hypersecretion of ACTH or GH at increased risk of myocardial injury if tight hemodynamic control not maintained during the transient, intense stimulations assoc with transsphenoidal surgery

Placenta Previa

Stacie N. Woods
Paul W. Shabaz
Karen S. Lindeman

Risk

- Incidence: 3.5–4.5 per 1000 births
- Highest incidence: Multiparous deliveries, repeat C-section, previous placenta previa, advanced maternal age

Perioperative Risks

- Maternal mortality: <1%
- Fetal mortality: ~20%
- Life-threatening hemorrhage of mother or fetus
- Fetal hypoxia

Worry About

- Blood loss, hypovolemia
- Full-stomach considerations due to pregnancy or recent oral intake

- Placenta accreta, increta, and percreta, predisposing to hemorrhage and possibly the need for hysterectomy
- Fetal compromise from inadequate intervillous blood flow
- Preterm labor

Overview

- Placental implantation in proximity to or obscuring the cervical os and in advance of fetal presenting part; mode of delivery depends on relationship between placenta and cervical os
- Often presents as painless vaginal bleeding or bleeding assoc with uterine contractions
- Dx confirmed by US, esp. transvaginal, or exam of cervical os under double setup conditions

- Concomitant tocolytic therapy can alter hemodynamic responses to hemorrhage.

ICD-9-CM Code: 641.1

Etiology

- Unknown

Usual Treatment

- Expectant management
- Vaginal delivery may be attempted on a case-by-case basis
- Delivery by C-section for persistent hemorrhage or when fetus is mature in pt with total placenta previa

ASSESSMENT POINTS

System	Effect	Assessment by Hx	PE	Test
HEENT	Airway edema	Pregnancy	Mallampati class	
CARDIO	Hypovolemia, anemia	Amount of bleeding	Tachycardia, hypotension	Hct
RESP	Reduced FRC	Pregnancy		
GI	Full stomach, decreased lower esophageal sphincter tone	Reflux symptoms		

Key Reference: Smith KA, Spielman FJ. Antepartum and postpartum hemorrhage. In: Chestnut DH, ed. *Obstetric anesthesia*. St. Louis: Mosby; 2009:811–836.

Perioperative Implications

Preoperative Preparation

- Nonparticulate oral antacid premedication
- Assess volume status
- Crossmatch blood and consider transfusion
- Large-gauge IVs (2)
- Consider regional anesthesia if hemodynamically stable

Monitoring

- Routine monitors
- Consider arterial and/or central venous catheter if hemodynamically unstable.

Airway

- Airway edema may make intubation more difficult.
- Full stomach

Preinduction/Induction

- Preoxygenate with four vital capacity breaths of O_2.
- Consider awake or rapid-sequence induction.
- Induction with thiopental or ketamine, depending on hemodynamics, plus succinylcholine

Maintenance

- Low-concentration inhalational agent 0.5–0.75 MAC before delivery
- Use of NO before delivery of baby is controversial.
- Can use NO with IV opioid and consider benzodiazepine after delivery
- Restore intravascular volume

Extubation

- Extubate awake; greatest risk is pulm aspiration of gastric contents

Adjuvants

- Oxytocin, methylergonovine, prostaglandin $F_2\alpha$ to enhance uterine contraction and decrease bleeding after delivery

Postoperative Period

- None

Anticipated Problems/Concerns

- Intrapartum and/or postpartum hemorrhage
- Full stomach
- Urgent induction of anesthesia
- Fetal distress

Pneumocystis Carinii Pneumonia (PCP)

Neal H. Cohen

Risk

- Resp infection in severely immunocompromised pts
- Pts with both acquired and congenital immunodeficiency syndromes
- Seen in all age groups
- Frequently assoc with pts with advanced AIDS, particularly if not treated with highly active antiretroviral therapy (HAART)

Perioperative Risks

- Resp failure often necessitating mechanical ventilatory support with high airway pressures
- Hemodynamic instability assoc with induction of anesthesia, positive pressure ventilation
- Pneumothorax
- Persistent expiratory airflow reduction after resolution of acute infection
- Bronchiectasis, lung cysts

Worry About

- Progressive resp failure
- Pneumothoraces, either spontaneous or assoc with positive pressure ventilation
- Persistent pulm dysfuntion
- Common cause of non-productive cough, dyspnea, fevers in immunosuppressed pt
- Assoc with other opportunistic infections, particularly CMV
- Toxicity from treatment, incl methemoglobinemia, anemia, leukopenia, and severe skin rashes
- Increasing incidence of drug resistance

Overview

- Indolent disease that can progress to severe resp failure
- May be cause for non-productive cough in high risk pt
- High incidence of spontaneous pneumothoraces
- Extrapulm sites of infection rare, but should be considered in critically ill pt
- May be assoc with other infections (tuberculosis, bacterial, viral, fungal) and malignancies (Kaposi's sarcoma, lymphoma) in immunosuppressed pts

ICD-9-CM Code: 136.3

Etiology

- *Pneumocystis jiroveci* (previously *carinii*), originally characterized as a parasite, now classified as fungus
- Organisms reside in lungs, usually as latent infection; activated in immunosuppressed host
- High prevalence of antibodies to *Pneumocystis jiroveci* in nonimmunosuppressed humans, suggesting that most are colonized early in life
- Human-to-human transmission has not been documented

Usual Treatment

- Trimethaprim/sulfamethoxazole (TMP-SMX)
- Pentamidine
- Primaquine
- Corticosteroids
- Prophylactic therapy with aerosolized pentamidine, oral TMP-SMX, or dapsone
- Supportive resp care

ASSESSMENT POINTS

System	Effect	Assessment by Hx	PE	Test
HEENT	Oropharyngeal lesions	Fever, chills, sweats	Circumoral, acral, and mucous membrane lesions	
CARDIO	Intravascular volume deficits Cardiomyopathy	Fluid intake, syncopy, resp rate	Hemodynamic lability Neck veins distended Heart sounds	Orthostatic BP changes
RESP		Cough, usually nonproductive Progressive dyspnea Hemoptysis	Tachypnea Breath sounds, prolonged expiratory phase Exam often normal	ABGs PFTs Transbronchial biopsy Gallium scan of lung LDH
GI	Hepatopathy Bowel lesions	Often assoc with wt loss, other infections causing diarrhea, GI Sx	Hepatosplenomegaly	LFTs
HEME	Anemia, leukopenia Coagulopathy			CBC Clotting studies
RENAL	Nephropathy, oliguria	Oliguria		BUN, Cr
CNS	Encephalitis, meningitis	CNS changes	Abn mental status	

Key Reference: Travis TJ, Hart E, Helm J, Duncan T, Vilar J. Retrospective review of *Pneumocystis jirovecii* pneumonia over two decades. *Int J STD AIDS.* 2009;20:200–201.

Perioperative Implications

Preoperative Preparation

- Ensure adequacy of oxygenation, ventilation, acid-base balance
- Assess pulm function, particularly expiratory phase of respiration
- Evaluate for evidence of other opportunistic infections
- Review CXR for evidence of infiltrates, abscesses, cystic lesions or cavitations, bullae, pneumothorax, effusions

Monitoring

- Confirm presence or absence of methemoglobinemia, if treated with sulfa drugs
- Interpret SpO_2 with caution, if metHb present; measure SaO_2 by co-oximeter

Airway

- Minimize airway pressures, TV
- Increased airway reactivity

Induction

- Maintain adequate PaO_2
- Minimize airway pressures, risk of pneumothorax
- Hypotension assoc with myocardial depressants, vasodilators, positive pressure ventilation
- Ensure adequate intravascular volume

Maintenance

- Ensure adequate oxygenation, ventilation
- Minimize airway pressures
- Administer bronchodilators

Extubation

- May be delayed
- Prolonged ventilatory support often required

Postoperative Period

- Ensure adequate oxygenation, ventilation
- Minimize airway pressures using low TV ventilation
- Maintain intravascular volume; optimize myocardial function
- Continue anti-*Pneumocystis* therapy, consider other antiviral agents

Anticipated Problems/Concerns

- Deterioration of resp status, prolonged resp failure
- Pneumothorax; may require surgical repair if tube thoracotomy unsuccessful
- Nosocomial infections, assoc viral infections
- Difficulty monitoring oxygenation with pulse oximeter, if pt treated with dapsone, primaquine
- Drug resistance

Post Transplant Lymphoproliferative Disease

Tamas Seres

Risk

• 2–3% of all allograft organ transplants, highest risk in intestinal or multiorgan transplants
• Major risk factors are the degree and type of immunosuppression (OKT3, ATGAM induction or prolongerd exposure to high doses of tacrolimus) as well as the EBV serostatus of the recipient (EBV negative recipients of EBV positive donor organs).
• Additional risk factors are the time after transplant (first year), recipient age (<25 y), and ethnicity (Caucasians).
• Overall survival rates ranging between 25–35%

Perioperative Risks

• Increased risk of airway or bowel obstruction and hemodynamic compromise
• Increased risk of dysfunction of the transplanted organs
• Increased risk for infection and CNS involvement

Worry About

• Enlarged tonsils and cervical adenopathy increasing difficulty of airway
• Thoracic adenopathy complicating intubation, ventilation, and cardiac output
• Pulm involvement causing decreased oxygenation and/or ventilation
• Dysfunction of the transplanted kidneys, liver, or heart
• GI involvement may manifest in N/V or bowel obstruction
• CNS involvement may manifest in mental staus change or increased ICP
• Immunosuppression causing an increased rate of infection

Overview

• Lymphoproliferative disorders are among the most serious and potentially fatal complications of chronic immunosuppression in organ transplant recipients.
• These tumors are mostly B-cell type large-cell lymphomas. Extranodal involvement is occurring in 30–70% of the cases as a localized tumor in either the transplanted organ or another site, such as the GI system, lungs, skin, liver, and CNS.

ICD-9-CM Code: 202.8 (Non-Hodgkin's lymphoma)

Etiology

• B lymphocytes are activated by EBV in the setting of chronic immunosuppression.
• A defect in cytotoxic T cell function due to immunosuppression, resulting in a disturbed equilibrium between cell division and death of EBV-infected B cells promoting the development of PTLD.

Usual Treatment

• Reduction of immunosuppression, interferon α, rituximab, cytotoxic T cell infusions and radiation (CNS)
• Surgery may be necessary to debulk large masses and relieve bowel obstructions.
• Chemotherapy for disseminated unresponsive disease

ASSESSMENT POINTS

System	Effect	Assessment by Hx	PE	Test

HEENT	Cervical adenopathy
	Pharyngitis
	Enlarged tonsils with
	  pseudomembranous appearance
	Otitis media
	Sinusitis
	Laryngeal edema
		Difficulty swallowing
		Sore throat
		Headache
		Facial pain, ear pain
		Difficulty talking, breathing
			Lymphadenopathy
			Tonsillar enlargement
			Spotty, erythematous tonsils
			Otitis media
			Tenderness over sinuses
			Drooling, tripod position
			Difficulty of breathing
				CT
				H and P
				Serological test for
				  EBV

RESP	Lung nodules Pleural effusions Hilar and mediastinal adenopathy	SOB Orthopnea	Decreased breath sounds Crackles, egophony	CXR CT
CARDIO	HF	SOB, tires easily Edema	New murmur, crackles Pitting edema	ECHO ECG
GI	Liver dysfunction Bowel obstruction Bowel perforation Tumors anywhere in GI tract	N/V Abd pain and discomfort Distention Swelling, tenderness over graft site	Jaundice Abd distention Tenderness over graft Rebound tenderness	LFTs Abd x-ray CT US
RENAL	Renal insufficiency or failure	Decreased UO Swelling	Pitting edema Crackles	BUN, Cr, electrolytes
ID	Mononucleosis syndrome Generalized lymphadenopathy Sepsis	Fatigue, fever	Elevated temp	CBC, serology for EBV
CNS	Brain tumors	Headache Loss of consciousness Seizure	Stupor, coma Seizure	CT, MRI

Key Reference: Hammer GB, Cao S, Boltz MG, Messner A. Post-transplant lymphoproliferative disease may present with severe airway obstruction. *Anesthesiology.* 1998;89(1):263–265.

Perioperative Implications

Preoperative Preparation
• Difficult airway techniques and consider GE reflux precautions
• Evaluate the needs for blood products and specific antibiotics
• Evaluate the function of the transplanted organs
• Consider stress dose steroids if receiving steroids

Monitoring
• Consider invasive monitoring in organ failure or mediastinal mass.
• Consider ICP monitor as indicated for CNS involvement.

Airway
• Consider awake fiberoptic techniques if upper airway edema or masses or mediastinal masses

Preinduction/Induction
• Mediastinal mass can compress aorta and SVC, leading to significant hypotension if supine. Consider sitting or semi-sitting induction.
• Consider lower extremity for volume resuscitation if a large mediastinal mass

Maintenance
• Keep the pt breathing spontaneously in case of significant airway obstruction.
• If a mediastinal mass, keep in semi-sitting position and turn to lateral or prone position if hemodynamics become compromised.

Extubation
• Risk of airway obstruction if manipulated during surgery

Postoperative Period
• Airway edema can become a problem
• Continue stress dose steroids

Anticipated Problems/Concerns

• Airway obstruction and hemodynamic compromise
• Dysfunction of transplanted organs
• Mental status change or increased ICP in CNS involvement

Postoperative Encephalopathy, Metabolic

Steven Roth

Risk

- Pts undergoing any surgical procedure are at risk. Esp. of concern following brain or cardiac surgery, or interventional neuro-radiology procedures, pts with COPD, cancer, renal or hepatic failure, and those with electrolyte abn
- No gender predominance

Perioperative Risks

- Aspiration, fluid and electrolyte imbalances, circulatory failure, hypoxia, insulin use

Worry About

- Suspect in any pt who fails to awaken or awakens more slowly than expected following GA
- Evaluate for presence currently or earlier in periop period of severe hypotension, hypoxemia, fluid and electrolyte disorders, pts with cancer, renal or liver dysfunction, thyroid abn
- Seizures, increasing intracranial pressure; persistent coma may result

Overview

- Altered state of consciousness that becomes apparent in periop period
- Pts may fail to awaken after GA for these reasons: Anesthetic-induced: narcotics, inhalational anesthetics, benzodiazepines, hypnotics may impair consciousness; brain injury: direct surgical intervention (e.g., occlusion of major intracranial vessel, intracranial hemorrhage, edema) may result in impaired consciousness; or embolization to a major artery may occur (e.g., during or after cardiac surgery, interventional neuroradiology procedures)
- Metabolic abn: Circulatory failure, hypoxia, insulin use, hepatic and renal insufficiency, electrolyte abn can result in failure or slowness to awaken. In all cases, Dx should proceed quickly in order to treat underlying cause before severe brain injury results.

ICD-9-CM Code: 348.3 (Encephalopathy)

Etiology

- Anoxic-ischemic encephalopathy
- Hypercapnic encephalopathy ($Paco_2$ >70 mmHg)
- Hypoglycemic encephalopathy (glucose ≤30 mg/dL)
- Hyperglycemic coma (glucose ≥450 mg/dL; Osm >319 mOsm/mm³)
- Acute hepatic encephalopathy: Liver failure
- Uremic encephalopathy: Renal failure
- Other brain injuries: SIADH, seizures
- Lyte imbalance: Hypokalemia or hyponatremia, hypercalcemia
- Endocrine: Thyrotoxicosis, hypothyroidism
- Drug and/or toxin exposure (use a drug and/or toxicology screen)

Usual Treatment

- Depends upon the etiology—see Assessment Points

ASSESSMENT POINTS

Etiology	Examples	Diagnosis	Treatment
ENDO	Hyperthyroid Hypothyroid	Thyrotoxicosis Myxedema	PTU Thyroid hormone replacement
ANOXIC-ISCHEMIC	Cardiac arrest Prolonged shock Hypoxemia	Obvious from clinical course	Reverse acute event Then, ↓ cerebral edema, maintain BP, ↓, temp??, prevent seizures
HYPERCAPNIC	Narcotic-induced Severe COPD, sleep apnea	↑ Heart rate and BP ↑ End-tidal or arterial Pco_2	Reverse narcotic Mechanical vent to ↓ Pco_2
HYPOGLYCEMIC	Insulin overdose Ethanol ingestion Neonatal (idiopathic)	No IVF or PO ingestion From Hx and alcohol level ↓ Blood glucose	IV glucose (D50)
HYPERGLYCEMIC	Hyperosmolar nonketotic coma Ketoacidosis	Suspect in known diabetic Ketones in blood, urine Acidosis	Insulin, correct acidosis and fluid volume deficit
ION DISTURBANCES	↓ Na^+ ↓ K^+	Serum Na^+ <125 mmol/L (e.g., SIADH) Serum K^+ <2.5 mEq/L Severe muscle weakness	Hypertonic saline (caution) NaCl and diuretics K^+ replacement
RENAL	Renal failure		
HEPATIC	Hepatic encephalopathy		

Key Reference: Bozbora A, Coskun H, Erbil Y, Ozbey N, Orham Y. A rare complication of adjustable gastric banding: Wernicke's encephalopathy. *Obes Surg.* 2000;10:274–275.

Perioperative Implications

- Correct ion and fluid disturbances
- Normalize blood glucose

- Optimize organ function (e.g., renal, hepatic)
- Adequate hormone replacement

- Search for drug/toxin exposure (sedative/hypnotics; ethanol and its street substitutes such as ethylene)

Prader-Willi Syndrome

Navil F. Sethna

Risk

- Prevalence: 1: 25,000.
- Incidence: 1:10,000– 15,000
- Racial prevalence: None
- Gender predominance: Similar frequency in both sexes and all races
- Morbidity increases with 2° complications from obesity
- Annual death rate is 3% primarily due to resp arrest

Perioperative Risks

- Infantile hypotonia, hypoventilation, and breathing difficulty
- Potential difficult intubation and aspiration risk
- Worsening of obstructive/central sleep apnea and abn ventilatory responses to hypoxia and hypercarbia and bronchospasm
- Bradycardia, ventricular arrhythmias (PVCs)
- Postop resp insufficiency
- Potential risk of rhabdomyolysis with succinylcholine
- Aberrant thermoregulation: Hyperthermia and MHS-like syndrome
- Glucose intolerance or DM

Worry About

- Abn of short and restricted neck mobility, limited mouth opening and difficult intubation
- Poor vascular access and intraop positioning
- Systemic and pulm Htn, conduction defects RBBB and cor pulmonale. Dilated cardiomyopathy.
- Restrictive lung disease (obesity, kyphoscoliosis) and reactive airways

Overview

- Presents in two stages: Infantile central hypotonia, FTT, and delayed developmental milestones. Childhood stage presents with obesity (BMI> 97th percentile in a child and ≥30% in an adult), skeletal abn (dysmorphic, short stature, short hands and feet, scoliosis), hypogonadism, and hypothalamic dysfunction
- Restrictive pulm disease results from muscle weakness, obesity and kyphoscoliosis. It starts in early childhood and is present in 80–90% of pts over 30 y
- CV system: Htn in 17–32% and myocardial hypotrophic hypokinetic syndrome

- Central thermo dysregulation: May develop hyperpyrexia
- Cognitive problems: Mild–moderate mental retardation. Mean IQ 60s–70s; some have normal intelligence.
- Behavior problems of oppositional behavior, emotional lability, aggressive and violent behavior, and obsession and compulsion to eat. Psychosis in 5–10% of adults.
- High threshold for pain

ICD-9-CM Code: 759.81

Etiology

- A leading cause of genetic obesity, caused by paternally derived deletion of long arm of chromosome 15 at 15q11–13. GH deficiency.

Usual Treatment

- Early intervention and education: Physical, occupational, speech, and behavioral therapies
- Wt and dietary management; low calorie diet and regular physical therapy
- GH replacement therapy
- Nighttime CPAP ventilatory support for severe OSA

ASSESSMENT POINTS

System	Effect	Assessment by Hx	PE	Test
CRANIO-FACIAL ANOMALIES	Facial dysmorphia, poor mask fit	Snoring, nystagmus, viscous and sticky saliva	Dental crowding and caries Micrognathia, short neck with limited movement	Imaging scans
CVS	Htn	Headache	High diastolic BP	EKG, CXR, renal function EKG, CXR
	Pulm Htn Cor pulmonale	Exertional and at rest dyspnea Dyspnea, exertional intolerance	Lung rales	EKG, CXR EKG, CXR, ECHO
	Cardiomyopathy	Dyspnea, exertional intolerance	Tachypnea, orthopnea, systemic venous congestion, gallop sounds	EKG, CXR, ECHO
RS	Alveolar hypoventilation Increase airway responsiveness Increase work of breathing Upper airway obstruction	Snoring and interrupted sleep, day time somnolence, exertional dyspnea, wheezing	Fatigue, limited upper airway access, short neck, limited mobility of neck	PFT, room air ABG CXR Polysomnography for severe OSA Difficult airway scoring
DIABETES TYPE I OR II	Increased risk for CVS, CHF and autonomic dysfunction	Hyperglycemia/hypoglycemia osmotic diuresis	Dysfunction of CVS, renal and peripheral neuropathy	Periop blood glucose Other test related to end-organ involvement

Key Reference: Chen C, Visootsak J, Dills S, Graham Jr JM. Prader-Willi syndrome: An update and review for the primary pediatrician. *Clin Pediatr (Phila)*. 2007;46:580–591.

Perioperative Implications

Preoperative Preparation

- Only a well-supervised pt should be considered NPO
- Oral metoclopramide and cimetidine
- Assess airways difficulty, CV and pulm status
- Effective premedication to ensure a cooperative pt during awake/sedated intubation and induction of GA

Monitoring

- Standard ASA monitors. Consider direct intra-arterial BP measurement if the non-invasive cuff does not fit. Continuous temp monitoring for instability
- Frequent ABGs, UO, and central venous or pulm artery pressure for major surgery

Airway

- Elective awake intubation if difficult airway is anticipated; increasing neck circumference, a Mallampati score of ≥3, micrognathia, and limited mouth opening

Induction

- Gastric regurgitation due to delayed gastric emptying and hiatal hernia
- Be prepared to manage a situation where ventilation and/or intubation are not possible. The degree of obesity is only one factor among others that makes glottis visualization problematic
- Semi-sitting position improves FRC and preoxygenation
- Slow IV induction with propofol and remifentanil or fentanyl with or cisatracurium to facilitate intubation

Maintenance

- Sevoflurane or desflurane with remifentanil infusion and cisatracurium. These inhaled agents are least soluble and allow rapid recovery from general anesthesia. No specific drug or combination is recommended; the aim is rapid emergence. Avoid long-acting opioid and substitute with IV NSAIDs.
- Regional anesthetic techniques are desirable alone or to supplement GA and provide postop analgesia to reduce the need for opioids.

Extubation

- Decision is dictated by the severity of obesity, assoc risks such as OSA and the extent of surgical procedure. Early tracheal extubation is desirable.

Adjuvants

- Hydrophilic drugs (e.g., muscle relaxants are calculated by lean body mass). Lipophilic drugs (e.g., fentanyl) are calculated in mg/kg body weight.

Postoperative Period

- Severe obesity is assoc with more atelectasis during, immediately, and for 24 hr longer after general anesthesia compared to non-obese pts. CPAP or BiPAP may be necessary to maintain patent airways, particularly during sleep and for those with severe OSA. High sensitivity to opioid-induced resp depression.

Anticipated Problems/Concerns

- Monitor for OSA and alveolar hypoventilation in ICU/PACU. Monitor hyper- and/or hypoglycemia, hyperthermia, and arrhythmias
- Early ambulation and thromboembolic precautions

Preeclampsia

Shobana Bharadwaj
Andrew M. Malinow

Risk

- 6–8% of all pregnancies
- Young, nulliparous, or multiparous with previous preeclampsia/eclampsia Hx, obesity
- May be increased with Hx of other microangiopathy (e.g., chronic Htn, diabetes, renal disease, SLE)
- Lower socioeconomic status; malnutrition; no prenatal care

Perioperative Risks

- Increased risk of fetoplacental or maternal deterioration necessitating (often operative) delivery
- Preeclampsia and eclampsia account for about 20% of maternal and perinatal deaths

Worry About

- Hypertensive crisis leading to intracerebral bleed or LV failure
- Increased interstitial volume leading to edema
- Maternal hypotension producing placental hypoperfusion
- Renal dysfunction progressing to acute renal failure
- Thrombocytopenia may contraindicate regional anesthetic
- Eclampsia (or seizure in a severely preeclamptic patient) necessitating difficult tracheal intubation

Overview

- Marked by Htn, proteinuria, edema
- Maternal vasoconstriction: Possibly leading to acute cardiorespiratory deterioration
- Proteinuria: Sign of deteriorating renal function and widespread endothelial damage
- Edema: Increasing total body water, proteinuria, Htn lead to increasing interstitial edema and decreasing intravascular volume
- Hematologic: Widespread endothelial damage often leads to thrombocytopenia,
- Epigastric/RUQ pain an ominous sign of liver subcapsular edema and possible rupture. Delivery should be urgently effected.
- HELLP (Hemolysis, Elevated Liver enzymes, Low Platelet count) a poor fetoplacental prognostic sign.
- Headache: seizure may be impending

ICD-9-CM Codes: 642.4 (Mild); 642.5 (Severe); 642.7 (With preexisting hypertension); 760.0 (Affecting fetus or newborn)

Etiology

- Acquired disease of unknown etiology
- Imbalance in circulating mediators of vascular tone and response (e.g., thromboxane vs. prostacyclin) from endothelial damage
- Pregnant pts who later manifest the disease have been shown to have demonstrated hyperdynamic CV response early in pregnancy compared with pts who do not go on to manifest disease.
- Microangiopathy leading to endothelial change, plt consumption, hemolysis

Usual Treatment

- Prevention with daily low-dose aspirin beginning in 2nd trimester has had limited success
- Delivery becomes cure
- In-hospital therapy incl: Antihypertensives, seizure prophylaxis, and support of maternal perfusion, with magnesium sulfate (therapeutic blood levels = 5–7 mg/dL), and intravascular rehydration
- Analgesia, esp. epidural analgesia for labor, reduces catecholamine response to pain, increasing placental perfusion

ASSESSMENT POINTS

System	Effect	Assessment by Hx	PE	Test
HEENT	Edema		Airway exam	
CARDIO	Systemic vasoconstriction ↓ Intravascular volume		Rales JVD BP UO	ECG CXR ECHO Hct
RESP	Pulm edema	Dyspnea Chest discomfort	Rales/rhonchi Cyanosis	SaO$_2$ CXR ECHO
GI	Hepatic subcapsular edema	Epigastric/RUQ pain	Enlarged liver edge	LFT
HEME	Thrombocytopenia	Easy bruising	Petechiae, gingival bleed	Plt count
RENAL	↑ Capillary permeability	Wt gain	Nondependent edema UO	Urinary protein Cr clearance Serum uric acid
CNS	Seizure Intracerebral hemorrhage Cerebral edema	Headache Blurred vision Seizure	Retinal edema CNS exam Deep tendon reflexes	CT scan
OB	↓ Placental perfusion		FHR—lack of variability or bradycardia	FHR monitoring BPP Doppler velocimetry
	Placental abruption	Vaginal Bleeding		FHR monitoring

Key Reference: Gogarten W. Preeclampsia and anaesthesia. *Curr Opin Anaesthesiol.* 2009;22(3):347–351.

Perioperative Implications

Antepartum Management
- Optimize maternal perfusion while lowering systemic diastolic BP <110 mmHg
- Ensure therapeutic blood magnesium sulfate level
- Replenish intravascular volume
- Avoid aortocaval compression

Monitoring
- Consider intra-arterial catheter for extremes of BP
- Consider CVP or PA catheter for oliguria or pulm edema
- Fetal heart monitoring

Airway
- Often difficult 2° to edema
- Prepare for emergent airway

Preinduction/Induction
- Epidural analgesia/anesthesia induces venodilation. Maintain maternal perfusion with judicious use of intravascular volume and (often) small, incremental prn doses of IV ephedrine, or low-dose phenylephrine, by bolus or infusion
- Rapid-sequence induction of anesthesia, titrating infusions of IV antihypertensive drugs or rapid-acting opioids to blunt pressure response to intubation

Maintenance
- Hemorrhage at delivery may lead to dramatic hypotension
- Titrate antihypertensive agents

Extubation
- Extubate awake, control pressure response

Adjuvants
- Magnesium sulfate for seizure prophylaxis and increased UBF; IV antihypertensive drugs (most often hydralazine, labetalol, nitroprusside, or nicardipine antepartum); rarely (but esp. in postpartum) dopamine to increase renal perfusion; finally, other inotropic support if demonstrable LV dysfunction

Postoperative Period
- Risk for developing pulm edema due to previous (appropriate) intravascular hydration
- Effective postcesarean analgesia beneficial in BP control

Anticipated Problems/Concerns

- Maternal Htn causes maternal morbidity/mortality; maternal hypotension causes fetoplacental hypoperfusion
- Eclampsia assoc with CNS residua

Pregnancy, Ectopic

Joseph Rosa III

Risk

- Implantation of fetus or blastocyst outside uterus
- Overall incidence, 1/90. More common in non-whites in 35–44 y; ⅓ – ½ have no identifiable risk factors
- Risk factors incl pelvic inflammatory disease, IUD, tubal surgery, prior ectopic, tubal ligation, smoking.

Perioperative Risks

- Second leading cause of maternal mortality (leading cause in 1st trimester), accounting for 14.7% of all maternal deaths; nearly 2× greater in nonwhites
- 85% of deaths due to hemorrhage, 5% due to infection, 2% due to anesthetic complications
- Highest mortality assoc with intra-abdominal and interstitial tubal pregnancies, 2° to larger size at time of Dx and therefore increased blood supply, and thus increased hemorrhage.

Worry About

- Hemorrhagic shock, decreasing intravascular volume
- Blood availability—may need type-specific or O neg blood
- Full-stomach/aspiration risk
- Consider physiologic changes of pregnancy if Dx made late in gestation, esp with intra-abdominal location (see Pregnancy, Intra-abdominal, in Diseases Section)

- If laparoscopic approach, consider effects of CO_2 insufflation and steep Trendelenburg position on ventilation. (see Laparoscopy, Gynecologic, in Procedures section)

Overview

- Primary concerns with ruptured ectopic are intravascular volume, and airway management
- Approach similar to a trauma with profound hypovolemia
- Differential Dx of abd pain: Appendicitis, any intra-abdominal infection or process. Dx made by Hx and physical—95% have pelvic pain, 75% amenorrhea, 60–80% uterine bleeding.
- β-hCG—elevated in 100% of ectopics, US to rule out intrauterine pregnancy. Laparoscopy useful in Dx of acute pelvic pain and to rule out ectopic.

ICD-9-CM Code: 633

Etiology

- Mechanical factors: Salpingitis, peritubal adhesions, previous ectopic, prior tubal surgery, multiple prior abortions
- Functional factors: External ovum migration, menstrual reflux, altered tubal motility

Usual Treatment

- Surgical
  - 70% of ectopics diagnosed before rupture; an acutely ruptured ectopic is a surgical emergency and thus an anesthetic emergency

- Salpingo-oophorectomy—advocated by some if the other adnexa appear normal and future pregnancy desired
  - Salpingectomy is most common treatment
  - Salpingostomy used to salvage unruptured tube
  - Laparoscopy: Diagnostic and can be used to remove small ectopic; associated with decreased morbidity and hospital stay
- Medical
  - Methotrexate used for unruptured small ectopics. Surgery avoided and possibly increased potential for future fertility.
- Combined surgical/medical management: Direct injection of methotrexate into fallopian tube
- Expectant management: Primarily used for small ectopics, follow β-hCG
- Prognosis: 40% of pts will never conceive again. Of the 60% who do conceive, 12% will have repeat ectopics and 15–20% will spontaneously abort.

ASSESSMENT POINTS

System	Effect	Assessment by Hx	PE	Test
HEENT		Snoring/difficult airway	Airway exam	
CV	Hypovolemia 2° to hemorrhage	Orthostatic dizziness	Vitals, neck veins, orthostatic vital signs Weak, thready pulse Cold legs and arms of vasoconstriction	
HEME	Blood loss 2° to rupture Hemoperitoneum/vaginal bleeding	Vaginal bleeding Orthostatic dizziness	Orthostatic vital signs	Hct
CNS	Hypoperfusion causing mental status changes and decreased urine production	CNS Hx	CNS exam	BUN/Cr UA

Key Reference: Current Mukul LV, Teal SB. Management of Ectopic Pregnancy. *Obstet Gynecol Clin North Am.* 2007;34:403–419.

Perioperative Management

Preoperative Preparation

- Assessment of volume status using clinical and laboratory measures
- 2 large bore peripheral IVs
- Blood availability—at least O neg; type-specific preferable
- Consideration of full stomach

Anesthetic Technique

- GA: Preferable in unstable pt with ruptured ectopic, if laparoscopy to be used or contraindication to regional
- Regional anesthesia: Spinal or epidural T2–T4 level needed; consider in hemodynamically stable pts

Monitoring

- Routine; once ectopic bleeding stopped, fluid resuscitation for replacement only; too zealous replacement can lead to pulm edema
- Consider arterial line placement in the hemodynamically unstable

Airway

- If difficult airway, awake fiberoptic; otherwise rapid-sequence induction and intubation

Induction/Maintenance

- If unstable, consider etomidate or ketamine, maintenance with O_2, inhalational, and narcotic with muscle relaxants
- Choice of drugs less important than anesthetic management

Surgical Stages

Induction

- Possible CV instability 2° to uncorrected hypovolemia, as well as full-stomach/aspiration potential
- Skin incision
  - Laparotomy for ruptured ectopic, hemoperitoneum and hypotension with uncontrolled bleeding. Upon opening abdomen, a release of tamponade may result in decreased BP.
    - Incision: Pfannenstiel or low midline
    - Laparoscopy: Infraumbilical and 1–4 suprapubic incisions. Peritoneal insufflation: Monitor

$ETCO_2$ and intraperitoneal pressures—should be <18 mm Hg. Potential for CO_2 embolus or intra-abdominal injury during introduction of the Veres needle.
- Dissection: Minimal to extensive depending on location of ectopic and degree of bleeding

Definitive Surgery

- Salpingectomy, ipsilateral oophorectomy—used for ruptured ectopic hysterectomy; may be necessary if interstitial implantation
- Salpingotomy
  - Technique of fallopian tube conservation
  - Can be performed via laparoscope; used to remove small ectopic <2 cm; preferred technique for unruptured ectopic
- Approximate duration: 1–2 hr
- Fluid shifts can be large with ruptured ectopic
- Closure: Minimal if laparoscopy; low midline or Pfannenstiel 15–20 min

Extubation

- Awake

Postoperative Period

- Blood loss may be extensive; check Hct
- Pain score: 4–6 laparoscopy, 5–8 laparotomy
- PCA or neuraxial narcotics; local anesthetics if regional ± neuraxial narcotics

- CV: Instability from massive hemorrhage from ruptured ectopic
- Potential for pulm edema, fluid overload in postop period due to massive crystalloid infusion and subsequent mobilization of third space fluid
- Postop shoulder and chest pain from unabsorbed gas and peritoneal irritation—30%
- Gastric dilation 3%, thrombophlebitis 3%, pulm embolism 2%, ureteral injury/stenosis 1% with laparotomy
- Postop infection, abscess

Pregnancy, Intra-Abdominal

Theodore G. Cheek

Risk

- Incidence in USA: 11/100,000 live births
- Higher incidence in African-Americans, Asians, and immigrant populations from Third World countries
- Higher incidence following in vitro fertilization procedures
- Maternal mortality 100 times that of intrauterine pregnancy

Perioperative Risks

- Usually misdiagnosed at the time of laparoscopy or exploratory laparotomy
- Exsanguinating hemorrhage possible preop, intraop, or postop

Worry About

- Severe hemorrhage

Overview

- Pt usually has a normal early pregnancy and presents with midtrimester abdominal pain, N/V, shock, partial bowel obstruction, and vaginal bleeding
- Correct Dx is made preoperatively in approx 10% of cases
- Differential Dx includes abruptio placentae, placenta previa, pelvic inflammatory disease, and bowel obstruction. MRI is better than US diagnosis
- Exsanguinating intra-abdominal bleeding can occur at any time.
- Cases of twin fetuses, one intrauterine and one extrauterine, have been described. Perinatal survival 5–25%.

ICD-9-CM Code: 761.4

Etiology

- Often results from a missed ruptured tubal ectopic pregnancy
- Fertilized ovum may implant anywhere in the peritoneal cavity, incl uterine surface, adnexa, and bowel

Usual Treatment

- Volume resuscitation
- Emergency diagnostic laparoscopy or exploratory laparotomy with delivery of the fetus. Excision of the placental implantation site complicated by life-threatening hemorrhage. Leaving in situ however may lead to infection.

ASSESSMENT POINTS

System	Effect	Assessment by Hx	PE	Test
CV	Hemorrhage	Postural dizziness	Hypovolemia, hypotension	Hct
GI	Bowel obstruction GI bleed if bowel implantation	N/V	GI bleed	Abd x-ray, CT, MRI, abd US falsely negative
CNS			Decreased consciousness if massive hemorrhage	

Key Reference: Gaither K. Abdominal Pregnancy – An obstetrical enigma. *South Med J.* 2007;100:347–348.

Perioperative Implications

Preoperative Preparation

- Assess volume status
- Fluid/blood resuscitation

Monitoring

- Arterial and central venous lines valuable if Dx known

Airway

- Rapid-sequence induction

Induction

- Rapid-sequence using ketamine or etomidate
- Two or three large venous access lines prior to induction

Maintenance

- Ensure vascular stability

Extubation

- May need to delay extubation for postoperative care
- Extubate awake

Adjuvants

- None

Postoperative Period

- May require intensive care if large fluid shifts or periop severe hypotension/hypoxia

Anticipated Problems/Concerns

- Hemorrhage, DIC

Pregnancy, Maternal Physiology

Stephanie R. Goodman

Risk

- Incidence in USA: Estimated 6.4 million pregnancies resulting in 4.1 million live births per year
- Pregnancy rate of 103 pregnancies per 1000 women between the ages of 15 and 44 y

Perioperative Risks

- Maternal mortality rate: 15 deaths per 100,000 live births in USA, 400 deaths per 100,000 live births in the world
- Hemorrhage and embolic disorders are two leading causes of maternal deaths.
- Risks of maternal mortality incl advanced maternal age, obesity, multifetal pregnancies, cesarean delivery and African-American race.

Worry About

- Difficult airway incl inability to intubate and ventilate due to maternal wt gain, breast enlargement, and swelling of oropharyngeal tissues (incidence of failed intubation 1:280 vs. 1:2230 in nonpregnant patients)
- Hypoxemia occurs more quickly during periods of apnea due to decreasing FRC and increasing O_2 consumption
- Aortocaval compression causing decreased uteroplacental perfusion and FHR late decelerations
- Hypercoagulability causing DVT/PE
- Aspiration pneumonitis

Overview

- Physiologic changes occur during pregnancy to allow maternal adaptation to the demands of the growing fetus, supporting placental unit, and ultimately to facilitate labor and delivery.
- These changes affect almost every organ system and influence the anesthetic and periop management of the pregnant woman.

- Adjust drug doses and administration schedules to compensate for increased volume of distribution, decreased peak plasma drug concentration, increased elimination $T_{1/2}$, and increased renal excretion

ICD-9-CM Code: v22.2 (Pregnancy)

Etiology

- Profound increases in hormonal concentrations, esp. progesterone
- Mechanical effects of an enlarging uterus
- Increased metabolic demand
- Presence of the low resistance placental circulation

Usual Treatment

- Normal spontaneous vaginal delivery
- C-section

ASSESSMENT POINTS

System	Effect	Assessment by Hx	PE	Test
HEENT	Capillary engorgement/swelling of nasal and oral pharynx, larynx, trachea Vocal cords and arytenoid edema	Epistaxis Voice changes Difficult nasal breathing/congestion	Careful airway exam Temporomandibular distance Mallampati class Neck ROM	
CARDIO	CO, SV, HR, ejection fraction↓ SVR, BP ↓ 3rd and 4th heart sounds Systolic ejection murmur Tricuspid and pulmonic regurgitation Peripheral edema	Palpitations Dizziness/pre-syncope	Auscultation of heart Pulse BP	EKG, ECHO, PA catheter (all rarely needed)
RESP	Tidal volume, resp rate ↑ FRC ↓ — *make sure to preoxygenate* Minute and alveolar ventilation ↑ *WELL!* PaO_2 ↑, $PaCO_2$ ↓ Elevated diaphragm	Dyspnea		CXR, ABG, PFTs (all rarely needed)
GI	↓ Lower esophageal sphincter tone ↓ Gastric emptying—only in labor ↓ Gallbladder emptying	GE reflux *more likely* Gallstones		RUQ US
RENAL	↑ RBF, GFR, Cr clearance ↓ Bicarbonate	↑ Drug clearance		↓ BUN, Cr, bicarbonate
HEME	↑↑ Plasma volume, ↑ RBC volume ↑ Coagulation factors (I, VII, VIII, IX, X, XII), ↑ clotting ↑ Plt turnover, fibrinolysis ↓ Albumin, $α_1$ acid glycoprotein	Physiologic anemia Leg pain, dyspnea Gestational thrombocytopenia	Pale, nail beds Homan's sign for DVT	Hg, Hct PT/PTT, lower extremity Doppler, V/Q scan, spiral CT Plt count, TEG
CNS	↓ MAC ↑ Pain threshold			
ENDO	↑ Insulin resistance Enlarged thyroid, ↓ TSH		Palpation of thyroid gland	Glucose Normal free T3 and T4
MS	↑ Lumbar lordosis ↑ Joint mobility	Back pain		

Key Reference: Gaiser R. Physiologic changes of pregnancy. In: Chestnut DH. *Obstetric anesthesia principles and practice.* 4th ed. Mosby; 2009:15–36 [Chapter 2].

Perioperative Implications

Preoperative Preparation

- Large-bore IV, consider a second IV if pt is at increased risk for bleeding
- Consider use of nonparticulate antacids and metaclopramide to decrease gastric acid and volume
- Keep pt with left uterine displacement to relieve aortocaval compression
- Good oropharynx exam to assess likelihood of difficult intubation
- Recommend NPO 6–8 hr prior to elective surgery

Monitoring

- Routine

Preinduction/Induction

- Need access to difficult airway equipment incl FOB, LMAs, and jet ventilation

- Use a short or stubby-handled laryngoscope, esp. in obese parturients
- Avoid nasal intubation due to increased risk of bleeding
- Preoxygenate with 100% O_2 at high-flow rates
- Use rapid sequence induction and cricoid pressure (Sellick maneuver) to decrease passive regurgitation of gastric acid into oropharynx
- ETT preferred to LMA to adequately protect against aspiration
- Pseudocholinesterase activity reduced, but recovery from succinylcholine usually not prolonged
- Decreased doses of induction agents needed

Maintenance

- Adjust ventilation to maintain $PaCO_2$ around 30 mmHg

- Decreased minimum alveolar concentration (MAC) for inhalation anesthetics.
- Avoid high dose inhalation agents due to uterine atony.
- High doses of opioids and/or benzodiazepines given prior to delivery can cause resp depression in the neonate.

Extubation

- Awake without residual NM blockade

Regional Anesthesia

- Spinal, epidural, combined spinal-epidural all possible techniques and usually preferred over GA for surgical delivery, esp. in the obese pt or one with apparent difficult airway
- Decreased dose of spinal or epidural local anesthetic achieves same dermatomal level as higher doses in nonpregnant adults

- Pharmacologic sympathectomy can cause severe hypotension at term
- Reduced response to vasopressors

Postoperative Period
- Pain can be treated with a combination of NSAIDs and preservative-free spinal or epidural morphine or PCA if GA is used

- Use compression stockings and early ambulation to lower the risk of DVT/PE
- Most physiologic changes of pregnancy resolve 6–8 wk postpartum

Anticipated Problems/Concerns
- Mallampati scores worsen during the progress of labor so the airway must be examined immediately prior to induction of GA

- Uterine artery blood flow 500 mL/min at term so obstetric hemorrhage can become life-threatening very quickly
- Increased risk of C-section with obesity, a common and increasing problem

Pregnancy-Induced Hypertension

Susan K. Palmer

Risk

- (PIH) incidence not known because Dx may not be made in hospital discharge summary unless it progresses to preeclampsia (PE) and/or eclampsia (EC)
- PE may occur in 5% of all pregnancies, but is more frequent in some pt populations.

Perioperative Risks

- Htn remains a top cause of maternal mortality.
- Progression to PE and/or EC is unpredictable and may occur up to 7 d postpartum.

Worry About

- Decreasing IVF volume in pts with interstitial volume overload
- Hyperresponsive to endogenous and exogenous vasopressors
- Decreased uteroplacental perfusion despite raised maternal BP
- Edema in larynx and airway

Overview

- Blood-borne placental factors activate maternal vascular endothelium, which then directly affects vascular smooth muscle (VSM) tone/growth, causing Htn; endothelium also regulates the adherence and transmigration of WBCs (inflammation) and stimulates the aggregation of plts (coagulation cascade); endothelium controls access to the interstitium throughout the body (permeability, edema).
- PIH: BP >140/90 *after* 20 wk gestation in previously normotensive pt; BP must show this elevation at least twice >6 hr apart and not assoc with uterine contraction
- PE: Above BP rise, plus evidence of other organ system involvement, e.g., proteinuria, nondependent edema, increased liver enzymes, decreased plt count, CNS dysfunction, low albumin
- Severe PE: *Either* BP >160/110 *or* proteinuria >5 g/24hr, *or* evidence of consumptive coagulopathy (DIC), *or* liver swelling and/or failure (epigastric or RUQ pain), *or* pulm edema (desaturation), *or* evidence of CNS edema (severe headache)
- Eclampsia: PIH and/or PE plus seizure; can occur up to 1 wk postpartum

ICD-9-CM Code: 642.11

- See also Eclampsia in Diseases section and Preeclampsia in Diseases section

Etiology

- Causation unknown, no animal models. Placental factors initiate maternal endothelial malfunction, which causes failure of normal CV adjustments needed for successful pregnancy and normal fetal growth.

Usual Treatment

- Control of BP, maintenance or improvement of uteroplacental perfusion, and prevention of seizures are primary goals.
- Epidural analgesia may relieve vasospasm and improve uteroplacental perfusion.
- Seizure prophylaxis can be accomplished with $MgSO_4$, benzodiazepine, barbiturate, or phenytoin.
- Delivery of fetus and all of placenta usually, but not always, followed by amelioration of symptoms

ASSESSMENT POINTS

System	Effect	Assessment by Hx	PE	Test
CARDIO	Vasospasm, ↑ CO (usually) ↓ IVF	↓ Exercise tolerance ↓ UO	Is there dyspnea at rest? BP check frequently	UA, 24-hr output BUN, uric acid, Cr, albumin
RESP	Swelling, edema in airway	"Hoarse" voice	Nasal obstruction?	Airway exam
HEME	↑ Hct, ↑ or ↓ plt ↓ Albumin ↑ BUN, Cr, uric acid			CBC Albumin, BUN, Cr Note than "normal" values for BUN/CR during pregnancy are ½ of non-pregnant values
RENAL	Oliguria Proteinuria			Oxytocin induction can cause IADHS ↓ UA, 24-hr quantified proteinuria
HEPATIC	↑ Enzymes	RUQ pain, jaundice		Liver enzymes
CNS	Cerebral edema	Anxiety, headache Hyperreflexia (DTR) Optic disc edema		

Key Reference: Roberts J, Redman CWG. Pre-eclampsia: More than pregnancy-induced hypertension. *Lancet* 1993;341:1447–1451.

Peripartum Implications

Preoperative Preparation

- PIH can go directly to EC, esp if BP is much higher than nonpregnant baseline. Before delivery, control BP using mostly vasodilators, since large doses of β-blockers raise intrauterine pressure, compromising fetoplacental circulation.
- Rapid-onset regional or general anesthesia may cause severe hypotension due to intravascular fluid deficit.

Monitoring

- Consider arterial line for BP management for severe PE or malignantly increasing BP
- Periop fluid challenge with plain balanced electrolyte solutions (with or without albumin) should increase renal output and improve fetal status. If no improvement, CVP/PA catheter may identify pts with low (<150% nonpregnant) cardiac output

(CO) who need both vasodilation and cardiac contractility improvement.
- Mg^{2+} blood levels or repeated exam of DTRs necessary to prevent overdosage in pts who may develop renal failure during labor

Airway

- Edema may obscure normal structures, making rapid-sequence intubation difficult or impossible
- Mask ventilation may be difficult if face, lips, tongue also swollen
- Awake, surface anesthetized, fiberoptic ETT tube placement recommended if airway is swollen or looks difficult. Avoid unopposed α-agonist in nasal spray because of systemic Htn.

Maintenance

- Pregnancy lowers MAC by 30% for all inhalation agents.

- All inhalation anesthetics cause uterine relaxation. May require greater than normal oxytocin infusion to contract uterus after delivery.

Extubation

- Extubate only when awake and strong, because half of maternal aspirations occur during emergence. Ensure that the airway will not become obstructed by increased edema.

Adjuvants

- Nerve stimulator can be used to monitor Mg^{2+}-potentiated effects of nondepolarizing muscle relaxants

Post Delivery

- Diuresis of interstitial fluid should occur
- Still at risk for progression to PE and EC for up to a wk

Preterm Infant

Jessica Miller

Risk

- Incidence in USA: <37 wk gestation, 12.8% of pregnancies; <34 wk gestation, 3.66%; <28wk gestation, 0.76% of all births in 2006
- Prematurity frequently correlates with birth wt. As birth wt declines, mortality in the first year increases. Low birth wt births comprised 8.3% of total births.
- VLBW (<1500 g) represented 1.5% of births in 2006 in USA
- ELBW (1000–1500 g), make up 0.7% of U.S. births.
- Micropremie (500–750 g): 50% survival rate

Perioperative Risks

- Inadequate oxygenation and ventilation, atelectasis, pneumothorax, tube displacement, O_2 toxicity, barotrauma
- Hypotension, limited ability to compensate for hypovolemia, risk of CV collapse
- Ductus arteriosus may shunt right to left with hypoxia, hypercapnia, hypervolemia, acidosis, hypothermia
- Hypoxic ischemic CNS injury due to poor perfusion and inadequate O_2 supply
- Intraventricular hemorrhage (IVH) common
- Apnea and bradycardia increases after exposure to anesthetic gases and sedation.
- Bleeding due to inadequate coagulation factors, spontaneous liver hemorrhage, thrombocytopenia
- Immature liver function resulting in altered drug metabolism, reduced albumin
- Hypothermia
- Elevated stress response worsening co-morbidities
- Electrolyte disturbances due to immature renal function

Worry About

- Resp status: Reduced reserve, presence of chronic lung disease (CLD), postop apnea
- Volume status and/or presence of anemia
- Normalize electrolytes and glucose levels preop
- Coagulation status: Thrombocytopenia, coagulation factor levels
- Adequate vascular access and ability to place invasive monitors

Overview

- Incidence of prematurity continues to increase, but mortality has decreased due to use of surfactant, perinatal steroid administration, specialization of NICU, and improved mechanical ventilation strategies.
- Immature organ systems present many challenges to delivery of anesthesia care.
- Pulmonary: Low lung volumes, decreased compliance, lack of surfactant production. V/Q mismatch, barotrauma, O_2 toxicity, and hypoxia. Long-term consequences: Bronchopulmonary dysplasia (BPD), chronic lung disease, reactive airway disease, O_2 requirement.
- Immature resp control leads to poor response to hypoxia and hypercarbia resulting in central apnea. Anatomic structures predispose to obstructive apnea. Increased risk of apnea with decreased gestational age and Hct <30%.
- Cardiac: CO dependent on HR. Structure of heart results in decreased ability to increase contractility, dependence on extracellular Ca^{2+}, poor response to catecholamines. Small blood volumes, impaired autoregulation, and anesthetic blunting of baroreceptors increases risk of CV collapse. High frequency of PDA causing pulm Htn and CHF.
- CNS: Watershed regions (periventricular white matter) are prone to hypoxic-ischemic injury during hypotension, low CO, hypoxemia, and hypocarbia. Incidence of IVH increased with pts with RDS, seizures, pneumothoraces, hypoxemia, acidosis, hypocarbia, use of vasopressor infusions. Long-term consequences of CNS injury incl developmental delay, behavioral abn, hearing and visual deficits, and cerebral palsy. Management of stress responses and pain reduce physiologic stress.
- CNS: Recent animal data regarding neuronal cell apotosis with exposure to anesthetic agents prompts considering avoidance or delay of elective surgeries in all infants.
- Retinopathy of prematurity (ROP) is common, incidence inversely proportional to birth wt and gestational age. Exposure to variations in arterial oxygenation and exposure to bright light play a role.

- GI/Liver: Preterm infants more susceptible to bilirubin encephalopathy due to immature neuronal protective mechanisms, hypoxia, infection. Cholestatic jaundice common with TPN use
- Renal: Immature kidneys can result in hyponatremia, elevated K^+ levels, and slower to achieve normal Cr clearance
- Endocrine: Prone to hypoglycemia due to decreased glycogen and body fat, and hyperglycemia due to insulin resistance, TPN, steroids, and poor insulin production
- Prone to hypothermia due to decreased keratin in epithelium, little fat, large surface area to mass ratio, poor thermoregulation. Hypothermia can result in bradycardia, coagulopathy, acidosis.
- Immature immune system, prone to sepsis
- Common surgeries in premature infants incl: Treatment of necrotizing enterocolitis, ligation of PDA, treatment of ROP, and inguinal hernia repair. In the unstable premature infants requiring HFOV or high level ventilatory support, may be preferable to perform surgery in the NICU. Surgical, nursing and anesthetic teams must be well coordinated to adapt to management in this environment.

ICD-9-CM Code: 765.x (Premature infant)

Etiology

- Multiple risk factors incl maternofetal endocrine activity, anatomic uterine factors, local or systemic inflammation, placental hemorrhage

Usual Treatment

- Optimization of care prior to surgery: Early surfactant use, antenatal glucocorticoids, appropriate nutrition, reduction of physiologic stress (handling, pain management).
- Minimizing inspired O_2 concentration and peak insp pressures, utilization of PEEP, maintain oxygenation at lowest safe level (90–95%), maintain ventilation with reduced I:E to minimize air trapping and barotrauma.
- Judicious fluid and colloid administration. Transfusion when appropriate based on O_2 supply and demand.
- Intracranial/intraventricular hemorrhage (IVH) incidence and severity reduced in pts receiving sedation with opioids, antenatal glucocorticoids, or indomethacin. Avoid rapid fluctuations in CBF, CBV, and cerebral venous pressure.

ASSESSMENT POINTS

System	Effect	Assessment by Hx	PE	Test
HEENT	Difficult airway	Assoc with common difficult airway syndromes, Hx in NICU	Morphology of airway esp. jaw, evaluation of breathing mechanics (stridor)	Not typically required unless obvious abn, x-ray, head and neck CT, MRI
	Intracranial bleed	Intracranial hemorrhage	Fontanel	Cranial US
	ROP		Ophthalmology exam	Optho exam under anesthesia
RESP	RDS/ BPD	Risk factors, use of supplemental O_2	Resp rate (>60 abn)	CXR
	Resp failure	Hx/frequency of apnea	Intercostal retractions	Blood gases
	Pneumonia	Intubated and/or ventilated	Grunting	
	Pneumothorax	Fever curves, increasing O_2 requirement	Rales or rhonchi	
			Absent/decreased breath sounds, SubQ emphysema	
CVS	Hypovolemia	Vital signs chart	HR (120–160), murmur	ECG, ECHO
	Hypervolemia	Wt chart	Bounding pulses (PDA), BP normal	CXR
	PDA	UO	Liver enlarged (CHF), edema: feet or eyelids	
	CHF	Inotropes infusing		

Continued

System	Effect	Assessment by Hx	PE	Test
HEME	Anemia	Precipitous delivery, placental bleeding	Tachycardia, hypotension, poor growth rate	CBC, retic count
	Sepsis	Perinatal exposures	Recent change in physiologic status-activity, resp function, CV stability, peripheral perfusion	WBC and differential, Plt count
	Coagulopathy	Birth asphyxia (low factors) Vitamin K given Bleeding	Purpura, occult bleeding	PT, INR, fibrinogen
METAB	↑ or ↓ glucose, ↑ Temp Hypocalcemia, hypomagnesemia Hyperbilirubinemia Na^+ or K^+ disturbance	Review charts and reports	Twitching Seizures Hypotension	Serum electrolytes, Ca^{2+}, Mg^{2+} Blood glucose, indirect bilirubin levels

Key Reference: Henderson-Smart DJ, Steer P. Postoperative caffeine for preventing apnea in preterm infants. *Cocrane Database Syst Rev*. 2000;CD000048.

Perioperative Implications

Preoperative Preparation
- Reassess cardiopulmonary and volume status
- Correct metabolic status
- Treat coagulopathy (Vitamin K, FFP, cryo, plt)
- Warm the OR, prepare warming devices, maintain temp during transport
- NPO: 2-hr fast for clear fluids, 4-hr fast for breastmilk and/or formula
- Assess IV access
- Determine location of surgery: ICU vs. OR
- Prepare appropriate dilute vasopressor solutions, IV calcium, epinephrine, atropine.

Monitoring
- Precordial or esophageal stethoscope
- Preductal and postductal SpO_2, ECG, BP cuff, temperature
- $ETCO_2$, arterial line for major procedures
- Make sure all monitors and/or lines are secure

Airway
- Large tongue, small mouth may lead to difficulty
- Anesthetize prior to intubation to avoid elevated ICP
- Prepare multiple sizes of ETT to account for possible subglottic stenosis

- With pre-existing ETT: Reassess position, suction to clear of secretions, position to minimize kinking

Induction
- Inhalational induction (uncommon except for outpatients with minor surgery): Careful titration of sevoflurane, monitor BP carefully, anticipate challenging IV access
- Alternatively, thiopental (1–2 mg/kg) plus fentanyl 5–10 µg/kg followed by relaxant
- In minor surgery: IV caffeine can reduce postop apnea

Maintenance
- Low concentrations of inhalational agent, fentanyl to control hemodynamics, paralytic to optimize surgical and ventilatory parameters, control ventilation but avoid hyperventilation
- BP is most reliable to indicate hypovolemia
- Infuse glucose at 4–6 mg/kg/min and monitor blood glucose levels with a glucometer
- Monitor hemoglobin if bleeding present. Administration of blood products frequently accompanied by IV Ca^{2+} due to myocardial dependence on extracellular Ca^{2+} and inability of liver to rapidly metabolize citrate. Monitor K^+ levels carefully.

- Monitor acid-base status, lactate production. Lower threshold to treat metabolic acidosis due to myocardial sensitivity to acidosis, consider THAM versus sodium bicarbonate.

Extubation
- Longer recovery time due to drug metabolism. Likely to need slow weaning from resp support.

Postoperative Period
- Continue cardiorespiratory monitoring, temp maintenance, NICU care
- Minor surgery: Pts <56 wk PCA should be placed on apnea monitor and observed for 24 hr, need to be apnea free at least 12 hr prior to discharge. Anemia increases risk of apnea and/or bradycardia. Extreme caution in discharging formerly preterm infants <60 wk PCA to home if opioids required for pain control.

Anticipated Problems/Concerns
- Risk of massive hemorrhage in major surgeries, can be difficult to obtain surgical control.
- Hypothermia
- Postop apnea
- Pain control necessary, monitor for affects on ventilation, hemodynamics

Protein C Deficiency

Charles Weissman

Risk

- Congenital deficiency: Homozygote is estimated at 1/500,000–1/750,000 live births. Occurs when gene coding for Protein C on both chromosomes #2 are affected.
- Heterozygote ~0.2–0.4% of healthy population; 2–5% of pts with DVT
- Acquired deficiency also seen

Perioperative Risks

- Pts with Protein C deficiency are at risk for venous thrombosis and pulm embolism (immobility, endothelial damage, and decreased blood flow during periop period may be triggers)

Worry About

- Increased incidence of thrombophlebitis and pulm embolism
- Thrombosis of other vessels, such as intracerebral and coronary arteries, can occur

Overview

- Protein C is a vitamin K–dependent protein found in blood and synthesized in liver.
- Protein C activated after forming complex with thrombin on endothelial cell receptor thrombomodulin; facilitated by binding to endothelial cell Protein C receptor
- Inhibits blood coagulation by proteolytic inactivation of factors V and VIII
- Protein S is a cofactor of Protein C
- Stimulates fibrinolysis possibly by neutralizing plasminogen activator inhibitors
- Deficiency causes hyperthrombotic state
- During systemic inflammatory response syndrome (SIRS) and sepsis there is decreased synthesis of Protein C.

ICD-9-CM Code: 286.9 (Coagulation factor deficiency)

Etiology

- Inherited: Autosomal dominant with variable expressivity
- Homozygotes develop life-threatening visceral vessel thrombosis or purpura fulminans (massive cutaneous necrosis) in early neonatal period.
- Heterozygotes may develop venous thrombosis and thromboembolism (rare prior to age 20 y); Protein C levels 35–65% of normal)
- Acquired causes: Hepatic dysfunction, vitamin K deficiency, DIC

Usual Treatment

- Heterozygotes
  - If acute thrombosis; start heparinization (heparin or high dose LMWH)
  - Long-term anticoagulation with warfarin in pts with Hx of thrombosis. (Heparin therapy continued until warfarin is at therapeutic levels to prevent skin necrosis.)
  - With acute thrombosis may need transfusions of FFP to increase Protein C levels
  - Pregnancy: Treat with LMWH during and for a few weeks after delivery.
- Homozygotes
  - Periodic FFP or purified Protein C concentrate transfusions to provide Protein C
- Acquired
  - Vitamin K deficiency: Parenteral vitamin K
  - DIC: Treatment of underlying cause

ASSESSMENT POINTS

System	Effect	Assessment by Hx	PE	Test
HEENT	Retinal vein thrombosis	Hx of vision problems	Ophthalmoscopic exam	
CARDIO	MI Angina Peripheral arterial disease	Hx of MI, angina Peripheral vascular thrombosis	Peripheral pulses	ECG
RESP	Pulm embolism	Hx of previous pulm embolism		
GI	Mesenteric thrombosis	Hx of bowel infarction		
HEME	Thrombophlebitis	Hx (and family Hx) of thrombophlebitis, pulm embolism	Exam of veins in legs, evidence for lower extremity postthrombotic syndrome	Screen for hypercoagulable state: PTT, Protein C & S; factor V Leiden; antiphospholipid antibody, antithrombin 3.
RENAL	Renal vein and artery thrombosis	Hx of renal problem		BUN/Cr Urine protein
DERM	Necrosis	Cutaneous necrosis after warfarin is begun	Cutaneous necrosis	
CNS	Intracerebral artery thrombosis	Hx of CVA, TIA	Neurologic exam	

Key Reference: Goldenberg NA, Manco-Johnson MJ. Protein C deficiency. *Haemophilia*. 2008;14:1214–1221.

Perioperative Implications

Preoperative Preparation

- Homozygotes and symptomatic heterozygotes: FFP and Protein C concentrates can be administered to increase protein C levels.
- Warfarin can be stopped a few days before surgery to allow PT to return to normal range and heparin administered until surgery.
- Intermittent pneumatic compression stocking can be placed prior to induction of anesthesia.

Airway

- Some have suggested that the ETT cuff not be inflated to prevent tracheal venous thrombosis.
- In neonates, there should be an audible leak.

Preinduction/Induction

- Regional anesthesia may be preferable, if possible.

Maintenance

- Special attention can be paid to positioning to reduce venous and arterial stasis.
- FFP and/or Protein C concentrates should be given to pts with prior thrombotic manifestations and for prolonged operations.

Adjuvants

- Intermittent pneumatic compression stockings can be used.
- Postop heparinization should be started as soon as deemed safe.

Anticipated Problems/Concerns

- Increased risk of thrombosis, esp. thrombophlebitis and pulm embolism
- When switching from heparin anticoagulation to warfarin, heparin should be continued until warfarin has achieved therapeutic effect to decrease risk of skin necrosis.

Pulmonary Atresia

Nirvik Pal

Risk

- Pulm atresia with intact ventricular septum (PA/IVS) happens in 3% of all congenital heart diseases (CHD) and prevelence of 0.07/1000 live births.
- Pulmonary atresia with ventricular septal defect (PA/VSD) happens in 3.4% of all CHD and about 20% of all tetralogy of Fallots' (TOF).
- Males are affected more than females.

Perioperative Risks

- RV failure (volume overload, pressure overload or both)
- Hypoxemia (metabolic acidosis)
- Myocardial ischemia

Worry About

- RV-dependent coronary circulation (rapid boluses of fluid through central line may precipitate myocardial ischemia)
- Maintaining a patent ductus arteriosus (continue prostaglandin infusion)
- Suicide RV (sudden release of PV obstruction leading to hyperdynamic RV and subpulmonic obstruction of RV outlet. Treatment: β blockade)

- Hyperventilation and hyperoxia: Excess pulm steal and low cardiac output syndrome and necrotizing colitis (maintain O_2 saturation to 70–80%)

Overview

- Assoc with other cardiac lesions, e.g., patent foramen ovale, patent ductus arteriosus, possible VSD, ASD
- High-risk infant
- PA and/or IVS is often assoc in varying extent to RV maldevelopment, TV hypoplasia and stenosis and RV-dependent coronary blood flow. Severe form of PA and/or IVS is another extreme of same spectrum as critical PV stenosis.
- PA and/or VSD on the other hand is an extreme form of tetralogy of Fallot. Due to the presence of VSD, these pts may not have a maldeveloped RV but present with multiple major aorto-pulmonary collateral arteries (MAPCA) trying to compensate for the maldeveloped PA.

ICD-9-CM Code: 424.3

Etiology

- Congenital

Usual Treatment

- Prostaglandin E_1 infusion
- Systemic to pulm shunt
- Infective endocarditis prophylaxis
- Palliative therapy

Surgical Treatment

- PA with VSD (usually RV well developed):
  - Blalock-Taussig shunt (BTS) followed by VSD closure and valved conduit (Rastelli's procedure)
  - If multiple MAPCAs present then unifocalization, followed by VSD closure and valved conduit (Rastelli's procedure)
- PA with IVS (often under-developed RV and coronary artery obstruction):
  - Extent of coronary artery obstruction:
    a) None: Radiofrequency perforation of inter-atrial septum and balloon dilatation, followed by staged BTS, Glenn shunt and total cavopulmonary connection (TCPC), and/or heart transplant.
    b) Minimal: Staged surgery with BTS, Glenn shunt, TCPC, and/or heart transplant.
    c) Severe: Heart transplant.

ASSESSMENT POINTS

System	Effect	Assessment by Hx	PE	Test
CARDIO	RV failure Hypoxemia Metabolic acidosis	SOB	Cyanosis Metabolic acidosis	ECG—RA enlargement, ECG-QRS axis 30-90° CXR—Left- or right-sided arch CXR—↓ pulm vascular markings ABGs ECHO—PV annulus size, flow across PV, TV size and function, infundibular atresia, ductus arteriosus, PA branches and size Cardiac cath—confirm ECHO findings and detect state of coronary blood flow, MAPCAs
RESP	↓ Pulm blood flow	SOB	Tachypnea	ECHO, cardiac catheterization
SYSTEMIC	Signs of RV failure	Hepatomegaly		

Key Reference: Lake CL; Booker PD. *Pediatric cardiac anesthesia.* 4th ed. 2005.

Perioperative Implications

Preoperative Diagnosis
- PA/IVS versus pulm valve stenosis or PA and/or VSD versus TOF

Preoperative Considerations
- Catheterization suite intervention vs. surgical intervention
- Patency of PDA
- Reduced pulm blood flow
- Avoid hyperoxia and hyperventilation
- RV hypoplasia
- RV-dependent coronary circulation
- Type of shunt to be performed
- Which systemic artery is to be used for shunt? Don't stick it during CVP attempts.
- Degree of hypoxemia, metabolic acidosis

Monitoring
- Standard ASA monitors
- A-Line
  - Umbilical artery if good trace
  - Radial artery: Opposite side of shunt
  - Could clamp (partially) subclavian artery: Same implication for pulse oximeter placement
- CVP for resuscitation drugs

- Temp/warmers
- Bubble precaution

Airway
- ET

Preinduction/Induction
- Do not be rushed
- Continue prostaglandin infusion (0.03–0.1 µg/kg/min). Patent ductus arteriosus needs to be open, as it may be keeping baby alive
- Inhalational preferred: May help relax RV infundibulum
- Intubation: Smooth and quick by experienced individual
- $ETCO_2$ significantly underestimates $PaCO_2$
- Goals: Decreased PVR, increased SVR, adequate preload, normal HR, normal contractility (maintains flow through pulm circuit)
- Hypoxemia, bradycardia disastrous
- Avoid increase in pulm vascular resistance (coughing, bucking; increased PEEP; increased CO_2; decreased Po_2)

Maintenance
- Hemodynamically stable anesthetic, e.g., ketamine plus low-dose narcotic or inhalational agent

- Normal heart rate: Avoid bradycardia, tachycardia
- Normothermia
- Normal filling volumes
- Normal myocardial contractility
- Aiming for early extubation

Extubation
- As early as reasonably safe

Postoperative Care
- Provided in the area where most physicians and nurses are thoroughly experienced in pediatric care
- Prostaglandin infusion maintained

Anticipated Problems/Concerns

- Palliative surgery only
- Definitive procedure later, e.g., Fontan, Rastelli
- Hypoxemia progressing: Inadequate shunt/ductus closing
- Tachypnea worsening: Hypoxemia, laryngeal swelling, pneumothorax (small chest tube easily occluded)

Pulmonary Embolism

Ronald G. Pearl

Risk

- Incidence in USA: 600,000/y
- No racial predilection
- Risk factors are those for deep venous thrombosis

Perioperative Risks

- Risk for hypoxemia and right heart failure
- Periop mortality of ~90% for acute thromboendarterectomy, of ~10% for chronic thromboendarterectomy
- Postop pulm embolism in up to 1% of surgical pts
- Pulm embolism accounts for 20–30% of deaths assoc with pregnancy

Worry About

- Recurrent pulm embolism (30% mortality if not treated)
- Right heart failure and CV collapse
- Hypoxemia
- Hemorrhage in pts on anticoagulants or thrombolytics

Overview

- Pulm embolism found in ~20% of autopsied pts
- Clinical presentation may range from asymptomatic to chest pain and hypoxemia to CV collapse depending on magnitude of the embolus
- Signs (tachycardia, tachypnea, calf swelling) and symptoms (dyspnea, pleuritic chest pain, calf pain) have low sensitivity and specificity
- Most pts have DVT (surgical pts may have pelvic vein thrombi).
- Dx involves a combination of clinical suspicion, ventilation-perfusion lung scan, evaluation of the deep venous system of the legs, and spiral lung CT scan; pulm angiogram rarely required
- Negative D-dimer test excludes Dx in selected pts

ICD-9-CM Code: 415.1

Etiology

- Acquired disease
- Risk factors present in almost all pts: age >40 y, obesity, malignancy, recent surgery, trauma, pregnancy, immobilization, estrogen use, prior Hx of DVT, hypercoagulable state (factor V Leiden, deficiency of Protein C, Protein S, or antithrombin III)

Usual Treatment

- Therapy decreases mortality from 30% to <5%
- Heparin (PTT 1.5–2.5 × normal) followed by warfarin sodium (INR 2–3) for most pts; LMWH and fondaparinux are at least as effective as dose-adjusted continuous IV unfractionated heparin
- Thrombolytic therapy for massive pulm embolism
- Vena caval filter if massive pulm embolism or if cannot receive anticoagulants
- Surgical or catheter thrombectomy in selected cases of acute massive pulm embolism
- Surgical thromboendarterectomy in selected cases of chronic thromboembolic pulm Htn

ASSESSMENT POINTS

System	Effect	Assessment by Hx	PE	Test
CARDIO	RV failure	Syncope Dyspnea Palpitations	↑ JVP; RV heave Hypotension Tachycardia Hepatojugular reflux	ECG ECHO
RESP	Pulm infarction V/Q abn Pain from pleural irritation	Hemoptysis Chest pain Shoulder pain Dyspnea Orthopnea	Tachypnea Pleural rub Wheezing	CXR, SaO_2 ABGs Lung V/Q scan Spiral CT scan Pulm angio
CNS	Syncope	Syncope		
MS	Phlebitis	Hx DVT Leg edema Leg pain	Leg edema Inflammation Palpable cord	Compression ultrasonography Impedance plethysmography Venography CT scan (combined with lung)

Key Reference: Konstantinides S. Clinical practice. Acute pulmonary embolism. *N Engl J Med.* 2008;359:2804–2813.

Perioperative Implications

Preoperative Preparation

- Preop Rx with heparin/LMWH and sequential compression devices, which decrease incidence of periop DVT and PE
- If active DVT, consider preop vena caval filter.

Monitoring

- Consider PA catheter.
- TEE may demonstrate RV dysfunction and PA thromboembolism.

Airway

- None

Preinduction/Induction

- May develop hypotension due to RV failure

Maintenance

- Adequate preload essential to RV function
- Systemic vasoconstrictors for hypotension due to RV failure
- Inhaled vasodilators (NO, prostacyclin) for refractory RV failure

Extubation

- None

Regional Anesthesia

- Appropriate, esp. if compatible with continued anticoagulation

Postoperative Period

- Resume anticoagulation as soon as possible (or use IVC filter)

Anticipated Problems/Concerns

- RV failure with systemic hypotension may be initial presentation of PE or may develop with recurrent PE
- Consider PE in all postop pts with unexplained hypoxemia or hypotension

Purpura, Immune Thrombocytopenic (ITP)

Evan G. Pivalizza
Olga Pawelek

Risk

- Rare
- Children, M:F ratio: 1:1
- Adults, M:F ratio: 2–4:1 (pregnancy 1/1000 deliveries, 5% of thrombocytopenia in pregnancy, esp. if present in first trimester)

Perioperative Risks

- Hemorrhage (mortality for splenectomy 1%, one-third of which related to bleeding)
- Infection and thrombocytosis postsplenectomy

Worry About

- Preop corticosteroids, immunosuppressives
- Splenectomy
- Hemorrhage (mucosal when plt <20,000 × 10^3/mm³, severe risk (incl intracranial hemorrhage) with plt <10,000 × 10^3/mm³).

Overview

- Acute, intermittent, or chronic immune-mediated thrombocytopenia (accelerated destruction with appropriate megakaryocyte response); dermal, mucosal, and CNS hemorrhage (most critical)
- Obstetric implications incl risk of transient neonatal thrombocytopenia

ICD-9-CM Code: 287.3

Etiology

- Antiplatelet IgG auto-antibodies target pH membrane glycoproteins. Leads to premature removal by spleen and RES.

Usual Treatment

- Corticosteroids: Initial therapy (1 mg/kg/d) with 30–60% response rates (up to 80% initially)
- IV immunoglobulin G (0.4–1 g/kg/d)
- Anti-D (if Rh⁺ pt) cheaper, easier than IV IgG
- Splenectomy: Defer as long as possible in children. Increasingly laparoscopic (requires disruption of spleen into bag before extraction to prevent splenosis). In chronic disease, indicated if steroids cannot be tapered or poor response to therapy. In acute disease, indicated for failed medical response and plt transfusion.
- Other second line: Azathioprine, vincristine, rituximab
- Platelets: Although have very short survival, may temporarily elevate pH count

ASSESSMENT POINTS

System	Effect	Assessment by Hx	PE	Test
HEENT	Airway manipulation—potential hemorrhage	Oral bleeding		
CVS	Vascular access			
HEME	Thrombocytopenia	Hemorrhage	Petechiae	Platelets <20–50,000 × 10^3/mm³ (depending on author), megakaryocytes, antiplatelet antibody
CNS	Hemorrhage in acute disease			Radiology if indicated
OB	Controversy predicting neonate at risk (10–15%) and mode of delivery			

Key Reference: Choi S, Brull R. Neuraxial techniques in obstetric and non-obstetric patients with common bleeding disorders. *Anesth Analg.* 2009;109:648–660.

Perioperative Implications

Preoperative Preparation

- Consult with hematology. Consider steroids, IV IgG ± anti-D to raise plt count
- Steroid supplement if already receiving
- Premedication: Avoid IM injections
- Pneumococcal, meningococcal vaccine (+ *Haemophilus* in children)

Monitoring

- Routine
- Protect pressure points and mucosal surfaces

Airway

- Avoid nasal ET intubation
- Careful instrumentation, esp. with plt count <50,000 × 10^3/mm³

Induction

- Avoid hypertensive response to ET intubation, esp. with plt count <10-20,000 × 10^3/mm³ (CNS risk)

Platelets

- If required, transfuse after splenic pedicle ligation. Intraop monitoring of plt function (e.g., thrombelastography) may be useful guide to replacement therapy (case reports).

Extubation

- As above: Care of mucous membranes and hemodynamic response

Adjuvants

- Although recombinant factor VIIa traditionally requires adequate plt count to facilitate generation of thrombin burst, case reports and in vitro data of successful use in pts with thrombocytopenia and ITP (20-30,000 × 10^3/mm³).
- Individual analysis of risk-benefit for neuraxial technique, esp. in parturient. Authors recommend plt count range >50 – 100 × 10^3/mm³ pt with reports of point-of-care testing (e.g., thromboelastography) in decision making. If time, consider steroids, IV IgG ± anti-D to raise plt count.

Postoperative Period

- Risks of thrombocytosis not as crucial as TTP

Anticipated Problems/Concerns

- Massive surgical hemorrhage
- CNS and airway hemorrhage

Purpura, Thrombotic Thrombocytopenic (TTP)

Evan G. Pivalizza
Omonele O. Nwokolo

Risk

- Rare (1/1 million), adult, pregnancy may be predisposing factor, 80% 6-mo survival

Perioperative Risks

- Pt for splenectomy with failed medical therapy. Risks of microthrombi with CNS and renal dysfunction combined with thrombocytopenia

Worry About

- Preop drugs and therapies
- CNS, renal dysfunction
- Thrombocytopenia (although usual quantitative plt triggers do not apply)

Overview

- Severe microvascular occlusive disease characterized by thrombocytopenia, microangiopathic hemolytic anemia, multisystem organ involvement (particularly CNS and kidney), considered part of spectrum of disease with hemolytic uremic syndrome (HUS)

ICD-9-CM Code: 446.6

Etiology

- Assoc with ultra-large von Willebrand factor (vWF) proteins (congenital or acquired deficiency of protease to cleave large vWF), which promote plt aggregation and endothelial damage, all leading to thrombotic occlusion of microcirculation.
- May be assoc with ticlopidine, malignancy
- Has been described post-cardiac, vascular, and abd surgery

Usual Treatment

- Parity of RCTs, combination of therapies:
- Plasmapheresis (exchange): More NB than plasma infusion *primary* therapy (plt-poor FFP) usually with rapid clinical response
- Plt aggregator inhibitors once plt count >50 × 10³/mm³ (aspirin, dipyridamole)
- Steroids: Adjuvant (methylprednisolone 1 g/day)
- Immunosuppression second line: Vincristine (risk of neurotoxicity, abn ADH secretion),
- Splenectomy: For failed medical response, prevention relapse
- Avoid plt transfusion

ASSESSMENT POINTS

System	Effect	Assessment by Hx	PE	Test
HEENT	Airway manipulation, potential hemorrhage			
CARDIO	Rare conduction pathway involvement		Baseline MAP for perfusion CNS/kidney Vascular access	ECG
RESP	Rare infiltrates causing hypoxemia			CXR
RENAL	Proteinuria, hematuria, ARF <common than HUS			BUN, serum Cr, urine sediment
HEME	Thrombocytopenia	Hemorrhage	Petechiae Jaundice	Plt 8000–44,000 × 10³/mm³; PT, PTT, fibrinogen, antithrombin usually normal. Fragmented RBCs (Hgb 8–9 g/dl); ↑ LDH, bilirubin
CNS	Fluctuating course	Spectrum—headache, seizures, coma		Lumbar puncture, EEG, neuroradiology studies
OB	May precipitate episode or relapse	Differentiate from HELLP/PIH (> CNS, < hepatic involvement, not improved post partum)		

Key References: Kam PCA, Thompson SA, Liew ACS. Thrombocytopenia in the parturient. *Anaesthesia.* 2004;59:255–264.
Benington SR, McKillop A, Macartney I, Burns S. TTP following TURP. *Anaesthesia.* 2009;64:1018–1021.

Perioperative Implications

Preoperative Preparation

- Steroid supplement if receiving
- Premedication: Not IM, caution with CNS involvement
- Pneumococcal, meningococcal (*Haemophilus* for children) if for splenectomy

Monitoring

- Protect skin, mucous membrane (NIBP cuff, esophageal probe, pressure points)
- Usually have central access for plasma exchange If required, avoid subclavian if possible (difficulty compressing hematoma).
- Theoretical risk of radial arterial line with thrombotic process

Airway

- Avoid nasal ETT. Careful instrumentation, esp. if plt count <50,000 × 10³/mm³.

Induction

- Avoid sympathetic intubation response (CNS disease spectrum), maintain MAP > CNS, renal autoregulatory thresholds (>50–60 mmHg)

Maintenance

- Theoretical advantage of inhibitory effect volatile anesthetics on plt aggregation

Fluids

- Do NOT transfuse plt unless life-threatening thrombocytopenia: Reports of deterioration due to further microthrombi
- Bleeding managed with RBCs (>48 hr old to avoid active plts) and FFP (plt-poor)

Extubation

- As above: Care of mucous membranes and hemodynamic response

Adjuvants

- Individual analysis of risk benefit for neuraxial technique in thrombocytopenic pt (if in remission)

Postoperative Period

- Mobilize early: Precipitous increase in plt count and viscosity with risk of thrombotic events

Anticipated Problems/Concerns

- Hemorrhage if life-threatening thrombocytopenia (no plt transfusion until then)
- Microthrombi with CNS dysfunction

Pyloric Stenosis

Inna Maranets

Risk

- Incidence: 1/300–1/1000 of all live births
- Children of affected parents have higher incidence (3–5%)
- Male predominance

Perioperative Risks

- Similar to other abd procedures in pts of same age
- Some association with GU anomalies
- Some have elevated unconjugated bilirubin related to decreased glucuronyl transferase activity; returns to normal after correction of stenosis

Worry About

- Full stomach. Recurrent emesis leads to dehydration, electrolyte imbalance, and alkalosis
- Typically hypochloremic, hyperkalemic metabolic alkalosis

Overview

- Reduced size of gastric outlet impedes emptying of contents, which can cause abn nutrition, gastric distension, repeated vomiting, and dehydration
- Onset of symptoms 3–6 wk of age
- Usually surgically cured

ICD-9-CM Code: 750.5 (Congenital)

Etiology

- Almost exclusively genetic in infants
- Can be acquired in adults

Usual Treatment

- Normalize fluid/electrolyte status: This is not a surgical emergency
- Surgical: Pyloromyotomy can usually be undertaken within 2–24 hr of admission (unless fluid derangements are severe)
- Short procedure (<1 hr): Open or laparoscopic

ASSESSMENT POINTS

System	Effect	Assessment by Hx	PE	Test
GI	Gastric outlet obstruction	Nonbilious projectile emesis	Pyloric "olive" palpable in upper abd	Contrast study Abd us

Key Reference: Schapiro F, Litman RS. Pyloromyotomy. In: Litman RS, ed. *Pediatric anesthesia practice.* Cambridge University Press, 2007:173–175.

Perioperative Implications

Preoperative Preparation
- Correct fluid and acid-base deficits
- Pyloric stenosis is not a surgical emergency

Monitoring
- Routine

Airway
- Full stomach

Preinduction/Induction
- IV atropine 0.02 mg/kg/min dose 0.15 mg
- Empty stomach with orogastric tube or suction catheter
- Consider awake intubation or IV rapid-sequence induction, esp. if pt received barium contrast.
- Hypoxemia is common during rapid-sequence induction; ventilate with cricoid pressure.

Maintenance
- No technique is absolutely contraindicated by pyloric stenosis alone.
- Inhalational agent in O_2 and air or N_2O, short or intermediate-acting muscle relaxant
- Avoid opioids
- Local infiltration with bupivacaine or ropivacaine by surgeon
- IV fluids should be warmed
- Replacemnt fluids: LR 1–2 mL/kg/hr
- May consider using D5W, if the procedure lasts more than 1 hr

Extubation
- Potential of full stomach; suction stomach prior to extubation
- Reverse NM blocking agent
- Awake extubation
- Delayed awakening is common

Adjuvants
- Consider potential of assoc liver and GU abn

Postoperative Period
- Potential for central apnea and reactive hypoglycemia
- Pulse oxymetry/apnea monitoring for the first 12–24 hr
- Continue IV glucose until adequate PO intake
- Pain score: 2–5, acetaminophen is usually sufficient

Anticipated Problems/Concerns

- Potential for full stomach
- Need to correct fluid and/or electrolyte imbalances preop
- Delayed awakening is common

Q Fever

Thomas A. Russo
Paul R. Knight, III

DISEASES

Risk

- Greatest after direct or indirect exposure to infected cattle, sheep, or goats; particularly at parturition
- Less from a variety of other animals, rarely from blood products
- Abattoir workers, veterinarians, and other animal workers at greatest risk
- Pts with immune impairment are at a higher risk (e.g., HIV, steroids)
- Mortality 2.4% overall, chronic infection ~16%

Perioperative Risks

- Decreased resp reserve 2° to pneumonia
- Decreased myocardial reserve 2° to endocarditis
- Further increase in hepatocellular injury if there is liver involvement

Worry About

- 2° resp complications
- Decreased myocardial performance and emboli with endocarditis
- Hepatic or neurologic involvement

Overview

- Acute infection: Asymptomatic (~50%) to moderate severity (2% hospitalized)
- Acute symptomatic disease presents as non-specific febrile syndrome ± pneumonitis (~50%), hepatitis (80% +), pericarditis and/or myocarditis (<5%), neurologic disease (<5%)
- Chronic disease occurs in <1% of infections, usually without fever
- Chronic disease, primarily endocarditis (particularly abn or prosthetic valves) and occasionally bone

ICD-9-CM Code: 083.0

Etiology

- *Coxiella burnetii* is a fastidious, obligate, intracellular bacterium
- Spore stage can withstand harsh environmental conditions for prolonged periods, facilitating indirect transmission
- Highly infectious (1–10 organisms) primarily by inhalation, unpasteurized milk, or tick bite
- Incubation period ~20 d (range, 3–40 d)
- Bacterium targets reticuloendothelial cells, and develops into granuloma

Usual Treatment

- DX: Epidemiologic circumstance and serology (positive in 2–4 wk)
- Acute disease: Doxycycline or quinolones for 2–3 wk hastens resolution
- Chronic disease: Doxycycline and rifampin for 1–3 y, ± valve replacement with endocarditis

ASSESSMENT POINTS

System	Effect	Assessment by Hx	PE	Test
CARDIO	Endocarditis Immune-complex vasculitis Microthromboembolism	Rash, ↓ exercise tolerance	Clubbing, rash, murmurs, petechiae	ECHO ECG, culture negative
RESP	Atypical pneumonia, asymptomatic pneumonia, rapidly progressive pneumonia, interstitial pulm fibrosis	Pleuritic chest pain, cough, dyspnea	Consolidation, rales, pleural effusions	CXR, sputum cultures
GI	Acute hepatitis	N/V, fatigue, diarrhea, sweats and chills	Hepatomegaly or hepatosplenomegaly	SGOT, SGPT, bilirubin, granulomas on liver biopsy
HEME	Hyperglobulinemia, anemia, thrombocytosis-cytopenia	Easy fatigue, bleeding tendency	Pallor; purpuric eruptions	Sedimentation rate, Hct/Hgb, plt
OB	Immune-complex vasculitis			Microscopic hematuria
REPROD	Q fever complications 2° to reactivation of infection during pregnancy	↑ Spontaneous abortions		Isolation of *C. burnetii* from placenta
CNS	Meningoencephalitis Optic neuritis	Weakness, seizures, meningismus, blurred vision, headache	Focal deficits, sensory loss	↑ Monocytes and protein in CSF; normal glucose
MS	Immune-complex vasculitis, vertebral osteomyelitis	Myalgia	Point tenderness	X-ray

Key Reference: Marrie TJ. In Mandell GL, Bennett JE, Dolin R, eds. *Principles and practice of infectious diseases*. 5th ed. New York: Churchill Livingstone; 2000;2043–2050.

Perioperative Implications

Preoperative Preparation

- Continue or initiate antibiotic therapy and optimize any organ system dysfunction.
- Only emergency surgery should be performed.
- Assess resp and cardiac reserve and hepatic and neurologic status.
- With chronic Q fever, subacute endocarditis prophylaxis may be appropriate.
- Monitoring
- Arterial line may be necessary if pneumonia present.
- Myocardial valvular disease may require PA line or other invasive hemodynamic monitors.
- Increased arterial line complications due to vasculitis (rare)

Airway
- None

Induction
- Pneumonia may cause rapid desaturation.
- Hypotension and CV instability if cardiac valvular injury present

Maintenance
- If acute hepatitis, avoid drugs that require hepatic metabolism or decrease blood flow to liver

Extubation
- Resp status and CV stability need to be considered.

Adjuvants
- Depends on hepatic or renal impairment

Postoperative Period

- Monitor resp and/or myocardial status carefully, ICU monitoring may be required.
- Liver enzymes should be followed if hepatic involvement.

Anticipated Problems/Concerns

- Emergent surgical pts who present with an acute infection might require extended antibiotic therapy to prevent persistent *C. burnetii* infection.

Raynaud's Phenomenon

Stephan J. Cohn

Risk

- 1.9% of population (based on reporting of color changes on exposure to cold)
- Almost all with disease are 15–40 y; almost all with 2° phenomenon are over 40 y
- Often assoc with scleroderma, SLE, and/or primary pulm Htn

Perioperative Risks

- Rare morbidity

Worry About

- Arterial thrombosis
- Low blood flow states (e.g., prolonged hypotension or use of tourniquet) can lead to gangrene of extremities

Overview

- Abn sensitivity of small arteries and arterioles to vasoconstrictive stimuli
- Often manifested in a bilateral symmetric pattern, with hands being affected more often than feet
- Pts exhibit triphasic color pattern in affected areas: Pallor, then cyanosis due to small arterial occlusion, followed by erythema and edema as vessels suddenly reopen

ICD-9-CM Code: 443.0

Etiology

- Unknown
- Likely hypothesis: Hyperactive sympathetic nervous system with excess neurotransmitter and/or little or no inactivation of norepinephrine

Usual Treatment

- Prevention is most effective. Avoid prolonged exposure to cold, avoid cigarette smoking.
- IV regional blocks with lidocaine at regular intervals. Reserpine, bretylium, and guanethidine all used as additives to lidocaine in IV regional blocks.
- In severe cases, surgical sympathectomy an option but not always beneficial (see also Systemic Lupus Erythematosus in Diseases section)

ASSESSMENT POINTS

System	Effect	Assessment by Hx	PE	Test
RESP	Assoc with primary pulm Htn	Chest discomfort DOE Weakness	JVD Pulmonic ejection click	CXR—right cardiomegaly, dilated pulm artery, ECG—right atrial enlargement, renal vascular Htn
MS	Impaired joint mobility due to pain or scleroderma	Joint mobility		
VASC	Small arterial occlusion	Triphasic color pattern	Often assoc with numbness and diaphoresis	

Key Reference: Nay PG, O'Brien K. Acute vasospastic attack after extradural block in a patient with Raynaud's disease. *Anesth Analg.* 2000;90:1417–1418.

Perioperative Implications

Preoperative Preparation

- Keep warm
- Assess for co-existing disease

Monitoring

- Assess risk-benefit ratio if considering arterial cannulation because of danger of thrombosis.
- Monitor pt's temp and check pressure points and distal pulses frequently.
- Airway
- Reduced TMJ mobility if assoc with scleroderma

Induction

- General or regional anesthetic options acceptable

Maintenance

- Use of tourniquet controversial

Adjuvants

- When using regional anesthetic, consider avoiding epinephrine.

Postoperative Period

- Keep as warm as possible.
- Check pulses in all extremities.

Reflex Sympathetic Dystrophy (Complex Peripheral Pain Syndrome)

David Bandola

Risk

- Incidence of 5.5 per 100,000 person years at risk
- Prevalence of 21 per 100,000 person years at risk
- M:F ratio: 2–4
- Mean peak ages 37–50 y
- CRPS I incidence 1–2% post fractures; 12% post brain lesions; 5% post MI
- CRPS II incidence 1–5% post peripheral nerve injury

Perioperative Risks

- Increased pain flare postop if procedure on affected extremity
- Increased tolerance and/or requirements of opioids if managed with chronic opioids
- Increased incidence of co-omorbid anxiety, depression

Worry About

- Pain exacerbation with manipulation of affected extremity
- Careful positioning of affected extremity
- Interactions and/or end organ effects of chronic pain medications
- IV access and/or tourniquet placement on affected extremity possibly intolerable due to pain

Overview

- Spontaneous, intractable, burning pain; allodynia; hyperalgesia
- Edema, autonomic (vasomotor/sudomotor) abn, trophic signs
- Significant decrease of normal function of affected limb
- Symptoms not limited to region of single nerve
- Pain disproportionate to inciting event
- DX largely based on pt Hx and clinical criterion
- No diagnostic gold standard test

ICD-9-CM Codes: 337.20 (Reflex sympathetic dystrophy—unspecified site); 337.21 (Reflex sympathetic dystrophy—upper limb); 337.22 (Reflex sympathetic dystrophy—lower limb); 337.29 (Reflex sympathetic dystrophy—other specified site)

Etiology

- Pathogenesis of CRPS is unknown
- Classically assoc with antecedent trauma, surgery, MI, stroke
- Likely involvement of peripheral, autonomic, and central nervous systems; myofascial dysfunction; altered psychological states
- Many proposed mechanisms
  - Abn sympathetic outflow and/or adrenergic receptor sensitivity
  - Abn spinal and/or central neuronal sensitization
  - Abn and/or exaggerated inflammatory process
  - Hypoxia
  - Psychologic and/or psychogenic factors
  - Genetic predilection with HLA-DR/DQ polymorphisms

Usual Treatment

- Early DX and multidisciplinary treatment assoc with best outcomes
- Physiotherapy most important component of rehabilitation to achieve optimal functional restoration
- Psychological intervention, cognitive-behavioral therapy
- Typical first line oral medications incl:
  - Antidepressants
  - Antiepileptics
  - NSAIDs
- Long-term, chronic opioids controversial
- Oral corticosteroids employed if prominent inflammatory component
- Other adjuvant, second line therapies incl:
  - NMDA antagonists (ketamine, memantine)
  - GABA agonists (intrathecal baclofen)
  - Bisphosphonates
  - Free radical scavengers (DMSO, NAC)
  - Alpha-2 agonists (epidural clonidine)
- Interventional therapies incl:
  - Sympathetic ganglion blockade
  - Chemical/surgical sympatholysis
  - Regional IV infusion therapy (lidocaine, reserpine, guanethidine)
- Neurostimulation (SCS, TENS, deep brain stimulation)

ASSESSMENT POINTS

System	Effect	Assessment by Hx	PE	Test
DERM	Skin/hair/nail changes	Changes in limb appearance Increased/decreased hair growth	Thickened/thin skin Glossy, waxy skin Increased/decreased hair growth Thickened/brittle nails	Serial physical exams Comparative exam photos
MS	Muscle mass/strength change Stiffened joints Bone changes/osteoporosis	Subjective weakness Decreased ROM	Muscle atrophy Objective weakness Decreased active/passive ROM	3 phase bone Scintigraphy Radiographs
PNS	Spontaneous pain Allodynia/hyperalgesia Motor changes	Spontaneous pain Pain to non-noxious stimuli Exaggerated pain to noxious stimuli	Allodynia Mechanical/thermal hyperalgesia Tremor/dystonia	Quantitive sensory testing (thermal/thermal/pain/vibratory)
ANS	Vasomotor/sudomotor abn	Hyper/hypohidrosis Temp changes Swelling	Moist, clammy, cool skin Edema, skin color changes Skin temp asymmetry of limbs	QSART Infrared thermometry/thermography Thermoregulatory sweat test

Key Reference: Stengel M, Binder A, Baron R. Update on the diagnosis and management of complex regional pain syndromes. *Adv Pain Manage.* 2007;1:96–104.

Perioperative Implications

Preoperative Preparations

- Preop PE and notation of pain symptoms, location and neurologic and/or MS deficits
- Careful planning of pt positioning
- Consider combined regional/GA for periop and postop pain control
- Detailed plan for postop pain control strategies

Monitoring

- Standard ASA monitors
- Avoid BP cuff, pulse oximetry, other monitors on affected extremity

Induction

- Possible increased induction agent dosage (chronic opioid pts)
- Consider regional blockade and/or catheter infusion

Maintenance

- Possible increased anesthetic and periop opioid requirements (chronic opioids)
- Diligent assessment of affected limb position and temp

Adjuvants

- Continuation of all neuropathic pain medications if possible
- NMDA antagonist infusion (ketamine) and/or other neuropathic meds can possibly avoid central sensitization (wind-up)

Postoperative Period

- Continue regional anesthesia and/or analgesia postop if feasible
- Resume preop pharmacologic regimen (home medications)
- Possible increased pain medication requirements (chronic opioids)
- Consider pain medicine consultation if pt admitted postop

Renal Failure, Acute (ARF)

Robert N. Sladen

Risk

- Incidence in USA: 1% of all hospital admissions (community-acquired), 5% of all general hospital pts (hospital-acquired), 10–30% of ICU pts
- Population with highest prevalence: Elderly (>65 y)

Perioperative Risks

- Overall mortality of periop ARF: 60–90%
- Hyperkalemia (and arrhythmias), metabolic acidosis, acute pulm edema
- Aspiration
- Bleeding (plt dysfunction)

Worry About

- Metabolic acidosis and hyperkalemia (pH decrease of 0.1 causes K^+ increase of 0.5 mEq/L)
- Ventricular arrhythmias (may occur without warning)
- Encephalopathy (aspiration risk, increased sensitivity to all sedatives and anesthetics)
- GI symptoms and aspiration (N/V, bleeding and encephalopathy)

- Coagulopathy (plt dysfunction) and surgical bleeding
- Hemodynamic intolerance of hemodialysis, peritoneal dialysis compromises FRC

Overview

- Elective surgery is contraindicated with new-onset ARF; procedures are urgent or emergency
- Regional anesthesia relatively contraindicated (plt dysfunction, encephalopathy)
- Repetitive hemodynamic insults markedly impair renal recovery
- Dialysis partially controls thrombocytopathy and enteropathy, but does not decrease risk of sepsis and poor wound healing

ICD-9-CM Codes: 584 (Acute); 977.5 (Due to procedure)

Etiology

- Ischemic ATN
  - Shock (hemorrhagic, cardiogenic, septic)
- Nephrotoxic ATN

- Hemolysis, rhabdomyolysis, radiocontrast nephropathy (RCN), drugs
- Vascular injury (thromboembolism, occlusion, compartment syndrome)
- Systemic disease (atherosclerotic embolism, acute vasculitis, sickle cell crisis)
- Acute interstitial nephritis, acute glomerulonephritis
- Acute in chronic kidney disease (CKD)

Usual Treatment

- Treat underlying cause (shock, rhabdomyolysis, etc.)
- Medical therapy
  - Fluid and electrolyte restriction, loop diuretics
  - Hyperkalemia: beta-adrenergic agonists, hyperventilation, bicarbonate, Ca^{2+}, insulin-glucose, kayexalate enema
- Dialysis (renal replacement therapy [RRT]): periop continuous venovenous hemodialysis (CVVHD) is treatment of choice

ASSESSMENT POINTS

System	Effect	Assessment by Hx	PE	Test
HEENT	Edema Coagulopathy	Epistaxis, GI bleeding	Airway edema Petechial hemorrhages	
CARDIO	VTach, VFIB Pericardial effusion	Syncope, cardiac arrest Dyspnea, pleuritic chest pain	Muffled heart sounds	ECG, serum K^+, Mg^{2+} ECG, CXR, TTE
RESP	Pulm edema	Dyspnea, orthopnea	Frothy sputum, crackles	CXR
GI	Reflux Ileus Serositis Ulceration, bleeding	Reflux Abd discomfort Acute abdomen Hematemesis, melena	Absent bowel sounds, tympany Tenderness, guarding Same	Esophagogram KUB series KUB, CT scan Stool guaiac, endoscopy
HEME	Plt dysfunction	Excessive bleeding	Petechial hemorrhages	
RENAL	AKI	Oliguria, anuria	Edema	Urinalysis, BUN, Cr, Cr clearance Renal US, scintigraphy
CNS	Encephalopathy	Confusion, disorientation, coma	Same + asterixis	EEG CT scan
MS	Rhabdomyolysis	Crush injury, limb ischemia	'Red urine'	Urine myoglobin Serum CK

Key Reference: Mehta RL. From acute renal failure to acute kidney injury: emerging concepts. *Crit Care Med*. 2008;36:1641–1642.

Perioperative Implications

Preoperative Preparation
- Dialysis to control fluid overload, hyperkalemia, metabolic acidosis, acute uremia
- Consider metoclopramide, H_2-blocker, rapid sequence induction to reduce reflux risk
- Consider DDAVP 0.3 $\mu g/kg$ to enhance plt function (effective 8–12 hr)
- Regional techniques may be contraindicated by coagulopathy

Monitoring
- ECG for arrhythmia detection
- Consider PA catheter or TEE for large fluid shift operations with or without LV dysfunction

Airway
- Consider awake intubation with airway edema
- Avoid nasal intubation (epistaxis)
- Treat as for full stomach: Head up, cricoid pressure
- Succinylcholine is relatively contraindicated (avoid if K^+ conc $\geq$ 5.0 mEq/L)

Preinduction/Induction
- Manage induction and/or replacement fluids as if renal function were normal (risk of hypovolemia)

- Anticipate enhanced pharmacodynamic effects of all sedative and/or anesthetic agents (encephalopathy)

Maintenance
- Restrict maintenance fluids; replace losses appropriately guided by hemodynamic monitoring
- Avoid morphine, meperidine, pancuronium
- Consider agents independent of renal elimination (volatile anesthetics, propofol, fentanyl, remifentanil, cisatracurium, esmolol, clevidipine)
- Increase minute ventilation to compensate for metabolic acidosis; sedative-hypnotic administration may lead to acidosis by eliminating compensatory resp alkalosis in spontaneously breathing pt
- Anticipate increased volume of distribution but decreased clearance of most drugs
- Check ABGs, serum K^+

Extubation
- Anticipate delayed emergence, vomiting, aspiration
- Treat as for full stomach
- Neostigmine elimination is delayed in ARF

- Consider short period of postop mechanical ventilation if pt has intraop acidosis (will not be able to generate adequate spontaneous resp compensation)

Postoperative Period
- Careful assessment of CV, resp status; check ABGs, serum K^+
- Morphine, meperidine have active metabolites that are renally excreted: Use with caution
- May require ultrafiltration and/or CVVHD for excess fluid and/or hyperkalemia in early postop period

Anticipated Problems/Concerns

- Major concerns are always hyperkalemia, acidosis, pulm edema
- Hyperkalemic arrhythmias may occur without premonitory ECG signs.
- Rapid K^+ flux more ominous than stable high serum K^+

Renal Failure, Chronic

Donald S. Prough

Lee A. Fleisher

Risk

- Incidence in USA and worldwide: >100 cases of end-stage renal disease (ESRD)/1 million population
- Racial prevalence: African-Americans ~200 cases/1 million; Hispanics ~100/1 million; Caucasians ~50/1 million

Perioperative Risks

- Overall periop mortality of pts with ESRD: 4%
- Overall periop morbidity of pts with ESRD: 50% (hyperkalemia, infections, hypotension/Htn, bleeding, dysrhythmias, clotted fistulas)
- Adjusted odds ratio assoc with renal failure was 3.56 in one study

Worry About

- Periop progression from chronic renal insufficiency (CRI), not requiring dialysis, to dialysis-dependent ESRD
- Hypovolemia and hypokalemia (esp if recently dialyzed)
- Hypervolemia, metabolic acidosis, and hyperkalemia (esp. if not recently dialyzed)
- Autonomic dysfunction (excessive hypotensive responses)
- Exaggerated hypertensive responses to noxious stimuli
- Prolonged responses to renally excreted drugs and metabolites (e.g., vecuronium, pancuronium, narcotics)
- Impaired immune status
- Occult CAD

Overview

- Decreased excretory and other functions of kidneys related to long-standing disease; with dialysis, a disease that can persist for many years
- Assoc with multiple complications of failed renal excretory function, incl volume overload, accumulation of products of catabolism (e.g., K^+ and hydrogen ions), plt dysfunction, and side effects of dialytic therapy, incl hypovolemia
- Associated with complications of concurrent diseases (e.g., DM, Htn)
- Volume status and electrolyte balance related to how recent dialysis has been

ICD-9-CM Code: 585

Etiology

- Htn (15% Hispanics; 20% Caucasians; 40% African-Americans)
- DM (20% Caucasians; 30% African-Americans; 37% Hispanics); represents 43.8% of all 2° cases
- Glomerulonephritis (12% African-Americans; 22% Hispanics; 25% Caucasians)
- Other causes: Polycystic disease, collagen-vascular disease, pyelonephritis

Usual Treatment

- CRI: Fluid restriction, protein restriction, diuretics, antihypertensives
- Peritoneal dialysis or hemodialysis; continuous venovenous hemofiltration or continuous venovenous hemodialysis while hospitalized
- Renal transplantation (often combined with pancreatic transplantation in diabetics)

ASSESSMENT POINTS

System	Effect	Assessment by Hx	PE	Test
CARDIO	CHF LVH Dysrhythmias	Exercise intolerance Htn Palpitations	Crackles; S_3, S_4 Pulse, auscultation	CXR ECG
GI	N/V, anorexia GI bleeding	N/V, anorexia Melena, rectal bleeding	Malnutrition	Positive occult blood
HEME	Plt dysfunction Anemia	Easy bruising Fatigability	Ecchymoses Pallor	Bleeding time Hgb
RENAL	↓ Concentrating ability (CRI)	Nocturia, frequency		Urine Osm BUN, Cr
CNS	Encephalopathy Autonomic dysfunction	↓ Mental acuity, disorientation Postural hypotension	Mental status Tilt table test: ↓ BP, ↑ HR when tilted	
PNS	Peripheral neuropathy	Paresthesias, burning, itching of lower extremities	Excoriations	

Key Reference:. Craig RG, Hunter JM. Recent developments in the perioperative management of adult patients with chronic kidney disease. *Br J Anaesth.* 2008;101(3):296–310.

Perioperative Implications

Preoperative Preparation

- Assess adequacy of dialytic therapy, volume and acid-base status, Hgb conc, CV status, serum K^+.
- If not dialysis-dependent, assess renal reserve, CV status.
- Consider issues of vascular access.

Monitoring

- Temp, ECG (rhythm, rate, hyperkalemia)
- Pulse oximeter, capnometer, peripheral nerve stimulator
- Consider arterial catheter if chronically hypertensive; consider PA catheter for high-risk surgery in pts with cardiac dysfunction.

Airway

- Gastroparesis precautions if diabetic

Preinduction/Induction

- Reduce dose of thiopental
- Higher doses of propofol required to achieve same level of BIS index
- Exaggerated response to benzodiazepines
- Consider avoiding renally excreted NM blockers (vecuronium, pancuronium)
- Use narcotics cautiously
- If not dialysis-dependent, theoretical concerns about sevoflurane, although do not appear clinically relevant
- Exaggerated BP swings with induction and intubation
- Reduce dose of local anesthetics if metabolic acidosis present or if sedatives will cause resp acidosis

Maintenance

- Precise volume management; titration of agents
- Propofol infusions assoc with faster eye opening

Extubation

- Ensure adequate reversal of NM blockers
- Evaluate airway reflexes

Adjuvants

- Avoid renally excreted NM blockers

Postoperative Period

- Use dialysis if necessary.
- Monitor for frequent causes of postop morbidity (see above).

Anticipated Problems/Concerns

- Hyperkalemia: Treatment with $CaCl_2$, insulin/glucose, or $NaHCO_3$ may be necessary; intraop dialysis occasionally required
- Balancing intraop volume requirements with need for postop fluid removal
- Exaggerated drug effects

Respiratory Distress Syndrome

Shawn M. Cantie
Edgar J. Pierre

Risk

- Mortality rates range from 10–90%, with an average of 50%
- Race and/or gender prominence: None

Perioperative Risks

- Frequent complication of trauma and surgery with a high morbidity and mortality
- Develops in 25% of pts with Gram-negative sepsis, 90% of those with Gram-negative septic shock, and 34% of pts who aspirate
- Large-volume crystalloid and blood product resuscitation

Worry About

- Decreased oxygenation
- Decreased pulm compliance

Overview

- Severe arterial hypoxemia
- Contributes to prolonged mechanical ventilation and lengthened stay in the ICU
- Reduced lung compliance
- Acute lung injury is defined as a PaO_2/FIO_2 below 300 mm Hg and pulm artery occlusion pressure less than 18 mm Hg if measured or not.

- ARDS is defined as a PaO_2/FIO_2 below 200 mm Hg and a pulm artery occlusion pressure less than 18 mm Hg if measured or not.

ICD-9-CM Code: 641.2

Etiology

- Direct lung injury: Pneumonia, aspiration, pulm contusion, fat emboli, near-drowning, inhalation injury
- Indirect lung injury: Sepsis, trauma, assoc shock, multiple blood transfusions, cardiopulmonary bypass, drug overdose, acute pancreatitis
- Increased intravascular volume and decreased colloid oncotic pressure can increase severity.

Usual Treatment

- Alleviation of hypoxemia utilizing lung protection strategy to ventilate
- Avoid large TVs that lead to alveolar overinflation (volutrauma assoc with high peak pressures >35 cm H_2O)
- Use PEEP so that functional residual capacity > closing capacity to reduce tendency towards alveolar collapse and worsening hypoxemia

- Inverse-ratio ventilation: Characterized by prolonged inspiratory:expiratory time. Used successfully to oxygenate and ventilate pts with lung injury but does not change outcome. Risks incl barotrauma and development of auto-PEEP as expiratory time is shortened.
- High frequency ventilation: Delivers a small tidal volume (1 to 5 mL) that generates smaller pressure swings, avoiding barotrauma. Can augment ventricular ejection if synchronized with systole
- Inhaled NO is a potent endogenous vasodilator that, when given by inhalation, selectively vasodilates the pulm circulation. It improves oxygenation by 50–70%.
- Providing CV and nutritional support
- Treatment of underlying cause, e.g., appropriate antibiotic therapy

ASSESSMENT POINTS

System	Effect	Assessment by Hx	PE	Test
CARDIO	Decreased O_2 delivery	SOB Decreased peripheral perfusion	Tachycardia Ischemia	ECG Arterial line PAOP Cardiac output/SVO_2
RESP	Decreased oxygenation, CO_2 accumulation	Dyspnea and tachycardia	Rales	CXR, ABGs
CNS	Agitation Confusion	Disorientation Confusion		Level of consciousness

Key Reference: Brower RG, Ware LB, Berthiaume Y, et al. Treatment of ARDS. *Chest.* 2001;120:1347–1367.

Perioperative Implications

Preinduction/Induction/Maintenance
- Use of an ICU ventilator in the operating room
- Preop use of pressure control ventilation
- PIP >50 cm H_2O with high flows >50 L/min
- High preop PEEP values or an increased A-a gradient (PaO_2/FIO_2<100)
- Coexisting expiratory obstruction (autoPEEP)
- Expecting large volume shifts

Monitoring
- Oxygenation monitored by pulse oximetry and blood gas analysis
- Peak and plateau inflation pressures
- Pulm catheter to manage fluid status, cardiac output and mixed venous saturation

Airway
- Maintain airway protection with intubation and mechanical ventilation
- High FIO_2 and PEEP
- Low airway pressures

Maintenance
- Intubation should be performed early and electively.
- If hypoperfusion is present, O_2 delivery may be compromised not only by hypoxemia but by inadequate cardiac output.
- Ventilator settings of low tidal volumes and PEEP with a goal of achieving maximal lung recruitment, and to achieve adequate oxygenation and avoid toxic levels of FIO_2

Extubation
- The pt should remain intubated at end of procedure in the majority of cases
- Maintain plateau pressure ≤30 cm H_2O

Postoperative Period
- Anticipate keeping pt intubated and mechanically ventilated
- Reduction of extravascular lung water if there is large volume shift
- If paralysis required, sedation is always necessary

Adjuvants
- It may be necessary to maintain paralysis in postop period.
- Muscle relaxation may improve gas exchange.

Anticipated Problems/Concerns
- Oxygenation will almost always worsen following surgery.
- CO_2 elimination may be a problem with worsening lung compliance.

Rett Syndrome

Catherine R. Bachman

Risk

- Almost exclusively females
- Incidence 0.4–0.7 per 10,000

Perioperative Risks

- Abn control of ventilation, with periods of apnea and hyperventilation
- May have GE reflux
- Multiple orthopedic and motor movement disorders

Worry About

- Risk of periop apnea not known
- Risk of succinylcholine-induced hyperkalemia not known
- Aspiration due to GE reflux and swallowing disorder
- Cardiac: Prolonged QTc, abn autonomic regulation, increased incidence of sudden death
- Intraop positioning because of spasticity and contractures

Overview

- DX based on clinical characteristics with inclusion and exclusion criteria, mutations in *MECP2* gene
- Normal development for the first 5–6 mo of life followed by rapid loss of acquired cognitive, verbal, and motor skills with eventual severe impairment in all areas
- Abn EEG; nonspecific changes
- Pathognomonic stereotyped hand movements, tortuous hand-wringing or other hand automatisms
- Seizures very common
- Resp abn when awake, hyperventilation alternating with hypoventilation or apnea and hypoxemia
- Orthopedic and movement disorders such as scoliosis, spasticity, ataxia, loss of locomotion

- ANS dysfunction with increased sympathetic tone
- Cachexia

ICD-9-CM Code: 330.8

Etiology

- Mutations in the *MECP2* gene, mechanism not yet determined
- DX made by Hx and clinical features (inclusion and exclusion criteria established)

Usual Treatment

- Supportive only, no specific therapy
- Aimed at improving quality of life, seizure control, nutrition, PT, possible surgery for orthopedic problems

ASSESSMENT POINTS

System	Effect	Assessment by Hx	PE	Test
HEENT	Nonspecific Spasticity may make airway difficult		Neck ROM Airway exam	Neck X-rays if indicated
CARDIO	Possible prolonged QTc Peripheral vasomotor disturbances		Extremities cool Trophic changes	EKG
RESP	Abn control of ventilation when awake with hyperventilation, apnea, cyanosis Lung changes due to scoliosis or aspiration	Hx of apnea, cyanosis Hx of scoliosis, aspiration	Observation Chest exam	O_2 saturation CXR
GI	GE reflux possible, swallowing difficulties, constipation Growth failure	Hx of GE reflux, feeding difficulties	Thin, small for age	Studies for GE reflux
CNS	Severe developmental delay Seizures Ataxia, loss of locomotion	Developmental level, seizure activity	Assessment of cognitive and movement disorders	EEG
MS	Hypotonia (early); spasticity (late); ataxia Secondary orthopedic manifestations: Scoliosis, joint contractures	Progress and extent of MS abn	Chest exam for scoliosis Limb and joint positions	X-rays

Key Reference: Acampa M, Guideri F. Cardiac disease and Rett syndrome. *Arch Dis Child*. 2006;91:440–443.

Perioperative Implications

Preoperative Preparation

- As for any pt with developmental delay
- Optimize resp status
- Assess resp control
- Minimize aspiration risk

Monitoring

- Routine
- More invasive depending on procedure

Airway

- Normal face
- Spasticity may make positioning difficult

Preinduction/Induction

- Risk of hyperkalemia following succinylcholine unknown
- Possible aspiration risk due to GE reflux

Maintenance

- Resp control abn; unknown if spontaneous ventilation under anesthesia assoc with significant apnea
- Attention to body temp because of thin body habitus and peripheral vasomotor disturbances

Extubation

- Possible aspiration risk
- Assess resp control

Postoperative Period

- Resp control abn
  - Effect of anesthetic agents
  - Duration of resp monitoring
  - Effect of narcotics versus local anesthetics for pain control

Adjuvants

- None

Anticipated Problems/Concerns

- Resp control abn not well understood. Therefore, effect of anesthetic agents intra- and postop on respiration not known. Need for postop monitoring for apnea unknown.

Reye's Syndrome

Mary A. Keyes

Risk

- Incidence prior to 1990: 0.3–0.6/100,000
- 1987-1993: 0.03-0.06/100,000; 2 cases reported/y since 1994
- During early 1980s, association between aspirin and Reye syndrome was recognized and incidence dramatically declined. In 1986, a warning label on all aspirin containing products was mandated in the USA.

Perioperative Risks

- Surgery (all but life-and-death emergencies) contraindicated during Reye syndrome
- Following recovery, repeat liver function tests

Worry About

- Unrecognized inborn errors of metabolism that produce Reye-like syndromes such as fatty-acid oxidation defects, carnitine deficiency, and amino and organic acidopathies
- Recurrent liver dysfunction
- Permanent neurologic sequelae

Overview

- An acute, noninflammatory encephalopathy with hepatic dysfunction predominantly in children; typically starts several days after viral illness, usually influenza or varicella
- Encephalopathy heralded by protracted, severe vomiting, with abn behavior and combativeness that may progress to coma
- Dx made by unexplained encephalopathy with one or more of following: Serum transaminases elevated to at least 3× normal; blood ammonia levels at least 3× normal; or hepatic microvesicular fatty infiltration on liver biopsy. There should be no other reasonable explanation for the cerebral or hepatic abnormalities.
- The CDC uses a Stage 1–6 classification of progressive disease severity. Mortality has decreased from 50% to 20% as a result of recognition in early phases and aggressive treatment.
- Prognosis depends on severity and duration of cerebral dysfunction. Severe disease may lead to subtle neuropsychological defects.

ICD-9-CM Code: 331.81

Etiology

- Abn reaction to viral illness modified by exogenous toxin in susceptible host
- Most frequently linked with influenza A and B and varicella. Exogenous toxin is aspirin in majority of cases. Salicylates were detectable in >80% of cases.

Usual Treatment

- Early recognition of mild cases and maintenance of fluid, electrolyte, acid-base, UO, and glucose balance.
- ET intubation may be required to ensure airway protection and control of ventilation to reduce ICP.
- Fluids restricted in pts with cerebral edema; ICP monitoring aids in improving cerebral perfusion pressure and managing ICP.
- Mannitol to induce cerebral dehydration and barbiturates to decrease cerebral metabolic demand.
- Coagulopathies treated with vitamin K and/or FFP.

ASSESSMENT POINTS

System	Effect	Assessment by Hx	PE	Test
GI	Hepatic dysfunction	Severe vomiting	Hepatomegaly	Hepatic transaminases, ammonia levels Liver biopsy PT, PTT
CNS	Delirium Combative behavior Seizures Lethargy Coma	Alteration in mental status	No focal signs	CT scan ICP monitor

Key Reference: Goetz CG. Aminoacidopathies and organic acidopathies, mitochondrial enzyme defects, and other metabolic errors. In *Textbook of clinical neurology*. 3rd ed. Saunders; 2007.

Perioperative Implications

- Surgery not undertaken except in life-and-death emergencies

Adjuvants

- Ondansetron to decrease vomiting
- Treat seizures with phenytoin
- Correct hyperammonemia with sodium phenyl-acetate/sodium benzoate

Anticipated Problems/Concerns

- Hepatic dysfunction
- Neurologic sequelae
- Underlying inborn errors of metabolism, particularly in children under 5 y

Rheumatoid Arthritis

Nathan Kudrick
Pedro Orozco

Risk

- Incidence in USA: 1% of population
- M:F ratio: 1:2

Perioperative Risks

- Risk of neurologic injury is increased due to occult cervical spine damage
- Assoc cardiac disease may be present but is not clinically apparent
- Pulm complications arise 2° to possible pulm fibrosis and restrictive lung disease

Worry About

- Visualization of glottis and tracheal intubation may be difficult 2° to rheumatoid-assoc damage of the cervical spine
- Former successful ET intubation does not reliably eliminate existing airway abn

- Occult pericardial effusion, pericardial thickening, rheumatoid nodules in the cardiac conduction pathway, valvular fibrosis
- Iatrogenic injury to the cervical spinal cord during laryngoscopy and tracheal intubation
- Chronic corticosteroid use may necessitate intraop steroid administration

Overview

- Chronic inflammatory disease involving diffuse joints and organ systems
- Systemic effects incl pericardial effusion, tamponade, pleural effusion, pulm fibrosis, anemia, and keratoconjunctivitis, and renal failure

ICD-9-CM Code: 714.0

Etiology

- Autoimmune disorder triggered by an antigen in genetically predisposed persons
- Clinical variability may stem from differences in triggering antigens and immune response
- Pathology: Synovial cellular hyperplasia, synovial infiltration by lymphocytes, plasma cells, and fibroblasts leading to degeneration of cartilage and articular surfaces

Treatment

- Aspirin and NSAIDs: Ibuprofen, indomethacin, naproxen, piroxicam, sulindac, and tolmetin
- Immuno-regulating drugs: Methotrexate, hydroxychloroquine, sulfasalazine, azathioprine, penicillamine, and gold

ASSESSMENT POINTS

System	Effect		Assessment by Hx	PE	Test
HEENT	Edematous mucosa		Epistaxis	Friable mucosa	Direct laryngoscopy
	Arthritis of larynx		Hx of voice change	Voice, airway exam	
CARDIO	LV dysfunction	*Most common valve lesion in RA; Aortic regurg*	Dyspnea	S_3	ECG
			Orthopnea	Rales	Stress ECG
	Aortis		Reduced exercise	Diastolic mumur (A1)	ECHO
	Pericarditis		Reduced exercise	Distant heart sounds	ECHO
			Dyspnea	Friction rub	ECHO
RESP	Fibrosis		Dyspnea	Dry rales	CXR, PFTs
GI	Peptic ulcer		Epigastric pain, N/V		
RENAL	Renal dysfuntion		Drug induced		Cr
CNS	Spinal cord compression		Neck pain	Sensory deficits	Radiography
	Neurologic dysfunction		Numbness	Motor deficits	
				ROM of neck	
MS	Arthritis		Joint pain	Swelling	Radiography
				Pain with motion	
				Restricted motion	

Key Reference: Lisowska B, Rutkowska-Sak L, Maldyk P, Cwiek R. Anaesthesiological problems in patients with rheumatoid arthritis undergoing orthopaedic surgeries. *Clin Rheumatol.* 2008;27(5):553–556.

Perioperative Implications

Preoperative Evaluation

- Thorough airway evaluation is a priority. If atlantoaxial instability exists, flexion of neck can compress the spinal cord. Radiating pain to occiput may be indication of cervical cord involvement. Imaging such as X-ray, CT, MRI may be indicated if amount of cervical involvement is not known.
- Cardiopulmonary status needs to be evaluated. If severe restrictive lung disease is suspected, preop pulm function tests may be indicated. Anticipation of postop ventilatory support to be considered.
- Adequate knowledge of pt's current medications. Stress dose corticosteroid supplementation may be indicated for pts being treated chronically with these drugs. Antiinflammatory medications, aspirin, and other rheumatoid drugs can interfere with plt function, clotting, as well as RBC formation.
- Joint mobility and restrictions should be assessed to determine appropriate intraop positioning.

Monitoring

- Standard monitors
- Further invasive monitoring dependent on pt's disease state and anticipated procedure

Airway

- Presence of atlantoaxial instability involvement assessed. Cervical collar placement to minimize movement during direct laryngoscopy considered. Awake fiberoptic laryngoscopy may be best method.
- TMJ disease can limit mouth opening and ability to adequate perform direct laryngoscopy.
- Cricoarytenoid involvement can decrease glottic inlet size and necessitate use of smaller ETT.

Preinduction/Induction

- Preinduction and induction agents/techniques dependent on pts specific assoc co-morbidies

Maintenance

- CV effects from induction agents and volatile anesthetics potentially more pronounced. Risks of hemodynamic instability, cardiac conduction abn, and myocardial ischemia increased.
- Pulm disease may be assoc with restrictive changes leading to decreased lung volumes and vital capacity, V/Q mismatch and poor arterial saturation.
- Hematologic abn such as anemia can be evident intraop.
- Appropriate extremity positioning, padding and manipulation assessed throughout procedure

Extubation

- Post extubation laryngeal obstruction 2° to edema and erythema possible from cricoarytenoid involvement
- Postop ventilatory support anticipated with severe restrictive lung disease

Adjuvants

- Regional and neuraxial techniques can be utilized assuming no significant thoracic, lumbar, and sacral spine involvement as well as normal coagulation studies

Anticipated Problems/Concerns

- Tracheal intubation difficulties 2° to cervical spine and TMJ involvement
- Intraop CV instability and restrictive pulm disease issues
- Assoc side effects of current drug therapy, e.g., anticoagulation, anemia, poor wound healing, etc.
- Multi-organ system involvement
- Intraop positioning concerns 2° to advanced joint involvement and decreased ROM
- Potential for postop ventilatory support

Rocky Mountain Spotted Fever

Sinisa Markovic
Paul R. Knight III

Risk

- Incidence in USA: In every state, most common in southeast and south central, ~ 250–1200 cases/y
- Exposure to tick-infested terrain or dogs
- Severe infection, young and healthy, men over 40 and G6PD deficiency at risk for death
- Mortality 20% untreated, 3–9% even with early treatment (within first 5 d)
- Mortality increases with delay in DX, older age (over 60 y), male sex, very young (< 4 y), black race, chronic alcohol abuse, G6PD deficiency

Perioperative Risks

- Increased mortality 2° to CV instability and noncardiogenic pulm edema
- Increased risk of organ injury due to compounded insults
- Increased bleeding tendency

Worry About

- Severe intravascular volume depletion leading to shock
- Electrolyte disturbances

- Cardiac arrhythmias
- Microvascular hemorrhage
- Consumptive coagulopathy
- Intraop resp and renal failure

Overview

- Uncommon but severe, pathophysiology primarily due to endothelial cell infection resulting in ↑ vascular permeability, edema, hypovolemia, and ischemia
- Initial symptoms in 1–3 d: Nonspecific, mimicking a viral syndrome, specific symptoms in 2–14 d, most in 5–7 d
- Rash appears in 3–5 d, after the onset of fever, initially as maculopapular progressing to petechiae; usually centripetal progression; rash absent in 10–15%
- Disease progression (more likely with delay in treatment) results in multi-organ involvement: noncardiac pulm edema, CNS signs, myocarditis, hepatitis, bleeding (2° to thrombocytopenia and direct vessel damage), and acute renal failure

ICD-9-CM Code: 082.0 (Spotted fevers)

Etiology

- *Rickettsia rickettsii* transmitted in saliva of ticks after 6–10 hr of attachment and feeding or by exposure to infected tick hemolymph, during the removal of ticks
- Incubation period ~7 d (2–14 d)
- Obligatory intracellular bacterium that replicates in the vascular endothelial cells, causing direct cell injury with loss of vascular integrity

Usual Treatment

- Dx difficult, primarily clinical and epidemiologic (potential tick exposure), biopsy of skin lesion to confirm or serologic testing
- Doxycycline, chloramphenicol (pregnant women), importance of early therapy within first 5 d (mortality 6.5 vs. 22.9)
- Correct hypovolemia, coagulation defects, thrombocytopenia, provide intensive, supportive care for various organ system failures

ASSESSMENT POINTS

System	Effect	Assessment by Hx	PE	Test
CARDIO	Extensive microvascular leak; interstitial myocarditis	Rash, swelling	Rash, edema, arrhythmias	ECG, CXR Lytes, BP
RESP	Noncardiac pulm edema; interstitial pneumonitis	↓ Exercise tolerance, dyspnea, cough	Rales by auscultation	CXR, spirometry
GI	Gastroenteritis; liver, spleen, and pancreatic microvascular hemorrhage and edema	N/V, abdominal pain, diarrhea	Abd tenderness Hepatosplenomegaly	SGOT, bilirubin
HEME	Thrombocytopenia, anemia	Easy bleeding, malaise	Rash	Hct/Hgb, plt/PT, PTT
RENAL	Microvascular hemorrhage and edema, interstitial nephritis, prerenal azotemia	Lumbar pain		BUN, Cr Lytes
CNS	Meningoencephalitis	Focal defects, deafness, confusion, meningismus, photophobia, seizures		CSF: ± ↑ WBC, ↑ protein
MS	Microvascular hemorrhage and edema	Myalgia, arthralgia	↓ ROM	

Key Reference: Walker DH, Raoult D. In: Mandell GL, Bennett JE, Dolin R, eds. *Principles and practice of infectious diseases.* 6th ed. Philadelphia: Churchill Livingstone; 2005:2288–2292.

Perioperative Implications

Preoperative Preparation

- Antibiotic therapy and correction of underlying organ system dysfunction
- Surgery only for emergency
- Assess volume, resp, renal status

Monitoring

- Consider PA catheter, arterial line, UO
- Intraop ABGs and lytes
- Plt and other coagulation variables

Airway

- Severe edema of oropharynx and increasing bleeding tendency can lead to difficult intubation

Induction

- Hypovolemia can cause hypotension.

- Microvascular leak in lung can cause rapid desaturation.
- Increased cardiac arrhythmias

Maintenance

- Owing to CV instability, volume status is key.
- Possibility of resp failure and constant volume resuscitation should be anticipated when selecting anesthetic technique.

Extubation

- Oropharyngeal edema and ↑ bleeding tendency may make reintubation very difficult

Adjuvants

- Vasoactive drugs used in acute resuscitation should be readily available.
- Lidocaine for treatment of cardiac arrhythmias

Postoperative Period

- Intravascular volume shifts; coagulation defects, resp failure, CV instability, renal failure

Anticipated Problems/Concerns

- Owing to the possibility of multisystem failure, prolonged postop ICU management may be required.
- Because early treatment with antibiotics is curative and highly successful in preventing complications, high index of suspicion, e.g., after tick exposure in endemic areas, is needed.

Sarcoidosis

Andrew D. Rosenberg

Risk

- Varies: ≤1–80/100,000 with highest incidence in Sweden; in USA 30/100,000
- Presenting ages 20–40 y in USA
- More common in African-Americans than Caucasians in USA
- Females > males

Perioperative Risks

- Severity depends on degree of airway, lung, cardiac, and CNS involvement

Worry About

- Airway granulomas distorting and obstructing anatomy risking obstruction with sedation and making intubation potentially difficult

- Degree of lung involvement and pulm fibrosis
- Cardiac involvement, heart block, arrhythmia, CHF
- CNS involvement

Overview

- Multisystem granulomatous disorder with widespread noncaseating epithelioid cell granulomas
- Lung most frequently affected organ
- Airway abn 2° to granulomas
- Local organ distortion can result in symptoms
- Mononuclear inflammatory cells: T-helper cells + mononuclear phagocytes lead to formation of granulomas

ICD-9-CM Code: 135.0

Etiology

- Unknown disease due to exaggerated cellular immune response involving mononuclear phagocytes and T lymphocytes

Usual Treatment

- Steroids: Oral prednisone (inhaled steroids have not been shown to be consistently effective)
- NSAIDs incl salicylates
- Chloroquine or hydroxychloroquine for mucocutaneous sarcoidosis
- If steroids ineffective: Methotrexate or immunosuppressive agents

ASSESSMENT POINTS

System	Effect	Assessment by Hx	PE	Test
HEENT	Involvement of nares, polyps with distorted anatomy; larynx granulomas, epiglottis, arytenoid involvement	Dyspnea Breathing difficulty	Nasal stuffiness, wheezing, hoarseness, stridor	Laryngoscopy
CARDIO	Heart block Cor pulmonale 2° to RV enlargement	Palpitations	Arrhythmia Rales	ECG
RESP	Pulm granulomas, airway obstruction Bilateral hilar lymphadenopathy (eggshell calcifications of hilar nodes); pulm fibrosis; interstitial disease	Dyspnea Wheezing, cough	Dry rales Wheezes	CXR PFTs (↓ vital and diffusing capacities) ABGs CT if airway obstrucion considered an issue
GI	Liver involvement			↑ LFTs; ↑ alkaline phosphatase
ENDO	DI	Thirst		
RENAL	↑ Ca²⁺ resorption			BUN/Cr
CNS	Nerve involvement DI	Space-occupying lesions Seizures Psychiatric examination	Focal nerve deficits	

Key Reference: Klippel JH, Crofford LJ, Stone JH, Weyland CM. *Sarcoidosis in primer on rheumatoid diseases.* 12th ed. Arthritis Foundation Atlanta; 2001:455–458 [Chapter 28].

Perioperative Implications

Preoperative Preparation

- Adequate steroid coverage
- For pulm and airway, determine if airway obstruction exists and degree of pulm involvement. Evaluate for Hx of SOB and dyspnea. Obtain CXR, consider PFTs and preop ABG based on symptoms and Hx. If airway obstruction suspected, obtain CT to better define issues.

Airway

- Distortion or obstruction 2° to granulomas
- Hypoxia 2° to lung disease

Monitoring

- Observe for heart block
- Arrhythmia

Anticipated Problems/Concerns

- Airway problems 2° to distorted anatomy
- Pulm problems 2° to lung involvement

Sarcoma

Stephan P. Nebbia
Douglas R. Bacon

Risk

- Incidence in USA
- Osteosarcoma: 1:100,000; 2000 new cases/y; second most decade (mean age 15)
- Soft tissue sarcoma: >20 types, 5500 new cases/y in USA, peak incidence in children and adults age 45–50 y
- Equal in male and female, all races

Perioperative Risks

- Morbidity and mortality related to surgical procedure
- Metastatic vital organ involvement, esp pulm, hepatic
- Mass effect, direct compression of organs, vascular structures

Worry About

- Adriamycin-induced cardiotoxicity (global LV hypokinesis)
- Mitomycin-induced acute pulm toxicity, pulm fibrosis, ARDS with increased FIO_2
- Immunosuppression, hemorrhagic cystitis, renal failure induced by antineoplastic chemotherapeutic agents

Overview

- Malignant tumors derived from embryonic mesoderm
- Multiple types in connective tissue, muscle, fat, vasculature, neural and other tissues
- Spread aggressively by local invasion and early hematogenous spread, esp to lung

ICD-9-CM Code: 171 (Depends on type)

Etiology

- Genetic factors, high-dose radiation, carcinogens (dibenzanthracene, methylcholanthrene), Maloney sarcoma virus may predispose to sarcoma
- von Recklinghausen's disease: 10–12% develop neurofibrosarcomas
- Paget's disease: 0.9% develop osteosarcoma
- Kaposi's sarcoma in AIDS pts and immunodeficient pts

Usual Treatment

- Wide surgical resection
- Antineoplastic chemotherapeutic agents
- Radiation

ASSESSMENT POINTS

System	Effect	Assessment by Hx	PE	Test
CARDIO	Atrial myxoma—ball-valve effect	Sx CHF, pulm edema	Rales S_3	CXR ECHO
	Vena caval obstruction	RV failure, CV collapse	Possible caput medusae, venous engorgement, edema	Angio
	SVC syndrome	Head, airway edema $\uparrow$ ICP	Venous congestion of head and neck	Angio V/Q scan
RESP	Pulm embolus	Dyspnea		CXR, angio
GI	Gastroparesis	Early satiety		
	Bowel obstruction	Vomiting	Abd distention	Plain film of abd
	Hepatic metastases	Obstructive jaundice	Jaundice	EGD, bilirubin
	Sarcoma of ampulla of Vater	Hepatic dysfunction		
HEME	Hypercoagulable	Alopecia		PT/PTT
	Immunosuppressive chemotherapy			CBC
	Anemia, due to GI hemorrhage		Gross rectal bleeding	Guaiac
RENAL	Compression of ureters by retroperitoneal tumor	Sx uremia		BUN/Cr Renal US
CNS	CN compression	Various symptoms Dysphagia Loss of sensation, motor function	Neurologic exam	EMG
MS	Bone sarcomas	Hypercalcemia	Chvostek's sign	Blood Ca^{2+}
	Limb loss			Albumin

Key Reference: Makela J, Kiviniemi H, Laitinen S. Prognostic factors predicting survival in the treatment of retroperitoneal sarcoma. *Eur J Surg Oncol.* 2000;26:552–555.

Perioperative Implications

Preoperative Preparation
- Metoclopramide, sodium citrate, ranitidine in pts with gastroparesis
- Assess end-organ impairment 2° to antineoplastic chemotherapeutic agents

Monitoring
- Arterial line and CVP or PA catheter for resection of large tumors

Airway
- Risk of aspiration with large abd mass, or brainstem compression

Induction
- Caution: With cardiac involvement, caval compression may have hemodynamic instability

Maintenance
- Potential CV instability

Extubation
- Awake, if at risk for aspiration

Adjuvants
- Altered pharmacokinetics with hepatic or renal involvement

Postoperative Period
- Pulm embolism, coagulopathy

Anticipated Problems/Concerns

- Adverse effects of chemotherapeutic agents (see Drugs section)
- Resp compromise due to pulm metastases
- Mass effect and/or organ compression and functional impairment
- Effects of prolonged anesthesia
- In prolonged abd cases; hypothermia, complications of massive transfusion

Schizophrenia

Jane C. Ahn
Sharon L. Lin

Risk

- Most common psychotic disorder with a lifetime worldwide prevalence of 1%.
- Increased risk of suicide 5–10%

Perioperative Risks

- Marked deterioration of function and self care
- Exacerbation of psychosis with abrupt discontinuation of medications

Worry About

- Uncooperative, combative, or catatonic pt
- Increased morbidity and mortality due to poorly controlled co-existing systemic disease and increased incidence of alcohol and substance abuse
- Drug interactions and side effects

Overview

- Schizophrenia is a psychiatric disorder that may be characterized by thought disorders, hallucinations, and fixed false beliefs.

- Antipsychotic medications are the mainstay treatment for schizophrenia.
- Antipsychotics have anticholinergic effects (dry mouth, blurry vision, urinary retention, constipation, tachycardia), histamine antagonism (sedation), and α1 antagonism (orthostatic hypotension).
- First generation antipsychotics have strong dopamine antagonism leading to extrapyramidal side effects (EPS) such as tardive dyskinesia.
- Second generation or atypical antipsychotics have serotonin antagonism and less dopamine antagonism leading to less EPS.
- EPS can be treated with anticholinergics such as benztropine 2 mg or diphenhydramine 50–100 mg.
- Neuroleptic malignant syndrome (NMS) is a rare but potentially fatal syndrome occuring after exposure or abrupt D/C of antipsychotic medications. The syndrome is marked by muscle rigidity, hyperthermia, and autonomic instability. It is clinically similar to malignant hyperthermia and may be related to dopamine blockade.

- Treatment of NMS includes hydration and cooling measures, IV dantrolene, and dopamine agonists.
- Avoid dopamine antagonists, such as metoclopromide, if NMS is suspected.

ICD-9-CM Code: 295

Etiology

- Functional hyperactivity of dopamine transmission may play a role
- Genetic and environmental factors are unclear and controversial.

Usual Treatment

- Antipsychotic medications
- Psychotherpay
- ECT

ASSESSMENT POINTS

System	Effect	Assessment by Hx	PE	Test
CARDIO	QT, PR prolongation Torsades de pointe MI Postural hypotension Tachycardia	Dizziness Palpitations	Orthostatic hypotension Arrhthymia	EKG
RESP	Significant increased incidence of smoking		SOB, wheezing	
GI	Paralytic ileus (Postop) Liver dysfunction due to meds			Abd XR LFTs
HEME	Agranulocytosis due to meds			CBC
ENDO	DM due to meds Hyperlipidemia due to meds			Blood glucose Lipid profile test
NEURO	Sedation Extrapyramidal side effects 1. Tardive dyskinesia 2. Akithisia 3. Dystonia 4. Parkinsonism		Somnulence 1. Choreathoid movements of head, limbs, trunk 2. Subjective discomfort causing agitation and restlessness 3. Slow sustained bodily contractions 4. Catatonia, rigidity, akinesia	
GENERAL	Neuroleptic malignant syndrome (NMS)	Antipsychotic use (usually increase in dose) or abrupt discontinuation	Hyperthermia, rigidity, autonomic instability, cardiac arrhythmia	WBC, body temp monitoring, creatine kinase, UA (myoglobinuria)

Key Reference: Kudoh A. Perioperative management for chronic schizophrenic patients. *Anesth Analg.* 2005;101:1867–1872.

Perioperative Implications

Preoperative Preparation
- Hx may be unreliable or unatainable
- Continue antipsychotic medications preop

Monitoring
- Routine

Airway
- Routine considerations

Preinduction/Induction
- No specific technique clearly superior

Maintenance
- Hypotension
- Tachycardia, arrhythmia
- Increased risk of thermodysregulation and hypothermia. Monitor temp and warm pt appropriately.

Extubation
- Usual criteria

Postoperative Period
- Decreased reports of pain
- Increased incidence of severe postop ileus
- Increased risk of postop confusion
- Increased postop mortality

Regional Anesthesia
- Contraversial, but epidural analgesia may decrease incidence of postop ileus

Anticipated Problems/Concerns

- Cardiac arrhythmia
- Hemodynamic instability and hypotension
- Hypothermia
- Potential for neurolytic malignant syndrome

Scleroderma

Lee A. Fleisher

Risk

- Incidence: 9/1 million/y
- Prevalence: 240/million
- M:F ratio: 1:3–7, highest in young African-American women
- More severe in Native Americans and African-Americans
- 10-y survival: 55–60%, presence of pulm Htn is major prognostic predictor

Perioperative Risks

- Severe hypotension 2° to hypovolemia
- Hypoxia 2° to pulm Htn and restrictive disease
- Failed intubation

Worry About

- GI reflux
- Obliterative vasculopathy leading to pulm Htn
- Restrictive lung disease
- Renal crises
- Intraop hypothermia-induced vasospasm

Overview

- Onset 35–50 y
- Chronic, systemic disease that targets skin, lungs, heart, GI, kidneys, and MS system
- Three features: Tissue fibrosis, small blood vessel vasculopathy, autoimmune response
- Two major classifications: Limited and diffuse cutaneous scleroderma
- May have overlap syndromes with other rheumatic diseases

ICD-9-CM Code: 710.1 (Diffuse), 701.0 (Localized)

Etiology

- Autoimmunity, genetics, hormones, environmental factors may all play role
- Autoantibodies: Antitopoisomerase in diffuse forms, anticentromere in limited form
- Twin studies suggest limited genetic role

Usual Treatment

- Begin during early inflammatory stage, strategies are target-organ specific; incl antifibrinolytic agents, anti-inflammatory drugs, immunosuppressive therapy, vascular drugs
- Skin thickening can be treated with numerous experimental drugs or interventions (D-penicillamine, interferon-gamma, mycophenolate mofetil, cyclophosphamide, photopheresis, allogeneic bone marrow transplantation

ASSESSMENT POINTS

System	Effect	Assessment by Hx	PE	Test
HEENT	Cutaneous fibrosis		Masked facies Small oral aperture Atrophy of gums Hyperpigmentation	
CARDIO	Pericardial disease Myocardial fibrosis Conduction abn	DOE CHF Arrhythmia Syncope	Rales	ECHO ECG, Holter
RESP	Fibrosing alveolitis Obliterative vasculopathy Pulm Htn	Dyspnea Nonproductive cough		CXR PFT Bronchoalveolar lavage ECHO
GI	Esophageal fibrosis/colonic dysmotility	Difficulty chewing Dysphagia Bloating Diarrhea	Weight loss	UGI/endoscopy
RENAL	Intrinsic renal vessel disease		Malignant Htn	Proteinuria Hematuria BUN or Cr
DERM	Cutaneous fibrosis		Fibrosis of limbs Sweating Atrophy and contractures Telangiectasis	
MS	Raynaud's disease	Excessive cold sensitivity Pain	Cyanosis of digits	

Key Reference: Roberts JG, Sabar R, Gianoli JA, Kaye AD. Progressive systemic sclerosis: Clinical manifestations and anesthetic considerations. *J Clin Anesth.* 2002;14(6):474–477.

Perioperative Implications

Preoperative Preparation
- Proton pump inhibitors to reduce gastric acid
- Consider metoclopramide for early disease
  - Less effective for late disease

Monitoring
- Invasive arterial monitoring relatively contraindicated in pts with Raynaud's disease because of risk of digit ischemia, but ABG may be indicated
- BP may be difficult because of reduced forearm blood flow
- Consider PA catheter if pulm Htn
- Skin temp may be significantly lower (1.5°C) than core temp

Anesthetic Technique
- Regional anesthesia may be preferable considering pulm problems
- Regional technique may be assoc with prolonged block in the presence of epinephrine because of severe vasoconstriction
- May see vasomotor instability

Airway
- Pt may have severe decrease in oral aperture
- Consider awake FOB intubation
- May require nasal intubation

Preinduction/Induction
- Pt may be hypovolemic due to vasoconstriction
- Consider volume expansion
- May initially observe Htn followed by vasodilation and hypotension

Maintenance
- Usually requires mechanical ventilation because of restrictive lung disease
- Intraop hypoxemia may develop 2° to pulm Htn

Extubation
- May require postop ventilation if significant pulm compromise
- Pain control important for pulm status

Anticipated Problems/Concerns

- Difficult airway
- Hypoxemia
- Hypotension

Scoliosis and Kyphosis

Choendal Martin

Chris C. Lee

Risk

- Scoliosis is a lateral and rotational deformity of the spine that occurs in 1–4% of adolescents.
- Idiopathic scoliosis is the most common etiology making up about 70% of cases, followed by congenital (Marfan's, neurofibromatosis and Scheuermann's disease) and NM disorders (e.g., Duchenne's muscular dystrophy).
- F:M ratio: 4:1 with severe curves occurring predominantly in females
- Kyphosis is usually classified as postural, congenital, and Scheuermann's kyphosis.

Perioperative Risks

- CV dysfunction 2° to underlying pathology and scoliosis distortion of the mediastinum causing a restrictive pulm defect. Cor pulmonale may develop from chronic hypoxia and pulm Htn.
- Neurologic injury
- Hemo: Massive blood loss (>50% of blood volume), and coagulopathy
- Vision loss most commonly due to ischemia of the optic nerve
- Resp: Atelectasis, pneumonia, PE, and resp impairment
- Ileus mostly due to pain and narcotics
- Superior mesenteric syndrome

Worry About

- Neurologic injury due to direct contusion by instrumentation, decreased spinal cord blood flow, distraction injury of the spinal cord, and epidural hematoma
- Fluid management and blood transfusion
- Vascular injuries
- Postop pulm decline requiring postop ventilation

Overview

- Scoliosis is the deformity of the lateral curvature. Idiopathic scoliosis involves the thoracic and lumbar spine with rotation of the vertebra and rib cage deformity. With increased curvature, rotation progresses and the chest cavity becomes more narrowed causing restrictive lung disease. With severe curves, V/Q mismatch occurs and pulm Htn causes cor pulmonale over time.
- Kyphosis is the posterior curvature deformity, which can be assoc with scoliosis.
- Scoliosis assoc with NM disorders usually involves the thoracolumbar spine and the underlying disease may compromise the resp function due to cough dysfunction, aspiration risk, and reduced ventilation capacity. NM disorders may also be assoc with cardiomyopathy.
- Cobb method is used to measure the severity of the curvature. A parallel line is drawn to the superior border of the caudal most vertebral body which tilts to the concavity of the curve, then a second line is drawn parallel to the inferior border of the cephalad most vertebral body that tilts to the concavity of the curve. Perpendicular lines are drawn from these two lines and the angle made by the intersection is measured as the Cobb angle.
- Surgery is indicated in idiopathic scoliosis with curve progression >40 degrees with nonop treatment, curves with >40–45 degrees in pts of skeletal immaturity, and curves >50 degrees in skeletal mature pts. Severe resp compromise occurs in pts with curves >100 degrees (See Overview in Scoliosis and Kyphosis Surgery).

ICD-9-CM Codes: 737.30 Scoliotic (idiopathic); 754.2 (congenital); (acquired) Kyphosis 737.10 (postural); 756.19 (congenital)

Etiology

- Idiopathic scoliosis is the most common etiology (70%) and occurs in up to 4% of the population.
- Scoliosis is assoc with congenital (spina bifida) or NM disorders (muscular dystrophies, cerebral palsy), neurofibromatosis, mesenchymal diseases (dwarfism, Marfan's, and Scheuermann's disease), and trauma.
- Scheuermann's kyphosis occurs in 0.4–8.3% with male predominance. Its cause remains unclear. Mechanical factors and trauma have a significant role in the pathogenesis. Congenital kyphosis, like congenital scoliosis, is caused by a failure of segmentation vs. formation of part or all of the vertebral body.

Usual Treatment

- Treatment goal is prevention of curve progression and correction of deformity.
- Bracing techniques are used for mild curves. For severe curves, spinal fusion with instrumentation of rods, pedicle screws, and/or laminar hooks are placed surgically to correct the deformity. Bone graft is applied to the fused area.
- Surgery may be approached posteriorly or via a combined anterior/posterior approach. The procedure may be staged over 1 or 2 wk to decrease morbidity and mortality. Anterior approach requires a thoraco-abdominal incision and retroperitoneal dissection. One lung ventilation (OLV) may be needed for thoracic exposure.

ASSESSMENT POINTS

System	Effect	Assessment by Hx	PE	Test
AIRWAY	Potential for difficult airway management	Prior difficult intubations, neck movement restrictions, glossal hypertrophy or aspiration risk 2° to DMD	Airway and neck exam	Cervical lateral spine, CT scan
HEME	Coagulation disorders	Hx of easy bruising or bleeding disorders		CBC, PT, PTT, Plt function, cross match, CMP
CV	Pulm Htn, cardiomyopathy 2° to underlying muscular dystrophies or mediastinal distortion	Functional status by exercise tolerance		ECG, ECHO, pulm arterial pressure
RESP	Restrictive pulm defect, severity of functional impairment related to curve severity	Functional status by exercise tolerance		CXR, ABG, spirometry, PFT with bronchodilator reversibility
GI	Poor nutrition	Feeding difficulty		Albumin, serum protein

Key Reference: Raw DA, Beattie JK, Hunter JM. Anesthesia for spinal surgery in adults. *Br J Anaesth*. 2003;91(6):886–904.

Perioperative Implications

Preinduction/Induction/Maintenance

- Premedication with bronchodilator may help to optimize the pt's resp status.
- The use of succinylcholine should be avoided in pts with muscular dystrophies due to the risk of hyperkalemia causing cardiac arrest.
- Boluses of IV induction agents cause a reduction of amplitude of evoked potential responses (cortical responses), but do not interfere with somatosensory potential (SSEP) or transcranial electrical motor evoked potentials (TCeMEP).
- Maintenance of stable anesthetic depth is necessary to provide effective monitoring of SSEPs or MEPs. Volatile anesthetics and propofol decrease SSEPs and MEP in a dose-dependent fashion. Ketamine and etomidate may enhance EP monitoring. Opioids have little effect on monitoring.
- For SSEP monitoring an anesthetic technique with less than 0.5 MAC volatile anesthetic plus propofol infusion with moderate/high dose opioid can be used.
- For MEP monitoring, remifentanil combined with propofol infusion is preferred.

Perioperative Implications

- Major blood loss is assoc with scoliosis correction. Preparation includes large-bore IV access, strategies for transfusion reduction (hypotension, antifibrinolytic agents, preop erythropoietin, cell saver, preop autologous donation, and hemodilution).

Monitoring

- Routine
- Consider arterial line and CVP line
- SSEPs, MEPs and EMG
- Consider BIS monitor
- Estimate blood loss from suction canister contents, cell-saver device and sponges
- Urinary catheter

- Consider O_2 sat pulse oximetry on big toes during anterior exposure of the lower lumbar spine to assess amount of iliac artery compression.

General Anesthesia

- Positioning for posterior fusion is prone with the abd free and in reverse Trendelenburg to reduce venous pressures at the surgical site and bleeding. Special care should be taken to ensure peripheral nerves are padded to prevent compression neuropathies, and eyes should be protected to avoid vision loss/corneal abrasions.
- Thoracic approaches may require a lateral position with a double-lumen ETT for OLV. DLT position should be verified by fiberoptic bronchoscopy.
- Wake up test (WUT) provides intraop testing of the lower limb motor for early detection of neurologic injury after instrumentation. This test requires the cooperation of the pt and carries the risk of unintentional extubation or IV access loss.

WUT requires the lighting of sedation and having the pt complete motor activity on command.

Postoperative Period

• Postop ventilation made necessary for some pts. Factors that suggest the need for postop ventilation incl NM disorder, severe restrictive pulm defect, congenital cardiac abn, RHF, obesity, prolonged surgical procedure, thoracotomy, and significant blood loss.

• Pain management requires a multimodal technique incl spinal/systemic opioids, local anesthetics, and NSAIDs.

• Ileus can be minimized with utilization of a multimodal pain management regimen.

• Fluid management with UO monitoring and replacement is necessary. ADH levels may be high postop requiring treatment/monitoring.

• Atelectasis, pneumonia, and decreased pulm function may occur postop.

Anticipated Problems/Concerns

• Resp complications (atelectasis and pneumonia)
• Neurologic injuries (spinal cord, nerve roots and peripheral nerves)
• Blood loss
• Wound infection
• Continued pain
• Vision loss
• Pulm embolism (PE)

Seizures, Epileptic

Benjamin K. Scott
W. Andrew Kofke

Risk

- Incidence of epilepsy estimated to be 0.5–2%
- 20–40% of pts with epilepsy will develop intractable seizures (greater than 1 per mo, unresponsive to two or more medications)
- Approx 400,000 people in USA have medically uncontrolled epilepsy

Perioperative Risks

- Many rare syndromes are assoc with epilepsy, which can involve disturbances in major organ systems
- Various psychiatric disorders are assoc with epilepsy; anti-epileptic drugs may cause mood, behavior, or cognition disturbances
- Sudden unexpected death reported with epilepsy, poorly understood, incidence is estimated at 2 cases per 1000 pt-years
- Many anti-epileptic drugs are hepatic enzyme inducers or inhibitors which may affect blood levels of drugs such as warfarin, tricyclic antidepressants, statins, chemotherapeutic agents, and antivirals.

Worry About

- Proconvulsant (as well as anticonvulsant) properties of anesthetics
- Antiepileptic drug therapy-induced resistance to NMBs and fentanyl
- Anticonvulsant-induced blood dyscrasia (carbamazepine and others), hepatitis (valproate and others), Stevens-Johnson syndrome, toxic epidermal necrolysis (lamotrigine and others; 10× greater risk for carbamazepine with Chinese ancestry), hyponatremia (oxcarbazepine)
- Rapid IV administration of IV phenytoin can cause profound hypotension

Overview

- Poorly controlled epilepsy results in inability to maintain normal lifestyle.
- Intellectual and social deficits can result from brain-damaging effect of uncontrolled recurrent seizures, negative attitudes of society, or side effects of antiepileptic drug therapy.
- Newer AEDs are generally better tolerated, but most still have potential idiosyncratic adverse effects.

- Seizures are categorized as partial (simple, complex, or with generalization) or generalized (convulsive or nonconvulsive), non-epileptic (pseudoseizures), or unclassified. Up to 56% of comatose neurologic ICU pts have seizure activity.

ICD9-CM: 345 (Epilepsy and recurrent seizures)

Etiology

- Congenital often assoc with other syndromes such as tuberous sclerosis, neurofibromatosis, multiple endocrine adenomatosis, Jervell-Lange-Nielsen syndrome
- Acquired assoc with traumatic brain injury, stroke, brain tumor, Alzheimer's, or idiopathic causes

Usual Treatment

- Antiepileptic drugs as monotherapy or in combination, incl phenytoin, phenobarbital, benzodiazepines, carbamazepine, and newer agents such aslevitiracetam, lamotrigine, topiramate, oxcarbazepine, and many others
- 13% of epileptic pts are thought to be candidates for epilepsy surgery, but only about 1% actually undergo surgery.

ASSESSMENT POINTS

System	Effect	Assessment by Hx	PE	Test
HEENT	Gingival hyperplasia	Phenytoin use		
CARDIO	Cardiac tumors with tuberous sclerosis ↑ Incidence of sudden death with epilepsy (anesthetic implications unknown)	Tuberous sclerosis	Murmur possible	ECHO
RESP	Pulm involvement with neurofibromatosis	Neurofibromatosis	Cor pulmonale	CXR ECG
GI	Anticonvulsant-induced hepatitis	Anticonvulsant use	Jaundice, tender RUQ	LFTs if symptomatic
ENDO	Hyponatremia	Carbamazepine use (rare)		Na+
CNS	Tolerance to fentanyl, psychiatric disturbances	Anticonvulsant use		Assess effects of preop sedatives
MS	Tolerance to NMBs	Anticonvulsant use		Train-of-four monitoring in OR

Key Reference: Kofke WA. Anesthetic management of the patient with epilepsy or prior seizures. *Curr Opin Anaesthesiol*. 2010;23(3):391–399.

Perioperative Implications

Preoperative Preparation

- Assess neuropsychiatric status.
- Determine antiepileptic drug Hx and review potential drug interactions.
- Assess for signs of concurrent disease, such as murmur suggestive of myocardial tumor (tuberous sclerosis) or stigmata of neurofibromatosis.

Monitoring

- For seizure surgery EEG may be placed intraop.

Airway

- Routine considerations

Preinduction/Induction (for Epilepsy Surgery)

- GA propofol or ultrafast-acting thiobarbiturate such as thiopental. If intraop EEG, etomidate or methohexital suitable alternative
- For conscious analgesia craniotomy: Position determined with protection of pressure points. O₂ delivered by nasal prongs or facemask with capnography. Airway adjuncts immediately available. Analgesia/sedation using fentanyl or remifentanil, and propofol or dexmedetomidine. Local anesthetic (scalp block) before surgical incision.

Maintenance

- If intraop EEG not planned, use an anticonvulsant anesthetic maintenance regimen such as desflurane with or without NO, propofol, or moderate-dose opioid.
- For GA with intraop EEG, low dose (less than 0.5 MAC) inhalational agent with opioid, low dose propofol. Methohexital, 25–50 mg, alfentanil, 50–100 μg, and remifentanil, 2.5 μg/kg, have been used as activating agents.
- For conscious analgesia continued titrated of sedation/analgesia during painful parts of procedure
- Consider "asleep-awake-asleep" anesthetic plan

Extubation

- NMB agents and narcotics may not last as long as expected, with unanticipated coughing as procedure comes to close.

Adjuvants

- Muscle relaxants: Decreased effect with some antiepileptic drugs
- Opioids: Tolerance with antiepileptic drug therapy

- Most anesthetics have potential to precipitate seizures during or after surgery.
- Antiepileptic drug levels can be significantly affected by anesthetics, changes in body physiology, and prolonged NPO status.

Postoperative Period

- Blood levels of antiepileptic drugs can be unpredictable, and parenteral antiepileptic drugs such as phenytoin, valproate, or levitiracetam may be required.
- Numerous case reports of postop seizures with a variety of anesthetics suggest ongoing concern for this possibility.

Anticipated Problems/Concerns

- Blood levels of antiepileptic drugs can be significantly affected by anesthetics, changes in physiology, and prolonged NPO status; may also affect non-AED drug levels as a result.
- Opioid tolerance may result in increased need for pain medication.

NEVER check BG after seizure. False ↑. WAIT At least 2hrs post-seizure.

Seizures, Grand Mal (Tonic-Clonic)

Marek A. Mirski

Risk

- Incidence in USA: 500,000–1,000,000 with recurrent tonic-clonic seizures
- 10–20 million at risk to have one tonic-clonic seizure 2° to alcohol withdrawal, febrile convulsions (in children), CNS pathology, metabolic disturbances

Perioperative Risks

- Intraop and postop seizures
- Status epilepticus (unrecognized intraop)
- Physical injury
- Delayed awakening
- Todd's paralysis
- Pulm aspiration
- Transient hypoxemia, tachycardia, Htn
- Elevated intracranial pressure

Worry About

- Check serum anticonvulsant levels preop, consider free versus total serum phenytoin equivalent levels (pt receiving fosphenytoin) in nutritionally depleted pts. May be best to normalize if serum levels are low preop.
- Somnolence
- Caution with intraop IV phenytoin or fosphenytoin (hypotension, $50\,\mu g/min$ and $150\,\mu g/min$ limit respectively) or phenobarbital

- IV levetiracetam (Keppra) often used in intraop settings owing to lack of hemodynamic disturbance and limited drug-drug interactions.
- Prudent to avoid drugs that may lower seizure threshold: Tricyclics, etomidate, ketamine

Overview

- Although typically a benign event, trauma to head or extremities is common if precautions not taken (padded hospital bed). May lead to status epilepticus, a life-threatening condition requiring active and immediate intervention to terminate attack before cerebral injury results (30–60 min). Subtherapeutic anticonvulsant serum levels and alcohol withdrawal most commonly provoke status epilepticus.
- During seizures and postictally, airway reflexes are typically preserved—intubation not indicated unless aspiration is strongly suspected.
- Postictally, enhancement of previous neurologic motor deficit is common (Todd's paralysis) for hours after seizure.

ICD-9-CM Code: 345.3

Etiology

- Leading cause (30%) is idiopathic; undetermined fraction have genetic predisposition

- Acquired: 2° to congenital defects, perinatal asphyxia, trauma, hypoglycemia, CNS infection, drug withdrawal (alcohol most common), metabolic pathology resulting in low Na^+, Ca^{2+}, or Mg^{2+} or increased BUN

Usual Treatment

- For one seizure, no therapy necessarily required. Check serum anticonvulsant levels if there is a Hx of epilepsy determines underlying cause.
- Rule out hypoxia, STAT determination of serum glucose, electrolytes, and serum Ca^{2+}.
- For recurrent or prolonged seizures: IV lorazepam 1–5 mg, midazolam 5–10 mg, diazepam 5–10 mg. Alternatively, thiopental 1–2 mg/kg, propofol 1 mg/kg. Ventilatory assistance should be available for greater dosage requirements.
- To prevent recurrence, IV anticonvulsants (fosphenytoin, levetiracetam, sodium valproate) should be considered to reach appropriate serum or dosage (levetiracetam) target level.
- STAT EEG is mandated in pts who do not emerge within 10–5 min to expected preseizure neurologic state in order to rule out continued seizures (nonconvulsive status epilepticus).

ASSESSMENT POINTS

System	Effect	Assessment by Hx	PE	Test
HEENT	Gingival hyperplasia (phenytoin) Seizure-induced oral trauma		Oral exam	
CARDIO	Drug-induced SIADH (carbamazepine) Hypoglycemia, hypocalcemia Thrombocytopenia, bone marrow suppression (several drugs)			CBC, electrolytes
RESP	Hypoxia Aspiration pneumonia	O_2 SOB, fever, supplemental	Auscultation	ABGs, O_2 sat CXR, sputum culture
GI	Poor absorption of anticonvulsant Drug-induced increase of hepatic P450 Drug-induced transaminase elevation	Low serum levels Increase dosage requirement of various drugs		Drug levels
CNS	Postictal somnolence Non-convulsive status epilepticus Possible multiple CNS abn	Developmental Hx	Disturbed sensorium Delayed emergence Cognitive, motor deficits	EEG
MS	Seizure-induced focal injury			

Key Reference: Mirski MA, Varelas PN. Seizures and status epilepticus in the critically ill. *Crit Care Clin.* 2008;24:115–147, Review.

Perioperative Implications

Preoperative Preparation
- Ensure therapeutic anticonvulsant levels
- Provide protection from injury should seizure occur

Monitoring
- Routine
- EEG postop if poor emergence observed

Airway
- Evaluate for past seizure-induced oral trauma
- Gingival hyperplasia (phenytoin)

Induction
- Standard induction drugs provide anticonvulsant action
- Benzodiazepines useful adjunct

Maintenance
- CV changes may be indicative of seizure

Extubation
- Extubate awake if possible
- Delayed emergence could signal postictal state or status epilepticus, EEG suggested

Adjuvants
- Anticonvulsants for acute seizure: IV benzodiazepines, propofol, barbiturates
- Load with phenytoin or barbiturate; oral drugs less reliable absorption
- Muscle relaxant doses altered by some anticonvulsants

Postoperative Period
- Check serum anticonvulsant levels
- EEG indicated if postop level of arousal not as expected

Anticipated Problems/Concerns

- Clinical seizure preinduction: Injury and aspiration risk if sedative drugs given
- Intraop seizure with consequent delayed emergence
- Subclinical or convulsive status epilepticus

Seizures, Intractable

René Tempelhoff

Risk

- Incidence in USA: 600,000 epileptics/y have uncontrolled seizures
- Racial predominance: None

Perioperative Risks

- Sudden death
- Status epilepticus
- Seizure-mediated cardiac dysrhythmias

Worry About

- Liver toxicity from anticonvulsants (on the decline with the new drug generation)
- Periop trauma from convulsions
- Sudden death
- Status epilepticus postop
- Altered pharmacologic responses due to chronic drug therapy

Overview

- Neurologic disease assoc with birth, congenital malformation, trauma, CNS pathology, idiopathic
- Periop risks increased for acquired seizure disorder, but furthermore some epilepsy and/or congenital malformations carry their own anesthetic risks
- Check type of seizures, clinical manifestations, duration, frequency
- Anticonvulsant therapy and side effects (liver function, level of consciousness)

ICD-9-CM Code: 780.3 (Seizure, recurrent)

Etiology

- Congenital (e.g., tuberous sclerosis and/or infantile seizure)
- Idiopathic
- CNS pathology: Trauma, tumor, hemorrhage

Usual Treatment

- Anticonvulsant and diet
- Surgery for ablation of foci
- GA regarded as a last resort for seizure that is unresponsive to sedative-hypnotics and resulting in decrease in consciousness or significant (<7.28) metabolic acidosis

ASSESSMENT POINTS

System	Effect	Assessment by Hx	PE	Test
HEENT	Tongue biting/swallowing		Airway assessment	
CARDIO	Cardiac dysrhythmias	Syncope Tachycardia		ECG ECHO Holter
RESP	Hyperventilation due to metabolic acidosis			ABGs
GI	Altered liver function Anticonvulsant toxicity Tuberous sclerosis		Jaundice	LFTs Anticonvulsant levels
ENDO	Assoc multiple endocrine adenomatosis			Glucose Ca^{2+}, thyroid function tests
RENAL	Renal dysfunction Tuberous sclerosis			Cr
CNS	Psychiatric problems CNS pathology			
MS	Occult trauma from seizures		Check joints, bones Examine tongue	

Key Reference: Kofke WA, Tempelhoff R, Dasheiff RM. Anesthesia for epileptic patients and epileptic surgery. In: *Anesthesia and neurosurgery.* 3rd ed. St. Louis: Mosby; 1994:495–520.

Perioperative Implications

Preoperative Preparation

- Usual anticonvulsant regimen

Monitoring

- Routine monitors
- $ETCO_2$: Increase in CO_2 production could be indirect sign of seizure
- Consider EEG monitoring

Induction

- Have sodium thiopental and/or benzodiazepines to treat possible seizures
- Significantly higher requirement for nondepolarizing muscle relaxants and narcotics

Maintenance

- Avoid proconvulsants (ketamine, etomidate, enflurane, and probably sevoflurane)

- Continue scheduled anticonvulsants
- GA is sometimes used as treatment for status epilepticus

Extubation

- To be delayed in case of doubt or situation such as:
    - High $ETCO_2$ despite adequate ventilation can be a sign of active seizure
    - Pt nonresponsive
    - Obvious convulsions
- Consider adding anticonvulsant (benzodiazepines) and ordering EEG

Adjuvants

- See specific anticonvulsant used

Postoperative Period

- Watch $ETCO_2$ on awakening, as high production may indicate seizure activity
- Resume anticonvulsants
- Treat seizures ad lib

Anticipated Problems/Concerns

- Seizures on induction and awakening are treated with first-line benzodiazepine Rx (e.g., lorazepam load) rather than long-acting anticonvulsants. The latter (e.g., phenytoin +/-leveteracetam) to be used after the seizure has been controlled.
- Evolution to status epilepticus: GA
- Sudden death (ventricular arrhythmias)

Seizures, Petit Mal (Absence)

Marek A. Mirski

Risk

- Incidence in USA: Approx 75,000–100,000
- Pure cases almost exclusively a risk in children, with age at onset 4–10 y

Perioperative Risks

- Risk of transition of petit mal absence seizures into tonic-clonic seizures or status epilepticus is exceedingly low.

Worry About

- Maintenance of serum anticonvulsant levels
- Inducing seizures with hyperventilation

Overview

- Relatively common seizure of childhood

- Seizure typified by brief absence (5–20 sec) with impairment of consciousness, 3/sec spike-wave EEG, mild facial motor manifestations
- Attacks may be few or occur >100/d
- Return to pre-seizure state without confusion and/or somnolence as typical with either temporal lobe or grand mal seizures
- Hyperventilation and bright flickering lights are common triggers.
- Atypical absence seizures may have more motor features and be of longer duration.
- Trauma from seizures rare, axial posture almost never affected
- No postictal sequelae; EEG and level of awareness return immediately

- Spontaneous resolution frequent in adolescence (25–30%); ~50% go on to develop tonic-clonic seizures

ICD-9-CM Code: 345.2

Etiology

- Strong genetic predisposition in otherwise normal children
- Structural lesions in adults

Usual Treatment

- Valproic acid (VPA) or ethosuximide (ESM) is drug of choice
- No emergent therapy required unless other seizure type present

ASSESSMENT POINTS

System	Effect	Assessment by Hx	PE	Test
CARDIO	Mild thrombocytopenia (VPA) Pancytopenia (ESM)			CBC with platelet count
RESP	Hyperventilation may induce seizure			
GI	↑ Liver enzymes (ESM, VPA) GI upset (VPA) Hepatotoxicity (VPA—rare >age 2 y)	GI Sx		SGPT, SGOT
CNS	EEG typically normal between seizures Normal development is rule			EEG
MS	Mild myoclonic movements		Movements	

Key Reference: Ren WH. Anesthetic management of epileptic pediatric patients. *Int Anesthesiol Clin.* 2009;47:101–116. Review.

Perioperative Implications

Preoperative Preparation

- Continue anticonvulsant therapy
- Verify adequate anticonvulsant levels: ESM 40–100 μg/mL, VPA >50 μg/mL (variable)

Monitoring

- No issues

Airway

- No issues

Preinduction/Induction

- Avoid bright flashing lights and hyperventilation

Maintenance

- Normocarbia unless otherwise indicated

Extubation

- Normocarbia

Adjuvants

- Muscle relaxant action is affected by some agents used to treat petit mal seizures

Postoperative Period

- Pain management beneficial if it results in avoidance of stress-induced hyperventilation

Anticipated Problems/Concerns

- Major periop morbidity rare
- Major concern is to document if other seizure types, such as tonic-clonic seizures, occur. Other seizure types would affect periop risk.

Septic Shock, Hyperdynamic; Systemic Inflammatory Response Syndrome (SIRS)

Peter Schulman

Risk

• Incidence in USA: Approx 750,000. Severe sepsis and septic shock is the tenth leading cause of death, and most common cause of death among critically ill pts in non-coronary ICUs
• Mortality rates are approx 25% for severe sepsis, 50% for septic shock
• Increased prevalence with advanced age, male gender, non-white ethnic origin, co-morbid diseases (COPD, cancer, chronic renal and liver disease, DM)

Perioperative Risks

• Hemodynamic and resp instability
• Thrombocytopenia and DIC
• End-organ ischemia and worsening multisystem organ dysfunction

Worry About

• Rapid hemodynamic deterioration following induction of anesthesia 2° to limited physiologic reserve
• Blunted response to vasopressors and inotropes
• Early and appropriate initiation of antibiotics (initial choice is wrong in up to 20% of cases, and mortality increases with each hour of ineffective antimicrobial therapy)
• Multidrug-resistant bacteria (up to 25% of cases of severe sepsis and septic shock)
• Multisystem organ failure (mortality increases with each successive organ failure)

Overview

• Syndrome is a continuum from *SIRS* to *Sepsis* to *Severe Sepsis* to *Septic Shock* resulting in worsening inflammation and widespread tissue injury

and ultimately leading to multisystem organ dysfunction
  • SIRS: Dx based on alterations in temp, HR, RR, WBC
  • Sepsis: SIRS plus suspected or proven infection (1992 Consensus Conference), or infection plus one clinical criteria or laboratory abn (2001 Consensus Conference)
  • Severe sepsis: Sepsis plus acute organ dysfunction
  • Septic shock: Severe sepsis plus hemodynamic instability (hypotension not reversible with fluid resuscitation)
• Prompt Dx and appropriate treatment is critical for survival
• Signs and symptoms of septic shock are non-specific and presentation is based on initial source of infection.

ICD-9-CM Code: 785.52

Etiology

• Environmental factors (exposure to infecting pathogen) plus possible genetic predisposition result in abn immune, coagulation, and inflammatory responses
• Gram-positive bacteria (MRSA, VRE, streptococcus) have become the most common causative pathogens. Other causative pathogens are gram-negative bacilli (*Escherichia coli*, Pseudomonas), and fungi (Candida)
• Most common site of infection is resp tract (pneumonia). Other common sites are genitourinary, abd, skin and soft tissue, device related (central lines), CNS, endocarditis.

• Also consider noninfectious causes of SIRS (burns, acute pancreatitis, trauma, thromboembolism, surgery)

Usual Treatment

• Speed and appropriateness of treatment administered affects outcome.
• General approach is triad of broad spectrum *antimicrobial therapy* (ideally within 1 hr of Dx), *hemodynamic resuscitation* (EGDT during first 6 hr) to maintain adequate perfusion pressure and optimize O_2 balance, and *source control*.
• Key considerations
  • Blood cultures ideally before antibiotic therapy
  • Imaging studies if warranted to confirm potential source of infection
  • Reassessment of antibiotic therapy to narrow coverage when appropriate
  • Vasopressors to maintain MAP>65 if fluid resuscitation is inadequate
  • Target Hb 7–9 in absence of tissue hypoperfusion, CAD, or acute hemorrhage
  • Lung protective ventilation strategy for ALI or ARDS
• Other considerations
  • Stress dose steroids (hydrocortisone preferred) in septic shock only if BP has been poorly responsive to fluid and vasopressor therapy
  • Activated protein C (Caution: risk of bleeding) in severe sepsis or septic shock and clinical assessment of high risk of death
  • Addition of low-dose vasopressin infusion in refractory septic shock

ASSESSMENT POINTS

System	Effect	Assessment by Hx	PE	Test
NEURO	Altered mental status	Level of consciousness, delirium	Somnolent, obtunded, confused	Head CT if focal deficit
CARDIO	Vasodilation, hypovolemia, acidosis, hypocontractility, circulatory failure	Signs of end-organ hypo-perfusion	Tachycardia, hypotension, wide pulse pressure, warm (or cold) extremities, low SVR, high CI, low SVO_2	Invasive hemodynamic monitoring, ECHO
PULM	Hypoxemia, hyperventilation, resp failure	Tachypnea, dyspnea	Use of accessory muscles, rapid and shallow breathing, cyanosis	CXR, ABG
RENAL	Oliguria, acute kidney injury, ATN	UO	Signs of hypovolemia, rising Cr, BUN	UO, Cr, BUN, urine lytes, UA
ID	Infection	Fever, chills, rigors	Hyper- or hypothermia	WBC with differential, cultures, radiographic imaging
HEME	Hemolysis, thrombocytopenia, DIC		Bleeding	CBC, D-Dimer, INR, PTT, fibrinogen

Key Reference: Dellinger RP, Levy MM, Carlet JM, et al. Surviving Sepsis Campaign: International guidelines for management of severe sepsis and septic shock. *Crit Care Med.* 2008;36(1):296–327.

Perioperative Implications

Preoperative Preparation

• Septic pts are often extremely unstable and have limited physiologic reserve.
• Surgery should be postponed until sepsis is treated unless underlying cause requires surgical intervention (source control).
• If surgery is urgent consider whether pt's condition may be optimized before proceeding to the OR.

Intraoperative

• Goal for induction is hemodynamic stability
• Invasive monitoring is generally indicated
• Inotropes and vasopressors should be readily available
• Target goal directed resuscitation to MAP >65, CVP 8–12, adequate UO, Normal pH, SVO_2 >70
• Consider steroids for refractory shock
• Consider need for pt to remain intubated post-procedure

Postoperative Period

• Need for ICU care and possible prolonged mechanical ventilation

Anticipated Problems/Concerns

• Hemodynamic and resp instability
• Worsening metabolic acidosis, low central or mixed venous O_2 sat
• Multisystem organ dysfunction
• Prolonged ICU stay
• High morbidity and mortality

Shy-Drager Disease

Brad J. Hymel
Don D. Doussan

Risk

- More common in men than women
- Symptoms begin in 5th–7th decades

Perioperative Risks

- Autonomic dysfunction with CV collapse due to decreased sympathetic outflow
- Aspiration risk

Worry About

- Orthostatic hypotension and intraop BP fluctuations particularly during induction
- Obstructive sleep apnea—found in advanced stages
- Vocal cord paralysis—found in advanced stages
- Response to sympathomimetic drugs is unpredictable and may be extreme due to denervation hypersensitivity

Overview

- A parkinsonism-plus syndrome. 80% of pts present with Parkinson's Disease.

- Clinical manifestations incl parkinsonian symptoms, urinary and bowel dysfunction, impaired potency and libido, decreased sweating and supine Htn with severe orthostatic changes.
- Previous autopsies have revealed widespread degeneration of the central and peripheral autonomic systems in addition to involvement of the corticobulbar and corticospinal tracts as well as the basal ganglia and cerebellum.
- Irreversible progressive neurodegenerative disease primarily with autonomic failure
- Death often occurs 7–8 y after onset of symptoms.
- Difficult to treat the parkinsonian symptoms as dopaminergic drugs may exacerbate orthostatic hypotension. One case report describes the use of vasopressin to treat intraop hypotention unresponsive to fluids, ephedrine, and pheny-lephrine.

ICD-9-CM Code: 333.0

Etiology

- Unknown

Usual Treatment

- Symptomatic relief of orthostatic hypotension
- Liberal salt intake
- Fludrocortisone
- Elastic stockings
- Midodrine—peripheral α-adrenergic agonist
- Sympathomimetics—ephedrine
- Prostaglandin inhibitors—indomethacin, ibuprofen
- MAO inhibitors
- Common to also receive antiparkinsonian drugs

ASSESSMENT POINTS

System	Effect	Assessment by Hx	PE	Test
HEENT	Vocal cord paralysis	Obstruction; apnea episodes; stridor particularly during sleep	Midline postion of the cords after induction	Direct laryngoscopy
	Obstructive sleep apnea	Snoring; dysphonia; dysarthria	Neck circumference	Polysomnograph
CARDIO	Orthostatic hypotension	Syncope; dizziness; supine Htn with positional hypotension	Postural changes in BP	Tilt table test ECG
	Fixed HR			Palpation
RESP	Irregular resp			Auscultation; visualization
GI	Gastroparesis Fecal incontinence, diarrhea, constipation, sodium loss	Early satiety, dysphagia	Loss of rectal sphincter tone	Electrolytes/BMP
GU	Urinary incontinence Atonic bladder Sexual dysfunction	Nocturia; stress/overflow incontinence Sexual impotence		
CNS	Parkinsonian symptoms Anhidrosis Heat intolerance		Cogwheel rigidity Shuffling gait Anisocoria Horner's syndrome	
MS	Osteoporosis and aseptic necrosis (may be assoc with autonomic dysfunction)		Muscle atrophy Fasciculations	

Key Reference: Niquille M, Van Gessel E, Gamulin Z. Continuous spinal anesthesia for hip surgery in a patient with Shy-Drager syndrome. *Anesth Analg.* 1998;87:396–399.

Perioperative Implications

Preoperative Preparation

- Reduce venous pooling; increase peripheral vascular resistance; increase plasma volume. Care must by taken using these techniques in the attempt to decrease postural hypotension, as fluid overload can occur. Avoid drugs that cause excessive decreases in peripheral vascular resistance and sympatholytics during induction.

Monitoring

- Arterial and central venous catheters if fluid shifts likely to guide fluid replacement
- Temp—reduced sweating may lead to elevations in temp

Airway

- Vocal cord paralysis and dysautonomia with gastroparesis may make awake intubation the more

desirable choice. Direct laryngoscopy allows the anesthesiologist to diagnose sublclinical vocal cord abductor paralysis by observing the position of the cords.

Preinduction/Induction

- Consider steroid supplementation if on fluodrocortisone
- Consider effects of MAO inhibitors
- Avoid agents that may cause a decrease in cardiac output, decrease in HR, or vasodilatation, as profound hypotension may occur due to decreased sympathetic outflow.

Maintenance

- IPPV may cause a decrease in venous return and exaggerate hypotension.
- Norepinephrine stores at the nerve endings may be reduced. Therefore, the response to adrenergic

drugs may be reduced or exaggerated: Use direct-acting drugs in small doses titrated to effect. Vasopressin has been used successfully in case reports when hypotension is not responsive to other sympathomimetics.

- Atropine may not increase the HR owing to parasympathetic deficiency

Extubation

- Awake

Postoperative Period

- Autonomic dysfunction. Continue invasive monitoring.

Anticipated Problems/Concerns

- Autonomic dysfunction with CV collapse
- Aspiration risk

Sick Sinus Syndrome (SSS)

Pranav Shah
Erin A. Sullivan

Risk

- Highest incidence in patients older than 60 y
- Common in pts who have had congenital heart defect repair surgery
- Sinus node dysfunction (SND) is the most common indication for pacemaker implantation in North America.

Perioperative Risks

- Syncope, cardiac arrest
- Angina, CHF exacerbation, or acute onset HF

Worry About

- Sinus bradycardia that can be poorly responsive to atropine, and require a pacer intraop
- Tachy-brady event where an atrial tachycardia occurs, and its termination leads to a prolonged bradycardia or asystole.
- Tachy-brady event can lead to demand myocardial ischemia, and can precipitate heart failure in pt with related co-morbidities

Overview

- A significant portion of elderly pts with SSS frequently have other cardiac co-morbidities such as CAD.

- SSS incl several abnormalities: (1) non-iatrogenic persistent spontaneous sinus bradycardia which is inappropriate for physiological circumstance, (2) sinus arrest or exit block, (3) combination of SA nodal and AV conduction disturbance, (4) alterations of paroxysmal atrial tachyarrhythmia (often fibrillation or flutter) and period of atrial or ventricular bradycardia — "tachy-brady" syndrome. Bradycardia occurs due to the overdrive pacing of SA node during the preceding tachycardia.
- Class I indication for pacemaker insertion in SSS: SND with documented symptomatic bradycardia, or sinus pauses; SND as a result of essential long-term therapy; SND with symptoms of chronotropic incompetence.
- A significant portion of pts with chronotropic incompetence (defined as the inability to achieve 80% of age predicted HR during physiological stimulus) also have SND.

ICD-9-CM Code: 427.8(1) (Sinoatrial node dysfunction)

Etiology

- Numerous and not clearly defined
- Elderly: Likely due to fibrosis of SA node, and hypersensitivity to autonomic changes
- Adults with congenital heart disease (esp. with ASD repair, or extensive atrial reconstruction): Likely due to surgical (direct or inflammatory) trauma to SA node.

Usual Treatment

- Undiagnosed until an episode of bradycardia in the OR: Atropine (0.5 mg–2 mg) and epinephrine (2–10 µg/min); pacing (external or transvenous). Pts with SSS often have a poor response to atropine.
- Diagnosed preop (i.e., ECG changes with symptoms): Pacemaker. Theophylline has been used to raise the resting heart rate. Pacemaker does not control tachyarrhythmia, but instead it allows antiarrhythmic therapy for tachycardia by pacing during bradycardia caused by the therapy.
- Anticoagulation with warfarin is used if continuous ECG monitor detects paroxysms of atrial tachyarrhythmia since this subset of pts has an increased thromboembolic risk.

ASSESSMENT POINTS

System	Effect	Assessment by Hx	PE	Test
CARDIO	Low cardiac output Tachy-brady event	Syncope, presyncope, lightheadedness, decreased exercise capacity, dyspnea on exertion, fatigue, confusion, memory loss, CVA (esp. in elderly) Palpitation, angina, CHF symptoms	Bradycardia, tachycardia	ECG Continuous ECG monitor with symptom diary
RENAL	Accentuate SSS	--	--	Potassium (hypokalemia)

Key Reference: Brignole M. Sick sinus syndrome. *Clin Geriatr Med*. 18 2002; 211–227.

Perioperative Implications

Preinduction/Induction

- Factors that alter autonomic balance can produce sinus bradycardia: Eye surgery, increased ICP, severe hypoxia, cervical/mediastinal tumors
- Optimize extrinsic factors that can decrease heart rate: Hyperkalemia, hypoxia, hypothermia, ICH, hypothyroidism
- Volatile anesthetics, propofol, vecuronium all decrease sinus node activity in a dose dependant fashion
- Standard monitors (pulse oximetry, ECG)
- In pt population that is dependent on their atrial systole for sufficient cardiac output (such as those with ischemic cardiomyopathy, aortic stenosis, or diastolic dysfunction), an atrial tachyarrhythmia (as part of the tachy-brady phenomenon) can lead to hypotension.
- MAC or elective general anesthesia in a pt with known SSS (i.e., with pacemaker)
- Consider using fentanyl, propofol, dexmedetomidine instead of inhaled anesthetics.

- If episode of tachycardia occurs, use normal agents for control of arrhythmia as pacemaker should rescue bradycardia.
- Emergent general anesthesia in pt with suspected SSS but without pacemaker, or first manifestation of SSS
- Consider transcutaneous pacing pads on pt prior to induction, or placing an introducer in preparation for a transvenous pacing wire if needed.
- Consider arterial BP monitoring.
- If asystole or bradycardia, can attempt therapeutic medications: Atropine 0.5–1 mg IV q 3–5 min up to 0.04 mg/kg (max 3 mg), or ephedrine 5–5 mg IV bolus, or dopamine 5–20 µg/kg/min IV, or epinephrine 2–10 µg/min IV, or isoproterenol 2–10 µg/min. Electrical pacing is most likely to succeed.

Regional Anesthesia

- Case reports show that SSS may manifest from several types of blocks incl a regional block that leads to sympathectomy, stellate ganglion blockade, thoracic epidural, and spinal anesthesia.
- Standard monitoring is recommended.

- If Hx is strongly suggestive of SSS, can consider having pacing pads in room.

Postoperative Period

- If SSS manifests in pt without pacemaker intraop, consult cardiology for evaluation for pacemaker.

Anticipated Problems/Concerns

- An episode of atrial tachyarrhythmia that terminates in asystole or significant bradycardia
- Atrial tachyarrhythmia in a susceptible population (aortic stenosis, diastolic dysfunction) may itself compromise cardiac output.
- Symptomatic sinus bradycardia may not respond robustly (or at all) to atropine. It may need a pacing if a second agent (isoproterenol, epinephrine, ephedrine, or dopamine) does not work.

Sickle Cell Disease

Risk

- Affects persons with ancestors from areas endemic for *P. falciparum* malaria: Greece, Turkey, Italy, Arab Peninsula, India, Africa
- Incidence in USA: 1/500 African-Americans (0.2%) have sickle cell anemia
- Early mortality: Median age of death in men is 42 y and in women is 48 y

Perioperative Risks

- Pts have 30% overall complication rate; risk decreases with increased levels of fetal Hgb
- Complications incl anemia, stroke, acute chest syndrome, myonecrosis, heart failure, MI, hepatic or splenic sequestration, retinal hemorrhage, hematuria, renal failure, atelectasis and pneumonia, new-onset tonic-clonic seizure, intraop stasis and hypotension, wound infection, UTI, unexplained death

Worry About

- Degree of anemia, dehydration, sepsis, stress, acid-base status, hypoxemia
- Percentage of HbSS-containing cells
- Postop atelectasis and pneumonia
- Previous renal or heart failure
- Precipitation of vaso-occlusive crisis

- Risk of hemolytic transfusion reaction due to alloimmunization

Overview

- Lifelong cause of painful vaso-occlusive episodes
- Average rate of painful episodes per pt-year is 0.8
- 5.2% of pts with 3–10 episodes/y account for 33% of all episodes
- Mortality positively correlates with increased pain rate in adults.
- Only Hct and percentage of fetal Hgb have predictive value in defining risk of painful crisis
- End-organ damage due to vaso-occlusion causes morbidity and mortality. Key conditions are pregnancy, heart failure, MI, CVA, acute chest syndrome, sequestration crisis, and severe anemia.
- Enhanced O_2 delivery by sickle Hgb causes rightward shift (P50 = 31 mmHg) of oxyhemoglobin dissociation curve
- Inherited hemoglobinopathy permits deoxygenated Hgb molecules to polymerize into rigid insoluble intraerythrocytic fibers, resulting in sickled cells.

- Organ damage is due to vaso-occlusive ischemia, which occurs because the sickled cells are unable to traverse narrow capillary beds, leading to distal blood flow impairment. Also, there is an enhanced tendency for sickle cells to adhere to the endothelium and cause release of vasoactive substances.

ICD-9-CM Code: 282.60

- See also Sickle Cell Trait in Diseases section

Etiology

- Molecular lesion is on β-chain of Hgb at position 6 Glu → Val
- Sickle erythrocytes are more fragile with shortened life span, which leads to chronic hemolysis and anemia

Usual Treatment

- Vaccines against pneumococcus and *Haemophilus influenzae* type b, and prophylactic penicillin therapy effective in autosplenectomized pts
- Palliative care for painful crisis
- Simple and exchange transfusions
- Hydroxyurea to increase fetal Hgb

ASSESSMENT POINTS

System	Effect	Assessment by Hx	PE	Test
HEENT	Hypoxemia due to sleep apnea	Snoring or sleep apnea Hx	Tonsillar hypertrophy	ABGs
CARDIO	MI; LV and RV dysfunction; CHF	Angina Sx; poor exercise tolerance; dyspnea	Displaced PMI S_3, S_4	ECG, exercise ECG; ECHO, Hct
RESP	Acute chest syndrome; lung and rib infarction; pneumonia	Previous acute chest syndrome; dyspnea	Point tenderness over rib; rales; crackles	CXR
GI	Gallstones; sickle girdle syndrome (mesenteric ischemia); hepatic sequestration crisis	RUQ pain; abd pain	Jaundice; RUQ tenderness	Bilirubin
HEME	Sickle pain crisis; asplenia or splenic sequestration crisis; anemia; infection	Pain in affected areas; fatigue; sepsis	Pallor; splenic enlargement; flank tenderness; fever	Hgb, Hct, WBC, % HbSS Electrophoresis
RENAL	Renal failure and insufficiency	Hematuria; hemodialysis Hx		UA, BUN, serum Cr
REPROD	Preterm labor and delivery; perinatal mortality; placenta previa; abruptio placentae	Vaginal bleeding		US
CNS	Stroke; intracranial hemorrhage; pneumococcal meningitis; retinopathy and hyphema; seizure	Previous CNS Sx (weakness, TIA, or neurologic dysfunction); headache; vomiting or altered mental status	Focal deficits, stupor or coma; nuchal rigidity	Head CT; EEG
MS	Leg ulcers; myonecrosis; myofibrosis; infant hand-foot syndrome; shoulder or hip avascular necrosis; osteomyelitis	Pain in affected areas	ROM; skin changes; fever	WBC, UA, x-ray

Key Reference: Firth PG. Anesthesia and hemoglobinopathies. *Anesthesiol Clin.* 2009;27:321–336.

Perioperative Implications

Preoperative Preparation

- Latest data suggest there is no benefit in exchange transfusion preop. Rather, transfuse to an Hgb of 10 g/dL, independent of HbSS percent, with HbAA erythrocytes using extended matched transfusions (minor group E, K, C, Fya).
- Alkalinization has no benefit.
- Autotransfusion: Predonated units and Hgb-based O_2 carriers remain of unestablished efficacy
- Venous access may be difficult and a central line or implantable reservoir is useful.
- Preop hydration for 12 hr preceding surgery is controversial and many have abandoned excessive hydration.

Monitoring

- Routine
- Avoid central lines unless absolutely indicated given increased risk of infection

- If PA catheter indicated due to co-morbidity and surgical setting, an oximetric catheter is useful in providing continuous mixed venous blood Po_2 sat for assessment of O_2 utilization and delivery.

Airway

- None

Induction

- Avoid oversedation, which may decrease respiration and lead to hypoxemia
- Avoid hypovolemia
- Retrobulbar blocks appear safe
- No differences in morbidity or mortality shown among various anesthetic agents or between regional and GA techniques

Maintenance

- Cardiopulmonary bypass presents special problems causing dilutional anemia, mechanical hemolysis, hypothermia, low-flow state, and plt activation

- Tourniquet use is relatively contraindicated, but unproven to show increased risk for sickle pts

Extubation

- Analgesic-induced resp depression at extubation may contribute to atelectasis, pulm infections, and hypoxemia

Postoperative Period

- Adequate hydration; analgesia; pulm toilet, incl incentive spirometry; supplemental O_2 therapy for 12–48 hr postop

Anticipated Problems/Concerns

- All blood transfusions in these pts carry high risk for hemolytic reaction due to previous exposure
- Avoid all situations leading to hypoxemia, hypovolemia, or stasis

Sickle Cell Trait

Michael F. Roizen

Risk

- Incidence in USA: 2.5 million; 300 million in world
- Race with highest prevalence: African-Americans

Perioperative Risks

- Increased risk of complications following CABG
- Periop mortality rate in published cases of SA trait is 0.8%
- Some increased risk of CVA and pulm infection but not well quantified

Worry About

- Increased risk of vaso-occlusive phenomenon with hypoxia and stress
- Sudden death with stresses such as vigorous exercise make one worry as recovery from surgery may be considered a similar stress as vigorous exercise

Overview

- Is not a disease
- Is not a cause of abn in blood count
- Does not produce vaso-occlusive symptoms under physiologic conditions—painful crisis not a hallmark or concomitant of condition

- Does not adversely affect individual's life expectancy
- Dx established by Hgb electrophoresis

ICD-9-CM Code: 282.5

- See also Sickle Cell Disease in Diseases section

Etiology

- Heterozygous in which individual has one beta S and beta A globin gene (SA disease)

Usual Treatment

- None, except iron supplementation (debated)

ASSESSMENT POINTS

System	Effect	Assessment by Hx	Test
RESP	Pulm embolism		
HEME	Hgb level usually 13–15 g/dL	Hx SOB: poor exercise tolerance 10–40% of Hgb S—same cells as Hgb A	Hgb
GU	Painless hematuria and bacteriuria; pyelonephritis (esp. with pregnancy) RO polycystic kidney disease		UA (culture if prosthesis planned)
CNS	Stroke	Migraine headache	

Key References: Djaiani GN, Cheng DC, Carroll JA, Yudin M, Karski JM. Fast track cardiac anesthesia in patients with sickle cell abnormalities. *Anesth Analg*. 1999;89:598–603. Tsaras G, Owusu-Ansah A, Boateng FO, Amoateng-Adjepong Y. Complications associated with sickle cell trait: a brief narrative review. *Am J Med*. 2009;122:507–512.

Perioperative Implications

Preoperative Preparation
- Warm room
- Consider prehydration

Monitoring
- Temp

Airway
- Occasionally distorted anatomy 2° to extramedullary erythropoiesis
- Sinusitis possible
- Prehydrate liberally if CV status will tolerate

Induction
- Routine

Maintenance
- Keep warm
- Keep vasodilated
- Keep without stasis
- High O_2 content

Extubation
- Keep warm

Adjuvants
- Vary if hepatic or renal insufficiency exists

Postoperative Period
- Aggressively prevent pain, hypovolemia, and hypothermia

Anticipated Problems/Concerns

- Stroke and/or pulm emboli or infection have been reported after CPB. Five of 544 pts in literature of sickle trait disease died periop.

Silicosis

Alexander A. Vitin
Karen B. Domino

General Risk

- Silicosis is irreversible fibronodular lung disease caused by inhalation of dust, containing crystalline silica alpha-quartz or silicon dioxide, during occupational exposure
- Currently, >1,000,000 workers exposed; 200–300 deaths/y; protection devices decrease incidence
- Mostly older than 65 y
- Males>females
- No racial predilection

Perioperative Risks

- Hypoxemia, bronchospasm, pneumothorax, atelectasis, mycobacterium (30-fold increased risk for TB) and fungal infection, bacterial pneumonia, chronic bronchitis exacerbation
- Periop resp failure, esp. following thoracic and upper-abd surgery
- Pulm Htn; cor pulmonale
- Renal insufficiency (tubular nephropathy)
- Steroid-induced diabetes (in cases of chronic steroid treatment)

Worry about

- In cases of assoc scleroderma and /or rheumatoid arthritis, possible difficult intubation
- Bronchospasm, chronic bronchitis exacerbation
- Resp failure
- Cor pulmonale

Overview

- Silicosis-pulm fibrosis commonly occurs after 4–5 y (acute, very rare), 5–10 y (accelerated), or >10 y (chronic) of occupational exposure
- In advanced stage, both obstructive (graduate loss of FEV_1, FVC and decrease of FEV_1/FVC ratio) and restrictive ventilatory defects, as well as decreases in diffusing capacity, are common; exertional dyspnea is the predominant symptom.
- CO_2 retention, pulm Htn, cor pulmonale late in the course
- Assoc TB, lung cancer, connective tissue diseases (scleroderma, rheumatoid arthritis, Sjögren's syndrome), nephritic syndrome, and renal failure

ICD-9-CM Codes: 502 (Nodular); 503 (Non-nodular)

Etiology

- Prolonged occupational exposures incl mining, stone cutting, sandblasting, abrasive industries, granite quarrying, packing silica flour causes dose- and time-related development of pulm fibrosis
- Alveolar macrophages engulf inhaled free silica particles and enter lymphatics and interstitial tissue. The macrophages cause release of cytokines (tumor necrosis factor-α, IL-1), tumor growth factor-β, and oxidants, stimulating parenchymal inflammation, collagen synthesis, and ultimately, fibrosis
- Initial lesions are silicotic nodule mostly located near the resp bronchiole. The nodule is composed of refractile particles of silica surrounded by whorled collagen in concentric layers, with macrophages, lymphocytes, and fibroblasts in the periphery. Emphysematous blebs surround the silicotic nodule, esp. in the subpleural area. Bleb and bulla formation, airways and vascular bed distortion by these nodules complicate advanced disease.

Treatment

- D/C occupational exposure
- In some cases, oral corticosteroids
- Empiric use of bronchodilators and inhaled corticosteroids for obstruction
- Sometimes, whole lung lavage; rarely, lung transplantation
- Prophylaxis for complicating infections (pneumococcal and influenza vaccines, TB treatment)
- Smoking D/C
- No cure so far

ASSESSMENT POINTS

System	Effect	Assessment by Hx	PE	Test
CARDIO	Pulmonary Htn Cor pulmonale	Dyspnea Exercise tolerance Leg swelling	S_3 Peripheral edema Distended neck veins	ECG CXR ECHO
RESP	Pulm fibrosis Bulla/bleb formation	Cough Sputum production Dyspnea Exercise tolerance	Rales, rhonchi Wheezing Cyanosis Use of accessory resp muscles RR	CXR ABGs PFTs Inspir force Diffusing capacity Lung biopsy/lavage fluid microscopy
GI/ENDO	Wt loss Hyperglycemia (in chronic steroid treatment)			Body wt monitoring Blood glucose
MS	Generalized weakness			
RENAL	Renal insufficiency		Htn Peripheral edema Oliguria	Serum creatinine, BUN, K$^+$ Creatinine clearance
IMMUNO	Hilar adenopathy (eggshell calcification) Increased susceptibility to infection, esp. pulm	Cough Fever Sputum production		CXR Sputum culture and sensitivity

Key Reference: Horan BF, Cutfield GR, Davies IM, et al. Problems in the management of the airway during anesthesia for bilateral sequential lung transplantation performed without cardiopulmonary bypass. *J Cardiothorac Vasc Anesth*. 1996;10(3):387–390.

Perioperative implications

Preoperative Preparation

- Lung condition optimization: Treat bronchospasm (if present), bronchitis, other pulm infections; possible lung lavage
- Consider steroids (short course)
- Stop smoking at least 24 hr before surgery

Monitoring

- Pre- and postop: Consider repetitive ABGs, lung mechanics (RR, TV, MV, FVC, NIP, etc.)
- Intraop: Arterial line; CVP is controversial. Consider PA catheter if pulm Htn is present and/or significant fluid shifts are expected

Preinduction/Induction

- Caution with IV agents that depress ventilation and regional techniques that affect accessory muscles of respiration (e.g., high epidural and interscalene blocks)
- Maintain adequate preload, optimize cardiac output. Avoid hypoxemia, hypercapnia, and acidosis (both resp and metabolic), as these may increase PA pressures and worsen cor pulmonale

Airway

- In case of difficult airway, consider techniques with spontaneous respiration preservation (e.g., awake FOI)

Maintenance

- Consider pressure-controlled mode of ventilation, for poor lung compliance may require increased airway pressures to reach the adequate TV. Observe for spontaneous pneumothorax, esp. in severe disease
- Optimize volume status, while avoiding crystalloids' overload; rather, use colloids. If possible, minimize blood products use to avoid lung injury.
- Avoid hypotension. Treatment may incl low doses of vasopressin that decrease PA pressures while maintaining systemic BP, rather than norepinephrine, which increases PAP and promotes acidosis
- For severe metabolic acidosis treatment, consider THAM. Bicarbonate should be avoided because of excessive CO_2 production and hypernatremia.

- Consider use of remifentanil. Caution with long-acting opioids.
- For muscle relaxation, short- and medium-acting agents titrated to effect may be preferred. Consider cisatracurium or rocuronium.
- Any of inhalational agents are adequate options.

Extubation
- Consider temporary postop mechanical ventilation, esp. for upper abd and thoracic surgery, until stringent criteria are met.

Postoperative Period
- Pain management is critical for adequate respiration and to avoid pulm Htn

Adjuvants
- Bronchodilators, supplemental O_2, incentive spirometry may improve ability to wean

Anticipated Problems/Concerns
- Increased risk of resp failure and complications esp. after upper abd and thoracic surgery
- Pts with cor pulmonale at increased risk of cardiac complications

Single (Including Common) Ventricle

Jamie McElrath Schwartz
Daniel Nyhan

Risk

- Hypoplastic left heart syndrome (HLHS) is the most common single ventricle (SV) congenital cardiac malformation.
- HLHS accounts for 7.5% of newborns with CHD.
- Male predominance for HLHS

Perioperative Risks

- Risk of paradoxical emboli
- Risk of complications of chronic hypoxemia: Hyperviscosity, ↓ coagulation factors and plts
- Risk of surgical shunts—narrowing of vessels anastomosed, obstructed shunts
- Hypovolemia-induced poor pulm blood flow or shunt occlusion
- Additional risk specific to anatomy and planned procedure

Worry About

- Impact of changes in PVR, SVR, and cardiac function on blood flow, cardiac output and O_2 sat
- Diastolic pressure and coronary perfusion
- Atrioventricular (AV) valve regurgitation
- Systolic and diastolic dysfunction
- Assoc anomalies

Overview

- Wide variety of lesions usually assoc with atresia of the ipsilateral AV or semilunar valve resulting in SV physiology
  - Tricuspid atresia (TA) is the prototypic single left ventricle. See TA in Diseases section.
  - HLHS with mitral and aortic stenosis/atresia is the prototypic single right ventricle
- Other anatomies incl unbalanced AV canal, some double inlet or double outlet ventricles, some heterotaxies.
- Initial lesion requires mixing of systemic and pulm venous return at atrial (ASD) or ventricular (VSD) level. The SV output is divided between pulm and systemic circulations.

- Single ventricle anatomy may be assoc with hypoplasia of a great vessel (pulm artery or aorta) and prior to initial palliation; systemic or pulm blood flow may be dependent on ductus arteriosus patency.
- Balance of blood flow in each circulation (Qp:Qs) is governed by the relative resistance to flow as determined by both anatomic and vascular resistance considerations.
- Goal throughout all stages is to balance the Qp:Qs at 1:1
  - With complete mixing, Qp:Qs at 1:1 results in sat of 75–80% at FIO_2 0.21
- FIO_2, CO_2, and pH management can be used to manipulate the Qp:Qs.
- Qp:Qs > > 1 results in pulm overcirculation/pulm vascular congestion and potentially hypoperfusion to end organs.
- Qp:Qs < < 1 results in hypoxemia

ICD-9-CM Code: 746.7 (HLHS)

Etiology

- Congenital defect, unclear etiology

Usual Treatment

- Series of palliative procedures with following goal: Creation of reliable systemic and pulm blood flow
- Staged connection of systemic venous return directly to pulm artery, dedicating the SV to systemic circulation
- First, stable blood flow to systemic and pulm circulations are established and balanced.
  - For TA, a Blalock-Taussig (BT) shunt is placed (See BT Shunt in Procedures section)
  - For HLHS, a stage I Norwood procedure is performed
- For other SV lesions, BT shunt or PA banding as dictated by anatomy
- Complete intracardiac mixing of blood is imperative.

- Stage I Norwood
  1. A neoaorta is created from hypoplastic aortic arch and native PA tissue, connecting the SV to systemic circulation.
  2. A BT shunt provides pulm blood flow, connecting branch of neoaorta to ipsilateral pulm artery.
  3. An atrial septectomy is performed for to ensure complete intracardiac mixing of systemic and pulm venous blood.
- At completion of the stage I Norwood, the SV provides cardiac output to the systemic circulation via the neoaorta and the pulm circulation via the BT shunt.
- The second stage is the first of two procedures to direct systemic venous return to the pulm artery.
  - The SVC is connected to the ipsilateral PA, which remains connected to the PA confluence.
  - This procedure is referred to as a cavopulmonary connection, Bi-directional Glenn or hemi-Fontan and is commonly performed around 6 mo of age.
- Low PVR is necessary to promote pulm blood flow, which is passive.
- The final stage, Fontan completion, is typically done 18 mo–5 y.
  - The IVC blood is directed to the ipsilateral PA, either intracardiac via lateral tunnel or extracardic via graft.
  - This effectively separates the circulations and reduces volume workload on SV; systemic venous return now flows passively to the PA without interposed pumping chamber.
  - A small fenestration from the IVC-PA conduit to the atrium is sometimes created. The fenestration ensures preload to the systemic circulation even when PA pressures fluctuate, maintaining cardiac output but at the expense of decreased O_2 sat via right-left shunt.

ASSESSMENT POINTS

System	Effect	Assessment by Hx	PE	Test
CARDIO	CHF	Dyspnea, tachypnea, feeding difficulties	S_3, rales, wheeze, enlarged liver, metabolic acidosis	CXR, pulse oximeter, ABGs ECHO
	Hypoxia Arrhythmia	Dyspnea, tachypnea, feeding difficulties cyanosis	Cyanosis	CXR, pulse oximeter, ABGs ECG
HEME	Polycythemia	See above	See above	Hgb, Hct

Key Reference: Leyvi G, Wasnick J. Single-ventricle patient: Pathophysiology and anesthetic management. *J Cardiothorac Vasc Anesth.* 2009;Oct 26.

Perioperative Implications

Preoperative Preparation

- Depending on the stage of the palliative process (Norwood stage I, Glenn/hemi-Fontan, completion Fontan), optimize hemodynamics.
- Cardiac catheterization is typically performed prior to Glenn/hemi-Fontan to measure PVR and coil any collateral venous vessels.
- Higher O_2 sat can ↓ O_2 delivery to the tissues by facilitating overcirculation to the lungs, particularly when pulm blood flow is via BT shunt.

Monitoring

- Arterial BP
- CVP monitoring via IJ is controversial due to SVC thrombosis risk and implications for subsequent staging, which requires patency of these vessels.
- Consider TEE

Preinduction/Induction

- Dependent on exact anatomy and stage of palliation
- Induction technique should consider impact of PVR and SVR changes on myocardial, systemic, and pulm blood flow.

Airway

- ET intubation and PPV
- Minimize intrathoracic pressures where possible to encourage pulm blood flow.

Maintenance

- IV or inhalational agents are acceptable.
- Body temp as dictated by potential use of cardiopulmonary bypass

Extubation

- Following stage I Norwood, pt requires mechanical ventilation for >2 d.
- Early extubation is recommended to facilitate pulm blood flow after stage II (Glenn or hemi-Fontan) or the completion Fontan. High intrathoracic pressure from PPV impedes venous flow to the pulm circulation, while negative intrathoracic pressure (spontaneous respiration) enhances flow.

Anticipated Problems/Concerns

- Overcirculation
- Hypoxemia
- New anatomy post-procedure will necessitate a reassessment of desired PVR and SVR to optimize flow to both circulations.
- Postop low cardiac output syndrome

Sleep Apnea, Central and Mixed

Andreas M. Ostermeier
Michael F. Roizen

Risk

- Incidence in USA: 2 to 9% of middle-aged adults (increased 3-fold in last 10 y, presumably due to increase in obesity) M:F ratio: 2:1; obstructive or mixed
- Risk increases with male sex, upper middle age (55 to 64), obesity, Hx of snoring with impaired daytime performance
- In elderly, risk is 2× higher for African-Americans

Perioperative Risks

- Increased risk of central and mixed (central and obstructive) apnea. In mixed SAS, obstructive apnea component can mask central apnea.
- Risk for resp depression also in intubated, tracheotomized, and awake pts
- Increased risk with sedative-hypnotic narcotics, postop with any form of pain relief

Worry About

- See medical records for previous problems.

- Look for related medical disorders (e.g., cor pulmonale, cardiac arrhythmias, erythrocytosis, disordered cognition, daytime somnolence)
- Apnea even several hours postop possible, esp after epidural anesthesia
- When administering O_2, think of possible dependence of ventilation on hypoxic drive

Overview

- Central implies failure of resp rhythmogenesis. In SAS pts, at least 30 periods of apnea, defined as cessation of airflow for ≥10 sec, are found during normal nocturnal sleep.
- Obstructive sleep apnea relates to a failed or inadequate resp activation of upper airway muscles, resulting in lack of airflow
- In central apnea, hypoventilation persists despite relief of obstruction
- Central apnea is unaccompanied by any resp effort, in contrast to obstructive sleep apnea
- Related to central alveolar hypoventilation syndrome (CAHS), also known as Ondine's curse

ICD-9-CM Code: 306.1 (Psychogenic apnea)

Etiology

- Central: Familial basis is evident in some cases, possible relation to neurologic disorders (e.g., encephalitis in childhood, damaged resp centers, autonomic neuropathy in diabetes)
- Mixed: Has obstructive component. Upper airway narrowing superimposed on co-existent abn of neurologic control or function of upper airway muscle tone or ventilatory control.
- Assoc with obesity, nasal obstruction (polyps, rhinitis, deviated septum, acromegaly, hypothyroidism, Htn)

Usual Treatment

- Continuous positive airway pressure (CPAP), bring to hospital and OR/PACU
- Tracheotomy and mechanical vent at night
- Diaphragmatic pacing, esp. at night
- Surgery to remove obstruction
- For central/mixed apnea, additional medical treatment with protriptyline, progesterone
- For mixed apnea, also wt loss and physical aids
- Avoid narcotics, benzodiazepines, alcohol

ASSESSMENT POINTS

System	Effect	Assessment by Hx	PE	Test
HEENT	Obstructive apnea	Snoring, partner gives Hx of pt's awakening at night with grunts	Visualization of uvula and tonsillar pillars	
CARDIO	Htn	Dyspnea at rest, DOE Poor exercise tolerance, angina	Cardiomegaly S_3/S_4 murmur	ECG, ECHO
RESP	Right-sided heart dysfunction, snoring, resp dysfunction, DOE	Awakening at night with grunts	Venous engorgement Rapid resp rate Cardiomegaly	SaO_2 supine ECG, CXR, ABGs, Hct Polysomnogram
GI	Hepatic dysfunction Full stomach NIDDM	Jaundice, bleeding disorders, ascites, heartburn, hiatus hernia, polydipsia, polyuria	Hepatomegaly, ascites, spider nevi, jaundice	LFTs, PT, PTT Fasting glucose
ENDO	Obesity Hypothyroidism Acromegaly		Mental function reflexes BMI	Free T4 estimate TSH, GH levels
HEME	Polycythemia		Plethora, clubbing, cyanosis	O_2 sat, Hct
CNS	Disturbed sleep, impaired daytime performance, morning headache, memory problems, irritability	Daytime sleepiness, complaints of disrupted sleep Ask for encephalitis, autonomic neuropathy, brainstem damage		Polysomnogram

Key References: Ostermeier AM, Roizen MF, Hautkappe M, Klock PA, Klafta JM. Three sudden postoperative arrests associated with epidural opioids in patients with sleep apnea. *Anesth Analg.* 1997;85:452–460. Somers VK, White DP, Amin R, et al. Sleep apnea and cardiovascular disease: An American Heart Association/American College of Cardiology Foundation Scientific Statement from the American Heart Association Council for High Blood Pressure Research Professional Education Committee, Council on Clinical Cardiology, Stroke Council, and Council on Cardiovascular Nursing. In collaboration with the National Heart, Lung, and Blood Institute National Center on Sleep Disorders Research. *Circulation.* 2008;118:1080–1111.

Perioperative Implications

Preoperative Preparation

- Take sleep Hx, if possible from bed partner
- If a question of sleep apnea, can use home sleep apnea tests (helmet, or wrist—two distinct types now exist) as a screen—do not need sleep lab for this screen. If positive refer to sleep lav preop.
- Avoid preop sedation with benzodiazepines and narcotics
- Examine airway carefully
- Consider metoclopramide 10 mg, cimetidine 300 mg PO the night before and IV preop.
- Assess myocardial and volume status.
- Initiate CPAP therapy over periop period, and in recovery room.

Monitoring

- Routine; consider arterial line
- UO, possible CVP or PA catheter if volume status likely to be significantly altered

Airway

- Airway control necessary if prominent central component and sedation mandatory
- Awake, sitting, fiberoptic intubation may be indicated if difficulty anticipated.

Induction

- Pt may need to remain semi-sitting if SaO_2 drops when supine. Preoxygenation should be complete throughout lung.

Maintenance

- Oxygenation may deteriorate with upper abd surgery or increased intra-abdominal pressure
- Consider the use of short-acting substances (e.g., propofol, remifentanil)
- Minimize postop sedation

Extubation

- Extubate as soon as pt maintains normocapnia and responds to command.
- Consider close monitoring after extubation.

Adjuvants

- Initial dose of induction agent and narcotics calculated on a mg/kg basis and muscle relaxants calculated on estimated lean body mass
- Subsequent doses of sedatives, hypnotics, relaxants, and narcotics calculated on estimated lean body mass

- Regional anesthesia if physically possible and if pt can use accessory muscles to help with breathing

Postoperative Period

- Pain control with opioids only when NSAIDs and/or regional anesthesia is contraindicated and/or insufficient, as (sudden) complete pain relief may increase risk of resp arrest
- Some think epidural or narcotic indicated and others think relatively contraindicated
- Extended resp monitoring
- Stabilize ABGs to adequate levels
- Pain control necessary. PCA acceptable in sleep apnea, but not in continuous mode.

Anticipated Problems/Concerns

- Resp insufficiency and pneumonia postop; use devices and/or CPAP in immediate and long-term pre- and postop periods
- Postop thromboembolic phenomena
- If problems occur, inform pt before discharge with written instructions, esp. for further anesthetic interventions.

Sleep Apnea, Obstructive

Charles Ahere
Claude Brunson
Michael F. Roizen

Risk

- Incidence in USA: 2–9% of whole population (increased 3-fold in last 10 y, presumably due to increase in obesity)
- M:F ratio: 2:1
- Race with highest prevalence: Unknown

Perioperative Risks

- Increased risk of pulm Htn, RV failure, systemic Htn
- Some pts may be polycythemic and have an increased risk of CVA
- Complications assoc with obesity, and craniofacial and upper airway soft tissue abn
- Increased risk in supine position of sudden arrest postop

Worry About

- Airway obstruction with sedating drugs: Need for awake, sitting intubation without sedation if obstructs when supine
- Increased sensitivity to sedating drugs
- Difficult airway management: Mask ventilation and intubation
- Aspiration risk in morbidly obese
- Postop airway obstruction or resp depression

- Nasal obstruction from NG tubes, e.g., may lead to resp compromise
- Have pt bring CPAP or other apparatus with them to hospital and to OR/PACU

Overview

- Apnea refers to cessation of airflow at the mouth for >10 sec
- Sleep apnea: Repetitive episodes of upper airway occlusion during sleep, often with O_2 sat to 85%, nearly always assoc with loud snoring. Episodes of apnea often terminate with a snort or gasp.
- Upper airway obstruction from relaxation of muscles of oropharynx
- Frequent periods of apnea lead to hypoxia and hypercarbia, which could lead to cor pulmonale.
- Polycythemia may result from chronic hypoxia.
- Nocturnal cardiac arrhythmias are common.
- Monitoring depth and quality of sleep along with cardiopulmonary variables in those with severe symptoms
- Other name is Pickwickian syndrome assoc with morbid obesity (see also Morbid Obesity in Diseases section)

ICD-9-CM Codes: 780.57, 278.0 (Morbid obesity)

Etiology

- Cessation of airflow due to complete obstruction of upper airway
- Narrowing due to enlarged tonsils, adenoids, uvula, low soft palate, or craniofacial abn superimposed on co-existent abn of upper airway muscle tone and/or neurologic control
- Obesity exacerbates upper airway obstruction
- Structural abn such as tonsillar hypertrophy, enlarged tongue, and micrognathia may contribute to airway obstruction

Usual Treatment

- Wt loss in overweight pts
- Avoidance of alcohol and sedatives before sleep
- Nasal CPAP
- Physical aids such as devices to detect and prevent snoring, keep pt off back while sleeping (e.g., tennis ball sewn on nightshirt)
- Nasopharyngeal or oropharyngeal airway
- Uvulopalatopharyngoplasty
- Tracheotomy in extreme cases
- Electrophrenic pacing for central sleep apnea

ASSESSMENT POINTS

System	Effect	Assessment by Hx	PE	Test
HEENT	Obstructive apnea	Snoring; partner gives Hx of pt's awakening with grunts at night	Visualization of uvula and tonsillar pillars	
CARDIO	Htn	Dyspnea at rest and on exertion Poor exercise tolerance	Rapid resp rate ↑ BP, cardiomegaly	ECG; ECHO
RESP	Right-sided heart dysfunction Restrictive dysfunction	Snoring; partner gives Hx of pt's awakening with grunts at night DOE	Venous engorgement, rales, S_3 and S_4, cardiomegaly	Pulse oximetry on room air while supine ECG, CXR, ABGs, Hct, polysomnogram
GI	Hepatic dysfunction Full stomach NIDDM	Angina Jaundice, bleeding disorders, ascites Heartburn; hiatus hernia Polydipsia, polyuria	Hepatomegaly, ascites, spider angiomas, jaundice	LFTs, PT, PTT Fasting glucose
ENDO	Obesity Hypothyroidism Acromegaly		Mental function Reflexes BMI	Free T_4 estimate TSH level; GH level
HEME	Polycythemia		Plethoric clubbing; cyanosis	Hypoxemia Hct
CNS	Disturbed sleep Memory problems Irritability	Daytime sleepiness Complaints of disrupted sleep		Polysomnogram

Key References: Fletcher EC, Proctor M, Yu J, et al. Pulmonary edema develops after recurrent obstructive apneas. *Am J Respir Crit Care Med.* 1999;160:1688–1696.
Epstein LJ, Kristo D, Strollo PJ, et al. Clinical guideline for the evaluation, management, and long-term care of obstructive sleep apnea in adults. *J Clin Sleep Med.* 2009;5:263–269.

Perioperative Implications

Preoperative Preparation

- Avoid sedatives
- Assess CV status
- Histamine H_2 blockers, metoclopramide, and antacids for morbidly obese pts
- Have pt bring CPAP or other apparatus with them to hospital and to OR/PACU

Monitoring

- Routine
- Volume status if RV dysfunction present
- Consider arterial catheter if BP cuff doesn't fit or takes too long to inflate

Airway

- Airway obstruction with induction—see HEENT
- Awake intubation in those with potentially difficult airway
- Consider elevating shoulders on bolsters

Induction

- Airway obstruction
- Exacerbation of pulm Htn by hypoxemia and hypercarbia

Maintenance

- Volume status may change precipitously with position change
- Oxygenation may deteriorate with upper abd surgery or increased abd pressure

Extubation

- Only when pt is fully awake
- Airway obstruction from residual anesthetics
- Avoid opioids and sedatives
- Monitor for airway obstruction and apnea

Adjuvants

- Very sensitive to CNS-depressant drugs
- CPAP or other apparatus for use in PACU and hospital or home recovery periods

Anticipated Problems/Concerns

- Airway obstruction at induction and after extubation
- 13% risk of periop complications esp. of pneumonia; avoided by minimal sedation, appropriate pain control, early ambulation
- Worsening pulm Htn and right-sided heart failure
- Aspiration risk in morbidly obese
- Postop thromboembolism
- Poor motivation resulting in poor ambulation. Avoided by intensive preop teaching and postop coaching.

Spasmodic Torticollis

Todd A. Bromberg
Richard Boortz-Marx

Risk

- Estimated prevalence of 9 cases per 100,000
- Spasmodic torticollis (ST), also known as cervical dystonia, is the most common form of focal dystonia
- Peak incidence in the fifth decade
- Two times more common in females
- 80% of cases are sporadic or primary
- 20% of cases are 2° to an underlying brain lesion or trauma

Perioperative Risks

- Dysphagia
- Aspiration
- Consider co-morbid neurologic problems such as seizures, cranial nerve palsies, hemiplegia, etc.

Worry About

- Difficult pt positioning 2° to sustained muscle contractions
- Difficult intubation as a result of poor extension of the cervical spine and diminished mouth opening

Overview

- ST is defined as twisting of the neck caused by involuntary muscle contractions.

- Idiopathic ST is a slowly progressive disease that manifests between the third and fifth decades. Idiopathic ST is likely caused by abn of the basal ganglia circuitry.
- The dystonia typically progresses over 3 to 5 y before it plateaus.
- Pain occurs in 75% and contributes to disease disability.
- If ST occurs acutely, must rule out causes related to trauma, medications (metoclopramide, haldol, phenothiazines), intracranial abn (tumors, AVMs, hemorrhages), and neck pathology (retropharyngeal abscess).
- The sternocleidomastoid and trapezius muscles are most commonly involved, but extracervical dystonia may occur in 20%.
- Jerking of the head and head tremors are common features.
- Head positioning determines the type of torticollis
  - Rotational torticollis: Rotation of the head around the long axis of the neck with the chin turned toward a particular side
  - Anterocollis: Head tilts forward with neck flexion
  - Retrocollis: Head tilts backward with neck extension

- Laterocollis: Head tilts to one side with the ear pulled towards the shoulder

ICD-9-CM Code: 333.83 (Spasmodic torticollis)

Etiology

- Likely a genetic component that contributes to the development of spasmodic torticollis.
- Trauma, medications, and intracranial pathology can cause focal dystonic reactions such as torticollis.

Usual Treatment

- Chemical denervation with botulinum toxin is the mainstay of therapy. Botulinum toxin is injected into overactive muscles in the neck that are responsible for the dystonia. It usually takes a week to take effect and lasts up to 3 mo before a repeat injection must be performed.
- Pharmacological therapy with anticholinergics, benzodiazepines, and baclofen are used as adjuncts to botulinum toxin.
- Surgical options incl mechanical denervation of affected muscles, deep brain stimulation, and intrathecal baclofen if spasticity is prominent.

ASSESSMENT POINTS

System	Effect	Assessment by Hx	PE
HEENT	Head deviation	Twisting, pulling sensation	Hypertrophic SCM and trapezius
PULM	Restrictive lung disease	Dyspnea	
GI	GERD	Food regurgitation; pain after meals	
CNS	Diplopia Difficulty with transfers Aspiration risk	Vision deficits Coughing with food Use of walker, cane, wheelchair	Abn eye movements; facial droop; depressed gag; tremor; spasticity of muscles; weakness

Key Reference: Mac TB, Girard F, McKenty S, et al. A difficult airway is not more prevalent in patients suffering from spasmodic torticollis: A case series. *Can J Anaesth*. 2004;51(3):250–253.

Perioperative Implications

Preinduction/ Induction/ Maintenance

- Routine considerations
- Consider the use of nondepolarizing muscle relaxants.
- NMB may have no effect on muscle contractures, which are permanently shortened muscles that result from structural muscle changes.
- Anticipate the use of fiberoptic intubation.

Preoperative Considerations

- Consider preop Botox injections at least 1 wk prior to anesthesia.
- It is imperative to preop evaluate the range of cervical spine extension, maximal mouth opening, and integrity of the temporomandibular joint.

Monitoring

- Routine

General Anesthesia

- Propofol is likely to be safe with all dystonias.
- General anesthesia with thiopental, succinylcholine, atracurium, isoflurane, and fentanyl are thought to be safe in spasmodic torticollis.

Regional Anesthesia

- Limited reports available but thought to be safe
- Postop period
- Risk of aspiration

Anticipated Problems/ Concerns

- Anticipate difficult intubation 2° to fixed head turning from muscle contractures that do not respond to muscle relaxants.
- Be aware of cervical spine pathology that may result from prolonged torticollis.
- Neurologic conditions such as cranial nerve dysfunction and seizure disorders may accompany 2° spasmodic torticollis caused by an underlying intracranial lesion.
- Spasmodic torticollis can cause head tremors, which should not be confused with hyperkinetic movement disorders.

Subclavian Steal Syndrome

Dolores B. Njoku
Sapna R. Kudchadkar

Risk

- Uncommon entity with a variably reported clinical significance
- M:F ratio: 2:1

Perioperative Risks

- Stroke from a plaque originating from vertebral artery system

Worry About

- Worsening neurologic symptoms

Overview

- Retrograde blood flow from vertebral artery to distal subclavian 2° to proximal ipsilateral subclavian or innominate artery stenosis or occlusion
- Presence of other extracranial arterial disease is a prerequisite to development of symptoms
- Criteria for diagnosis: Must be symptomatic
  - Cerebral ischemia causing neurologic symptoms assoc with ipsilateral arm exercise
- Decreased BP or arm claudication in ipsilateral arm 2° to occlusion or stenosis of subclavian artery proximal to vertebral artery
- Ratio of left-sided to right-sided subclavian steal phenomenon (SSP) is 3:1; left subclavian artery at increased risk for atherosclerosis 2° to more acute angle of take-off and turbulent flow
- More acutely angled left subclavian artery most commonly atherosclerotic branch of aortic arch 2° to turbulent flow—affected 3 times as often as right subclavian artery.
- Symptoms may be obscured by concomitant carotid insufficiency.
- Spontaneous resolution of vertebrobasilar symptoms may be related to the establishment of extracranial collaterals to the subclavian circulation.

ICD-9-CM Code: 435.2

Etiology

- Most commonly atherosclerosis
- Other causes incl Takayasu's arteritis, tumor, Hx of aortic stenting/grafting for aneurysm, and previous surgery
- Rare causes incl congenital atresia of first portion of left subclavian, hypoplastic arch with severe coarctation, or stenosis of left subclavian at old suture site of a coarctation repair

Usual Treatment

- Surgical
  - Common carotid to subclavian artery bypass graft
  - Subclavian-to-subclavian artery bypass graft
  - Axillary-to-axillary artery bypass graft
- Nonsurgical
  - Percutaneous transluminal angioplasty and stent placement

ASSESSMENT POINTS

System	Assessment by Hx	PE	Test
CARDIO	Claudication	Bruit	Difference in brachial systolic BP of at least 20 mm Hg
			Bruit at base of neck or supraclavicular area on affected side (proximal subclavian artery)
			Reactive hyperemia: Temporary cuff inflation causes peripheral vasodilation distal to cuff, when released results in increased demand leading to neurologic symptoms
			Color Doppler ultrasound: Ipsilateral vertebral artery flow reversal with a parvus tardus waveform in the ipsilateral subclavian artery confirms the diagnosis of SSP
			Vascular structures well demonstrated by contrast-enhanced MRA
			Flow reversal well demonstrated by flow-encoded MRI
CNS	Vertigo		Retrograde catheter
	Rarely cortical visual disturbances, ataxia, syncope, dysarthria		Angiogram
MS	Paresis/paresthesias		See CV

Key Reference: Wood RJ, Walmsley AJ. Subclavian artery stenosis and blood pressure control. *Anaesthesia.* 2006;61(4):409–410.

Perioperative Implications

Preoperative Preparation
- Bilateral upper extremity BP in pts undergoing surgery characterized by large variations in hemodynamic status or in pts with previous internal mammary-coronary bypass grafts

Monitoring
- Consider arterial catheterization since BP maintenance may be essential for cerebral perfusion
- Consider CVP monitoring and/or PA catheterization if contributing factors in pt

Maintenance
- Consider maintaining arterial BP and heart rate near preop levels to facilitate cerebral perfusion

Extubation
- None

Postoperative Period
- Neurologic evaluation at end of surgery

Anticipated Problems/Concerns

- Pts with internal mammary grafts may experience a similar syndrome of coronary-subclavian steal: There is a gradient in systolic brachial blood pressure of 60 mm Hg. In such situations myocardial ischemia that is refractory to medical management may occur.

Subphrenic Abscess

Betsy Ellen Soifer

Risk

- Prior abd surgery, either open or laparoscopic
- Blunt or penetrating trauma
- GI perforation (malignancy, appendicitis, diverticulitis)
- Inflammatory bowel disease
- Immunocompromised pt

Perioperative Risks

- Developing sepsis

Worry About

- Resp compromise (pleural effusion, atelectasis, V/Q mismatching, ARDS)
- Preop ileus/bowel obsrtuction; aspiration risk
- Sepsis incl septic shock and assoc renal failure and/or coagulopathy
- Increased capillary permeability (hypovolemia)
- High-output cardiac failure/LV dysfunction
- Electrolyte and acid-base disturbances

Overview

- Classic findings incl fever, leukocytosis, and abd pain
- Assoc findings incl atelectasis, pleural effusions, elevated diaphragm, ipsilateral shoulder pain, and/or hiccups 2° to diaphragmatic irritation
- May be right- or left-sided, or both; above or below the liver or spleen
- Fistulas may form to any abd or thoracic organ incl pericardium or bronchi
- Disease severity ranges from mild to moribund

ICD-9-CM Code: 567.22

Etiology

- Primary; Assoc with perforated viscus such as duodenal ulcer, diverticulitis, appendicitis, primary liver abscess, immunocompromised state. (Pathogens incl *Escherichia coli*, *Enterococcus* spp, *Bacteroides fragilis*, *Clostridium* spp and are often polymicrobial.)
- Secondary: Following surgical intervention, critical illness, or blunt abd trauma. (Pathogens incl *Candida* spp, *Enterococcus* spp, *Enterobacter* spp, *Staphylococcus epidermidis*, *E. coli* and are often polymicrobial with anaerobic bacteria outnumbering or equal to aerobic bacteria in all but postbiliary surgeries.)

Usual Treatment

- Broad-spectrum antibiotics +/- antifungals. Narrow coverage after cultures obtained based on culture and sensitivity
- Percutaneous or surgical abscess drainage (80–90% successful resolution)
- Supportive therapy: Appropriate monitoring, nutrition, oxygenation, hydration, vasopressors as indicated using the surviving sepsis recommendations

ASSESSMENT POINTS

System	Effect	Assessment by Hx	PE	Test
CARDIO	*Early*: Hyperdynamic state, high cardiac output assoc with low SVR *Late*: Septic shock, low output assoc with high SVR, LV dysfunction		Tachycardia Bounding pulses Warm, ruberous skin Tachycardia Diminished pulses Cool integument Peripheral cyanosis	ECG CVP *or* PA catheter ECHO
RESP	Atelectasis, elevated diaphragm, pleural effusion, abd distention, pain, or ARDS ↓ Diaphragm excursion	Dyspnea Ipsilateral shoulder pain	Tachypnea Cyanosis ↓ Or abnormal breath sounds, dullness to percussion	CXR; fluoroscopy ABGs CT scan
HEME	Anemia due to suppressed marrow Coagulopathy assoc with sepsis	Fatigue	Pallor Oozing around old incisions or IV sites Petechiae Ecchymoses	Hgb, Hct Plt count PT/APTT Fibrinogen, FSPs, D-dimer Thromboelastogram
GU	↓ Perfusion due to hypovolemia or sepsis		↓ UO	BUN, Cr Lytes Acid-base balance
CNS	Mental status changes assoc with sepsis		Range from mild confusion to coma	Must exclude other possible causes (e.g., CVA, CNS infection)

Key Reference: Dellinger RP, Levy MM, Carlet JM, et al. Surviving Sepsis Campaign: International guidelines for management of severe sepsis and septic shock: 2008. *Crit Care.* 2008;36:296–327.

Perioperative Implications

Preoperative Preparation

- Appropriate broad spectrum antibiotics
- Restore intravascular volume
- Optimize resp function: PEEP, bronchodilators, rarely thoracentesis
- NG tube for ileus and/or obstruction
- Tenuous CV status may require central venous access for monitoring/access or vasopressor and/or inotrope infusion
- Assess coagulation status

Monitoring

- Tailor to severity of illness

Airway

- Rapid-sequence induction or awake fiberoptic intubation (aspiration risk)

Preinduction/Induction

- Titrate agents to severity of disease

Extubation

- Tenuous pulm status and/or septic deterioration may require prolonged mechanical ventilation

Postoperative Period

- NPO until intestinal function returns
- Analgesia important for adequate resp function
- Monitor for postinterventional complications (transient sepsis, organ injury, hemorrhage, pneumothorax, peritonitis, wound dehiscence)

Anticipated Problems/Concerns

- Drainage will need to be prolonged (often greater than 10 days)
- Recurrent abscess formation or sepsis (57% in high-risk pts)
- At risk for MODS (resp/ARDS, renal, hepatic, GI bleed)
- High mortality rate (23–50%) in the presence of multiple organ dysfunction
- Periop pneumonia/empyema/pleural effusion
- Fistula formation

Supratentorial Brain Tumors

Tod B. Sloan

Risk

- Highest incidence age 3–12 and 55–65 y
- $^2/_3$ of adult tumors: ~29,000 adults (USA) new tumors in 2005
- $^1/_3$ of childhood tumors: ~0.8–1/100,000 children–600–1000 new tumors in in USA.

Perioperative Risks

- Increased ICP: Headache, seizures, neurologic deficit/dementia, visual and hearing changes, focal neurologic changes (hemiparesis, numbness, ataxia)
- Endocrinopathy and/or visual deficits if pituitary tumor

Worry About

- Seizure medications: Dilantin, keppra, tegretol
  - Need adequate levels to avoid postop seizures
- Raised ICP and brain edema: May lead to herniation (transtentorial [dilate ipsilateral pupil], subfalcine (leg weakness), tonsillar (neck stiffness, spasticity, extensor-plantar response), upward transtorial (small pupils, extensor rigidity)
  - Dexamethasone Rx may lead to hyperglycemia
  - Hyperglycemia may cause more retractor-induced ischemic injury to adjacent brain tissues

- Endocrinopathy, particularly diabetes insipidus if near pituitary

Overview

- Portion of brain superior to tentorium cerebelli
- 13,000 deaths per year, third leading cause of death in 15–34 y old (2.5% all deaths due to cancer)
- Brain edema surrounding malignant tumors causes initial Sx; often improve initially after corticosteroids
- Seizures due to local neuronal irritation, 30–70% incidence related to tumor type, cortical most common
- Obstructive hydrocephalus if tumor near 3rd ventricle or foramen of Monro

ICD-9-CM Code: 239.6 (Tumor, brain)

Etiology

- Adult: 85% are primary tumors in anterior $^2/_3$ of cortex (most benign): glioma (45–50%), medulloblastoma, ependyoma, low-grade lymphoma (children: astrocytoma, medulloblastoma). 15% mengiomas. Common presentation age 55–65 (1% all cancers)

- Many supratentorial tumors are metastases (20–30%): melanoma, breast cancer, small-cell lung, non-Hodgkin's lymphoma, colon, renal, nasal/throat, 50% have multiple mets (25% of all pts with cancer have brain mets)
- Assoc Dx: Neurofibromatosis, von-Hippel-Lindau
- Brain tumor rarely metastasize outside brain
- Pediatric (uncommon > age 2) <1 y present when large (pliable skull, glioma 50% (astrocytoma), most low-grade and deep midline, others ependymoma, medulloblastoma, PNET (primitive neuroectodermal tumors)

Usual Treatment

- Dexamethasone for initial Sx (vasogenic edema)
- Usually surgery with almost all tumors for diagnostic biopsy/resection/debulking
- Radiation/Gamma knife (common with metastasis), chemotherapy
- Radioactive implants, antibodies against tumor-specific antigens or radiosensitizing agents may be used.
- Children may need anesthesia for Gamma knife, linear accelerator, and proton-beam treatments.

ASSESSMENT POINTS

System	Effect	Assessment by Hx	PE	Test
HEENT	Cartilaginous overgrowth in acromegaly		Acromegalic features / 3rd nerve palsy, papilledema, vision changes, hearing changes, macrocrania, bulging fontanel (infant)	Lat neck x-ray
CARDIO	Age effect: CHF, ASCVD, chemotherapy cardiomyopathy, inc ICP	DOE, edema, angina	Gallop, rales, jugular distention, Htn, bradycardia	CXR, ECG, ECHO
RESP	COPD: Primary lung tumor with cerebral metastases	Dyspnea, cough, sputum	Signs of COPD, altered breathing pattern	FEV_1, FVC (if indicated) ABGs CXR
RENAL, GI	Dehydration, SIADH	Mannitol, diuretics, decreased intake, vomiting (esp. children)	Dry mucous membranes	Urine SG, sodium, creat
ENDO	Iatrogenic Cushing's syndrome due to decadron, infertility	Improved level of consciousness with decadron	Cushingoid appearance	Glucose levels
HEME	Anemia, paraneoplastic syndrome, increased thromboembolism	Occult GI bleeding caused by primary tumor	Pale conjunctiva, positive occult fecal blood	Hct, Hgb, T&C
CNS	Seizures (50% as presenting symptom), somnolence, hydrocephalus	Headache, confusion, ataxia, Neck stiffness	Altered consciousness, personality changes, memory loss, speech changes	MRI, CT
PNS	Hemiparesis	Clumsiness	Weakness, numbness, hemiparesis, tingling, spasticity, or rigidity	Nerve conduction velocity

(handwritten: atherosclerotic CV disease; dyspnea on exertion)

Key Reference: Drummond JC, Patel PM. Neurosurgical anesthesia. In: Miller RO, ed. *Anesthesia*. 5th ed. Philadelphia: Churchill Livingstone; 2000:1895–1933.

Perioperative Implications

Preoperative Preparation

- Neurologic exam: Level of consciousness evaluation: is pt candidate for awake stereotaxic surgery?
- Focal neurologic symptoms, new weakness w/in 1 y (avoid succinylcholine)
- Is there elevated ICP to start with? (headache, N/V, loss of vision or diplopia) (? Delayed gastric emptying or N/V with inc ICP)
- Dexamethasone: May lower ICP initially, but ICP on knee of curve at time of operation
- Head scan report:
  - Temporal lobe lesion with impending herniation?
  - Massive peritumor edema with shift of midline?
  - Antiseizure drugs adequate? Beware postop seizure.
- Assess volume status (? Dehydrated)

Monitoring

- Consider arterial line: BP control, frequent ABGs, glucose, avoid dec. PaO_2

- Monitor CPP (MAP-ICP), (MAP at ear level)
- $ETCO_2$ as rough guide only, rely on $Paco_2$, avoid inc. CO_2
- ICP:
  - If lumbar CSF drains are used, connect to transducer, leave closed until head open and surgeon ready, then drain slowly as need by surgeon
  - ICP monitors for postop measurement
  - Optimize hyperventilation (25–30 mm Hg $PaCO_2$), mannitol Rx
  - Diagnostic if pt slow to awaken from anesthetic
- NMB: Increased receptor density in paretic extremities gives false twitch data: Use nonparetic arm/leg
- EEG used if surgery to treat seizure disorder
- Positioning occipital and pineal tumors): mild head up, if sitting then monitor for air embolism (precordial Doppler, CVP, etc.)

Airway

- Cushingoid facies may result in difficult mask ventilation
- Acromegaly causes laryngeal compromise by cartilaginous overgrowth. Anticipate difficult

intubation. Consider lateral neck x-ray for airway abn such as enlarged epiglottis, narrowed cricoid ring.

Preinduction/Induction

- Induction with agents that act to ↓ cerebral blood flow (avoid ketamine)
- Opioids prn to avoid hemodynamic responses early on
- Avoid ↑ BP with intubation/head pins
- Avoid brain swelling due to venous outflow occlusion: Do not permit overflexion or excessive rotation of neck
- Eye protection from prep solution and pressure while face covered by drapes, instruments
- Use soft bite block (esp. with MEP)

Maintenance

- Goal normovolemia, normotension
- Normonatremic fluids, replace diuresis if needed
- Avoid hyperglycemia, hypo-osmolality (<290 mosm/kg)
- Low intrathoracic pressure
- Monitor $PaCO_2$, esp. with COPD
- Mannitol: 0.5–1 gm/kg per surgeon

- No painful structures below dura: Minimal anesthetic requirement with brain manipulation; low-dose inhalation agent and/or propofol infusion
- Avoid hyperthermia, hyperglycemia
- Avoid N_2O, use inhalational agent <1 MAC <½ MAC if SSEP, TIVA if MEP monitored
- Avoid NMB with MEP monitoring
- Maintain good cerebral perfusion but not Htn
  - Antibiotics, redose at appropriate interval

Extubation
- Extubate in head up position to dec bleeding
  - Awake: Normocarbia, early neuro assessment (risk of coughing, straining, possible hematoma formation. Risk ↑ postop Htn)
  - Deep: Avoids coughing, may be Htn (transient $PaCO_2$ about 50 mm Hg until pt awakens, use deep ext. only if no brain edema during craniotomy and no anticipated airway problems)
- Consider postop intubation/ventilation with preop poor mental status

Adjuvants
- Decadron, mannitol, lasix
- Muscle relaxants
  - Profound paralysis: May minimize need for inhalation agents
  - Expect nondepolarizing NMB will be shorter acting if pt taking dilantin, most other antiseizure medications (except keppra)
- Regional and local drugs
  - Expect hemodynamic effects from epinephrine in local infiltrated into scalp incision site
- Antiemetics (differentiate PONV vs. Inc ICP)
- Vasoactive compounds

- Consider treatment with labetalol
- Consider cerebral vasodilators: Hydralazine, sodium nitroprusside if severe Htn

Anticipated Problems/Concerns
- Intraop brain swelling (head up, dec. CO_2, inc. venous drainage, dec. inhaled anesthesia, propofol/barbiturates
- Air embolism with tumors near dural sinuses and sitting position
- Intracranial bleeding (dural sinuses, vascular tumors)
- Postop inc. ICP due to loss autoregulation
- Delayed awakening, esp. with depressed consciousness preop
- Postexcision brain swelling; seizures
- Postop arterial Htn/bleeding

Supraventricular Tachycardia (Tachyarrhythmias)

Gina Whitney

Risk

- SVT is assoc with advancing age, significant cardiac and pulm disease.
- PSVT is assoc with WPW, congenital heart disease, and mitral valvel prolapse. It is more common in younger pts. Mechanism is re-entrant in nature.
- Atrial tachycardia (AAT) may be automatic, triggered, or re-entrant. It is seen more commonly in children and those with a Hx of prior atrial surgery. In adults it is rare, though can be assoc with digitalis toxicity and hypokalemia.
- Multifocal atrial tachycardia (MAT) is seen in adult pts with critical illness or advanced pulm disease.

Perioperative Risk

- Myocardial ischemia assoc with tachycardia and resulting coronary insufficiency
- Circulatory compromise
- Increased risk of atrial thrombus
- Chronic sustained tachycardia can result in irreversible cardiomyopathy.

Worry About

- Electrolyte and acid-base balance (K, Mg, alkalosis)
- Digitalis toxicity

Overview

- Tachycardia (HR>100 in adults) with origin above the bundle of His in sinus node, atrial or junctional tissue. It may be re-entrant, automatic or triggered in origin.
- SVT may be paroxysmal (PSVT) or gradual in onset (sinus tachycardia, atrial tachycardia, or multiform atrial tachycardia). Tachycardia mechanisms vary (re-entrant vs. triggered and automatic) and treatment varies accordingly.
- PSVT is a re-entrant arrhythmia usually seen more commonly in children. The re-entrant circuit usually involves an accessory conducting pathway and the AV node.
- AAT is more commonly seen in the pediatric population 2° to the enhanced automaticity seen in children.

ICD-9-CM Code: 427.0 (Paroxysmal supraventricular tachycardia)

Etiology

- PSVT is due to re-entry, which generally involves the AV node and an accessory pathway. Accessory pathways are relatively common in children. Also assoc with WPW and Lown-Ganong-Levine Syndrome (LGL).

- AAT is much more common in children and thought to be due to areas of enhanced automaticity of sites, which are usually found at the mouth of either atrial appendage, the orifices of the pulm veins, or the crista terminalis.

Usual Treatment

- PSVT: Drugs, which alter the refractoriness of tissue within the re-entrant circuit, may terminate tachycardia. Adenosine IVP is commonly used to terminate tachycardias. Other agents that may be used incl procainamide, propafenone, amiodarone, sotalol, esmolol, and verapamil.
- PSVT may be terminated by cardioversion or rapid atrial pacing as well.
- AAT may be treated using amiodarone, sotalol, flecainide, and beta blockers.
- MAT may be managed using beta blockers or Ca-channel blockers to slow the ventricular rate and improve cardiac function. Underlying cardiopulmonary disease must be addressed as well.

ASSESSMENT POINTS

System	Effect	Assessment by Hx	PE	Test
CARDIO	Arrhythmia	Palpitations, pre-syncope or syncope, angina, dyspnea Failure to thrive (pediatrics)	Regular (PSVT, AAT) or irregular pulse (MAT)	ECG, Holter, EP study
	LV function	CHF, evercise intolerance	Signs of CHF (S_3, rales, edema, wheezing)	CXR, ECHO
	Ischemia	Angina	Diaphoresis	Angio Scintigraphy
RESP	CHF, COPD	Dyspnea, orthopnea, cough	S_3, rales, wheezing	CXR, PFT's
GI	Hypoperfusion	Abd discomfort, diarrhea		
RENAL	Hypoperfusion	Oliguria, polyuria	UOP	BUN/Cr, FENa

Key Reference: Thompson A, Balser JR. Perioperative cardiac arrhythmias. *Br J Anaesth.* 2004;93:86–94.

Perioperative Implications

Preoperative Preparation

- PSVT: Adenosine, esmolol, and amiodarone should be available.
- AAT: Check and optimize electrolyte (K, Mg) and acid-base status. Rule out digitalis toxicity.
- MAT: Optimize status of various organ systems incl cardiac, pulm, renal, and metabolic.

Monitoring

- ECG, ST segment analysis
- Consider arterial pressure or PAC monitoring depending on anticipated case and pt status.

Induction

- In the setting of LV dysfunction or cardiomyopathy aim for hemodynamically stable induction.

- AAT and MAT: Use caution with medications or situations which increase pt's heart rate (ketamine, pancuronium, desflurane, beta-agonists, light anesthesia)

Maintenance

- Volatile agents are not thought to increase incidence of PSVT, AAT, MAT with the possible exception of desflurane.
- Prophylactic beta-blockade may be useful intraop if the pt is able to tolerate them.

Extubation

- Avoid excess sympathetic stimulation around the time of extubation as this increases the incidence of tachyarrhythmias. Strategies aimed at mitigating airway stimulation and hyperdynamic circulation are helpful in this regard.

Adjuvants

- Avoid use of beta agonists and histamine-releasing drugs if at all possible.

Postoperative period

- Ensure adequate sedation and pain control.
- Use of beta-blockers as tolerated will reduce incidence of MAT, AAT postop.
- Optimize cardiopulmonary and metabolic status.

Anticipated Problems/Concerns

- PSVT: Be prepared to treat afib/aflutter with RVR or ventricular fibrillation with cardioversion and/or defibrillation, particularly in pts with WPW or LGL
- Cardioversion of AAT or MAT may result in life-threatening arrhythmias.

Swallowing Disorders

Shiroh Isono

Risk

- More than 10% of elderly individuals have an absent gag reflex
- Pts with bulbar paralysis of any etiology

Perioperative Risks

- Malnutrition and dehydration due to inadequate oral intake
- Presence of pneumonia due to chronic aspiration
- Increased risk of aspiration pneumonia postop
- Increased retained bronchial secretions

Worry About

- Aspiration pneumonia

Overview

- Condition usually assoc with impairment of any part of swallowing reflex arc, such as sensory receptors in pharynx and larynx, afferent nerves, CNS, efferent nerves, muscles
- High risk for aspiration pneumonia pre- and postop can be evaluated by video fluoroscopy
- Assoc with abn hygiene of upper and bronchial airways

ICD-9-CM Code: 787.2 (Dysphagia)

Etiology

- Depressed CNS by sedation, sleep, coma, or light anesthesia
- NM disorders such as polymyositis, progressive MD, MS, myasthenia gravis, Eaton-Lambert syndrome
- Regional anesthesia to upper airway
- Tracheotomy or prolonged ET intubation; surgery on the head and neck, cardiac surgery
- Precurarization
- Peripheral nerve disorders such as Guillain-Barré syndrome, acute porphyria, laryngeal nerve injury; parkinsonism; advanced age

Usual Treatment

- Control for underlying disorders if possible
- Cricopharyngeal myotomy sometimes indicated
- Nasogastric balloon tube reported useful

ASSESSMENT POINTS

System	Effect	Assessment by Hx	PE	Test
HEENT	Aspiration	Cough	Check gag reflex Chest exam	Videofluoroscopy
CARDIO	Dehydration	Skin, orthostatic vital signs	UO	
RESP	Pneumonia	Dyspnea, sputum production	Fever	CXR, ABGs
GI	Dysphagia	Salivation Repeated pneumonia	UA inspection Laryngeal movement	Fluoroscopy, manometry CT, MRI, endoscopy
	GE reflux	Heartburn		
CNS	Cranial nerve IX or X or others dysfunctional	Eating/swallowing pattern	Cranial nerve examination	

Key Reference: Barker J, et al. Incidence and impact of dysphagia in patients receiving prolonged endotracheal intubation after cardiac surgery. *Can J Surg.* 2009;52:119–124.

Perioperative Implications

Preoperative Preparation

- Control underlying disorders and complications (pneumonia, dehydration).
- Correct malnutrition and dehydration by tube feeding, gastrostomy, or parenteral alimentation.
- Consider metoclopramide or domperidone as a part of preop medication to treat prolonged retention of stomach contents.
- H_2 blocker or proton pump inhibitor to decrease effects of silent regurgitation due to use of anticholinergic drug
- Avoid deep sedation

Monitoring

- Routine + quantitative acceleromyographic monitoring

Airway

- Tracheal intubation with cuffed ETT
- Suction of secretions above the tracheostomy tube
- Do not apply local anesthetics to upper airway

Preinduction/Induction

- Rapid induction/intubation of trachea after cricoid pressure
- Avoid precurarization, possibly leading to severe dysphagia or pharyngeal obstruction

Maintenance

- Minimize NMB

Extubation

- Aspirate stomach contents and clear the oronasal cavity before extubation
- Eliminate or reverse residual anesthetics and muscle relaxants before extubation
- Check recovery of swallowing reflex

Possible Drug Interactions

- Light sedation may impair swallowing reflex
- Precurarization and residual muscle relaxants can severely impair swallowing
- Possible synergistic effect of low concentration of inhalational anesthetics and partial paralysis on impairment of upper airway muscles
- Regional anesthesia impairs other upper airway protective reflex (closure of the larynx, cough reflex)

Postoperative Period

- Fowler position if possible
- Prophylaxis of and/or treat N/V
- Evaluate for presence of aspiration pneumonia

Anticipated Problems/Concerns

- Aspiration pneumonia (chemical or infectious)

Syndrome of Inappropriate Antidiuretic Hormone Secretion (SIADH)

Shalin Patel
Albert T. Cheung

Risk

- Elderly pts
- Nursing home residents
- Planned major operations, esp. neurosurgical procedures
- Central nervous system disorders incl psychiatric diseases
- Cancer, esp small-cell lung cancer
- Lung disease

Perioperative Risks

- Hyponatremia
- Cerebral edema causing altered mentation, seizures, and coma
- Acute water intoxication and fluid overload

Worry About

- Other causes of hyponatremia such as heart failure, liver failure, renal failure, or pseudohyponatremia (e.g., hyperglycemia) (see Hyponatremia)
- Acuity and magnitude of hyponatremia influences the risk of CNS complications
- Central pontine and extrapontine myelinolysis caused by rapid correction of hyponatremia

Overview

- Hyponatremia is the most common electrolyte disorder in hospitalized pts (affects 15%) and SIADH is the most frequent cause of hyponatremia, but other causes of hyponatremia should be excluded before making a Dx of SIADH
- Normally, increased serum osmolarity, hypovolemia, or hypotension triggers thirst and ADH release. ADH increases aquaporin-2 channels on the luminal surface of the distal tubules and collecting duct and acts to promote free water reabsorption. Thirst, free water intake, or hypotonic fluid administration combined with ADH-induced free water retention causes hyponatremia.
- Dx of SIADH: Serum osmolarity <275 mOsm/L, urine osmolarity >100 mOsm/L, urine sodium >40 mEq/L, euvolemia, normal thyroid and adrenal function, and absence of diuretic therapy
- SIADH can be classified as: Type A is unregulated secretion of ADH; Type B is elevated basal secretion; Type C is reset osmostat; Type D is undetectable ADH.

ICD-9-CM Codes: 259.3 (Ectopic); 259.6 (Neurohypophysial)

Etiology

- Malignant diseases causing ectopic ADH secretion: Lung cancer (esp. small-cell and mesothelioma); brain tumors, cancer of the duodenum, pancreas, head and neck, GU tract, lymphoma, and sarcomas
- Pulm disorders: Infections, asthma, cystic fibrosis
- CNS disorders: Infection, masses, head trauma, intracranial bleed, MS, Guillain-Barre syndrome, Shy-Drager syndrome, delirium tremens, acute intermittent porphyria
- Drugs: Incl, but not limited to, chlorpropramide, carbamazepine, cyclophosphamide, SSRIs, TCAs, clofibrate, nicotine, NSAIDs, antipsychotics, narcotics, arginine vasopressin analogues: desmopressin (DDAVP), oxytocin, vasopressin
- Major surgery: Pain, stress, general anesthesia, PPV, neurosurgery
- Hereditary: Mutation of gene for renal vasopressin-2 receptor; mutation for gene affecting osmolarity sensing in hypothalamus

Usual Treatment

- Decision to treat depends on acuity and severity of hyponatremia or the presence of symptoms
- Treat underlying causes for SIADH when possible
- Water restriction to 500–1000 mL per day for asymptomatic or chronic SIADH
- Normal saline (0.9%, 154 meq/L) infusion and furosemide (20 mg) for hyponatremia of unknown duration or moderate CNS symptoms. Goal is to increase [Na+] by 8–10 mEq/L in first 24 hr. Measure [Na+] every 4 hr.
- Hypertonic saline (3%, 513 mEq/L) at 1–2 mL/kg/hr infusion and furosemide (20 mg) for acute hyponatremia assoc with coma or seizures. Goal is to increase [Na$^+$] by 2 mEq/L/hr until symptoms improve. Measure [Na$^+$] every 2 hr.
- Demeclocycline 300–600 mg po bid to diminish responsiveness of collecting tubule to ADH for persistent hyponatremia unresponsive to other therapy
- Vasopressin-receptor antagonist such as conivaptan (20–40 mg IV qd) or tolvaptan (15–60 mg PO qd) as an adjunct to increase free water clearance and [Na$^+$]
- Urea, 30 g PO qd, to enhance water excretion in chronic SIADH
- Infusion rate (mL/hr) = [TBW x ([Na]$_{target}$ – [Na]$_{current}$) / ([Na]$_{infusion}$)] * (1000 mL / L) * (1 / t)
- Where: TBW = total body water (0.6 x body weight); [Na]$_{target}$ = target [Na$^+$];
- [Na]$_{current}$ = current [Na$^+$]; [Na]$_{infusion}$ = [Na$^+$] of saline infusion; t = time to achieve target [Na$^+$] in hr

ASSESSMENT POINTS

System	Effect	Assessment by Hx	PE	Test
CNS	Cerebral edema	Headache, confusion, coma, seizures, difficulty concentrating, lethargy	Decerebrate posturing, altered level of consciousness	CT (brain) MRI (brain) EEG
GI	Increased free water intake	N/V, anorexia		
RENAL	Free water retention	Concentrated urine	No edema	Serum [Na$^+$] < 130 mEq/L, serum Osm <275 mOsm/L, urine Osm >100 mOsm/L, Urine [Na$^+$] >40 mEq/L
NM	Fatigue, lethargy	Muscle cramps, falls	Motor weakness	

Key Reference: Ellison DH, Berl T. Clinical practice. The syndrome of inappropriate antidiuresis. *N Engl J Med.* 2007;356:2064–2072.

Perioperative Implications

Preoperative Preparation
- Medical evaluation for duration and other causes of hyponatremia
- Neurologic assessment for symptomatic hyponatremia

Monitoring
- Periop measurement of serum [Na$^+$]
- CVP or pulm artery catheter if necessary to maintain euvolemia

Induction
- Avoid drugs that may potentiate SIADH

Maintenance
- Hyponatremia reduces MAC
- Avoid hypotonic IV fluids

Extubation
- Symptomatic hyponatremia may contribute to delayed emergence from anesthesia
- Hyponatremia can cause obtundation and diminished ability to protect the airway

Adjuvants
- Normal saline (0.9%, 154 meq/l) and furosemide to maintain euvolemia and normal [Na$^+$]

Postoperative Period
- Free water restriction, avoid hypotonic fluids
- Monitor serum [Na$^+$]
- Assess for CNS signs of hyponatremia: lethargy, confusion, seizures

Anticipated Problems/Concerns

- Major surgery causes increased ADH release
- Acute symptomatic postop hyponatremia is a medical emergency
- Practice of using hypotonic maintenance fluids in pediatrics is controversial
- Most reported cases of central pontine and extrapontine myelinolysis were assoc with rapid correction of hyponatremia at rates over 12 mEq/L per day, but may occur at slower rates of correction.

Syndrome X

James A. Ramsey

Risk

- True incidence unknown, characterized by angina with or without ST changes, with or without reversible perfusion defects on stress test, with normal coronary ateriograms.
- Postmenopausal or posthysterectomy women most often at risk
- Common cause of chest pain in women with angiographically normal coronary arteries
- No diagnostic test; mortality risk low, morbidity high due to recurring angina and readmission.

Perioperative Risks

- Acute withdrawal of sex hormone replacement can potentially lead to symptoms.
- Preop angina can delay procedures.

Worry About

- D/C of medications (HRT) could precipitate symptoms.

Overview

- Poorly understood multifactoral etiology makes specific treatment difficult.
- Multimodal approach to reducing oxidative stress and improving endothelial function may be beneficial.

ICD-9-CM Code: 413.9

Etiology

- Etiology unproved, but thought to be due to endothelial dysfunction, +/- vasospasm, with systemic inflammation (increased CRP) playing a role
- Bioavailablity of NO plays a role
- Acute withdrawal of estrogen appears to be more significant factor than chronic withdrawal

Usual Treatment

- Beta blockade, Ca++ channel blockers, statins, folate found to be beneficial and should be continued periop.
- Estrogen patch has been found to significantly improve exercise tolerance and alleviating chest pain.

ASSESSMENT POINTS

System	Effect	Assessment by Hx	PE	Test
CV	Angina (chest pain) Inflammation	Hx of exertional angina Hx of evaluations leading to catheterization Hx of hormone replacement therapy		Normal coronary angiogram in presence of chest pain Elevated CRP

Key Reference: Lim TK, et al. Therapeutic development in cardiac Syndrome X: A Need to Target the underlying pathophysiology, *Cardiovasc Ther.* 2009;27(1):49–58.

Perioperative Implications

Preoperative Preparation

- Estrogens are withdrawn due to threat of procoagulant activity. Pts with this syndrome may experience significant angina upon such withdrawal.
- Distinguish chest pain due to this syndrome from chest pain due to coronary insufficiency from other causes.
- Continue preop meds, with appropriate thromboembolic prophylaxis.

Monitoring

- ST-segment analysis, usual ASA monitors.
- Invasive as appropriate for procedure.

Preinduction/Induction

- Contingent upon type of surgery; may consider maintaining usual medications, with use of beta blockers as appropriate.
- No data as to preferred anesthetic technique, agents.

Anticipated Problems/Concerns

- Angina pre- or periop in a pt with known clear coronary arteries
- Continuation of HRT can increase coagulability.
- Continuation of beta blockers and calcium channel blockers can lead to expected use of vasopressors.

Systemic Lupus Erythematosus

Sharon L. Lin
Jane C. Ahn

Risk

- Prevalence: 1/2500 in Northern Europeans; 1/500 in African-American population
- 90% of pts with lupus are female.
- 65% of SLE pts are diagnosed between ages 16 and 55; 20% of SLE patients present prior to age 16

Perioperative Risks

- Increased lupus activity is assoc with surgery and stress
- Infections can initiate lupus or cause a relapse

Worry About

- CV: Htn, CAD, Libman-Sacks endocarditis with mitral insufficiency, myo-carditis
- Pulm: Restrictive lung disease with decreased diffusion capacity
- Renal: Lupus nephritis and renal insufficiency
- Endo: Adrenal insufficiency 2° to chronic corticosteroid use

- Heme: Increased risk of thromboembolism in pts with antiphospholipid antibodies or severe nephrotic syndrome; thrombocytopenia and anemia
- Neuro: Peripheral neuropathy, delirium, stroke due to thromboembolism
- Neonatal lupus syndrome: Fetal heart block from maternal autoantibodies that cross placenta

Overview

- Autoantibody-mediated tissue damage results in multisystem organ damage
- Biopsy demonstrates inflammation, deposition of autoantibodies and complement in skin and kidneys
- 15-y survival with lupus is 80%
- Procainamide, hydralazine, quinidine, clonidine, enalapril, isoniazid, or captopril may cause drug-induced lupus variant
- Mechanism of increased lupus activity with surgery is unclear, but may be related to release of antigens into the bloodstream that bind to circulating antinuclear antibodies to form immune complexes

ICD-9-CM Code: 710.0

Etiology

- Genetic contribution (major histocompatibility complex gene) is important but not sufficient to cause lupus
- Ultraviolet radiation is strongest environmental factor linked to lupus

Usual Treatment

- Lack of specific therapy for SLE
- NSAIDs are first-line therapy for musculoskeletal symptoms and serositis
- Antimalarials are second-line agent for arthritis and may alter induction of autoimmunity
- Immunosuppressive medications incl glucocorticoids, azathioprine, cyclophosphamide, and mycophenolate

ASSESSMENT POINTS

System	Effect	Assessment by Hx	PE	Test
CARDIO	Htn, ↑ CAD, pericarditis, endocarditis, myocarditis, CHF, conduction blocks, pulm hypertension	Chest pain Palpitations Dyspnea	Murmur Pericardial friction rub Peripheral edema	ECG ECHO CXR
RESP	Restrictive lung disease, alveolar hemorrhage, pleural effusion, pulm edema	Pleuritic chest pain Hemoptysis Cough Dyspnea	Pleural rub Cyanosis ↓ Lung volume Rales, crackles	CXR PFTs ABGs
GI	Gastritis/PUD 2° to medications, lupoid hepatitis, SLE vasculitis resulting in colitis, pancreatitis, and bowel ischemia	N/V Abd pain Ileus	Hepatomegaly Splenomegaly Jaundice	LFTs PT/PTT/INR
HEME	Thrombocytopenia, leukopenia, anemia, thromboembolism (lupus "anticoagulant" prolongs aPTT in vitro, but pts have prothrombotic tendency)	Bruising Thrombosis	Lymphadenopathy Splenomegaly	CBC/platelet PTT
RENAL	Glomerulonephritis, nephrotic syndrome, renal insufficiency, renal failure	Fever, hematuria Polyuria Oliguria	Costophrenic tenderness Edema	Urinalysis BUN, Cr, TP, albumin Renal U/S or scan
CNS	Peripheral neuropathy, stroke, psychosis, fatigue, seizures	Numbness Hemiparesis Paranoid states Hyperirritability	Psychosis Nystagmus, ptosis, diplopia Aphasia	EMG/NCS MRI CT scan EEG
MS/ DERM	Vasculitis and ulceration Arthritis, myalgias, myositis, Raynaud phenomenon	Photosensitivity Ecchymosis or purpura Joint pain or immobility	Malar or butterfly rash Perioral ulcerations	X-ray ANA

Key Reference: Rahman A, Isenberg DA. Systemic lupus erythematosus. *N Engl J Med.* 2008;358:929–939.

Perioperative Implications

Preoperative Preparation

- Consider hydrocortisone 100 mg IV prior to induction if on chronic steroid therapy
- Antibiotic prophylaxis if valvular disease present

Monitoring

- Caution with arterial line in pts with Raynaud phenomenon
- Consider PA catheter for pulm Htn or CHF
- Consider Foley catheter and CVP/PA catheter for fluid titration if renal involvement

Airway

- Occasionally reduced TMJ ROM and cricoarytenoid arthritis manifesting as hoarseness, stridor, or airway obstruction; consider fiberoptic intubation

Preinduction/Induction

- Consider stress dose corticosteroid therapy

Maintenance

- No specific agents indicated or contraindicated; consider myocardial function
- Regional acceptable if no coagulopathy
- Avoid renally excreted drugs and renal toxins if renal insufficiency is present.
- Cyclophosphamide inhibits plasma cholinesterase and may cause prolonged response to succinylcholine.

Adjuvants

- Corticosteroids, supplemental O_2, careful titration of fluids with renal involvement

Extubation/Postoperative Period

- Reassess resp, renal, CV status prior to extubation

Anticipated Problems/Concerns

- Adrenal insufficiency from chronic steroid suppression
- Postop infections and pulm compli-cations
- Postextubation laryngeal edema or stridor
- CAD, CHF and arrhythmias
- Renal insufficiency and volume status
- CNS dysfunction, seizures, neuropathy
- Thrombocytopenia, anemia, and thromboembolism
- Lupoid hepatitis

Tetanus

Kirk Lalwani

Risk

- A major public health problem in the developing world, responsible for 200,000–300,000 deaths/y; of these, approx 180,000 were neonatal deaths (in 2002).
- Incidence in USA: 0.16 cases/million population (1998–2000).
- Highest incidence in USA is among the elderly (>60 y), persons of Hispanic ethnicity, older adults with diabetes, and parenteral drug users.

Perioperative Risks

- Difficult airway or intubation in the presence of masseter spasm, neck rigidity, or opisthotonus.
- Autonomic instability with sudden fluctuations in BP, arrhythmias, cardiac failure, and cardiac arrest

Worry About

- Spasms of the laryngeal and resp muscles can be life-threatening as a result of airway obstruction or chest wall rigidity respectively, and may mandate urgent ET intubation.
- Resp failure may require NM paralysis in addition to sedation for effective PPV in the presence of severe spasms.
- Autonomic instability: Tachycardia, bradycardia, Htn, hypotension, arrhythmias, cardiac failure, repeated cardiac arrest
- Pneumonia, sepsis, myoglobinuria, pulm embolism, bony fractures, hyperthermia

Overview

- Infection of penetrating wounds or devitalized tissue with spores of anaerobic gram-positive bacillus *Clostridium tetani*; enter the CNS via peripheral nerves and spread via retrograde intraneuronal transport to disable inhibitory pathways in the spinal cord and brain (glycine and GABA).
- CNS disinhibition characteristically begins with spasms of the masseter muscles ('risus sardonicus', lockjaw) and progresses to involve rest of the body, incl spasms of resp muscles ('resp convulsions') that cause glottic spasm, airway obstruction, hypoxia, and resp failure.
- Autonomic instability is a hallmark of the disease and may cause fatal cardiac arrest.
- The initial injury may be insignificant or unnoticed by the pt.
- Neonatal tetanus typically presents 6–8 d after birth with trismus and inability to feed.
- Tetanus may follow surgery (usually intra-abd or on contaminated tissues), burns, gangrene, dog bites, chronic infection, parenteral drug use, dental infection, abortion, and childbirth.

ICD-9-CM Code: 037

Etiology

- Infection of penetrating wound or devitalized tissue by spores of anaerobic, Gram-positive bacillus *Clostridium tetani*; they proliferate and produce a potent exotoxin, tetanospasmin.
- Tetanospasmin is taken up by motor nerve endings and spreads to other neurons in skeletal muscle, the spinal cord, and brain, where it principally inactivates inhibitory interneurons in glycinergic and gamma-aminobutyric acid pathways.

Usual Treatment

- Neutralize circulating toxin with IV human antitetanus globulin.
- Eradication of the organism by wound care, surgical debridement, and antimicrobial therapy.
- High dose metronidazole or penicillin G (erythromycin if penicillin allergy) therapy IV for 10 d is effective at eradicating spores and bacilli.
- Control muscle spasms by sedation, other muscle relaxants, and NM paralysis.
- Supportive therapy incl ventilatory support, treatment of autonomic instability, nutritional support, prophylaxis of DVT, and prevention of nosocomial infection, particularly ventilator-assoc pneumonia (VAP).

ASSESSMENT POINTS

System	Effect	Assessment by Hx	PE	Test
AIRWAY	Laryngospasm and glottic obstruction	Dyspnea, noisy breathing	Stridor, retractions of accessory muscles, limitation of mouth opening and ROM of neck	
CNS	Generalized or localized muscle rigidity and spasms	Dysphagia, drooling, spasms	Opisthotonus, trismus, 'risus sardonicus', onset of spasms with minimal stimuli, bony fractures	
CARDIO	Cardiac failure, myocarditis, arrhythmias, Htn, hypotension, cardiac arrest	SOB, palpitations	Episodic fluctuations in BP, heart rate, arrhythmias, signs of cardiac failure	ECG, ECHO
RESP	Hypoventilation, apnea, resp failure, pneumonia	Dyspnea	Hypoventilation, limited chest excursions, decreased breath sounds, rhonchi, cyanosis	ABG, CXR
RENAL	Rhabdomyolysis	Pink or red urine	Hematuria	Urinalysis, serum creatine kinase

Key Reference: Cook TM, Protheroe RT, Handel JM. Tetanus: A review of the literature. *Br J Anaesth*. 2001;87(3):477–487.

Perioperative Implications

Preinduction/Induction/Maintenance

- Adequate sedation with benzodiazepines to control spasms; muscle relaxants may be necessary.
- Minimize environmental stimuli.
- Difficult airway or intubation: Consider fiberoptic intubation.
- Avoid pancuronium and desflurane (sympathetic stimulation).
- Resistance to multiple non-depolarizing agents has been described.

Monitoring

- EKG for dysrhythmias.
- Echocardiography (CV decompen-sation).
- Arterial line for continuous BP measurement and arterial blood gas measurement.
- NM monitoring with nerve stimu-lator.

General Anesthesia

- Magnesium sulfate can be useful in controlling spasms, decreasing autonomic instability, and decreasing the requirements for sedative drugs.
- Watch for S-T segment and T-wave changes that may indicate toxic myocarditis.
- Hypotension and bradycardia may be indicative of brainstem involvement and a poor prognosis.
- Elective tracheostomy recommended for long-term ventilator support and pulm toilet.
- Consider pulm embolism in the event of sudden decompensation during anesthesia.
- Maintain alkaline diuresis in the event of myoglobinuria.

Regional Anesthesia

- Consider adding epidural anesthesia for autonomic hyperreactivity.

Postoperative Period

- Endotracheal intubation or tracheostomy needed for assisted ventilation on ICU with sedation and NMBs.

- Magnesium sulfate, benzodiazepines, opioids, clonidine, and intrathecal baclofen may help control spasms; magnesium also decreases autonomic instability and the need for sedation.
- Nutritional support via enteral or parenteral feeding.
- DVT prophylaxis to prevent pulm embolism

Anticipated Problems/Concerns

- Sudden CV instability or cardiac arrest may occur.
- Propranolol, labetalol, and phentolamine are assoc with increased risk of cardiac arrest.
- Mortality in USA averages about 10%, rising to 50% in pts >60 y of age.
- Abn neurologic findings may persist for up to 2 y following recovery.

Tetralogy of Fallot (TOF)

Veronica C. Swanson
Norah Janosy

Risk

- Occurs in 1 in 3000 live births
- Most common cyanotic CHD
- Slightly more common in males than females

Perioperative Risks

- If unrepaired: Tet spells >RVH>RV failure> death (50% in first year of life)
- Mortality after TOF repair: 5–8% in first 2 y post repair (if uncomplicated anatomy)
- Increased mortality if co-existing PA hypoplasia, atresia, or major AP collaterals

Worry About

- Decrease in SVR resulting in increased R → L shunt
- Increase in PVR resulting in increased R → L shunt
- Crying and agitation leading to tet spell, more hypoxemia, hypercarbia, acidosis
- Air bubbles in IV tubing
- Polycythemia and assoc thrombocytopenia
- RV failure after inadequate or late repair
- Arrhythmias following repair

Overview

- Anatomy: Tetralogy
  - RV outflow tract obstruction (RVOTO)
  - (Infundibular narrowing, pulmonary stenosis, PA hypoplasia, pulm atresia). May have bicuspid pulm valve.
    - VSD: Single or multiple; outlet.
    - Overriding aorta (<50%)
- RV hypertrophy (5%) have anomalous origin of LAD from right coronary artery: Must confirm before OR.
- 25% have right aortic arch.
- Degree of R → L shunting determined by fixed factors (degree of infundibular obstruction, size of pulm valve annulus, size of PA) and dynamic factors (infundibular muscle bundle spasm, PVR, SVR)
- Fixed factors determine amount of chronic cyanosis
- Dynamic factors determine tet spells
- Pink tets have minimal amount of PS
- Avoid hypoxia, acidosis, high airway pressures, excitement, agitation
- Dx by ECHO, cardiac catheterization, and/or MRI

- Assoc with chromosome 22 deletions and diGeorge syndrome, VACTERL, CHARGE, and velocardiofacial syndrome

ICD-9-CM Code: 745.2

Usual Treatment

- Primary repair: See TOF: Procedure chapter
- If not immediately operable (low birth weight, prematurity, other disease processes): Palliative shunts to increase pulm blood flow (Blalock-Taussig shunt, aortopulmonary shunts)
- β-blockers to decrease infundibular spasm and spelling
- Treatment of tet spell
  100% O$_2$ (pulm vasodilator)
  - Sedation (morphine/fentanyl)
  - Increased SVR (squatting, phenylephrine)
  - Propranolol (decreased contractility of infundibulum; decreased RVOTO)
  - Bicarbonate to correct metabolic acidosis

ASSESSMENT POINTS

System	Effect	Assessment by Hx	Test
GENERAL		FTT, Clubbing	Growth charts
CHEST	RVH	Signs of right heart failure	CXR with boot-shaped heart
CARDIO	See Overview: Anatomy	Frequency and severity of tet spells	ECHO/cath/MRI ECG-RVH, RA
HEME	Polycythemia from chronic hypoxemia Plt count may be low from polycythemia	Chronic cyanosis	HCT, plt count

Key Reference: von Ungern-Sternberg BS, Petak F, Hantos Z, Habre W. Changes in functional residual capacity and lung mechanics during surgical repair of congenital heart diseases: Effects of preoperative pulmonary hemodynamics. *Anesthesiology.* 2009;110(6):1348–1355.

Perioperative Implications

- Heavy premedication to avoid agitation, crying
- Phenylephrine appropriately drawn up and diluted.

- Avoid increase in PVR and decrease in SVR
- Consider IM ketamine if no IV present. Caution if Hx of tet spells
- Narcotics may be used

- See TOF Procedure chapter for detailed periop implications.

Thalassemia

Anna Jankowska
Ronald S. Litman

Risk

• Worldwide, 15 million people have clinically apparent thalassemia. Small percentage of that resides in USA.
• Affects primarily children of Mediterranean, African, and Southeast Asian descent.
• In endemic areas with highest frequency, carrier status is present in as many as 1 in 7 individuals and thalassemia major can occur in 1 in 158 live births.

Perioperative Risks

• Severe anemia and its complications (e.g., CHF)
• End-organ effects of hemochromatosis from chronic iron therapy: Cardiomyopathy, cirrhosis, endocrinopathies (e.g., diabetes, hypopituitarism)
• Airway difficulties; maxillofacial abn 2° to bone marrow expansion
• Coagulation abn; hypercoagulopathy in asplenic pts, and coagulopathy in pts with cirrhosis
• Alloimmunization 2° to multiple blood transfusions. Obtaining appropriately cross-matched blood may require prolonged testing

Worry About

• Difficult airway 2° to maxillary deformation
• Cardiac arrhythmias or CHF
• Coagulopathy

Overview

• Thalassemia is a heterogeneous group of inherited microcytic anemias that result from a genetic mutation causing a defect in the synthesis of one or more globin chain subunits of the adult hemoglobin tetramer (HbA), which is normally composed of two alpha and two beta chains (β2α2)
• Thalassemia is classified according to the genotype which correlates with clinical severity.

• Alpha thalassemia: Alpha globin gene deletion leads to a decrease in alpha chain production relative to beta chain production. This leads to formation of β4 tetramers which causes RBCs to be more rapidly removed leading to anemia
• Alpha thalassemia silent carrier: One gene absent (aa/a-); healthy except occasional mild anemia
• Alpha thalassemia trait: Two genes absent (a-/a- or aa/--); mild anemia
• Alpha thalassemia intermedia = Hgb H disease: Inactivation of three genes (a-/--); mild to moderately severe anemia, splenomegaly, icterus, abn RBC indices; Heinz bodies = beta chain tetramers
• Alpha thalassemia major: Complete deletion of all alpha chain genes; incompatible with life, hydrops fetalis unless intrauterine blood transfusions.
• Beta thalassemia: Decreased beta chain production relative to the alpha chain production as a result of mutation resulting in either absence (beta o) or decrease (beta +) in the production of beta globin. Alpha chains precipitate leading to inadequate erythroid maturation. In most severe forms this leads to splenomegaly, anemia, massive expansion of medullary and extramedullary erythropoetic tissue leading to skeletal, growth, and metabolic abnormalities.
• Beta thalassemia silent carrier (beta/ beta+); shows no clinical symptoms except for low RBC counts
• Beta thalassemia trait (beta / beta +) = beta thal minor: Mild anemia, abn RBC indices, hypochromia, microcytosis
• Beta thalassemia intermedia (beta/beta o, beta+/beta+, beta+/beta o): A compound heterozygous state; profound anemia which periodically may require transfusion support and occasionally splenectomy

• Beta thalassemia major (beta o/beta o) = Cooley's anemia – transfusion dependent anemia, massive splenomegaly, bone deformities, growth retardation and abn facies. As a result of chronic anemia and ineffective erythropoesis, bone expansion and extramedullary erythropoesis may develop in liver and spleen, and marrow space expansion at sites such as the cranium and paravertebral areas can lead to disfiguring bony changes.

ICD-9-CM Code: 282.4

Etiology

• Genetic mutation assoc with ancestry in areas endemic to malaria

Usual Treatment

• Alpha thalassemia carriers (aa/-a) and those with alpha thalassemia trait (a-/a- or --/aa) are usually asymptomatic and require no treatment.
• Alpha thalassemia intermedia (--/-a): folic acid, transfusions and possible splenectomy for progressive anemia, avoidance of oxidant drugs
• B thalassemia minor (beta/ beta+) usually does not require treatment.
• B thalassemia intermedia and major: Treatment is symptomatic and supportive
• Transfusion support with leukoreduced blood when Hb <7 g/dL; transfuse up to Hb 11–13 g/dL
• Splenectomy usually needed around age 6–7 y or in adolescence when transfusion treatments required are at 1.5 times normal (e.g., >200 mL/kg/y)
• Iron chelation therapy; deferasirox po or desferoxamine IV
• Hematopoietic stem cell transplantation

ASSESSMENT POINTS

System	Effect	Assessment by Hx	PE	Test
HEENT	Malar hypoplasia with relative mandibular hyperplasia	Prior difficulties with intubation	Airway evaluation	
CV	Cardiomyopathy Arrhythmias Pericarditis	Exercise tolerance H/o palpitations	Dyspnea Dysrhythmias Murmurs	ECG, annual ECHO, CXR, Halter
RESP	Restrictive lung disease	Exercise tolerance		PFTs
HEME	Anemia Splenomegaly Alloimmunization Coagulopathy	Exercise tolerance H/o splenectomy Blood transfusion reactions	Tachycardia Splenomegaly	CBC Type and screen Coagulation studies
HEPATIC	Cirrhosis		Hepatomegaly	LFTs, coagulation studies, hepatitis serologies
ENDO	Diabetes mellitus Hypothyroidism Adrenal insufficiency	Cold intolerance, lethargy, depression, decreased metabolism		Fasting glucose Glucose tolerance test Thyroid function test Cortisol determination

Key Reference: Rodgers GP. *Hemoglobinopathies: The Thalassemias in Cecil medicine.* 23rd ed. Chapter 166.

Perioperative Implications

• Thalassemia minor, in general, does not create anesthetic problems. In pts with thalassemia major, consideration has to be given to problems derived from the severity of the anemia itself, but also those related to transfusion therapy, and to bony malformations.

Preinduction

• Detailed airway evaluation

• Cardiac function evaluation
• Hemoglobin level should be determined and preop transfusion considered
• Cross-matched blood should be available (antibody matched, leukocyte reduced for frequently transfused children); high degree of alloimmunization in this population exists.
• Evaluation for endocrine dysfunction (e.g., DM, hypopituitarism, hypothyroidism) and adequacy of treatment

• Hepatic function evaluation in light of risk of cirrhosis and iron or viral-induced damage
• Coagulation studies
• Presplenectomy antibiotics and immunizations (when appropriate)

Monitoring

• Consider the need for a Swan-Ganz catheter and measurements of CI, CO, mixed-venous oxygenation

- Consider arterial catheter and frequent hemoglobin, lactate, and blood gas analysis

Induction/Maintenance
- Preparation for possible difficult airway
- Close attention to the positioning in light of demineralization and scoliosis
- Careful monitoring of CV function; incl post-splenectomy Htn
- Beware of the effects of laparoscopy on circulatory and resp function
- Thromboembolism prophylaxis; SCD and/or pharmacotherapy when applicable
- Consider cell salvage

General Anesthesia
- Facial abn can present a difficult airway

Regional Anesthesia
- Osteoporosis, osteopenia, scoliosis are common
- Vertebral bodies maybe of reduced height as a result of osteoporosis; the segmental portion of conus medullaris may be lower than predicted
- Extramedullary hematopoesis is uncommon in the intraspinal location, but if symptoms of spinal compression are suspected, MRI should be performed prior to regional anesthesia
- Consider epidural versus spinal in pts who need a regional anesthetic, but have CV pathology
- Evaluate closely coagulation studies prior to regional anesthesia
- Periop thromboembolism prophylaxis, esp. in post-splenectomy pts
- Spinal and epidural techniques have been performed safely in parturients

Postoperative Period
- Postop monitoring dependent on the preop status
- Prophylaxis for thromboembolism (post-splenectomy pts in particular)

Anticipated Problems/Concerns

- Intubation difficulties
- CV instability 2° to severe chronic anemia, cardiomyopathy, and endocrinopathies
- Coagulation abn: hyper- or hypo-coagulable
- Impaired drug metabolism 2° to cirrhosis
- Adrenal insufficiency complications
- Difficulty in obtaining cross-matched blood due to alloimmunization

Thrombocytopenia

Risk

- Common in both adults and children
- Often assoc with systemic illness and pathologic conditions of pregnancy
- Heparin-induced thrombocytopenia (HIT) occurs in ~5% of pts exposed to heparin

Perioperative Risks

- Bleeding assoc with invasive procedures (both anesthetic and surgical)

Worry About

- Excessive periop bleeding
- Concurrent anemia, hypovolemia, and hemodynamic instability
- Potential need for blood and plt transfusions
- Underlying cause for thrombocytopenia

Overview

- Definition: <150,000 plt/mm^3
- Hemostasis is adequate with plt counts >100,000/mm^3 unless concurrent plt dysfunction is present (e.g., antiplatelet agents, cardiopulmonary bypass).
- Plt transfusion may be necessary for plt counts between 50,000 and 100,000/mm^3 to prevent/treat bleeding, depending on site and extent of invasive procedure

- Spontaneous bleeding does not generally occur unless plt count <20,000/mm^3
- Generalized petechiae, purpura, and bleeding from mucous membranes denotes high risk of bleeding from other sites
- Diagnosing cause of thrombocytopenia is key to successful treatment; begins with CBC, PT/PTT, fibrinogen, and D-dimer
- Bleeding time does not correlate with risk of surgical bleeding

ICD-9-CM Code: 287.5

Etiology

- Increased plt destruction, immune: Drug-induced, idiopathic thrombocytopenic purpura (ITP), rheumatologic disorders, post-transfusion purpura, neonatal immune thrombocytopenia, hemolytic uremic syndrome (HUS)
- Increased plt destruction, nonimmune: Infection with or without overt DIC, preeclampsia/HELLP syndrome, thrombotic thrombocytopenic purpura (TTP)
- Decreased plt production: Marrow failure, chemo- or radiation-therapy, ethanol

- Hypersplenism: Cirrhosis, portal or splenic vein thrombosis
- Dilution: Plt counts usually maintained until intravascular replacement >1.5–2 blood volumes

Usual Treatment

- Treat underlying cause
- D/C offending drug, treat infection, splenectomy
- HIT treatment incl a direct thrombin inhibitor (e.g., bivalirudin, argatroban) to prevent/treat thrombosis in addition to D/C of heparin
- ITP generally responds to corticosteroids (plus IgG therapy in severe cases); TTP requires exchange transfusion or plasmapheresis
- Decision to transfuse plts depends on etiology of thrombocytopenia and relative risks of bleeding vs. transfusion; not useful for thrombotic syndromes (e.g., HIT, TTP)
- Each unit of transfused plts should raise count ~10,000/mm^3 but increases risk of future thrombocytopenia (alloimmunization occurs in 50% of pts transfused with plts)

ASSESSMENT POINTS

System	Effect	Assessment by Hx	PE	Test
HEENT	Mucosal hemorrhage		Petechiae, purpura, and ecchymoses of skin, oral mucosae, and conjunctivae	
CARDIO	Hypovolemia, anemia, pericardial effusion	Lightheadedness, syncope, palpitations	Tachycardia, hypotension, orthostasis, pericardial friction rub, pulsus paradoxus	ECG, CXR
RESP	Pulm hemorrhage	Cough, hemoptysis		CXR
GI	GI bleeding	Hematemesis, hematochezia, melena		Stool guaiac
RENAL	Potential prerenal or renal azotemia, glomerulonephritis with specific disease entities	UO		BUN, Cr, urinalysis
CNS	Intracranial hemorrhage	Change in mental status	Mental status, focal motor weakness	Head CT

Key Reference: Levy JH, Hursting MJ. Heparin-induced thrombocytopenia, a prothrombotic disease. *Hematol Oncol Clin North Am.* 2007;21(1):65–88.

Perioperative Implications

Preinduction/Induction/Maintenance

- Assess volume status and Hct
- Determine bleeding risk from physical exam, extent of thrombocytopenia, and type of surgical procedure
- Ensure that blood bank has adequate cross-matched blood and plts available
- Plt transfusion immediately prior to surgical procedure if plt count <50,000/mm^3

- Vigilance to volume status and blood/fluid replacement is essential
- Hespan administration can impede plt function

Monitoring

- Routine

General Anesthesia

- Nasal intubation relatively contraindicated

Regional Anesthesia

- Epidural and spinal anesthetics can be safely administered with plt counts ≥100,000/mm^3

- Regional techniques are relatively contraindicated with plt counts <100,000/mm^3; however, a few dozen cases of epidural anesthesia have been reported by retrospective review without neurologic sequelae.

Anticipated Problems/Concerns

- Bleeding from anesthetic or surgical procedures
- Potential for blood and plt transfusions

Thyroid Neoplasms

Alisa C. Thorne

Risk

- Incidence in USA: 23,500 new thyroid cancer cases/y
- Approx 1% of new cancer diagnoses each year
- Hispanics, African-Americans, lower rate; Caucasians, moderate rate; Japanese, Chinese, Hawaiian, Filipinos, higher rate
- Overall incidence 3 × higher in women than in men, peaks in third and fourth decades of life

Perioperative Risks

- Large thyroid mass may produce airway compression, deviation, or vocal cord paralysis
- Decreased BP, decreased HR, asystole with manipulation of carotid sinus
- Postop complications: Phrenic nerve injury, pneumomediastinum, pneumothorax, tracheomalacia and tracheal collapse post extubation, hematoma or laryngeal edema leads to airway compromise; bilat laryngeal nerve injury calls for tracheotomy; superior laryngeal nerve injury leads to aspiration
- Accidental removal and/or injury of parathyroid glands causes decrease in Ca^{2+}

Worry About

- Occult pheochromocytoma: bilateral lobe medullary thyroid cancer is assoc with MEN IIA and IIB

Overview

- 4 types: Papillary (80%), follicular (10%), medullary (5–10%), 1° thyroid lymphoma (rare) and 1° thyroid sarcomas (rare)
- Prognosis of well-differentiated papillary cancer excellent, esp. for age <40 y with small tumors
- Prognosis worsens for large tumors with poorly differentiated, anaplastic histology
- Age at Dx, tumor burden, gender, extrathyroidal invasion, and distant metastases: important prognostic factors
- Latest research: Define subcellular and molecular prognostic factors, genetic studies
- BRAF mutation most common mutation in papillary thyroid cancer and is assoc with disease aggressiveness

ICD-9-CM Code: 193

Etiology

- Factors incl previous radiation, dietary iodine deficiency, goitrogens (chemical or dietary), pre-existing benign thyroid disease, and genetic factors (Gardner's syndrome, Cowden's disease)
- Association between primary thyroid cancer and ↑ incidence of subsequent breast cancer

Usual Treatment

- Surgery initial therapy of choice
- Lobectomy with or without isthmectomy, near-total or total thyroidectomy as indicated
- Radioiodine scanning and ablation commonly used after thyroidectomy in well differentiated tumors
- Radical debulking procedure (palliative) for large tumors invading airway and causing esophageal obstruction and bleeding
- Recurrences usually treated with surgery
- Combined chemo- and radiation therapy for poor prognosis cases
- Doxorubicin: Most active single agent; medullary thyroid cancer responds poorly

ASSESSMENT POINTS

System	Effect	Assessment by Hx	PE	Test
HEENT	Vocal cord dysfunction Tracheal obstruction	Dysphonia SOB, DOE Wheeze/stridor	Neck mass	Indirect laryngoscopy CXR CT of neck
CARDIO	Mediastinal mass	SOB, DOE Wheeze, may be asymptomatic	Facial swelling	CXR CT/MRI
RESP	Lung metastases Lower airway obstruction	SOB, DOE Wheeze, hemoptysis		CXR CT/MRI
GI	Esophageal obstruction Liver metastases	Dysphagia		LFTs
ENDO	MEN IIA/IIB pheochromocytoma	HTN, esp. episodic Flushing Palpitations, episodic Sweating		CT/MRI 24 h urine epinephrine ↑ Epinephrine/norepinephrine
	Hyperparathyroidism			↑ Ca^{2+}
	Ganglioneuromatosis	Colic Cramping Diarrhea Obstruction	Mucosal neuromas in tongue, subconjunctival areas, or GI tract Thickened lips Marfanoid features	Hypercalciuria provocative test for calcitonin release
MS	Bone metastases PTH-induced bone disease	Bone pain		Bone scan

Key References: Vriens MR, et al. Diagnostic markers and prognostic factors in thyroid cancer. *Future Oncol.* 2009;5(8):1283–1293. Snyder SK, et al. Local anesthesia with monitored anesthesia care vs. general anesthesia in thyroidectomy: A randomized study. *Arch Surg.* 2006;141(2):167–173.

Perioperative Implications

Preoperative Preparation

- Assess thyroid gland and/or tumor size
- Assess larynx and/or trachea compression
- May need smaller or armored ETT to prevent kinking (check CT scan)
- Record description of voice preop
- Correct abn Ca^{2+}, TFTs prior to surgery
- Check serum calcitonin level if medullary cancer suspected; rule out pheochromocytoma

Monitoring

- Routine

Airway

- Anticipate difficult airway

Induction

- Consider awake fiberoptic intubation for large thyroid masses

Maintenance

- No one agent or technique shown superior
- CV instability may occur with manipulation of carotid sinus

Extubation

- May develop tracheomalacia
- May require reintubation owing to hematoma

Postoperative Period

- Metabolic: Decreased Ca^{2+}, hypoparathyroidism
- Nonmetabolic: Unilateral or bilateral nerve injury, hemorrhage, airway obstruction

Adjuvants

- May be performed under local anesthesia with IV sedation in selected cases
- Antiemetics, incl dexamethasone, effective in reducing postop N/V

Anticipated Problems/Concerns

- Pts with medullary thyroid cancer: Rule out occult pheochromocytoma
- Thyroid tumor can invade larynx, trachea, pharynx, or esophagus
- If esophageal wall invaded, reconstruction often by free microvascular jejunal transfer or gastric pull-up

Transfusion-Related Acute Lung Injury (TRALI)

Sheela S. Pai

Risk

- All pts receiving blood or blood products incl plts, plasma, and cryoprecipitate
- Overall incidence probably <1%, increasing awareness of the syndrome has resulted in improved recognition.
- Use of leukodepleted blood has decreased the incidence of packed red cell–related lung injury.

Perioperative Risks

- Noncardiogenic pulm edema usually within 2–6 hr after transfusion
- Mortality reported, but rare

Worry About

- O_2 toxicity
- Barotrauma or volutrauma 2° to PPV

- Should be suspected in the face of persistent hypoxemia in the absence of volume overload

Overview

- Classic presentation is acute development of resp compromise indistinguishable from ARDS.
- Symptoms usually begin within 1–2 hr after transfusion and may be manifested by 2–6 hr.
- There are typically severe hypoxemia, hypotension, fever, and bilateral infiltrates on chest radiograph.
- Dx is one of exclusion (rule out fluid overload, CHF, sepsis)

ICD-9-CM Code: 999.8 (Transfusion, complication)

Etiology

- Classically, has been attributed to the presence of leukocyte antibodies in the plasma of multiparous donors directed against recipient WBCs.
- Alternatively, effect from biologically active lipids in stored cellular blood components
- Pulm edema arises from capillary injury rather than volume overload.

Usual Treatment

- Supportive care: Ventilation if required, supplemental O_2. No clear indications for steroids. Generally resolves within 1–4 d with appropriate care and no supervening complications.

ASSESSMENT POINTS

System	Effect	Assessment by Hx	PE	Test
CARDIO	Pulm edema		S_3, S_4	PA catheter, ECHO
RESP	Pulm edema	Recent transfusion	Rales, hypoxemia	CXR—bilateral infiltrates, SpO_2
HEME	Leukoagglutination			Agglutination of recipient leukocytes by donor plasma: Contact blood collection agency

Key Reference: Rizk A, Gorson K, Kenny L, Weinstein R. Transfusion-related acute lung injury after the infusion of IVIG. *Transfusion*. 2001;41:264–268.

Perioperative Implications

Perioperative Concerns

- Acute resp compromise that may occur shortly after transfusion in healthy pt, but more typically 2–4 hr after transfusion

- Usually related to massive transfusion although on occasion may happen after a single unit transfusion.

Monitoring

- PA catheter may aid in the exclusion of cardiac etiology

Postoperative Considerations

- Most require ventilatory support for several days
- Ventilator management appropriate for ARDS

Anticipated Problems/Concerns

O_2 toxicity and barotrauma

Transverse Myelitis

John A. Ulatowski

Risk

- Incidence: 1–1.7/1 million

Perioperative Risks

- Few data available (usually grouped with MS; demyelinating disease)
- Anesthetic effect (worsening) unknown, causative only question
- Sequelae of hypotension or Htn
- Urinary retention and UTI
- Delayed gastric emptying

Worry About

- Autonomic dysfunction (midthoracic lesion and above)
  - Acute: Hypotension from spinal shock
  - Chronic: Htn and bradycardia from mass reflex (autonomic dysreflexia)
- Hyperkalemia from succinylcholine; prolonged NM blockade rarely

Overview

- Inflammatory disease of spinal cord causing demyelination/necrosis
- Ascending paralysis and sensory level; T8–12 assoc with pain and urinary retention
- Spinal cord swelling; increased CSF protein, WBC 10–200 (higher if culture positive)
- Onset over hours to days
- Antecedent febrile illness (33%)
- Variable recovery
- MS (subsequent demyelinating lesions) occurs in 5–10% of cases

ICD-10-CM Code: G 37.3 (Acute transverse myelitis)

Etiology

- Viral (polio, HSV, HIV)
- Bacterial, fungal, parasitic
- Noninfectious (postinfectious, postvaccine, lupus, immune compromise)

Usual Treatment

- High-dose steroids; immune globulin antibodies recently reported, stem transplant tried
- Acute antibiotics if infectious; long-term antibiotics if frequent UTI
- Chronic pain treated with spinal cord stimulator
- Avoid noxious stimuli below level of the lesion

ASSESSMENT POINTS

System	Effect	Assessment by Hx	PE	Test
HEENT	Eyes (MS, Devic's syndrome)	↓ Visual acuity	Optic neuritis, ophthalmoscopy	Visual EPs
CARDIO (acute) CARDIO (chronic)	↓ BP, tachy- or bradycardia ↑ BP, bradycardia	Syncope Headaches, flushing, sweating	BP changes Flushed skin above level of lesion, blanched skin below lesion	Orthostasis Stop stimuli below lesion
RESP	Pulm embolism	Dyspnea, tachycardia	DVT, cord signs	Doppler, V/Q scan
GI	Gastric atony	N/V, dyspepsia, early satiety	Tympany, CXR	Stomach bubble
CNS	Brain Spine	Encephalitis Spinal level (sens/motor)	Mental status changes Paraplegia	MRI (brain) MRI (spine, LP)
RENAL	Bladder paralysis (acute) Bladder spasticity (chronic)	Retention, oliguria Frequent urination	Palpation, catheterization	UA, bladder scan Residual urine volumes

Key Reference: Krishnan C, Kaplin AI, Pardo CA, Kerr DA, Keswani SC. Demyelinating disorders: Update on transverse myelitis. *Curr Neurol Neurosci Rep.* 2006;6(3):236–243.

Perioperative Implications

Preoperative Preparation
- Relieve gastric ileus, treat as full stomach

Monitoring
- Routine, unless dysautonomia

Airway
- Avoid succinylcholine, hyperkalemia

Induction
- Adequate hydration because of vasorelaxation acutely and dysautonomia chronically

Maintenance
- GA preferred or epidural; TM has been described after all anesthetics
- Spinal with caution, possible toxicity with usual doses; usually avoided
- Follow Train-of-4; variable response to NM blockers

Extubation
- Return of airway reflexes if demyelinating lesions in brain/brainstem

Adjuvants
- Resistance and sensitivity to nondepolarizing muscle relaxants reported
- Dysautonomia reported assoc with use of dexmedetomidine

Anticipated Problems/Concerns

- Unstable hemodynamics
- Possible hyperkalemia following succinylcholine
- Worsening of baseline symptoms and neurologic signs after anesthesia (transient)

Treacher Collins Syndrome

Arlyne Thung
Inna Maranets

DISEASES

Risk

- Incidence of 1/25,000–50,000 live births

Perioperative Risks

- Difficult airway management

Worry About

- Difficult mask ventilation and intubation
- Acute airway obstruction
- Hx of obstructive sleep apnea and cor pulmonale

Overview

- Also known as mandibulofacial dystosis and Franceschetti-Zwahlen-Klein syndrome
- Clinical features incl various degrees of mandibular hypoplasia, high arched or cleft palate, malar hypoplasia, ophthalmic abn (downward slant of palpebral fissures, lower lid coloboma, partial to total absence of lower eyelashes, visual loss), microtia and middle ear hypoplasia.
- Fishlike facies
- Choanal atresia may occur
- Conductive hearing loss due to ear abn is universal with varying degrees of severity.
- Airway compromise may occur due to maxillary hypoplasia (narrows nasal passages resulting in choanal stenosis or atresia) and mandibular hypoplasia (tongue base is retropositioned thereby obstructing oropharyngeal and hypopharyngeal spaces)
- Limited orophayngeal and hypopharyngeal space may lead to obstructive sleep apnea, pulm Htn and in severe cases cor pulmonale
- Affected newborns and infants may have feeding difficulties

ICD-9-CM Code: 756.0

Etiology

- Abn bilateral first and second branchial arch development due to mutation in TCOF1 gene on chromosome 5 (60% spontaneous/40% familial)
- When inherited shows autosomal dominance with variable penetrance and expression
- TCOF1 mutation results in a deficiency of neural crest cells leading to failed development of cartilage, bone, and connective tissues particularly in the head and neck region.

Usual Treatment

- Prenatal detection of micrognathia and dysmorphic facial features on fetal US may prompt genetic testing and counseling if Treacher Collins is suspected
- Evaluation of airway and assessment of swallowing and feeding difficulties at birth. Some pts require ET intubation in delivery room
- Severe airway compromise and feeding issues may require tracheostomy and gastrostomy tube placement. Mandibular distraction procedures can be used to relieve airway obstruction and facilitate tracheal decanulation.
- Evaluation and correction of hearing and visual impairment. Early use of hearing aids (bone conduction) allows for proper development of speech. Surgery for bone anchored hearing aids placement may improve the quality of sound transmission.
- Oral-motor physical and speech therapy for speech clarity.
- Detailed assessment and imaging to determine the extent of craniofacial involvement during the first year of life. Repeated imaging may be needed prior to reconstructive procedures.
- Staged zygomatic, orbital, maxillomandibular and nasal reconstruction
- Surgical repair for cleft palate, choanal atresia
- Staged external ear reconstruction. Very few TCS pts are candidates for external ear canalplasty to restore hearing.

ASSESSMENT POINTS

System	Effect	Assessment by Hx	PE	Test
HEENT	Limited airway	Hx of stridor, dyspnea, snoring, obstructive sleep apnea	Micrognathia, retrognathia, limited pharyngeal area	
	Hearing loss	Hearing difficulties	External/middle ear atresia	Hearing evaluatiom
CARDIO	Cor pulmonale Pulm Htn	Easy fatigability	S_3, hepatomegaly ↑ Jugular venous pulsations Heart murmur	ECG: Right axis deviation P waves in II, IIIa, VF ECHO/ cardiac cath
GI	Difficulty feeding	Difficulty swallowing, chewing, poor Po intake	Poor wt gain	
	GERD, esp. in pts with tracheostomy	Frequent regurgitation, discomfort after meals		Upper endoscopy
RESP	Obstructive sleep apnea	Loud snoring, intermittent complete obstruction, frequent arousal, daytime hypersomnolence or hyperactivity		Polysomnography

Key Reference: Posnick JC, Tiwana PS, Costello BJ. Treacher Collins syndrome: Comprehensive evaluation and treatment. *Oral Maxillofac Surg Clin North Am.* 2004;16:503–523.

Perioperative Implications

Preoperative Preparation
- Thorough airway assessment and review of previous anesthetics
- Review of pertinent labs, studies, and imaging
- Medical Hx inquiring about obstructive sleep apnea or cor pulmonale
- Antisialogogue for airway preparation

Monitoring
- Standard monitors
- Invasive monitoring for lengthy reconstructive procedures with anticipated blood loss

Airway
- Assume difficult intubation and prepare anesthetic plan in a case by case situation (ease of intubation with previous anesthetics may not guarantee ease of intubation with current anesthetic)
- Back up airway devices (fiberoptic bronchoscope, glidescope, bullard laryngoscope, LMA) and surgical airway preparation

Preinduction/Induction
- Avoidance of sedatives if Hx of severe OSA is present
- Inhaled sevoflurane induction with maintenance of spontaneous ventilation during laryngoscopy

Maintenance
- Avoidance of excessive opioids to minimize risk of postop resp depression

Extubation
- Strict extubation criteria
- Airway devices and staff support in case pt requires re-intubation

Postoperative Period
- Acute airway obstruction
- Consider steroids, racemic epinephrine to decrease airway swelling

Anticipated Problems/Concerns

- Obstructive sleep apnea, pulm Htn and cor pulmonale
- Difficult airway

Tricuspid Atresia

Jimmy Windsor

Risk
• Uncommon. Occurs in 0.056 per 1000 live births.

Perioperative Risks
• Hypoxia caused by limited pulm blood flow.
• Reliable systemic and pulm blood flow in these pts depends on existence of an unobstructed atrial level right to left shunt, an unobstructed left to right ventricular septal defect and intact pulm artery
• There is obligatory mixing of systemic venous blood return to the heart from the vena cavas (lower O₂ sat) and blood return to the heart from the pulm veins (higher O₂ sat).

Worry About
• Inadequate ability of systemic venous and pulm venous blood to mix caused by restrictive atrial septal defect (rare additional problem, but vital).
• Inadequate pulm blood flow caused by restrictive ventricular septal defect, pulm artery stenosis, pulm subvalvular obstruction or pulm atresia.
• Less common is the pt that presents with too much pulm blood flow and CHF (completely unobstructed pulm blood flow).

Overview
• Defined by the lack of a connection between the right atrium and hypoplastic (could be practically nonexistent) right ventricle.
• The tricuspid valve may be completely absent or there may be a rudimentary valve-like structure on the floor of the right atrium that is not patent.
• Basically, three major types
• Tricuspid atresia with normally related pulm artery and aorta (70%–80%). There are three subtypes.

Ia Tricuspid atresia with normally related great vessels, pulm atresia and no ventricular septal defect (pulm blood flow completely dependent on the maintainence of a patent ductus arteriosis in the immediate period after birth).
Ib Tricuspid atresia with normally related great vessels, hypoplasia of the pulm artery and a small ventricular septal defect.
Ic Tricuspid atresia with normally related great vessels, no hypoplasia of the pulm artery and a large ventricular septal defect.
• Tricuspid atresia with transposition of the great arteries (pulm artery arising from the left ventricle and the aorta arising from the hypoplastic right ventricle—20%–30%). There are three subtypes.
IIa Tricuspid atresia with transposed great arteries, atresia of the pulm artery arising from the left ventricle, and a ventricular septal defect allowing systemic blood flow to occur through the aorta arising from the hypoplastic right ventricle (pulm blood flow completely dependent on the maintainence of a patent ductus arteriosis in the neonatal period).
IIb Tricuspid atresia with transposed great arteries, hypoplasia of the pulm artery arising from the left ventricle and a ventricular septal defect.
IIc Tricuspid atresia with transposed great arteries, no hypoplasia of the pulm artery and a ventricular septal defect.
• Tricuspid atresia with congenitally corrected transposition of the great areteries. The pt can have varying degrees of pulm, subpulmonary, or subaortic stenosis. Also, can be assoc with other lesions like atrioventricular septal defect.

ICD9-CM: 746.1 (Tricuspid atresia and stenosis, congenital)

Etiology
• Cause is unknown.
• Although specific genetic causes of the malformation have not been determined in humans, data indicate that the FOG2 gene may be involved in the process.

Usual treatment
• Limited pulm blood flow makes the neonatal pt dependent on Prostin (PGE1) to maintain the patency of the ductus arteriosis and requires surgical creation of a systemic arterial to pulm arterial shunt.
• Rarely, if the atrial level shunt is limited then this will impede adequate mixing of blood return from the vena cavas and the pulm veins. An atrial balloon septostomy may be required.
• Rarely, if pulm blood flow is unrestricted then a surgical banding of the pulm artery may be needed.
• These pts are usually treated with two more operations intended to separate the blood returning to the heart via the vena cavas (with lower O₂ sat) from the blood returning to he heart via the pulm veins (with higher O₂ sat). This will then mimic normal physiology. A pathway is first created directly from the superior vena cava in the right pulm artery (Bidirectional Glenn Procedure). Then a pathway is created from the inferior vena cava to the right pulm artery (Fontan Procedure).

ASSESSMENT POINTS

System	Effect	Assessment by Hx	PE	Test
CV and RESP	More common, limited pulm blood flow causing hypoxia and possibly resp acidsosis	Possibly requiring intubation or supplemental O₂	Cyanosis, holosystolic murmur, possible thrill	SpO₂ ABG ECHO
	Rare, over-circulation of pulm vessels causing unacceptably high pO₂	Signs of poor systemic arterial blood flow like metabolic acidosis, necrotizing enterocolitis, poor wt gain	Tachypnea, tachycardia, hepatomegaly	CXR SpO₂ ABG
CNS	Stroke due to single ventricle physiology	Pt may have received a balloon septostomy	Varying levels of consciousness Varying degrees of hemiplegia	CT MRI

Key Reference: Bailey Jr PD, Jobes DR. The Fontan patient. *Anesthesiol Clin.* 2009 27(2):285–300.

Perioperative Implications

Preopartive Preparation
• Maintain PGE1 preop if needed.
• Have drugs and blood products available to maintain BP, pre-load and contractility to maintain pulm blood flow in ductal or systemic to pulm shunt–dependent pt.

Monitoring
• Routine
• Recommend placement of arterial catheter and central venous catheter for surgery to create systemic arterial to pulm arterial shunt.

Airway
• Consider keeping the pt intubated postop after systemic arterial to pulm shunt creation. This is

usually the period when the Prostin is weaned off and the transition is made to pulm flow being purely maintained by the newly created shunt.

Preinduction/induction
• Careful titration of induction drugs to maintain adequate afterload, preload, contractility, heart rate, and heart rhythm.

Maintenance
• Maintain preload.
• If possible, a hemoglobin level of approx 13.5–15 g/dL, is desirable to maintain adequate systemic O₂ delivery with a single ventricle.
• Maintain adequate sedation to prevent rises in pulm vascular resistance.

Adjuvants
• Heparin, usually 100 units/kg (more may be necessary), to maintain an activated clotting time of at least 200 sec during the creation of the surgical shunt. May require redosing, depending on the length of the procedure.
• Inotropes to maintain adequate contractility and systemic vascular resistance.

Anticipated Problems/Concerns
• A thorough understanding of how to balance and maintain as close to equal the pulm arterial and systemic arterial blood flow from a single ventricle (parallel physiology) is required.

Trigeminal Neuralgia (TIC Doloureux)

L. Jane Easdown

Risk

- Trigeminal neuralgia (TN) has an incidence of 4/100,000
- More common in women, pts >50 y
- 1–5% of pts with MS have TN, and 2–4% of pts with TN have tumors in the posterior fossa. It is rarely seen in pts with Charcot-Marie-Tooth disease.

Perioperative Risks

- Evaluate co-morbidities with pts with MS
- Liver enzyme induction with use of anticonvulsant and/or antiepileptic drugs

Worry About

- Severe bradycardia with manipulation of the fifth nerve in the posterior fossa or with balloon ablation
- Oversedation and management of the airway in RFA procedures
- Postop exacerbation of MS

Overview

- TN is characterized by recurrent episodes of intense; lancinations pain over the distribution of the fifth cranial nerve more commonly the V2 and V3 divisions. Pain can be spontaneous or set off by stimuli in the trigger zones: light touch, cold air, talking or drinking. Pain is described as brief, like an electric shock, shooting or stabbing and terminates abruptly. Pt may have bouts over weeks or months with some spontaneous remissions up to 6 mo. Usually the bouts become more frequent and the pain more sustained. Pts with MS rarely have remissions.

- No specific tests exist for diagnosis of TN. Imaging techniques such as MRI and MRA are used to evaluate nerve decompression, and to rule out MS and tumors.
- Neurologic exam is normal in most pts with the exception of a minimal amount of sensory loss over the affected area.

ICD-9-CM Code: 350.1

Etiology

- The pathophysiology responsible for the signs and symptoms of TN is unknown but several theories exist
- **Idiopathic:** More than 90% of cases are idiopathic with evidence of focal demyelination of trigeminal sensory fibers within the nerve root or within the brainstem. Usually due to compression by an aberrant artery or vein which results in close apposition of axons and absence of intervening glial processes. This favors ectopic impulses and ephaptic conduction to adjacent fibres. In the area of the trigeminal nerve entry zone demyelination would lead to ephaptic conduction between fibers for light touch and those for pain explaining the sensitivity of trigger zones.
- **Symptomatic:** These pts have less classical features of TN. Primary demyelinating disorders such as MS will lead to demyelination and plaque formation in the root enrty zone but they may also have nerve compression by a vascular structure. Rarer presentations would incl compression by tumor, infiltration by tumor or amyloid, small infarcts or angioma in the brainstem.

Usual Treatment

- **Pharmacologic:** Despite few randomized trials, the mainstay of treatment is with anticonvulsant/antiepilepsy drugs. Initial response in over 70% of pt occurs with carbamazepine (Tegretol). Polypharmacy with other medications is common: baclofen, gabapentin, lamotrigine and oxcarbazepine. Pain or inability to tolerate these medications limits their use.
- **Procedural:**
  - **Radiofrequency ablation (RFA):** Under fluoroscopic control, a radiofrequency electrode is advanced into the foramen ovale and the pt awakened to describe the location of the parasthesia. The lesion made in cycles of 45–90 secs at temps 60–90° C. Glycerol, ethanol, and cryotherapy have been used to create a nerve lesion by this approach. Balloon compression of the ganglion for 1–6 min has been employed under general anesthesia.
  - **Microvascular decompression (MVD):** The posterior fossa is approached through a suboccipital craniotomy. The fifth nerve is identified and decompressed from the artery or vein and a surgical felt is interposed to protect the nerve. This procedure is performed under general anesthesia.
  - **Stereotactic radiosurgery:** The trigeminal nerve root at the pons is targeted with a "Gamma knife" radiosurgery, a focused array of 201 intercepting beams of gamma radiation produced by separate cobalt sources. Few centers offer this treatment and long-term outcomes are yet unknown.

ASSESSMENT POINTS

System	Effect	Assessment by Hx	PE	Test
CNS	Cranial nerve involvement, sensory loss	Pain Hx and distribution	Full neurologic exam	MRI, MRA

Key Reference: Nurmikko TJ, Eldridge PR. Trigeminal neuralgia-pathophysiology, diagnosis and current treatment. *Br J Anaesth*. 2001;87:117–132.

Perioperative Implications

Preinduction/Induction/Maintenance

- If the procedure calls for pt assistance in identifying the area for ablation then minimal sedation is used esp. longer-acting benzodiazepines
- NPO status must be observed.
- If the pt has MS then neurological status preceding the procedure should be documented.
- Pts on anticonvulsant/antiepilepsy medications will be less responsive to induction agents and metabolize liver metabolized agents more quickly.
- Must take special care to avoid trigger zones when placing mask, nasal prongs

Perioperative Implications

Monitoring

- For MAC or GA for ablation procedures: Usual ASA monitors
- For posterior fossa craniotomy: ASA monitors, invasive arterial and venous lines, precordial Doppler for venous air embolism detection, nitrogen analysis, all depending on the position of the pt
- Consider means to pace the heart: Transesophageal pacemaker, transthoracic noninvasive pacer (Zoll pads)

General Anesthesia

- All usual considerations for posterior fossa craniotomy incl pt positioning, detection of air embolism, brainstem, and cranial nerve, manipulation resulting in bradycardia, asystole, tachyarrythmias and hyper- or hypotension
- Avoid succinylcholine in MS pts with extensive motor involvement.
- Expect rapid metabolism of opioids, nondepolarizing muscle relaxants in pts managed with anticonvulsants medications (cytochrome P-450).
- Surgeons may monitor BAERS for eighth nerve function.
- Arousal and extubation will require careful management of BP, HR.
- If manipulation of lower cranial nerves has occurred, the pt may not be able to protect the airway and delayed extubation may be planned.
- Surgeons will expect the pt to respond to commands before leaving the OR.

Regional Anesthesia/Monitored Anesthesia Care

- Judicious use of sedation required such that level can be increased during painful lesioning but the pt can be aroused for consultation. Agents used: Remifentanil, fentanyl, methohexital, propofol, dexametatomodine

- Nasal prongs, careful assessment of patent airway, oxygenation, and ventilation esp. in the elderly and obese.
- Head and airway may be at a distance from the anesthesiologist.
- Probe alone may be painful, may need to convert to GA.

Postoperative Period

- Same day surgery is possible with cases under sedation alone
- Posterior fossa craniotomy postop care will require a monitored unit. for overnight neuro vital signs.

Anticipated Problems/Concerns

- Surgical problems: Infarct, hemorrage, cranial nerve paralysis, masseter muscle weakness, eighth nerve injury, CSF leak, dysaesthesia
- Anesthesia problems
- For GA: Positioning problems—skin, joints, nerve compression, eye injuries in prone position
- For MAC care: Oversedation, loss of airway

Truncus Arteriosus

Manchula Navaratnam
Chandra Ramamoorthy

Risk

- Uncommon congenital heart defect; <3% of all congenital heart defects
- No gender predilection

Perioperative Risks

- CHF
- Volatile agents may cause myocardial contractile depression and lower SVR.
- Inadvertent hyperventilation resulting in reduced PVR with excess PBF and worsening CHF
- Infective endocarditis
- Risks of CPB

Worry About

- Difficult intubation due to assoc with velocardio facial syndrome (e.g., DiGeorge)
- Air embolus (VSD almost always present)
- Hyperoxia and hyperventilation result in pulm overcirculation.
- CV collapse at induction due to diastolic run off and assoc truncal regurgitation with resulting coronary steal and myocardial ischemia
- Hypocalcemia due to parathyroid hormone dysfunction

Overview

- Single great artery arising from heart; supplies systemic, pulm and coronary circulations

- VSD almost always present; ASD in two-thirds
- Abn truncal valve; 50% are regurgitant
- Anomalies of coronary artery and aortic arch may be present.
- Pulm circulation arises directly from systemic circulation.
- Dominant physiology is a left to right shunt driven by relative lower resistance of the pulm vascular bed.
- Runoff from systemic circuit into PA during diastole may compromise myocardial perfusion.
- Primary goal is to balance PVR and SVR so that Qp:QS is close to unity.
- Early development of pulm vascular obstructive disease due to excessive pulm blood flow. Preferred repair in early neonatal period before onset of pulm Htn.
- 30–40% of pts with TA have 22q11 deletion. Phenotypes incl DiGeorge syndrome and Sphrintzen syndrome.
- Uniformly fatal without surgical correction (50% die by 1 mo and 80% within 1 y)
- Approx 30% have 22Q11 deletion resulting in phenotypic variants such as DiGeorge and Sphrintzen syndrome

ICD-9-CM Code: 745.0

Etiology

- Cono-truncal defect
- Embryonic truncus arteriosus fails to separate into a pulm and aortic trunk.
- Partial or complete absence of cono-truncal septum
- Single arterial trunk arising from both ventricles
- Classified into four types
- Maternal diabetes predisposes to cono-truncal abn

Usual Treatment

- Medical therapy is temporizing (digoxin, loop diuretics, inotropes) to treat CHF and usually only to optimize status before surgery. Should not delay surgery for an extended period of time.
- Surgical repair in the neonatal period is the definitive treatment. On hypothermic CPB, the pulm trunk is separated from the truncal artery. VSD is closed, RV-to-PA (Rastelli) conduit is placed for pulm blood flow. PFO is left open.

ASSESSMENT POINTS

System	Effect	Assessment by Hx	PE	Test
HEENT	Difficult laryngoscopy and intubation		Small mandible, small mouth	
CARDIO	CHF—truncal valve regurgitation Pulm Htn	Difficulty feeding Sweating during feeds FTT	Cyanosis ± single S$_2$ Murmur—systolic or diastolic	Pulse oximeter, ECG, ECHO, cardiac cath ±
RESP	CHF—excessive pulm blood flow	Difficulty breathing	Tachypnea retraction	CXR ($\uparrow$ pulm markings, cardiomegaly)
ENDO	Parathyroid hypoplasia	Seizures, tetany		Serum ionized Ca^{2+}, parathyroid hormone level
IMMUNO	Cellular immunodeficiency	Recurrent infections Chronic diarrhea	70% of 22q11 pts are immunosuppressed.	CBC, T-cell function
MS	Dysmorphic facies		Hyperteleorism, low-set ears	

Key Reference: *Anesthesia for left to right shunt lesions* in *Andropoulos, Stayer, Russell, Mossad: Anesthesia for congenital heart disease.* 2nd ed. Blackwell Futura; 2010, pp. 386–387.

Perioperative Implications

Perioperative Preparation

- Treat CHF
- If intubated transport and ventilate with FIO$_2$ 21% aiming for SpO$_2$ 75–80% and appropriate hypoventilation to maintain PaCO$_2$ 45–50 mmHg and pH 7.25–7.35
- Avoid hyperventilation: Increase PBF and may compromise systemic and coronary perfusion.
- Check serum electrolytes, Ca2$^+$, and Hct.

Airway

- High index of suspicion for difficult airway with appropriate precautions if velocardiofacial syndrome present.
- Maintain FIO$_2$ at 21% but may give a few breaths at 100% just prior to intubation.
- Once intubated return to FIO$_2$ 21% and avoid hyperventilation.

Preinduction/Induction

- Meticulous air bubble exclusion
- Preop antibiotics
- Consider inotropic support (e.g., dopamine at 3–5 mcg/kg/min) if MAP low prior to induction.
- Obtain baseline EKG prior to induction. Monitor for myocardial ischemia (best detected with EKG leads II and V) due to PA runoff.

- Volume infusion is unlikely to increase diastolic BP unless the pt is significantly volume depleted. Consider 1–2 mcg/kg bolus of phenylephrine for low MAP.
- Pts are usually ventricular volume overloaded and aggressive volume resuscitation will further elevate ventricular end-diastolic pressure compromising subendocardial perfusion.
- Balance PVR and SVR so Qp/Qs approaches unity. Key: Maintain SVR; keep SpO$_2$ below 90%
- Surgeon must be in the OR prior to induction and prepared for sternotomy.
- For persistent hypotension rapid sternotomy followed by partial occlusion of PA to elevate MAP and reduce pulm overcirculation.

Monitoring

- Intra-arterial catheter and CVP. May have in situ umbilical arterial and/or venous lines.
- TEE valuable to assess truncal valve function, VSD patch leak, ventricular function and pulm artery pressure.
- Intraop LA line placement for postop management of preload.
- NIRS monitoring useful esp. during low flow CPB and DHCA

Maintenance

- Usually fentanyl infusion 2–4 mcg/kg/hr
- Deep hypothermia and circulatory arrest or low-flow CPB
- Inotropic drugs commonly used to facilitate weaning from CPB incl dopamine (3–5 mcg/kg/min), milrinone (0.5–0.75 mcg/kg/min) and low dose epinephrine (0.03–0.05 mcg/kg/min), calcium chloride (20–30 mg/kg/hr)
- Inhaled NO should be available in the OR for the post CPB period as high risk of pulm vasoreactivity.

Extubation

- Postop ventilation usually required for at least 24 hr as pulm hypertensive crisis may occur. Not suitable for fast-tracking.

Postoperative Period

- Poor RV function (right ventriculotomy and Rastelli conduit placement): maintain appropriate inotropic support, afterload reduction and adequate preload for RV. Mechanical ventilation with minimal mean aiway pressure.
- LV dysfunction (circulatory arrest, long bypass time, myocardial ischemia, truncal valve abn)

- Increased PVR and pulm Htn (low CO and low SaO$_2$) responds to hyperventilation, metabolic alkalosis, vasodilators (milrinone, PGE$_1$, NO), sedation (analgesia, paralysis).
- If PA pressures are high need to exclude residual VSD and RV outflow tract obstruction in addition to treating pulm Htn.

- Right to left shunting across PFO facilitates systemic cardiac output at the expense of SaO$_2$ in the face of RV dysfunction and elevated PA pressures.
- AV block requiring pacemaker.
- Bleeding
- Cardiac tamponade

Anticipated Problems/Concerns

- CHF
- Truncal valve regurgitation and/or stenosis
- Pulmonary Htn
- Infective endocarditis

Tuberculosis (TB)

Muhammad B. Rafique

Risk

- Incidence in USA: 4.2 cases per 100,000 persons in 2008; worldwide over 9 million cases every year.
- Incidence of TB is decreasing in USA every year since 1992.
- Risk of TB is higher among homeless, elderly, Asian and Latin American immigrants, minorities and prisoners. Also immunosuppression (e.g., HIV infection, transplant recipients, CRF) increases the risk of TB infection.
- TB is the leading cause of death among HIV infected pts.

Perioperative Risks

- Risk to the pt and risk to medical personnel
- Pt risk depends on extent of pulm disease, other organ systems involvement, and overall health.

- Elective surgery is recommended to be delayed until pt is determined either noninfectious or not have tuberculosis.

Worry About

- Overall health status of the pt, infectiousness of the pt, cross contamination through anesthesia machine and effects of anti-TB therapy on organ systems.

Overview

- Mycobacterium tuberculosis is the causative organism of TB.
- Pulm TB is the most common form of TB but other organ systems could be affected (e.g., intestine, spine and bones, kidneys, and brain).
- TB could be fatal if untreated.

ICD-9-CM Codes: 010–018

Etiology

- TB is transmitted by droplet nuclei produced by coughing, sneezing, or talking.
- TB does not spread by casual contact (e.g., shaking hands, sharing food or drink, or touching bed linens).
- Primary infection could be reason for up to one third of the cases.

Usual Treatment

- 2 mo therapy with isoniazid, rifampin, pyrazinamide, and ethambutol and then 4 mo therapy with only the first two drugs. All medicines taken orally.
- All four drugs are recommended in drug-resistant cases of TB for 6 mo.
- AIDS/HIV pts need a longer duration (9–12 mo).

ASSESSMENT POINTS

System	Effect	Assessment by Hx	PE	Test
GENERAL		Night sweats, wt loss	Fever	Tuberculin skin test and in vitro T-cell release of IFN-gamma assay (IGRAS)
RESP	Hilar or mediastinal lympadenopathy, apical infiltrate or necrosis	Cough and hemoptysis	None or inspiratory rales in affected area	CXR, sputum culture
CARDIO	Pericardial effusion, constrictive pericarditis	SOB	Signs of tamponade, muffled heart sounds	ECG, ECHO
CNS	TB meningitis	Listlessness, headache, seizures, coma	Altered mental status, cranial nerve abn	LP, CSF analysis
GI	Peritonitis, enteritis	Abdominal pain, obstruction	Palpable mass, ascities	Endoscopy and biopsy, ascitic fluid analysis/culture
GU	Chronic cystitis, epididymitis, hydronephrosis, female genital tract disease	Late appearance of pyuria, hematuria	May have thickened epididymis	Urine analysis and culture, cystoscopy
Skeletal TB	Wt bearing joints (e.g., spine, hip, knee)	Pain, kyphosis	Spine tenderness	X-ray, CT, bone biopsy

Key Reference: CDC website www.cdc.gov/tb/, Langevin P, Rand K. The potential for dissemination of mycobacterium tuberculosis through the anesthesia breathing circuit. *Chest.* 1999;115:1107–1114.

Perioperative Implications

Preoperative Preparation

- Evaluate for anti-TB therapy toxicity. Plt count, ALT, AST, and serum bilirubin. Visual symptoms (optic neuritis), peripheral neuropathy.
- Properly fitted N95 mask use by the care team.
- Schedule TB and/or suspected TB pts at the end of the day to maximize time for cleaning and minimize spread.
- Use OR that has an anteroom; otherwise keep the doors closed, minimize traffic and use additional air cleaning (e.g., UVGI)

- Use disposable equipment, add bacterial filter (0.3 μm) to expiratory side or at Y-connection of anesthesia circuit.
- After use stop all gas flow through the anesthesia machine for at least 1 hr to avoid cross contamination.

Monitoring

- Standard ASA monitors
- Consider case by case according to co-morbidities and type of surgery.

Postoperative Care

- Postop recovery in an AII room (AII room—an isolation room with single occupancy, negative pressure in the room, airflow rate at 6–12 ACH or equivalent).
- If AII room not available, air cleaning technologies (e.g., HEPA filtration and UVGI) can be used.

Ulcerative Colitis, Chronic

Patrick J. Forte
Kathleen E. Barrett

Risk

- Incidence in USA and Northern countries of 35-100/100,000, incidence of 11/100,000/y with 2- to 4-fold increased frequency in Jewish populations
- Mortality highest in early years of disease, or with prolonged disease due to risk of colon cancer, 2 peaks for age of onset: 15–30 and 60–80
- M:F ratio: 1:1, smokers-nonsmokers 0.4:1, former smokers-nonsmokers 1.7:1. Up to 20% with positive family Hx.

Perioperative Risks

- Inflammatory mediators activate coagulation cascade in local blood vessels
- Chronic steroid use can cause adrenal insufficiency, delayed wound Hx

Worry About

- Diarrhea causing metabolic acidosis, hypokalemia, electrolyte abn, intravascular volume depletion
- Defects in bleeding or clotting due to activation of coagulation cascade

- Bowel distension precluding use of NO and increasing risk of perforation
- Extracolonic manifestations: Primary sclerosing cholangitis and/or cirrhosis of liver: choose appropriate anesthetics, analgesics, and NMBs; ankylosing spondylitis: limited cervical range of motion, restrictive pulm mechanics

Overview

- Indications for surgery incl toxic megacolon, colonic perforation, massive hemorrhage, obstruction, and cancer prevention or resection. If pt is presenting for surgery, disease is in progressive stage and operation can be urgent/emergent in nature.
- Pts may have steroid dependence, hypovolemia, electrolyte imbalance, malnutrition, hypoalbuminemia, anemia, bleeding
- Sulfasalazine is mainstay of treatment for all stages of disease. Side effects incl blood dyscrasias, aplastic anemia, hemolytic anemia, hepatitis, pancreatitis, nephrotoxicity, hypersensitivity pneumonitis, impaired folate absorption

ICD-9-CM Code: 556

Etiology

- Etiology unknown
- Genetics, exogenous factors, host factors, and specific environmental factors are all hypothesized to play a role

Usual Treatment

- Mild: Sulfasalazine or other 5-aminosalicylates (5–ASA)
- Moderate: 5-ASA + glucocorticoid oral and enema, electrolyte repletion, parenteral nutrition
- Severe: 5-ASA, glucocorticoid enema, glucocorticoid PO or IV
- Fulminant: Glucocorticoid IV, cyclosporine IV, azathioprine PO, 6-mercaptopurine PO, infliximab IV

ASSESSMENT POINTS

System	Effect	Assessment by Hx	PE	Test
CARDIO	Hypovolemia		Tachycardia, hypotension, orthostatic vital signs, delayed capillary refill	BUN/Cr
HEME	Anemia, thrombocytosis	Passing fresh blood	Pallor	CBC
RENAL	Metabolic acidosis, electrolyte abn		Tachypnea, oliguria	Electrolytes, BUN/Cr, ABG
RESP	Restrictive pulm mechanics (if ankylosing spondylitis) Hypersensitivity pneumonitis from 5-ASA	SOB, DOE	Cyanosis, SpO$_2$	CXR, PFTs
GI	Diarrhea, bowel obstruction/perforation Hepatic steatosis, PSC/cirrhosis	Diarrhea, no bowel movements	Abd pain only present with toxic colitis Hepatomegaly	Electrolyes Abd X-ray Abd CT

Key Reference: Kasper B, Fauci H, Longo J. *Harrison's Principles of Internal Medicine*. 16th ed. vol. II. McGraw-Hill, 2005:1776–1788.

Perioperative Implications

Preinduction/Induction/Maintenance

- Fluid, electrolyte, volume repletion
- Stress dose steroids if needed
- Special attention to airway if ankylosing spondylitis
- Careful choice of anesthetics if hepatic or renal dysfunction
- Aggressive volume replacement

Monitoring

- Standard monitoring
- Monitor urine output
- Consider arterial line if electrolyte abn
- Consider CVP if hypovolemic or anticipating large fluid shifts.

General Anesthesia

- Consider renal function for opioid dosing
- Consider renal, biliary function for NMB dosing
- Monitor ventilator settings carefully if restrictive pulm mechanics or toxic megacolon
- Beware of NO for risk of perforation

Regional Anesthesia

- Caution with local anesthetic esters: May decrease action of sulfasalazine

Postoperative Period

- Maintain normothermia for wound healing and coagulation
- Early parenteral nutrition

Anticipated Problems/Concerns

- Complicated operations with adhesions, obstructions, perforation risk
- Large intraop fluid requirement
- Need for stress dose steroids
- Correct electrolyte abn
- Risk of hemorrhage

Upper Respiratory Infections

Selina Read

DISEASES

Risk

• Most adults will suffer one upper resp tract infections (URTI) per year, this incidence jumps to approx six episodes per year in the pediatric population. Approx 95% of the infections have a viral etiology.
• URTIs are generally self-limiting, however, airway hyperreactivity may persist for several weeks.
• Adults are less likey to have URTI due to larger airways enabling them to compensate with edema and increased secretions.
• Those with underlying disease, esp. diseases afflicting the airways, are more likely to have complications following anesthesia when confounded with URTI.

Perioperative Risks

• Complications incl bronchospasm, subglottic edema, stridor, desaturations, apneas, and atelectasis.
• A pt with a fever, purulent rhinitis or productive cough should have elective surgery cancelled.

Worry About

• Lung specific: Bronchospasm, desaturations, apnea, and atelectasis
• Cancellation of surgery and prolonged hospital stay.

Overview

• To cancel or not to cancel; that has been the dilemma of many anesthesiologists who are confronted with a pt that has recently, or currently has an URTI, who is scheduled for elective surgery.
• Several studies have linked URTIs to possible morbidity; however, none have linked it to increased mortality.
• Retrospecive studies: Children with a recent URTI were at higher risk for laryngospasm, bronchospasm, and stridor. Children with URTI had a two to seven times greater incidence of resp complications. The complication risk increased to 11-fold if the trachea was intubated.
• Prospective studies: Children who developed laryngospasm were twice as likely to have a URTI.

ICD-9-CM Code: 465.9

Etiology

• Affect the airway by making them esp. susceptible to touch or chemical irritation, such as airway management and inhalational anesthetics.
• Postulated that viruses release neuroaminidases which damage the M2 muscarinic receptors, increasing acetylcholine released at NM junctions setting off vagally mediated bronchoconstriction.

• Viruses also cause the release of chemical mediators, such as bradykinin, prostaglandins, and histamine that contribute to bronchospasm.
• URTIs increase airway secretions intensifying intraop atelectasis, decreasing diffusion capacities and increasing closing volumes.

Usual Treatment

• Postponing an elective case if the pt has a fever, purulent rhinitis, or productive cough.
• Laryngospasm is treated with PPV or small dose muscle relaxation.
• Bronchospasm treated by deepening the anesthetic, administering IV bronchodilators or inhaled beta-agonists.
• Hypoxemia treated with supplemental O_2
• Atelectasis can be decreased with incentive spirometry or sigh breaths intraop.
• Increased secretions can be managed by frequent suctioning.

ASSESSMENT POINTS

System	Effect	Assessment by Hx	PE	Test
CARDIO	Tachycardia due to infection	Assess for possible CHD which can complicate the picture	Auscultation: BP, HR	None
RESP	Increased secretions, bronchospasm	Quantify cough, secretions	Auscultation: wheezes, ronchi	CXR ABG in severe cases
RENAL	Dehydration	Poor intake, UO	Skin turgor, sunken fontanelles	BMP

Key Reference: Tait A, Malviya S. Anesthesia for the child with an upper respiratory tract infection: Still a dilemma? *Anesth Anal.* 2005;100:59–65.

Perioperative Implications

Preinduction/Induction/Maintenance

• Evaluate whether symptoms are severe or likely due to infectious etiology. Examples are copious secretions and fever. If so, consider postponing.
• Minimize secretions, deep suctioning after pt deeply anesthetized.
• Avoid airway stimulation if possible, consider LMA or bag masking.
• IV necessary for adequate hydration and potential medications if bronchospasm encountered.
• Optimization of resp status is of utmost importance.

Monitoring

• Standard ASA monitors absolutely necessary: Heart rhythm, pulse oximiter and BP
• Have ABG monitoring available.

General Anesthesia

• Depending on the procedure, may be the best option to allow for deep anesthesia during stimuli, helping to prevent bronchospasm
• Agent used for induction can have effect on chance of bronchoconstriction: Propofol and sevoflurane best, thiopental worst.

Regional Anesthesia

• Useful as an adjunctive anesthetic.

Postoperative Period

• Almost all of the complications cited as a possible cause to cancel surgery can easily be treated by an experienced and diligent anesthesiologist along with proper monitoring and rapid response in the recovery room.
• Must monitor heart rate and pulse oximetry.

Anticipated Problems/Concerns

• Must have all available airway equipment such as ETTs and LMAs.
• Have rescue medications available and the ability to administer them in a variety of ways, esp. beta-agonists.

Urinary Lithiasis

Peter A. Nagi

Risk

- Annual incidence of stone disease: 16.4/10,000
- 12% of all individuals will experience calculous disease
- M:F ratio: 1.3–1.6:1
- Race with highest prevalence: Caucasians; rare in North American Indians and African-Americans
- Peak incidence: Third to fifth decade of life
- Recurrence rate after first stone: 15% at 1 y, 35–40% at 5 y, 50% at 10 y

Perioperative Risks

- Morbidity and mortality very low

Worry About

- Decreased renal function from partial or complete renal obstruction
- Sepsis, possibly septic shock, if surgical procedure performed in presence of UTI
- Perinephric hematoma if bleeding diathesis
- Pregnancy testing of women of child-bearing age because urologic procedures often use radiation, and lithotripsy is contraindicated during pregnancy

Overview

- Urolithiasis refers to abn concretions occurring anywhere along collecting system of urinary tract
- Most stones seen in industrialized countries contain calcium oxalate (75%); remainder are composed of uric acid, struvite, or cystine
- If properly treated, urolithiasis does not adversely affect life expectancy
- Calculi <4 mm in diameter usually pass without intervention
- ~20% of stones cause enough symptoms to require surgical removal

ICD-9-CM Codes: 592.0 (Calculus of kidney); 592.1 (Calculus of ureter)

Etiology

- Intrinsic factors: Renal tubular acidosis, cystinuria, primary hyperparathyroidism
- Gout, Lesch-Nyhan syndrome, Dent's disease
- Extrinsic factors: Increased environmental temp resulting in increased perspiration and hyperconcentration of urine (southeast and southwest regions of USA); low-intake drinking habits resulting in low UO; diet rich in calcium, animal fat (uric acid), or leafy vegetables (oxalate); immobility, incl sedentary occupations, obesity

Usual Treatment

- Observation, hydration, and symptomatic pain relief until spontaneous passage
- Medical expulsive therapy (MET) using nifedipine or tamsulosin can facilitate earlier stone passage
- If surgical intervention necessary (20%), choice based on stone size and location
- Shock wave lithotripsy
- Flexible ureteroscopy and Holmium laser lithotripsy
- Percutaneous nephrolithotomy
- Retroperitoneal laparoscopy

ASSESSMENT POINTS

System	Effect	Assessment by Hx	PE	Test
CARDIO	↑ Heart rate or BP 2° to pain		Tachycardia Htn	
RESP	Grunting respiration during renal colic		Normal chest exam	
GI	Abdo pain	N/V Moving irritation in abd	Tenderness to deep palpation of abd	
RENAL	Renal colic characterized by unusually severe pain localizing to affected flank; pain may radiate to groin or abd	Sudden onset of flank pain	Flank tenderness to palpation over affected kidney	UA (hematuria), BUN/Cr Non-contrast CT scan (gold standard) plain film (KUB), intravenous pyelography (IVP)

Key References: Drach GW. Urinary lithiasis: Etiology, diagnosis and medical management. In: Walsh PC, Retik AB, Stamey TA, Vaughan Jr ED, eds. *Campbell's urology.* 6th ed. Philadelphia: Saunders; 1992:2085–2156. Curhan GC, Aronson MD, Preminger GM. *Diagnosis and acute management of suspected nephrolithiasis in adults.* UpToDate version 17.3; Sept 30 2009.

Perioperative Implications

Preoperative Preparation

- If obese, require acid aspiration prophylaxis and airway evaluation

Monitoring

- Routine
- Temp monitoring during immersion lithotripsy essential because water temp may produce hyperthermia or hypothermia
- Shock waves synchronized to ECG to avoid dysrhythmias

Preinduction

- Adequate padding to avoid nerve damage

Induction

- Sedation may be adequate for lithotripsy and minor ureteroscopy procedures. GA, spinal or continuous lumbar epidural with T8 level epidural are all acceptable depending on type of procedure, co-morbid diseases and pt preference.

Maintenance

- Central blood volume increases
- May become hypotensive 2° to warm water decreased SVR
- Vital capacity decreased and work of breathing increased
- Pleural effusion or hydropneumothorax may occur during percutaneous renal procedures

Adjuvants

- Visualization of stone may require iodine-containing contrast material
- Anticholinergic agents (glycopyrolate) occasionally given to shorten lithotripsy treatments; however, tachycardia can occur, resulting in myocardial ischemia in high-risk pts
- Most pts receive prophylactic antibiotics prior to urinary tract procedures

Anticipated Problems/Concerns

- Peroneal nerve compression from lithotomy position
- Allergic reactions in 5% receiving IV contrast media
- Steinstrasse, ureteral obstruction by fragmented calculi, may cause ureteral colic following lithotripsy
- Htn may occur following lithotripsy
- Septic complications occur in 1% after lithotripsy
- Ureteral injury occurs in 9% of ureteroscopy procedures, with 1.6% requiring further surgical intervention
- Bladder perforation may present as shoulder pain, unexplained Htn, tachycardia in PACU

Urticaria, Cold

Lyndia Jones
Lesley Lirette

Risk

- Prevalence is very low, < 1/100,000.
- Appears in all races and genders, reported between ages 3 mo and 74 y but seen typically at 18–25 y

Perioperative Risks

- Can develop urticaria or angioedema with skin cooling and rewarming
- Shock-like reactions can occur with whole body cold exposure
- Cooling with cardiopulmonary bypass can induce symptoms

Worry About

- Cold exposure of pt (e.g., cold room, cold fluids, cold instruments or devices to cool skin)

Overview

- Characterized by appearance of urticaria or angioedema after cold exposure
- Can be familial or acquired (most common). Acquired can be idiopathic or 2° to an underlying disease (e.g., malignancy, cryoglobulinemia, or infection).
  - In 2° syphilis, it is caused by the Donath-Landsteiner antibody.
  - Disease course varies widely. Symptoms may resolve after several months or can last 5–9 y or more. Symptoms in 2° cold urticaria usually regress with treatment of underlying disease.
- Dx by cold stimulation test (e.g., the ice cube test)

ICD-9-CM Code: 708.2

Etiology

- 1° cold urticaria appears related to skin mast cells sensitized to cold by a serum factor, very likely antibodies
- Sensitized skin mast cells (not blood basophils) release histamines on interaction with cold
- Similar activation by cryoglobulins appears in 2° cold urticaria

Usual Treatment

- Antihistamines, both H_1 and H_2, successful at reducing occurrences even for hypothermic cardiopulmonary bypass.

ASSESSMENT POINTS

System	Effect	Assessment by Hx
SKIN	Urticaria or angioedema	Hx of cold reactions
RESP	Angioedema	Hx of swelling on cold exposure

Key Reference: *Middleton's allergy. Chapter 61: Urticaria and angioedema from Adkinson: Middleton's allergy: principles and practic.* 7th ed. Edinburgh: Mosby; 2009.

Perioperative Implications

Preoperative Preparation

- Antihistamines H_1 and H_2 only if a cold challenge anticipated during surgery

Monitoring

- Temp, skin condition

Maintenance

- Warm IV fluids; keep room and pt warm

Anticipated Problems/Concerns

- Localized areas of urticaria and/or angioedema not of great concern, but serious widespread edema can compromise the airway or lead to fluid extravasation or shock
- Maintain temp
- Pretreatment with antihistamines if cold is unavoidable

Uterine Rupture

Matthew Fiegel

Risk

- Incidence varies: 1/1280–1/3000 for all vaginal deliveries
- Incidence of uterine rupture in women with unscarred uterus approx 0.01% in industrialized countries
- Incidence of rupture with prior C-section ranges from 0.2–0.8%.
- In women with previous upper uterine surgery (myomectomy), incidence of rupture can be as high 1.7%.
- Risk factors incl prior uterine scar; rapid, tumultuous labor; prolonged, augmented labor; trauma; and grand multiparity, polyhydramnios

Perioperative Risks

- Potentially catastrophic for mother and fetus. Maternal morbidity is ~0.1% and incl hemorrhage, shock, and hysterectomy. If fetus delivered within 30 min, fetal morbidity improved but still incl hypoxemia and/or acidosis, depressed apgar scores, and admission to neonatal ICU.
- Maternal mortality greatly increased in pts with traumatic or spontaneous rupture likely 2° to delayed suspicion and/or Dx and treatment.

Worry About

- Massive hemorrhage in mother
- Fetal hypoperfusion and hypoxemia

Overview

- Due to a breach in the myometrium, which is often 2° to a separation of a previous C-section scar, uterine rupture can occur antepartum, intrapartum, or postpartum. The lower uterine segment, at term, contains mostly connective tissue and little placental tissue. Therefore, most ruptures are asymptomatic and do not result in maternal and/or fetal compromise. However, if placental tissue is involved, massive bleeding with resultant need for emergent C-section and/or laparotomy can occur.
- Vaginal delivery is preferred over C-section as maternal blood loss and maternal morbidity are decreased.
- ACOG advocates trial of labor after delivery in pts with previous low transverse uterine scar. Mothers with classical C-sections and/or inductions with prostaglandins are both discouraged by ACOG as risk of rupture is greatly increased. As well, trial of labor after C-section is discouraged in hospitals where emergency C-sections cannot be performed within 30 min.

- Fetal bradycardia is most common presenting symptom (~70%). Other Sx incl vaginal bleeding, abd and/or shoulder pain, hypotension and/or shock. Abd pain is still a reliable sign in the presence of an epidural if low-dose concentration local anesthesia is used.

ICD-9-CM Code: 665.1 (Uterine rupture during labor)

Etiology

- Separation of scar from previous C-section, often during trial of labor
- Rupture of myomectomy scar (highest incidence of rupture)
- Weak or stretched uterine muscles due to grand multiparity, polyhydramnios, or multiple gestations
- Precipitous labor or prolonged labor with oxytocin augmentation
- Traumatic rupture

Usual Treatment

- When occurring antepartum or during labor, urgent and/or emergent laparotomy with C-section and uterine repair or hysterectomy is the only treatment. Urgency is determined by speed of Dx and maternal and fetal stability.
- If diagnosed incidentally postpartum, mother may undergo close observation without surgery.

ASSESSMENT POINTS

System	Effect	Assessment by Hx	PE	Test
CARDIO	Tachycardia, hypotension, shock		BP, HR, orthostasis	
RESP	Discomfort with breathing due to diaphragmatic irritation		Tachypnea, labored breathing	
GU	Vaginal bleeding	Abd pain, shoulder pain, absence of contractions	Abd tenderness, presenting fetal parts	HCT
FETUS	Category 2 or 3 fetal distress			FHR monitor

Key Reference: Bucklin BA. Vaginal birth after caesarean delivery. *Anesthesiology*. 2003;99(6):1444–1448.

Perioperative Implications

Preoperative Preparation

- In trial of labor after C-section, monitor fetal heart rate tracing continuously. Continuous labor epidural can be advantageous in that it can provide surgical anesthesia if repeat caesarean is indicated. Use combination low-dose local anesthetic and opioid.
- If epidural is not present or time for dosing is inadequate, use GA for emergent repeat C-section and/or suspected uterine rupture.
- Anesthetic management of suspected or confirmed uterine rupture incls:
  - Large bore IV access
  - Available blood products
  - Arterial line
  - Large bore central line if peripheral access is poor
  - Fluid warmer
  - Quick access to laboratory values (istat, blood gas lab)

Monitoring

- ASA monitors, arterial catheter, and with or without central venous catheter

Induction/Airway

- If mother grossly unstable or no epidural, proceed to GA
- Rapid sequence induction with cricoid pressure
- If severely hypovolemic, transfuse with induction. As well, use minimal vasodilating and/or negative inotropic induction agents to spare BP.

Maintenance

- If mother stable, may use continous epidural for procedure
- If GA, 100% FIO_2 predelivery, volatile anesthetic at 0.5 MAC or less if maternal BP tolerates.
- Restore blood volume to keep Hgb >7 gm/dL and BP stable
- After delivery, if stable, consider titrating opioids.
- Fetus may require intensive resuscitation (neonatologists present).

Extubation

- Normal extubation criteria: Pt awake, strong, hemodynamically stable, no continuous bleeding, fairly normal acid/base, electrolyte status

Postoperative Period

- Consider ICU overnight
- EBL: 3000–6000 mL, check Hct, coags frequently
- Pain score: 6–8, consider IV PCA or postop epidural if coagulation status normal

Anticipated Problems/Concerns

- Other more common causes of antepartum hemorrhage incl placenta previa and placental abruption
- Pregnant mothers who hemorrhage can go into DIC quite quickly. Monitor coags, plts.
- Symptoms of rupture may be misleading. Must possess high index of suspicion to diagnose in a timely fashion.
- Rupture of classic scar or previous upper uterine surgery scar much more likely to result in severe hemorrhage

Varicella-Zoster Virus

Lee A. Fleisher

Risk

- Prevalence: <10% of adults seronegative
- Usually contracted during childhood

Perioperative Risks

- Minimal additional risk to pt unless immuno-compromised
- Risk of infection to caregivers

Worry About

- Encephalitis in immunocompromised pt
- Potential nosocomial transmission
- Acyclovir-induced nephrotoxicity
- Transmission to pregnant woman

Overview

- Viral cause of varicella (chickenpox) and herpes zoster (shingles)
- Both nosocomial transmission and direct contact
- Development of herpes zoster common in immunocompromised pt and may be forerunner of AIDS
- Zoster is reactivated form of varicella from neural ganglion cells and can be assoc with severe pain
- May lead to congenital abn if contracted during 1st trimester of pregnancy.

ICD-9-CM Code: 053.9

Etiology

- Herpes group of viruses

Usual Treatment

- Varicella immune globulin
- Vaccine available but controversial
- Antiviral medications decrease the duration of symptoms and the likelihood of postherpetic neuralgia, esp. when initiated within 2 d of the onset of rash.
- Most common is acyclovir; valacyclovir, penciclovir, and famciclovir, are also available.
- Corticosteroid controversial for postherpetic neuralgia in pts with herpes zoster, controlled-release oxycodone was superior to placebo in the early period of pain.

ASSESSMENT POINTS

System	Effect	Assessment by Hx	PE	Test
RESP	Pneumonia	Dyspnea	Rhonchi	CXR
HEME	Thrombocytopenic purpura	Bleeding		Plts
DERM	Rash		Erythematous macules, papules, vesicles	
RENAL	Acyclovir nephrotoxicity			Cr
CNS	Encephalitis Optic neuritis; transverse myelitis	MS changes Vision changes		CT scan
PNS	Zoster shingles		Shingles in single dermatome Multiple dermatomes in immunocompromised	
IMMUNO	Assoc with AIDS			HIV tests; CD4 titer

Key Reference: Christo PJ, Hobelmann G, Maine DN. Post-herpetic neuralgia in older adults: Evidence-based approaches to clinical management. *Drugs Aging.* 2007;24(1):1–19.

Perioperative Implications

Preoperative Preparation
- Consider isolation precautions

Monitoring
- Routine

Airway
- Routine

Induction/Maintenance
- Routine
- May require modification of periop pain management regimen if treatment for post-herpetic neuralgia

Extubation
- Routine

Anticipated Problems/Concerns

- Multiple dermatomes may indicate immunocompromised individual
- Avoid exposing pregnant individuals to virus

Ventricular Fibrillation

Sheela S. Pai

Risk

- VFIB/VTach: Most frequent rhythm in sudden cardiac arrest
- At risk are the 1.5 million/y in the USA who have acute MIs: About 540,000 will die, 350,000 before they reach hospital (this incls death from dysrhythmia and myocardial failure)
- 1-y mortality in near-sudden death survivors: 20–30% if nonresponsive to antiarrhythmics (20–50% of near-sudden death survivors)

Perioperative Risks

- 1° VFIB, if assoc with acute infarction, when treated promptly with defibrillation, may not affect prognosis
- 2° VFIB (preceded by pump failure or hypotension) assoc with 75–80% mortality during hospitalization

Worry About

- Hypoxemia, hypercarbia, hyper- or hypo-kalemia, ischemia hypomagnesemia, digitalis toxicity, acid-base abn
- Antiarrhythmic drug levels
- Availability of defibrillator, myocardial ischemia and early revascularization

Overview

- Asynchronous, chaotic contraction of ventricles characterized by no organized ventricular depolarization and therefore no QRS; no cardiac output
- Coarse VFIB indicates recent onset, readily correctable with prompt defibrillation
- Fine VFIB (coarse asystole) indicates delay since collapse; successful resuscitation more difficult

ICD-9-CM Code: 427.41

Etiology

- Usually ischemic, often assoc with LV aneurysm
- Idiopathic cardiomyopathy
- Coronary spasm esp. in the immediate postop period
- Hypothermia
- Long QT syndrome is assoc with VTach, esp. torsades de pointes (one type of polymorphic VTach; other types not assoc with long QT)

Usual Treatment

- Definitive emergency Rx is always electrical defibrillation: External—either manual or automatic (AEDs)—or internal: Internal may be implanted (ICDs)
- Time to defibrillation is a major determinant of survival, with chances of success reduced by 10% each minute
- Early bystander CPR and early defibrillation are the only factors that have increased, the rate of return of spontaneous circulation (ROSC) and decreased mortality.
- Vasopressors such as epinephrine and vasopressin are indicated after three successive countershocks fail to terminate VFIB. Vasopressors improve coronary and cerebral perfusion pressures; increased coronary perfusion pressure is assoc with increased likelihood of ROSC.
- Vasopressin may have fewer side effects than epinephrine, while being equally or more effective, particularly in acidotic pts. Vasopressin's longer duration of action (10–20 min) has led to the recommendation of a single, one-time dose for VFIB.
- Amiodarone is the only antiarrhythmic assoc with improved resuscitation rates from VFIB; it is recommended after 3 successive shocks, an IV vasopressor (epinephrine or vasopressin), and a subsequent 4th shock are unsuccessful in restoring a perfusing rhythm
- Prospective trials of lidocaine and bretylium in VFIB pts have shown no benefit on outcome. However, based on historical use and the lack of side effects, lidocaine is considered an alternative to amiodarone in VFIB.
- Due to inconsistent availability, side effects, and lack of confirmed benefit, bretylium is no longer recommended for VFIB
- Evidence supporting procainamide use in VFIB is limited, while the need for slow infusion makes it less than ideal
- Magnesium may be beneficial in torsades de pointes (polymorphic VTach assoc with prolonged QT), but routine use does not improve outcome.

ASSESSMENT POINTS

System	Effect
HEENT	Right radical neck dissection assoc with increasing QT interval
CARDIO	No effective cardiac output
RESP	Apnea should be anticipated
CNS	Glucose administration may worsen CNS outcome

Key Reference: ECC Committee, Subcommittees and Task Forces of the American Heart Association. 2005 American Heart Association Guidelines for Cardiopulmonary Resuscitation and Emergency Cardiovascular Care. *Circulation.* 2005;112(suppl 24):IV1–IV203.

Perioperative Implications

Preoperative Preparation

- Antiarrhythmic drug levels in optimal therapeutic range
- If for EPS, ablation, or ICD, antiarrhythmic drugs withdrawn on ECG monitoring
- Avoid anticholinergic premedication or sympathetic stimulation
- For pts with prolonged QT syndrome consider β-blockers or prophylactic left stellate ganglion block

Monitoring

- Consider ECG and pulse oximetry en route to OR.
- Consider arterial catheter for transport and in OR.

Airway

- Apnea expected with acute VFIB; ventilation should be supported with 100% O_2
- Airway secured with ETT if 3 successive countershocks fail to restore perfusing rhythm

Induction

- Avoid ketamine; intubate after adequate depth of anesthesia

Maintenance

- Suppress sympathetic responses to stimulation

Extubation

- Suppress sympathetic stimulation; extubate when spontaneous ventilation with oropharyngeal reflexes has been restored
- Reversal of NMBs acceptable
- Regional: Serum levels of local anesthetics given epidurally may affect intraop defibrillation threshold testing during ICD placement
- Defibrillator should be available with sterile defibrillator paddles on surgical field; pharmacologic therapy for dysrhythmia conversion/maintenance, for treating Htn and tachycardia, which frequently follow defibrillation; bradycardia may require pacing.

Postoperative Period

- Cardiac monitoring; resumption of preop antiarrhythmics, maintaining adequate oxygenation and ventilation
- Avoid and treat promptly electrolyte abn
- Post-defibrillation pain score: 1–3 from chest wall and psychic disturbances
- Psychiatric counseling if disturbed by shock or "out of body" experience

Anticipated Problems/Concerns

- PA catheter insertion may induce VTach or VFIB in dysrhythmia-prone pts; if PA catheter necessary consider central venous placement with advancement after ventricular dysrhythmia procedure completed
- For pts with prolonged QT syndrome avoid drugs that prolong the QT interval (class Ia antiarrhythmic drugs such as quinidine and procainamide)
- Psychic disturbances from defibrillation in aware state

Ventricular Preexcitation Syndrome

Risk

- A premature activation of ventricular myocardium via anomalous accessory pathways (AP) without physiologic delay in AV junction. Depending on the type of AP, several variants of preexcitation syndrome have been described.
- Wolff-Parkinson-White (WPW) syndrome is caused by abn AP assoc with classical AV pathways (bundle of Kent), is found in 0.1–0.3% of the population, is more prevalent in males, and is characterized by short P-R interval (<0.12 s), widened QRS (>0.10 s) and delta waves, and episodes of tachyarrhythmias.
- Anomalous pathways other than accessory AV pathways may cause preexcitation or participate in reentry tachycardia, but they are rarely diagnosed.
- Lown-Ganong-Levine (LGL) syndrome usually reflects abn antegrade and retrograde conduction through the "James bundle" (atria to bundle of His)—intranodal or paranodal fast pathway. This syndrome is characterized by a short PR interval, normal QRS and no delta waves. It manifests itself through intermittent reentrant-type PSVT or paroxysmal atrial fibrillation or flutter. The frequency of LGL is up to 0.5% in adults. LGL is more prevalent in women.
- Mohaim type, a less common form of preexcitation, is assoc with the presence of *Mahaim fiber* (accessory connections running into the right ventricular muscle) and is characterized by normal PR, long QRS and delta wave, may trigger episodes of AFIB and SVT. Prevalence is unknown.
- Pregnancy, through an unknown mechanism, may predispose to exaggerate symptoms of WPW-related PSVT.

Perioperative Risks

- Asymptomatic forms of WPW (ECG pattern) may present no added risk. Symptomatic individuals with WPW are prone to PSVT (up to 80%), less commonly to AFIB (15–30%) and AFLT (5%) with a rapid ventricular rate which may occasionally deteriorate to VTachor, even VFIB.
- There is a danger that WPW patterns of ECG will be mistaken for: a bundle branch block, due to the wide QRS, an MI, due to the negative delta waves simulating pathologic Q waves, other tachyarrhythmias (incl V-Tach). All prompt inappropriate treatment.
- General anesthesia may unmask asymptomatic WPW syndrome due to precipitating conduction in the pre-existing anomalous AP by volatile agents (particularly Halothane).
- Drugs used to suppress AV conduction (to slow the ventricular rate in treatment of AFIB /AFLT) may dangerously accelerate the rate in WPW.

Worry About

- Hyperadrenergic states, over stimulation and other interactions that may provoke or aggravate tachyarrhythmias
- High spinal anesthesia may be assoc with an effective block of the sympathetic cardiac accelerator nerve and suppression of normal AV conduction. Along with relative parasympathetic predominance, it may further facilitate conduction by the AP, resulting in preexcitation and tachyarrhythmias.
- Effects of both inhalation and IV agents may suppress normal conduction pathways and increase conduction of AP, resulting in preexcitation.
- Some CV medications may have unfavorable effects, e.g., Ca^{2+}-channel blockers (diltiazem, verapamil) and digitalis slow AV nodal conduction and may enhance conduction over AP, worsening WPW-related tachyarrhythmia.
- Potential of WPW-related PSVT to deteriorate into AFIB/AFLT, with danger of extremely rapid ventricular rates ensuing VTach/VFIB.

Overview

- SVT in pts with pre-excitation is generally owed to a reentrant mechanism, in which the AP plays an essential role. Re-entrant SVT involves the presence of dual conducting pathways between the atria and the ventricles: natural AV nodal His-Purkinje tract and AV accessory (or bypass) tract, such as Kent fibers, James bundle, or Mahaim fibers.
- Re-entrant orthodromic tachycardia during PSVT may produce normal looking narrow QRS complex in the absence of δ wave since normal pathway is used for ventricular depolarization. The AP, alternatively, is used for the retrograde conduction essential for the reentry mechanism. PVCs may also initiate orthodromic PSVT.
- Less common antidromic tachycardia may produce wide QRS complex with δ waves. In this case, a shorter refractory period in the AP may cause a block of ectopic atrial impulse in the normal pathway, with antegrade conduction down the accessory tract and then retrograde reentry of the normal pathway with ventricles activated via accessory pathways.
- Orthodromic and antidromic PSVT account for 70–80% of all paroxysmal tachycardia in pts with preexcitation syndrome, up to 30% of AFIB and up to 10% of AFLT. Primary VTach/VFIB is rare, but they may occur as a result of rapid SVT.
- The first episode of PSVT in many pts (regardless of ECG markers of pre-excitation during sinus rhythm) appears before the age of 20, rarely in middle age, and infrequently after the age of 50. The frequency of episodes of PSVT increases with age in pts with WPW.
- The rate of paroxysmal SVT may be faster in pts with LGL syndrome compared to pts with normal P-R intervals. In addition, the capacity for more rapid conduction may have an effect during AFIB/AFLT.

ICD-9-CM Codes: 426.7 (WPW); 426.81 (LGL)

Etiology

- Both WPW and LGL may be congenital or hereditary in nature.
- May be assoc with congenital cardiac defects (e.g., Ebstein anomaly)
- May be assoc with certain acquired cardiac defects, such as cardiomyopathy, idiopathic hypertrophic subaortic stenosis, or asymmetric septal hypertrophy.

Usual Treatment

- Caution should be exercised when treating WPW syndrome tachycardia. Agents with an AV node blocking effect, such as adenosine, Ca^{2+}-channel blocker (diltiazem, verapamil) or digitalis, increase the chance of worsening existing tachycardia and precipitating AFIB/AFLT. Digitalis generally is not recommended in adult pts with WPW, particularly in treatment of AFIB/AFLT.
- Initial treatment of choice in WPW pts with hemodynamically unstable tachyarrhythmias (incl AFIB/AFLT) is direct-current synchronized electrical cardioversion. Minimum effective energy (100 joules) should be used initially; energy should be titrated to minimize potential injury to myocardium.
- Treatment of AFIB/AFLT and wide-complex tachycardia assoc with WPW syndrome is necessarily different from the treatment of AFIB/AFLT in pts with a normal heart. In hemodynamically stable pts, AP suppressing agents would be the treatment of choice, e.g., procainamide (class IA agent) and propranolol (class II beta-blocker). Amiodarone and sotalol, that influence both the AV node and the AP conduction, may also be used, particularly if VTach cannot be excluded. It is advisable to avoid lidocaine since it does not prolong refractoriness in the AP and may increase ventricular response.
- In termination of stable narrow-complex PSVT (reentrant type), vagal maneuver may be carefully attempted initially, followed by cautious introduction of adenosine or diltiazem. An external cardioverter-defibrillator should be immediately available in case AFIB occurs as a result of attempted treatment. In some cases amiodarone or a β-blocker may be considered since neither facilitates AP conduction.
- In long-term pharmacologic maintenance, agents that prolong refractoriness in APs and encourage AV conduction are recommended, such as disopyramide, procainamide, and quinidine, and newer generation antiarrhythmics such as flecainide, propafenone, and moricizine. Amiodarone may be the treatment of choice in some pts since it also prevents recurrences of AFIB/AFLT and deterioration to V-Tach.
- For most pts with recurrent symptomatic tachyarrhythmias, the definitive treatment is catheter ablation of APs by delivering electrical or RF energy subsequent to EP studies and localization/mapping of APs.

ASSESSMENT POINTS

System	Effect	Assessment by Hx	PE	Test
CARDIO	Arrhythmia	Palpitations, dizziness, syncope or near-syncope, angina, chest pain, cardiac arrest; sometimes asymptomatic	Monitor BP; variable S_1-pulse amplitude; fast regular, irregular, and/or weak pulse; S_3; rales	12-lead ECG, Holter ECG, cardiac EP study, ECHO and possible further study
	LV function	Weakness, lassitude, exercise intolerance, CHF		

Key Reference: Tarditi DJ, Hollenberg SM. Cardiac arrhythmias in the intensive care unit. *Semin Respir Crit Care Med*. 2006;27(3):221–229.

Perioperative Implications

Preoperative Preparation

• Cardiology consultation involving an electrophysiologist is necessary to determine pt's status, specific type of arrhythmia, risk of symptomatic arrhythmia and management

• Regional anesthesia (provided hemodynamic stability) may have an advantage over GA owing to avoidance of multiple triggering drugs and noxious stimuli of airway instrumentation.

• A variety of antiarrhythmic drugs should be readily available, as well as cardioverter-defibrillator with synchronization capability.

Monitoring

• Standard ASA monitoring (incl ECG strip-chart recorder), an arterial line if pt is at high risk for unstable tachyarrhythmias

Induction

• Smooth non-triggering induction is warranted to avoid unnecessary tachycardic response. Adequate depth of anesthesia, pain, and stress control with opioids and β-blockers prior to airway instrumentation may reduce the risk of tachyarrhythmias.

• In rare cases of ventricular dysfunction due to tachycardiomyopathy, the dose of induction agent should be appropriately titrated; etomidate and balanced anesthetic techniques may be considered.

• If neuraxial anesthesia is chosen, efforts should be made to avoid BP swings on induction since they may cause compensatory tachycardia. Vasopressors for BP correction should be used with caution to avoid tachycardic response.

Maintenance

• Some volatile agents (e.g., Halothane) may precipitate conduction via AP and should be avoided, whereas isoflurane and sevoflurane have no such effect or may even suppress AP conduction.

• Agents that can precipitate tachycardia should be used with caution or avoided. Among these are ketamine, pancuronium, atropine, and oxytocin. Fentanyl and droperidol, on the other hand, have been shown to be beneficial since they increase AP refractoriness.

Extubation

• Efforts should be made to avoid adrenergic hyperactivity on emergence and/or extubation. Adequate pain control with opioids or a regional block and β-blockers may be useful.

Adjuvants

• Agents that may suppress or enhance AV conduction should be avoided.

• Drugs that directly or indirectly increase adrenergic response should be used with caution.

Postoperative Period

• Adequate pain control is essential to reduce the likelihood of paroxysmal tachycardia.

Anticipated Problems/Concerns

• Possibility of unmasking WPW syndrome-related tachyarrhythmias under GA in previously asymptomatic pts.

• Risk of dangerous ventricular rates with AFIB/AFLT, with early deterioration into VFIB.

• Wide QRS complex of WPW patterns during antidromic PSVT or AFIB/AFLT mistaken for V-Tach/VFIB.

Ventricular Septal Defect (Congenital)

Alexander J.C. Mittnacht
David L. Reich

Risk

- Incidence is ~2–6/1000 live births

Perioperative Risks

- Mortality higher in older children, elevated PVR, and (>7 Wood's units), and surgery complicated by complete heart block.

Worry About

- Worsening of L→R shunt with hyperventilation and increased FIO_2
- Paradoxical embolization
- Hypothermia
- Post-CPB pulm Htn and RV failure

Overview

- Small defects asymptomatic, present with murmur, usually close spontaneously, observation only
- Larger unobstructed defects result in CHF symptoms, poor wt gain, and URIs beginning at 3–12 wk of age, as decreases in PVR cause increase in L→R shunting.
- Untreated large L→R shunting may result in fixed pulm Htn (Eisenmenger's syndrome) in some pts.

ICD-9-CM Code: 745.4 (Ventricular septal defect)

Indications/Usual Treatment

- 75% of small defects close spontaneously and require only antibiotic prophylaxis.
- Medical therapy for symptoms of CHF incl digoxin, ACE inhibitors, and furosemide.
- Surgery is indicated when CHF not amenable to medical treatment, or if failure to thrive
- Surgical repair contraindicated if PVR >10 Wood's units, unless reactive to selective pulm vasodilators.

ASSESSMENT POINTS

System	Effect	Assessment by Hx	PE	Test
CARDIO	Low forward cardiac output due to L→R shunt Pulmonary Htn due to excessive flow	CHF symptoms, FTT Age of pt	Loud holosystolic murmur and thrill Cyanosis	Auscultation, ECHO, cardiac cath
RESP	Congestion/edema due to L→R shunt	Frequent URI	Rhonchi	CXR
HEME	Anemia in massive L→R shunt; polycythemia in R→L shunt	Pallor or cyanosis	Paleness or plethora	Hct
MS	Chronic hypoxemia due to late reversal of shunt flow (Eisenmenger's syndrome)	Cyanosis	Clubbing of digits	Pulse oximetry

Key Reference: Scully BB, Morales DL, Zafar F, McKenzie ED, Fraser Jr CD, Heinle JS. Current expectations for surgical repair of isolated ventricular septal defects. *Ann Thorac Surg.* 2010;89:544–549; discussion 550-1.

Perioperative Implications

Preoperative Preparation

- Digoxin and furosemide until day of surgery, ACE inhibitors controversial, but vasoplegic syndrome following CPB less common in pediatric pts.
- May not be possible to delay operation until free of upper resp symptoms

Anesthesia

- Limit FIO_2 to minimum necessary prior to CPB to restrict excessive pulm blood flow
- Maintain normal to slightly high $Paco_2$ to restrict excessive pulm blood flow
- Pts typically receive inhalational anesthetic for induction, if peripheral IV in place IV drugs can be administered alternatively.
- Avoid N_2O to prevent sequelae of paradoxical air embolization

Monitoring

- Indwelling arterial catheter for invasive monitoring in all pts.
- Central venous access and pressure monitoring in most pts undergoing surgery with CPB.
- Standard ASA monitoring, incl pulse oximetry, ECG, capnometry, multiple-site temp monitoring.
- Transesophageal echocardiography

Induction/Maintenance

- Mask induction with sevoflurane in most cases, IV drugs if peripheral IV in situ, IM induction possible for uncooperative pts.
- High-dose opioid anesthetic technique rarely used

Surgical Stages

- Pre-CPB
  - Low FIO_2, normal to high $Paco_2$
  - Avoid hemodilution with large amounts of crystalloid and/or colloid prior to CPB.
- CPB
  - After pt's Hct has been obtained in the OR, dilutional Hct incl CPB prime is calculated. If calculated Hct is less than 25%, consider priming of CPB with whole blood or reconstituted whole blood (PRBC and FFP).
  - Inhalational anesthetic administration via CPB or continuous IV drug administration to allow for fast-tracking in most pts presenting for VSD repair.
- Post-CPB
  - Rule out residual shunting by transesophageal echocardiography.
- Maintain Hct >25–30%

Postoperative Considerations

- Most pts presenting for VSD repair can be extubated at end of surgery
- Consider mechanical ventilation and sedation in the immediate postop period in pts prone to pulm hypertensive crises (e.g., Down's syndrome)
- Infective endocarditis prophylaxis for 6 mo

Anticipated Problems/Concerns

- Imbalance in pulm to systemic blood flow ratio:
  - Excessive pulm blood flow results in high arterial saturation but with diminished tissue perfusion and metabolic acidosis
  - Diminished pulm blood flow results in good tissue perfusion but with cyanosis and potential injury due to hypoxia
- Postop ventricular dysfunction more likely with ventriculotomy
- Pulm Htn and/or right heart failure
- Coagulopathy, particularly in very small children.

Ventricular Septal Rupture (Defect), Post Myocardial Infarction

Gregory W. Fischer

David L. Reich

Risk

- Historically seen in 1–3% of MIs prior to era of acute revascularization
- Incidence 0.2% after lysis therapy or percutaneous intervention
- Majority occur within 1 wk; 20–30% in first 24 hr post MI
- Rarely occurs >2 wk post MI
- Medical management alone shows a mortality >90%

Perioperative Risks

- Accounts for 5% of MI-related deaths
- Without surgical therapy, survival is less than 10% at 1 month
- Surgical short-term survival 42–75%

- Increased mortality seen in the setting of urgent repair and posterior VSD
- Percutaneous device closure with GA and TEE have similar mortality

Worry About

- Assoc papillary muscle rupture
- Poor systemic perfusion and end-organ dysfunction
- Pulm congestion with massive L→R shunt

Overview

- Sudden onset of holosystolic murmur with thrill and hemodynamic deterioration (hypotension and pulm congestion)
- Despite advances in periop management, expect increased morbidity and mortality

- Expect complicated postop course with prolonged ICU stay

ICD-9-CM Codes: 429.71 (Acquired cardiac septal defect); 410.00–410.92 (Associated MI)

Usual Treatment

- Repair of new VSD with hemodynamic deterioration using pericardial or prosthetic patch material
- Support preop with inotropic agents/intra-aortic balloon counterpulsation
- Percutaneous device closure as an alternative to surgery

ASSESSMENT POINTS

System	Effect	Assessment by Hx	PE	Test
CARDIO	Low forward cardiac output due to massive L→R shunt	Sudden onset of hypotension and shock	Loud holosytolic murmur and thrill	ECHO, cardiac catheterization
RESP	Congestion/edema	Resp distress	Rales	CXR
RENAL/HEPATIC	Dysfunction due to cardiogenic shock	Anuria		ABGs Foley catheter

Key Reference: Jeppsson A, Liden H, Johnsson P, Hartford M, Rådegran K. Surgical repair of post infarction ventricular septal defects: A national experience. *Eur J Cardiothorac Surg.* 2005;27:216–221.

Perioperative Implications

Preoperative Preparation

- Consider elective tracheal intubation and PEEP
- Support cardiac output using inotropic agents
- Lower resistance to forward cardiac output using afterload reduction, incl intra-aortic balloon counterpulsation
- Obtain coronary angiogram. Concurrent revascularization can potentially improve outcome.

Anesthetic Technique

- High-dose opioid/muscle relaxant technique common
- Prior to CPB, use minimal FIO_2 and PEEP (maximizes PVR) to decrease L→R shunt across VSD

Monitoring

- Intra-arterial line
- Most use PA catheter due to pulm hypertension and for shunt quantitation. Step-up in saturation between right atrium and PA to measure degree of shunting.
- Thermodilution cardiac output falsely elevated.
- TEE to define anatomy, diagnose assoc papillary muscle rupture, monitor ventricular function (incl stroke volume), assess adequacy of surgical repair

Airway

- High airway pressures and frequent suctioning in the setting of pulm edema

Induction

- High-dose opioid technique to maintain hemodynamic stability. Avoid vasodilation assoc with volatile anesthetics

Maintenance

- If hypertensive, titrate low doses of volatile agent or benzodiazepines

Surgical Stages

- Pre-CPB
  - Median sternotomy with aortic and biatrial cannulation
  - May require vein or internal mammary artery harvest for concomitant myocardial revascularization
  - Lowest FIO_2 consistent with adequate oxygenation
- CPB
  - Maintain Hct using hemofiltration and transfusion
- Post-CPB
  - Inotropic support almost universally required for LV failure
  - RV failure common
  - Assess ventricular repair using TEE or right atrial-to-pulm O_2 sat ratio

- FIO_2: 1.00 to minimize PVR
- May require ventricular assist devices
- Blood loss/volume concerns
- Antifibrinolytic therapy (beginning pre-CPB)
- Transfuse coagulation factors based on results obtained from point of care testing (TEG, plt function analyzers)

Postoperative Considerations

- Postop renal/hepatic/neurologic dysfunction
- Postop LV, RV, or biventricular failure

Anticipated Problems/Concerns

- Cardiogenic shock with multi-organ dysfunction syndrome (MODS)
- Prolonged ventilatory dependency and ICU stay
- Course not dramatically improved with percutaneous device closure

Ventricular Tachyarrhythmias

Nasrin N. Aldawoodi
Jeffrey M. Berman

Risk

- Ventricular tachycardias (VT/VF) are uncommon but potentially fatal dysrrhythmias.
- Risk increases with age due to higher incidence of structural heart disease.
- Primary cause of sudden death; incidence in USA: ~300,000/y, similar in other developed nations.
- Males have greater risk (46% vs. 34%) correlating with higher incidence of CAD, right ventricular dysplasia (2-fold male predominance) and Brugada syndrome (8-fold male predominance).
- Pts under 30 y with hypertrophic cardiomyopathy, RV dysplasia, myocarditis, long QT syndrome at higher risk of VT/VF

Perioperative Risks

- Uncorrected electrolyte and/or acid-base imbalances.
- Uncontrolled sympathetic discharge
- Catecholamine-induced dysrrhythmias with halothane, enflurane, and to a lesser degree isoflurane.
- Use of class 1 and 3 antiarrhythmics, sympathomemetics, QT prolonging drugs.
- Placement of central venous catheters (CVC)

Worry About

- Electrolyte, acid-base, and metabolic disturbances esp. with ongoing myocardial ischemia.
- Cardiac function.
- Drugs: Sympathomemetics, antiarrhythmics (class 1 and 3), tricyclics, antipsychotics, drugs that >QT; organophospates
- Modulation of neuro-endocrine stress responses.
- More than three consecutive PVCs (considered VTach); duration >30 sec considered sustained VTach and should be treated.
- Six or more PVCs/min or multifocal PVCs

- R on T phenomenon
- Chest pain, SOB, palpitations, presyncope, altered mental status

Overview

- Ventricular tachyarrhythmias are characterized by QRS >120 msec, rates >120 bpm; can be monomorphic (MVT) or polymorphic (PVT).
- Monomorphic ventricular tachycardias (MVT) have a single QRS morphology; can evolve into polymorphic ventricular tachycardia.
- Polymorphic ventricular tachycardias (PVT) are rapid rhythms with varying QRS morphology. Several types: Long/short QT (acquired/congenital), catecholaminergic, torsade de pointes (TdP), Brugada syndrome
- TdP: Characterized by twisting of QRS around isoelectric baseline and assoc with long QT syndrome.
- VTach <150 bpm may be tolerated for protracted periods. >150 bpm usually impedes perfusion. Rates >220 bpm generally cause CV collapse.
- Significantly compromised perfusion requires urgent intervention, generally electrical cardioversion or if pulseless, CPR and/or defibrillation.
- Ventricular fibrillation: Non-perfusing rhythm; disorganized irregular complexes of varying morphology.

ICD-9-CM Code: 427.1 (Ventricular tachycardia); 427.41 (Ventricular fibrillation)

Etiology

- Structural heart disease, most commonly CAD and/or IHD and acute MI. Also, CHF, valvular disease, cardiomyopathy, myocarditis, RV dysplasia.
- Long QT (>450 msec) familial, idiopathic or acquired 2° to hypokalemia, hypocalcemia, hypomagnesemia.

- QT prolonging drugs incl class 1 and 3 antiarrhythmics, antihistamines, TCAs, lithium, antipsychotic drugs, certain analgesics such as methadone.
- Short QT (≤320 msec) syndrome
- Catecholaminergic MVT and/or PVT provoked by stress, exercise, cocaine, or infusion of catecholamines without QT prolongation or structural heart disease.
- Brugada syndrome: ECG right bundle branch-like conduction and ST elevation in right precordial leads without prolonged QT or structural heart disease.
- Electrolyte and acid base abn: Hyper- and/or hypokalemia, hypomagnesemia, acidosis, hypoxia, and hypercarbia
- Mechanical irritation 2° central lines, mechanical ventilation

Usual Treatment

- Hemodynamically unstable MVT with pulse: Urgent electrical cardioversion
- Pulseless MVT, unstable PVT, or VF: CPR, electrical defibrillation; epinephrine 1 mg q 3–5 min or vasopressin 40 IU.
- Hemodynamically stable MVT/PVT: Amiodarone 150 mg over 10 min; repeat if needed of start infusion. Alternative drugs are procainamide and lidocaine.
- Correct underlying acid base, electrolyte, metabolic disturbances.
- TdP: Also use $MgSO_4$ 1–2 g over 1–2 min.
- Chronic VT: ICD; RF ablation, PO antidysrhythmic drugs.

ASSESSMENT POINTS

System	Effect	Assessment by Hx	PE	Test
CARDIO	Ischemia, MI, decreased cerebral perfusion, decreased cardiac output	Angina, palpitations, anxiety, lightheadedness, syncope	Pallor, diaphoresis, heart murmur, tachycardia, JVD, cannon a waves, displaced PMI, S_3 gallop	12-lead EKG, TTE, TEE, Holter monitor, cardiac CT and cardiac MRI, cardiac catheterization (right or left heart), cardiac enzymes
PULM	Increased pulm venous pressure, pulm edema 2° to HF	Dyspnea, tachypnea, sleep apnea	Wheezing, course breath sounds, crackles	CXR, CT chest, PFTs, ABG

Key Reference: Amar D. Strategies for perioperative arrhythmias. *Best Pract Res Clin Anaesthesiol.* 2004;18(4):565–577.

Perioperative Implications

Preinduction/Induction/Maintenance

- Pt Hx of VT/VF or CAD; functional status optimized, treatment of heart disease.
- Congenital and/or acquired long QT: Avoid and/or stop causative drug(s);
- TdP: Correct K^+ & Mg^{++}. May require $MgSO_4$ or pacing to suppress TDP.
- Congenital TdP is best managed with beta blockade, RF ablation, and/or AICD.
- Minimize sympathetic response to stress; judicious choices of drugs to maintain adequate perfusion; avoid drugs that are sympathomimetic sensitizing.
- Nonsustained VT intraop without apparent cause needs postop evaluation. Sustained VT may need cardioversion (electrical/chemical), evaluation of acid-base status/electrolytes, and postop evaluation.

Monitoring

- Routine monitors incl ST segment trending and recorder.
- Arterial line for pts with cardiac disease, Hx of VT, or undergoing high-risk procedures.
- Consider TEE in pts with intraop hemodynamic turbulence, EKG changes, and/or MI.

General Anesthesia

- Avoid and treat electrolyte imbalances, esp. K and Mg.
- Check CVC if new PVCs occur after placement.
- Control/prevent sympathetic surges.

Regional Anesthesia

- Meticulous avoidance of intravascular injection
- Maintenance of adequate perfusion

Postoperative Period

- Adequate analgesia.
- Further workup and/or cardiology consult for episodes of periop VT

Anticipated Problems/Concerns

- SVT with aberrant conduction can be confused for MVT as it can be rapid and wide complex. Distinguishing the two rhythms may not be possible. Judicious use of adenosine helps with diagnosis. Pts with significant hemodynamic instability and a pulse with wide complex QRS tachycardia should be cardioverted.

Ventricular Tachycardia

Arvind Rajagopal

Kenneth J. Tuman

Risk

- Structural heart disease (most commonly chronic phase of MI). Predictor of sudden cardiac death after MI.
- Most common cause of mortality with CHF
- Cardiomyopathies, both hypertrophic and dilated are assoc with VTach
- Seen in genetic syndromes such as long QT sydrome, Brugada syndrome and arrhythmogenic right ventricular dysplasia

Perioperative Risks

- Endogenous or exogenous catecholamines trigger VTach in susceptible pts
- Central venous, pulm artery catheters and intubation can trigger VTach
- Hyperventilation may decrease serum K^+
- Precipitation of polymorphic VTach with agents that alter QT interval

Worry About

- Decreased vital organ perfusion related to low cardiac output
- Possible effect of antiarrhythmics on cardiac and pulm function
- Periop ventricular dysfunction and/or ischemia
- Progression of VTach to VFIB
- Reduction of LV function due to IV antiarrhythmic

Overview

- Defined as 3 or more consecutive ventricular beats (usually at a rate >100 bpm)
- Sustained VTach persists for >30 sec or requires an intervention for termination

- Nonsustained VTach is ≤6 consecutive beats terminating spontaneously within 30 sec
- Possible signs of VTach incl a wide QRS (>140 msec), presence of fusion beat, AV dissociation, LBBB morphology
- Must rule out SVT with aberrant conduction or pre-existing bundle branch block
- Torsades de pointes refers to VTach characterized by polymorphic QRS complexes that undulate in a regular fashion about baseline. Often assoc with prolonged QT interval.

ICD-9-CM Code: 427.42

Etiology

- CAD—acute myocardial ischemia or MI or old MI with LV scar or aneurysm
- Cardiomyopathies, esp. with ventricular dilation/enlargement
- Myocarditis
- Mechanical irritation (catheters)
- Metabolic (hypokalemia, hypomagnesemia)
- Hypertrophic cardiomyopathy or mitral valve prolapse may present with VTach
- Acquired polymorphic VTach (torsades) may result from electrolyte imbalances (K^+, Mg^{2+}) or drugs that prolong repolarization (phenothiazines, tricyclic antidepressants, class Ia antiarrhythmics, erythromycin, pentamidine, terfenadine, astemizole)
- Congenital QT prolongation may be assoc with left-sided cardiac sympathetic dominance
- Rare association with right radical neck dissection

Usual Treatment

- Removal or manipulation of intracardiac catheter if pt hemodynamically stable
- Chronic PO therapy incl Ia: quinidine, procainamide, disopyramide; Ib: mexilitene, tocainide; Ic: propafenone; II: β-blockers; and III: amiodarone, sotalol
- IV therapy incl amiodarone, procainamide, phenytoin, lidocaine, and bretylium (less commonly quinidine) as well as Mg^{2+} and/or K^+ when necessary. Amiodarone superior to other agents.
- Digoxin antibodies if digitalis-induced VTach
- Class I antiarrhythmics generally contraindicated in presence of polymorphic VTach (torsades de pointes)
- Electrical cardioversion for VTach with hemodynamic instability
- Nonpharmacologic management incl ablative techniques, myocardial revascularization, implantable cardioverter-defibrillators (recommended for recurrent VTach and structural heart disease with poor ventricular function) and left ventricular assist devices
- IABP may be used to improve myocardial perfusion and hemo-dynamics
- Treatment of torsades incl withdrawal of offending agent, correction of electrolyte abn (K^+, Mg^{2+}), and/or electrical defibrillation to terminate episode. Accelerating HR with isoproterenol or cardiac pacing may terminate rhythm. Empirical Mg^{2+} treatment may be lifesaving.
- Treatment of congenital QT prolongation incl β-blockade to blunt sympathetic activity, Mg^{2+}, and/or left cervicothoracic sympathectomy

ASSESSMENT POINTS

System	Effect	Assessment by Hx	Pe	Test
CARDIO	Myocardial ischemia Hypotension	Angina/anginal equivalent (syncope, SOB, palpitations, and exercise intolerance)	Cardiomegaly, JVD Cannon A waves; S_3, S_4	ECG, CXR Electrophysiologic studies
	Cardiac arrest	CHF		Ambulatory ECG
RESP	Pulm edema Amiodarone effects (fibrosis)	SOB	Rales (wet or dry)	CXR, PFTs (A-a)O_2 gradient
CNS	Syncope	Dizziness or loss of consciousness		

Key Reference:. Amar D. Strategies for perioperative arrhythmias. *Best Pract Res Clin Anaesthesiol.* 2004;18(4):565–577.

Perioperative Implications

Preoperative Preparation

- Ascertain etiology of VTach and assoc problems
- Evaluate for Hx of palpitations, SOB, VTach, dizziness, syncope, chest pain
- Evaluate ECG for morphology of PVCs, QT interval, underlying BBB (important for Dx and therapy of wide complex tachycardia)
- Review electrophysiologic studies to determine optimal treatment of VTach
- Assess K^+ and Mg^{2+} levels, digoxin level if indicated

- Pulm and thyroid function tests may be indicated for chronic amiodarone therapy
- Continue PO antiarrhythmic therapy
- Have defibrillator immediately available (near by) whenever inserting central venous catheters
- May need to have AICD deactivated for surgery to prevent firing with electocautery use

Monitor

- ECG for ischemia or QT prolongation
- Consider invasive hemodynamic monitor if suspect serious concomitant cardiac disease and major anesthetic/surgical intervention

Induction/Maintenance

- Avoid myocardial ischemia (maintain O_2 supply and minimize O_2 demand)
- Minimize surgical stimulus response and subsequent catecholamine release
- Avoid sympathomimetics, which may aggravate ventricular dysrhythmias
- Avoid hypokalemia, excessive hyperventilation

Postoperative Period

- Consider continuous arrhythmia monitoring.
- Continue parenteral antiarrhythmics until able to resume PO.
- Treat Mg^{2+} and K^+ deficits (common postop, esp. after major surgical procedures)

Vitamin B$_{12}$/Folate Deficiency

Donald D. Koblin

Risk

- 5–20% of elderly
- Predisposed by prolonged exposure to N$_2$O, ICU pts, ileal resections, chemotherapy with antifolates, ethanol abuse, AIDS, pregnancy

Perioperative Risks

- Worsening of pre-existing megaloblastic anemia and neuropathies after exposure to N$_2$O (infrequent)
- Anemia and limited O$_2$-carrying capacity
- Limb (positioning) injuries assoc with pre-existing neuropathy

Worry About

- Delayed onset of hematologic and neurologic abn after N$_2$O exposure—several weeks may pass before Sx develop
- Untoward outcomes (e.g., death, infection) in critically ill pts with megaloblastic anemia undergoing anesthesia and surgery

Overview

- Folate metabolism requires vitamin B$_{12}$-dependent enzyme methionine synthase, which converts methyltetrahydrofolate and homocysteine to free tetrahydrofolate and methionine and is rapidly inactivated (T$_{1/2}$ ~ 1 h) by N$_2$O
- Vitamin B$_{12}$ required for two enzymes in humans: Methionine synthase and methylmalonyl-CoA mutase (which converts L-methylmalonyl-CoA to succinyl-CoA)
- Tetrahydrofolate (in its free form and derivatives) needed for many metabolic processes, incl pyrimidine, purine, DNA synthesis; amino acid metabolism; formate elimination
- Vitamin B$_{12}$/folate required for synthesis and maturation of blood cells, integrity of CNS, GI function, growth of fetus and child
- Assoc with ↑ serum homocysteine levels and atherosclerosis

ICD-9-CM Codes: 281.0–281.2

Etiology

- Pernicious anemia (antibodies to gastric cells and lack of intrinsic factor) is most common cause
- Impaired nutritional intake, malabsorption (e.g., ileal resection), increased folate demand (e.g., pregnancy), treatment with antifolate drugs (e.g., methotrexate, prolonged N$_2$O exposure)

Usual Treatment

- Daily oral supplements of folate and/or weekly IM injections of vitamin B$_{12}$
- Folate treatment alone may produce partial hematologic remission due to vitamin B$_{12}$ deficiency but mask vitamin B$_{12}$ deficiency and result in irreversible neurologic abn
- Deficiencies assoc with N$_2$O exposure have been successfully treated with IM injections of vitamin B$_{12}$, IV administration of folinic acid, oral methionine

ASSESSMENT POINTS

System	Effect	Test
HEENT	Glossitis and painful tongue (infrequent)	
CARDIO	Angina and palpitations 2° to anemia DOE 2° to anemia	
GI	Anorexia, diarrhea	Schilling test for malabsorption of vitamin B$_{12}$
HEME	Megaloblastic anemia	Serum levels of vitamin B$_{12}$ and folate. RBC folate considered better indicator of tissue folate levels than serum folate. ↑ Urinary levels of methylmalonic acid in vitamin B$_{12}$ deficiency Hematologic variables may be normal or abnormal; anemia, ↑ mean corpuscular volume Hypersegmented neutrophils may be present
GU	Impotence	
CNS	Subacute combined degeneration of spinal cord Gait ataxia Romberg's sign, memory deficits, psychosis	
PNS	Diminished vibratory sense, proprioception, and sensation; paresthesias, loss of deep tendon reflexes	

Key Reference: Koblin DD. Toxicity of nitrous oxide (N$_2$O). In: Rice SA, Fish KJ, eds. *Anesthetic Toxicity*. New York: Raven Press; 1994:135–155.

Perioperative Implications

Preoperative Preparation

- If elective procedure, postpone to correct vitamin deficiencies and hematologic and/or neurologic abn

Monitoring

- Myocardial ischemia may occur with anemia and is assoc with increased homocysteine levels

Airway

- Large and painful tongue may be present

Induction/Maintenance

- Avoid NO if pt known to be vitamin B$_{12}$/folate–deficient and has hematologic and/or neurologic abn

Adjuvants

- Regional: Documentation of pre-existing neurologic deficits is required before proceeding with regional anesthesia

Postoperative Period

- Worsening of hematologic and neurologic abn may not occur until several weeks after N$_2$O exposure

Anticipated Problems/Concerns

- Anemia may result in impaired oxygenation of tissues and be assoc with myocardial ischemia
- CNS and PNS abn may exist.
- NO may exacerbate pre-existing hematologic/neurologic abn assoc with vitamin B$_{12}$ and/or folate deficiency.

Vitamin D Deficiency

Nancy C. Wilkes

Risk

- High prevalence of deficiency, much more than previously recognized.
- At risk: Dietary insufficiency, elderly, nursing home residents, inadequate sun exposure, latitudes higher than 38 degrees, institutionalized, premature infants of VLBW, blacks, Hispanics, obese
- Genetically predisposed: Rickets, osteomalacia

Worry About

- Vitamin D–deficient pts are probably hypocalcemic. Without vitamin only 10–15% of dietary calcium and approx 60% of phosphorous is absorbed. Low total body magnesium is also likely.
- Calcitrol influences muscle function, CV homeostasis and immune response.
- Deficiency assoc with Htn, myocardial infarction, CHF, and calcific aortic stenosis.
- Ample evidence to connect adequacy to risk and/or severity of certain cancers (colorectal, prostate, breast, leukemia) and autoimmune diseases (RA, MS, type 1 DM)
- Chronic vitamin D deficiency may lead to impaired mineralization of cervical spine (increased incidence of abn neck mobility; pediatric pts with deformed chest wall may experience lowered FRC; increased incidence of resp infections)

Overview/Pharmacology

- There are two main forms of vitamin D. Vitamin D_3 (cholecalciferol) is synthesized in the skin by exposure to ultraviolet (UVB) radiation. Vitamin D_2 (ergocalciferol) is obtained through irradiation of ergosterol in plants and subsequent dietary intake.
- Amount of vitamin D obtained through food sources is minimal compared to that from the sun.
- Vitamins D_2 and D_3 are hydroxylated in the liver to 25 vitamin D (calcidiol), the major circulating form. Further hydroxylation in the kidney produces the active metabolite 1, 25 vitamin D (calcitriol). Calcitrol and not 25 vitamin D is the active form.
- Involved in functioning of hemopoietic cells, skin cells, cancer cells of various origins, islet cells of the pancreas, immune response, as well as CV function (via serum Ca^{2+})

ICD-9-CM Code: 268.9

Etiology

- Inadequate sun exposure, dietary insufficiency
- Two types of vitamin D-dependent rickets. Type I: Inherited autosomal recessive trait (defect in the 25OH-D_3 conversion into calciferol [true vitamin D]). Type II: Autosomal dominant disorder, where single amino acid change in vitamin D receptor results in nonfunctional state.

- Osteomalacia: Metabolic disease with inadequate and/or delayed mineralization of osteoids in mature bone

Usual Treatment

- Now recognized as essential supplement for most adults, esp. ages >50.
- Dose: Recommended doses higher than previously thought. Most adults require intakes of 800–1000 IU/day. Adults over 50 benefit from 1000 IU/day. Up to 2000 IU/day is safe in adults without renal insufficiency. Food sources incl fortified milk and/or dairy products, salmon, mackerel, cod liver, tuna, fortified cereals, and egg yolks.
- Toxicity: Margin of safety is large. Prolonged intake of doses >40,000 IU/d promotes bone demineralization, leads to hypercalcemia and enhances CV calcification.
- Prescribed for rickets, osteomalacia
- Vitamin D insufficiency: Vitamin D 800–2000 IU/d + elemental calcium 1200 mg/d
- Vitamin D deficiency: Elemental calcium 1200 mg/d plus ergocalciferol 50,000 IU/wk for 8–12 wk, then 2000 IU/d vitamin D_3

ASSESSMENT POINTS

System	Effect	Assessment by Hx	PE	Test
MS	Impaired mineralization Increased arthritis due to bone spur formation Osteomalacia Osteoporosis	Bone pain, fracture Joint pain Weak antigravity muscles	Dry, scaly skin Brittle nails Coarse hair Neck immobility Osteoarthritis	Bone density X-ray
CARDIO	CHD CHF Irregular heart beat Orthostatic hypotension Htn Cardiac hypertrophy Vascular calcification Stroke	Angina Dyspnea Palpitations Fatigue	Auscultation	ECG BP Stress test Cardiac echo
CNS/PNS	NM irritability	Muscle stiffness, rigidity Numbness, paresthesias Muscle cramps Persistent, nonspecific musculoskeletal pain	Seizure	Calcium levels PTH (if severe)

Key Reference: Stechschulte S, Kirsner R, Federman D. Vitamin D: Bone and beyond, rationale and recommendations for supplementation. *Am J Med.* 2009;122:793–802.

Perioperative Implications

Preoperative Preparation

- Both PTH and vit D_3 (calcitriol) work to keep the level of ionized Ca^{2+} within tight range (±0.1 mg/dl).
- Cimetidine: This hepatic P450-mediated-metabolism inhibitor leads to decreased vitamin D plasma concentration
- Periop considerations are related to
  - Level of ionized Ca^{2+} (regulation of muscle contraction)
    - Neurotransmitter release
    - Blood coagulation

Monitoring

- ECG changes: Compare to previous tracing. Prolonged QT interval (adjusted to R-R interval; 2:1 intraventricular heart block)

- Easy availability of blood sample for immediate serum calcium assessment (art catheter vs. vein stick).

Maintenance

- $ETCO_2$: Avoid hyperventilation (alkalosis shifts ionized Ca^{2+} into the cells). Acute hypocalcemia increased chance of tetany.
- Monitor/replete Mg^{2+} as well

Extubation

- Laryngeal spasm on extubation in fully awake pt is also likely. Predictor may be distal extremity paresthesia.
- Antibiotics: Rifampin, isoniazid

Anticipated Problems/Concerns

- Chronic anticonvulsant Rx (phenobarbital/phenytoin) may lead to hypocalcemia ($\downarrow Ca^{2+}$ absorption from the intestine) and diminished vitamin D biosynthesis in the liver

- Vitamin D serum concentration is decreased when PTH is decreased (may occur with thiazide medications)
- Linked to Htn, CHD, vascular calcification, metabolic syndrome, autoimmune certain cancers
- Deficiency can be a result of deficient production of vitamin D in the skin, lack of dietary intake, impaired vitamin D activation or resistance to the biological effects of calcitriol
- Disorders of small bowel, hepatobiliary system, pancreas (bile salt deficiency, pancreas insufficiency, poor intestinal absorption of fat-soluble vitamins [A, D, K, E]) may cause maldigestion and/or malabsorption states
- Liver disease can impact CRI/ESRD (GFR < 25% of nml); moderate to severe impairment of renal phase synthesis of vitamin D with reduction of serum albumin

- Uremia, CRF, and nephritic syndrome suppresses vitamin D action on gut
- Chronic renal failure acidosis leads to negative calcium balance; typical pts have increased phosphorous and/or decreased calcium serum levels

- Nephrotic syndrome causes vitamin D deficiency related to chronic proteinuria (loss of circulating 25 vitamin D_3–binding globulin). Symptoms present are 2° hyperparathyroidism, low serum Ca^{2+}, osteomalacia.

- Vitamin D_3 (1,25 dihydroxycalciferol) directly facilitates Ca^{2+}, Mg^{2+}, and $(PO_4)^{3-}$ uptake by intestinal mucosa, their transport through intestinal cells and efflux.

Vitamin K Deficiency

Sameer Menda
Jeffrey Kirsch

DISEASES

Risks

• Vitamin K deficient bleeding (VKDB) from abn factors II, VII, IX, and X
• Controversy exists regarding whether vitamin K deficiency leads to osteoporosis, abn cartilage calcification, and possible arterial calcification resulting in CV disease.

Perioperative Risks

• Minor or massive hemorrhage unrecognized as VKDB.
• Long-bone fractures during positioning the anesthetized pt (particularly in women).

Worry About

• Pts with underlying risk factors demonstrating unexplained coagulopathy
• Intracranial hemorrhage in infants (30-60% infants with VKDB) and other occult bleeding sites such as retroperitoneal hemorrhage (more commonly in infants)
• Avoid IM dosing of vitamin K if bleeding is present
• Anaphylaxis with IV vitamin K replacement (extremely rare)

Overview

• Vitamin K is cofactor for a carboxylase enzyme in liver, which is essential for normal function of factors II, VII, IV, X and proteins C, S and Z.
• Coagulopathy manifests as prolonged PT and INR (normal or prolonged aPTT) with normal fibrinogen and factor 5 (both lowered in liver disease and DIC).

• Fat-soluble vitamin K is absorbed in small bowel and colon and synthesized in gut by bacteria.
• Poor oral intake alone not sufficient to cause vitamin K deficiency.
• Prevalence extremely rare in adults with adequate nutrition. Prevalence is as high as 30% in pts with chronic GI disorders. More frequent in infancy with classic VKDB occurring in 0–1.5% despite routine prophylaxis.

ICD-9-CM Code: 269.0

Etiology

• Inadequate nutrition (often combined with antibiotic therapy)
• Malabsorption diseases (IBD, celiac, short bowel syndrome)
• Total parenteral nutrition
• Parenchymal liver diseases (vitamin K supplementation will not likely correct coagulopathy)
• Biliary diseases
• Drugs (coumadin, salicylates, rifampin, antibiotics, sulfa drugs)
• Hemorrhagic disease of newborn or vitamin K deficient bleeding (VKDB)
  • Early stage (<24 hr) – drugs taken by mother during pregnancy and low placental vitamin K transfer
  • Classic (d 1–7) – inadequate formula intake or breastfeeding only
  • Late (wk 2–6 mo) – breastfeeding only or malabsortion disease (most often cholestatic)

Usual Treatment

• Vitamin K can be administeterd orally, intramuscularly, or intravenously with both route and dosage depending on urgency and degree of coagulopathy.
• Massive bleeding should promptly be treated with FFP, prothrombin complex concentrate, or factor VIIa along with IV administration of vitamin K (most sources recommend an adult dose of 10 mg IV and rarely more than 50 mg in first 6 hr)
• Labs for PT, INR, aPTT, fibrinogen, and plt count should be obtained in urgent situations to determine etiology of bleeding.
• When given IV, normalization of INR should be noted as soon as 30–120 min and no longer than 12 hr. If no correction noted or improvement in bleeding within 24 hr, an alternative etiology should be suspected, such as liver dysfunction or DIC.
• In non-urgent settings of prolonged INR w/o bleeding, other tests available incl serum vitamin K level or abn prothrombin level (most specific). If INR >9.0 recommend 5–10 mg oral vitamin K. If INR is between 5.0–9.0, recommended dosage is 2.5–5.0 oral vitamin K.
• Definitive diagnosis of vitamin K deficiency is made by correction of coagulopathy with vitamin K administration.
• For all routes of administration, sufficient serum vitamin K levels are present within 24 hr to reverse coagulopathy in most cases.

ASSESSMENT POINTS

System	Effect	Assessment by Hx	PE	Test
HEME	Insufficient Hemostasis/ Mucosal bleeding, acute or chronic anemia	Bleeding diathesis	Easy bruising, epistaxis, ICH (infants), retroperitoneal bleeding (infants)	Coagulation profile incl PT/INR, aPTT, fibringogen, Hct, platelets
GI/RENAL	Mucosal bleeding/ inadequate production of clotting factors/ inadequate absorption of vitamins	Inadequate nutrition/parenchymal liver disease/cholestatic disease/ malabsorption/bleeding diathesis	Hematuria/gastrointestinal bleeding/ wt loss/jaundice/pale stools/dark urine/	Urinalysis, endoscopy
UTERUS/ VAGINA	Mucosal bleeding	Bleeding diathesis	Vaginal bleeding	
MET/OTHER		Antibiotic therapy/coumadin/other drugs		

Key References: Merli Gj, Fink J, Vitamin K. Thrombosis. *Vitam Horm.* 2008;78;265–279.

Perioperative Implications

Preinduction/Induction/Maintenance

• Suspect vitamin K deficiency in pts with underlying risk factors and unexplained anemia, bruising/bleeding, or prolonged PT/INR.
• Providers should have low threshold to correct unexplained prolonged PT/INR with vitamin K supplementation periop. With no signs of bleeding or easy bruising, a 1-mg IV dose of vitamin K is reasonable.
• If VKDB is present, PRBCs and FFP should be available and IV vitamin K should be given concomitantly to promote synthesis of clotting factors. Prothromin concentrate, though less readily available, is more effective than FFP due to higher concentrations of factors II, VII, IX, and X.
• Large bore (16 gauge or larger in adults) IV access should be established prior to surgery to allow rapid volume resuscitation in the event of significant hemorrhage.

Perioperative Implications

Monitoring

• Anesthetic monitors recommended depend on degree of coagulopathy and signs of bleeding. Consider Foley catheter, and CVP to monitor for volume status, and invasive arterial pressure monitoring to assess beat-to-beat BP during hemorrhage.

General Anesthesia

• Significant coagulopathy can result in easy bleeding wih venipuncture, surgical incision, line placement, airway instrumentation.

Regional Anesthesia

• Prolonged PT and INR precludes neuraxial anesthetic 2° to risk of hematoma and subsequent neurologic injury.
• Prolonged PT and INR may result in hematoma formation during plexus anesthesia.

Postoperative Period

• Common setting for unrecognized vitamin K deficient coagulopathy given setting of inadequate oral intake and aggressive antibiotic therapy

Anticipated Problems/Concerns

• Oral vitamin K is often ineffective as supplementation in pts with GI disease or cholestatic disease.
• IV vitamin K should be administered in a dilutent such as 0.9% isotonic sodium chloride and administered at a rate no faster than 1 mg/min to reduce the risk of an adverse reaction.
• FFP will only temporize VKDB unless a supplemental source of vitamin K is provided.
• Prolonged PT/INR related to liver disease often will not correct with vitamin K supplementation.

Von Willebrand's Disease

Thomas M. McLoughlin, Jr.

Risk

- Incidence in USA: >1 million; 1% carry gene (severe disease 1/10,000–1 million)
- Race and gender with highest prevalence: None

Perioperative Risks

- Increased risk if hepatic dysfunction present
- Significant risk of bleeding if untreated

Worry About

- Excessive periop hemorrhage
- Concurrent antiplatelet agents or NSAIDs contributing to bleeding
- Adverse reactions to desmopressin therapy (seizures due to hyponatremia, hypotension, anaphylaxis)

Overview

- Coagulopathy characterized by quantitative/qualitative alterations in von Willebrand factor (vWF). vWF acts as a bridge between plts and vascular subendothelium, and stabilizes Factor VIII to prolong its circulating half-life.

- Presents as defect in primary hemostasis—mucocutaneous hemorrhage
- Highly variable severity; family Hx very helpful in predicting severity
- Diagnosed by prolonged aPTT, Factor VIII antigen and activity levels, vWF antigen, and ristocetin aggregation studies. Many disease subtypes further classified by band pattern of radiolabeled vWF after gel electrophoresis (multimeric analysis)
- Type I: Quantitative decrease in vWF of all sizes (most common, 70–80% of cases); Type II: Quantitative/qualitative alterations primarily in largest molecular weight vWF multimers, many subtypes exist (20–30% of cases), type IIB may be accompanied by thrombocytopenia; Type III: Severe quantitative reductions or absence of vWF (rare, 2° to homozygous inheritance)

ICD-9-CM Code: 286.4

Etiology

- Autosomal dominant trait; variable penetrance and expression leads to unpredictable clinical severity; most severe disease in homozygotes
- Rarely, acquired disorder due to autoimmune disease or induced alterations in vWF function

Usual Treatment

- Must know disease subtype prior to therapy
- Desmopressin acetate (DDAVP), 0.3 μg/kg IV, stimulates release of endothelial vWF, variably effective in types I and II disease
- Desmopressin absolutely contraindicated in type IIB
- Recombinant vWFs
- Pasteurized pooled factor VIII concentrates that preserve vWF (Humate-P) and solvent detergent heat-treated pooled concentrates (alphanate) are mainstays of therapy, if recombinant vWFs not available
- Cryoprecipitate best alternative if concentrates unavailable
- Antifibrinolytics often useful adjuncts

ASSESSMENT POINTS

System	Effect	Assessment by Hx	Test
HEENT		Epistaxis	
GI	GI bleeding	Melena, hematochezia	Stool guaiac
HEPAT	Requirement for transfusion therapy	Random donor exposures	LFTs, hepatitis panel
HEME	Coagulopathy, principal defect in primary hemostasis	Easy bruising, menorrhagia, epistaxis, pt or family experience during prior surgery or hemostatic challenge (e.g., dental extraction) vital to assessing periop risk, given variable severity of disease among individuals	PT, PTT, plt count often normal; platelet function assay; quantitative vWF antigen; ristocetin cofactor activity; multimeric analysis

Key Reference: Cameron CB, Kobrinsky N. Perioperative management of patients with von Willebrand's disease. *Can J Anaesth*. 1990;37:341–347.

Perioperative Implications

Preoperative Preparation

- Collaboration with consultant hematologist and blood bank
- Desmopressin 1 hr preop in all but IIB subtype
- Antifibrinolytics for dental procedures

Monitoring

- Bleeding time/vWF activity periodically in prolonged procedures; $T_{1/2}$ of administered vWF about 8–12 hr

Airway

- Laryngoscopy can lead to tissue trauma
- Nasotracheal route best avoided

Induction

- No specific recommendations

Maintenance

- Meticulous surgical hemostasis

Extubation

- Avoid coughing if possible; gentle orotracheal suction best performed under direct vision

Adjuvants

- Consider regional anesthetics with caution
- Repeat desmopressin doses likely to be less effective than initial; reaccumulation of endothelial stores takes time

Anticipated Problems/Concerns

- Excessive intraop and postop blood loss
- Increased likelihood of infectious bloodborne disease

Waldenström's Macroglobulinemia

Amy C. Robertson

Risk

- Rare hematologic neoplasm (accounts for 1–2% of hematologic malignancies)
- In USA, age-adjusted incidence of 3.4 per million among males and 1.7 per million among females. Median age 63–68 y
- Racial preponderance: Caucasians >> African-Americans
- Median survival ranges between 5 and 10 y; age >65 y, anemia, and organomegaly assoc with poor prognosis

Perioperative Risks

- Consequences of hyperviscosity
- Anemia and coagulopathy

Worry About

- Anemia
- Coagulopathy
- Hyperviscosity
- Hypervolemia
- Hepatosplenomegaly and lymphadenopathy in 15–25% of pts

- Cryoglobulinemia with Raynaud's syndrome and vasculitis
- Symmetric sensorimotor peripheral neuropathy

Overview

- Uncommon B-cell lymphoproliferative disease characterized by bone marrow infiltration and production of monoclonal immunoglobulin M (IgM)
- Symptoms attributable to tumor infiltration and/or excessive IgM production
- Anemia most common finding, caused by combination of factors: decrease in red cell survival, impaired erythropoiesis, hemolysis, plasma volume expansion, blood loss from GI tract
- Potentially severe adverse neurologic, hematologic, CV problems periop
- Anesthetic concerns similar to those in multiple myeloma except that hypercalcemia and bone lesions are rare; renal failure and proteinuria less common

ICD-9-CM Code: 273.3

Etiology

- Unknown
- Probable genetic predisposition, reported familial associations with other immunologic disorders
- Role of environmental factors remains to be clarified

Usual Treatment

- Alkylating agents (chlorambucil, cyclophosphamide, melphalan), purine analogues (cladribine, fludarabine), and monoclonal antibody (rituximab)
- Plasmapheresis to treat hyperviscosity symptoms

ASSESSMENT POINTS

System	Effect	Assessment by Hx	PE	Test
CARDIO	Hyperviscosity (high output cardiac failure, valvular dysfunction, MI)	Angina Dyspnea Fatigue	Venous thrombosis Fluid overload	Serum viscosity >4 centipoise (cP) (normal ≤1.8 cP)
RESP	Pulm involvement	Dyspnea	Hypoxia	CXR (pleural effusion, diffuse pulm infiltrates)
HEME	Coagulopathy (multifactorial)	Episodic epistaxis, mucosal and gum bleeding		Coagulation studies
	Anemia (multifactorial)	Fatigue	Pallor	CBC (normocytic, normochronic anemia)
	Cryoglobulinemia	Cold intolerance Raynaud's syndrome Arthralgia	Purpura	Cryoglobulin assay
	Lymph node involvement		Lymphadenopathy	
RENAL	Glomerulonephritis	Dehydration Uremic symptoms		BUN/Cr Urinalysis (proteinuria)
CNS	Leukoencephalopathy Abn cerebrovascular permeability (hyperviscosity)	Headaches Blurred vision	Mental status changes Retinal hemorrhage, papilledema	
PNS	Demyelinating peripheral neuropathy		Symmetric, distal sensorimotor neuropathy, ataxic gait	
GI	Organomegaly secondary to IgM infiltration		Hepatomegaly Splenomegaly	

Key Reference: Fonseca R, Hayman S. Waldenstrom macroglobulinemia. *Br J Haematol.* 2007;138:700–720.

Perioperative Implications

Preinduction/Induction/Maintenance

- Consider plasmapheresis and transfusion
- All drugs: Theoretical unpredictable pharmacokinetics due to alterations of relative proportions of globulins in blood and expanded plasma volume
- Judicious fluid management

Monitoring

- Normothermia to prevent cryoglobulin precipitation

General Anesthesia

- Macroglossia if amyloidosis (rare)

Regional Anesthesia

- Relative contraindication in presence of peripheral neuropathy

Postoperative Period

- Transient postop paresis due to disease rather than anesthetic management

Anticipated Problems/Concerns

- Hyperviscosity symptoms (20–30% incidence)
  - Excessive amounts of circulating IgM impair transit of blood cells resulting in microvascular congestion and decreased tissue perfusion
  - Capillary blood flow impaired, leading to decreased O_2 delivery through microcirculation and tissue ischemia
  - Classic triad of symptoms incl neurologic abn, visual changes, and bleeding
  - CV manifestations 2° to expanded plasma volume: Angina, high output cardiac failure, valvular dysfunction, or MI
  - Plasmapheresis is fastest, most effective method to reduce plasma viscosity

- Anemia
  - Hgb value may be artificially reduced by 2 g/dL 2° to increased plasma volume
  - Transfusion may precipitate CHF or hyperviscosity syndrome (by increasing serum viscosity) and potentially decrease O_2 delivery
  - Consider plasmapheresis before transfusion
- Coagulopathy
- Cryoglobulinemia (5% risk)
  - Precipitation of cryoglobulins at cold blood temp triggers complement activation which results in immune complex vasculitis and ischemia
  - Raynaud's syndrome, arthralgia, purpura, peripheral neuropathy, hepatic dysfunction, and renal failure may develop

Wilms' Tumor

Peter J. Davis

Risk

- Most common malignant renal tumor in childhood
- 6% of all childhood malignancies
- 5–7.8 / million children <15 y
- M = F
- Peak age 1–3 y
- 5% bilateral
- Relapse-free survival rate at 2 y, 90%
- Pts with favorable staging 80–90% chance of cure. Pts with metastasis have 50% long-term survival.
- Overexpression of HER-2 oncoprotein good predictor of survival

Perioperative Risks

- Increased intra-abdominal pressure
- Immunocompromised
- Tumor extension into renal vein, IVC, and heart
- Some treated with chemo prior to surgery
- Assoc Htn

Worry About

- Anomalies
  - Aniridia 1%, hemihypertrophy 2%
  - Neurofibromatosis
  - Beckwith-Wiedemann syndrome
  - GU abn, horseshoe-shaped kidney, cryptorchidism, gonadal dysgenesis, hypospadias, duplication of collecting systems
- Metastatic disease
  - Lymph nodes, lung, liver, brain

Overview

- Most common abd tumor of childhood; prognosis related to staging
- Because of location of tumor, blood loss can be significant
- Tumor is also assoc with other congenital abn, which may affect anesthetic and/or surgical management
- Tumor extension into IVC and heart carries increased morbidity and mortality

ICD-9-CM Code: 189.0

Etiology

- Embryonal neoplasm
- No consistent chromosome abn, although abn in chromosomes 1 and 11 are common
- 3 genes assoc with Wilms'
  - 11p13 interstitial deletion assoc with Wilms'-aniridia-growth retardation
  - 11p15.5 deletion assoc with Beckwith-Wiedemann syndrome
  - Third locus not determined assoc with familial Wilms'

Usual Treatment

- Chemotherapy (with vincristine, actinomycin D, and adriamycin)
- Radiotherapy
- Surgical removal of tumor. If tumor bilateral, surgery has focused on nephron-sparing procedures. (Procedure incl biopsy followed by chemo and delayed definitive resection.)

ASSESSMENT POINTS

System	Effect	Assessment by Hx	PE	Test
HEENT	Beckwith-Wiedemann syndrome	Obstructive airway 2° to large tongue	Direct exam	Blood glucose levels
CARDIO	Htn Tumor extension into heart	Asymptomatic	Htn	ECG CT abd US renal vein/IVC Cardiac ECHO
RESP	Resp compromise	Abd distention Metastatic disease Tumor embolization	↑ RR Hypoxemia	Pulse oximetry CT abdomen US renal vein/IVC Possible cardiac ECHO
GI	Gastric reflux	↑ Intraop pressure Hx of reflux	Abd distention	Review CT scan

Key Reference: Whyte SD, Mark Ansermino J. Anesthetic considerations in the management of Wilms' tumor. *Paediatr Anaesth*. 2006;16(5):504–513.

Perioperative Indications

Preoperative Preparation

- Htn-controlled
- R/O renal vein and/or IVC tumor involvement

Monitoring

- Arterial catheter may be indicated
- CVP catheter may be needed esp. if IVC and tumor extend mid-heart
- Pre-existing hematuria. Foley catheter to aid in fluid balance.
- IV catheters above diaphragm, large-bore catheters preferable
- ETCO$_2$ to rule out air and/or tumor embolus

Airway

- May be a problem if Beckwith-Wiedemann syndrome present

Preinduction/Induction

- Age-appropriate use of sedation
- Rapid-sequence if increased intra-abdominal pressure
- Regional anesthesia; epidural for postop pain
- Pre-existing chem may have cardiac depressant effect
- IV access above diaphragm

Maintenance

- Prolonged procedure
- Avoid N$_2$O
- Maintain temp
- Increased third space fluid requirements
- Procedure may be assoc with large blood loss
- Pulm function may be compromised, 2° to metastasis and/or tumor embolization, abd distention, and/or surgical traction

Extubation

- Expected if temp maintained and pt hemodynamically stable

Postoperative Period

- Pain control
- Third space fluid requirements
- Htn may still be present

Anticipated Problems/Concerns

- Risk of tumor and/or air embolus. If tumor extends into renal vein, IVC may have to be cross-clamped, the IVC opened, and the tumor removed.
- Intraop blood loss can be extensive
- Periop implications

Wolff-Parkinson-White (WPW) Syndrome

Oliver Panzer
Tricia Brentjens

Risk

• WPW pattern (asymptomatic) prevalence: 0.15–0.25% in general population, increases to 0.55% in pts with a 1° relative with WPW.
• WPW syndrome (ECG pattern and arrhythmia): prevalence: 0.005–0.07% in general population, approx 2% out of pts with WPW

Perioperative Risks

• Atrioventricular reentry tachycardia (AVRT) (80% of pts WPW syndrome): rapid heart rate impairs left ventricular (LV) filling, which may cause hemodynamic instability and/or myocardial ischemia esp. if LV failure, LV hypertrophy, aortic stenosis, or mitral stenosis is present.
• Atrial fibrillation (AFib) (15–35%), increasing incidence with age. Major concern is rapid ventricular response due to antegrade conduction over accessory pathway (AP)
• Atrial flutter (5%)
• Ventricular fibrillation (VFib)/sudden death (0–0.4%): Out of rapid ventricular response due to antegrade conduction over AP in Afib/AVRT
• Myocardial ischemia in pts with CAD if SVT or AFib occurs

Overview

• Definition: WPW syndrome is a preexitation syndrome. Ventricular depolarization occurs in part via an accessory pathway (AP) directly connecting the atrium and ventricle and thus capable of conducting electrical impulses into the ventricle bypassing the AV-His Purkinje conduction system. The AP in WPW syndrome is called the bundle of Kent and connects atrial and ventricular myocardium and is not connected to the conduction system.
• The accessory pathways electrical conduction may occur in an antegrade or retrograde fashion and is faster than the AV node and therefore the PR interval is shortened (<0.12 sec). Additionally the myocardium around the AP insertion in the ventricle is activated earlier, i.e., pre-excitation. The impulse then spreads slowly from muscle fiber to muscle fiber until it joins the regular conduction system. This results in a slurred upstroke and widening of the QRS complex on the ECG (fusion complex from early but slow ventricular excitation

via AP and rapid activation via the normal conduction system). These abn in the QRS complex may vary in magnitude and depend on relative contribution of normal AV nodal system and AP to ventricular depolarization.
• PSVT results from a re-entrant circuit involving the AV node and AP. The QRS complex during PSVT matches the usual QRS morphology when conduction is antegrade through the AV system and retrograde through the AP, i.e., orthodromic. 5–10% of the time, conduction through the AP is antegrade, i.e., antidromic in the re-entrant circuit, producing a wide QRS complex. This rhythm may be confused with VTach.
• AFib and/or AFLT is more common in pts with WPW. Usually, but not always, AFib is precipitated by an episode of PSVT. Rapid (≥300 bpm) ventricular rates may occur in pts with APs with short refractory periods. These pts are at risk for developing VFIB and hemodynamic collapse.

ICD-9-CM Code: 426.7 (Anomalous atrioventricular excitation)

Standard Therapy

• With severe hemodynamic compromise: Synchronized DC cardioversion (50–100 J)
• AVRT and/or narrow complex tachycardia: Apply vagal maneuvers or IV adenosine (6–12 mg IV). A small incidence of induction of AFib with adenosine therapy for PSVT in WPW has been described.
• AFib: Agents that reduce the accessory bundle refractory period (digoxin, Ca²⁺-channel blockers, β-blockers, and adenosine) increase the risk of causing VFib and hemodynamic collapse in pts with WPW and AFIB and should therefore be avoided.
• Broad complex tachycardia, i.e., antidromic AVRT: It should be treated with IV procainamide or amiodarone.

Perioperative Implications

Preoperative Preparation
• If pre-excitation on ECG or Hx of WPW, consider cardiology evaluation
• If symptomatic, consider electrophysiologic study and catheter ablation.

Monitoring
• ECG for detection of periop PSVT or AFib
• Consider arterial line and CVP catheter if LV dysfunction or valve disease as these pts have a high dependence on preload and atrial kick.
• For emergency surgery, consider placement of defibrillator pads prior to induction.

Induction/Maintenance/Extubation
• Volatile anesthetics and IV induction agents such as propofol and benzodiazepines seem to have no influence on the conduction system and are safe to use. Enflurane and isoflurane as well as medications that enhance vagal tone (e.g., opioids, propofol infusion) actually decrease conduction via the AP and are safe to use as well.
• However increased sympathetic tone may decrease the refractory period and therefore accelerate the conduction in the AP and AV node. This may facilitate the precipitation of AVRNT, AFib, and/or VFib
• Limit the use of vagolytic agents such as pancuronium and atropine, use α-1 agonists (phenylephrine) instead of ephedrine to avoid positive chronotropy and arrhythmias.

Postoperative Period
• Pain management to avoid catecholamine excess
• If the delta wave appears in periop period, rule out myocardial infarction (decreased AV conduction second to ischemia facilitating increasing AP conduction).

Anticipated Problems/Concerns

• AV nodal blockers (digoxin, Ca²⁺-channel blockers, adenosine, and β-blockers) may shorten refractoriness in the AP and thereby provoke VFIB in WPW pts with AFIB.
• Hemodynamic collapse may occur when verapamil or β-blockers are used in the treatment of antidromic (wide-complex) PSVT in pt with WPW that is mistaken for VTach.

ASSESSMENT POINTS

ECG Criteria:

ECG	P wave & PR interval	QRS	Comments
Classic (Type A)	Shortened PR interval, typically <0.12 secs (left-sided bypass track)	Slurred upstroke (delta wave), widened QRS complex	The faster the AP conduction the more prominent the delta wave and the wider the QRS
Atypical (Type B)	Shortened PR interval (right-sided bypass track)	Q waves (inverted delta wave) in V1	May be confused with MI
Concertina effect	Periodically progressive shortening of the PR interval, with the P wave disappearing in QRS	The shorter the PR interval, the more pronounced is the delta wave (wider QRS)	This is the result from a periodically ↑ conduction via the AP
Intermittent WPW	May be mistaken for frequent ventricular premature beats, if it persists for several beats may be held for accelerated idioventricular rhythm		

Key Reference: Wheeler DW, Sayeed RA, Ritchie AJ. Unsuspected Wolff-Parkinson-White syndrome causing arrhythmias after cardiac surgery. *J Cardiothorac Vasc Anesth*. 2002;16(3):354–356.

SECTION II

Procedures

Abdominal Aortic Aneurysm Repair

Qianjin Liu

Ivan Kangrga

Risk

- AAA affects approx 5% of males and 1.7% females over 65 y
- Risks: Smoking, males, age, white race, family Hx, Htn, atherosclerosis
- Risk of rupture: Female sex, diameter >5.5 cm, low FEV1, smoking, high MAP.
- Rupture: 80% mortality, approx 4500 deaths annually in the USA
- Incidence in USA: About 45,000 AAA repairs annually, resulting in 1400 deaths

Perioperative Risks

- Open repair (OR): Mortality is 4–8 % for elective and 25–60% emergent/ruptured AAAs. Risks are higher in women, pts with more co-morbidities and emergencies
- Morbidity: Renal 5% of infra-and 13% of suprarenal AAAs; MI 4–15%, resp 10%, ischemic bowel 3–4%, and paraplegia <1% for infrarenal and 1–5% for supraceliac AAAs
- Endovascular aneurysm repair (EVAR): 1–2% 30-d mortality but significant periop complications: MI 7%, resp 10%, ARF 5.5% (dialysis < 0.4); conversion to open 1.6%, ischemic bowel 1.0%, bleeding requiring re-intervention 0.8%, thromboembolic 0.5 to 1.5%

Worry About

- OR: Massive blood loss, hypovolemia, anemia, electrolyte and coagulation abn
- OR: Ischemia-reperfusion with acid-base derangement, hypothermia, and multi-organ injury
- OR: Myocardial ischemia/infarction and renal insufficiency/failure
- EVAR: Contrast nephropathy, myocardial ischemia/infarction

Overview

- High incidence of co-morbidities: Htn, CAD, renal insufficiency, cerebrovascular disease
- Emergent repair has much higher assoc mortality and morbidity
- Need for invasive monitoring and significant IV access

AAA ICD-9-CM Code: 441.4   OR AAA ICD-9-CM Code: 38.44 EVAR ICD-9-CM Code: 39.71

Indications

- Elective repair is indicated for AAA≥5.5 cm in absence of serious co-morbidities
- Surveillance and medical management is recommended for pts with AAA≤5.4 cm
- Urgent repair for all symptomatic AAAs and emergent (OR or EVAR) for ruptures

Usual Treatment

- OR: Transperitoneal or retroperitoneal approach. The latter is favored in AAA with juxtarenal or visceral extension, inflammation, horseshoe kidney and hostile abdomen.
- EVAR comprises more than 50% repairs; periop mortality is lower then with OR but 2-y outcomes are similar. Vascular anatomy unsuitable for EVAR in 30% pts.

ASSESSMENT POINTS

System	Effect	Assessment by Hx	PE	Test
CARDIO	CAD, MI, CHF, arrhythmias	Orthopnea, SOB, PND angina, palpitations	Pedal edema, JVD, S_3	Noninvasive if >3 of: CHF, CVA, DM, Cr>2, MET<4; Revasc.: STMI, unstable angina, 3-v dis
RESP	COPD	SOB, cough	Distant BS, wheeze	CXR, ABGs, PFTs, CT
RENAL	Renal insufficiency	Reno-vascular Htn	Generalized edema	Serum Cr, creatinine clearance
CNS	CV disease	TIA, stroke, syncope	Focal deficits, bruits	Neuro assessment, carotid US

Key Reference: Chaikof EI, et al. SVS practice guidelines for the care of patients with an abdominal aortic aneurysm: Executive summary. *J Vasc Surg.* 2009;50(4):880–896.

Perioperative Management

Preoperative Preparation
- ACE-inhibitors and ARBs held the day of surgery
- β-blockers, ASA and statins continued
- Thoracic epidural should be considered for OR postop analgesia.
- Large-bore IV access is essential.

Monitoring
- Invasive arterial pressure monitoring in both OR and EVAR
- OR: CVP for all. PAC or TEE for poor LVEF and active CAD, and/or high clamp

Anesthetic Technique/Induction
- OR: General anesthesia with epidural for postop pain
- EVAR: Neuraxial or MAC anesthesia may be assoc with better outcomes than GA; anesthetic choice is based on team experience, complexity of repair and pts' co-morbidities.

Surgical Stages: Open Repair

- **Dissection**
  - IV access and ability to transfuse blood products are essential
  - Normotension is the goal of BP control to prevent premature rupture
  - Mannitol (12.5–25 g) is a useful free radical scavenger but not a proven renoprotectant
  - Heparinization (75–100 U/kg) 5 min prior to aortic cross clamp; optimal ACT >250s
- **Aortic Clamping**
  - Hemodynamic goals: Avoid excessive Htn above the clamp but maintain adequate pressures below the clamp to ensure spinal, bowel perfusion. One strategy is MAP at 20% increase from baseline with good heart rate control
  - For excessive Htn with infrarenal clamp the first choice is an afterload reducer (i.e., nicardipine), and for supraceliac a preload reducer (i.e., nitroglycerine).
  - Lactic acidosis below the clamp provides rationale for $NaHCO_3$ administration: Higher base deficit and $NaHCO_3$ requirements in supraceliac clamp.
- **Aortic Unclamping**
  - Hemodynamic challenge: Reperfusion hypotension, arrhythmias, hyperkalemia, hypothermia
  - Optimize preload, afterload; maintain NSR; $CaCl_2$ $NaHCO_3$ and vasopressors ready to use
  - Closing: Normalization of hemodynamics and coagulation, warming, dosing of epidural

Postoperative Considerations
- ICU for continued hemodynamic and coagulation monitoring, possibly ventilatory support
- Pain is significant; effective epidural promotes early extubation and pulm rehabilitation

EVAR

- Bilateral groin dissection, insertion of an introducer sheath, and arteriogram
- Stent is inserted over a guidewire, position confirmed radiologically, and deployed. Temporary balloon insufflation may be used to promote the seal.
- Conversion to OR is rare (<2%) but assoc with higher morbidity and mortality
- Postop considerations: Lower extremity embolism, myocardial ischemia, renal insufficiency. Endoleaks are late complications. Routine EVAR requires an overnight stay.

Anticipated Problems/Concerns

- In the setting of potential blood loss early intraop epidural dosing is not advisable.
- Temp management is difficult in OR as lower body warming cannot be used.
- Renal protection remains elusive. OR: Keys are short clamp time and maintenance of intravascular volume and CO. In EVAR, evidence additionally supports administration of $NaHCO_3$ and acetylcysteine or use of CO_2 contrast to attenuate contrast-induced nephropathy.
- High prevalence of CAD predisposes AAA pts to periop myocardial ischemia.

Abdominoperineal Resection

David W. Miller

Risk

- About 40,000 cases of rectal cancer per year (abdominoperineal resection used in 18–27% of cases; remainder involve sphincter-preserving low-anterior resections)
- Average age at diagnosis is 67 (less than 4% of cases under 40 y)
- Slight male predominance (poorer prognosis)
- Slower progression in elderly
- African-Americans have highest incidence and mortality in USA

Perioperative Risks

- Periop mortality 2–3%
- Mortality related to pre-existing cardiac and pulm disease
- Significant impotence or urinary dysfunction 10–60%
- Urinary retention ~30%
- Perineal wound infection 16%; breakdown 7%

- Pelvic/abdominal abscess, ostomy problems, abd wound issues also occur

Worry About

- Hypovolemia periop related from bowel prep and 3rd spacing
- Presacral bleeding during pelvic dissection
- Urologic complications (bladder or ureteral injury)
- Nerve/compression injury from pt positioning in lithotomy; brachial plexus injury from steep Trendelenburg position
- Hemodynamic changes with changes in bed position and surgical stimulus

Overview

- Pts may have had preop chemotherapy or radiation
- Anemia may be masked by hypovolemia

- Procedure involves removal of the distal colon, rectum, closure of anus, and creating a permanent colostomy

ICD-9-CM Code: 154.1 (Malignant neoplasm of rectum)

Indications and Usual Treatment

- Rectal adenocarcinoma involving levator ani muscle
- Inability to completely resect distal rectal cancer from abd approach
- Recurrent anal squamous cancer
- Tumors of anus too large to locally resect
- Decreasing in popularity in favor of low anterior resection and local excision of tumors
- Some pts with poor sphincter control benefit from APR instead of low anterior resection

ASSESSMENT POINTS

System	Effect	Assessment by Hx	PE	Test
CARDIO	Hypovolemia	Bowel prep, N/V/D	Hypotension, UO	Othostatics/ EKG
RESP	Metastases	Cough, SOB		CXR, CT scan
GI	Hepatic metastases	Pain	Tenderness	CT scan
	Bowel obstruction	N/V, no flatus	Abd distension and tenderness	Abd x-ray and/or CT scan
RENAL	Metabolic alkalosis if NGT	High NG output	Mental status	ABG and electrolytes
	Obstruction	Pain, oliguria		BUN Cr, IVP or other imaging
ENDO	Malnutrition	Wt loss	Muscle wasting	Albumin, electrolytes
HEME	Anemia	GI bleeding, fatigue	Pallor	CBC

Key Reference: Perry WB, Connaughton JC. Abdominoperineal resection: How is it done and what are the results? *Clin Colon Rectal Surg.* 2007;20:213–220.

Perioperative Management

Preoperative Preparation

- Assess pre-existing conditions and volume status, electrolytes; aspiration premedication with H$_2$ blockers, metoclopramide (contraindicated in obstruction), and sodium citrate
- Consider insertion of epidural catheter for periop pain control

Monitoring

- Routine monitors
- Arterial line in pts with significant pre-existing cardiopulmonary disease
- Insertion of CVP or PA cath for significant co-morbidities; not usually necessary
- Foley to monitor UO; assess hydration and urologic complications

Anesthetic Technique/Induction

- General endotracheal anesthesia; general/regional

Airway

- Pts at high risk for aspiration should undergo awake technique or rapid sequence induction; can still perform cricoid if pt has NG tube

Maintenance

- Prevention of hypothermia through the use of forced warm air, warm IV fluids, and warmed humidified gas to avoid postop wound infection and bleeding

Surgical Stages

Dissection

- Replacement of fluid deficit from bowel prep and NPO time; anticipate large 3rd-space losses; attempt to maintain euvolemia
- Lower midline incision on abd
- Abd portion of case involves mobilization of rectum, sigmoid colon, and creation of a descending colostomy with the pt in a modified lithotomy position
- During the abd phase steep Trendelenburg is usually needed for dissection. Watch for hemodynamic changes with pt position; ensure proper padding and securing of pt to OR table
- High peak airway pressures can occur in steep Trendelenburg

- Perineal portion of case involves removal of the anus, the anal sphincters, and the distal rectum; can be done simultaneously as abd portion if two teams used
- Stoma has to be matured and incision closed after perineal portion of case if single team approach used; watch for hypotension
- EBL: 300–1000 mL

Postoperative Considerations

- Extubation at end of case is typically routine
- Pain score: 7–8
- Postop analgesia: IV PCA or epidural
- Consider ICU admission

Anticipated Problems/Concerns

- Hypovolemic pts prone to hypotension when epidural used
- Male pts have narrower pelvis making dissection more difficult; watch for bleeding during pelvic dissection
- Watch for hypoventilation and hypoxemia postop

Adrenalectomy for Pheochromocytoma

Michael F. Roizen

Risk

- People within USA: 0.03%–0.04% (~100,000) by autopsy of nonselected individuals; 0.1%–0.3% of individuals with sustained Htn
- Race with highest prevalence: Caucasian

Perioperative Risks

- Major goal to avoid pheo crisis; preop, intraop goals of management of extra-adrenal surgery no different from those of adrenal surgery; if α blockade not present before surg, try to delay operation until degree of α blockade judged appropriate by:
  - No BP >165/90 mmHg for 48 hr
  - Presence of orthostatic hypotension, but BP on standing should not be <80/45 mmHg
  - An ECG free of ST-T changes due to cardiomyopathy
  - Absence of Sx of catecholamine excess; and signs of α blockade (e.g., nasal stuffiness)
- If emergency use α-blockers, β-blockers, nitroprusside; keep in ICU till most painful time has passed or adrenergic control attained
- Increased risk of Htn crisis with bleeding into myocardium, brain, kidney or ischemia
- Mortality rate to 3% even with appropriate preparation for tumor resection, in good hands
- 25–50% of those who die in hospitals of pheo crisis do so during induction of anesthesia/stressful periop periods, or in labor, delivery
- Assoc with cholelithiasis, renal stones

Worry About

- Catecholamine crisis with hemorrhage/infarcts in vital organs, hypotension due to ↓ levels of catecholamines postop (uncommon more than 3 d postop if all pheo tissue removed)

Overview

- Tumor of catecholamine-producing tissue (90% in adrenals): painful (stressful) events often cause exaggerated stress response
- For pts with pheo, even small stresses can lead to blood catecholamine levels of 2000–20,000 pg/mL; infarction of tumor, with release of products on retroperitoneal surfaces, surgical, or other pressure causing release of products, can result in blood levels of 200,000–1 million pg/mL
- Need α-blockers before β blockade unless vasoconstrictive effects of latter go unopposed, causing increased risk of dangerous Htn. β blockade suggested if persistent arrhythmias or tachycardia not resolving α-adrenergic effects or when aggravated by α-adrenergic effects.
- If appropriate, α blockade preop can lower risk of crisis by >90%

ICD-9-CM Code: 194.0

Indications and Usual Treatment

- 90% spont arise; 10% familial (autosomal dominant genetics involving chromosome 7 implicated)
- Assoc with MEA IIA (medullary thyroid cancer, 1° hyperparathyroidism), IIB (medullary thyroid cancer, mucosal neuromas; assoc with neurofibromatosis, von Hippel-Lindau syndrome, and retinal and cerebellar hemangioblastoma, ataxia-telangiectasia, Sturge-Weber syndrome)
- Prehydrate liberally over 6–60 d if CV status tolerates; expand with high salt and/or fluid diet while increasing α blockade over 7–60 d period

ASSESSMENT POINTS

System	Effect	Assessment by Hx	PE	Test
HEENT		Nasal stuffiness (from α-adrenergic blockade)		
CARDIO	Htn, dysrhythmias, AFIB, sinus tachycardia, mitral valve prolapse, CHF, myocardial fibril necrosis or myocarditis	SOB, exercise tolerance, palpitations, Htn (50% sustained, 40% paroxsymal)	Standard exam plus measurement of BP q1min in stressful environment plus orthostatic maneuvers with BP/HR measurement q1min	ECG, ECHO (if cardiomyopathy suspected)
GI	90% tumors adrenal or abd wt loss, diarrhea, dehydration		Be careful when palpating abdomen not to trigger pheo crisis	No different from normal
HEME		Mild polycythemia, thrombocytopenia		Hgb (way to judge volume expansion)
CNS	↑ Catecholamine effects	Headache, tremor, anxiety, ↓ pain threshold, fatigue		
METAB	Assoc with hyperparathyroidism	Glucose intolerance due to α-adrenergic gluconeogenesis, ↓ insulin secretion		Glucose often ↑ (insulin Rx prescribed before correct Dx of cancer made)

Key References: Roizen MF, Fleisher L. Pheochromocytoma in anesthetic implications of concurrent disease. In: *Miller's anesthesia*. 7th ed. New York: Churchill Livingstone; 2010:1084–1087. Tauzin-Fin P; Sesay M; Gosse P; Ballanger P. Effects of perioperative alpha-1 block on haemodynamic control during laparoscopic surgery for phaeochromocytoma. *Br J Anaesth*. 2004;92:512–517.

Perioperative Management

Monitoring
- Temp
- Art line placement before induction difficult
- Consider TEE if CV system severely affected; CVP rarely used

Anesthetic Care/Technique
- No technique assoc with better or worse outcome; use of droperidol controversial. Agents that block catecholamine reuptake (ketamine) or cause release might be avoided.

Induction/Maintenance
- Prehydrate liberally if tolerated
- Gentle induction with nitroprusside available
- Dopamine infusion in reserve
- Painful or stressful events often cause exaggerated stress response caused by release of catecholamines from nerve endings loaded by reuptake

Surgical Stages

Initial Dissection
- Trans abd incision preferred if localization does not exclude bilat tumors; flank/post approach with nephrectomy/jackknife position if unilateral adrenalectomy without paraganglionoma exploration planned
- Laparoscopic approach assoc with same intra- and postop CV events. Faster bowel recovery. Most now done laparoscopically, many thru single belly button approach

Adrenal Removal
- Dissection to secure venous drainage, double ligature with transection between; then arterial supply; then complete mobilization, liberation
- After predominant tumor removed, palpation of paraganglionic chain with observation to monitor for sudden increasing in BP or HR
- Goal in resection is securing venous supply from tumor(s). Pressure on tumor causing release can result in blood levels of 200,000–1 million pg/mL (ask for temporary stay of surgery while nitroprusside infusion increased).
- Good communication essential
- Relative hypotension often develops after venous drainage of tumor or its removal. If perfusion adequate can let BP stay at 80/40. Massive infusions of catecholamines occasionally required.

- EBL: 100–400 mL; cell saver use not advised
- Often hypovolemic if <2–3 wk has been allowed for increased titration of α-blocking drugs; guide volume replacement with PCWP or TEE vol estimates

Postoperative Considerations
- Postop, do not force high UO with crystalloid infusions, as pts have tendency to CHF
- Postop, ~50% remain hypertensive for 1–3 d, when all but 25% become normotensive
- Usually use epidural, PCA, IV narcotics for 2–4 d postop (1 d if laparoscopic)

Anticipated Problems/Concerns
- Pheo crisis a life-threatening illness, manifest by increased temp, increased HR, alterations in consciousness

Laparoscopic Adrenalectomy

Madhavi Naik

Risk

- Pheochromocytoma when it is a well-defined tumor, maximum diameter of 7–8 cm, with good preop BP control.
- Aldosteronoma, nonfunctioning adenoma, cortisol producing adenoma, Cushing's disease, cysts, myelolipoma and metastatic adrenal tumor, when tumors are less than 10–12 cm in size.
- For adrenal cancer, open adrenalectomy is preferred esp. if the tumor is large.

Perioperative Risks

- Depend on tumor type and severity of symptoms.
- Main co-morbidities
  - Pheochromocytoma: Htn, cardiomyopathy, acute pulm edema, cardiac arrhythmias, myocardial ischemia or infarction
  - Adrenal adenoma and aldosteronoma: Htn, hypokalemia, hyperglycemia
- Hemodynamic fluctuations during tumor manipulation may occur and when severe, can increase periop morbidity.
- During laparoscopic resection of a pheochromocytoma, pressure on the tumor caused by insufflation of gas can cause release of catecholamines from the tumor.

- Pts undergoing bilateral adrenalectomy are at risk for developing acute adrenal insufficiency

Worry About

- Pt position in lateral with head up/head down. Osteoporosis (from excess cortisol secretion) is a consideration when positioning pts with adrenal adenoma.
- The cardiorespiratory effects of pneumoperitoneum and systemic absorption of carbon dioxide:
  - Increased SVR, increased PVR, decreased CO, increased BP, increased HR. In pts with pheochromocytoma, these could be worsened by the effects of circulating catecholamines. Myocardial ischemia can occur in pts with CAD.
  - Increased intra-abdominal pressure opposes diaphragmatic descent and causes decreased FRC. This, coupled with reduced CO, results in V/Q mismatch.
  - Hypercapnia from systemic absorption of CO_2 requires ↑ minute ventilation and high-peak inspiratory pressures, increasing the risk for barotrauma. If unacceptably high peak pressures are needed to maintain normocapnia, it may be necessary to allow a mild degree of hypercapnia and resp acidosis to prevent barotrauma.

Overview

- Safe and effective procedure for removal of small benign adrenal neoplasms
- For pts with pheochromocytoma, periop morbidity from adrenergic crisis can be greatly reduced by adequate preop medical management

ICD-9-CM Code: 194.0 and 227.0

Indications and Usual Treatment

- Aldosteronoma: Initial treatment with potassium supplementation, competitive aldosterone inhibitor (spironolactone) and antihypertensive drugs.
- Adrenal adenoma: Antihypertensives and drugs to control blood sugar, treatment of electrolyte imbalances.
- Pheochromocytoma
  - Alpha blocker (phenoxybenzamine) to lower BP, combined with beta blocker to treat cardiac arrhythmias.
  - A beta blocker should not be used as the initial or sole therapy as profound vasoconstriction from unopposed alpha receptor stimulation may lead to a hypertensive crisis or pulm edema.
  - Calcium channel blocker (nicardipine) can be used instead of alpha blockers for BP control

ASSESSMENT POINTS

System	Effect	Assessment by Hx	PE	Test
CARDIO	Htn Hypovolemia Dysrhythmias cardiomyopathy	Palpitations SOB, orthopnea	Standard BP measurement Orthostatic hypotension	 EKG ECHO
Electrolyte imbalance	Hypokalemia (alsosteronoma, adrenal adenoma)	Muscle weakness, cramps		EKG Serum K level
METAB	Hyperglycemia (adrenal adenoma, ↑ cortisol) (pheochromocytoma, α_2 mediated inhibition of insulin release)			Serum glucose level

Key Reference: Sprung J, et al. Anesthetic aspects of laparoscopic adrenalectomy for pheochromocytoma. *Seminars in Anesthesia, Perioperative Medicine and Pain.* 2002;21(1):35–45.

Perioperative Management

Preoperative Preparation

- Assess co-existing morbidities and optimize their medical management.
- Supplemental steroid therapy for those at risk for developing adrenal insufficiency.
- Continue alpha and beta blockade for pheochromocytoma

Monitoring

- Routine
- Arterial line and large-bore IV access.
- Central venous catheter to infuse fluids and vasopressors when needed. Position and pneumoperitoneum affect absolute valve of the CVP
- Pulm artery catheter in pts who have preexisting cardiac co-morbidities (catechola-mine induced cardiomyopathy, LVH, myocardial ischemia, CAD) and severe pulm disease
- TEE for pts with significant left ventricular dysfunction
- Close monitoring of serum electrolyte and blood glucose concentration

Anesthetic Technique

- Adequate preop sedation and/or anxiolysis to prevent catecholamine release for anxiety.
- Midazolam is a good choice.
- Consider adding fentanyl for line placement before induction.
- Induction technique to prevent swings in heart rate and BP.
- Isoflurane, fentanyl, and vecuronium are good choices for maintenance. Isoflurane is a vasodila-

tor and does not sensitize the myocardium to the effects of catecholamines. Desflurane is not the agent of choice because it may cause sympathetic stimulation. The use of sevoflurane is questionable if hypokalemic nephropathy and polyuria are present (hyperaldosteronism).
- Introp hyperventilion can potentiate hypokalemia, resp acidosis may increase the risk for arrhythmias.
- Treatment of intraop Htn with sodium nitroprusside, nicardipine, nitroglycerin
- Treatment of tachycardia with esmolol or labetol
- Ligation of the adrenal vein and resultant sudden decrease in circulating catecholamines can cause hypotension needing fluid resuscitation, vasopressors (phenylephrine) and inotropic agents (dopamine, epinephrine, norepinephrine)
- Hypoglycemia may result (from decrease in catecholamines and reduction in the α-adrenergic suppression of insulin secretion) and must be treated.
- Blood loss during laparoscopic adrenalectomy is generally lower than with open, however the potential for massive blood loss does exist and the anesthesiologist must prepare for it.

Surgical Stages

- Positioning: Right or left lateral decubitus, the OR table is flexed to open up the area between the costal margin and iliac crest, the kidney bridge is elevated. For bilateral adrenalectomy, the pt may need repositioning or the surgeon may choose to use supine position.

- Pneumoperitoneum is established with CO_2 insufflation to 15 mm Hg via a Veress needle placed in the midclavicular line below the costal margin.
- Approaches: The transperitoneal approach is the most commonly used and provides the best access to the adrenal gland. A retroperitoneal approach may also be used, however because of the limited space in the retroperitoneum, this may be technically more difficult.
- The adrenal veins are ligated early to prevent spillage of catecholamines into the circulation (pheochromocytoma)
- Left laparoscopic adrenalectomy: Three trocars are placed along the costal margin. After mobilization of the splenic flexure and the spleen, the adrenal gland is exposed and the adrenal vein is clipped and divided. After further dissection and clipping or cauterization of all blood vessels, the adrenal gland is freed and extracted in a sterile endocatch bag through the most anterior trocar.
- Right laparoscopic adrenalectomy: A fourth trocar is needed to retract the liver. After mobilization of the hepatic flexure, the adrenal gland is exposed. The right adrenal vein empties directly into the IVC and dissection to expose this may be difficult when the adrenal gland is enlarged. The vein is either clipped, or when short and broad, stapled and divided. After further dissection, the gland is freed and extracted.

Postoperative Considerations

• Hemodynamic monitoring and treatment of any CV instability may require admission to the ICU, esp. in cases of pheochromocytoma.

• PONV and shoulder pain can be treated with antiemetics, NSAIDs and IV or PO narcotics.

Generally, the need for postop pain medications is significantly lower after laparoscopic adrenalectomy than open.

Anticipated Problems/Concerns

• Most serious periop complications are myocardial ischemia and infarction, acute pulm edema, acute right heart failure, cerebrovascular accident, rupture of intra-abdominal or cerebral aneurysm

Advanced Cardiac Life Support (ACLS)
Alan Jay Schwartz

Risk

- Incidence in USA: Based on data from the Resuscitation Outcomes Consortium, emergency medical services treat >294,000 out-of-hospital cardiac arrests annually
- On average, 31% of out-of-hospital cardiac arrests receive bystander CPR
- CHD caused about one of every five deaths in USA in 2005; the largest single killer of American males and females
- Nine risk factors: Cigarette smoking, abn blood lipid levels, Htn, diabetes, abd obesity, a lack of physical activity, low daily fruit and vegetable consumption, alcohol overconsumption and psychosocial index

Perioperative Risks

- 1.7 cardiac arrests/10,000 anesthetics

- Assoc pathology: Ischemic, valvular, or hypertensive heart disease; congestive cardiomyopathy
- Uncommon assoc conditions: Preexcitation syndromes, hereditary or acquired prolonged QT disorders, metabolic abn, adverse drug reactions

Worry About

- Cardiac pathology
- Periop ischemic changes, metabolic abn
- Subsequent episodes postresuscitation
- Postresuscitation end-organ ischemic damage

Overview

- Morbidity and mortality decreased when ACLS initiated promptly
- Outcome dismal if initiation of ACLS is delayed >8 min or lasts >30 min

- Other factors assoc with decreased survival: age >70 y, unwitnessed arrest, sepsis, cancer, renal failure, prearrest hypotension
- Survival rate for in-hospital cardiac arrest to discharge is 15%.

Indications and Treatment

- ACLS indicated for treatment of life-threatening/fatal arrhythmias or cardiac arrest, e.g., supraventricular bradycardias and tachycardias, ventricular fibrillation (VFib), bradyasystole and electrical mechanical dissociation
- Treatment depends on the arrhythmia or cause of cardiac arrest and the hemodynamic stability of pt.
- The quicker the restoration of normal rhythm, the more likely survival. Defibrillate early.

ASSESSMENT POINTS

System	Effect	Assessment by Hx	PE	Test
CNS	Arrhythmia may cause hypotension	Syncope	CNS exam	ECG, MRI
CARDIO	Arrhythmia, Htn, valvular disease	CV status, Hx angina, SOB, palpitations	CV exam	ECG, ECHO
RESP	Pulm edema	SOB, orthopnea	Chest exam	SaO_2, CXR

Key Reference: 2005 American Heart Association Guidelines for Cardiopulmonary Resuscitation and Emergency Cardiovascular Care. http://circ.ahajournals.org/content/vol112/24_suppl/.

Intraoperative Implications

Monitoring

- Routine; confirm ETT position using qualitative $ETCO_2$ indicator, capnographic, capnometric and esophageal detector devices
- Invasive monitoring as indicated by the pts condition

Management

- Dependent upon type of rhythm and hemodynamic status
- Emergency drugs, incl epinephrine, lidocaine, and atropine, must be immediately available
- Cardiac defibrillator and means of cardiac pacing must be available.
- Initiate BLS with attention to maintenance of airway, ventilation, and circulation via chest compressions until definitive treatment established
- Supraventricular bradyarrhythmias
  - Treat if significant decrease in BP or cardiac output or in the presence of PVCs; atropine 0.5 mg IV, may repeat to total of 3 mg; transcutaneous or transvenous pacing; dopamine or epinephrine infusion; isoproterenol infusion used with extreme caution
- Supraventricular tachyarrhythmias
  - Paroxysmal supraventricular tachycardia (PSVT) with severe hypotension and atrial fibrillation (AFib) or flutter with hemodynamic compromise
  - If stable in PSVT, vagal maneuvers followed by adenosine 6 mg IV, then adenosine 12 mg IV after 1–2 min if PSVT persists, treat recurrence with diltiazem or β-blockers.
  - If stable in AFib or atrial flutter, consider diltiazem or β-blockers.

- If unstable, cardioversion with a biphasic defibrillator at 120–200 J (360 J with a monophasic defibrillator)
  - Atrial flutter often responds to lower energy
- Ventricular bradyarrhythmias
  - Heart block with slow idioventricular escape rhythm and signs and/or symptoms of poor perfusion treated with transcutaneous or transvenous pacing
  - Atropine 0.5 mg IV or an epinephrine 2–10 mcg/kg or dopamine 2–10 mcg/min infusion until pacing is available; use of isoproterenol may precipitate VT or VFib
  - Unstable pt-immediate synchronized cardioversion (biphasic waveform recommended) (recommended starting dose)
    - AFib 100–200 joules (J)
    - Atrial flutter 50–100 J
    - VT and VFib 120–200 J (360 J with a monophasic defibrillator)
- Stable pt
  - Narrow QRS (≤0.12 sec) (supraventricular tachycardia [SVT]) and regular rhythm-vagal maneuvers, adenosine 6 mg rapid IV, if no conversion 12 mg rapid IV, diltiazem or β-blockers
  - Narrow QRS and irregular rhythm (probable AFib, atrial flutter)-diltiazem or β-blockers
  - Wide QRS (≥0.12 sec) and regular rhythm (VT)—amiodarone 150 mg IV over 10 min to a maximum of 2.2 g/24 hr
  - Wide QRS (≥0.12 sec) and irregular rhythm (if AFib)-diltiazem or β-blockers
  - Torsades de pointes—magnesium 1–2 g over 5–60 min followed by a magnesium infusion
- Premature ventricular beats
  - Look for treatable cause
  - Suppress with lidocaine 1.0–1.5 mg/kg IV; may repeat 0.5–0.75 mg/kg every 5–10 min to total of 3 mg/kg

- VT
  - If stable, lidocaine 1.0–1.5 mg/kg IV; may repeat 0.5–0.75 mg/kg every 5–10 min to total of 3 mg/kg; amiodarone 150 mg IV over 10 min to a maximum of 2.2 g/24 hr
  - If unsuccessful or hemodynamically unstable, cardioversion
- VFIB
  - Rapid defibrillation 120–200 J biphasic defibrillator (360 J with a monophasic defibrillator)
  - If persistent, intersperse defibrillation with epinephrine 1.0 mg IV, vasopressin 40 U IV, then lidocaine 1.0–1.5 mg/kg IV followed by amiodarone, magnesium, and procainamide
- Bradyasystole
  - High mortality, suspect hypoxia
  - Consider immediate transcutaneous pacing
  - Epinephrine is drug of choice along with atropine
  - Defibrillation may be tried as asystole may be unrecognized VFib
- Pulseless electrical activity (PAE)
  - Caused by acute derangements in preload (hypovolemia, cardiac tamponade, tension pneumothorax), afterload (pulm embolism), myocardial performance (acidosis, hypoxemia)
    - Treatment dependent on cause
    - Epinephrine and atropine may be given

Anticipated Problems/Concerns

- Following resuscitation, continued support of vital organ function required: CNS insult may cause increase in ICP or seizures; myocardial damage may result in persistent dysrhythmias or decreased contractility; renal damage may result in acute renal failure.

Amputation, Above-Knee (AKA)

Caridad Bravo-Fernandez

Risk

- 9 to 23 per 100,000 person y, depends on study. Ratio AKA/BKA = 3/2 in some centers
- Mean age 70 y, incidence increases with age between 45 and 85.
- M:F ratio: 3–5:1 with 3:1 up to age 85; >85 male to female is 5:1
- Causes: DM, ESRD, vascular insufficiency, malignant neoplasm, trauma
- DM followed by ESRD, dominant underlying medical condition leading to limb ischemia

Perioperative Risks

- Operative mortality 3–5% (within 30 d), as high as 30% 1-y mortality
- Morbidity incl cardiac disease (myocardial ischemia, infarction, CHF, arrhythmias), renal failure/replacement, advanced age, emergency admission, nursing home admission
- Pulm emboli: 6–10%
- Nonhealing, infection common surgical problems

Worry About

- Underlying disease leads to AKA; 20% conversion from BKA to AKA
- Assoc infection, gangrene, tissue loss
- Cardiac disease
- Periop pulm emboli, thromboembolism, stroke
- Flexion contractures of involved limb, postop ambulation
- Decubiti
- Phantom limb pain and/or stump pain

Overview

- Assoc with high periop mortality
- Vascular insufficiency to limb limits viability, increased risk of sepsis and complications of immobility; viability evaluated by Doppler, blood flow studies to determine level of amputation
- Preop epidural narcotics to eliminate rest pain
- Regional anesthesia, postop analgesia frequently used; contraindicated in pts receiving anticoagulants

- Rehabilitation more difficult with AKA than below knee amputation (BKA)

ICD-9-CM Codes: 747.64 (PVD); 897.2 (Trauma); 250.0 (DM); 585.6 (ESRD); 195.5 (Tumor)

Indications and Usual Treatment

- Amputations for trauma done early to decrease contamination
- Control infection, sepsis with antibiotics
- Control blood sugar with regular insulin in diabetic pts
- Smoking should be D/C 1 wk before operation or on admission
- Consider revascularization to improve changes for good results
- Below-knee amputation preferred for better rehabilitation
- Early management of systemic complications

ASSESSMENT POINTS

System	Effect	Assessment by Hx	PE	Test
CARDIO	CAD, Htn, hyperlipids	CV status, chest pain, previous MI, SOB	CV exam	ECG, stress test ECHO
RESP	Emphysema, COPD	SOB, smoking, exercise tolerance	Chest exam	O_2 sat, CXR, ABGs, PFTs
ENDO	DM	Polyuria, polydipsia, cardiomyopathy, neuropathy Autonomic neuropathy Delayed gastric emptying	Sensory exam	Glucose, orthostatic BP Hgb A1C
HEME	Thrombophlebitis, bleeding	Pain, bruising, bleeding	Ulcerations, ecchymoses	PT, PTT, Hct, INR, WBC
RENAL	Renal insufficiency/failure	Dialysis, transplant		BUN/Cr, K+
CNS	CVA, TIA	CNS deficits	CNS exam	Carotid studies
PNS	Poor circulation Posterior cerebral circulation	Claudication	Peripheral pulses Neck extension	Doppler, flow studies, angio
INFECTION	Malaise, swelling, gangrene	Fever, chills	Extremity ulcers, swelling, calor, rubor	Temp, cultures for organism

Key Reference: Johannesson A, Larsson G, et al. Incidence of lower-limb amputation in diabetic and non-diabetic general population. *Diabetes Care*. 2009;32(2).

Intraoperative Management

- Volume status monitoring: Blood loss without tourniquet

Preoperative Preparation
- Antibiotics for trauma
- Ensure availability of blood products

Anesthetic Technique
- Either regional or GA appropriate in normal coagulation status

Monitoring
- Routine monitors incl ST-segment analysis
- Consider arterial line (FloTrac), CVP, or PA line if long surgery, depending on CV status

Airway
- In trauma, diabetes, dialysis, consider full stomach

Surgical Stages

Induction
- Spinal or epidural acceptable in pts with normal coagulation profile
- If GA, worry about myocardial ischemia and ventricular dysfunction

Skin Incision
- Circular incision at the level of amputation
- Observe blood loss; need for ligation of large vessels

Dissection
- Identify femoral artery, vein for clamping, division, ligation; sciatic nerve for ligation
- Assessment of viability of tissue by observing bleeding and/or blood loss

Definitive Surgery/Closure
- Femur is divided with a saw, filed
- Wound closed in 2 layers
- Sterile dressing applied
- Immediate postop prosthesis can be applied; more common BKA > AKA
- Approx duration: 1–2 hr
- EBL w/o tourniquet: 250–500 mL

Postoperative Considerations
- Blood loss may continue; replace as indicated by Hct/Hgb
- Venous thrombosis assoc with prolonged hospitalization, immobilization, venous stasis

- Aggressive pulm toilet to prevent atelectasis, pneumonia
- Phantom limb sensation in 100% of pts; usually resolves in 1 y
- Pain score: 5–10
- Pain relief by PCA if epidural is contraindicated

Anticipated Problems/Concerns

- CV morbidity, mortality common 5–30%
- Amputation for acute ischemia has higher co-morbidities

Amputation, Lower Extremity (LEA)

Ryan P. Ellender
Kirit M. Patel

Risk

- Over 100,000 pts undergo LEA annually
- Approx 50% are the result of vascular disease
- Estimated that two-thirds of these pts are also diabetic
- Other etiologies incl trauma, malignancy, and congenital anomalies
- Incidence increases with age, more predominant in males, esp. in trauma pts

Perioperative Risks

- Highest morbidity: Cardiac (10%) followed by resp (pneumonia)
- Increased risk of arrhythmias, MI, CHF
- Most common cause of death: Cardiac, followed by resp failure
- Overall 30-d mortality around 9%; worse for AKA (17%) than BKA (6%)
- Survival in elderly diabetic amputees less than 50% at 3 y
- Long-term survival dismal for pts with DM and ESRD undergoing AKA

Worry About

- Periop cardiac morbidity and/or mortality
- Blood glucose control in diabetics
- Emotional stress assoc with limb loss, pt may experience depression
- Phantom limb pain common after LEA

Overview

- Major LEAs incl hip disarticulations, AKA, BKA, and ankle (Syme's)
- Most performed for PVD, often complicated by infections (osteomylitis) and/or chronic pain
- High incidence of morbidity and mortality
- Co-existing diseases common: DM, CAD, Htn, CHF, ESRD, sepsis

ICD-9-CM Code: 433.9 (PVD)

Indications and Treatment

- Open (guillotine) amputations common in severe infection and/or gangrene; require extensive revision
- Below-knee-above-knee amputation ratio in USA is around 3:1
- Revisions can infrequently convert BKAs into AKAs
- Preservation of knee joint important for more efficient ambulation; less energy expenditure
- Adequate stump flap essential for weight bearing on prosthesis
- Over two-thirds of BKA pts are rehabilitated with prosthesis versus less than one-third of AKA pts

ASSESSMENT POINTS

System	Risk Factors/Effect	Assessment by Hx	PE	Test
CARDIO	CAD, MI, CHF Autonomic neuropathy	SOB, angina, stents, Sx Syncope	JVD, rales, S_3 Orthostasis	ECG, enzymes, ECHO Holter, tilt-table
RESP	Asthma Obesity, sleep apnea COPD	Smoking Difficult intubation SOB/bronchospasm	Wheezing Airway exam Auscultation	PFTs CXR
GI	Gastroparesis	GERD, early satiety	N/V, NG tube	
ENDO	Diabetes	DKA or hypoglycemia	AMS may be 2/2 ↓ glu	Accucheck, UA
HEME	Pts on anticoagulants Anemia	Bleeding Transfusion	Bleeding, bruises Pallor	PT, INR, PTT Type and cross
GU	ESRD	Dialysis	Fistula, graft, or vas cath	Electrolytes: K, Cr
MS	Infections/sepsis Rhabdomyolysis	Antibiotics, cultures Crush injury, ischemia	VS, wound Hematuria	WBC with diff, Cx CPK

Key Reference: Aulivola B, Hile CN, Hamdan AD, et al. Major lower extremity amputation: Outcome of a series. *Arch Surg.* 2004;139:395–399.

Perioperative Management

Preoperative Preparation

- CV assessment
- Diabetic pts: Control glucose, preserve renal function, provide prophylaxis against aspiration
- Know hemodynamic status for trauma pts (Hb/Hct)

Anesthetic Technique

- Can be performed with regional, general, or combined anesthetic techniques
- Regional anesthesia may be contraindicated if pts septic and/or on antithrombotic Rx
- Pts with contaminated wounds needing serial I & Ds may benefit from a continuous epidural catheter
- Postop phantom limb pain may decrease with use of continuous regional anesthesia and/or analgesia

Monitoring

- Rarely need a-line, CVP, or PA catheter, except in pts with severe heart disease

Airway

- Consider possibility of difficult airway in diabetics
- Preoxygenation, sniffing-position, shoulder ramp to facilitate intubation in obese pts

Induction/Maintenance

- Vigilant control of hemodynamic variables and fluids shifts in pts with heart disease

Operation

- Procedure length, blood loss and morbidity depend on type of amputation
- Hip disarticulation: 3–4 hr, 1,000–2,000 mL blood loss, ICU postop care
- More distal procedures are generally faster, with less bleeding, and PACU postop
- Use of a tourniquet also significantly affects the amount of blood loss
- Access for pain during dissection of musculature and bone
- Monitor for major bleeding during dissection of vasculature
- Clean wounds will be covered with a flap then closed
- Contaminated wounds often left open (Guillotine) and a vacuum dressing is placed

Postoperative Considerations

- If significant heart disease consider need for postop monitored care for 24–48 hr
- Blood glucose control in diabetic pts may be difficult to achieve
- 26% of vascular pts undergo subsequent amputation within 1 y
- Early as well as late postop pain issues common

Pain after Amputation

- Phantom sensation refers to any sensation of the missing limb except pain
- Almost universal in the first month after surgery, usually not debilitating
- Stump pain reported in up to 50% of pts and results in disuse of prosthesis in 50% of pts
- Fewer than 10% of amputees have severe incapacitating phantom limb pain
- Risk factors: Bilateral amputation, lower limb amputation
- Incidence of phantom limb pain increases with more proximal amputations
- Pain often localized in distal parts of the missing limb
- Commonly intermittent, burning, aching, or cramping
- Pain usually remains the same or improves gradually, assoc with a poorer quality of life
- Treatment focused on medical therapy, interventional therapies are more controversial
- Antidepressants, esp. tricyclics (TCA) and sodium channel blockers commonly improve pain.
- Pts also benefit from anticonvulsants, esp. carbamazepine and gabapentin.

Aneurysm Coiling

Allan Gottschalk

Risks

• Prevalence of intracranial aneurysms is approx 2.3% in the general population. At least 5.4% of these have multiple aneurysms. Aneurysms may develop from a congenital abn of the arterial wall, are more common in those with connective tissue disorders and those with polycystic kidney disease and may be seen in association with other vascular defects such as arteriovenous malformations. Cerebral injury, infections, and tumors have also been assoc with aneurysm formation. Smoking, Htn, atherosclerosis, and drug abuse (esp. cocaine) are also risk factors. Oral contraceptives have been postulated as a risk factor to explain the slightly increased prevalence in women.

• The annual risk of subarachnoid hemorrhage (SAH) from aneurysmal rupture is 1.3% per year. The risk of rupture increases with the size of the aneurysm, is greater for those located in the posterior cerebral circulation, and is more likely for those who have already experienced the rupture of an intracranial aneurysm at another location. Other risk factors for aneurysmal rupture incl Htn, smoking, alcohol abuse, drug (cocaine) abuse, a family Hx of cerebrovascular disease and features related to aneurysmal shape.

• The 30-d mortality rate for SAH from aneurysmal rupture is 30–40%, and only one third of those who survive remain functionally independent. Additional aneurysmal events are assoc with even higher mortality.

Perioperative Risks

• Rupture of the aneurysm from procedural manipulation or Htn during the intervention

• Cerebral infarction due to thrombosis, misplaced embolic material, interruption of flow from vessels originating from the aneurysm neck or dome, or vasospasm

• Complications related to anticoagulation which generally incl heparin and some type of antiplatelet therapy. These can result from hemorrhage in the brain or other sites, reactions to heparin (heparin-induced thrombocytopenia) and reactions to protamine when it is used to reverse heparin.

Worry About

• Contrast reactions which can range from direct cardiac depression to anaphylactoid reactions. Although the use of non-ionic contrast agents has not decreased the incidence of fatal contrast reactions, it has decreased that of mild to moderate ones.

• Contrast nephropathy, Risk factors incl DM the large dye loads that are common during prolonged endovascular procedures, volume depletion, pre-existing renal dysfunction, and concurrent administration of other nephrotoxic medications.

• Hypothermia

• Radiation exposure of pt and caregivers

• Distance from pt's airway due to interposed imaging equipment and radiation shields.

Overview

• Endovascular approaches are used to secure both intact aneurysms and those assoc with prior SAH in order to prevent additional events and their resulting morbidity. Endovascular approaches may be advantageous for aneurysms whose location is not anatomically favorable for surgical interventions, such as the posterior cerebral circulation. Endovascular approaches generally favor aneurysmal geometry where the neck is narrow relative to the dome. Overall, as endovascular technique advances, the available literature appears to demonstrate the noninferiority of endovascular approaches for equivalent lesions.

• The 1° technique involves the use of multiple platinum coils advanced through a microcatheter placed at the opening of the aneurysm and detached from the pusher wire. Coil dimensions refer to the length and diameter of the coil. Detachment of the coil once it is in place occurs by passing an electrical current through the insulated pusher wire to initiate electrolysis of the junction between it and the coil. Coils are packed into the aneurysm until contrast dye no longer opacifies the aneurysmal lumen. The placement a fenestrated stent over the aneurysmal orifice makes endovascular treatment possible for aneurysms with wider necks where the coils would be otherwise expelled. To date, there is no consensus as to whether various bioactive coatings on the coils facilitate or contribute to the effectiveness of the intervention.

• To facilitate manipulation of the microcatheter and coil placement a "roadmap" is generated by subtracting the background image obtained from a scout film, and then superimposing the image of the vascular anatomy obtained by an injection of contrast dye on the fluoroscopic image. Clearly, such a technique requires immobility, often to the point where respiration must be suspended for short periods of time.

• Access to the arterial circulation is generally obtained through a sheath in one of the femoral arteries. However, access can also be obtained through the brachial and carotid arteries.

• Anticoagulation therapy is an important component of endovascular therapy and is generally comprised of longer-term antiplatelet therapy initiated prior to the procedure and heparin administered during the procedure which is later reversed with protamine. An exception to this may be when treating an aneurysm assoc with prior SAH. Then, anticoagulation is often held until successful placement of the initial coil(s), an indication that the aneurysm will eventually be secured. At that time antiplatelet medications can be administered by gastric tube or per rectum, and heparin can be administered IV.

ASSESSMENT POINTS

System	Effect	Assessment by Hx	PE	Test
HEENT	Ability to maintain airway while supine and during sedation	Obstructive sleep apnea	Airway adequacy	
CARDIO	SAH is assoc with ECG changes and left ventricular dysfunction Fluid shifts assoc with contrast dye administration may lead to congestive failure	Exercise tolerance, angina	Signs of congestive failure	ECG, cardiac echocardiogram, cardiac enzymes
RESP	Pulm edema is common following SAH	Exercise tolerance, prior smoking Hx	Rales	CXR, ABGs
RENAL	Assessment of risk for contrast nephropathy	Diabetes mellitus	Evidence of decreased intravascular volume and electrolyte abn that may accompany SAH	Cr, serum glucose, Na$^+$, K$^+$ Ca^{2+}, Mg^{2+}
CNS	Determination of prior SAH. Baseline exam for post-procedure comparison, and, if prior SAH, prognostication via SAH grading scales (see chapter on Cerebral Aneurysm Clipping)	Headache, or established history of prior aneurysmal rupture	Nuchal rigidity, level of consciousness, cranial nerves, focal deficits	Prior cerebral imaging
HEMAT	Pts frequently will have anticoagulants administered during the procedure, thrombocytopenia following SAH does occur		Bruising, bleeding from other sites	Plt count, PT, PTT
IMMUNE	Contract reaction, protamine allergy, heparin allergy	Prior Hx of contrast reaction, allergies to protamine or heparin		

Key Reference: Lakhani S, Guha A, Nahser HC. Anaesthesia for endovascular management of cerebral aneurysms. *Eur J Anaesthesiol.* 2006;23:902–913.

Perioperative Management

Preoperative Preparation

- Antiplatelet therapy (e.g., aspirin and clopidogrel bisulfate) for those with intact aneurysms.
- Prophylaxis for those with contrast dye allergy (e.g, for scheduled procedures: Prednisone 50 mg, orally 13, 7 and 1 hr prior to procedure with diphenhydramine 50 mg po and ranitidine 150 mg po 1 hr prior to procedure; for emergent procedures: hydrocortisone 200 mg IV with diphenhydramine 50 mg IV and ranitidine 50 mg IV).
- Prophylaxis for those at risk for contrast nephropathy (e.g., sodium bicarbonate 154 mEq/L, 3 mL/kg for 1 hr prior to procedure then 1 mL/kg for 6 hr and acetylcysteine 600 mg bid po prior to procedure)

Monitoring

- Standard ASA monitors
- Arterial catheter for those with SAH and those at high risk of rupture. Many would place an arterial catheter even in those presenting for elective procedures to facilitate management in the event of a rupture and to permit ongoing assessment of the extent of heparinization. The catecholamine surge that accompanies rupture can sometimes produce vasospasm so marked that radial artery catheters are unreliable, and arterial pressure monitoring from the femoral artery should then be provided by the interventionalist.
- A urinary drainage catheter is necessary given the large fluid shifts and uo that accompany the large dose of contrast dye.
- NMB monitoring is essential for techniques using NMB in order to render the pt immobile without excessively prolonging the time until emergence.

Anesthetic Technique/Induction

- Anesthetic techniques can range from local, to sedation, to general anesthesia. The level of noxious input is primarily from catheter insertion and is comparable to that for diagnostic angiography for which general anesthesia is rarely necessary. If general anesthesia is not used, the patient must be capable of lying flat, and sedation should not be such that the pt becomes uncooperative, or so deep that resp artifacts from airway obstruction become significant. The use of nasal airways to relieve airway obstruction can be problematic in an anticoagulated pt. Although the ability to monitor the neurologic exam is lost with general anesthesia, it provides a level of immobility which facilitates the procedure. Sedatives that might later interfere with the neurologic exam are best avoided with any technique.
- For general anesthesia, almost any technique with IV or inhalational anesthetics is appropriate as long as the induction is smooth, the response to laryngoscopy blunted, the emergence is crisp and immobility is assured. In pts with unruptured aneurysms, a decreased transmural pressure (proportional to cerebral perfusion pressure) is desirable. However, for those with vasospasm following SAH, it may be necessary to maintain higher Bps to provide adequate cerebral perfusion. Despite its benefit in facilitating rapid emergence, concern exists about the capacity of NO to increase the size of microbubbles introduced into the cerebral circulation.

Surgical Stages

Procedure

- Access of arterial system
- Detailed angiography to plan the embolization
- Stent placement if dictated by anatomy
- Coil placement to opacity the aneurysm
- Exit from arterial system. The sheath is often left in place or a vascular closure device is used, obviating a prolonged period of pressure to the groin at the conclusion of the procedure.

- Although the treated aneurysm is considered secure, if other lesions are present the impact of their rupture would be compounded by ongoing anticoagulation. In these instances, it is essential to avoid Htn during emergence.
- A detailed neurologic exam should be performed prior to transfer from the procedure table.

Postoperative Considerations

- The pt should be in a situation permitting frequent neurologic assessments.
- Pts are encouraged to remain supine without flexion of the joint adjacent to the vascular access site.

Anticipated Problems/Concerns

- Aneurysmal rupture during the procedure can be catastrophic with mortality similar to unwitnessed SAH. The incidence is reported to be 3–5% and is more common with lesions of the posterior circulation, but may be less in experienced hands. Rupture is generally accompanied by a massive Cushing's response. If technically feasible, the ruptured aneurysm is packed with coils. Further treatment consists of controlling intracranial pressure and systemic BP. Placement of an intraventricular catheter may be beneficial. It will be necessary to reverse any heparin with protamine, and administer working plts if the pt received antiplatelet therapy.
- Thrombus formation may be revealed during the procedure, or during angiography administered in response to a neurologic deficit upon emergence from anesthesia. Thrombolytic therapy administered directly to the thrombus may necessitate resumption of general anesthesia. Regardless, an increase in cerebral perfusion pressure is desirable.

Anterior Cervical Discectomy and Fusion (ACDF)

Milad Sharifpour

Laurel E. Moore

Risk

- ACDF is one of the most commonly performed spine procedures with an 8-fold increase in prevalence from 1990–2004
- M:F ratio: 3:2

Perioperative Risks

- <1% in hospital postop mortality assoc with cervical spine surgery
- Postop airway complications in 6% of cases of anterior cervical spine surgery
- Incidence of recurrent laryngeal nerve (RLN) injury: 5%

Worry About

- Airway management in pts with limited cervical spine mobility resulting in increased risk of difficult intubation.
- Pts at risk for postop airway complications incl those with prolonged procedures; exposure of more than three vertebral levels; involvement of C2, C3, or C4; and more than 300- mL EBL. These risks (and thus complications) more commonly assoc with complex corpectomy and fusion procedures rather than 1–2 level ACDF.

- Surgical complications incl RLN paralysis, esophageal perforation, cerebrospinal fluid leak, injury to vertebral artery, carotid artery, jugular vein, postop dysphagia, and pharyngeal edema or hematoma.
- Pts having previously undergone ACDF may have unrecognized pre-existing RLN injury. If contralateral approach planned, preop fiberoptic exam of cord function should be considered.

Overview

- Indications incl cervical radiculopathy and/or myelopathy 2° to degenerative disc disease and/or spondylesthesis
- The clinical outcome of this procedure is good or excellent in the majority of cases.
- Anterior approach provides good access to vertebral bodies and transverse processes of C2–C7
- Right anterior approach assoc with increased risk of damage to RLN but decreased risk of damage to thoracic duct.
- Anterior plate almost always used, thus securing intervertebral graft placement
- Although fusion rate is greater with autograft (iliac bone) vs. allograft (cadaveric fibula or iliac bone), morbidity assoc with taking bone graft plus improved fusion rates with anterior instrumentation have made the use of allografts for ACDF the standard at most centers. Titanium cages also utilized for interbody fusion and corpectomy/fusion.

Indications and Usual Treatment

- Cervical herniated disk or spur
- Degenerative or traumatic hypermobility or subluxation
- Radiculopathy with foraminal stenosis
- Decreased AP diameter of spinal canal
- Compressive myelopathy
- Degenerative kyphoscoliosis
- Alternative Rx incl posterior cervical approach and conservative management with NSAID, rest.

ASSESSMENT POINTS

System	Effect	Assessment by Hx	PE	Test
HEENT	Access limited 2° to pain, anatomy, prior fusion, neurologic Sx	↑ Neurologic Sx or pain with movement	Oral opening, cervical ROM, thyromental distance, neuro exam	Review of cervical imaging studies
PNS	Radicular Sx, myelopathy	Onset of pain, numbness, weakness, bowel or bladder Sx	Motor, sensory assessment, single root vs. cord compression	Review of cervical imaging studies (X-ray, MRI, CT, myelogram)

Key Reference: Daniels AH. Adverse events asssociated with anterior cervical spine Surgery. *J Am Acad Orthop Surg.* 2008;16:729–738.

Perioperative Management

Preoperative Preparation

- Careful exam of the airway incl evaluation of cervical mobility
- Consider awake fiberoptic intubation (FOI) or having immediate access to glidescope or Bullard laryngoscope in those pts with potentially difficult airways.
- Surgical positioning generally requires greater neck extension than required for routine direct laryngoscopy.
- In pt with traumatic spine injury or evidence of unstable spine consider awake FOI and positioning.

Monitoring

- Generally routine
- Consider invasive monitoring if multiple levels involved and/or significant co-morbidities
- Arms and neck inaccessible during procedure so invasive monitoring is placed prospectively. Consider placing a second IV catheter for this reason.

- Neurophysiologic monitoring frequently utilized, particularly for more invasive corpectomy and fusion. May incl somatosensory monitoring and/or motor-evoked potential monitoring (MEP).

Anesthetic Technique

- General endotracheal due to poor access to airway and surgical traction on trachea, esophagus
- Pt is placed supine with the neck extended
- Consider narcotic-based anesthesia to assist with neurophysiologic monitoring
- Muscle relaxation assists in distraction of the cervical spine but may interfere with MEP monitoring

Surgical Stages

Dissection

- Trachea and esophagus retracted medially
- Carotid artery retracted laterally
- RLN retracted inferiorly
- Superior laryngeal and hypoglossal nerves retracted superiorly
- Vertebral artery ascends via foramina of transverse processes.

Other Intraoperative Considerations

- Cervical traction occasionally requested of the anesthesiologist to facilitate graft placement
- Coughing or bucking on the ETT at conclusion of case may rarely lead to anterolateral expulsion of the graft in the absence of anterior plating.
- EBL and third space losses are generally small.

Postoperative Considerations

- Postop dysphagia is the most common complaint 2° to traction on esophagus.
- If iliac bone graft is harvested this can be more painful than surgical site (pain score: 6–8). Discomfort can be attenuated with local anesthetic injection pre-emergence.

Anticipated Problems/Concerns

- Airway management in pts with limited cervical spine motion
- Post-operative airway compromise 2° hematoma formation, soft tissue swelling, or neurologic deficit (RLN injury)
- Failure of fusion now rare given instrumentation, rates range from 2–10%.

Aortic Valve Replacement

Matthew A. Klopman
James G. Ramsay

PROCEDURES

Risk

- Incidence in USA: 27,000 operations in 2005
- M:F ratio: 3:2

Perioperative Risks

- For isolated AS, 3–8% periop mortality for pts <70 y, 3–16% for pts >70 y
- Mortality for elective AVR in pts with chronic AR is 4–10%
- Increased mortality with emergency surgery, advanced age, AI, decreased LV function, CAD, HTN, preop pacing, dialysis-dependent renal failure, infective endocarditis
- Morbidity incl heart block, CVA

Worry About

- Maintaining optimal hemodynamic variables for valvular lesion
- Decreasing LV function preop, esp. with AR
- Arrhythmias

- Myocardial preservation in hypertrophied ventricle during bypass
- De-airing before D/C of CPB

Overview

- Operative mortality for isolated AVR <5%, increased mortality with increasing age, decreasing LV function, co-existing CAD, and decreasing exercise tolerance
- Pts with AS generally have better prognosis than those with AR, esp. when decreasing LV function present
- Choice of porcine bioprosthesis or mech valve based on pt's expected longevity, risks of chronic anticoagulation
- Homograft valve is alternative if active infection, young woman desiring pregnancy, or anticoagulation is contraindicated

- Arrhythmias and/or heart block—atrial contribution to CO very important after AVR, esp. in hypertrophied heart. Bundle of His prone to injury; atrial, ventricular pacing wires often used.

ICD-9-CM Codes: 424.1 (AS); 424.1 (AR); 35.22 (AVR—other)

Indications and Usual Treatment

- Symptomatic AS (angina, syncope, CHF) or AR (fatigue, DOE, CHF)
- Asymptomatic AS with aortic valve area <0.7 cm² or pressure gradient >50 mmHg at rest (with normal LV function)
- Acute severe AR
- Optimal timing in chronic AR controversial; benefit greatest before onset of LV dysfunction

ASSESSMENT POINTS

System	Effect	Assessment by Hx	PE	Test
HEENT	Co-existing dental infection—↑ risk for postop endocarditis	Oral hygiene	Oral exam	
CARDIO	Aortic valve dysfunction Arrhythmia Ischemia LV dysfunction	Angina, syncope, CHF Palpitation, syncope Angina DOE, fatigue	CV exam – Rhythm – Murmur – Gallop	ECG ECHO Cardiac cath
RESP	Pulm vascular congestion from ↑ LVEDP	Dyspnea Orthopnea PND	Rales S₃	CXR SaO₂
RENAL	Renal insufficiency			BUN, Cr
CNS	TIA, RIND, CVA Syncope	Chronic AFIB Endocarditis Carotid disease	Carotid bruit Neuro deficit	Carotid Doppler TEE (atrial thrombus, valvular vegetations)

Key Reference: Augoustides JG, Wolfe Y, Walsh EK, Szeto WY. Recent advances in aortic valve disease: Highlights from a bicuspid aortic valve to transcatheter aortic valve replacement. *J Cardiothorac Vasc Anesth.* 2009;23(4):569–576.

Intraoperative Management

Preoperative Preparation

- Cautious premed; prevent anxiety but avoid acute changes in HR, preload, and afterload
- Adequate vascular access, blood products available

Anesthetic Technique—AS

- Periop hemodynamic goals: Maintain preload, afterload, avoid lowering BP (coronary perfusion pressure essential with LVH), maintain sinus rhythm, normal rate, aggressive Rx for dysrhythmias (loss of atrial kick/rapid rate poorly tolerated) may require synchronized cardioversion

Anesthetic Technique—AR

- Periop hemodynamic goals: Maintain preload, maintain arterial dilation (nitroprusside, nicardipine, clevidipine), avoid significant myocardial depression, maintain high-normal HR (90–100/min); bradycardia results in increasing regurgitation leading to increased LVEDP, inotropic support frequently required post bypass if decreased LVEF
- IABP contraindicated in presence of AR

Monitoring

- A-line, ECG with ST-segment analysis
- CVP vs. PAC (CVP may grossly underestimate LVEDP, but placement of PAC has potential for dysrhythmias, PA rupture)

- Consider TEE to monitor LV filling, contractility, regional wall motion, adequacy of de-airing, and postop valve function
- Consider external defibrillation pads with capability of transthoracic pacing
- Consider esophageal stethoscope with atrial pacing capacity if no PAC pacing available

Surgical Stages

Induction/Prebypass

- AS
  - Maintain preload, afterload (phenylephrine)
  - Avoid lowering BP: Coronary perfusion pressure essential with LVH (CPP = diastolic BP – LVEDP)
    - Maintain sinus rhythm, normal rate
    - Aggressive Rx for dysrhythmias
    - Surgeon and perfusionist available
- AR
  - Maintain preload
  - Afterload reduction to improve forward flow (nitroprusside, nicardipine, clevidipine)
    - Avoid significant contractile depression
    - Maintain high-normal HR (90–100/min); bradycardia results in increased regurgitation
    - IABP contraindicated in presence of AR

Cardiopulmonary Bypass

- Cardioplegia: Antegrade ± retrograde to allow infusion without interruption
- In AR, prevent LV distention at initiation of CPB by maintaining sinus rhythm:
  - IV esmolol 1–2 mg/kg
  - IV lidocaine 1–1.5 mg/kg
  - Defibrillation or urgent aortic cross-clamping/LV venting poss necessary
- Evacuate air and assess valve function with TEE before D/C CPB
- Inotropic support frequently required post bypass if decreasing LVEF (AR)

Postoperative Considerations

- Compliance of hypertrophic ventricles after AVR unchanged, need adequate preload + NSR
- Control Htn to avoid bleeding and dissection
- Anticoagulation for mechanical valves; coumadin usually begun 2–3 d postop

Anticipated Problems/Concerns

- Decreased preop LV function may require support
- AFIB/AFLT poorly tolerated with LVH; consider low-dose β-blocker to prevent arrhythmias
- Heart block can develop on postop day 1. Atrial, ventricular pacing wires recommended. Bundle of His prone to injury, permanent pacemaker possibly required.

401

Aortopulmonary Window

Scott Watkins

Risk

- 0.2–0.6% of congenital HD
- Assoc with secundum ASD, PDA, VSD, aortic origin of right PA, interrupted aortic arch/coarctation (25%), tetralogy of Fallot, anomalous origin of coronary arteries
- Assoc with 22q11 chromosome deletion
- No gender predilection

Perioperative Risks

- Periop mortality rate <3%
- Classic defect just above the sinus of Valsalva, near left main coronary artery orifice, which can be damaged during repair

Worry About

- Increasing pulm flow 2° to left to right shunt preop
- Development of preop CHF
- Pulm Htn with assoc reactive pulm vascular bed of concern when presenting late, >3 mo of age

Overview

- Manifests similarly to VSD or PDA with over circulation of pulm vascular bed
- Sx of CHF incl FTT, diaphoresis, dyspnea, recurrent resp infections

ICD-9-CM Code: 745.0

Indications and Usual Treatment

- Surgical correction indicated in most cases using CPB with patch closure (Dacron or glutaraldehyde-treated pericardium) via transaortic approach
- Children presenting beyond 3 mo of age may require cardiac cath to assess reversibility of pulm vascular resistance
- Assoc congenital heart lesions may result in postop problems unrelated to the aortopulmonary window repair
- Eisenmenger's syndrome with physiologic changes from long-standing left to right shunting only contraindication to surgical closure

ASSESSMENT POINTS

System	Effect	Assessment by Hx	PE	Test
CARDIO	CHF, pulm Htn, Eisenmenger's syndrome	Exercise intolerance, dyspnea, cyanosis	CV exam, bounding pulses, harsh systolic murmur, cardiomegaly, PA sat > RV sat	ECG, ECHO, CXR Cath, MRI
RESP	Reactive pulm vascular bed	Tachypnea, cyanosis	Auscultation	O$_2$ sat, CXR

Key Reference: Fraser CD. Aortopulmonary septal defects and patent ductus arteriosus. In: Nichols DG, et al. *Critical heart disease in infants and children*. Philadelphia: Mosby; 2006:663–668.

Perioperative Implications

Anesthetic Technique

- General anesthesia with narcotic-based technique usual
- Avoid increases in PVR in the neonatal pt or those with reactive pulm vascular bed
- Excessive diastolic runoff may exist during periods of hypotension, resulting in reduced coronary perfusion, ischemia, and arrhythmias

Monitoring

- Arterial line
- Two peripheral IVs or CVL
- Right and left atrial lines placed by surgeon at conclusion of CPB for monitoring

Airway

- No assoc airway anomalies

Induction

- If IV access available can use opioids, benzodiazepine, ketamine, or etomidate
- If pt is without IV access, sevoflurane mask induction is acceptable
- Use principles applied to VSDs, PDAs, other L → R shunting lesions

Surgical Stages

Dissection

- Under CPB through midline sternotomy

Definitive Surgery

- Involves placement of pericardial or Dacron patch
- Performed under moderately hypothermic conditions

- Rarely, deep hypothermic circulatory arrest may be required in certain situations
- Modifications of reconstruction may occur in pts with assoc coronary anomalies
- Consider use of aminocaproic acid

Postoperative Considerations

- Reactive pulm vascular bed with assoc pulm. Htn is a major concern
- Efforts to reduce PVR should be considered; adequate sedation/analgesia, mild hyperventilation, and avoidance of hypoxia
- Postop blood loss 2° to CPB
- Packed RBC, plts, cryoprecipitate, and/or FFP replacement as indicated
- Significant postop pain (Pain score: 6–8)

Appendectomy

Joseph Rosa II

Risk

- Consider in any pt with abd pain.
- Rare in infants, more common in childhood; max incidence in teens, 20s; thereafter declines; 1 in 7 sometime in their lifetime
- Incidence in USA: 15%
- M:F ratio: 3:2
- Etiology: 60%, hyperplasia of submucosal lymphoid follicles; 35%, fecal stasis (fecalith); 4%, other foreign bodies; 1%, tumors

Perioperative Risks

- Mortality: Overall, <1/100,000; in acute but not gangrenous, <0.1%; gangrenous, 0.6%; perforated, 5%
- Morbidity: Pelvic, intra-abd, subphrenic abscess with perforation, ~20%; wound abscess, <5%; fecal fistula, <1%; wound hematoma, <0.5%; ileus, variable
- Greater morbidity and mortality in children, due to absence of fully developed omentum, with subsequent spread of infection, and development of peritonitis after perforation

Worry About

- Intravascular volume status due to poor oral intake, vomiting, third spacing with peritonitis
- Full stomach, aspiration; ileus
- Electrolyte abn due to vomiting
- Periop sepsis
- If laparoscopic, usual concerns with pneumoperitoneum, CO_2 insufflation
- Differential Dx: Consider more catastrophic etiologies of abd pain, incl rupturing abd aortic aneurysm, intestinal ischemia, acute pancreatitis, acute diverticulitis, bowel obstruction or perforation, bowel carcinoma
- Postop infection, sepsis

Overview

- Obstruction of appendiceal opening
- Periop infection a concern with perforated appendix, peritonitis
- Increased morbidity, mortality with perforation and immunocompromised
- Fewer normal appendixes removed since US, laparoscopy, CT, and MRI used for Dx

ICD-9-CM Code: 540

Indications and Usual Treatment

- Suspected appendicitis
- Differential Dx in young children: Acute gastroenteritis, mesenteric lymphadenitis, pyelitis, Meckel's diverticulitis, intussusception, pneumonia
- Dx In teenagers and adults depends on gender: in females, ruptured ectopic pregnancy, mittelschmerz, endometriosis, salpingitis, regional enteritis; in males, regional enteritis, renal calculi, testicular torsion, acute epididymitis
- Differential Dx in older adults: Diverticulitis, perforated ulcer, acute cholecystitis, pancreatitis, intestinal obstruction, perforating cecal cancer, torsion of ovarian cyst, mesenteric vascular occlusion, rupturing abd aortic aneurysm
- Differential Dx made easier with US, spiral CT, or MRI
- Urine 5-hyroxyindolacetic acid (U-5-HIAA) increases significantly in the early stages of acute appendicitis.
- LRG (leucine-rich α-2 glycoprotein): Elevated in the urine of children with acute appendicitis – [LRG] increased with severity of appendicitis

ASSESSMENT POINTS

System	Effect	Assessment by Hx	PE	Test
CARDIO	Age-related considerations; dehydration 2° to fever, emesis; ↓ PO intake	CV status, Hx of angina, SOB, exercise tolerance	CV exam	ECG if indicated, orthostatics to assess vol
RESP	Resp impaired 2° to abd pain/splinting in elderly; tachypnea, hyperpnea may suggest perforation/sepsis; full-stomach considerations		Chest exam	CXR if indicated
HEME	Leukocytosis, with left shift hemoconcentration; 4% of pts have normal WBC, differential			CBC with differential
RENAL/CNS	Mental status changes assoc with dehydration; electrolyte abn, early sepsis; ↓ UO 2° to ↓ IV vol	UO, mental status	CNS exam	UA

Key Reference: Green JM. When is faster better? Operative timing in acute care surgery. *Curr Opin Crit Care.* 2008;14:423–427.

Perioperative Management

Preoperative Preparation
- Restore IV vol temp management

Anesthetic Technique

- GA generally indicated for laparoscopic appendectomy
- General endotracheal anesthesia: Rapid-sequence induction and intubation with Sellick's maneuver or awake if difficult airway
- Regional: Spinal vs. epidural if no absolute contraindications, pt adequately hydrated, and cooperative; high abd exploration unlikely – most often used with open appendectomy
- Small surgery, but can be fraught with unexpected findings and complications. Be prepared.

Monitoring
- Routine, or determined by pt pathophysiologic indicators.

Airway
- Routine

Induction
- Consider IV volume status when choosing induction agents
- Consider possibility of myopathy in children esp. males, in choosing muscle relaxant

Maintenance
- Usually volatile agent ± N_2O, narcotic, relaxant, use N_2O cautiously in laparoscopy

Surgical Stages

Skin incision
- McBurney's incision (RLQ)

Dissection
- Extent depends on appendix location, degree of inflammation; third space volume a consideration
  - Retrocecal position, 65%
  - 30% tip in pelvis

Closure
- Perforated ± skin closure if abscess present, surgeon may place drain; minimal if laparoscopic
- EBL: <75 mL
- Vol requirements
- Replace deficit and 5–8 mL/kg/hr with normal saline or lactated Ringer's solution
- Transgastric — laparoscopic assisted appendectomy: Undergoing clinical trials

Postoperative Considerations
- Pain score: 5–7; PCA for postop pain

Anticipated Problems/Concerns

- Similar for open versus laparoscopic appendectomy
- Sepsis, paralytic ileus, atelectasis
- Aspiration risk, esp. during emergence
- Prolongation of NMB drugs 2° to interaction with antibiotics, esp. aminoglycosides

Atrial Fibrillation Ablation

Nabil Elkassabany
Sanjay Dixit

PROCEDURES

Risk

- Incidence in USA: More than 2.5 million Americans have atrial fibrillation. It is the most common cardiac cause of stroke.
- Predominantly a disorder of the elderly pts and is more frequent in males.
- Assoc co-morbidities: Htn, sleep apnea, valvular heart disease, congestive failure, chronic obstructive and/or restrictive lung disease
- Antiarrhythmic drugs (AADs) are usually only 60% effective in maintaining long-term sinus rhythm (SR) and so radiofrequency ablation has become a popular alternative in the management of this arrhythmia.

Perioperative Risks

- Procedure related risks incl bleeding, infection (at site of vascular access), cardiac perforation and/or pericardial effusion with or without tamponade, thrombo-embolic complications incl stroke, pulm vein stenosis, damage to the phrenic nerve, esophageal injury with or without development of atrio-esophageal fistula and death. Radiation exposure poses another hazard for the health care providers and the pt.
- Pt related risk factors: pts undergoing AF ablation often have co-morbidities, which can place them at higher risk for development of periop complications
- Anesthesia related factors incl the risks assoc with delivering anesthesia in a remote location, usually the electrophysiology (EP) lab, and caring for pts with multiple co-morbidities.

Worry About

- If the case was done under monitored anesthesia care (MAC)
  - The need to immobilize pt throughtout the course of a relatively long procdure (4–5 hr).
  - Limited access to the airway of the sedated pt because of the tight space and bulky x-ray equipments.
  - Sedative agents can influence mapping by increasing the threshold for arrhythmia induction.
  - Hypoventilation and hypercarbia in sedated pts.

- If the case was done under general anesthesia (GA):
  - Fluctuations in the hemodynamics during induction and maintenance of general anesthesia
  - Motion of the ablation catheter through the resp cycle with higher tidal volumes during PPV. Few centers have recently adopted the use of high frequency jet ventilation (HFJV) as a mode of ventilation to minimize resp motion and hence have a relatively stable position of the ablation catheter during ablation.
- Use of paralytic agents can compromise ability to assess proximity of ablation lesion to phrenic nerve – done by pacing at ablation site and detecting movement of the ipsilateral diaphragmatic muscle
- Pts can be fully anticoagulated (on Coumadin and IV heparin) at the time of the procedure.
- Air embolism, development of intracardiac thrombus, thromboembolic complications (incl stroke and/or peripheral arterial compromise), development of cardiac tamponade, pulm vein stenosis, esophageal thermal injury

Overview

- Since its original description in 1998, AF ablation procedure has become a popular treatment strategy. It involves creation of serial circumferential radiofrequency ablation (RFA) lesions around PV ostium (os) to electrically isolate it from rest of the left atrium (LA). This is accomplished by demarcating the PV os either with the help of a circular multipolar mapping catheter (Lasso) and/or utilizing 3-dimensional mapping to define the PV /LA junction..
- To accomplish this, multipolar catheters are inserted percutaneously via the right and left femoral veins into the right atrium. Via transseptal puncture, the Lasso and the mapping/ablation catheter are advanced into the LA.
- Using a combination of orthogonal fluoroscopy, intracardiac US and 3-D mapping (aided by CT or MRI segmented anatomy), the pulm vein/left atrial junction is identified. RFA involves the delivery of energy via the generator to the tip of the ablation catheter which is moved sequentially around individual or ipsilaterl PV os (typical RF

duration 20–40 sec; power 20–40 watts). After completion of PV isolation, standard stimulation protocol (decrememtal overdrive pacing with and without isoproterenol infusion) is performed to assess AF inducibility and unmask any remaining non PV triggers of AF.

- After completion of the ablation protocol, catheters and sheaths are withdrawn into the RA, intracardiac echocardiography (ICE) is utilized during the course of the procedure to monitor for development of any pericardial effusion and periodically assess flow velocities across the PV os.
- At the end of the procedure all catheters are removed, heparin is stopped and if there are no contraindications then a small dose of IV protamine is administered. The sheaths are left in place and removed subsequently once the activated clotting time is ≤180 sec.
- Pts are subsequently monitored on telemetry and stay on bed rest for 6 hr after sheath removal following which heparin is restarted (without bolus) and all previous medications (incl Coumadin and AADs) are resumed.
- A follow-up transthoracic ECHO is performed within 24 hr of the procedure and pts are typically discharged home within 48 hr.

ICD-9-CM Codes: 427.31 (A FIB); 427.2 (Paroxysmal atrial tachycardia, unspecified)

Indications and Usual Treatment

- As per the AF consensus statement, AF catheter ablation is indicated in pts with symptomatic paroxysmal and/or persistent AF that have failed and/or are intolerant to ≥1 membrane stabilizing antiarrhythmic drug. In rare clinical situations, it may be appropriate to perform AF ablation as first line therapy. Selected symptomatic pts with heart failure and/or reduced ejection fraction. The presence of a LA thrombus is a contraindication to catheter ablation of AF.

ASSESSMENT POINTS

System	Effect	Assessment by Hx	PE	Test
CARDIO	Myocardial ischemia LV dysfunction Rate, LA thrombus	Angina symptoms Exercise tolerance, DOE	S_3, rales Irregular irregularity	ECG, pharmacologic or exercise stress testing ECHO, cardiac cath EPS, ambulatory ECG, Holter monitor
RESP	Pt co-morbidities may incl COPD, obstructive sleep apnea (OSA), and amiodarone toxicity	Exercise tolerance, DOE		CXR, sleep study, PFTs, ABGs
RENAL	Renal insufficiency		Edema	BUN, Cr
NEURO	CV disease	Stroke, TIAs	Bruits	Carotid duplex
LYTES	Reversible causes of arrythmias	Diuretic Rx		Serum K^+ and Mg^{2+}

Key Reference: HRS/EHRA/ECAS Expert Consensus Statement on Catheter and Surgical Ablation of Atrial Fibrillation. Recommendations for personnel, policy, procedures and follow-up. A report of the Heart Rhythm Society (HRS) Task Force on Catheter and Surgical Ablation of Atrial Fibrillation. *Heart Rhythm.* 2007;4(6):816–861.

Perioperative Management

Anesthetic Technique

- Options for anesthesia incl: MAC or GA or a combination of both.
- The mapping is usually done under MAC with minimal sedation to minimize interference with the stimulation protocol.
- The choice of agent for sedation depends on the discretion and judgment of the anesthesia provider. Midazolam and fentanyl are commonly used.

- Local anesthetic infiltration of the site for percutaneous vascular access.
- General anesthesia is used frequently for the ablation part of the procedure.
- Induction of general anesthesia is usually done after successful accomplishment of transseptal access and basic assessment of neurologic status.
- Propofol and etomidate are the most commonly used induction agents.
- Support of ventilation and oxygenation is provided with PPV.
- All EP labs in the authours institution are equipped with anesthesia machines. Some centers

have recently adopted the use of HFJV to minimize resp movement for better contact between the ablation catheter and the target area for ablation.
- When HFJV is used, inhalation anesthetic delivery is often unreliable and in these cases, total IV anesthesia is the approach of choice. A combination of propofol and remifentanyl infusion has been used for maintenance of anesthesia. The driving inspiratory pressure, resp motion, and $PaCO_2$ should be monitored during HFJV.

Monitoring
- ASA standarad monitors
- Invasive BP monitoring
- Intracardiac ECHO
- Frequent measurements if ABGs
- Activated clotting time (ACT)

Airway
- Endotracheal intubation for the majority of the procedure; airway instrumentation equipments should be readily available during sedation and before induction of general anesthesia at the time of percutaneous access.
- If HFJV is used, the ETT cuff may be left deflated to minimize barotrauma, thereby creating an open system. This approach, however, results in greater entrainment of room air. Lung atelectasis may develop and frequent recruitment maneuvers are necessary.

Surgical Stages
- Surgical preparation and draping of the operative site (both groins and infrequently the right neck for internal jugular vein access).
- Infiltration of the skin with local anesthetic
- Obtaining venous access through both femoral veins. Confirm venous access cannulation using fluoroscopy.
- Placement of multiple sheaths: Typically two 8F sheaths in the right femoral vein, two 7F sheaths and one 9F sheath in the left femoral vein; intrarterial access for invasive BP monitoring is achieved either via a radial or 5F left or right femoral arterial sheath.

- After sheaths are in place, 2 decapolar catheters are advanced via the 7F sheaths in left groin and positioned in the posterior RA and CS. The ICE catheter is advanced via the 9F sheath and positioned in the mid RA. The 8F sheaths are replaced serially by a deflectable 12F and long 8F sheaths and in each instance using a Brockenbrough needle, transseptal puncture is performed. The mapping/ablation catheter and the Lasso catheter are then deployed in the LA via the 12F and 8F sheaths respectively.
- A detailed shell of the LA (incl the PVs) is created on the 3-D mapping system and merged with the segmented anatomy of the chamber obtained from the CT or MRI scan.
- With the ablation and Lasso catheter positioned in the left and right sided veins, stimulation protocol is performed to identify PV arrhythmogenecity.
- With the Lasso catheter positioned at PV ostia, RF lesions are targeted at the PV-LA junction encircling the veins (either individually or as ipsilateral common) to achieve electrical isolation (loss of PV entry and exit), which is reassessed 30–60 min after initial ablation. Next, the stimulation protocol is repeated to identify and target any non-PV triggers.
- After achieving successful PV isolation and if necessary targeting non-PV triggers, catheters are withdrawn, heparin is D/C, individual PV flow velocities are assessed, and protamine is administered.

- Sheaths are eventually removed (usually 1–2 hr later when ACT is ≤180 sec) and the pt is kept on bed rest for 6 hr. Heparin is then started (without bolus) and all prior medications incl Coumadin and antiarrhythmic drugs are resumed.

Postoperative Considerations
- Common problems in PACU incl postop pain, N/V, and hypothermia.
- Pts with Hx of obstructive sleep apnea should be subject to extended periods of monitoring for desaturation and apneic episodes.
- Typically postprocedure pts are kept in the hospital for 24–48 hr during which they are monitiored on the telemetry and are maintained on IV unfractionated heparin.
- A transthoracic echocardiogram is obtained the following day to assess chamber dimensions, valve function, and pericardial effusion.

Anticipated Problems/Concerns
- Complications of percutaneous vascular access incl bleeding, hematoma, development of arteriovenous fistula, and development of pseudoaneurysm.
- Procedural complications incl pericardial effusion/tamponade, development of PV stenosis, thrombo-embolic complications incl cerebrovascular accidents, formation of intracardiac thrombus, injury to the phrenic nerve, and damage to the esophagus, which can potentially result in the development of atrio-esophageal fistula.

Atrial Septal Defect, Repair of

Joshua D. Stearns
Charles W. Hogue, Jr.

Risk

- ASD is the most common congenital heart defect.
- *Ostium secundum* represents 7% and 40% of all congenital heart disease in children and adults, respectively
- M:F ratio: 1:2, except for *ostium primum* ASD, for which ratio is 1:1

Perioperative Risks

- Risk dependent on age, degree of reversibility of increased PVR; mortality usually <1%
- Supraventricular arrhythmias incl atrial flutter, AFib
- AV conduction block possible if ASD close to AV node

Worry About

- Paradoxical venous embolism
- Right heart volume overload with RV dysfunction
- MVP and mitral regurgitation assoc with *ostium secundum*

- Partial anomalous pulm venous drainage assoc with *sinus venosus* defect
- Cleft anterior mitral valve leaflet associated with *ostium primum* defect
- Endocarditis prophylaxis
- Left to right shunt leading to pulm Htn and eventual Eisenmenger's syndrome (right to left shunt); concern greater with large defects (>1 cm diameter)

Overview

- Classified by location: *Ostium secundum* (70% of ASDs) involves midseptal fossa ovalis; *sinus venosus*, may occur near RA/SVC or RA/IVC junction; *ostium primum*, in inferior septum, represents an endocardial cushion defect
- Unless heart murmur heard, usually not diagnosed until symptomatic in third or fourth decade of life
- Degree of left to right shunting dependent on size of ASD, relative compliance of ventricles, relative SVR, PVR

- MVP in 10–30% of pts; may be 2° to shift of interventricular septum from RV volume overload; usually reversed with closure of ASD
- RV diastolic dimensions increased, interventricular septum shifted; normal resting but decreased LVEF with exercise possible

ICD-9-CM Code: 745.5

Indications and Usual Treatment

- Surgical closure for uncomplicated ASD with pulm-to-systemic flow ratio >1.5
- Optimal age of repair may be <5 y
- PVR at rest >8 U/m^2 that fails to lower to <7 U/m^2 with pulm vasodilators usually contraindication to surgery
- Lung Tx considered with correction of ASD or heart and lung Tx for irreversibly raised PVR
- Transcatheter closure possible in some centers

ASSESSMENT POINTS

System	Effect	Assessment by Hx	PE	Test
CARDIO	Pulm Htn, RHF	SOB, DOE, fatigue	↑ RV impulse, JVD	ECG (R axis deviation in *ostium secundum* vs. L axis deviation in *ostium primum*)
			Fixed split S_2, hepatomegaly, ascites, edema	ECHO (RAE, RVE; paradoxical septal motion; Qp:Qs calculation from R- and L-sided stroke volumes; color-flow Doppler; check for anomalous pulm veins and MVP/mitral valve regurgitation), cardiac catheterization
RESP	Infection	Cough, sputum	Rhonchi, wheezing, consolidation	CXR, CBC, cultures
HEPAT	Passive edema		Hepatomegaly, jaundice, ascites	Liver enzymes, albumin, PT, PTT

Key Reference: Vistarini N, Aiello M, Mattiucci G, et al. Port-access minimally invasive surgery for atrial septal defects: A 10-year single-center experience in 166 patients. *J Thorac Cardiovasc Surg.* 2010;139(1):139–145.

Perioperative Implications

Anesthetic Technique
- General

Monitoring
- CVP
- Arterial line
- Consider TEE with color-flow Doppler, LAP

Induction/Maintenance
- Anesthetic technique guided by preferences, age, condition; extubation early after surgery in most pts
- Maintain HR, preload, contractility
- Avoid large increases in PVR or large decreases in SVR to minimize R → L shunt

Surgical Stages

- Median sternotomy most common approach, but anterior lateral thoracotomy, and cosmetic submammary incision becoming more common
- Cardioplegic arrest
- Direct suture (primary) closure if ASD small, pericardial patch closure for larger defects. Dacron graft, Gore-Tex CV patch suitable substitutes for pericardial patch in some cases.
- Anomalous pulm venous drainage repaired with pericardial patch "baffle," redirecting pulm venous flow into LA
- Mitral valve repair for some pts with *ostium primum* and subsequent mitral cleft

Postoperative Considerations

- LAP/PCWP may be high, 2° to MR, LV diastolic dysfunction from co-existing disease or shift of I-IV septum
- RV dimension, hemodynamics improve shortly after surgery
- Supraventricular arrhythmias incl AFib/flutter
- Reoperation uncommon, but occasional dehiscence of atrial baffle
- Pulm and peripheral thromboembolism with AFib (warfarin commonly started second day after surgery for 8–12 wk).
- Risk of heart block, esp. in *ostium primum* repairs and in primary closer of atrial defect

AV Graft for Hemodialysis

Randall F. Coombs

Risk

- Incidence in the USA: 26 million Americans have chronic kidney disease
- End stage renal disease (ESRD) is defined as either a glomerular filtration rate less than $15 mL/min/1.73 m^2$ or a need for dialysis or renal transplantation.
- >355,000 on hemodialysis in the USA

Perioperative Risks

- Periop mortality is low related to complications of ESRD (electrolyte-induced arrhythmias, cardiac decompensation)
- Fistula failure rate is 10–20% due to thrombosis or inadequate flow through graft.
- Other surgical complications: Infection, venous aneurysm, venous Htn, vascular steal

Worry About

- Adequate preop Rx of Htn, CAD, and
- DM. More than 70% of diabetic ESRD pts have CHF, and almost 70% have CAD. In nondiabetic ESRD pts, CHF and CAD occur just more than 40% for both diagnoses. CV disease is the number one cause of mortality in pts with kidney failure.
- Hypovolemia and hypokalemia (esp. if recently dialyzed)
- Hypervolemia, hyperkalemia, and acidosis (esp. if not recently dialyzed)
- Possible marked Htn in response to surgical stimuli under general anesthesia
- Adequate intravascular volume and BP to preserve graft patency

Overview

- Causes of ESRD: Glomerulonephritis, diabetes, Htn, pyelonephritis, polycystic disease, collagen diseases, reflux or obstructive nephropathy, renal vascular disease, drug toxicity
- Manifestations of chronic renal failure (*Stoelting's anesthesia and co-existing disease* 5th ed., 2008)
  - Electrolyte imbalance: Hyperkalemia, hypermagnesemia, hypocalcemia, increasing phosphate
  - Metabolic acidosis
  - Unpredictable intravascular fluid volume status
  - Anemia: Increased cardiac output, oxyhemoglobin dissociation curve shifted to the right
  - Uremic coagulopathies: Plt dysfunction
  - Neurologic changes: Encephalopathy, peripheral neuropathies
  - Cardiovascular changes: Htn, CAD, CHF, attenuated
  - Sympathetic nervous system activity due to treatment with antihypertensive drugs
  - Renal osteodystrophy
  - Pruritus
  - Autonomic dysfunction (e.g., Stokes-Adams attacks)
  - Poor nutritional state: Fatigue, general malaise, and anorexia

Indications and Usual Treatment

- ESRD: Cr clearance ≤5 mL/min or serum Cr > 1200 μmol/L
- Methods of dialysis: Peritoneal dialysis (PD) versus hemodialysis (choice depends on the pt's general condition and preference)
- PD preferred in young children, elderly, difficult vascular access, pt's preference for independent self-care
- Contraindications to hemodialysis
  - Absolute: CHF or hemodynamic instability,
  - Relative: Psychosis and/or severe mental retardation, carcinomatosis, multiple nonrenal complications, e.g., blindness, diabetic neuropathy
  - AV fistula created 1–2 mo prior to expected start of hemodialysis to allow time for maturation of shunt

ASSESSMENT POINTS

System	Effect	Assessment by Hx	PE	Test
CARDIO	CAD, CHF, LVH, arrhythmias	Chest pain, exercise tolerance, Htn, palpitations	Heart exam: S_3 murmur, irregular rhythm? BP, jugular venous distention	ECG, CXR
RESP	Pulm edema	SOB, orthopnea, PND	Rales, respiratory rate and pattern	CXR
GU	↓ Concentrating ability, uremia, electrolyte/acid-base abn, oliguria/anuria	Anorexia, N/V, diarrhea, malaise	Wt	K, Cr, BUN, HCO_3^-
ENDO	↑ Glucose, ↓ glucose after treatment	Hx DM?, daily glucose values	Evidence of PVD and/or poor healing	Hemoglobin A1C, blood glucose
HEME	Anemia Platelet dysfunction	Fatigue, SOB, bruising	Pallor, bruising	Hgb/Hct Plt count
CNS	Encephalopathy	↓ Mental acuity, somnolence	Mental status exam, sedation assessment	
PNS	Peripheral neuropathy	Weakness, numbness, paresthesias	Motor and sensory neurologic exam	
GI	↓ Gastric emptying	Reflux symptoms?		

Key Reference: Laskowski IA, Muhs B, Rockman CR, et al. Regional nerve block allows for optimization of planning in the creation of arteriovenous access for hemodialysis by improving superficial venous dilatation. *Ann Vasc Surg.* 2007;21(6):730–733.

Perioperative Management

Anesthetic Techniques
- Monitored anesthesia care (MAC)
  - Local anesthesia by surgeon with IV sedation by anesthesiologist
  - Best when surgical dissection is minimal (i.e. radial-cephalic anastomosis at the wrist)
- Regional (brachial plexus block)
  - Vasodilation helps surgeon identify best vein to anastomose to
  - Increased blood flow decreases incidence of periop thrombosis
  - Better hemodynamic stability and less N/V than with GA
  - Contraindications: pt objection, anticipated technical difficulty
- General anesthesia (GA)
  - Better for uncooperative pt
  - Potential for prolonged drug effects and drug interactions
  - Potential for complications related to electrolyte/acid-base abn
  - Potential for airway problems and resp depression
  - May see hypotension 2° to anesthetic medications
  - May see Htn 2° to surgical or airway stimulation

Monitoring
- Place IV, BP cuff, pulse oximeter on nonop arm
- Five-lead electrocardiogram
- Temp (skin or esophageal)
- $ETCO_2$ for MAC and plexus block as well as GA if sedative drugs given

Fluids
- Non-K^+-containing, careful fluid balance monitoring
- Large volume of NS leads to ↑ metabolic acidosis and thus higher K^+ than when equal volume of LR is given

Induction/Maintenance
- Decreasing plasma proteins lead to prolonged and increased effect of highly protein-bound drugs
- Acidosis increases non-ionized, unbound drug (active portion of drug is non-ionized)
- Uremia inhibits the sympathetic nervous system, thus decreasing compensatory vasoconstriction
- Increased CNS effects of anesthetic induction drugs due to uremic disruption of the blood brain barrier
- Maintenance of general anesthesia
  - Inhalation agents (sevoflurane, isoflurane, desflurane) all acceptable
  - Total IV anesthesia (remifentanil, propofol, and cisatracurium) also acceptable
- Muscle relaxants
  - Avoid succinylcholine if K^+ ≥5.5 (K^+ may increase by 0.5–1.0 mEq/L after succinylcholine)
  - Delayed excretion of pancuronium, thus increasing the duration of action
  - Duration of action of vecuronium, and rocuronium are not significantly prolonged
  - Clearance of mivacurium, atracurium, and cisatracurium is independent of renal function
- Opioids
  - Increase magnitude and prolonged duration (decrease protein binding and delayed clearance)
  - Accumulation of morphine metabolite, morphine glucuronide leads to resp depression
  - Fentanyl may be given judiciously (large doses accumulate and prolonged effect)
- Local anesthetics
- Increase susceptibility to toxicity due to reduced protein binding, metabolic acidosis, and delayed elimination

Surgical Stages

Location
- Should be easily accessible for dialysis
- First fistula: As far distal as possible (adequate size of vein is the determining factor)
- Non-dominant arm if possible
- Wrist: Radial artery to cephalic vein
- Forearm (most common first site): Radial, ulnar, or brachial artery to brachial vein
- Upper arm: Brachial artery to basilic or axillary vein

Blood Flow
- 200–300 mL/min immediately after anastomosis formed
- 200 mL/min required to complete dialysis in 3–4 hr
- Doppler often used during closure to check shunt for patency

Types of Access
- Fistulas: Side of artery to side of vein, or side of artery to end of transected vein
- Prosthetic graft: Usually Teflon (polytetrafluoroethylene)

Procedure Duration
- Variable, ~ 1–3 hr

Blood Loss
- Usually minimal (depends on access and ease)

Postoperative Considerations
- Medical management
  - Monitor and manage co-existing diseases (i.e., DM, CAD, CHF, and Htn)
  - Assess fluid volume status and serum electrolytes (esp. serum K^+)
  - Consider early postop dialysis (but not via new fistula).
- Operated arm
  - Elevated for several hours and avoid constrictive clothing since arm may swell
    - Avoid venipunctures and BP measurements.
  - Monitor fistula blood flow (palpate thrill, auscultate, Doppler).
  - Early surgical revision for inadequate fistula blood flow
- Pain management
  - Medication initially unnecessary if brachial plexus block was performed
    - PO analgesia usually adequate
- Maturation of fistula
  - Blood flow increases with time (up to 1200 mL/min)
  - Venous wall thickens (prevents venous tears)
  - Maturation period is variable but generally takes longer for smaller vessels.

Anticipated Problems/Concerns
- IV access can be difficult in these pts. Central venous line may be necessary.
- Avoid fistula use for initial 3 wk to prevent aneurysm formation
- Thrombosis is the most common complication: up to 20% in first few weeks after surgery.
- Infection: Higher incidence with graft fistulas

Prognosis
- Fistulas have a finite life span. Revisions and repeat procedures are common.
  - Less than 50% patent at 1 y, less than 40% patent at 2 y
- Renal transplantation is the optimal treatment for ESRD in suitable pts

Blalock-Taussig Shunt (BTS)

Aris Sophocles
Mark Twite

Risk

• Indicated for infants with congenital heart lesions resulting in either severely reduced pulm blood flow (PBF) (e.g., tetralogy of Fallot, pulm and tricuspid atresia) or as the first stage of single ventricle palliation (e.g., hypoplastic left heart syndrome [HLHS])

Perioperative Risks

• Fewer BT shunts are performed now compared to previous decades and operative mortality has fallen despite a higher percentage of pts with single ventricle physiology.
• Periop complications incl Horner's syndrome, chylothorax, phrenic nerve damage and acute arm ischemia with classic BTS.

Worry About

• BTS for decreased PBF keep PVR as low as possible (high FIO_2, avoid hypercarbia and acidosis)
• BTS for single ventricle staged palliation essential to balance SVR and PVR (often requires FIO_2 0.17 - 0.21 and normocarbia)

Overview

• One of multiple types of systemic to pulm shunts to increased PBF
• Familiarity with underlying anatomy and physiology is essential to management.
• Subclavian artery (opposite side of arch to limit kinking) to PA anastomosis performed directly (classic BTS), or most common is using a Gore-Tex tube graft (modified BTS)

• Advantages of modified BTS incl: preservation of subclavian artery, technically easier anastomosis and later take down, greater PA growth with less distortion of PAs and low shunt failure rate
• Goal: Adequate but not excessive PBF
• Nonconfluence of PAs, distal PA stenosis and single ventricle lesions require cardiopulmonary bypass (CPB) and more extensive surgery

ICD-9-CM Code: 745.2 (Tetralogy of Fallot)

Indications and Usual Treatment

• Infants with decreased PBF who are unable to have a 1° surgical correction of their congenital heart lesion may have a BTS to improve PBF and allow PAs to grow.
• Infants with single ventricle physiology have a BTS as part of a three-stage surgical palliation (Stage 1 Norwood procedure).

ASSESSMENT POINTS

System	Effect	Assessment by Hx	PE	Test
HEENT	↑ Incidence of craniofacial defects	Other congenital abn	Airway	FISH for DiGeorge syndrome Chromosomes
CARDIO	CHD Single ventricle physiology Qp:Qs	FTT, tachypnea	Heart murmur Rales	ECHO Cardiac cath
RESP	↓ Pulm blood flow	'Tet' spells (hypercyanotic episodes from dynamic RVOT narrowing in tetralogy of Fallot)	Cyanosis	O_2 sat, Hct ABGs CXR

Key Reference: Williams JA, Bansal AK, Kim BJ, et al. Two thousand Blalock-Taussig shunts: A six-decade experience. *Ann Thorac Surg.* 2007;84:2070–2075.

Perioperative Management

Preoperative Preparation

• Pts often already intubated, consider placing a nasal ETT for infants under 12 mo (tube more stable and makes placement of TEE probe easier)
• Arterial line: For cardiac lesions with ↓ PBF place A-line in contralateral radial artery from BTS or in the femoral artery. For single ventricle lesions place an A-line in right radial artery if low flow cerebral perfusion technique to be used for Stage 1 Norwood and/or in the umbilical or femoral artery.
• Central venous line: All cases for inotropes. Consider co-oximetry central venous catheter.

Intraoperative Period

• May use inhalation induction. Single ventricle pts often have IV access.
• Infants with tetralogy of Fallot may have tet spells due to worsening RVOT obstruction.
• Lateral thoracotomy classic approach: Anticipate worsened hypoxia with PA clamping, blood product transfusion usually not required
• Sternotomy and CPB for complex and single ventricle cases

Postoperative Period

• Goal is adequate but not excessive pulm blood flow; shunt should be slightly restrictive to avoid CHF. Calculate Qp:Qs.

• Cyanosis or clotting possible if shunt too small, hypotension, or systemic vessel kinks
• CHF or pulm edema possible (may be unilateral) if pulm blood flow is too great

Prognosis

• Ultimate prognosis depends on underlying congenital defects
• Current surgical techniques allow many pts to undergo primary complete repair of their cardiac lesion (e.g., tetralogy of Fallot), avoiding BTS

Blood Components

Samuel A. Cherry, III

Risk

• One out of every 10 hospitalized pts receives a transfusion
• Approx 29 million components transfused annually

Perioperative Risks

• Transfusion-transmitted infection (HIV, hepatitis, West Nile, etc.)
• Hemolytic transfusion reactions (acute and delayed)
• Nonhemolytic reactions (fever, allergy, anaphylaxis, transfusion-related acute lung injury)
• Immunosuppression (increased infection rate, cancer recurrence)

Worry About

• Pt willingness to accept transfusion
• Presence of RBC antibodies detected on antibody screen
• Availability of components from blood bank

Overview

• The U.S. blood supply is dependent on volunteer donations
• Whole blood donations are processed into the various components (RBC, FFP, cryoprecipitate, and Plts). Components can also be collected individually via apheresis.
• Citrate is the anticoagulant in all components.
• Preservative solutions are added to RBC units to extend the shelf-life up to 42 d

Indications and Usual Treatment

• RBC: Given to increase O_2 carrying capacity due to acute blood loss or chronic anemia. Dose: 1 unit, expect increase in Hgb by 1 g/dL or Hct by 3% in adults.
• Plt: Given to prevent or treat bleeding due to thrombocytopenia or plt dysfunction. Dose: Whole blood-derived plt 1 unit/10kg, expect each unit to increase plt count 5000/μL; Apheresis plt 1 unit, expect 1 unit to increase plt count 30,000–60,000/μL.
• FFP: Given to prevent or treat bleeding due to depletion and/or deficiency of multiple coagulation factors, incl urgent warfarin reversal, DIC, massive transfusion. Dose: 10–20 mL/kg, expect factor levels to increase by 20%.
• Cryo: Given to treat bleeding in hypofibrinogenemia or dysfibrinogenemia. Second line therapy to treat Hemophilia A only when Factor VIII concentrate is not available, and von Willebrand's disease only when pt is not DDAVP-responsive, and vWF concentrate is not available. Dose: 1 unit/7–10 kg, expect fibrinogen levels to increase by ~50 mg/dL.

ASSESSMENT POINTS

Component	Effect	Assessment by Hx	PE	Test
RBC	O_2 delivery	Anemia; blood loss; chemotherapy; cardiopulmonary reserve	Pallor; acute blood loss; hypotension; tachycardia	Hgb, Hct, O_2 extraction ratio
PLT	Coagulation	Mucosal bleeding; diseases or drugs affecting plt function; blood loss ≥1 blood volume	Microvascular bleeding, petechiae, purpura	Plt count; plt function testing
FFP	Coagulation	Personal/family Hx of bleeding; ecchymoses; liver disease; warfarin therapy; blood loss ≥1 blood volume	Microvascular bleeding	PT, PTT
CRYO	Coagulation	Personal/family Hx of bleeding; vWF disease; congenital dysfibrinogenemia; blood loss ≥1 blood volume	Microvascular bleeding	Fibrinogen

Key Reference: American Society of Anesthesiologists Task Force on Blood Component Therapy. Practice guidelines for blood component therapy. *Anesthesiology.* 1996;84:732–747.

Perioperative Management

Preoperative Preparation

• Type and screen: ABO/Rh type, and detection of clinically significant RBC antibodies
• Type and crossmatch: Same as above, plus testing to demonstrate compatibility between donor and recipient
• ABO compatibility is important for all components; Rh compatibility is important for RBC and plt components
• Coagulation testing is not advocated in pts with no Hx or exam suggestive of abn

Induction/Maintenance

• Hypotension can further compromise O_2 delivery in anemic pts
• Periop cell salvage and acute normovolemic hemodilution can reduce allogeneic RBC transfusions
• Massive blood loss (>1 blood volume) will likely require transfusion of RBC, FFP, plt, and cryo; ideally, component therapy is driven by laboratory and clinical assessment

Postoperative Considerations

• Continued blood loss may necessitate additional transfusion

Anticipated Problems/Concerns

• Risk of transfusion and/or transmitted infection is lower now than at any other time
• Some pts refuse transfusion based on religious beliefs. An in-depth discussion with the pt can elucidate what he/she will allow/refuse. This should be thoroughly documented.
• The blood bank will need additional time to find compatible RBC units for pts with antibodies. A discussion with the blood bank can provide insight regarding the relative ease or difficulty in finding compatible units based on the antibody(ies) present.

Blowout Orbital Fracture

Kathryn E. McGoldrick

Risk

- Rare
- Pts subjected to blunt trauma assoc with battery, motor vehicle accidents, and sports injuries with a nonpenetrating object (e.g., fist)
- Racial predominance: None

Perioperative Risks

- In absence of serious assoc injuries, rare periop mortality (<0.1%)
- Postop risk of visual disturbances, incl blindness, infection, and cosmetic deformity

Worry About

- Intraocular damage (ruptured globe rare in isolated orbital blowout fracture owing to release of compressive forces into the maxillary sinus)

- Assoc nonophthalmic injuries (intracranial injury, cervical spine fracture or subluxation, Le Fort fractures with basilar skull fracture)
- Prolapse and incarceration of orbital soft tissues
- Preop systemic steroids (to distinguish NM edema or related motility disturbance from true entrapment, unmask enophthalmos, and reduce discomfort) predispose to sinus-orbital infections
- Hemostasis for delicate surgery

Overview

- Fractures of orbital floor are repaired by various surgical approaches
- Intraop infiltration with lidocaine with 1:100,000 epinephrine for hemostatic effect
- Entrapped tissues freed with care taken to avoid infraorbital neurovascular tissue trauma

- Autologous or alloplastic implant material placed over fracture site; reconstruction typically done with mesh, implants, or solvent-preserved bone graft

ICD-9-CM Code: 802.6

Surgical Indications/Usual Treatment

- The three standard indications for surgical intervention are enophthalmos, motility disturbance 2° to entrapment, hypo-ophthalmos
- Timing of surgical intervention depends on assoc injuries and pt's age, general health, and preference; often preferable to delay in order to permit some resolution of edema and bleeding; technical ease and functional result typically enhanced by surgery in 5–14 d or longer; rarely considered urgent unless muscle entrapped and possibly ischemic

ASSESSMENT POINTS

System	Effect	Assessment by Hx	PE	Test
HEENT	Trauma may produce orbital subcutaneous emphysema, restriction of globe motility, globe ptosis, enophthalmos, retinal or choroidal injury		Inspection Palpation Funduscopic exam	CT scan
CNS	Trauma may produce head injuries	CNS Hx	CNS exam	CT scan
MS	Trauma may produce assorted MS and organ injuries	Pain	Palpation	Plain films as indicated

Key Reference: Parbhu KC, Galler KE, Li C, Mawn LA. Underestimation of soft tissue entrapment by computed tomography in orbital floor fractures in the pediatric population. *Ophthalmology*. 2008;115(9):1620–1625.

Perioperative Implications

Preoperative Preparation
- Children with a trap door injury may require treatment for vagal reactions, incl nausea and syncope, caused by trapped parasympathetic nerve fibers that travel with the injured muscle.

Anesthetic Technique
- GA usual; also local

Monitoring
- Routine

Airway
- Other facial injuries may complicate airway management

Induction/Maintenance
- Without assoc injuries, few hemodynamic perturbations
- Avoid Htn (to minimize bleeding)
- Adequate depth of anesthesia to prevent pt movement during delicate surgery
- Consider anti-emetic prophylaxis

Surgical Stages

Dissection
- Minimal blood loss

Definitive Surgery
- Minimal blood loss (<100 mL) and fluid shifts
- Approximate duration: 2 hr

Postoperative Considerations
- Mild postop pain
- IV PCA usually not necessary
- Without other injuries, discharge on day of surgery

Anticipated Problems/Concerns

- Blindness
- Infraorbital paresthesia
- Implant extrusion
- Diplopia and delayed extraocular muscle restriction
- Obstructive sinus disease
- Infection
- Return to potentially violent environment

Bone Marrow Transplantation (Harvest Procedure)

Charles D. Boucek

Risk

- Autologous: Pts with certain malignancies that respond to chemotherapy with need for marrow reconstitution and for cell-based therapies (experimental treatment for acute MI, refractory CHF)
- Allogeneic: HLA-matched healthy donor for recipient with malignancy or marrow failure as alternative to peripheral blood–stem cell transplant

Perioperative Risks

- Postop morbidity is high 2° to underlying disease of autologous donor.
- Life-threatening complications extremely rare (0.27%) for allogeneic (healthy) donor

Worry About

- Volume status and/or blood loss
- Position-related injuries (prone)
- Anesthetic drug interactions with prior chemotherapy; decreased adrenal reserve
- Puncture of intrathoracic structures if sternal harvest necessary; peripheral (tibia) marrow is often replaced by fat in adults.

Overview

- Multiple (often 100–200) needle punctures of posterior iliac crest (occasionally other sites) made to obtain stem cells for reinfusion following marrow ablative chemotherapy for malignancy or as protocol directed for cell-based therapy.
- Operating physician may be a hematologist (not surgeon)

ICD-9-CM Code: V59.3 (Bone marrow donor)

Indications and Usual Treatment

- Marrow failure, hematologic malignancy, selected chemotherapy-responsive solid tumors
- Recipient anticipates prolonged hospitalization in major medical center, aggressive support for anemia, thrombocytopenia, neutropenia, GVHD
- Autologous transplantation may follow first or subsequent remission for hematologic malignancy or be performed prior to chemotherapy for solid tumor of sites remote from bone marrow stores
- Cell-based therapy (protocol-driven) uses bone marrow stem cells for experimental treatment of acute MI and refractory CHF. (Smaller quantities of marrow may be harvested under local anesthesia.)

ASSESSMENT POINTS*

System	Effect	Assessment by Hx	PE	Test
CARDIO	CHF, dysrhythmias	Doxorubicin, pericardial effusions	CV exam	ECG, consider ECHO/MUGA
GI	Electrolyte imbalance	Vomiting, melena	Edema, orothostasis	Na^+, K^+, Ca^{2+}
HEME	Blood loss, infection	Recent chemotherapy	Petechiae, ecchymosis	CBC, platelets

*Applies primarily to autologous donors with malignancy.

Key Reference: Koca E, Champlin RE. Peripheral blood progenitor cell or bone marrow transplantation: Controversy remains. *Curr Opin Oncol.* 2008;20(2):220–226.

Intraoperative Management

Monitoring

- Large-bore IV (×2); meticulous sterile technique
- Consider CVP, if access difficult
- Check availability of irradiated blood
- Urinary cath may be necessary (large fluid shifts)
- Arterial access may result in hematoma (thrombocytopenia); useful if BP is labile
- Pulse oximetry may guide O_2 requirements: Acutely reduced $ETCO_2$ may indicate embolism from marrow space

Induction

- Decrease the dose of induction agent if there is Hx of cardiotoxic chemotherapy

Surgical Stages

- Establishment of adequate venous access
- Induction of general anesthesia (spinal or epidural possible for allogeneic donors)
- Establish prone position
- Supine to prone position change requires minimum of 4 persons
- Wt supported on chest/pelvis with arms extended on armboards
- Avoid pressure on eyes, throat, genitals
- Abd position for free excursion
- Aspiration of marrow
- Cell count of marrow determines volume needed
- Return to supine position
- Duration 2–4 hr
- Postop pain score 1–4; usually PO drugs (acetaminophen with codeine) adequate

Anticipated Problems/Concerns

- Familiarity with pt's specific chemotherapy and protocols
- Volume replacement with crystalloid, albumin
- Avoid starch (interferes with processing of marrow)
- Avoid non-irradiated RBCs (potential engraftment of random donor nucleated cells)
- Prior steroid Rx may result in reduced adrenal reserve
- Avoid unnecessary O_2 enrichment if prior chemotherapy incl bleomycin
- Air and/or O_2 may be used (N_2O inhibits methionine synthetase resulting in marrow toxicity)

Bowel Resection

Mark C. Phillips

Risk

- Incidence depends on disease process
- Person living in North America has an average lifetime risk of 6% of developing colorectal cancer
- Crohn's disease has an annual incidence of 4 cases per 100,000

Perioperative Risks

- Periop mortality 0.5-5% mainly due to underlying disorder and other co-morbidities
- Periop morbidity: Prolonged ileus 5–10%; anastomotic leak 2–4%; wound dehiscence 1–2%, bleeding 1%

Worry About

- Decreased intravascular volume and electrolyte abn, esp. hypokalemia due to bowel prep

- Bowel obstruction, esp. in the small bowel can lead to bowel necrosis, perforation, and development of septic shock
- Risk for aspiration with bowel obstruction
- Contamination of peritoneum with bowel perforation
- Development of PTE

Overview

- Bowel resection of the large and small bowel is performed for a variety of reasons
- Crohn's disease most common surgical disease of the small intestine
- Small bowel resection involves varying amounts of mesentery
- Large bowel resection requires mobilization prior to resection; 1° anastomosis vs. colostomy depends on several factors—inflammation, prepped vs. unprepped bowel, local ischemia

- Laparoscopic approaches are being increasingly used for surgery on both the small and large bowel.

ICD-9-CM Codes: 153.9 (Neoplasm, large intestine); 555.9 (Crohn's disease)

Indications and Usual Treatment

- Small-bowel resection: Obstruction, volvulus, intussusception, tumors, trauma, Crohn's disease
- Large-bowel resection: Colon cancer, diverticular disease, Crohn's disease, ulcerative colitis, GI bleed, trauma
- Medical treatment varies depending on the underlying disease process.

ASSESSMENT POINTS

System	Effect	Assessment by Hx	PE	Test
HEENT CARDIO	Hypovolemia	Dizziness	Orthostatic BP	Electrolytes, Hct
RESP	Aspiration risk Hypoventilation and hypoxemia	N/V Splinting	Bowel distention Auscultation	ABG, O_2 saturation, CXR
RENAL	Renal insufficiency		Signs of hypovolemia, dry mucus membranes	Electrolytes, BUN, Cr
GI	Diarrhea, N/V	Nausea	Orthostatic vital signs	Electrolytes

Key Reference: Evers B. Small intestine. In: Townsend C, Beauchamp R, Evers B, Mattox K, eds. *Sabiston textbook of surgery*. Philadelphia: Saunders/Elsevier; 2008:1278–1332.

Perioperative Management

Preoperative Preparation

- Volume replacement and correction of electrolytes prior to induction
- Aspiration prophylaxis with sodium citrate and H_2 antagonist
- Avoid metoclopramide in pts with bowel obstruction or perforation
- Appropriate antibiotic prophylaxis

Monitoring

- Routine monitors
- Consider CVL if significant co-morbidities or pt has difficult venous access
- Consider arterial line for continuous BP measurement and blood sampling
- Foley catheter to monitor urine output

Anesthetic Technique

- General anesthesia
- Consider combined GETA/epidural for postop analgesia
- Avoid LMA due to risk of aspiration
- Large bore IV access
- Monitor hemodynamics and airway pressures closely during abd insufflation if laparoscopic approach

Airway

- Increased incidence of gastric aspiration due to bowel obstruction or emergency surgery
- Consider placement of NG tube prior to induction to suction gastric contents

Induction

- Often RSI due to aspiration risk
- Consider awake intubation
- Induction agents depend on volume status and assoc co-morbidities

Maintenance

- Avoid NO in cases of bowel obstruction
- Relaxation with non-depolarizing agent is often needed in order for surgeon to have optimal working conditions

Surgical Stages

Dissection

- May have extensive adhesions if previous surgeries
- Hypotension with manipulation of perforated or strangulated small bowel
- May have hypotension after peritoneum opened, esp. if intra-abdominal bleeding has been tamponaded

Definitive Surgery

- Large third-space loss, depends on degree and duration of bowel exposure, may require extensive crystalloid and colloid
- Risk of hypothermia when large amounts of bowel exposed
- Risk of ureteral injury during mobilization of pelvic colon
- Suction enterostomy of obstructed bowel will lead to additional fluid requirements

Postoperative Considerations

- Consider epidural analgesia or IV PCA for pain
- Hypoventilation and hypoxemia due to splinting, consider supplemental O_2 during postop period
- Ileus from bowel manipulation and narcotics

Anticipated Problems/Concerns

- Aspiration on induction due to bowel obstruction
- Hemodynamic instability due to hypovolemia from bowel prep
- Septic shock if bowel perforation preop

Brain Cortex Resection (for Epilepsy)

Patricia H. Petrozza

Risk

- Incidence in USA: 300,000
- 3000 ablative operations/y
- Racial predilection: None

Perioperative Risks

- Depends on procedure—potential unintentional interruption of neural pathways
- Combined morbidity, mortality rates <5% for epileptogenic focus resection, <11% for corpus callosotomy, <17% for functional hemispherectomy
- Blood loss diathesis (functional hemispherectomy)
- Risk of craniotomy incl hypercoagulable state (PE, thromboembolism), intracerebral hemorrhage, air emboli, infection

Worry About

- Intraop seizures
- Aspiration; airway obstruction

- Tailoring anesthetic technique for appropriate intraop testing, responsiveness
- Favorable cranial conditions
- N/V
- Blood loss diathesis
- Appropriate pt sedation

Overview

- Used for intractable seizures
- Requires discussion with surgeons and neurologists; concerns about intraop electrocorticography (ECoG), and functional testing when elegant brain cortex is at risk
- Concerns about seizures, possible status epilepticus
- Concerns about craniotomy, incl blood loss, adequate operating conditions, postop responsiveness
- Pt may have co-morbid conditions—e.g., psychiatric disorders, tuberous sclerosis, neurofibromatosis, obesity

- Pts on anti-epileptic drugs often require larger doses of narcotics, muscle relaxants than expected; adverse risks of anti-epileptic medications
- Hepatic enzyme induction and drug interactions are common

ICD-9-CM Code: 345.91

Usual Treatment

- Pts recommended for cortical resection for epilepsy have met these criteria:
  - Have focal seizure not responding to adequate trial of antiepileptic agents
  - Seizures significantly interfere with pt's overall function
  - Surgery appears to offer reasonable opportunity for improvement of overall function
- Preop testing likely incl Wada's test to determine hemispheric dominance, functional MRI testing, and both invasive and non-invasive EEG localizations

---

ASSESSMENT POINTS

System	Effect	Assessment by Hx	PE	Test
CARDIAC	Arrhythmias	Rx with carbamazepine and phenytoin	Clinical cardiac exam	ECG
	Wt gain	Valproic acid	Calculate BMI	
HEENT	Gum hypertrophy	Phenytoin	Airway exam	
	Acute myopia and 2° narrow angle glaucoma	Topiramate, eye pain, vision less	May require specialized ophthalmologic exam	
	Diplopia	Carbamazepine	Cranial nerve exam	
	Peripheral field vision loss	Vigabatrin	Visual field exam	
GI/HEPATIC	Hepatitis, pancreatitis	Most commonly with valproic acid, trimethadione, mephenytoin, lamotrigine, felbamate (more common in females), abd pain	Hepatomegaly, jaundice	Routine biochemical monitoring (ALT, AST, GGT amylase) is NOT indicative of extent of liver damage. Blood lipase levels if pancreatitis suspected.
HEME	Blood dyscrasias related to antiepileptic drugs	Weakness, fatigue, Rx with carbamazepine, ethosuximide, mephenytoin, phenytoin, trimethadione, lamotrigine, phenobarbital, valproic acid, felbamate	Petechiae, rash	CBC
RENAL	Nephritis	Trimethadione therapy		BUN, Cr, Na, Bicarb, ABG
	Hyponatremia	Carbamazepine, oxcarbazepine		
	Metabolic acidosis	Zonisamide, topiramate		
NEURO	Lethargy, depression, insomnia, dizziness, etc., related to anticonvulsants	Rx lamotrigine, topiramate (decreased attention, memory impairment), zonisamide, valproic acid	MS exam	
	Tremor	Carbamazepine	Neurologic exam	
ORTHO	Osteoporosis	Phenytoin, carbamazepine, barbiturates, valproic acid		
	Factures			
SKIN	Rash	Highest risk: Phenytoin, lamotrigine, carbamazepine; may occur with all anti-epileptic drugs	Skin exam	

Key Reference: Erickson KM, Cole DJ. Anesthetic considerations for awake craniotomy for epilepsy. *Anesthesiol Clin.* 2007;25:535–555.

Perioperative Management

• Cortical resection under general anesthesia is most frequently performed for temporal lobe operations where structural lesions have been identified and intraop testing of speech, motor and other functions is unnecessary.

Intraoperative Electrocorticography/ Conscious Sedation

• Discussion by surgeon, anesthesiologist about specific pt's suitability for an awake craniotomy
• Work to establish rapport with the pt; preop orientation to intraop testing
• Pts position themselves as comfortably as possible; O_2 delivered by nasal prongs
• Avoid benzodiazepines if intraop ECoG or serial neurocognitive testing is planned

Monitoring

• Anesthesiologist's continuous awareness of pt's well being
• Capnography by nasal prongs
• Urinary cath
• 1 large-bore IV line
• Arterial line placement based on co-morbidities

Airway

• Careful inspection mandatory: Difficult intubation anticipated in lateral position with pre-existing airway abn
• Rigid pinion fixation may be used; fiberoptic equipment should be available.
• Some centers use LMA in an "asleep/awake/asleep" technique.

Induction

• If intraop ECoG, general anesthesia chosen, induction can be with propofol, maintenance with N_2O, propofol, narcotic technique supplemented with low-dose isoflurane 0.25%. Avoid N_2O if craniotomy for electrode placement within previous 2 wk.
  • LMA with spontaneous breathing
  • Anesthesia maintenance with remifentanil (0.01 to 0.05 µg/kg/min) infusion often satisfactory for intraop ECoG recording
  • D/C propofol and/or inhalation agents 20 min prior to ECoG
• Narcotic requirements may be increased
• During closure of craniotomy, care must be taken to avoid Htn, movement by pt
• For craniotomy, conscious sedation under local anesthesia, two generally accepted techniques: Remifentanil 0.03 to 0.09 µg/kg/min and propofol 30 to 180 µg/kg/min or dexmedetomidine 0.3 µg/kg bolus and infusion at 0.2 µg to 0.7 µg/kg/hr with occasional fentanyl 50 µg bolus
• Infusions D/C 20 min before pt needs to be responsive to ECoG recordings
• Consider glycopyrrolate prior to dexmedetomidine bolus
• Local infiltration of scalp by surgeons (careful attention to local anesthesia overdose)
• Consider addition of morphine 5–10 mg for postop analgesia

Surgical Stages

• Scalp incision: Should be comfortable with adequate local anesthesia
• Removal of bone flap: Pt may be bothered by drilling (should be warned)
• Stripping of dura: May cause N/V
• Meningeal vessel manipulation: May cause pain
• Blood loss: While usually not great, replaced to avoid hypovolemia
• N/V: Can be controlled with metoclopramide 5–10 mg or ondansetron 4 mg
• Pt at risk for seizures
  • Often eliminated by cold saline applied to cortical surface
  • May require therapy with propofol, IV methohexital 0.5–1.0 mg/kg if ECoG anticipated; following ECoG, benzodiazepines acceptable.

Postoperative Considerations

• Fluctuating blood levels of anticonvulsants
• Possible postop agitation
• Control of hemodynamics, possibility of recurrent seizures
• Pain score ~5–10; careful narcotic titration

Anticipated Problems/Concerns

• Difficulties with seizure control
• Possible brain swelling or intracranial hematoma related to resection
• Pt anxiety related to lengthy operation time
• Intraop N/V

Breast Biopsy

Victoria Smoot

Risk

- 80% breast lumps are benign
- 1% breast cancers are in males
- Postmenopausal breast cancer 1.5× more likely in obese women

Perioperative Risk

- Mortality low
- Morbidity
  - Seroma common
  - Hematoma <10%
- Increased risk of PONV; reported as high as 80%

Worry about

- Allergic reaction to dye if injected for sentinel lymph node biopsy
- Dislodging wire if needle localization performed
- PONV
- Airway management in obese pts

Overview

- Palpable mass, nipple discharge, or abn finding on mammogram indication for surgery
- Excisional biopsy removes benign lesion in entirety
- Lumpectomy removes cancerous tissues with sufficient tumor-free margins
- Sentinel lymph node biopsy performed by injecting marker (blue vital dye or low radioactive tracer) for lymphatic mapping. Node closest to location of breast cancer has 97% accuracy in predicting metastasis of tumor to nonsentinel nodes. Nondiagnostic sentinel node biopsy mandates auxiliary dissection. Positive node greater than 0.2 mm requires complete auxiliary dissection.

ICD9-CM: 174 (Malignant neoplasm of female breast)

Indications and Usual Treatment

- Non OR diagnostic procedures may incl US guided, mammographically guided, MRI-guided biopsy or stereotactic core biopsy.
- Open breast biopsy, breast biopsy with sentinel lymph node biopsy are OR procedures
- Excisional biopsy for benign lesions
  - Palpable lesions (e.g., fibroadenomas)
  - Non-palpable lesions (e.g., nipple discharge from intraductal papillomas)
- Needle localized biopsy for potentially malignant, nonpalpable abn seen on screening mammograms
- Sentinel lymph node biopsy for small invasive breast cancers without clinical evidence of lymph node involvement

ASSESSMENT POINTS

System	Effect	Assessment by Hx	Test
HEENT	Obesity may make airway management difficult for sedation	OSA Prior difficult intubtaion	
GI	GERD	Reflux	
CNS	Ability to tolerate with sedation	Anxiety level	

Key Reference: Layeeque R, Siegel E, Kass R, et al. Prevention of nausea and vomiting following breast surgery. *Am J Surg.* 2006;191(6):767–772.

Perioperative Implications

- Preop preparation
  - Pts tend to be very anxious. Consider preop sedation
  - High incidence of PONV. Give appropriate prophylaxis

Anesthetic Technique

- Local anesthesia with IV sedation
- General anesthesia
- Paravertebral block

Monitors

- Routine monitors with attention to EKG lead placement
- IV and BP cuff on nonoperative side

Airway

- Surgical field may limit access to airway
- Supplemental O_2 via nasal cannula or face mask
- May need airway adjuncts for pts with OSA done under sedation. Consider GA with LMA

Induction and Maintenance

- IV sedation: Propofol infusion plus anxiolytic (e.g., midazolam) and/or short acting narcotic
- GA standard induction. Usually performed as outpatient procedure: any technique that allows rapid emergence. Mask or LMA in appropriate pts

Surgical Stages

- Dye injected to identify lymph nodes frequently causes transient drop in pulse oximeter reading
- Use of electrocautery may cause increased discomfort requiring deep sedation or GA
- Postop considerations
  - Pain score 2–5
  - Pain management PO analgesics
  - PONV may require rescue antiemetics

Anticipated Problems/Concerns

- Depth and size of mass may necessitate converting from local with sedation to GA
- Use of injectable dye may cause blue urine, emesis or stool for 24–48 hr. Reaction to isosulfan blue may incl itching, blue hives, decreased BP.

Bronchoscopy, Fiberoptic

Andranik Ovassapian

Risk

- First performed 1966 by Ikeda
- Is applied for evaluation of tracheobronchial tree
- Has virtually replaced rigid bronchoscopy
- Available in a range of sizes applicable to neonates and adult populations
- Better tolerated than rigid bronchoscopy

Perioperative Risks

- Increased risk in pts with cardiac disease, hypoxemia, and bleeding diathesis
- Depends on nature of disease for which bronchoscopy is performed

Worry About

- Coughing, breath holding, hypoxemia
- Increased airway resistance when performed through endotracheal or tracheostomy tube
- Postbronchoscopy airway irritation, coughing, airway obstruction, hypoxemia if not treated with O_2

Overview

- Fiberoptic bronchoscopy enables endoscopist to go deeper into bronchial tree for evaluation, biopsy of lesions not commonly accessible to rigid bronchoscopy
- Fiberoptic bronchoscopy assoc with repeated coughing, Htn, tachycardia often due to inadequate topical or general anesthesia
- Hypoxemia common when performed without supplemental O_2 Rx
- Blood loss from biopsy site of lower airway lesions can be troublesome.
- Tracheal and sometimes bronchial intubation, separation of lungs possibly necessary for major hemoptysis

ICD-9-CM Code: 162.9 (Lung cancer)

Indications and Usual Treatment

- Evaluation of upper, lower airway problems, Dx of pulm disease
- Most useful for diagnosis and staging of lung cancer
- Has diagnostic, therapeutic, and problem-solving indications
- Rx of acute atelectasis performed by saline lavage, aspiration of thick secretions
- Transbronchoscopic bronchial biopsy, brushing cytology, transbronchial needle aspiration biopsy, bronchoalveolar lavage performed
- Absolute contraindications incl acutely unstable CV system, current life-threatening cardiac arrhythmias, severe hypoxemia

ASSESSMENT POINTS

System	Effect	Assessment by Hx	PE	Test
HEENT	Upper airway obstruction due to tumor, edema Limitation of movement	Degree of compromise Airflow pattern Snoring Stridor	Mandibular subluxation Size of tongue Head and neck anatomy Mouth opening Neck ROM	Lateral x-ray CT scan Barium swallow Flow-volume loop
CARDIO	Ischemic CAD potential	CAD Hx: Chest pain CHF Sx	Heart rate and rhythm, S_3, rales	ECG with stress
GI	Aspiration potential	GE junction integrity by Hx of regurgitation Nighttime cough Sour nighttime taste	Evaluate nutritional status	Esophagoscopy Examination of larynx
CNS	Sleep dysfunction due to obstruction	Sleep Hx	CNS exam	MRI
RESP	Upper airway obstruction due to tumor	Tumor Hx	Wheezing Cyanosis Clubbing	Flow-volume loop, ABGs

Key Reference: Ovassapian A. *Fiberoptic endoscopy and the difficult airway.* 2nd ed. Philadelphia: Lippincott-Raven. 1996

Perioperative Management

Preoperative Preparation

- Depends on indication
  - If laryngeal tumors, evaluate for degree of airway compromise
  - If stridor present, closely observe, preferably in ICU. Humidified O_2 and steroids may be given to avoid severe and/or complete airway obstruction.

Monitoring

- Routine

Anesthetic Technique

- Topical anesthesia and light sedation for most adults and some children
- General anesthesia with laryngeal mask airway in children.
- Laryngeal mask airway provides open airway and easy access for bronchoscope
- Short-acting IV drugs (e.g., alfentanil, midazolam, esmolol) may provide analgesia and attenuate CV response to rigid laryngoscopy
- Blood loss negligible

Postoperative Concerns

- CV hyperactivity
- Status of upper airway

Anticipated Problems/Concerns

- Hypoxemia in immediate postop period
- Acute ventilatory failure

Bronchoscopy, Rigid

Andranik Ovassapian

Risk

- First performed by Killian in 1895. Its use has declined continuously after introduction of fiberoptic bronchoscope.
- Performed for removal of foreign body, massive hemoptysis, to dilate tracheobronchial strictures, laser resection of airway tumors, and stent placement

Perioperative Risks

- Depends on nature of disease
- Cardiac arrhythmias, hypoxemia, increased BP and HR, myocardial infarction
- Incidence of reintubation reported at 0.39% when panendoscopy performed for upper airway path

Worry About

- Ventilation, oxygenation in pts with chronic lung disease, airway pathology
- Endoscopist, anesthesiologist share airway, complicating ventilatory management
- Massive hemorrhage
- Postbronchoscopy ventilatory failure

Overview

- Assoc with severe CV response manifested with tachycardia, Htn
- Bleeding from biopsy site could be troublesome
- Level of the lesion critical
- Ventilation performed through side arm
- Requires communication with surgeon throughout procedure

ICD-9-CM Code: 146.9 (Oropharyngeal cancer)

Indications and Usual Treatment

- Removal of foreign bodies
- Management of major hemoptysis
- Establishing emergency airway
- Dilation of tracheobronchial stricture
- Laser resection of airway tumors
- Bronchoscopy in infants, small children
- Bronchoscopy, esophagoscopy, laryngoscopy for staging of oropharyngolaryngeal malignant lesions
- Biopsy of endobronchial lesion
- Evaluation of the lower airway
- Placement of stent

ASSESSMENT POINTS

System	Effect	Assessment by Hx	PE	Test
HEENT	Airway compromise	Wheezing, stridor	Lung, airway exam	CXR
CARDIO		Exercise intolerance, angina, Hx of CV disease	S_3, rales	ECG Stress test
RESP		Wheezing, exercise tolerance impairment, Hx of smoking	Clubbing, cyanosis, wheezing	PFTs ABGs CXR
AIRWAY	Tumors Infections Compressions	SOB Hemoptysis	Wheezing Use of accessory muscles	X-ray studies PFTs ABGs

Key Reference: Morris IR. Anesthesia and airway management of laryngoscopy and bronchoscopy. In: Hagberg C, ed. *Benumof's airway management*. 2nd ed. Philadelphia: Mosby; 2007:859–888.

Perioperative Management

- Usually done as outpatient procedure with pt in sitting or supine position
- Antisialagogue (glycopyrrolate 0.2 mg IV or 0.4 mg IM) to minimize secretions, enhance topical anesthesia of airway
- Appropriate size bronchoscope, ancillary equipment should be available

Monitoring

- Routine

Anesthetic Technique

- Usually done under sedation, topical anesthesia
- Lidocaine 4% spray of oropharynx followed by translaryngeal injection of 3 mL 4% lidocaine provides excellent topical anesthesia

- Spray-as-you-go technique used to anesthetize rest of bronchial tree
- General anesthesia for children
- Short-acting IV drugs used during fiberoptic bronchoscopy
- Jet ventilation can be applied through fiberscope but not commonly practiced

Postoperative Concerns

- Hypoxemia treated with supplemental O_2
- Irritable airway, coughing, tachycardia, Htn common during early recovery
- Bleeding from biopsy site may necessitate repeating the procedure

Anticipated Problems/Concerns

- Inadequate ventilation, hypoxemia with heavy sedation
- Airway obstruction, hypoxemia, barotrauma of lungs possible
- Consider precautions to minimize fire hazards during laser surgery

Burr Hole

Risk

- Often indicated for cranial decompression, esp. traumatic brain injury
- Annually, 470,000 people sustain traumatic brain injury.

Perioperative Risks

- Depending on pathology and severity of injury, mortality ranges 24–50%.

Worry About

- Proper maintenance of CPP (MAP-ICP)
- Compromised CBF because of altered cerebral autoregulation

- If trauma pt, worry about other injuries, esp. assoc cervical spine injury (2–5%)
- Air embolism, esp. if burr hole over or near major sinus.
- If traumatic brain injury, prevention of 2° injury.

Overview

- Burr hole often placed to decompress hematoma. Two major types: Subdural hematoma (24% of closed head injuries) is a crescent-shaped lesion resulting from torn bridging veins. Epidural hematoma (6% of CHI) is a biconvex lesion arising from arterial bleeding (usually middle meningeal artery).

- Improved pt survival if early surgical evacuation
- Depending on pt's level of consciousness and urgency, Burr hole may be performed with local or MAC (monitored anesthetic care) or under general anesthesia.

Indications and Usual Treatment

- Hematoma evacuation
- Pneumocephalus and hydrocephalus evacuation
- Drainage suprasellar cysts
- Placement of intraventricular drain
- Evacuation subdural empyemas
- EEG electrode placement

ASSESSMENT POINTS

System	Effect	Assessment by Hx	PE	Test
HEENT	C-spine injury creating difficult airway	Mechanism of injury (blunt vs. penetrating)	Airway exam but assume unstable neck	CT, C-spine series
CARDIO	Autonomic dysfunction, blunt chest trauma concerns (PTX, hemothorax), pre-existing cardiac arrhythmias	Hx atrial fibrillation requiring anticoagulation	Auscultation	CXR, EKG
RESP	Brainstem injury, Cushing's reflex, blunt chest trauma concerns (PTX, hemothorax)	Abn respiration	Bilateral breath sounds, wheezing	ABGs, pulse oximetry, CXR
HEME	Anemia may compromise cerebral O_2 delivery	Hx anticoagulation (warfarin)		CBC, PT/INR, plts
GU	ARF due to hypotension. Electrolyte abn—hyperkalemia, hyponatremia, hyperglycemia)	Recent osmotic diuretic, hypertonic saline, steroid administration		Na^+, K^+, BUN, Cr, serum, urine osmolality
CNS	Impaired LOC, increased ICP	Glasgow coma scale assessment	Gross neuro exam, CN exam, pupil exam	CT, MRI

Key Reference: Gopinath SP, Robertson CS. Management of severe head injury. In: Cottrel JE, Smith DS, eds. *Anesthesia and neurosurgery.* 3rd ed. St. Louis: Mosby–Year Book; 2001:663–691.

Perioperative Management

Preoperative Preparation

- CT/MRI scans to confirm side of lesion. Assess midline shift and ventricular compression.
- Routine medical management: Avoid hypoxemia, hypotension, hypercapnia. Elevation of head 15–30 degrees, mannitol (0.25–1 g/kg), neutral head position, antibiotics.
- Prophylactic hyperventilation (PaCO$_2$ of 25 mm Hg or less) is not recommended.
- Correct underlying coagulopathy, esp. if Hx of warfarin.

Anesthetic Technique

- Local anesthesia, MAC, or GA

Monitoring

- Consider large-bore IV access. Central line may be necessary if mannitol, hypertonic saline indicated.
- Consider arterial line, esp. if hyperventilation needed.
- Consider ICP monitoring, Foley catheter (esp. if osmotic diuretics administered).
- Nasal ETCO$_2$ monitoring with local/MAC technique.

Airway

- If trauma pt, RSI and inline stabilization for presumed C-spine injury.
- Since airway is not easily accessible, ensure ETT secured well.

Induction/Maintenance

- Avoid increased ICP. Avoid coughing due to light anesthesia. Turning head may obstruct venous drainage. Consider elevation HOB 30 degrees. If severe increased ICP, consider total IV anesthetic.
- Prepare for increased HR and BP during intubation and possible pin placement. Consider propofol, increased inhalational agent, and beta blockade.
- Hyperventilation should be limited in first 24 hr from injury because of decreased CBF, esp. if hypoxemia and hypotension also present.
- Avoid long-acting opioids to facilitate prompt neuro exam.
- Avoid secondary insult—hypoxia, hypercarbia, hyperglycemia.

Surgical Stages

Dissection

- Risk of accidentally tearing dura

- Beware sudden bleeding if sinus or middle meningeal artery encountered.
- Air embolism risk increased if venous sinus encountered and elevated HOB

Definitive Surgery

- Bradycardia if brainstem herniating.
- Observe surgical site for excessive brain swelling. Steroids not indicated.

Closure/Postoperative Considerations

- Prompt neuro exam to assist in management in ICU as well as determine need for additional surgery
- Low threshold to remain intubated if unable to assess CNS status
- EBL 50–200 mL

Anticipated Problems/Concerns

- Still concern for intracranial Htn, despite Burr hole drainage.
- Appropriate sedation to prevent postop Htn (>160 mm Hg) leading to increased CBF, ICP, bleeding, and cerebral edema
- Strongly consider specialized neuro ICU to detect neurologic changes.

PROCEDURES

Bypass, Femoral-Femoral

Alexandru Gottlieb

Risk

- Incidence in USA; ~10,000/y, number is decreasing; number of aortic and iliac stents is increasing.

Perioperative Risks

- Related to diffuse arteriosclerosis, CV disease
- Periop MI 3–10%
- Mostly geriatric pts with age-related risk factors and accompanying diseases: DM, COPD, Htn, renovascular
- Potential for improvement and/or more distal occlusion with risk of need for amputation

Worry About

- Thrombosis and embolism of leg or graft
- Blood loss

- The groin is considered a dirty location, rendering prosthetic graft infection relatively common

Overview

- Femoral-femoral bypass is suggested for pts too risky to undergo abd procedure (ABI, ABF)
- Done with prosthetic graft. This is a nonanatomic graft that might be fed by a nonoptimal vessel.
- Regional anesthesia can be beneficial in its effect on coagulation and graft patency
- Procedure sometimes can be performed also under monitored anesthesia care

ICD-9-CM Code: 440.2x (Atherosclerosis, Peripheral)

Indications and Usual Treatment

- An extra-anatomic procedure
- Performed in pts with lower extremity ischemia, gangrene, or severe short-distance claudication; in one limb more than the other
- Replace the standard anatomic bypass of ABI or ABF in pts with the following conditions:
  - S/P abd procedure
  - S/P extensive abd radiation
  - Intestinal stoma
  - Abd infection
  - Poor medical condition
  - S/P iliac: Aortic stent graft
  - Ischemic limb from thoracic dissection

ASSESSMENT POINTS

System	Effect	Assessment by Hx	PE	Test
RESP	High incidence of lung disease that could have caused this procedure to be selected	Smoking, chronic cough, dyspnea	Chest exam, wheezing, clubbing cyanosis	CXR, ABGs, spirometry
CARDIO	High incidence of CAD, myocardial ischemia, and/or infarction	Angina, MI, CHF, dysrhythmia, PCI (metallic/DE stents), CABG, exercise tolerance, activity level Anticoagulants Tx ? Antiplatelet Tx ?	Chest auscultation, VS	ECG, stress ECHO, dipyridamole, thallium or dobutamine test Cardiac cath Anticoagulation Antiplatelet
	Chronic HTN	BP Rx, drug interaction, LVH	BP	ECG, CXR, retinal funduscopy
RENAL	Renal insufficiency 2° to age, arteriosclerosis, and multiple dye studies	Hx edema and intolerance to salt load	Edema, anuria	Urea, Cr, electrolyts
CNS	Possible carotid disease	Syncope, stroke, or TIAs	Neuro exam Carotid bruit	Carotid angiogram, CT, MRI
ENDO	DM	Infections, stress/gestational DM, polydipsia, polyuria, coma/stupor, abn glucose	Skin infections	CNS exam, UO; glucose
HEME	Periop heparin, t-PA, or aspirin	Petechiae, nasal bleed	Petechiae or bruising	PT, PTT, ACT

Key Reference: Ellis JE, Roizen MF, Mantha S, Tzeng G, Desai T. Anesthesia for vascular surgery. In: Barash PG, Cullen BF, Stoelting RK, eds. *Clinical anesthesia*, Philadelphia: Lippincott Williams & Wilkins; 2000:929–968.

Perioperative Management

Perioperative Evaluation

- A detailed H & P, drug Hx, evaluation of CV status
- Dysrhythmias, CAD, CHF
- Hypertensive and valvular heart disease
- Noninvasive and invasive cardiac evaluation tests such as cardiac cath

Anesthetic Techniques

- General anesthesia, regional anesthesia, or MAC. Regional anesthesia preferred by some clinicians because of lack of systemic effect on the resp, CV, and GI systems. There is some positive effect of regional anesthesia on coagulation, preserving fibrinolysis and graft patency.

Monitoring

- ECG, arterial BP, UO
- Consider CVP or PA line in pts with severe CAD or severely ↓ EF.
- Monitoring for myocardial ischemia; ECG with continuous 3-lead ST-segment analysis, PA catheter, or TEE
- Monitoring of vol replacement: CO, CVP, PAOP, or with TEE

Surgical Stages

- Groin area should be thoroughly prepped and draped; procedure can be lengthy, 2–4 hr. Minimal third space or blood loss.
- Avoid decrease in BP—femoral-femoral bypass can thrombose easily with lack of flow

Postoperative Period

- Mild postop pain: 5–7
- Ischemic leg pain should improve
- Epidural extended for postop pain control

Anticipated Problems/Concerns

- High incidence of periop cardiac and resp complications
- Inappropriate blood flow from donor side tends to make the bypass not functional
- Infection of prosthetic graft at the groin is relatively frequent, compared to other prosthetic graft locations
- If the femoral-femoral bypass is not functional, a bypass such as axillary femoral-femoral or amputation may be needed

Bypass Graft Procedure, Infrainguinal

R. Yan McRae
Grace L. Chien

Risk

• 0.4–14% prevalence of intermittent claudication in adults; occurs most frequently in individuals age 50–75 y old; peripheral vascular disease asymptomatic in >50% of pts, identified only by noninvasive testing (ankle/brachial index; ABI)
• Co-existing conditions commonly incl: tobacco use, Htn, diabetes, CAD, COPD, renal insufficiency.

Perioperative Risks

• Mortality: 5.8% at 30 d, 16% at 1 y; approx half of periop deaths due to cardiac complications
• Common morbidity: 2–6.5% incidence of periop myocardial infarction; respiratory complications; poor wound healing

Worry About

• Reperfusion syndrome after prolonged ischemia: Hyperkalemia, metabolic acidosis, hypotension, transient increase of O_2 consumption, hypothermia
• Intra- and periop cardiac complications: Myocardial ischemia, myocardial infarction, dysrhythmias, CHF
• Graft thrombosis/failure
• Wound healing incl need for periop glycemic control

Overview

• Determine urgency of surgery (see Indications below)
• Consider the need for myocardial revascularization prior to infrainguinal revascularization (see Coronary Artery Revascularization Prophylaxis [**CARP**] Trial) if pt has an indication for myocardial revascularization based on ACC/AHA 2007 guidelines on periop evaluation for noncardiac surgery.
• Reduce risk of periop thrombosis in pre-existing coronary or vascular stents, or new graft, through coordinated anesthetic and surgical plan for periop antiplatelet or anticoagulant therapies
• Reduce periop risk of cardiac complications through initiation and/or continued periop administration of beta-blocker, clonidine, and/or statin therapy
• Manage intraop hemodynamics and hematocrit to maintain adequate myocardial O_2 supply/demand matching
• Provide tight glycemic control

• No definitive benefit of regional anesthetic over general anesthetic in reducing cardiac complication or increasing graft patency rates

Indications and Usual Treatment

• Two primary indications:
  • Claudication: Exercise-induced leg pain relieved with rest. Initially treated with trial of lifestyle modification, smoking cessation, exercise and medical management. Surgery primarily to improve quality of life, done when anatomy suggests possible durable, long lasting repair. Elective nature of procedure allows careful preop evaluation and treatment to reduce periop morbidity and mortality.
  • Critical limb ischemia defined as persistent, recurring ischemic rest pain. Ankle systolic pressures usually lower than 50 mmHg +/- visible tissue damage. Generally requires intervention despite operative risks and graft failure risks. Surgery may briefly be delayed to optimize pts with CHF, hemodialysis for volume or hyperkalemic issues, anticoagulation management, etc.

ASSESSMENT POINTS

System	Effect	Assessment by HX	PE	Test
CARDIO	CAD, previous MI, CHF, arrhythmias, upper extremity PVD	Angina, orthopnea, prior stents and stent types	Pedal edema, S_3, murmurs, discordant BP in arms	ECG, CXR, noninvasive cardiac testing, cardiac cath
RESP	COPD, pulm edema	Dyspnea, S_4 gallop	Crackles or wheezes, barrel chest	CXR/CT, PFTs, ABG
Renal	CRI, dialysis	Htn, timing of most recent dialysis, recent/anticipated IV contrast load	Fistula patency, edema, dyspnea	K+, BUN, creatinine
CNS	Carotid and cerebral atherosclerosis	Amaurosis fugax, TIA, stroke	Neurologic deficits, carotid bruits	Neuro exam, carotid US, CT/MRI

Key Reference: Norris EJ. Anesthesia for vascular surgery. In: Miller RD, ed. *Miller's anesthesia*. 6th ed. Philadelphia: Elsevier Churchill Livingstone; 2005:2051–2125.

Perioperative Management

Preoperative Preparation

• Evaluate severity of CV, pulm and other morbidities, and determine if surgery should be delayed for additional treatments or interventions to reduce surgical risks.
• Evaluate if pt is a candidate for regional technique based on coagulation issues, surgical site(s), anticipated length of procedure, and pt preference and/or tolerance. Carefully integrate the **ASRA consensus statement** for anticoagulated pts and the surgeon's anti-platelet and periop anticoagulation plans with any regional anesthetic plans.
• Ensure proper degree of beta-blockade, proper glycemic control, and need/availability of blood products.
• If a groin incision is to be used, then consider if prophylactic antibiotic coverage should be expanded to incl expected skin flora plus gram negative bacteria found in groin locations.

Monitoring

• Invasive monitoring should be guided by severity of co-existing diseases and not by procedure itself. Monitoring need may range from good peripheral IV access and ASA standard monitors only up to the addition of arterial line, CVP, PA catheter or TEE depending primarily on cardiac concerns.

Anesthetic Technique/Induction

A general or regional anesthetic may be appropriate and needs to be tailored to each individual pt and procedure. Spinal anesthetic is effective if expected operative times permit. Epidural allows easier control of duration of block and postop analgesia but postop anti-coagulation plans must be considered.

If a general anesthetic is chosen then hemodynamic stability at induction is important 2° to co-existing CAD, Htn, and CHF.

Surgical Stages

Dissection

• Often a very stimulating procedure at beginning due to long incisions and dissection but maintenance period may have much lower anesthetic requirements.
• Heparin usually given just prior to arterial clamping.

Arterial Clamping

• Clamping of artery, unlike more proximal arterial clamping, usually has little effect on overall BP or cardiac afterload.
• Blood loss usually well controlled, however, can be difficult to detect or quantify 2° to distant surgical sites and loss into absorbent drapes.
• Important to ensure adequate normovolemia, Hct and pt temp before a cold, ischemic leg is unclamped.

Arterial Unclamping

• Hypotension may occur when reperfusion of the ischemic limb allows venous return of acidic, hyperkalemic blood and various metabolic waste products.
• Possible hyperkalemia with reperfusion is esp. a concern in the settings of renal failure or extremely long ischemic time.
• Risk of increased blood loss at anastomosis sites at time of reperfusion
• Heparin reversal with protamine creates chance of significant allergic reaction
• Preparation for unclamping generally involves brief increase in minute ventilation, increase percentage O_2 delivered and ready availability of inotropic/pressor support.

Postoperative Considerations

• Important to continue tight BP and HR control in postop period as this is time most cardiac complications occur; risk peaking in postop d 2–3.
• Shivering after anesthesia 2° to hypothermia or as side effect of anesthesia should be prevented or treated to avoid increased metabolic demands on the cardiac system.
• Post-extubation pulm status may be compromised 2° to COPD and/or atelectasis resulting from prolonged GA.

• Disposition to ICU versus ward is highly dependent on need for graft/limb monitoring, and on preop cardiac and pulm status. Pt may require ICU or step-down unit care to monitor for cardiac ischemia or arrhythmias.

Anticipated Problems/Concerns

• Induction of general anesthetic or neuroaxial blockade may be assoc with profound hypotension $2°$ to a relative volume contraction due to chronic Htn or as an interaction of antihypertensive medications (e.g., ACE inhibitors, beta blockers) with the anesthetized state.

• Rebound tachycardia $2°$ to beta-blocker withdrawal must be avoided through peri- and intraop use of beta-blockers. However caution is advised as the POISE trial has recently demonstrated that acute high doses of beta-blockers may increase risk of stroke and death.

Carcinoid, Excision of

Mark Twite
Aris Sophocles

Risk

- Incidence: 1.5 cases/100,000/y; 1/300 appendectomies; 1/2500 proctoscopic exams
- Race and gender predominance: None
- Age with highest incidence: Fourth and fifth decades

Perioperative Risks

- The presence of carcinoid heart disease and high urinary 5-HIAA levels are significant risk factors for periop complications incl death
- 1.5–10% periop mortality reported before use of somatostatin analogue

Worry About

- CV: Carcinoid crisis (CV collapse 2/2 release of vasoactive mediators)
- Respiratory: Bronchospasm. Bronchial tumor leads to compression and/or obstruction of bronchi.
- Cardiac: Right heart involvement leads to tricuspid insufficiency or pulmonic valve stenosis.
- Autonomic: Stimulation (pain, hypercarbia, hypothermia) or sympathomimetics leading to tumor mediator release and carcinoid crisis
- GI: Increased motility and secretion of H_2O, NaCl, and K+ leading to fluid and electrolyte abn. Midgut (ileal, jejunal) carcinoids leading to fibrosis of mesentery. GI tumor leading to compression and/or obstruction of small bowel.

Overview

Pathophysiology

- Slow-growing malignancies capable of metastases. Derived from APUD cells of embryonic neuroectoderm capable of synthesizing and secreting peptide hormones and monoamines, most commonly serotonin (5-HT). Other neurohumoral agents involved in carcinoid syndrome incl dopamine, histamine, bradykinin, kallikrein, prostaglandins, gastrin, corticotropin, neuron-specific enolace, substance P, neurotensin, vasoactive intestinal peptide, and somatostatin.
- 75% originate in GI tract (from esophagus to rectum). Most common site is the appendix (rarely metastasize or produce carcinoid syndrome). Tumors in ileocecal region have highest incidence of metastases. Carcinoid tumors have also been reported to arise from lung, head and neck, gonads, breasts, and urinary tract. The liver is the most common site for metastases.
- Carcinoid syndrome is usually assoc with ileal carcinoid tumors that have metastasized to the liver (hypothesized that metastasis impair hepatic metabolism of mediators released by the tumor) or from a 1° tumor draining into the systemic circulation.
- 20–40% of pts with carcinoid syndrome have carcinoid heart disease. Vasoactive substances released by the tumor cause fibrosis of the heart valves leading to pulmonic stenosis, tricuspid insufficiency, and/or myocardial plaque formation. (Cardiac involvement is usually right-sided because mediators are cleared or inactivated in the lungs before reaching the left side of heart.)

Presentation

- Pts with nonfunctional tumors (or whose tumor mediators are inactivated by the liver) present with pain, GI bleeding, or intestinal obstruction
- Pts with carcinoid syndrome present with flushing 74%, intestinal hypermotility 68%, cardiac symptoms 41%, and wheezing 18%. Only 7% of pts with a carcinoid tumor have carcinoid syndrome.

Prognosis

- Related more to location and size of 1° than to pathologic findings
- Metastases rare if tumor <1 cm and more common if tumor >2 cm
- Pts with noninvasive appendiceal, rectal tumors <2 cm have 5-y survival rates near 100%; if tumor is >2 cm, survival declines to 40%; with liver metastases, 5-y survival 21–42%

ICD-9-CM Codes: 199.1 (Tumor); 259.2 (Syndrome)

Indications and Usual Treatment

- Indications for operation: 1° should be treated with resection regardless of metastases.
- Common procedures: Tumor debulking, relief of intestinal obstruction, "appendicitis," liver resection or transplantation for hepatic metastases, heart valve replacement, and thoracic surgeries for resection of lung or bronchial carcinoids
- Surgery only potentially curative Rx. With distant metastases, cure by resecting all tumor. When resection not possible, palliative procedures may be needed for obstruction or to debulk tumor, decreasing quantity of vasoactive peptides released, or replace heart valves.
- Medical Rx: Octreotide, a somatostatin analogue, inhibits synthesis, release, and binding of vasoactive peptides; can control Sx, retard tumor growth, and prolong survival by as much as 3 y. Steroids have been effective for treating the symptoms of bronchial carcinoid tumors.

ASSESSMENT POINTS

System	Effect	Assessment by Hx	PE	Test
CARDIO	Carcinoid crisis, right heart valve involvement, hemodynamic instability (usually hypotension), 5-HT has indirect positive chronotropic and ionotropic effects (mediated by norepinephrine) Arrhythmias	Hx carcinoid syndrome, fatigue, ascites, edema	Hemodynamic collapse; JVD, murmur, pulse	ABGs ECHO EKG
RESP	Bronchospasm, bronchial obstruction	SOB	Wheezing	O_2 sat
GI	Diarrhea +/- electrolyte disturbances	Abd pain, wt loss	Flushing	Electrolytes, urinary 5-HIAA
ENDO	10% MEN (hyperplasia of parathyroid, pancreas, pituitary) hyperglycemia	Ulcers, renal calculi	Lipomas	Ca^{2+}, PO_4^{2-}, prolactin, gastrin, blood glucose
CNS	Postop sedation (2/2 5-HT)			
NUTRITION	Hypoproteinemia and niacin deficiency (Pellagra) 2/2 tryptophan depletion	Diarrhea	Dermatitis, dementia	Serum protein Rx niacin

Key Reference: Holdcroft A. Hormones and the gut. *Br J Anaesth.* 2000;85(1):58–68.

Operative Management

Preoperative Preparation

- Evaluate for carcinoid syndrome and the extent of assoc multisystem disease: Urinary 5-HIAA (5-HT metabolite), imagining of 1° tumor and metastases (CT, MRI, abd US, barium GI x-ray films, radionuclide scans) echo to evaluate for carcinoid heart disease, CXR or broncoscopy for suspected bronchial carcinoids
- Correct CV instability, volume depletion, bronchospasm, hyperglycemia, and hypoproteinemia
- Premedication (aimed at minimizing tumor mediator release or activity): First line octreotide 100 ug SC (peak level in 30 min and half-life of 100 min) followed by octreotide infusion 50 µg/hr or 25–50 µg bolus prn and before tumor manipulation. Second-line drugs incl H1 & H2 receptor blockers, aprotinin, ketanserin, cyproheptadine. Consider endocarditis prophylaxis for pts with significant carcinoid heart disease.
- Avoid triggers of mediator release (anxiety, pain, hypoxia, hypercarbia, tumor compression) and drugs that cause histamine or catecholamine release.

Monitoring

- Arterial catheter
- Consider CVP cath for vol monitoring (substitute PA cath or TEE if valvular lesions)

Airway

- Gastric emptying may be delayed.
- Occasional laryngeal tumors

Anesthesia Technique

- Induction/maintenance: Etomidate or propofol appropriate for induction, maintenance with volatile agent (isoflurane)
- Paralysis: Caution with succinylcholine (may cause fasciculation of abd wall leading to mechanical compression of tumor and release of vasoactive peptides). Succinylcholine, atracurium, cisatracurium, and mivacurium stimulate the release of histamine.
- Analgesia: First line is fentanyl. Caution with morphine and meperidine, which stimulate the release of histamine, and light sedation, which increases the sympathetic response.
- Regional: With a neuraxial regional anesthetic, hypotension and reflex sympathetic stimulation can be minimized using titratable techniques such as epidural rather than spinal anesthesia.

- Carcinoid crisis:
  - Stop manipulation of tumor, 100% O₂, reduce concentration of volatile anesthetics if hypotensive, restore intravascular volume, administer drugs to decrease mediator release and effect
  - Rx: First line is octreotide, which is effective in controlling flushing, hypotension, diarrhea, and bronchospasm in 75% of pts (80% of tumors have somatostatin receptors.) Second-line therapies incl drugs with rapid onset and brief clinical effect for hemodynamic instability (phentolamine, esmolol, and phenylephrine) vasopressin and angiotensin for refractory hypotension, ketanserin (a 5-HT antagonist for Htn) H1 & H2 blockers, and aprotinin (inhibitor of kallikrein)
  - Avoid direct sympathomimetics (epinephrine, norepinephrine), drugs that cause reflex sympathetic stimulation 2/2 peripheral vasodilatation (nitroprusside) and histamine-releasing drugs (thiopental, succinylcholine, atracurium, cis-atracurium, mivacurium, morphine, merperidine)
- Bronchospasm
  - Usually responds to octreotide. Use corticosteroids, inhaled ipratropium bromide, and antihistamines as adjuvants.
  - Avoid beta-2 agonists, theophylline, and epinephrine, which can exacerbate bronchospasm.

Surgical Stages

- Skin incision-tumor resection
- Sympathetic and/or mechanical stimulation incl skin preparation, incision, and manipulation of tumor may release vasoactive substances leading to carcinoid crisis.
- Dissection may be extensive if small-bowel fibrosis has occurred.
- En bloc resection of ileal carcinoids justified due to frequent presence of multiple tumors

Closure and Postoperative Considerations

- About one third of pts with advanced (hepatic) disease require blood transfusions intraop
- Postop PCA usual
- SQ octreotide resumed with IV supplement for hypotensive episodes
- Pain score depends on location: abd 4–7

Anticipated Problems/Concerns

- Carcinoid crisis can result in abrupt CV collapse or severe bronchospasm
- When correcting for low cardiac output 2/2 tricuspid insufficiency, avoid drugs that increase pulm vascular resistance such as vasopressin and angiotensin. Acidosis, hypercapnia, and hypothermia can also increase pulm vascular resistance and should be avoided.

Cardiopulmonary Bypass (CPB)

Veronica A. Matei

Risk

- Over 2,000,000 CPB procedures are performed annually worldwide.

Perioperative Risks

- Dependent on pt preop status, emergent institution of CPB, duration of CPB
- Cardiac, renal, resp, and CNS complications contribute to CPB morbidity.
- Variable degrees of renal and neurologic deficits are common post-CPB. Incidence of stroke is 5%. Incidence of acute renal failure requiring dialysis is 4%.

Worry About

- Potential catastrophic events during CPB: Inadequate coagulation with clotting of CPB machine components, circuit disconnection with massive air embolism and /or exsanguination
- Communication among surgeons, perfusionist, and anesthesiologist is of vital importance.

Overview

- CPB technology temporarily replaces cardiac and pulm functions during surgery. CPB is a form of extracorporeal circulation.
- Full CPB requires an oxygenator and a blood pump. Systemic venous blood is drained (via venous canulla) to a venous reservoir. From the reservoir, the blood is pumped through an oxygenator and then returned (via arterial cannula) to the arterial system.
- Partial CPB requires a blood pump that supports only a portion of the body (usually the infra-diaphragmatic portion). The oxygenation can be accomplished by a mechanical oxygenator (femoral vein to femoral artery partial CPB) or by pt's lungs (left atrium to femoral artery partial CPB)

ICD-9-CM Code: 39.61

Indications

- Heart and great vessels surgery: CABG, valve surgery, heart transplant, congenital heart defects surgery, repair of aortic or cerebral aneurysms, removal of intracardiac and great vessel masses, pulm thromboendarterectomy
- Treatment of severe hypothermia
- Local anesthetic toxicity (bupivicaine)

ASSESSMENT POINTS

System	Effect	Assessment by Hx	PE	Test
CARDIO	Severity of cardiac disease dictates pre/post CPB management	Angina, CHF, arrhythmias, exercise tolerance	Cardiac	ECG, ECHO, cardiac cath
RESP	Prior resp dysfunction ↑ risk of "pump lungs"	Smoking Hx, dyspnea	Resp	CXR, PFTs, ABG
ENDO	CPB-induced hormonal stress response	Diabetes		Blood glucose
HEME	Prior anemia, plt dysfunction or coagulopathy ↑ chance for blood products transfusion pre/post CPB	Hx of bleeding disorders, antiplatelet or anticoagulant medication use		Ht, PT/INR, PTT, plt count
RENAL	Prior renal dysfunction ↑ risk of renal complications post CPB	Hx of renal dysfunction, diuretic use		BUN, Cr, UA, FeNa
CNS	Prior CVA/TIA ↑ risk of neurologic complications post CPB	Hx of CVA, TIA	Neuro exam	Carotid US

Key Reference: Kaplan JA, ed. *Cardiac anesthesia*. 5th ed. Philadelphia: Saunders; 2006:893–935.

Perioperative Management

Preoperative Preparation

- Assess co-existing morbidities and define anesthetic goals for individual cases.

Monitoring

- Standard ASA monitors (temp is monitored at multiple simultaneous sites)
- Invasive arterial pressure monitoring essential
- Large-bore vascular access mandatory. Central vascular access preferred for administration of vasoactive drugs.
- Laboratory parameters: Blood gases, Hct, serum potassium, ionized calcium, glucose measurement
- Adequacy of anticoagulation (ACT goal >400 sec)
- CVP. PAC if ventricular function compromised (LVEF <35%) or pulm Htn
- Cardiac output (via PAC or TEE), UO (goal >1 mL/kg/hr)
- Intraoperative TEE
- Additional monitoring during CPB: Pump flow rate, venous reservoir level, arterial inflow line pressure, blood and myocardial temp, in-line (arterial and venous) O_2 sat
- Surgical field monitoring essential

Anesthetic Technique/Induction

- All variations of carefully conducted anesthesia techniques can be employed.

Surgical Stages

- Skin incision, sternotomy, and pericardiectomy are stages of intense stimulation. Titration of anesthetic agents is necessary to avoid tachycardia and Htn
- Heparinization, ACT check
- Cannulation
- Arterial cannulation sites: Proximal aorta, femoral artery, axillary artery, descending aorta, apex of the heart. Reduce systemic BP (to 90–100 mmHg) during cannulation to prevent aortic dissection. Inspect the cannula for bubbles to avoid air embolism.
- Venous cannulation sites: Right atrium, SVC and IVC, femoral vein.
- Manipulation of the heart during venous cannulation can result in hypotension and dysrrhythmias
- CPB initiation: Venous return should be quickly assessed. If venous reservoir empties, massive air-embolism can occur.
- Hypotension 2° to hemodilution is frequent on CPB start. If persistent hypotension, rule out aortic dissection.
- Aortic cross-clamp placement
- Institution of hypothermia: Mild hypothermia (28C), deep hypothermia to 16–18C (deep hypothermic arrest) or maintenance of normothermia (descending thoracic aorta surgery).
- Delivery of cardioplegia through special cannulae inserted in aortic root (antegrade delivery), in coronary sinus (retrograde delivery), in coronary ostia, or in bypass grafts.
- Ventricular distension and electrical activity on ECG are evidence of poor myocardial protection and possible difficult separation from CPB
- Rewarming: Temp gradients should not exceed 10–12 C.
- Light anesthesia during this critical period can result in awareness and recall.
- Checklist for separation from CPB
  - Core temp >36.5 C
  - Stable HR and/or rhythm
  - Adequate de-airing of left heart (TEE)
  - Mechanical ventilation resumed
  - Acceptable labs
  - No bleeding at major sites (grafts, suture lines)
- Reversal of anticoagulation with protamine, ACT check. Watch for protamine-related adverse hemodynamic effects (pulm Htn, hypotension)
- Chest closure: Hemodynamic (hypotension) and /or ventilation disturbances (increased peak airway pressures) 2° to increased intrathoracic pressure
- Continued vigilance is mandatory after completion of procedure, particularly during transport to recovery room or ICU.

Anticipated Problems/Concerns

- Re-do surgery can result in massive bleeding during sternotomy. In some cases, initiation of CPB (via femoral-femoral cannulation) is achieved before sternotomy
- Heparin is an essential drug for CPB. For patient with Hx of HIT, alternative drugs are used for systemic anticoagulation.
- Controversies incl the use of pulsatile vs. non-pulsatile flow during CBP, acceptable arterial pressure during CPB, blood gas management (alpha-stat vs. pH-stat), need for routine use of PACs, BIS monitoring, optimal site for temp monitoring.

Cardioversion

Michael Hall
Andrew Oken

Risk

- Cardioversion risks vary and are influenced by the hemodynamic status of the pt, the underlying cardiac rhythm, whether the procedure is elective, urgent or emergent, and the pt's underlying co-morbidities.
- Mortality: 0.1% (elective cardioversion)
- Risks with cardioversion for atrial fibrillation
  - Embolic event 2% (increased risk with mitral valve disease)
  - Acute pulm edema: 1%
  - More serious arrhythmia: 1%
  - Myocardial damage: Unknown
  - Thermal injury: <15% first degree, 2% second degree.

Cardioversion Concerns

- Neurologic: Cardioembolic event and/or atrial clot (approx 2%)
- Pulmonary: Aspiration precautions, airway compromise, possible need for intubation
- CV: Arrhythmia, myocardial ischemia, CHF, failure to convert, hemodynamic instability: (large atrial size, mitral regurg, and duration of AFib all predict failure to respond to cardioversion)
- Endocrine: AFib from hyperthyroidism and other hyperadrenergic states
- GI: Aspiration precautions
- Hematologic: Need for anticoagulation?
- Laboratory: Tests as indicated from H & P, digitalis toxicity, electrolytes, etc.
- Other: Recall

Overview

- Brief procedure where either electrically or chemically an attempt is made to convert an abn heart rhythm to a normal rhythm. Electrical cardioversion is usually done for atrial fibrillation; however it can also be done for a flutter, supraventricular tachycardia, and ventricular tachycardia.
- Cardioversion from atrial flutter and v. tach usually requires a small amount of energy. Atrial fibrillation and ventricular fibrillation usually require a larger number of muscle fibers to be depolarized and thus a larger amount of energy.
- For supraventricular arrhythmias, cardioversion should be synchronized and occur during the R wave of the QRS cycle to prevent depolarization during the vulnerable period of the ventricle which could lead to a more unstable arrhythmia.
- Defibrillators currently used typically deliver energy in a variety of waveforms generally classified as monophasic or biphasic. Biphasic energy delivery requires lower energies and is assoc with greater first shock efficacy as compared with monophasic defibrillation. Monophasic defibrillation however is still in common use and quite effective and currently there are no data to suggest a clear clinical outcomes benefit of one over the other.

ICD-9-CM Code: 427.31 (AFib)

Indications and Usual Treatment

- AFib
- Cardioversion from AFib to NSR does not reduce the pt's risk for stroke but can improve the pt's symptoms. May also be necessary for acute rate control when rate or rhythm control medications have not succeeded. Particularly true if assoc with hemodynamic instability.
- In general, for AFib of duration less than 48 hrs, the risk of embolism with cardioversion is low (<1%) and cardioversion may be performed without anticoagulation. For AFib that has lasted longer than 48 hrs; 3 wk of anticoagulation with or without a consideration of TEE is recommended prior to cardioversion. TEE may also be used to assess for the presence of left atrial thrombus as an alternative to 3 wk of anticoagulation.

ASSESSMENT POINTS

System	Effect	Assessment by Hx	PE	Test
CARDIO	Hemodynamic instability CHF Acute ischemia	Cardiac symptoms functional status wt fluctuations	Heart and lung exam murmur, S3/4, edema venous stasis	ECG Consider ECHO CXR
RESP	↓ Pulm function OSA	Exercise tolerance Recent infection Tobacco use	Wheezes Crackles Rales	Room air SpO_2 Blood gas CXR poss PFTs
CNS	Potential ischemic/ embolic stroke	Functional status TIA/CVA	Neuro exam document deficits	Possible head CT/MRI

Key Reference: Go AS, Hylek EM, Phillips KA, et al. Prevalence of diagnosed atrial fibrillation in adults: National implications for rhythm management and stroke prevention: The Anticoagulation and Risk Factors in Atrial Fibrillation (ATRIA) Study. *JAMA*. 2001;285:2370.

Anesthetic Considerations

- Often a small bolus of IV sedative or a brief general anesthetic (GA) is employed to provide pt comfort and tolerance of the procedure. Each treatment and medicine choice carries its own relative risk/benefits profile and should be selected accordingly. The duration necessary for sedation/anesthesia will vary based on whether TEE is employed and number of defibrillation attempts required.
- An important initial treatment consideration is whether a GA with or without intubation is necessary. The procedure is typically brief and induction medications are titrated to loss of consciousness or deep sedation. Intubation may be necessary due to aspiration risk. Pts with a Hx of or risk factors for a difficult intubation or BMV should be approached with caution and appropriate rescue equipment should be available.

- Considerations for intubation incl
  - Full stomach and/or delayed gastric emptying
  - Limited CV and/or cardiopulmonary reserve
  - Known or anticipated difficult intubation and/or bag mask ventilation
  - Obesity
  - Pt compliance

Induction Agents

Some Advantages of Selected Induction Agents
- Propofol: Short duration, anti-emetic
- Etomidate: Hemodynamic stable
- Ketamine: Some pain control, potential for continued spontaneous respirations
- Benzodiazepines: Amnesia

Some Disadvantages of Selected Induction Agents.
- Propofol: Hypotension
- Etomidate: Myoclonus (making ECG reading difficult), adrenal suppression
- Ketamine: Myocardial ischemia, tachycardia, increased ICP
- Benzodiazepines, prolonged sedation

Postoperative Management
- Typically minimal, possible recall and/or pain etc. (see Periop Risk).
- Observation until awake and stable (institutional variation on postop management)

Anticipated Problems/Concerns

- CNS event: Immediate CNS evaluation necessary, recall possible, pain
- Cardiac: Possible myocardial ischemia, Htn, tachycardia, arrhythmia, hypotension
- Pulm: Acute pulm edema, airway difficulties, aspiration
- Dermatologic: Thermal injury

Carotid Endarterectomy

Andrea Vannucci

Ivan Kangrga

Risk

- Incidence in USA: About 100,000 CEAs performed annually
- Risk factors for carotid disease: Tobacco, DM, Htn, age, male sex, hypercholesterolemia, hyperlipidemia, obesity, family Hx
- Prevalence of significant carotid stenosis (60–99%) is 1%. TIA the most common presentation
- Annual stroke rate is about 2% for asymptomatic and 13% for symptomatic carotid stenosis
- Ulcerated plaque presents an increased risk of stroke independent of the degree of stenosis

Perioperative Risks

- Main periop risks are death, stroke and MI. All are higher in symptomatic pts.
- Mortality from 0.3–1%
- Stroke from 0.8–2.7%
- MI from 1.7 to 2.–3%
- Independent risks for postop mortality: TIA/stroke, age, CHF, obesity, CRF

Worry About

- CNS status: Asymptomatic versus symptomatic
- Degree of carotid stenosis and status of collateral/contralateral circulation
- Co-morbidities: CAD, Htn, COPD, renal disease
- Pt cooperativity for an awake procedure

- Postop: Monitored care, CNS assessment, BP control, hematoma/airway, nerve injury

Overview

- Carotid endarterectomy is a stroke-preventative surgery.
- Risk of cerebral ischemia during surgery due to embolism or hypoperfusion
- Risk of postop hyperperfusion cerebral injury
- Possibility of persistent postop cognitive decline
- Intermediate cardiac risk surgery, as per ACC/AHA 2007 Guidelines
- Periop mortality highest from cardiac event, followed by cerebrovascular event
- Anesthetic techniques incl general (GA) and regional anesthesia (RA)
- RA does not seem to improve cardiac and CNS outcomes or hospital stay, but may be assoc with more hemodynamic stability and lower vasopressor requirements
- Periop ASA and statins are CNS protective; beta-blockers per ACC/AHH Guidelines.

ICD-9-CM Code: 443.1 (Arteriosclerosis of carotid artery)

ICD-9-CM Code: 38.12 (Carotid endarterectomy)

Indications

- Indications are based on the degree of stenosis and symptoms.
- Symptomatic pts (RIND, TIA, or stroke) benefit from CEA when carotid stenosis is >70%. In stenosis of >50% risk reduction is lower. Maximum benefit is achieved when surgery is performed within 2 wk from the onset of symptoms.
- Asymptomatic pts: Carotid stenosis >60% in men. No benefit has been shown in asymptomatic women because of the high periop risk.
- Surgery is beneficial if stroke rates of the periop team are lower than 3% for asymptomatic pts, 5% for TIA and 7% for stroke pts.

Usual Treatments

- Surgical plaque removal by longitudinal or eversion endarterectomy, the former with or without a patch. A temporary shunt can be placed between the common and internal carotid artery to prevent and/or treat cerebral hypoperfusion during the carotid artery clamp.
- An alternative to surgery is endovascular angioplasty/stenting. Approx 7000 endovascular procedures are perfomed annually in the USA.

ASSESSMENT POINTS

System	Effect	Assessment by Hx	PE	Test
CARDIO	CAD, Htn, CHF, PVD Renovascular disease	Chest pain, MI, CHF, SOB, dyspnea, exercise tolerance	HR, BP both arms; S_3 or S_4 murmurs, dysrhythmia, bruits	ECG, ECHO stress test
RESP	Tobacco use COPD, OSA	SOB, cough, exercise tolerance, Orthopnea, use of CPAP, O_2	Decreased breath sounds, wheezing	CXR PFTs
ENDO	DM, obesity	Diet, PO meds or insulin control Duration, effectiveness of treatment	Wt, BMI Peripheral neuropathy	Serum glucose HbA1c
CNS	TIA, RIND, stroke	Tinnitus, dizziness, vision changes, weakness, slurred speech, paralysis	Motor, visual, or speech	US, CT, EEG Angio/MRI

Key Reference: AbuRahma AF. Process of care for carotid endarterectomy: surgical and anesthesia considerations. *J Vasc Surg.* 2009;50:921–933.

Intraoperative Management

Monitoring

- Standard ASA monitors. ECG incl leads II and V_5.
- Arterial line for continuous BP and blood sampling (ABGs, glucose, etc.)
- CNS function
  - Regional anesthesia: Mentation, speech, motor function
  - General anesthesia: EEG (raw or processed), SSEP, transcranial cerebral oximetry (rSO$_2$), transcranial Doppler (TCD), jugular venous oximetry
- Monitoring modalities have similar sensitivities and specificities. rSO$_2$ is gaining favor because of the ease of use and low failure rate. TCD differentiates hypoperfusion from embolic neurologic events, but is technically not feasible in 15–20%. There is no consensus on multimodal monitoring strategies.
- Stump pressure helps with the decision whether to shunt; cannot be monitored continuously.

CNS Protection

- Glycemic control
- Maintain normocarbia. Consider FIO$_2$ of 100% if neurologic deterioration.
- BP management: Preop ABP control, optimally <180/110 mmHg; intraop at baseline; during clamp most clinicians increase ABP by 20% or higher, guided by CNS monitoring; postop at baseline and/or normotensive, to avoid hyperperfusion injury.

- Mild hypothermia is not beneficial.
- There is no proven pharmacological brain protection
- Temporary shunt may be inserted to maintain cerebral perfusion. Risks are embolism or dissection. Shunting criteria during general anesthesia are not universal and practices differ.

Anesthetic Technique

- Regional: Superficial with/without deep cervical plexus block, interscalene block, or epidural. An awake pt under regional anesthesia is gold standard for neurologic assessment and selective shunting. Superficial block seems as effective as the combined block, and may be assoc with fewer complications. US guidance may improve success rate and decrease complications. Mild sedation reduces stress but prompt neurologic assessment is essential. Dexmedetomidine or low-dose propofol infusions are useful adjuncts.
- General: Mandates neurologic monitoring. Goals are maintaining hemodynamics, perfusion pressure, normocapnia and rapid post-emergence neurologic assessment.

Surgical Stages

- Intraop considerations
- Dissection: Concern is embolization from surgical manipulation. Blood loss usually not a concern.

- Cross-clamping: Follows heparinization (ACT>250s). Assess adequacy of cerebral perfusion if awake or by CNS monitors if asleep. Shunt, FIO$_2$, and BP control accordingly.
- Unclamping and reperfusion: Avoid Htn. Continue neurologic assessment.
- Closure: Ideally heparin should not be reversed

Postoperative Considerations

- Altered BP control and occasional bradycardia
- Hyperperfusion syndrome with Htn, esp. after repair of high-grade stenosis
- CNS deficit (ischemia, emboli, intimal flap, thrombosis, etc.)
- Hematoma with possible airway compromise
- Cranial n. injury (XII, recurrent, etc.) or persistent phrenic n. block from regional anesthesia

Anticipated Problems/Concerns

- Periop TIA or stroke
- Unstable BP and myocardial ischemia
- Resp impairment from upper airway obstruction or phrenic nerve paralysis
- Difficult neurologic assessment in oversedated awake pts or after general anesthesia
- Rare but potentially challenging urgent conversion from regional to general anesthesia

Carpal Tunnel Syndrome

O. Jameson Stokes

Risk

- M:F ratio: 1:3
- Incidence: 0.125%–1%
- Peak incidence around 55 to 60 y old
- Classically involves the thumb, index and middle fingers, and radial half of the ring finger
- Often bilateral, but dominant hand is involved initially
- Common causes incl occupational trauma, congenital predisposition, pregnancy, diabetes, and obesity

Perioperative Risks

- Burning, tingling, and/or numbness in the distribution of the median nerve distal to the wrist
- Loss of coordination and weakness in the affected hand
- Exacerbated with activity or work

Worry About

- Assoc with conditions with higher risk anesthetic implications incl gout, rheumatoid arthritis, diabetes, obesity, pregnancy, lupus, renal failure, hemodialysis, alcoholism, and acromegaly
- More susceptible to compression with edema (fluid retention) and sustained wrist flexion
- Sensory and/or motor deficits

Overview

- Accounts for approx 90% of all entrapment neuropathies
- Due to entrapment of the median nerve in the carpal tunnel at the wrist
- Most common symptom is burning pain assoc with tingling and numbness in the distribution of the median nerve distal to the wrist
- Symptoms often first appear during the night (nocturnal paresthesia), since many people sleep with flexed wrists
- Dx should be based on Hx, physical exam, and results of electrophysiological studies
- Gold standard test is nerve conduction studies
- Mild symptoms can be managed with conservative treatment, incl steroid injections
- Moderate to severe symptoms are treated via surgical intervention.

ICD-9-CM Code: 354.0

Etiology

- Two distinct types: Acute and chronic
- Acute type is uncommon and is due to rapid and sustained pressure in the carpal tunnel
- Acute type is assoc with burns, coagulopathy, fractures, infection, and injections
- Chronic type is common and slow in progression

- Chronic type is assoc with local (infection, trauma, tumors), regional (arthritis, gout), or systemic causes (pregnancy, diabetes, obesity, renal failure, etc.).

Usual Treatment

- Nonsurgical methods effective in mild to moderate carpal tunnel syndrome; i.e., pts with no muscle weakness or atrophy, absent denervation with EMG, and only mild abn on nerve conduction studies
- Nonsurgical treatments incl: Splinting of the wrist, hand brace, rest, ice, NSAIDs, local injections with corticosteroids, vitamin B6 (pyridoxine), US therapy, yoga, and workplace modifications
- Surgery is indicated in almost all pts with moderate to severe carpal tunnel syndrome
- An absolute indication for surgery is muscular atrophy
- Surgery consists of division of the transverse carpal ligament, which releases pressure on the median nerve by increasing the volume of the carpal tunnel
- Two different surgical approaches: Open and endoscopic release

ASSESSMENT POINTS

System	Effects	Assessment by Hx	PE	Test
NEURO	Pain with activity, sensory deficits, and motor deficits	Paresthesias, weakness, Hx of dropping objects, nocturnal sensory abn	Diminished pinprick, decreased hand grip, Thenar atrophy, Tinel's sign and Phalen's test	Nerve conduction study, US

Key Reference: Sinha A, Chan V, Anastakis D. Anesthesia for carpal tunnel release. *Can J Anaesth*. 2003;50(4):323–327.

Perioperative Management

Preoperative Preparation

- Evaluate for and/or optimize underlying causes such as diabetes, hypothyroidism, etc.
- Optimize volume status in order to decrease edema (diuretics, dialysis, etc.).
- Consider Hx of corticosteroid usage and NSAIDs prior to surgical intervention.
- Document musculoskeletal and neurologic exam prior to performing regional anesthetic.

Monitoring

- Standard ASA monitoring

Anesthetic Technique/Induction

- Goal: To maintain a bloodless operative field without anatomical distortion
- Options incl:
  - Local anesthetic infiltration
  - Advantages: Simple, economical, rapid onset, no motor block, good pt satisfaction
  - Disadvantages: Tourniquet pain, anatomical distortion
  - IV regional infiltration
  - Advantages: Simple, rapid onset
  - Disadvantages: Short post-block analgesia, local anesthetic toxicity, motor block
  - Peripheral nerve block

- Advantages: Tourniquet tolerance, no anatomical distortion, good postop analgesia
- Disadvantages: Time consuming, technically difficult
- General anesthesia
  - Advantages: Rapid anesthesia, no anatomical distortion, no tourniquet intolerance
  - Disadvantages: Postsurgical pain, dizziness, nausea, and vomiting

Surgical Stages

- Open carpal tunnel release surgery is easy to perform and leads to symptomatic relief in most pts. It is performed by making a curved longitudinal inter-thenar incision approx 4–5 cm in length. The subcutaneous tissue, superficial fascia, transverse carpal ligament, and 2–3 cm of distal forearm fascia is opened under direct vision. The canal is then inspected for mass lesions or anatomical abn.
- Endoscopic carpal tunnel release can be broadly divided into single portal and dual portal techniques depending on the number of ports used to access the carpal tunnel. A ½-inch incision is made in the wrist and palm through which a camera is inserted through a tube. The camera enables the surgeon to indirectly visualize and release the transverse carpal ligament.

- The Cochrane database group reviewed all available evidence comparing various alternative surgical techniques and found no strong evidence to favor endoscopic repair against the open technique. There was no conclusive evidence favoring either technique when assessing a pt's symptom relief and return to work.

Anticipated Problems/Concerns

- Early postsurgical complications: Incomplete release of the transverse carpal ligament, neuropraxia or injury to median or ulnar nerve, inadvertent entry to Guyon's canal (tunnel between pisiform and hamate bone and the ligament connecting both bones), injury to the palmar cutaneous or recurrent motor branch of the median nerve, and injury to the superficial palmar arch or ulnar artery
- Late post-surgical complications: Scar tenderness, loss of grip strength, pillar pain (tenderness in the thenar or hypothenar eminence), complex regional pain syndrome, and bow stringing of flexor tendons

Cataract ± Iol

Kathryn E. McGoldrick

Risk

- Incidence in USA: >1.5 million cataract operations/y
- Gender predominance: None
- Advanced age
- Direct trauma
- Response to other intraocular conditions, incl chronic uveitis, glaucoma, retinal detachment
- Systemic diseases (diabetes mellitus, myotonic dystrophy, galactosemia)
- Chronic use of topical or systemic corticosteroids
- Congenital (idiopathic, familial, assoc with prenatal infection)

Perioperative Risks

- Periop mortality exceedingly rare
- Surgical morbidity: Bleeding into anterior chamber; capsule rupture; posterior dislocation of lens into degenerative vitreous; loss of vitreous, producing retinal detachment and macular edema; expulsive hemorrhage

Worry About

- Anesthetic morbidity following retrobulbar block
  - Retrobulbar hemorrhage (1–3%)
  - Perforation of globe (0.1% or less)
  - Central spread of local anesthesia that may affect brainstem (0.1%)
  - Intra-arterial injection with immediate seizures (<0.1%)
  - Optic nerve injury (<0.1%)

Overview

- Removal of cloudy lens with small incision(s), with aspiration or ultrasonic fragmentation
- Assoc with extremely low mortality, although complications of retrobulbar block (e.g., brainstem anesthesia) can be life threatening
- Morbidity can incl blindness in operated eye

- Topical anesthesia for selected pts (cooperative and able to control eye movements, not photophobic, appropriate-size pupil) avoids potentially serious complications of needle-based techniques (i.e., retrobulbar or peribulbar block).. Topical anesthesia has become increasingly popular in recent years, as has sub-Tenon (episcleral) block.

ICD-9-CM Code: 366.9

Indications and Usual Treatment

- Based on degree of visual impairment in relation to visual needs of the individual, as well as anticipated visual improvement and risk of serious complications
- With congenital cataracts, risk of amblyopia dictates that surgery be performed within the first few months of life

ASSESSMENT POINTS

System	Effect	Assessment by Hx	PE	Test
OCULAR	Determination of lens power of intraocular implant			Ultrasonic measurement of axial length of eye; optical measurement of corneal curvature
CARDIOPULM	Impaired ability to lie flat; chronic coughing	SOB, orthopnea	Inspection, auscultation	
CNS	Impaired ability to follow instructions and remain motionless because of age, anxiety, claustrophobia, deafness, tremors	CNS Hx	CNS exam	

Key Reference: Ezra DG, Nambiar A, Allan BD. Supplementary intracameral lidocaine for phacoemulsification under topical anesthesia: A meta-analysis of randomized controlled trials. *Ophthalmology.* 2008;115(3):455–465.

Perioperative Implications

Preoperative Preparation

- None

Anesthetic Technique

- Can be performed under regional (peribulbar or retrobulbar), general, sub-tenon's, or topical anesthesia

Monitoring

- Routine
- Invasive monitoring seldom indicated

Regional Techniques

- Eye in neutral gaze to minimize risk of optic nerve injury
- Small-gauge needle, no longer than 31 mm (1¼ inch) to ↓ risk of globe perforation
- Consider general or topical anesthesia if high risk (e.g., extreme myopia; severe enophthalmos; staphyloma; previous ocular complications of regional anesthesia; severe vascular disease; bleeding diathesis; one-eyed pt) for complications assoc with retro- or peribulbar block
- Avoid deep orbital penetration
- Avoid heavy sedation

General Anesthesia

- Meticulously secure endotracheal tube or laryngeal mask airway to prevent intraop extubation
- NM paralysis with appropriate monitoring to avoid coughing or bucking that can cause loss of intraocular contents
- Consider prophylactic antiemetic

Surgical Stages

- The vast majority of cataract procedures are extracapsular because an intact posterior capsule may reduce posterior segment complications: retinal tear, retinal detachment, macular edema
- Incision for extracapsular procedure: With the pupil fully dilated, an anterior capsulotomy is performed
- **Definitive Surgery:** Central anterior capsule removed, with irrigation and aspiration of lens nucleus through wound. Alternatively, nucleus may be fragmented ultrasonically (phacoemulsification) behind iris plane to avoid corneal epithelial damage. Phacoemulsification is generally considered the preferred technique.

- Incision partially closed and every precaution taken to maintain normal anterior chamber depth (by air infusion, fluid infusion, or injection of viscoelastic solution) to prevent corneal endothelial damage during intraocular lens insertion
- Supporting loops of posterior chamber lens inserted into capsular bag or ciliary sulcus
- Minimal hemodynamic disturbance
- Approx duration: 1 hr or less

Postoperative Considerations

- EBL: Negligible
- Minimal postop pain
- Pts instructed to avoid bending, lifting, straining

Anticipated Problems/Concerns

- Ptosis
- Postop wound dehiscence
- Iris prolapse
- Infectious endophthalmitis
- Retinal tear or detachment
- Cystoid macular edema
- Delayed posterior capsule opacification

Cerebral AVM Repair

Armin Schubert
Logan S. Emory

Risk

- ~2000–3000/y
- More commonly diagnosed in pts age 20–40 y
- Risk of intracranial hemorrhage is 2–4%/y; 7–33% incidence of rebleeding
- Mortality 1%/y; 10–15% after first bleed
- Racial predominance: None
- Risk of hemorrhage is increased with male gender, size and location of lesion

Perioperative Risks

- Preop embolization decreases bleeding, facilitates resection, and decreases hyperemic complications
- 30-d operative morbidity 20–40%; worse with higher clinical grade
- 30-d mortality <5%
- Unique complication: Normal perfusion pressure breakthrough (NPPB) syndrome; overall risk 1–18%; at highest risk are high-flow lesions, border-zone AVM location, large AVMs (19–37% risk); lesions with severe hypoperfusion or steal around AVM; severe CNS deficit (may significantly improve over time)
- Postop CNS deficits may predispose to airway obstruction, aspiration

Worry About

- Blood availability
- Effect of preop embolization: New neuro deficit; bleeding; pulm embolus
- Emergence: To allow early CNS assessment
- Massive brain swelling; cerebral hemorrhage
- High-dose barbiturate Rx to prevent edema, intracranial Htn
- Tight BP control on emergence, early postop

Overview

- Congenitally abn connections between arterial and venous cerebral circulation, without intervening capillaries; 80% are supratentorial
- Mass of thin-walled vessels with abn vasomotor response, deficient muscularis layer, dilated veins, and chronically ischemic surrounding brain tissue
- Assoc with cerebral aneurysms in 5–10%; in neonates and infants, shunt usually causes high-output heart failure. Excision can be assoc with substantial blood loss.
- After extirpation of nidus, may get hyperemic brain swelling

ICD-9-CM Code: 747.81 (Cerebral AVM)

Indications and Usual Treatment

- Stereotactic craniotomy for smaller lesions (<3 cm); scalp flap with craniotomy and surgical excision for larger lesions (>3 cm) if resectable with low risk of deficit; progressive Sx; refractory seizures; <40 y
- Alternate Rx: Stereotactic radiosurgery or embolization for older population, location in eloquent area, symptom control. Embolization is palliative, not curative.

ASSESSMENT POINTS

System	Effect	Assessment by Hx	PE	Test
CARDIO	Hyperdynamic CHF in small children, FTT	Recurrent resp failure, prolonged ventilatory support Diaphoresis with feeding	Auscultation, hepatomegaly JVD, diaphoresis	CXR, ECHO
RESP	May aspirate during seizure, hemorrhage	Review with family; records from ER, ICU	Auscultation	CXR, pulm compliance, ABGs, oximetry
GU	Dehydration and/or mild renal insufficiency from multiple CNS imaging	Chart review		BUN, Cr
CNS	Seizures, chronic ischemia of brain surrounding AVM; hydrocephalus, intracranial Htn	LOC, headache, diplopia, nausea; family to describe Sx	MS CNS exam (esp. hemiplegia, cranial nerves)	MRI, angio, clinical AVM grade: Size, location, drainage (deep vs. superficial)

Key Reference: Bederson JB, et al. Guidelines for the management of aneurysmal subarachnoid hemorrhage: a statement for healthcare professionals from a special writing group of the Stroke Council, American Heart Association. *Stroke.* 2009;40(3):994–1025.

Intraoperative Management

Preoperative Preparation
- Avoid premedication if mental status impaired or ICP high
- Determine risk of NPPB

Anesthetic Technique
- Requirements incl brain relaxation, mildly decreased CPP, early emergence (or in pts at high risk for NPPB, high-dose barbiturates)
- Hyperventilation to Paco₂ of 25–30 mmHg to improve regional distribution of CBF
- Avoid glucose-containing fluid.

Monitoring
- Routine
- Direct arterial pressure prior to induction, placing transducer at level of head to reflect cerebral BPs; CVP for larger, deeper AVMs; PA catheter, ECHO for CV compromise
- Consider EPs
- Consider EEG for barbiturate effect
- ICP for emergence and postop

Surgical Stages

Induction
- Avoid succinylcholine with hemiplegia, increased ICP
- Maintain BP control; avoid coughing

Skeletal Fixation
- Avoid BP spike during fixation

Skin Incision
- Avoid Htn; may see effects of local anesthesia, epinephrine
- Consider beginning mannitol 0.5–2.0 g/kg

Dissection
- Arterial supply resected first; severe episodic bleeding, esp. if dural sinuses involved
- After resection, test for bleeding by normalizing BP
- Consider barbiturate infusion to prevent NPPB

Definitive Surgery
- May develop edema (NPPB) and hyperemia of surrounding tissue with occlusion of AVM

- Rx for NPPB: Hyperventilation, diuretics, propofol, mild hypothermia, BP control

Closure/Postoperative Period
- EBL: 300–2000 mL; depends on AVM size, location; no need for third-space allowance
- Careful BP control during emergence/postop period, consider fast-acting agents
- Assure normal coag status
- Controlled emergence to minimize coughing/bucking, sympathetic response to pain
- Rx small doses of IV opioid, if CNS status OK

Anticipated Problems/Concerns

- Intraop concerns: Bleeding, brain volume control; CNS assessment at end of procedure
- Postop concerns: Brain swelling (NPPB); bleeding into surgical site; hydrocephalus, seizure

Cervical Spine Fusion

Douglas Hester

Risk

- Age: 20 –85, usually 20–60
- Female > male, 2:1

Perioperative Risks

- 5%: Recurrent laryngeal nerve injury
- 1% or less: Nerve root injury, sympathetic chain injury, CSF leak
- 1% or less: Esophageal injury
- 1% or less: Massive blood loss: carotid or jugular injury
- 1% or less: Postop instability, instrument failure
- 1% or less: Resp problems

Worry About

- Difficult airway management

- Recurrent laryngeal nerve injury, myelopathy, or nerve-root injury
- Postop resp compromise (edema, hematoma, neurologic injury)
- Injury to non-neurological structures: Carotid artery, jugular veins, esophagus

Overview

- Various etiologies, usually a repair of cervical spinal cord compression from instability caused by traumatic, neoplastic, arthritic, degenerative, congenital, or infectious processes
- Various approaches: Anterolateral retropharyngeal, transoral, posterior midline (prone or sitting position)

- Blood loss: Usually less than 500 mL, unless corpectomy planned (can be up to 1000 mL)

Indications And Usual Treatment

- Upper cervical spine: Atlantoaxial or occipitoatlantal instability, odontoid fractures, congenital or neoplastic lesions; cervical instability, prior failed surgery, spinal tumor
- Mid and lower cervical spine: Herniated disks, spinal cord compression (myelopathy), cervical spondylosis, cervical radiculopathy (nerve-root compression), cervical instability; prior failed surgery, kyphotic deformities, spinal tumor

ASSESSMENT POINTS

System	Effect	Assessment by Hx	Pe	Test
HEENT	Limited mobility (pain or parasthesias, prior fusion)	Changes in pain or neurologic symptoms with movement	Oral opening, cervical flexion and extension, prior surgical scars (anterior and posterior), neurologic exam	Cervical imaging (X-ray, CT, MRI, other)
RESP	Acute trauma can impair ability to protect airway and cause resp insufficiency	Nature of injury	Neurologic exam	Vital signs, ABG
CNS	Radicular or myelopathic pain, weakness, or parasthesias	Onset of symptoms, progression, pain/weakness/paresthesias, GI/GU symptoms	Neurologic exam, muscle atrophy	Cervical imaging (X-ray, CT, MRI, other)

Key Reference: Langen KE, Jellish WS, Ghanayem AJ. Anesthetic considerations in spine surgery. *Contemporary Spine Surgery*. 2006;7(6):1–8.

Perioperative Management

Preoperative Preparation

- Sedation for either awake airway management or placement of neck traction prior to induction

Monitoring

- Usually routine monitors are sufficient
- Upper extremities inaccessible; consider needs for arterial catheter placement
- Large peripheral access sufficient; consider CVP and Doppler if pt will be in sitting position (VAE risk)
- Neurologic monitoring (SSEP, MEP)

Anesthetic Induction/Maintenance

- General endotracheal
- Monitoring may impact (e.g., SSEP might be optimized with narcotic-based technique)
- Stimulating parts of procedure incl: incision and initial dissection, retraction at neck, and bone graft harvesting (if done)

Airway Management

- Consider awake intubation
- Consider difficult airway equipment
- Airway will be difficult to access during case; consider wire reinforced ETT to avoid kinking/obstruction

Emergence

- Rapid emergence facilitates timely neurologic examination

Surgical Stages

Transoral Approach

- Pins, head brace, or Gardner-Wells tongs used to provide cervical traction (5–20 lbs)
- Dingman retractor used to facilitate access; soft palate also retracted via sutures; hard palate sometimes transected

Anterolateral Approach

- Neck is hyperextended; straps, brace or Gardner-Wells tongs used to provide cervical traction (5–20 lbs)

- Trachea, esophagus, carotid, and neural structures retracted to allow bone graft or plating

Posterior Approach

- Pt either prone or sitting (usually done in Mayfield pin system)

Postoperative Considerations

- Cervical collar often placed before emergence
- Airway edema
- Dysphagia
- Pain at autologous bonegraft donor site

Anticipated Problems/Concerns

- Airway management (resp insufficiency, hematoma, recurrent laryngeal nerve injury)
- Dysphagia
- Pain at autologous bonegraft donor site

Cesarean Section, Emergent

Denis Snegovskikh

PROCEDURES

Risk

- Incidence in USA: 30.3% of all deliveries
- 24.5% of all C-sections are performed for an emergent indication
- Racial predominance: Slight non-Hispanic black predominance
- Obesity is a risk factor for both elective (odds ratio 1.87) and emergency (odds ratio 2.23) cesarean delivery

Perioperative Risks

- In 2003, anesthesia was the 7th leading cause of maternal mortality in the USA.
- Most maternal anesthesia related death occurs during emergent C-section.
- Most frequent cause: Failed airway management during or just after emergence from general anesthesia or related to intubation for high neuroaxial block.
- Nonanesthetic risks: Embolism, hypertensive disorders, bleeding

Worry About

- Difficult airway
- Rapid desaturation
- Full stomach if in labor or exposed to any opioids (even neuroaxial)
- Hemodynamic instability
- Increased sensitivity of pregnant patients to effect of certain medications
- Maternal and/or fetal homeostasis
- Higher risk of awareness and recall under GA
- Coagulopathy
- Air and amniotic fluid embolism

Overview

- Classification of urgency of cesarean section:
  - Grade I, Emergency: Immediate threat to life of woman or fetus
  - Grade II, Urgent: Maternal or Fetal compromise that is not immediately life-threatening
  - Grade III, Scheduled: Needing early delivery but no maternal or fetal compromise
  - Grade IV, Elective: At a time to suit the woman and maternity team
- For urgent cesarean sections, anesthesia goal should be to permit the start of delivery within 30 minutes of the decision
- Number of deaths during cesarean section was 17 times higher with GA than with RA
- 1 min Apgar score lowers after general anesthesia than after regional, but no differences by 5 min.

- Keep mother and fetus adequately oxygenated while limiting fetal drug transmission and maintaining maternal comfort
- Uterine incision to delivery time is more important for neonatal outcome than is induction to delivery time.

ICD-9- CM Code: 656.31 (Fetal distress resulting in delivery)

Indications and Usual Treatment

- Maternal: bleeding (abruption placenta, placenta previa, aneurysm rupture), high risk of uterine rupture (laboring patient with history of classical incision for cesarean section or multiple low transverse cesarean section), uterine rupture, quick deterioration of maternal condition due to decompensation of comorbidities (CHF secondary to congenital heart disease, acute renal failure in a patient with chronic renal disease etc.) or progression of preeclampsia (HELLP, acute fatty liver)
- Fetal: prolapsed umbilical cord, shoulder dystocia, vasa previa, severe distress (category III tracing), laboring malpresentation

ASSESSMENT POINTS

System	Effect	Assessment by Hx	PE	Test
HEENT	Upper airway edema	Severe nasal congestion	MP – may increase by 1 class with labor	
CARDIO	Increased CO and total plasma volume, total blood volume=95ml/kg Biventricular hypertrophy, MR, TR, PI. Arrhythmias Aorto-caval compression	SOB, chest pain, peripheral, edema, palpitation, irregular heartbeats	Wide split S_1, possible S_3, 3/6 syst M of MR	ECG: Left axis deviation, S1Q3, inverted T in III and AVF, arrhythmias (SVT, nonsustain VT) ECHO: MR, TR, PI, aortic dilation RVH = 20% LVH = 6%
RESP	Hyperventilation, resp alkalosis, 20% increase in O_2 consumption (14) Decreased vertical size of the chest, increased diameter		Barrel shape chest High position of the diaphragm	MV increased 50%, FRC decreased 20% Normal ABG: pH = 7.44, $PaCO_2$ = 32mm Hg, HCO_3= 20 mmol/L, PaO_2=105mm Hg
OB	Preeclampsia, eclampsia, HELLP syndrome	Headache, RUQ pain, blurry vision	Elevated BP, severe per edema, petechia, jaundice, papilledema, seizures	Elevated creatinine and uric acid, proteinuria, elevated LFTs, thrombocytopenia, prolonged PT, PTT
GI	Decreased LES tone, poss. Increased acidity	Heartburn	Increased risk of aspiration of gastric content	

Key Reference: Haque MF, et al. Anesthesia for emergency cesarean section. *Mymensingh Med J*. 2008;17:221–226.

Perioperative Management

Preoperative Preparation
- Administer oral antacid (sodium citrate 30 mL), if not contraindicated otherwise, IV H2-blockers (famotidine), metoclopramide 10–20 mg
- Position the pt with left uterine displacement
- If pt is bleeding or has high risk of placenta accrete, use 2 large-bore IV

Monitoring
- Standard ASA monitoring, fetal HR monitoring, Foley catheter
- A-line if pt is bleeding or has high risk of placenta accreta
- CVP, PAP, BIS monitoring are rarely indicated. CVP or PA catheters—insertion of catheters in pregnant pts carries higher risk of complications.

Anesthetic Technique/Induction
- Modern U.S. data is unavailable.
- In United Kingdom, anesthetic technique for Grade I cesarean section
  - Primary GA: 35.5%
  - Converted to GA: 9%
  - Regional: 55.5%
- In Singapore: 90% of all Grade I cesarean section is performed under GA

Induction

- Don't induce until obstetrician is ready to make skin incision. Surgery can be started only after airway is secured. Instruct obstetrician to begin surgery after you say "cut", do not use words like "begin", "start", or "lets go"; can be confused with command to start the induction.

Medications

- Ketamine: 1 mg/kg. Hallucinations and emergence phenomena are dose-related and less frequent in obstetric pts. Sympathomimetic effect limits its use in preeclamptic pts.
- Thiopental: 3–7 mg/kg. Doses <4 mg/kg unlikely to cause fetal depression, doses >7 mg/kg are liable to do so.
- Propofol: 2.5 mg/kg propofol may cause severe bradycardia in combination with succinylcholine at 1–1.5 mg/kg.

- Although pseudocholinesterase activity is decreased about 24% at term, it does not cause clinically significant prolongation of paralysis after one dose of succinylcholine. Fasciculation may be absent, esp. in pts on magnesium therapy.
- Vecuronium/rocuronium: Avoid, if necessary titrate to effect, start with 20% of standard dose), esp. for pre-eclamptic pts on magnesium therapy or/and infected pts (chorioamnionitis) on gentamicin or clindamycin. Even defasciculating dose can cause total muscle paralysis.

Extension of Preexisting Epidural Block

- Lidocaine:2% + Epinephrine 1:200,000-18mL+ Bicarbonate2mLor2-Chloroprocaine3%-18mL+ Bicarbonate-2 mL.
- Spinal
  - More appropriate for Grade II-III C-section
  - Hyperbaric bupivacaine 0.75%–1.8 mL, may be mixed with fentanyl 10 mcg and preservative-free morphine–200 mcg for better pain control during and up to 15–18 hr after surgery.
- Spinal after failed epidural

- To minimize risk for high block perform intrathecal injection in sitting position, reduce dose of spinal bupivacaine by 20%, let pt sit for 60–90 sec after injection

Surgical Stages

Dissection Till Delivery
- Inhalation agent should be started after intubation. MAC is reduced in pregnancy by 25–40% (32). All volatile agents, except NO, are potent uterine relaxants.
- Hyperventilate the pt to maintain normal for term pregnancy resp alkalosis with pH = 7.4, $PaCO_2$=32, HCO_3 = 20. Normoventilation will cause acute resp acidosis
- Avoid opioids

Delivery of placenta, closing.
- Start oxytocin infusion 20–40 units in 1000 mL of LR.
- Uterus will contract in response to oxytocin if MAC is <0.8 (33). Reduce concentration or stop halogenated agent, give 50–70% NO in O_2 and midazolam/opioids combination.
- Uterine atony-\: Methergine 0.2 mg IM (contraindicated during preeclampsia), Hemabate 250 mcg IM (contraindicated for pts with asthma).
- If massive blood loss: Transfuse RBC/FFP/platelets-1:1:1. Cryoprecipitate to keep fibrinogen higher than 100 mg/dL

Postoperative Consideration
- None of maternal death happened during induction or maintenance of anesthesia, but all of them during the emergence or soon thereafter.

Anticipated Problems/Concerns

General Anesthesia
- Problems during induction
  - Rapid desaturation
  - Difficult airway
  - High risk of aspiration
  - Higher risk of intraop recall

Regional Anesthesia
- Local anesthetic toxicity
  - Use amiodarone to treat arrhythmia and vasopressin to treat CV collapse
- High block
- Hypotension
- Failed block
- Rate of failed block converted to GA: 14% (35); spinal to GA: 1.4–2.1 % (7, 48)

Cesarean Section, Planned

Andrew P. Harris

Risk

- Incidence in the USA increasing again: 1995, 785,000/y; 1998, 900,000/y; 2007, 1.37M/y
- Racial predominance: African-American higher, Hispanic lower rate

Perioperative Risks

- Periop pulm morbidity varies by type of anesthesia. GA is assoc with increased pulm morbidity
- Low mortality, but anesthesia (5–24/100,000) significant contributor to mortality

Worry About

- Inability to intubate
- Unintentional high regional block
- Unanticipated blood loss
- Spinal headache

Embolism

- Embolism: Thromboembolism, air embolism, amniotic fluid embolism
- Postop endometritis

Overview

- Significant other frequently accompanies pt to the OR
- Hysterotomy usually through the lower uterine segment
- Occasional uterine atony after delivery Rx with oxytocic agents, occasionally progressing to cesarean hysterectomy
- Exteriorization of the uterus during closure assoc with greater intraop discomfort if regional anesthesia

- Regional anesthesia preferred to avoid risk of airway mishaps and postop pulm morbidity

ICD-9-CM Code: V22.2 (Pregnancy)

Indications and Usual Treatment

- Maternal preference or conditions that would result in increased perinatal morbidity for mother or fetus if vaginal delivery attempted; most common examples incl Hx of classic (or maybe any) cesarean section, macrosomia, Hx of CPD, twin gestation
- May also be emergent (see Cesarean Section, Emergent, in Procedures section)
- Vaginal birth after C-section may be attempted in lieu of elective repeat cesarean, but now risks seem to be greater than benefits

ASSESSMENT POINTS

System	Effect	Assessment by Hx	PE	Test
AIRWAY	Engorgement of vessels and enlargement of breasts		Airway exam Mallampati class	
PULM	$\uparrow$ Minute ventilation $\uparrow$ O$_2$ consumption	SOB		
CARDIO	$\uparrow$ Cardiac output $\uparrow$ Dilutional anemia Vena caval obstruction	Cardiac failure Supine hypotensive syndrome		Hgb Antibody screen
GI	Delayed gastric emptying	Regurgitation		
MS	$\uparrow$ Back pain	Back pain, sciatica		

Key Reference: Hawkins JL. Epidural analgesia for labor and delivery. *N Engl J Med*. 2010;362(16):1503–1510.

Perioperative Management

Preoperative Preparation
- Antacids or H$_2$ blocker and/or metoclopramide
- Left uterine displacement

Anesthetic Technique
- Any: General, local, spinal, epidural, combined spinal/epidural; regional preferred due to potential airway problems

Monitoring
- Fetal HR monitoring during induction if possible or indicated

Airway
- Engorgement leads to easy bleeding, difficult intubation

- ~1/300 unanticipated difficult intubation
- Airway cart and/or equipment available

Induction/Maintenance
- 33% less local anesthetic required for regional anesthesia
- T4 level during regional anesthesia desirable
- If GA, D/C halogenated agents (if possible) after delivery to reduce blood loss
- Prophylactic antibiotic usually prior to incision
- Oxytocin, methylergonovine, carboprost available for uterine atony after delivery

Surgical Stages

- Skin incision to delivery: Amniotic fluid embolism possible

- Closure: Venous air embolism, uterine atony, or hemorrhage possible
- EBL: 750-1000 mL normal; can be much greater with uterine atony

Postoperative Considerations
- Uterine atony, hemorrhage possible
- Pain score: typically 4–8
- IV PCA or epidural PCA for 1–2 d

Anticipated Problems/Concerns

- Inability to intubate
- High block with hypotension, sudden bradycardia
- Hemorrhage
- Postop headache

Cholecystectomy, Laparoscopic

Stephen Aniskevich
Sorin J. Brull

Risk

- Incidence in the United States: 20 million with gallstones
- 600,000 cholecystectomies/y
- Prevalence increases with age; higher incidence in women, 17%; men, 8%
- Among Pima Indian women, 75% affected
- Incidence in African-Americans lower than in Caucasians

Perioperative Risks

- Periop mortality ~0.1%, morbidity 4–6× lower than in open procedure (2–9%)
- Most benefits derived from avoidance of large abd incision
- Shorter hospital stay (-3d), more rapid convalescence (-22d)

Worry About

- Intraop hemorrhage
- Visceral damage. Bile duct injury is an iatrogenic catastrophe with significant morbidity, mortality, and reduced quality of life.
- Bacterbilia, sepsis
- PE, arrhythmias (CO_2 absorption)
- SQ emphysema from improperly placed CO_2 insufflating needle
- Hemodynamic consequences of pneumoperitoneum
- CO_2 absorption, position changes; CO_2 embolism

Overview

- Laparoscopic procedure increasing in frequency
- Lower incidence of complications than with open but mortality is the same

- Frequently a short stay; outpatient procedure in appropriate pts

ICD-9-CM Code: 574.0 (Cholelithiasis)

Indications and Usual Treatment

- Indications: Chronic cholecystitis, symptomatic cholelithiasis
- Early contraindications: Large stones in common bile duct, acute inflammation, pregnancy, obesity, but now used in acute cholecystitis and pregnancy
- Considered technique of choice in octogenarians
- Alternative Rx: Open procedure, stone/contact dissolution, biliary lithotripsy, cholecystolithotomy

ASSESSMENT POINTS

System	Effect	Assessment by Hx	PE	Test
CV	Likely co-morbidities: PVD, CAD		CV exam	ECG
RESP	Co-morbidity likely: COPD (elderly) Sleep apnea		Chest exam Neck circumference	CXR O_2 sat, polysomnography
HEME	Intraop blood loss (cystic artery liver laceration)	Preop dehydration (N/V, elderly)	Orthostasis	Hct, electrolytes
GU	Impairment 2° to age, co-morbidity	CNS Hx	CNS	BUN/Cr

Key References: Cunningham AJ, Brull SJ. Laparoscopic cholecystectomy: Anesthetic implications. *Anesth Analg.* 1993;76:1120–1133.
Keus F, de Jong JA, Gooszen HG, van Laarhoven CJ. Laparoscopic versus open cholecystectomy for patients with symptomatic cholecystolithiasis. *Cochrane Database System Rev.* 2006;18:(4):CD006231.

Intraoperative Management

Monitoring
- Routine, UO (Foley catheter)
- $ETCO_2$ not good substitute for arterial Pco_2

Airway
- Change in position from head-up to head-down may displace ETT into endobronchial position

Anesthetic Technique
- GA, controlled ventilation with cuffed ETT (prevent aspiration during pneumoperitoneum); regional (axial) anesthesia not advocated

Surgical Stages

Induction
- CV instability if co-existing disease, elderly
- Trocar insertion: Injury to viscera
- Trendelenburg position
  - CV effects: Improves venous return, CO, BP; pulm effects: reduced VC, atelectasis, shunting
- Pneumoperitoneum creation
- SQ emphysema from poorly placed insufflating needle
  - CV effects: Intra-abd pressure <15 mmHg assoc with minimal CV changes (slight increase in MAP, no change in CO)
- Pulm effects: Hypoventilation, resp acidosis, hypoxemia, tension pneumothorax (via patent pleuroperitoneal canal), atelectasis, shunting; exogenous CO_2 insufflation—rapid absorption, necessitating controlled ventilation; arrhythmias,

catecholamine release; possible CO_2 pulm embolism, esp. at release of pneumoperitoneum

Definitive Surgery
- Postop N/V high (42%); prophylaxis recommended: Metoclopramide, droperidol, ondansetron
- Avoiding neostigmine, narcotic requirements by using NSAIDs (ketorolac) also effective
- Narcotic-induced sphincter of Oddi spasm reversed with narcotic antagonists, local anesthetic infiltration, glucagon
- Use of N_2O not recommended because of bowel distention, postop N/V
- Pre-emptive/adjuvant anesthesia with local anesthetic infiltration of skin, gallbladder bed may reduce postop pain
- Blood loss: Minimal
- Surgery Duration: ~1–3 hr
- Fluid shifts: Minimal
- Pain score: 2–5; same day or next day hospital discharge
- Long-term benefits of laparoscopic technique: lower incidence of bowel obstrucion

Anticipated Problems/Concerns

- Intraop: Tension pneumothorax, CO_2 absorption, arrhythmias, hemodynamic compromise from pneumoperitoneum, visceral damage from surgical trocar, CO_2 embolism
- Conversion to open procedure (1–7% incidence) due to technical factors

- Gasless (traction) laparoscopic techniques are less expensive and may help increase (or maintain) cardiac index.
- De Vinci surgical surgery is an emerging laparoscopic technology. Its benefits are yet to be established over traditional laparoscopic techniques.
- Miniport and single-incision (2-cm) laparoscopic techniques use smaller ports than the traditional 5- and 10-mm diameter ports, but their benefits have not been established.
- Ultrasonic energy dissection (Harmonic scalpel) may result in shorter operative time, lower gallbladder perforation risk, and shorter hospital stay than traditional electrocautery dissection techniques.
- Early laparoscopic cholecystectomy for acute cholecystitis appears safe and shortens total hospital stay.
- Low-pressure pneumoperitoneum procedures (intra-abdominal pressures < 12 mmHg) decrease postoperative pain and analgesic consumption.
- Natural-orifice trans-luminal endoscopic surgery (NOTES) technique provides an incisionless operation by insertion of operative instruments into peritoneal cavity through the GI tract (stomach) or urogenital tract (vagina). Advantages include less pain, no hernias, no surgical wound infection, and better cosmetic results.

Cholecystectomy, Open

David M. Corda
Sorin J. Brull

PROCEDURES

Risk

- Incidence in the USA: 20 million
- 600,000 cholecystectomies/y
- Prevalence increases with age; in women incidence is 17%, in men 8%
- Pima Indian women, incidence is 75%
- Incidence in African-Americans lower than in Caucasians

Perioperative Risks

- Periop mortality: 0–0.5% (0.1% in pts <50 y)
- In elderly: Up to 10%
- Morbidity: 5–25%, esp. 2° to impairment of pulm mechanics (abd incision)

Worry About

- Intraop hemorrhage
- Hepatic failure

- Bacterbilia, sepsis
- Open cholecystectomy techniques have mostly been replaced by laparoscopic techniques, leaving most newly trained surgeons with little experience with the open technique.

Overview

- Becoming rare mode of cholecystectomy. Roughly 5% of laparoscopic cholecystectomies converted to open 2° to technical difficulties.
- Antibiotic prophylaxis; midline, paramedian, or subcostal surgery incision
- Identification of cystic duct, common hepatic duct, common bile duct, cystic artery
- Operative cholangiogram performed for choledocholithiasis (adds 10 min to procedure)
- US ~98% sensitivity, specificity

ICD-9-CM Code: 574.0 (Cholelithiasis)

Indications and Usual Treatment

- Chronic cholecystitis and symptomatic cholelithiasis
- Biliary colic treated with parenteral narcotics; antibiotic therapy for pts over age 60 with chronic cholecystitis, and for pts with acute cholecystitis or with concomitant common duct stones
- NG suction and low-fat diet not proven beneficial
- Other Rx: Gallstone dissolution; percutaneous shockwave lithotripsy; contact dissolution; percutaneous cholecystolithotomy; laparoscopic cholecystectomy

ASSESSMENT POINTS

System	Effect	Assessment by Hx	PE	Test
CARDIO	Rule out angina vs. cholecystitis ECG changes and arrhythmias	Rule out CAD relief by nitroglycerin (relieves both angina and biliary colic)		ECG, coronary angio; exercise tolerance test if unable to differentiate
RESP	Co-morbidity likely: COPD (elderly)	Pulm reserve Exercise tolerance	Auscultation	CXR
GI	N/V	N/V	RUQ pain	

Key References: Nahrwold DL. The biliary system. In: Sabiston Jr DC, ed. *Textbook of surgery*. 15th ed. Philadelphia: Saunders; 1997:1126–1131.
Keus F, Gooszen HG, Van Laarhoven CJ. Systematic review: open, small-incision or laparoscopic cholecystectomy for symptomatic cholecystolithiasis. *Aliment Pharmacol Ther.* 2009;29:359–378.

Perioperative Management

Perioperative Evaluations

- Assess CV system, CAD: pulm system, predict postop resp issues

Anesthetic Technique

- GA
- Regional (axial) anesthesia may not be appropriate due to high level of sensory denervation required (at least T4)
- Local anesthesia for cholecystectomy
- Adjunct techniques: Paravertebral block, intercostal nerve block, interpleural cath
- Prophylaxis for postop N/V

Monitoring

- Routine

Airway

- May warrant rapid-sequence induction 2° to pain, ↓ gastric emptying, preop N/V

Induction

- Narcotic-induced sphincter of Oddi spasm reversed with narcotic antagonists, injection of local anesthetic, or glucagon

- Use of N_2O not recommended because of nausea, bowel distention

Surgical Stages

- Skin incision: Large, usually subcostal

Dissection

- Possible bleeding from cystic artery, liver laceration/damage
- Possible pneumothorax if diaphragmatic or pleural damage

Definitive Surgery

- Exposure, bowel manipulation/traction may lead to hypotension (release of vasoactive substances from gut and/or ↓ venous return)
- Approx duration: 0.5–3.0 hr
- Fluid shift: Can be marked if bowel exposed for long periods
- Hypothermia a concern if prolonged procedure, esp. in elderly
- EBL: 50–150 mL

Postoperative Considerations

- N/V: Consider prophylaxis
- Pain score: 6–10; narcotic requirements ↓ by "pre-emptive analgesia," adjunct techniques (paravertebral block, intercostal nerve block, interpleural cath), local anesthetic infiltration of gallbladder bed, postop NSAIDs for visceral pain

Anticipated problems/concerns

- Severe postop pain (incisional) may lead to ↓ ambulation; splinting ↓ cough, mobilization; atelectasis, pulm infection
- Open procedures assoc with longer hospital stay and convalescence.
- No difference in mortality between laparoscopic and open cholecystectomy techniques.
- The routine use of postop drains to prevent subhepatic abscesses or bile peritonitis results in higher abd wound and chest infection and is not recommended.

Circumcision

Stanley W. Stead

Risk

- ~2 million/y procedures are performed
- Generally performed in neonatal period

Perioperative Risks

- Considered minimal 0.2–0.6% (aspiration, bleeding, hematoma, malignant hyperthermia reported 1 series [2/476], postop fever); complications from local anesthesia rare
- Local skin necrosis after dorsal penile nerve block (<0.5%)

Worry About

- Complicated preop neonatal course: sepsis, hypospadias, immaturity

Overview

- Most common surgical procedure in USA. Uncommon in most other parts of the world. Religious followers of Jewish and Islamic faiths practice circumcision for religious and cultural reasons. Circumcision rates also vary among racial and ethnic groups, with whites being much more likely to be circumcised.
- Rate increased from 1985 to 1992; largest increment following 1989 American Academy of Pediatrics statement of "potential benefits and advantages" of procedure
- According to the Agency for Healthcare Research and Quality 56% of male infants were circumcised in 2005; however, some estimate the percentage in the mid- to high-60s. Risk from UTI in uncircumcised males is 4–10 times greater than in circumcised males, with the greatest risk in infants <1 y. Absolute risk of developing UTI in an uncircumcised male infant is low (~1%).

ICD-9-CM Diagnosis Codes: V50.2 (Circumcision [no medical indication, ritual, routine]); 605 (Phimosis); 607.1 (Balanitis)

ICD-9-CM Procedure Code: 64.0 (Circumcision, excision of the prepuce or part of it).

Indications and Usual Treatment

- Parental choice
- Coincidence with other surgery
- Recurrent balanoposthitis
- Difficulty retracting foreskin: "tight prepuce"
- UTIs
- True phimosis (obstruction of urine flow)
- Three methods used in the newborn male all use an assoc device: Gomco clamp, the Plastibell device, or the Mogen clamp. After the newborn period, a more formal surgical procedure is used, necessitating hemostasis and suturing of the skin edges; frequently performed with GA

ASSESSMENT POINTS

System	Effect	PE	Test
GU	Hypospadias Balanoposthitis, phimosis UTIs	Urethra ventral surface of penis Nonretractile prepuce or tight ring	UA, microscopic
OVERALL	Immaturity, sepsis		

Key Reference: American Academy of Pediatrics Task Force on Circumcision. Circumcision policy statement. *Pediatrics*. 1999;103:686–693 (Reaffirmed September 1, 2005).

Intraoperative Management

- Considerable evidence that newborns circumcised without analgesia experience pain and physiologic stress, manifested by changes in heart rate, BP, O$_2$ sat, and cortisol levels
- In the past, the procedure was performed without analgesia or anesthesia. Recommendations now emphasize procedural analgesia.
- Subcutaneous ring block: A SQ circumferential ring of 0.8 mL of 1% lidocaine without epinephrine injected at the midshaft of the penis was found to be more effective than either EMLA cream or dorsal penile nerve block (DPNB)
- 1–2 g of EMLA cream is applied to the distal half of the penis and wrapped in an occlusive dressing 60–90 min before the procedure. There is a risk of methemoglobinemia from a metabolite of prilocaine, which can oxidize hemoglobin to methemoglobin.

- DPNB: A 27-g needle is used to inject 0.4 mL of 1% lidocaine, administered at the 10- and 2-o'clock positions at the base of the penis. The needle is directed posteromedially 3–5 mm on each side until Buck's fascia is entered. After aspiration, the local anesthetic is injected. Bruising may be seen from the injection.
- GA may be preferred in children or adults.

Monitoring
- Routine

Airway
- Routine: Mask, laryngeal mask airway, intubation

Surgical Stages

Skin Incision/Definitive Surgery
- Two methods, sleeve or freehand, in which ring incision made around prepuce, or using a clamp (Plastibell, Gomco, or Mogen). In either, maximum surgical stimuli at this point; no dissection. Bleeding controlled with compression or electrocautery; suture placement rare.

- Commonly, petrolatum-based gauze used to dress wound edges, which are brought together
- Adult circumcisions are frequently performed without clamps and may require 4–6 wk to heal.

Postoperative Considerations
- Pain score: 2–4
- Pain relief by rectal acetaminophen in neonates
- Older individuals may require opiates

Anticipated Problems/Concerns

- Newborn infants experience pain manifested by physiologic changes (increase in BP, HR, sweating, decrease in oxygenation), behavioral changes, which persist for at least 22 hr; physiologic, behavioral effects attenuated by local or regional anesthesia
- Pain often undertreated
- Infection remains a possibility in neonates, because hygiene may be compromised.

Cleft Lip Repair

Risk

- 1/700 live births
- Racial predominance: Asian and Native American 1/500; Caucasian 1/1,000; African descent 1/2,500
- Gender predominance: Male 60–80%; female 20–40%
- Assoc with cleft palate in 70–85% of cases
- Cause of orofacial clefting is multifactorial: Genetic and maternal influences incl smoking, alcohol use, phenytoin, folate deficiency

Perioperative Risks

- Extremely low morbidity and/or mortality
- When assoc with cleft palate repair, the most significant risk is postop airway obstruction

Worry About

- Difficult airway when assoc with syndromes that cause craniofacial abn such as Pierre Robin, Treacher Collins, Downs, Goldenhar, Nager, or Apert
- 30% of pts with cleft lip and/or palate have other anomalies. Possible undiagnosed assoc congenital heart or renal disease
- Dislodgement of ETT during pharyngeal pack placement
- Timing of surgery coinciding with physiologic anemia of infancy
- Postop airway obstruction
- Assoc with cleft palate, risks of preop anemia due to poor feeding; intrainduction laryngospasm due to chronic otitis media, URI; intrainduction airway obstruction due to tongue wedged in cleft palate; postop airway obstruction due to lingual edema

Overview

- Congenital condition by 7th wk intrauterine life; unilateral left-sided cleft is most common
- Strong genetic influence; one-quarter of cases bilateral cleft lip
- Timing of repair follows "rules of ten": age >10 wk, wt >10 lbs, hemoglobin >10, WBC <10

ICD-9-CM Code: 749.10

Indications and Usual Treatment

- Single stage cleft lip repair, cheiloplasty, is performed if infant is appropriate surgical candidate
- Functional repair of lip and orbicularis oris muscle for feeding, facial expressions, normal facial growth, and speech development
- Cosmetic repair to facilitate parental bonding and social integration

ASSESSMENT POINTS*

System	Effect	Assessment by Hx	PE	Test
HEENT	Difficult airway	Snoring, grunting, difficulty with oral feeds	Airway exam: particular attention to head and neck mobility, palate, presence of mandibular hypoplasia	
	Otitis media	Ear pain, fever	Otoscopic exam	
CARDIO	Assoc CHD	SOB, cyanosis, poor growth	CV exam	ECG, ECHO
RESP	URI	Cough, fever, rhinorrhea	Auscultation, chest exam	CXR, ABGs
	Aspiration	Coughing with oral feeds, cyanosis		
GI	Impaired deglutition	Nasal regurgitation		Observe feeding
	Malnutrition	Poor growth		Albumin
HEME	Anemia	Malnutrition	Pallor	Hgb/Hct
GU	Assoc congenital defects	UTI		UA, BUN/Cr

*Inclusive for associated cleft palate.
Key Reference: Hardcastle T. Anaesthesia for repair of cleft lip and palate. *J Perioper Pract*. 2009;19(1):20–23. Review.

Perioperative Implications

Preoperative Preparation

- Identify and evaluate assoc birth defects
- Prepare for potentially difficult airway/intubation with a variety of of face masks, oropharyngeal airways, nasopharyngeal airways, laryngoscope blades, LMAs, and possibly a video laryngoscope or fiberoptic scope

Anesthetic Technique

- Mask induction with sevoflurane, oral intubation using appropriate-sized uncuffed RAE tube well secured to mandible, reinforce tape since very close to surgical field
- Maintenance with inhalational agent; NMB not needed
- Pain control with short-acting opioid titrated to effect, consider bilateral infraorbital nerve block

Monitoring

- Standard ASA monitors; Precordial stethoscope esp. important since intraop access to airway severely limited
- Temp monitoring, forced air warmers, and warming blankets critical in infants

Surgical Stages

- Placement of pharyngeal pack, potential for ETT displacement if pack is placed
- Surgical field block with local anesthetic with 1:200,000 epinephrine
- Tissue flap elevation followed by closure of mucosa, orbicularis oris muscle, and skin
- Procedure time: 45–90 min
- EBL: Minimal

Postoperative Considerations

- Confirm that pharyngeal pack has been removed before extubation.
- Avoid disrupting sutures and/or repair during suctioning, extubation, and postop airway interventions.
- If pt less than 55 wk postconceptual age consider oximetry and apnea monitoring for 24 hr
- Oral or rectal acetaminophen usually sufficient for pain control
- Oral feeding can start with clear liquids as soon as pt is awake

Anticipated Problems/Concerns

- Undiagnosed cardiac anomalies in neonate
- Postop airway obstruction due to congenital airway abn, forgotten pharyngeal pack or airway edema

Cleft Palate Repair

Elizabeth A. Hein
C. Dean Kurth

Risk

- Incidence of cleft palate is about 1/1000 live births
- Repaired before speech develops, usually at age 6–12 mo

Perioperative Risks

- Periop mortality rare in pediatric centers

Worry About

- Assoc deformities, their risks: Congenital heart disease (SBE prophylaxis, cyanosis, CHF), micrognathia (difficult intubation), retroglossia (difficult mask airway), upper airway congestion (laryngospasm)
- Airway: Difficult mask ventilation, difficulty placing oral airway, difficult intubation; tube occlusion, inadvertent extubation, endobronchial tube advancement during surgery
- Intraop arrhythmias and Htn
- Postop airway obstruction, non-use of oral airway

Overview

- Usually isolated deformity; it can also be part of syndrome (e.g., Pierre Robin)
- Repaired to separate oral, nasal cavities; improve feeding, speech; prevent middle ear disease, hearing loss; aspiration
- Surgical position: Supine, head extended, mouth open (Dingman gag), pharyngeal packs in
- Before incision, palate is infiltrated with epinephrine for hemostasis
- Surgery involves undermining tissues around defect to create flap to cover it; soft palate edema; opioid administration may contribute to postop obstructive apnea

ICD-9-CM Codes: 749.0; 749.2

Indications and Usual Treatment

- Defects are surgically repaired if life expectancy reasonable
- Bottle-fed with special nipple before defect closed; caloric intake, growth monitored
- Otitis media often occurs; antibiotic prophylaxis common preop
- Myringotomy tubes frequently placed concomitantly with repairs

ASSESSMENT POINTS

System	Effect	Assessment by Hx	PE	Test
HEENT	Palate defect, other deformities, rhinorrhea	Apnea, known syndrome	Defect size, airway exam, nasal secretions	
CARDIO	Cardiac defect	Slow feeding, diaphoresis	Murmur, liver size, cyanosis, HR, RR	ECG/CXR ECHO
RESP	Bronchitis, chronic aspiration	Cough, fever, feeding problem	Rhonchi, wheeze	O_2 sat CXR
HEME	Anemia	Age 3–9 mo	Pallor	Hct

Key Reference: Kharkov LV. Evolution of methods of uranostaphyloplasty exemplified by the analysis of 1118 primary operations for congenital palatal defects. *Br J Oral Maxillofac Surg.* 2000;38:104–106.

Perioperative Management

Preoperative Preparation

- Premedication: If no obstructive apnea, then midazolam PO, atropine if young infant
- Consider cross-match, depending on surgeon, pt's Hct

Anesthetic Technique

- No special techniques

Monitoring

- Routine incl forced air warmer

Airway

- Oral RAE tube secured tracheal tube at midline, flat against chin, bend of tube at lip; use water-resistant tape, maintain small leak or use low-pressure ETT
- Flex, extend head to check for bronchial intubation or inadvertent extubation

Surgical Stages

- Palate infiltrated with epinephrine before incision; keep dose <10 μg/kg
- Tissue on both sides of defect mobilized to create flap
- During dissection, observe wound for bleeding, but transfusion rarely required
- After defect, check palate for edema, gauge airway caliber
- At end, heavy ligature may be placed through tongue, or NP airway may be inserted
- Wound may be injected with bupivacaine for postop analgesia; keep dose <2 mg/kg
- Surgical duration: 2–4 hr
- Blood loss variable

Emergence

- Before extubation, ensure that the pharyngeal pack is gone and that the oral cavity is dry.
- Extubation best done when pt is awake
- Restrain arms to prevent child from pulling at oral suture line

Postoperative Considerations

- Analgesia with acetaminophen, or opioid (usually fentanyl); be careful with opioid dose to avoid obstructive apnea
- Pulse oximetry, cardiorespiratory monitoring recommended for 24–48 hr on floor unless other medical problems warrant ICU stay

Colostomy

George S. Tseng

Risk

- All colostomies 42–65,000/y; 10–15/100,00 for Ulcerative Colitis (UC); 7/100,000 for Crohn's
- M:F risk equal; increased incidence in non-Jewish and Jewish caucasian pts; Crohn's – M=F
- Colorectal Ca incidence per 100,000, all races male 57.3%, female 42.8%
- White male 56.9%, female 42.1%; black male 69.3%, female 53.5%
- Emergency surgery for obstruction and/or trauma, 10–15% have perforated, some resulting in ostomy

Perioperative Risks

- Risks are related to underlying disease process and surgical procedure.
- Mortality when a colostomy is an option is rare.
- Morbidity dependent on prior treatments, surgical procedure, and ongoing diseases: Wound healing problems and infections from irradiation or steroid use, perineal hernia from APR, stomal retraction, bleeding, common postop fecal incontinence, constipation, and pain

Worry About

- GI: Assessment of nutritional status, acid-base status, electrolytes, intravascular volume
- Renal: Assess electrolytes, acid-base, intravascular volume
- Intravascular volume: Bleeding, anemia, emesis, diarrhea, bowel prep, NPO status, anorexia
- Aspiration risk
- Steroid use: Htn, osteoporosis, infections, electrolytes, adrenal insufficiency
- TPN use: Liver problems, metabolic imbalances, bacteremia
- Metastatic disease to liver, lungs, brain from colon cancers.
- Trauma: Concurrent injuries and bleeding
- Smoking and/or heavy alcohol consumption

Overview

- Colostomy is a stoma that connects the colon to surface of the abd, can be permanent or temporary
- Transverse colostomy: 2 types, ascending and descending

- Sigmoid colostomy
- Type of surgery and colostomy dependent on surgical procedure and pathology
- Primary anastomosis also viable consideration for perforated traumas and bowel pathology

ICD-9-CM Code: 46.1 (Colostomy)

Indications and Usual Treatment

- Used to divert fecal matter proximally from distal pathology
- Used as blow-hole to decompress distal blockage
- Colon Ca: Resection with postop radiation or chemotherapy
- IBD: Sulfasalazine, steroids, bowel rest preop
- Trauma: Exploratory laparotomy with colostomy or 1° anastomosis
- Intestinal ischemia: Vascular surgery, bowel resection, colostomy, open abd
- Distal obstructions, fistulas

ASSESSMENT POINTS

System	Effect	Assessment by Hx	PE	Test
HEENT	Ankylosing arthritis	C-spine mobility and neurologic complaints	C-spine ROM, airway and neuro exam	CT scan and/or MRI if positive neurologic findings
CARDIO	Volume depletion, tachycardia, hypotension	Blood loss, emesis, diarrhea, anorexia, bowel prep, MET score, orthostasis	Vital signs, mental status	EKG, further testing as required in relation to urgency of surgery (stress test, troponin)
RESP	Pulm disease from metastases, smoking	Cough, hemoptysis, dyspnea, MET score	Auscultation, percussion	CXR, PFT, CT scan and/or MRI as time permits
GI	Aspiration risk	Obstruction, NPO status, GERD, pregnancy, trauma, N/V	Abd. exam, percussion, auscultation	KUB, FAST US, CT scan/MRI as time permits
HEME	Anemia	Orthostasis, pallor, exercise tolerance	Vital signs, cardiac exam	Hct

Key Reference: *Clinics in colon and rectal surgery.* 2009:22(1):1–72.

Perioperative Management

Preoperative Preparation

- Restoration of fluid deficits, correction of electrolyte and acid-base imbalances if feasible
- Mechanical bowel preparation less de facto practice
- Corticosteroid supplementation as needed
- H₂/PPI and promotility agents as needed
- SQ LMWH and/or fondaparinux for DVT prophylaxis
- Antibiotics IV prior to skin incision
- Discuss FastTrack anorectal surgery with surgeon if appropriate

Monitoring

- ASA monitors
- Foley catheter
- Consider CVC based on need for pressure infusion, postop access

- Consider noninvasive esophageal Doppler or impedence technology if anticipating third spacing, bleeding, volume status problems
- Consider arterial line for co-existing diseases, hemodynamic instability, bleeding

Anesthetic Technique/Induction

- GETA for airway protection and PPV when using muscle relaxants
- Epidural provides for postop pain relief, decreased blood loss, decreased incidence of postop DVT and PE
- RSI if risk for aspiration
- Maintenance
- Avoid N₂O
- Anticipate large fluid shifts, bleeding, problems from assoc trauma and electrolyte problems
- Keep pt warm
- Higher FIO₂ of 80% may help with wound healing and decrease anastomotic breakdown
- Optimize fluid resuscitation with noninvasive SV/intravascular volume monitoring

Postoperative Considerations

- SICU for pts with hemodynamic instability, extensive surgery requiring ongoing resuscitation, and severe co-existing disease
- Continue corticosteroid use if adrenal suppression is anticipated
- Establish pain control regimen with epidural catheter and/or PCA
- High FIO₂ supplementation may decrease wound infections and anastomotic breakdown
- Continue chemical DVT prophylaxis

Anticipated Problems/Concerns

- Postop resp problems with large fluid shifts or concurrent trauma injuries
- Postop pain control from surgery or concurrent trauma injuries

Coronary Artery Bypass Graft (CABG)

Paul L. Samm

Risk

- 500,000 CABG annually, although number has been declining
- Risk factors for CAD: Htn, DM, hyperlipidemia, lipoprotein a genotype, smoking, age, male sex, family Hx

Perioperative Risks

- Overall mortality 0.5–4 % (average 2%)
- Main cause of death during and after bypass is MI (2–10%)
- Mortality and/or complications increase with age >70, decreased EF, DM, COPD, chronic renal failure
- Stroke 1–2%, primarily elderly; 30–55% pts have less than perfect cognitive function postop; mental status changes decrease as time post surgery lengthens

- 3% require exploration 2° to bleeding lead to ↑ risk of chest infection and lung complications
- Mortality of female > male

Worry About

- Periop ventricular function
- Myocardial protection, periop ischemia, early graft closure
- Completeness of surgical revascularization
- Bleeding with reoperations

Overview

- Occluded or severely diseased coronary arteries bypassed with venous or arterial grafts
- Anesthesia technique, monitoring, postop ventilatory care affected by pt's physical condition

ICD-9-CM Code: 36.11 (aortocoronary bypass of one coronary artery) to 36.14 (aortocoronary bypass of four coronary arteries)

- Various approaches depend on bypass locations and surgical preferences; incl beating heart and arrested; minimally invasive and sternotomy; use of one or two internal mammary arteries now standard.
- Early extubation and discharge are goals if good preop condition.

Indications and Usual Treatment

- Disease of LMCA, LAD, LCX, and RCA
- Diffuse disease not amenable to treatment with PCI
- Pt with severe ventricular dysfunction or DM

ASSESSMENT POINTS

System	Effect	Assessment by Hx	PE	Test
HEENT	Plaques in other areas	Risk factor search: Smoking stain; hypercholesterolemic lesions	McArdle's earlobe	
CARDIO	↓ LV or RV compliance ↓ Pump function arrhythmias Autonomic pain Htn	SOB, DOE Angina ↓ Exercise tolerance Palpitations PND	HR/BP prior to and after 2-stair climb if stable enough to do so; S_3; rales; JVD; use character and rhythm	ECG, CXR, stress ECHO or dipyridamole thallium or ambulatory Holter
RESP		Nocturnal cough, orthopnea		
RENAL	Perfusion insufficiency	Nocturia		BUN/Cr
CNS	Autonomic pain syndromes Other atherosclerotic syndromes	Pain in neck or left arm Stroke/TIA Hx	CNS and cranial nerve exam; mental status exam	Carotid Doppler ANS testing

Key Reference: Aldea GS, Mokadam NA, Melford Jr R, et al. Changing volumes, risk profiles, and outcomes of coronary artery bypass grafting and percutaneous coronary interventions. *Ann Thorac Surg.* 2009;87:1828–1838.

Intraoperative Management

Preoperative Preparation

- Continue all preop medications, esp. aspirin, beta-blockers and statins
- Statins reduce early death, atrial fib, and stroke

Monitoring

- 5-lead for ST segment analysis
- Arterial (radial, ulnar, brachial, femoral) line
- Central venous access for assessing volume status, cardiac function, fluid, and vasoactive drugs administration
- Core temp and peripheral temp monitoring
- UO monitor
- TEE, if ↑ risk of hemodynamic complications during periop period, Category II, monitors left ventricle systolic function, hemodynamic/volume status, MR 4% assoc with CAD, assessment of viability, assess adequacy of cardioplegia distribution
- PAC (controversial) to measure pulm vascular resistance, filling pressures, and serial CO/CI

Anesthetic Technique

- Narcotics, volatile agents, benzos, muscle relaxants, Amicar
- Any technique is appropriate with concurrent monitoring of hemodynamics, setting of goals and keeping variables within desired parameters
- Technique can vary depending on whether beating heart or open circulatory arrest, and variants

Induction

- Avoid increased myocardial O_2 consumption
- Avoid decreased myocardial O_2 supply

Surgical Stages (Sternotomy Surgical Technique)

Skin Incision

- ↑ anesthesia to prevent ischemia during periods of ↑ stimulation (incision, sternotomy, sternal spreading)
- Worry a lot about errant vessels adhering to sternum in redo ops or ops after a prior sternotomy
- Harvesting of internal mammary and vein grafts
- Temp suspend ventilation during sternotomy to prevent injury to lung and right side of heart
- Heparin 300 units/kg given centrally, and monitor effectiveness prior to institution of bypass
- Venous cannula placed in RA or vena cava

CPB

- Act >400
- ↑ potential for recall anesthesia narcotics, benzo, propofol infusion, precedex infusion
- Pt cooled to approx 28°C
- Stop ventilation when CPB full flow
- Aortic cross clamp
- Cardioplegia blood or crystalloid given in aortic root proximal to cross clamp (anterograde) or directly into coronary ostia and through coronary sinus (retrograde)
- Repeat dose of cardioplegia depending on time and reappearance of electrical activity

- MAP 60–80 mm Hg cerebral autoregulation fail below cerebral perfusion pressure of 50–55 mm Hg
- Maintain MAP by ↑ arterial flow or give phenylephrine

Termination of CPB

- Normothermia
- Resume mechanical ventilation with 100% O_2
- SR with slightly ↑ rate; epicardial or transvenous pacing can be used
- Return blood to heart
- Calcium to treat hypocalcemia, hyperkalemia, ↑ SVR, enhance contractility
- CPB terminated with acceptable pressure IABP
- CI >2 for adequate organ perfusion
- TEE to evaluate RWMA, ventricular function, filling defects
- Stop Amicar
- Reverse heparin with protamine 1.3 mg/100 units slowly to prevent protamine reactions
- Suction to bypass machine stopped and vents removed with 50% protamine in ACT, ABG, electrolytes

Anticipated Problems/Concerns

- Myocardial infarction due to embolism, hypoperfusion or graft failure
- Postperfusion syndrome, or pump head
- Acute renal failure due to embolism or hypoperfusion
- Stroke 2° to embolism or hypoperfusion
- Extubation as soon as possible

Craniotomy

R. Alexander Schlichter

Risk

- Intracranial tumors
- Vascular abn (aneurysms, AVMs)
- Traumatic Brain Injury (TBI)
- Stroke
- Intractable seizure disorder
- Intracranial infections (abscess, CJD)

Perioperative Risks

- Tumors: Size and grade can effect neurologic outcome
- Vascular: Stroke, vasospasm, bleeding
- TBI: Cardiomyopathy, cervical spine trauma
- Infection: Meningitis, sepsis
- Overall: Risk of stroke, hemiplegia, coma, and seizure

Worry About

- CPP= MAP-ICP (or CVP). Increases in ICP need to be matched with increases in MAP. In TBI and lesions with edema, perfusion can be more of a challenge.

- In vascular lesions, maintaining normal pressure to not rupture lesion until clipped or ablated. Once clipped, increasing MAP to aid collateral perfusion and avoid ischemia.
- Once dura has been opened, optimitizing surgical field to avoid herniation
- ABG: Avoid hypoxia, hypercapnea. Follow osmolality. Tight glycemic control (80–160).

Overview

- Craniotomies are performed to correct intracranial lesions such as tumors, abscesses, aneurysms, AVMs. Can also be decompressive in cases of subarachnoid hemorrhage, TBI, or stroke.
- Autoregulation of ICP and MAP lead to good compensation in chronic neurologic disease. Acute changes such as subarachnoid hemorrhage, TBI, or stroke lead to rapid decompensation of neurologic status.
- Vital signs changes that can lead to decompensation incl increased ICP, hypercapnia, hypoxemia, and malignant Htn or prolonged hypotension.

ICD-9-CM Codes: 239.6 (Brain tumor); 437.3 (Nonruptured cerebral aneurysm); 854.x (Head injury)

Etiology

- Intracranial tumor: Benign mass, 1° malignancy, metastatic
- Vascular: Aneurysm, AVM, AV fistula
- Traumatic: TBI, subarachnoid hemorrhage, subdural hemorrhage, epidural hemorrhage
- Stroke: Thromboembolic, ischemic, hypertensive
- Infectious: Bacterial, fungal, prion

Indications and Usual Treatment

- Intracranial tumor: Benign mass, 1° malignancy, metastatic
- Vascular: Aneurysm, AVM, AV fistula
- Traumatic: TBI, subarachnoid hemorrhage, subdural hemorrhage, epidural hemorrhage
- Stroke: Thromboembolic, ischemic, hypertensive
- Infectious: Bacterial, fungal, prion

ASSESSMENT POINTS

System	Effect	Assessment by Hx	PE	Test
HEENT	TBI: Concurrent cervical/facial trauma Concussion/bleed can cause uneven pupils	Hx of acute trauma	Facial trauma Cervical trauma/c-collar Pupillary exam	CT scan of head and neck
CARDIO	TBI: Tachycardia/cardiomyopathy from catecholamines Aneurysms: Htn/bradycardia	Often have concurrent Htn/CAD/PVD	BP HR	ECG
RESP	Brainstem pressure causes apnea/resp depression	Agonal/Cheyne-stokes	Breath sounds Resp rate	CXR
GI	Arterial bleed 2° to steroids	Hx of steroid use	Melena, coffee ground emesis	EGD
CNS	Change in consciousness, seizure, weakness/dysarrthria	Acute vs. chronic changes in neurologic exam	Focal motor/sensory dysfunction; awake/lethargic/comatose Papilledema Seizure	MRI or CT of brain EEG Cerebral angiography

Key Reference: Todd MM, Weeks J. Comparitive effects of propofol, pentobarbital, and isoflurane on cerebral blood flow and blood volume. *J Neurosurg Anesthesiol.* 1996;8(4):267–355.

Perioperative Implications

Preoperative Preparation
- Emergent: Secure airway, hyperventilation, avoid hypoxia. Maintain MAP.
- Elective: Minimize preop sedation. Evaluate symptoms and radiologic imaging to determine anesthetic approach. Give steroids, diuretics (mannitol, lasix), and anticonvulsants.

Monitoring
- Intra-arterial BP
- Consider CVP in SAH
- UO
- EEG, SSEP, MMEP, cranial nerves (acoustic)

Airway
- TBI: May have cervical spine trauma
- Aneurysm: Treat Htn assoc with laryngoscopy
- Avoid hypoxia and hypercapnia

Preinduction/Induction
- IV induction with propofol, barbituate, or etomidate
- NMBA to prevent coughing, facilitate intubation. Use rocuronium if RSI is indicated.
- Avoid succinylcholine and ketamine due to increase in ICP.
- Treat hypotension with phenylephrine, Htn with nicardipine or labetolol

Maintenance
- Low dose volatile agent
- Consider propofol infusion with severe cerebral edema.
- NMBA unless MMEP, EMG, or CN monitoring
- Fentanyl bolus vs. sufentanil or remifentanil infusion
- Ventilate to a PaCO$_2$ of 26-30
- Propofol/barbituates decrease ICP, inhaled increases CBF, opioid no effect

Extubation
- Neurologic exam before extubation
- Smooth extubation with no coughing or bucking
- If unable to assess neurologic status, postop CT scan
- Low preop GCS should remain intubated

Anticipated Problems/Concerns
- Intraop: Bleeding, stroke, seizure, venous air embolism
- Postop: Hypo/Htn, stroke, seizure, cerebral edema, vasospasm, neurologic changes
- Postop neurologic changes necessitate physical exam and possible CT imaging.

Craniotomy, Awake

Letha Mathews

Indications

- Resection of tumor or vascular malformation
- Resection of epileptic focus
- Deep brain stimulation for Parkinson's disease, essential tremors or dystonia

Perioperative Risks

- Seizures
- Excessive sedation, resp depression, airway obstruction
- N/V, aspiration
- Disinhibition and lack of pt cooperation, agitation, postural discomfort
- Intracranial Htn and bleeding
- Hypercarbia and brain edema
- Venous air embolism
- Poor neurologic outcome

Worry About

- Resp depression and need for emergent airway control
- Hypercarbia leading to brain edema
- Pt movement, disorientation, and lack of cooperation

Overview

- Awake craniotomy performed for resection of space occupying lesions (tumors or vascular malformations) or epileptic foci or to place deep brain stimulation electrodes
- It is used when the pt's conscious response and cooperation is necessary for intraop functional testing such as speech mapping and motor mapping.
- Awake intraop mapping allows wider tumor excision and lower periop morbidity

- Allows early recovery and discharge

ICD-9-CM Code: 239.6 (Brain tumor)

Etiology

- Brain tumor
- Epileptic foci
- Parkinson's disease refractory to medical management

Indications and Usual Treatment

- Space occupying lesions in eloquent areas of the brain
- Craniotomy under general anesthesia with electrocorticography
- Deep brian stimulation improves function in 15% of pts with Parkinson's disease.

ASSESSMENT POINTS

System	Effect	Assessment by Hx	PE	Test
HEENT	Airway access, risk of aspiration	BMI, difficult airway, sleep apnea	Mallampati exam, neck mobility, neck circumference	
CARDIO	Htn and bradycardia if severe increase in ICP	PMH: Htn, CAD	BP, HR, rhythm	EKG, ECHO and functional studies as indicated
RESP		Sleep apnea, smoker, COPD	Chest exam	CXR
GI	GERD, gastric ulceration from steroid usage, N/V	Significant use of antacids, H_2 blocker or proton pump inhibitor use, steroid usage, Hx of postop N/V		
CNS	Level of consciousness, seizures, headache, focal deficits, speech	Seizures, focal deficits	Neurologic evaluation	Head CT/MRI

Key Reference: Bonhomme V, Franssen C, Hans P. Awake craniotomy. *Eur J Anaesthesiol*. 2009;26:906–912.

Perioperative Management

Preoperative Preparation

- Appropriate pt selection and very thorough explanation of procedures and expectation of pt. Pts with morbid obesity, OSA, severe mental retardation, extreme anxiety, claustrophobia, and pts with documented difficult airway may not be good candidates for awake craniotomy.
- Minimize preop sedation. Avoid and/or minimize benzodiazepines preop because of the risk of disinhibition. Antiepileptic drugs should be given on the day of surgery.
- Antacids and nausea prophylaxis may be indicated.
- Neurologic exam and documentation of baseline status.

Monitoring

- Standard ASA monitors plus invasive BP monitoring
- Electrocorticography and/or direct cortical stimulation (Ojemann stimulator)
- UO

Anesthetic Technique/Induction

- Sedation during with scalp infiltration or specific scalp blocks of branches of trigeminal nerve and cervical plexus with 0.5% bupivacaine or ropivacaine.
- Most common sedation drug combinations that have been used successfully incl a short-acting narcotic (fentanyl, sufentanyl or remifentanil) combined with propofol or dexmedetomidine.
- Dexmedetomidine alone administered as a bolus at 1 mcg/kg over 10 min followed by infusion at 0.2–0.7 mcg/kg/min provides sedation without resp depression.
- Asleep-Awake-Asleep technique: GA for craniotomy via LMA or ETT with inhalational agents and/or propofol for maintenance. The pt is awakened for functional testing and then asleep for closure of craniotomy.
- Local infiltration only with no sedation
- Hemodynamic management
- Normal BP or mild hypotension during brain exposure to minimize bleeding and brain swelling

- Normal BP during closure to achieve surgical hemostasis
- Prevention and aggressive treatment of Htn to prevent intracranial bleed

Intraoperative Functional Testing

- Electrocorticography
- Speech and motor mapping
- Testing may be done by anesthesiologists or electrophysiologists

Emergence

- Prompt emergence and extubation in asleep cases for neurologic exam
- Prevent or treat Htn at emergence with antihypertensive of choice.

Postoperative Considerations

- Frequent neurologic exam

Anticipated Problems/Concerns

- Postop brain edema
- Hypovolemia from intraop osmotic diuretics and fluid restriction
- Seizures

Craniotomy, Sitting Position

Thomas J. Toung

Risk

- Pts with infratentorial tumors (pineal, floor of fourth ventricle, pontomedullary junction, vermis, cerebellopontine angle)
- Trend decreasing, but still used in some institutions in USA, esp. for pineal surgery

Perioperative Risks

- Venous air embolism (as high as 80%)
- Paradoxical air embolism (probe patent foramen ovale in 25% of adult population)
- Hypotension
- Brainstem and/or cervical spinal cord ischemia
- Airway obstruction
- Tension pneumocephalus
- Macroglossia

Worry About

- Subdural hematoma due to major brain shift (excessive CSF drainage)
- Venous and/or paradoxical air embolism
- Brainstem, lower cranial nerve injury
- Poor cerebral venous drainage with acute flexion of head on neck

Overview

- Acoustic neuroma most common infratentorial tumor in adults
- 2 mmHg reduction in cerebral BP with every inch of elevation above heart
- Head, neck markedly flexed for better exposure
- Operation is performed around brainstem centers vital to respiration and circulation
- N_2O avoided during closure of dura

- Muscle relaxant avoided by some because of facial nerve monitoring; when used, 2–3 twitches of train-of-4 usually maintained

ICD-9-CM Code: 239.6 (Brain tumor)

Indications and Usual Treatment

- Surgical indications
  - Supracerebellar infratentorial approaches to pineal region, midline, 4th ventricular lesions, CP angle tumor
- Contraindications
  - Ventriculoatrial shunt in place and open
  - Cardiac diseases
  - Hydrocephalus
  - Autonomic dysfunction
  - Extremes of age
  - Cerebral ischemic disease (stroke)

ASSESSMENT POINTS

System	Effect	Assessment by Hx	PE	Test
HEENT	Dysphagia, facial paralysis	Choking, hoarseness	ENT exam	Cine x-ray
CARDIO	Patent foramen ovale predisposes to paradoxical air embolism	Easy fatiguability	Auscultation	CXR cardiac cath
RESP	Aspiration	Coughing	Auscultation	CXR
CNS	Ventriculoatrial shunt predisposes to venous air embolism, hydrocephalus predisposes to tension pneumocephalus	Shunt surgery	CNS exam	Head CT scan

Key Reference: Wong AY, Irwin MG. Large venous air embolism in the sitting position despite monitoring with transoesophageal echocardiography. *Anaesthesia.* 2005;60(8):811–813.

Perioperative Implications

Preoperative Preparation
- Antishock trouser (MAST suit)
- Precordial Doppler
- Multiorificed RA catheter
- Adequate hydration

Anesthetic Technique
- General with controlled ventilation

Monitoring
- PA catheter or CVP
- $ETCO_2$
- Precordial Doppler or TEE
- Direct intra-arterial BP: Transducer zeroed at head level
- SSEP and BAER
- EMG-facial muscle, tongue, shoulders

Airway
- ETT may be kinked by acute flexion of neck
- Allow at least 2 fingerbreadths between chin, sternum

Induction/Maintenance
- Isoflurane, N_2O, low-dose fentanyl most common technique
- Use of short-acting NMB (for quick reversal for facial nerve monitoring)

Surgical Stages

Dissection
- Sudden onset of tachycardia/bradycardia, PVCs, hypotension

Definitive Surgery
- Except for extra-axial lesions in cerebellopontine angle, surgery for pathologic Dx, and/or to reduce mass effect

- Blood loss usually not significant
- Chemo/radiation Rx

Postoperative Considerations
- Pain score: 0–5
- Minimize coughing, straining on ETT
- Cranial nerve dysfunction, esp. cranial nerve 7, 9
- Extubation determined by extent of surgery
- Postop Htn possibly caused by brainstem compression due to hematoma

Anticipated Problems/Concerns
- CV complications resulting from venous air embolism
- Tension pneumocephalus
- Cranial nerve paresis, aspiration
- Macroglossia
- Failure to awaken from anesthesia, possible brainstem or subdural hematoma

Electroconvulsive Therapy (ECT)

Laurel E. Moore

Risk

- Lifetime prevalence of major depressive disorder (MDD): 16.2%

Perioperative Risks

- Periop mortality rare
- Dysrhythmias and Htn common
- Cognitive dysfunction common post-treatment

Worry About

- Sympathetic stimulation producing myocardial ischemia and infarction
- Assoc between MDD and CHD
- Risk of dysrhythmia as a result of parasympathetic and sympathetic stimulation
- Cognitive dysfunction and short-term memory loss from Rx
- Adequate medical Hx frequently difficult to obtain from depressed pt

Overview

- ECT remains the most effective acute antidepressant intervention
- Induced seizures produce multiple neuroendocrine changes (increased ACTH, cortisol, epinephrine, norepinephrine, growth hormone, decreased GABA) and changes in serotonergic and dopaminergic receptor function in the brain; these and other effects of ECT are well-documented but which of these produce antidepressant effects is unclear and the mechanism(s) by which ECT affect mood remain unclear.

- Effectiveness of ECT related to positioning of electrodes (bilateral>right unilateral, RUL) and electrical dosage. Overall response rates range from 20–80%. Side effects of ECT incl (transient) cognitive decline and both retrograde and anterograde amnesia are assoc with bilateral lead position and increased electrical dosage. New data supports use of ultra-brief (0.3 ms) RUL suprasthreshold stimulus; this also assoc with decreased cognitive side effects.
- ECT course in USA is generally 3×/wk treatments for total of 15–18 treatments.
- Predictors of poor clinical response to ECT include chronicity of depression, prolonged depressive episode, medication resistance and comorbid borderline personality disorder.
- Use of antidepressants complicates anesthetic management:
  - Tricyclic antidepressants (TCA) block the reuptake of neurotransmitters and also cause their acute release, thus depleting noradrenergic stores. This results in an unpredictable response to indirect-acting sympathomimetics. Direct-acting sympathomimetics may produce an exaggerated response. Most TCAs have anticholinergic effects.
  - Monoamine oxidase inhibitors (MAOIs) form an irreversible complex with MAO, preventing breakdown of intraneuronal norepinephrine, serotonin, and dopamine. The use of an indirect-acting sympathomimetic can produce a hypertensive crisis; direct-acting agents may also produce an exaggerated response. MAOIs generally D/C prior to ECT.

- Lithium (Li) may prolong the effects of depolarizing relaxants, certain nondepolarizing relaxants, and sedatives (barbiturates). It may also increase the incidence of confusion and memory loss from ECT; Li is generally D/C before ECT.

ICD9CM Codes: 296.2 (Major depression, single episode); 296.3 (Major depression, recurrent episode); 311 (Depressive disorder, not elsewhere classified)

Indications and Usual Treatment

- Clinical indications
  - Failure to respond to conventional pharmacologic Rx
  - Medical contraindication to pharmacologic Rx (e.g., cardiac conduction defect)
  - Profound depression if delay in Rx places pt at unacceptable risk for suicide
  - Maintenance ECT (weekly to monthly) being used in pts at risk for relapse
  - More controversial indications incl schizophrenia, mania, eating disorders, and catatonia.
- Relative contraindications incl intracranial space–occupying lesion, recent MI, recent CVA, pheochromocytoma, long-bone fractures and pregnancy.
- Alternative therapies incl the use of antidepressants and psychotherapy. Recent advances in brain stimulation techniques such as transcranial magnetic stimulation, direct-current stimulation, and deep brain stimulation have not been shown to be superior to ECT in terms of response rates or speed of response.

ASSESSMENT POINTS

System	Effect	Assessments by Hx	PE	Test
CARDIO	CAD	Angina, prior MI		ECG or stress test as indicated
	↓ LV function	↓ Exercise tolerance PND, orthopnea	Enlarged heart JVD Rales	ECG/ECHO as indicated
	Dysrhythmia	Syncope or near syncope Medications	Rhythm	ECG or Holter as indicated
GI	GE reflux	Reflux Sx		
MS	Fracture or vertebral collapse	Pain or trauma	Palpation	X-ray, CT as indicated
NS	Confusion/delirium	Prior Hx	CNS exam	Routine workup for change in MS incl CT if indicated
PSYCH	Competent for consent			Determined by psychiatric team

Key Reference: Hooten WM, Rasmussen KG. Effects of general anesthetic agents in adults receiving electroconvulsive therapy: A systematic review. *J ECT*. 2008;24:208–223.

Perioperative Implications

- Pt comfort and amnesia
- Minimize risk of physical injury from generalized seizure
- Management of hemodynamic changes assoc with treatment
- Rapid return to conscious state
- Recent interest in evaluating anesthetic techniques which may ameliorate cognitive deficits inherent to treatment

Monitoring

- Routine incl ECG, pulse oximetry, capnography and NIBP
- EEG to determine adequacy, duration of seizure
- In high-risk pts consider invasive monitoring for initial treatments.

Induction/Maintenance

- GA, usually by mask
- IV induction
  - Methohexital (0.5–1.0 mg/kg): Decreased seizure threshold, increased seizure duration, rapid awakening
  - Thiopental (2–3 mg/kg): Increased seizure threshold, delayed awakening
  - Propofol (0.75–1.3 mg/kg): Decreased seizure duration, rapid awakening, limited data suggest improved CV stability versus methohexital or thiopental, limited data suggest improved cognitive outcome versus methohexital.
  - Ketamine (1–3 mg/kg): Increased seizure duration versus methohexital, shorter recovery versus methohexital, limited data suggested improved cognitive outcome versus methohexital

- Etomidate (.15–0.3 mg/kg): Increased seizure duration, improved hemodynamic stability; increased nausea and confusional states, generally used in pts refractory to stimulus
- Muscle relaxation achieved with small dose of succinylcholine (0.5–1.0 mg/kg) to decrease potential for injury from generalized seizure; mivacurium when succinylcholine contraindicated
- Hyperventilation with 100% O_2 by mask before stimulus produces reduced seizure threshold and may prolong seizure duration.
- Stimulus produces initial parasympathetic stimulation assoc with bradycardia and hypotension; transient asystole possible.
- Subsequent sympathetic stimulation assoc with increased HR, increased BP, increased CO, increased myocardial O_2 consumption; rate

pressure product (HR × SBP) increases 50–400%; regional wall motion abn common by TTE

• Other physiologic effects incl increased $CMRO_2$, increased CBF, increased ICP, increased intragastric pressure, increased IOP.

• Vasodilators (sodium nitroprusside, nitroglycerin) and β-blockers (esmolol, labetolol) effective for ameliorating hemodynamic effects of seizure

• Bradycardias rarely require Rx.

Management

• Waveform, frequency, and duration of stimulus adjusted to produce desired seizure

• Some psychiatrists utilize the isolated limb technique: Inflate BP cuff on extremity prior to succinylcholine administration to monitor motor response to seizure

• Seizures ideally 25–120 sec but controversial whether clinical efficacy actually related to seizure duration; prolonged seizures assoc with increased cognitive deficit

Anticipated Problems/Concerns

• Pts frequently have multiple co-morbidities and thorough preop interview may be difficult or impossible given psychiatric illness.

• Repetitive short anesthetics require efficient system to record medical Hx, allergies, drug dosages, complications, etc.

• Rx produces sympathetic activation in pt population deemed medically unfit to tolerate conventional pharmacologic Rx

• Pts commonly complain of headache or myalgias post ECT; this can be treated with acetaminophen or ketorolac.

Endoscopic Sinus Surgery (ESS)

Laura Cavallone

Risk

- Incidence in USA: Chronic rhinosinusitis affects nearly 15% annually
- Males and females equally affected
- Most frequently pts undergo bilateral surgery

Perioperative Risks

- Major complications (0.3% to 1%) incl CSF leak, meningitis, massive bleeding, visual impairment (to diplopia and blindness), stroke, death.
- Minor complications (<1% to 20%) incl periorbital emphysema and ecchymosis, middle turbinate adhesions, epistaxis, facial pain.

Worry About

- Periop control of asthma and airway reactivity
- Quantification of intraop blood losses and/or postop bleeding

- Aspiration of blood and secretions
- Postop N/V

Overview

- ESS is performed to restore normal sinus ventilation and mucosal function in the context of chronic sinusitis of the paranasal sinuses. Also utilized for tear duct surgery, orbital decompression, and drainage of mucoceles.
- Major risks are related to the possibility of perforation of the ethmoid sinus roof, orbital penetration through a dehiscence or fracture of the lamina papyracea, injury to the carotid artery and the optic nerve.
- Surgeon's knowledge of normal anatomy of the nasal cavity and its many variations is of paramount importance in avoiding major complications. Preop CT scans of the nasal cavity and paranasal sinuses are extremely useful to the surgeon as a diagnostic tool and to provide important landmarks for surgery.

Indications and Usual Treatment

- Failure of medical management of recurrent or chronic rhinosinusitis (steroids, antihistamine, antibiotics, decongestant)
- Chronic sinusitis assoc with obstructive nasal polyps
- Treatment of mucoceles
- Dx of neoplasms of the nasal cavity and paranasal sinuses and orbital cellulitis

ASSESSMENT POINTS

System	Effect	Assessment by Hx	PE	Test
HEENT	Postnasal drip	Persistent cough/aspiration	Airway	Laryngoscopy
CARDIO	CAD, toxicity from medications	SOB, exercise tolerance, Hx of palpitations and/or chest pain	CV exam	ECG/other testing as indicated per guidelines for non-cardiac surgery; theophylline level
RESP	Frequent assoc with asthma, allergies, bronchitis	Frequency of asthma exacerbations, hospitalizations with intubation, chronic steroids, known allergens	Chest, larynx (vocalization)	Spirometry
GI		N/V		Theophylline level
CNS	Rule out meningitis	Headache, fever, N/V, visual impairment, mental status, seizures	Neuro	Neuro tests as indicated by Hx/PE

Key Reference: Danielsen A, et al. Anesthesia in endoscopic sinus surgery. *Eur Arch Otorhinolaryngol*. 2003;260(9):481–486.

Perioperative Management

Preoperative Preparation
- Bronchodilator puffs prior to surgery
- Consider stress dose of steroids
- Oxymetazoline spray for topical decongestion

Monitoring
- Standard

Anesthetic Technique/Airway
- General anesthesia preferred technique
- MAC possible only for minor procedures
- Oral intubation +/- oropharyngeal packing or LMA

Induction/Maintenance
- TIVA with propofol and/or remifentanil proposed as better choice (N/V, hemodynamic stability)

- Eye protection with clear tape to allow for orbit inspection by surgeon
- Avoid histamine-releasing medications.
- Intraop anti-emetic drug indicated to prevent N/V
- Controlled hypotension to maintain clear surgical field and facilitate hemostasis not always necessary: always wt benefits against risks of cerebral and/or coronary hypoperfusion (age, co-morbidities).

Surgical Stages

- Lidocaine plus epinephrine injection may cause arrhythmia and/or tachycardia.
- When mucosa is removed from posterior ethmoid cell, risk of perforation of the roof of the ethmoid sinus. During exposure, risk of penetration of the lamina papyracea.
- Injuries to brain, optic nerve, and carotid artery may occur during sphenoidectomy.

Extubation/Postoperative Considerations
- Nasal packing placed after surgery
- Removal of oropharyngeal packing if present and suction of oropharynx/esophagus/stomach are of paramount importance before emergence and/or extubation.
- EBL is usually modest (even if difficult to quantify) unless arterial injury occurs
- Postop pain control is generally easily achieved with opiates and/or acetaminophen.

Endovascular Aortic Stent Repairs

Alexandru Gottlieb

Risk

• Incidence in the USA: About 15,000 aortic stents/y. The number is increasing dramatically (originally was reserved only for high-risk pt, is now indicated for all pts)

Perioperative Risks

• Mostly related to the diffuse arteriosclerotic CV disease, unknown long-term mortality and/or morbidity
• Periop MI: 3–10%
• Geriatric pts with age and other related risk factor: Htn, DM, and COPD
• Potential for thrombosis, embolization, occlusion, or bleeding

Worry About

• Failure of deployment and need to convert to open procedure
• Leak to aortic sack—repeat endovascular intervention
• Device cost may be limiting
• Dissection of the aortic wall.
• Organ ischemia, esp. with the new fenestrated and high thoracic repairs

Overview

• Open repair is still the gold standard. Aortic stent repair was initially suggested for high-risk pts, but successful enough that it is recommended for all reconstructive aortic pts, provided that they do not have contraindication for the operation (see Indications)

• MAC, regional or general anesthesia
• Applicability will be determined by safety, efficiency, durability, cost, and pt demand

ICD-9-CM Code: 44.4 (AAA [unruptured])

Indications and Usual Treatment

• Indication: AAA, occlusive disease, or aortic dissection
• Contraindications: Young pt (long-term prognosis—unknown); aneurysm neck: 4 cm long, >3.5 cm wide irregular, calcified, mural circumferential thrombus; iliac artery disease: occlusive, calcified; dominant inferior mesenteric artery

ASSESSMENT POINTS

System	Effect	Assessment by Hx	PE	Test
RESP	High incidence of lung disease that could have caused this procedure to be selected	Smoking, chronic cough, dyspnea	Chest exam, wheezing, clubbing, cyanosis, dyspnea	CXR, ABGs, spirometry
CARDIO	High incidence of CAD, myocardial ischemia, and/or infarction	Angina, MI, CHF, dysrhythmia PCI, stents, CABG, exercise tolerance, activity level Antiplatelet, anticoagulation Rx	Chest auscultation Vital signs	ECG stress test: ECHO, dipyridamole, thallium, dobutamine Cardiac cath monitor Antiplatelets/ anticoagulants
	Chronic Htn	BP Rx, drug interaction LVH	BP	ECG, CXR Retinal funduscopy
RENAL	High incidence of renal insufficiency 2° to age, arteriosclerosis, and multiple dye studies	Hx of edema and intolerance to salt load	Presence of edema Anurea	Urea, Cr, electrolytes
CNS	Possible carotid disease	Syncope, stroke, or TIAs	Neuro exam Carotid bruit?	Carotid angiogram CT, MRI
ENDO	High incidence of DM	Hx of infections Stress-related/gestational DM Polydipsia, polyuria, coma/stupor Hx of abnormal glucose	Skin infections	CNS exam Urine output Serum glucose
HEME	Some pts on periop heparin, t-PA, or aspirin	Hx of petechiae, nasal bleed	Presence of petechiae or clinical bleeding	PT, PTT, ACT

Key Reference: Baril DT, Kahn RA, Ellozy SH, Carroccio A, Marin ML. Endovascular abdominal aortic aneurysm repair: Emerging developments and anesthetic considerations. *J Cardiothorac Vasc Anesth.* 2007;21(5):730–742.

Perioperative Management

Perioperative Evaluation

• A detailed H & P of the CVS, and medication Hx
• Dysrhythmias, CAD, CHF
• Hypertensive and valvular heart disease
• Noninvasive and invasive cardiac evaluation tests such as stress test and cardiac catheterization

Anesthetic Techniques

• GA, regional anesthesia, or MAC can be performed. Regional anesthesia preferred by some clinicians because of lack of systemic effect on the resp, CV, and GI systems. There is some positive effect of regional anesthesia on coagulation, preserving fibrinolysis and graft patency. General endotracheal anesthesia is used more often lately, due to the development of newer more sophisticated fenestrated and aortic arch graphs, that might lead to bleeding and or organ ischemia.

• Set for possible immediate conversion to open procedure: IVs, arterial line, and CVP

Monitoring

• ECG, arterial BP, UO
• Consider CVP or PA line in pts with severe CAD or LV impairment
• Monitoring for myocardial ischemia: ECG with continuous 3-lead ST-segment analysis, PA catheter, or TEE
• Monitoring volume replacement, CVP, PAOP, cardiac output

Surgical Stages

• Percutaneous or open access to both groins (femoral artery) and/or L brachial artery.
• Thoroughly prep, drape area (2–4 hr, with minimal third space or blood loss)
• Involves multiple fluoroscopy and contrast injection

Postoperative Consideration

• Mild postop pain (3–4)
• Groin hematoma, seroma, or bleeding

Anticipated Problems/Concerns

• Periop cardiac, pulm complications
• Thrombosis and/or embolization of lower limb
• Leak around aortic stent
• Decreased UO
• Spinal ischemia

Pathology Findings

• Continuous persistent leak
• Potential for decreased renal function
• Long-term prognosis after stent repair unavailable

Esophagectomy

Ronald W. Pauldine

Risk

- Esophageal carcinoma: Worldwide sixth leading cause of cancer.
- Adenocarcinoma more common in western countries, among males; assoc with gastro-esophageal reflux and resulting Barrett's esophagus
- Squamous cell more common among African-Americans, males (3:1), tobacco abusers (4:1), alcohol abusers (6:1), Hx of achalasia, caustic burns to esophagus, Paterson-Kelly syndrome (iron-deficiency anemia, esophageal webs, glossitis)

Perioperative Risks

- Operative mortality less than 5% reported by some centers but may be as high as 10–14%
- Multiple risk factors reported for morbidity and mortality incl age, tumor stage, pulm dysfunction, smoking Hx, diabetes, cardiac dysfunction, hepatic dysfunction, and impaired functional status
- Periop complication rate of 10–27% incl anastomotic leak (risk for sepsis due to mediastinitis with intrathoracic anastomosis), pulm insufficiency, delayed emptying of intrathoracic stomach, diaphragmatic herniation of abd viscera, chylothorax, massive aspiration, pancreatitis, delayed splenic rupture, and dysrhythmia

Worry About

- Aspiration risk
- Hemodynamic effects of blunt dissection
- Consequences of N_2O technique if colonic interposition performed
- Recurrent laryngeal nerve injury if cervical anastomosis performed
- Consequences of periop TPN (hypoglycemia, increased CO_2 production)

Overview

- Midline laparotomy to explore for metastases
- Mobilization of stomach (Kocher's maneuver), pyloromyotomy
- Mobilization of esophagus: Depends on site of lesion, surgeon's preference; may occur via transhiatal approach, right (Ivor-Lewis) thoracotomy or three-incision approach with the addition of a left cervical incision.
- Reconstruction: Stomach is preferred conduit, but colon or jejunum may be used

- Minimally invasive endoscopic resection incl thoracoscopy, laparoscopy, and robot-assisted techniques are increasingly employed. Outcome benefit has not been convincingly demonstrated. Some surgeons employ prone positioning for mobilization of the esophagus.

ICD-9-CM Code: 150.9 (Esophageal carcinoma)

Indications and Usual Treatment

- Surgery only curative treatment (5-y survival as high as 70% if limited to stage I disease)
- At presentation disease is usually advanced with overall 5-y survival of only 25%
- Palliative Rx incl chemotherapy, combined chemo/radiation, or radiation alone
- Postop chemotherapy has not resulted in improved survival
- Preop (neoadjuvant) chemotherapy with irradiation may downstage tumors before resection; role in possible improved survival is controversial and not clearly established
- If albumin low, consider preop enteral nutrition

ASSESSMENT POINTS

System	Effect	Assessment by Hx	PE	Test
HEENT	Aspiration risk, esophagorespiratory fistula Tracheal compression	Dysphagia, heartburn, N/V		Barium swallow CT, flow loops
CARDIO	Chemotherapy-induced cardiomyopathy	DOE, PND, orthopnea, exercise tolerance	Auscultation JVD, edema, hepatojugular reflex	CXR, ECHO, MUGA
RESP	Chronic aspiration	Wheezing, dyspnea	Auscultation	CXR, spirometry
GI	Malnutrition GERD	Wt loss, fatigue Heartburn	Cachexia	Serum protein Albumin, pre-albumin
RENAL	Dehydration Electrolyte wasting Renal failure (nephrotoxic chemotherapy)		Orthostatic VS	BUN, Cr Serum electrolytes
HEME	Anemia Impaired immune function			CBC

Key Reference: Cense HA, Lagarde SM, de Jong K, et al. Association of no epidural analgesia with postoperative morbidity and mortality after transthoracic esophageal cancer resection. *J Am Coll Surg.* 2006;202:395–400.

Perioperative Management

Anesthetic Technique

- General or combined technique (thoracic epidural frequently employed, increasing experience with paravertebral techniques)
- Evidence suggests improved outcome with addition of thoracic epidural. However, concern for decreased perfusion of distal end of gastric tube reconstruction—may have implications for BP management
- If transhiatal or left thoracotomy approach, single-lumen ETT is adequate. Right thoracotomy approach requires placement of a double-lumen tube or bronchial blocker.
- Consider lung protective ventilation strategy – may have beneficial effect on postop SIRS

Monitoring

- Large-bore IV access
- Consider arterial catheter
- Consider central venous catheter

Airway

- Full-stomach precautions
- Possibility of tracheal compression if significant mediastinal lymphadenopathy

- Possible esophagorespiratory fistula (may need to maintain spontaneous ventilation)
- Use of gel lubricants on ETT cuff may decrease risk of aspiration intraop

Induction

- Potential for significant hypotension if dehydrated
- If esophagorespiratory fistula: Avoid PPV, vent stomach if necessary, isolate fistula with appropriate double-lumen ETT

Surgical Stages

Dissection

- Initial laparotomy
- Depending on approach may have right thoracotomy
- Cervical incision if cervical anastomosis to be performed (necessary with transhiatal approach, in addition to thoracotomy with three-incision approach)

Definitive Surgery

- Blunt dissection during transhiatal approach may result in compression of vena cava or heart with resultant hypotension or dysrhythmias

- Impaired gas exchange may occur during 1-lung ventilation if required
- EBL: 500–1500 mL

Postoperative Considerations

- High periop mortality due to cardiorespiratory complications, sepsis (related to anastomotic leak)
- Pulm complications common and strongly correlated with increased morbidity and mortality Significant postop pain, esp. with approaches employing thoracotomy
- Pain management may incl IV PCA, epidural PCA, epidural and subarachnoid narcotics, intrapleural techniques and paravertebral block
- Possibility of disruption of cervical anastomosis if reintubation required immediately postop. However early extubation appears safe and is assoc with decreased LOS in ICU. Delayed extubation can be considered for selected high-risk pts

Anticipated Problems/Concerns

- Possibility for unrecognized pneumothorax with transhiatal approach

Extracorporeal Membrane Oxygenation (ECMO)

Suanne M. Daves

Risk

- Proven utility in newborn resp failure
- Common causes of newborn resp failure are meconium aspiration, persistent fetal circulation, persistent pulm Htn (PPH), congenital diaphragmatic hernia, sepsis
- May be indicated in children and adults with potentially reversible resp failure unresponsive to conventional therapy
- Used for cardiac and pulm support after cardiac surgery in infants and children

Perioperative Risks

- Survival depends on the underlying condition
- Neonatal resp failure has an 80% survival for those thought to have a 20% survival without ECMO

- Survival after repair of CHD in infants is largely dependent on the severity of the underlying lesion (43–54% in TOF, 14% in HLHS)

Worry About

- Mechanical complications (cannula dislodgment, clot in circuit, air in circuit)
- Bleeding complications (particularly intracranial hemorrhage)
- Multisystem organ failure

Overview

- Provides total resp support with venovenous or venoarterial bypass
- Venoarterial bypass also provides total hemodynamic support

- Pt is anticoagulated to maintain an activated clotting time (ACT) of ~200 sec

ICD-9-CM Code: 756.6 (Congenital diaphragmatic hernia; 769 (RDS])

Indications and Usual Treatment

- Criteria vary among institutions
- Contraindications: Congenital abn not compatible with meaningful life, profound neurologic impairment, irreversible lung disease, prolonged ventilatory support (>7–10 d), estimated gestational age <35 wk, evidence of intracranial hemorrhage

ASSESSMENT POINTS

System	Effect	Assessment by Hx	PE	Test
CARDIO	Myocardial dysfunction	Hypoxemia, acidosis	CV exam	ECHO Hemodynamic variables ABGs
	PPH	Hypoxemia R → L shunt through PDA or PFO	CV exam	ECHO Hemodynamic variables ABGs
NEURO	Hemorrhage	Intracranial hemorrhage	Neuro exam	Cranial US

Key Reference: Rais-Bahrami K, Short BL. The current status of neonatal extracorporeal membrane oxygenation. *Semin Perinatol.* 2000;24:406–417.

Intraoperative Management

Monitoring

- ECG, temp, UO
- Arterial and central venous pressures
- Arterial and mixed venous blood gases
- Pulse oximetry if cardiac ejections present

Surgical Stages

Anesthetic Choice

- Cannulation often performed at the bedside in ICU with local anesthetic infiltration. Narcotics and muscle relaxants may be used and continued while cannulas in place.
- ECMO may be initiated in OR after failure to wean from CPB

Initiating ECMO

- Venoarterial ECMO can be done with extrathoracic cannulation (carotid artery and internal jugular vein or femoral artery and vein) or by transthoracic cannulation through a median sternotomy (aorta and right atrium)
- Original cannulation sites are used after failure to wean from CPB in OR
- Right internal jugular vein is commonly used for venovenous bypass
- Heparin (100–150 units/kg) is given and the vessels are cannulated
- Bypass is initiated slowly by increasing extracorporeal flow rate
- After reaching full flow rates, ventilate at nontraumatic settings

Ecmo Management

- Heparin to maintain ACTs at approx 200 sec. If bleeding occurs, the ACT can be maintained at lower levels (140–180 sec).
- Plts transfused to maintain 100,000/mm^3
- As cardiopulmonary function improves, the pump flow is decreased. Prior to decannulation, the pt is given a trial without ECMO support.
- After decannulation, the vessels are usually ligated.

Anticipated Problems/Concerns

- Hypoxia and hemodynamic instability prior to bypass
- Bleeding complications
- Multiorgan failure
- Mechanical problems with ECMO circuitry

Extracorporeal Shock Wave Lithotripsy (ESWL)

Peter T. Choi

Christopher D. Beatie

PROCEDURES

Risk

- Annual incidence of urolithiasis: 1.5/1000

Perioperative Risks

- Shock waves can trigger cardiac dysrhythmias if not delivered during ventricular refractory period.
- Shock waves can damage kidney resulting in perinephric hematoma, parenchymal injury with loss of renal function, hematuria, new-onset Htn.
- Shock waves can cause pancreatic, hepatic injury resulting in elevations in amylase, lipase, bilirubin, lactic dehydrogenase, transaminases, CK; changes are usually mild, transient.

Worry About

- Cardiac dysrhythmias
- Cardiopulmonary derangements resulting from immersion
- Electrical safety in water bath
- Renal insufficiency
- Plt dysfunction

Overview

- Shock waves propagated through body to pulverize urinary stones. First-generation lithotriptors require immersion in water bath, which complicate monitoring, airway management, and induce, changes in cardiopulmonary physiology; regional (usually epidural) anesthesia preferred for procedures in these machines.
- Second-generation "dry" lithotriptors eliminate these problems, generate less powerful shock waves, so lighter planes of anesthesia or sedation combined with topical anesthesia may be effective.
- Third-generation lithotriptors use piezoelectric crystals with smaller focal zone, are essentially painless; may also be used to pulverize gallstones.

ICD-9-CM Codes: N20.0 (Kidney stones); N20.1 (Ureteral stones); N20.9 (Urinary stones)

Indications and Usual Treatment

- Preferred choice for upper urinary tract stones <2 cm; lower stone-free rate compared to invasive methods, esp. with stones >1 cm. Absolute contraindications: Urosepsis, pregnancy, coagulopathy, uncorrected obstruction; relative contraindications: morbid obesity, renal malformations, intra-abd calcific processe (e.g., AAAs)
- Urolithiasis may also be Rx by alkalinization of the urine using potassium citrate.
- Urinary stones can be extremely painful; pts may be taking variety of analgesic drugs incl NSAIDs, opioids.

ASSESSMENT POINTS

System	Effect	Assessment by Hx	PE	Test
GI	Delayed gastric emptying, gastritis, PUD	Reflux Sx, dyspepsia, abd pain		Hgb, endoscopy, upper GI x-ray, stool heme
HEME	Anemia (due to renal failure, GI losses), Plt dysfunction (due to analgesia or uremia)	Fatigue, bruising, bleeding	Pallor, ecchymoses, petechiae	Hct, bleeding time
GU	Obstructive uropathy, analgesic nephritis	Oliguria, anuria, CHF Sx	Rales, edema	BUN/Cr, UA, CXR

Key Reference: Lee C, et al. Impact of type of anesthesia on efficacy of medstone STS lithotripter. *J Endourol.* 2007;21:957–960.

Intraoperative Management

Preoperative Preparation

- Evaluate renal function
- Evaluate plt function
- R/O anemia

Anesthetic Technique

- Regional anesthesia usually preferred for immersion-type lithotriptors
- Plt dysfunction may influence decision to use regional anesthesia.
- If GA used, small TV should be used to keep stone at focal point of shock wave.
- Pt position in gantry requires care to avoid peripheral nerve damage; pt can be prone on newer lithotriptors.
- Local anesthesia, topical anesthesia (e.g., EMLA) and/or IV sedation usually sufficient with newer lithotriptors

Monitoring

- Easier if pt arms not immersed
- Cover ECG leads with waterproof tape

- If BP cuff to be immersed, use clip-type cuff (Velcro will not work).
- Pulse oximetry probes may be placed on ear or nose if fingers immersed.

Airway

- Intubation or LMA indicated for GA

Induction/Maintenance

- Typically 1000–4000 shocks/Rx, 60 shocks/min
- If shock waves gated (synchronized) to ECG, bradycardia can prolong Rx.
- HR higher than lithotriptor's max firing rate also prolongs Rx by forcing shock waves to be triggered by every other QRS complex.

EBL/Volume Concerns

- Effects of immersion in water bath
  - Increased venous return due to hydrostatic pressure, resulting in increased CO
    - Afterload, FRC, TV decreased
  - Increased renin, ADH secretion result in diuresis, kaliuresis, natriuresis

- Hypotension possible on emergence from water bath
- Diuretics, hydration may be used to encourage passage of stone fragments.

Postoperative Considerations

- Pain scale: 1–3; NSAIDs usually sufficient
- Postop N/V common: Give appropriate prophylaxis intraop
- Hematuria frequent postop: Usually resolves spontaneously over several days

Anticipated Problems/Concerns

- Lithotripsy suite often noisy, dimly lit. Use caution to maintain adequate monitoring, pt safety

Eye Enucleation

Howard D. Palte

Risk

- Eye trauma
- Incidence in USA: >2 million/y; 8000–10,000 ablations/y
- Majority pts <30 y of age
- Most common cause of enucleation in children >3 y of age
- Ocular tumors <5/100,000 population

Perioperative Risks

- Age, co-morbidities and medications
- Hx of postop N/V (PONV)
- Assoc trauma
- Chemotherapy and/or radiation therapy
- Pt acceptance and/or psychological preparation

Worry About

- Oculocardiac reflex (OCR)
- Co-morbid illness
- PONV
- Hemorrhage

Overview

- Evisceration: Removal of the contents of the globe leaving the sclera and extra-ocular muscles intact
- Enucleation: Removal of the eye from the orbit with preservation of all other orbital structures
- Exenteration: Removal of the eye, adnexa, and portions of the bony orbit.

Etiology

- Intraocular malignancy (choroidal melanoma, retinoblastoma, other)
- Trauma (primary or sympathetic ophthalmia)
- Blind painful eye (endophthalmitis, uveitis, neovascular glaucoma, cosmetic)

ASSESSMENT POINTS

System	Effects	Assessment by Hx	PE	Test
HEENT	Sleep apnea Anxiety	Snoring Claustrophobia	Airway exam	
CARDIO	Htn, CAD Arrhythmia	Headache, angina Syncope, palpitations	BP Pulse rate/rhythm	EKG/ECHO
RESP	COAD	Chronic cough, exercise Tolerance	Chest auscultation	CXR O_2 sat

Perioperative Management

Preoperative Management

- Age, co-morbidities and medications
- Hx of postop N/V (PONV)
- Assoc trauma
- Chemotherapy and/or radiation therapy
- Corroboration of surgical necessity by second ophthalmologist
- Pt acceptance and psychological preparation (lesser importance in pts with blind painful eye)
- Anesthesia technique discussion (GA vs. RA+ MAC)
- Anxiolysis

Intraoperative Management

- Pt, site, and procedure verification ("TIME OUT")
- Standard ASA monitors
- Technique: General (GA) vs. regional (RA) and monitored anesthesia care (MAC)
- Evisceration: RA > GA (usually elderly, frail, ASA Status III-IV)
- Enucleation: RA = GA (trauma/painful eye, children, ASA Status I-II)
- Exenteration: GA (extensive resection + bony orbital wall components)

General anesthesia

- Endotracheal tube (ETT) versus supraglottic airway (LMA)
- Deep plane anesthesia during dissection of extra-ocular muscles and optic nerve
- Optic nerve difficult to dissect and sever: Beware of bradycardia and asystole.
- Request early alert from surgeon, and deepen anesthesia and/or sedation in a timely fashion
- Venous congestion and pt positioning (head-up and/or pressure points)

Regional Anesthesia

- Extraconal versus intraconal block
- Local anesthetic solution (intermediate vs. long-acting agent)
- Additives (hyaluronidase and/or epinephrine); consider benefit vasoconstriction vs. risk tachycardia.
- OCR (traction extra-ocular muscles and/or ablation optic nerve); consider anticholinergic agents
- PONV prophylaxis

Emergence

- Avoid coughing and/or straining
- Awake versus deep extubation

Postoperative Management

- Analgesia: Supplement GA with regional block (esp. children)
- Emesis control (consider use > 1 agent)
- Minimize venous congestion with head-up position
- Hemorrhage and/or apply firm dressing
- Visual hallucinations
- Psychological concerns and/or professional intervention

PROCEDURES

Gas Embolism

Richard E. Moon
Bryant W. Stolp

Risk

- Accidental injection of gas into a blood vessel during diagnostic or therapeutic procedures
  - Cardiopulmonary bypass
  - Cardiac catheterization, angiography
  - Hemodialysis
  - Pressurization of an IV bottle using air
- Entrainment of air into a vein during surgical procedures in which venous pressure at the wound site is subatmospheric (wound higher than heart)
  - Sitting craniotomy
  - Spine surgery
  - Total hip replacement
  - Dental implant surgery
  - Cesarean section
- Surgery in which gas could be injected into tissues
  - Intrauterine laser surgery
  - Laparoscopy
  - Arthroscopy
- Other forceful instillation of air into tissues
  - Injury due to industrial compressed air
  - Blowing air intravaginally during oral sex
- Pulm overexpansion, in which gas enters the pulm capillaries
  - Breath holding or regional gas trapping during ascent from a scuba dive
  - PPV
- Hydrogen peroxide irrigation or ingestion

Perioperative Risks

When NO is used, gas in blood vessels or tissues can expand to 2—4× its original volume, compounding the original injury.

Worry About

- Stroke, cerebral edema
- Myocardial infarction
- Pulm edema

Overview and Etiology

- Immediate effect: Obstruction of blood flow and tissue ischemia; pulm Htn if venous gas
- Secondary effect: Increased permeability of vascular endothelium, tissue edema (pulm edema from venous gas)
- Tertiary effect: Leukocyte accumulation on vascular endothelium, resulting in release of mediators and late reduction in blood flow
- While small venous gas emboli are prevented by the pulm capillary network from entering the arterial circulation, large volumes of gas can exceed its filtration capacity. Air can also enter the left heart via intrapulmonary or intracardiac right-to-left shunts, incl patent foramen ovale.
- Venous gas embolism can cause sudden hypotension, hypoxemia, pulm Htn or cardiac arrest. Awake individuals may experience dyspnea, tachypnea, or cough.
- Arterial gas embolism is manifested by altered consciousness, acute onset of focal neurologic deficit, arrhythmias, and ST segment elevation or depression.
- Venous gas emboli can be detected by a change in the cardiac sounds as detected using a precordial Doppler monitor, an immediate reduction in ETCO$_2$, mass spectrometer or Raman detection of nitrogen in the expired gas (when the inspired gas contains no air). Bubbles can also be detected using trans-thoracic or trans-esophageal echocardiography and transcranial doppler.

- Rarely, a "mill-wheel" murmur (a whoosh sound in both systole and diastole) can be heard by precordial stethoscope. The absence of this sign cannot be used to exclude the diagnosis.

ICD-9-CM Codes: 958.0; 999.1; 673.0

Usual Treatment

- If possible prevent further ingress of gas
- If surgical gas embolism:
  - Flood surgical field with fluid
  - Lower surgical site with respect to the heart
  - Elevate venous pressure (accomplishing this via application of PEEP can augment right-to-left shunt if the pt has an intracardiac defect, e.g., patent foramen ovale).
- 100% inspired O$_2$ to enhance oxygenation of ischemic tissues and increase the nitrogen diffusion gradient from bubble into blood.
- IV fluid administration to maintain intravascular volume
- Use hyperbaric O$_2$ to effect reduction in size and rapid resolution of bubbles. Hyperbaric O$_2$ (HBO) may also inhibit adherence of leukocytes to endothelium, thus minimizing the tertiary effects noted above. Immediate treatment with hyperbaric O$_2$ is most efficacious; delayed treatment can also be effective. Indications for HBO incl neurologic deficit, myocardial ischemia, residual left-sided intracardiac gas, or cardiovascular compromise. Pulm edema may also respond to HBO therapy.
- Radiographic imaging (e.g., brain CT, MRI) cannot be used to confirm the diagnosis and plays no useful role.

ASSESSMENT POINTS

System	Effect	Assessment by Hx	PE	Test
CARDIO	Filling of cardiac chambers with air ↑ Permeability of vascular endothelium Tissue edema		Hypotension Mill-wheel murmur	Echocardiography, precordial Doppler, ↓ PETCO$_2$, ↑ PETN$_2$, ECG (ST depression)
RESP	Pulm Htn Pulm edema	Dyspnea, tachypnea, cough	Crackles on auscultation of chest (commonly not heard)	PA pressure measurement CXR
CNS	Arterial gas embolism or transpulmonary/transcardiac passage of venous gas emboli	Acute onset of focal neurologic deficit, generalized encephalopathy, seizures	Neurologic exam	Brain imaging (CT, MRI) often normal, cerebral edema may be seen.

Key Reference: van Hulst RA, Klein J, Lachmann B. Gas embolism: Pathophysiology and treatment. *Clin Physiol Funct Imaging*. 2003;23:237–246.

Perioperative Implications

- Pts at high risk for venous gas embolism should receive appropriate monitoring, which may include
  - Direct arterial pressure monitoring
  - Continuous monitoring of PETCO$_2$, PETN$_2$
  - Precordial Doppler
  - TEE

- Consider avoiding the use of NO, and if pulm O$_2$ toxicity is not a concern, using 100% O$_2$
- If gas embolization is suspected, NO or nitrogen and/or O$_2$ gas mix should be immediately D/C and replaced with 100% O$_2$.
- Individuals requiring surgery, who have recently suffered gas embolism due to scuba diving, or decompression sickness (in situ gas formation due

to nitrogen supersaturation) from diving or compressed air exposure, should not be administered NO anesthesia.

Gastrectomy

Risk

- Adenocarcinoma of stomach: 21,000 new cases annually; ~11,000 deaths annually
- 1/113 people will be diagnosed in lifetime; most pts diagnosed after age: 65
- M:F ratio: 2:1
- Higher incidence in first-generation Asian-Americans; higher incidence in USA black men compared to white men
- Incidence of gastrectomy has been decreasing 2° to treatment of *Helicobacter pylori* infection, medical treatment of Zollinger-Ellison syndrome

Perioperative Risks

- In-hospital mortality 2–6% in more recent trials; 15–32% in slightly older trials with extended dissection; <2% for partial garstrectomy
- Worse nutritional status results in higher morbidity and mortality

- Pulm complications in 15% of pts
- Pulm emboli: 1%
- Pneumonia: 8%
- Postop bleeding: 6%
- Abd abscess: 7%

Worry About

- Periop hypovolemia
- Anemia
- Large third space losses
- Malnutrition

Overview

- Resection of all or part of the stomach for either malignant or benign diagnoses
- Bleeding can occur from spleen or blood supply to stomach
- Periop hypovolemia from blood loss, poor PO intake, or GI losses
- NGT can be accidently ligated; make sure it is properly pulled back prior to resection

ICD-9-CM Codes: 151.9 (Gastric cancer); 531 (Gastric ulcer)

Indications and Usual Treatment

- Total gastrectomy
  - Gastric cancer (adenocarcinoma, GIST, etc)
  - Uncontrollable hemorrhagic gastritis (less commonly currently with angiography and endoscopy)
  - Zollinger-Ellison syndrome (medical management more common currently with proton pump inhibitors and octreotide)
  - Severe gastroparesis after previous stomach surgery
- Partial gastrectomy
  - Gastric ulcers
  - Gastric cancer

ASSESSMENT POINTS

System	Effect	Assessment by Hx	PE	Test
CARDIO	Hypovolemia	N/V, diarrhea, poor oral intake	↓ BP, ↑ HR, ↓ UO, ↓ skin turgor	Orthostatics, EKG
RESP	Pulmonary aspiration	N/V, hypoxemia	Chest auscultation	CXR, ABG, pulse ox
GI	Obstruction	Abd pain or N/V	Abd exam	CT scan or Abd x-ray
HEME	Anemia	GI bleeding	Pallor, tachycardia	CBC; PT/PTT if coagulopathy suspected
GU	Renal dysfunction	Poor UO	Hydration status	BUN, Cr, electrolytes
ENDO	Malnutrion	Wt loss	Cachexia	Albumin, prealbumin

Key Reference: Murray P, Whiting P, Hutchinson SP, Ackroyd R, Stoddard CJ, Billings C. Preoperative shuttle walking testing and outcome after oesophagogastrectomy. *Br J Anaesth.* 2007;99(6):809–811.

Perioperative Management

Preoperative Preparation

- Assess pre-existing conditions and volume status, electrolytes consider periop beta-blockade in elderly
- Aspiration premedication with H₂ blockers, metoclopramide (contraindicated in obstruction), and sodium citrate
- Preop resuscitation; correct anemia appropriately, esp. with pre-existing cardiac disease
- Consider TPN to correct malnutrition prior to OR if albumin <2.1
- Consider insertion of an epidural for periop pain control and less pulm complication postop; test prior to induction to ensure correct placement

Monitoring

- Essential to have good measurement of volume status 2° to fluid shifts and periop hypovolemia
- Foley catheter to monitor UO
- Consider arterial line based on co-morbidities
- CVP may be helpful; PA cath is usually not needed

Anesthetic Technique/Induction

- Balanced general anesthetic; general/regional

- Consider awake techniques or rapid sequence induction with cricoid pressure for pts at high risk of aspiration
- Use forced air warmers, warmed IV fluids, and warmed humidified gases to prevent hypothermia
- NGT is often needed; discuss when to place with surgeon

Surgical Stages

- Incision: Upper midline; unilateral or bilateral subcostal
- Pt is positioned supine, thoracotomy is a possibility in proximal lesions; lung isolation should be planned through discussion with surgeon
- Some surgeons use laparoscopy to assess for metastasis prior to laparotomy
- Left lobe of liver is retracted and packs may be inserted near diaphragm; watch for increased peak airway pressures
- The greater and lesser omentum are part of surgical specimen; splenectomy is occasionally performed for total gastrectomy for cancer; distal pancreatectomy if pancreas involved with tumor
- Stomach is mobilized and blood supply ligated; duodenum and esophagus are transected

- Intestinal continuity restored, typically with roux-en-y esophagojejunostomy
- Drains inserted and abd closed
- EBL: >500mL for total gastrectomy
- Third space losses are around 10 mL/kg/hr

Postoperative Considerations

- Pain score: 8–9
- Pain control with IV PCA or epidural analgesia
- Consider ICU for pts with significant cardiopulmonary co-morbidities
- Postop mechanical ventilation may be needed uncommonly for diaphragmatic impairment, hemodynamic instability, or acidosis

Anticipated Problems/Concerns

- Anemia may be masked by hypovolemia
- Pulm complications are common (2° to decreased FRC from incisional pain)
- Consider use of SQ heparin for DVT prophylaxis pre-induction
- Re-operation most commonly for bleeding <6%

Gastric Bypass Stapling for Morbid Obesity

David Eckmann

Risk

- Incidence in USA: 65% of adult population (>200 million in USA)
- >300,000 deaths annually attributable to obesity
- Second to smoking as preventable cause of death
- Predominantly caused by long-term excess caloric ingestion

Perioperative Risks

- Depends on degree of obesity (superobese, obese class I–III)
- Mortality: 0.27% (laparoscopic), 0.81% (open)
- Morbidity: Strongly depends on co-existing disease: obstructive sleep apnea, metabolic syndrome, CV disease, renal dysfunction
- Wound, GI, pulm, and CV complication 1–5%

- Complication rates higher with open procedures
- Re-operation causes incl postop intra-abd bleeding, anastomotic leakage, suture line dehiscence, small bowel obstruction, deep wound infection
- DVT and pulm embolism

Worry About

- Pt positioning for airway management
- Maintenance of lung volume
- Anesthetic drug dosing

Overview

- High incidence of co-existing metabolic syndrome, obstructive sleep apnea, Type 2 diabetes, Htn, CAD
- Ease of airway management directly related to optimizing pt positioning

- Anesthesia goals are to maintain lung volume, manage airway safely, dose drugs and medications for obesity, optimize return to spontaneous ventilation in the face of obstructive sleep apnea

Indications and Usual Treatment

- Body mass index >35 kg/m²
- Failure of nonsurgical management of obesity
- Endocrine abn (metabolic syndrome, Type 2 diabetes) or other CV (Htn) or pulm (obstructive sleep apnea) pathophysiology present
- Restrictive (gastric banding) or malabsorptive (roux-en-y gastric bypass or sleeve) procedure to induce wt loss and aid resolution of endocrine and other abn

ASSESSMENT POINTS

System	Effect	Assessment by Hx	PE	Test
HEENT	Obstructive sleep apnea Excess oral and pharyngeal adipose tissue	Snoring, dyspnea, daytime somnolence	Large tongue, tonsils, uvula	Polysomnography
CARDIO	Htn, pulm Htn, CAD with possible ventricular dysfunction, LVH, RVH	Angina, PND	Pedal edema	Stress ECG, ECHO, dipyridamole thallium or dobutamine ECHO
RESP	Obstructive sleep apnea, diminished closing volume	Snoring, dyspnea, daytime somnolence	Dyspneic when supine	Polysomnography, PFTs, CXR, ABG
CNS	Neurovascular insufficiency	TIA, stroke	Cognitive impairment, neuro deficits	Neuro assessment

Key Reference: Gross JB, Bachenberg KL, Benumof JL, et al. Practice guidelines for the perioperative management of patients with obstructive sleep apnea: A report by the American Society of Anesthesiologists Task Force on Perioperative Management of patients with obstructive sleep apnea. *Anesthesiology.* 2006;104:1081–1093.

Perioperative Management

Preoperative Preparation

- Assess co-existing morbidities, plan to maintain homeostasis
- Consider epidural placement for open procedures for periop analgesia
- Consider inferior vena cava filter placement for superobese pts and discussion with surgeon regarding DVT for all

Monitoring

- Noninvasive monitoring, large-bore vascular access
- Invasive arterial pressure monitoring for pts with significant cardiac disease (LVEF < 35%, and/or proven significant CAD)
- Central venous access only if peripheral access cannot be established

Anesthetic Technique/Induction

- Pt carefully placed in ramped positioned for induction of general anesthesia following placement of epidural, if used
- Adequate preoxygenation using PEEP or pressure support
- All drugs dosed for total or ideal body weight, as appropriate
- Stable induction technique with full NMB achieved prior to intubation

- Perform lung volume recruitment maneuvers following intubation
- Avoid use of NO
- Careful positioning and padding of extremities
- Administration of DVT prophylaxis if pt lacks IVC filter

Surgical Stages

Dissection

- Maintain adequate NMB
- Provide appropriate level of mechanical ventilation, esp. in laparoscopic procedures during pneumoperitoneum
- Provide adequate IV fluids, esp. with use of steep reverse Trendelenberg position

Gastric Stapling

- Remove NG tube, esophageal temp probe prior to stapling
- For gastric pouch creation, advance and remove bougie carefully without disturbing ETT position
- Carefully reinsert NG tube into gastric pouch under surgical guidance and assess staple lines for leaks

Anesthetic Technique/Emergence

- Fully reverse NMB
- Establish adequacy of analgesia for immediate postop care

- Maintain mechanical ventilatory support until extubation
- Extubate pt from head-up position and immediately apply CPAP

Postoperative Considerations

- Maintain CPAP or BiPAP, supplemental O₂ and head-up positioning in recovery and on floor
- Postop analgesia: Epidural vs. IV PCA
- Monitor IV PCA use and undesired side effects increasing airway obstruction
- Use continuous pulse oximetry postop
- Clearly identify those pts who were difficult to intubate

Anticipated Problems/Concerns

- Use of IV PCA can be assoc with resp depression and exacerbation of airway obstruction symptoms requiring reintubation
- Pts may derecruit lung volume rapidly during any phase of the anesthetic care
- Controversies incl rapid sequence induction versus attempted mask ventilation after anesthetic induction; resp monitoring postop; requirement for high acuity nursing floor care

Gastroschisis Surgery

Peter J. Davis

Risk

- Rare abd wall abn
- Occurs in 1/20,000 births

Perioperative Risks

- Increased risk of infection
- 90–100% survival reported

Worry About

- Large fluid requirements
- Temp instability
- Cardiopulmonary compromise 2° to increase intraabd pressure
- Postop ventilation
- Postop nutrition
- Postop infection
- Other congenital abn

Overview

- Extrusion of abd contents through a defect to the right of the umbilical cord. Must be differentiated from omphalocele.
- True surgical emergency
- Abd contents not covered by sac
- Abd viscera matted together and thickened 2° to amniotic fluid exposure and chemical peritonitis
- 60% of pts are premature
- Assoc abn (other than GI) rare, but their presence may affect pt morbidity and mortality
- GI abn incl intestinal atresia and stenosis.

ICD-9-CM Code: 756.7 (Congenital)

Usual Treatment

- Medical management
  - Wrap exposed viscera in saline-soaked gauze
  - NG tube to decompress abd contents
  - Antibiotics
  - Treat CV and resp instability
- Increased fluid requirements, large 3rd space fluid losses
- Temp instability
- Surgery definitive treatment
  - Spring-loaded silo may obviate surgery

ASSESSMENT POINTS

System	Effect	Assessment by Hx	PE	Test
CARDIO	Impaired transitional circulation Hypotension 2° to hypovolemia	Cyanosis and acidosis Poor UO Poor tissue perfusion	Poor capillary refill Poor perfusion Poor UO	CXR, ECHO, SaO_2 BP ABGs
	Hypotension 2° to ↑ intra-abd pressure	Poor UO, poor tissue perfusion, cold lower extremities, vascular congestion, cyanosis		
RESP	Surfactant deficiency 2° to prematurity Restrictive lung disease 2° to ↑ intra-abdominal pressure	Tachypnea, hypoxemia	Auscultation	ABGs ↓ Pulm compliance
METAB	Large 3rd space fluid requirements Hyper-/hyponatremia	Review of volume replacement	Skin perfusion, UO	BP Electrolytes
TEMP	Hypothermia 2° to large heat loss from large 3rd space fluid requirements			

Key Reference: Raghavan M, Montgomerie J. Anesthetic management of gastrochisis—a review of our practice over the past 5 years. *Paediatr Anaesth*. 2008;18(11):1055–1059.

Perioperative Implications

Anesthetic Technique

- GA
- Endotracheal intubation
- Avoid N_2O

Monitoring

- Pulse oximeters on both the right upper extremity and a lower extremity
- Adequate venous access preferably above the diaphragm
- Consider arterial catheter
- Consider central venous catheter
- Foley catheter

Airway

- Expect usual neonatal variants
- Endotracheal intubation
- Avoid distention of bowel by bag and/or mask ventilation
- Muscle relaxation required

Induction

- CV instability 2° to hypovolemia
- Avoid N_2O

Surgical Stages

Dissection

- Care in bowel manipulation
- Blood loss 2° to adhesions
- Hypotension from bowel manipulation, blood loss, and large third space fluid requirements

Definitive Surgery

- Four surgical options
  - 1° fascial closure
  - Skin closure
  - Prosthetic silo with delayed closure, *or*
  - Insertion of Silastic spring-loaded silo
- All options assoc with increased intraabd pressure. With abd closure: If intragastric pressure >20 mmHg and CVP changes by >4 mmHg, consider silo. If intragastric pressure <20 mmHg and CVP changes <4 mmHg, consider 1° repair.
- All surgical closure options assoc with increased risk of sepsis
  - Spring-loaded silo may obviate surgery

Postoperative Considerations

- Need for mechanical ventilation
- Need for hyperalimentation
- In pts with silo, gradual reduction of abd contents, increased risk of sepsis, and prolonged ventilatory requirements

Anticipated Problems/Concerns

- Hypovolemia 2° to large third space–fluid requirements
- Instability 2° to increased intra-abdominal pressure following abd wall closure
- Decrease in lung compliance 2° to impaired diaphragmatic movement from reduced abd contents and increased intra-abd pressure
- Prolonged postop pain relief may be required
- Increased risk of necrotizing enterocolitis
- Long-term survival dependent on assoc abn
- Bowel obstruction common morbidity

Geriatric Surgery

Stanley Muravchick

Risk

- Major complications: 20% for vascular procedures, 10% for general surgery, 3% for minor procedures
- Periop (1 mo) mortality: About 3%

Perioperative Risk Factors

- Emergency procedures
- Increased acuity and severity of pre-existing disease
- Compromised physical status (ASA 3–4) and limited range of daily activity
- Extreme agedness (85 y or older)
- Surgery that will significantly limit postop mobility

Worry About

- Susceptibility to infection
- Fluid overload
- Renal insufficiency
- Prolonged drug effects
- Myocardial ischemia
- Disorientation and delirium
- Pressure points and tissue fragility

Overview

- Aging of healthy individuals reduces organ system functional reserve.
- Age-related disease exposes and exacerbates the decrease in reserve produced by aging.
- Polypharmacy for age-related co-morbidities further increases the risk of adverse periop outcome in older adults.
- Therefore, the severity of age-related disease is the most powerful predictor of periop complications and death in the elderly.

Choice Of Anesthetic Approach

- Anesthesia itself is not a major factor in periop morbidity and mortality.
- There is no objective evidence to support a "best" anesthetic approach for the elderly pt.
- Optimal periop outcome generally reflects aggressive preop disease management, meticulous attention to the details of intraop management, adequate control of periop pain and stress, and early ambulation.

Perioperative Management

Preoperative Preparation

- Careful clinical Hx and assessment of physical status with special scrutiny of ability to ambulate and exercise
- Limit preop "screening tests" to those areas with a clinical correlate (Hx or physical exam) that suggests presence of a definable disease process.
- Echocardiographic estimate of cardiac ejection fraction if adequacy of aerobic capacity not obvious
- Optimize control of significant pre-existing medical issues such as CAD, asthma, Htn, or diabetes.

Monitoring

- Standard ASA monitors usually adequate for short diagnostic procedures (e.g., endoscopy or cystoscopy) and surgery not involving major body cavity
- Consider arterial cannulas for pts having major surgery (i.e., intra-abdominal, -thoracic, -cranial) or for prolonged procedures requiring repeated arterial samples or continuous BP assessment
- Consider central venous catheters for pts with evidence of diffusely impaired ventricular function or those who do not have reliable peripheral IV access; consider pulm artery catheter if clear evidence of severe left ventricular compromise.

Altered Response to Anesthetics

- Prolonged circulation time dictates slow drug infusion to avoid overdosage
- Unconsciousness usually achieved with lower plasma levels of drug than in younger adults.
- Anesthetic maintenance requirements reduced 20–30% by the eighth decade of life
- Regional anesthesia is effective but slightly smaller segmental dose requirements and greater risk of sympathectomy-induced hypotension
- Expect reduced narcotic requirement and increased duration of clinical effect, but adequacy of analgesia must be carefully titrated.
- Usually little change in dosage required for NMB, but expect some prolongation of duration of clinical effect
- Complex intraop polypharmacy may produce unpredictable emergence phenomena, esp. if it alters central cholinergic receptors.

Postoperative Considerations

- Pay careful attention to adequate hydration and control of hemodynamics to maintain metabolic homeostasis and good tissue perfusion.
- Avoid excessive sympathoadrenal stress that can increase CV demands in excess of the age-related reduction in functional reserve.
- Avoid the CNS depression and coagulopathies assoc with hypothermia.
- Anticipate high likelihood of acute postop delirium, exacerbated by poor pain control, Hx of alcohol abuse, or pre-existing cognitive impairment.

Anticipated Problems/Concerns

- 1° causes of postop morbidity and mortality in this age group are infection, myocardial ischemia, and thromboembolism.
- From the middle adult years onward, increasing age is assoc with a significant risk (5–15%) of subtle and poorly understood long-term postop cognitive dysfunction (POCD). The risk does not appear to be reduced with any specific anesthetic approach.
- Long-term survival in elderly surgical pts appears to be enhanced when there are minimal complications in the acute postop period and the surgery itself improves the pt's mobility and physical independence.

Consequences of Aging	Anesthetic Implications	Clinical Adjustments and Therapies
Generalized loss of metabolically active tissue mass and reduced aerobic capacity	Decreased cardiopulmonary reserve; reduced hepatorenal capacity	Cautious dosing of anesthetic agents with myocardial- and respiratory-depressant properties; supplemental O_2 therapy; reduced dosage of anesthetic agents requiring hepatic or renal biotransformation; avoidance of aggressive volume loading with IV fluids
Reduced autonomic and immune homeostasis	Greater intraop variability of vital signs; increased risk of infection	Minimize periop sympathectomy due to neuraxial anesthesia; early treatment of abn BP or HR; antibiotic prophylaxis and meticulous sterile technique for invasive procedures; periop warming
Decreased neural tissue mass and neurotransmitter activity	Decreased anesthetic and analgesic requirement	Age-adjusted dosing of anesthetic agents and adjuvants; allow increased time for emergence and for recovery of NM transmission; increased risk of postop delirium and/or cognitive dysfunction
Increased co-morbidities and prevalence of age-related disease and polypharmacy	Complex periop polypharmacy; uncontrolled or inadequately-controlled cardiopulmonary or metabolic disorders; increased frequency of adverse drug interactions	Careful preop assessment of chronic disease and functional status; full review of routine medications and adverse drug episodes; selective use of pharmacy expertise and specialist consultants

Key Reference: Rosenthal RA, Kavic SM. Assessment and management of the geriatric patient. *Crit Care Med.* 2004;32(suppl 4): S92–S105.

GI Endoscopy/EGD, Non-Operating Room Anesthesia

Brian Rothman

Risk

- Varied risks depending on disease process

Perioperative Risks

- Risks are more dependent on the pt's co-morbid conditions.
- Aspiration risk: Minor
- Vagal response with insufflation
- Perforation leading to pneumoperitoneum or pneumomediastinum: Rare
- Dental injury
- Sore throat
- Bronchospasm and laryngospasm

Worry About

- Airway obstruction
- Bleeding
- Perforation of visceral structures

Overview

- Diagnostic and therapeutic procedures for Barrett's esophagitis, eosinophilic esophagitis, esophageal strictures and rings, mediastinal masses, gastric bypass screening, GI bleeding, pancreatic masses and cysts, chronic pancreatitis, lower GI tract strictures, cholelithiasis and choledocolithiasis, biliary cancer, Crohn's, ulcerative colitis, diverticulosis, colon and rectal cancer staging, polypectomies, colon cancer screening, follow-up for h/o colon polyps.
- Procedures incl esophogogastroduodenoscopy (EGD), colonoscopy, esophageal and rectal US, esophageal dilation, tissue biopsies, endoscopic retrograde cholangiopancreatography (ERCP), celiac plexus block, pancreatic cyst drainage, balloon assisted enteroscopy (BAE).

Indications and Usual Treatment

- Pts will present with recent, unexplained wt loss, nausea, emesis, abd pain, substernal and/or subcostal pain, dysphagia, a significant change in bowel habits, hematemesis or bloody stool, achalasia, radiation-induced strictures, radiation proctitis, or chronic conditions that require frequent follow-up (ulcerative colitis, Crohn's, etc.), or a combination of these.

ASSESSMENT POINTS

System	Effect	Assessment by Hx	PE	Test
HEENT	Airway obstruction and cannot intubate	OSA, obesity, difficult mask and intubation	Airway exam Poor dentition	
RESP	Bronchospasm and laryngospasm	Asthma and smoking	Auscultation	
GI	Aspiration risk	Hx of emesis, gastroparesis, gastric outlet syndrome	Active emesis or hematemesis	
HEME	Anemia	Hematemesis or melena	Tachycardia, pale skin and mucous membranes	PCV or CBC

Perioperative Management

Preoperative Preparation

- NPO guidelines must be followed unless emergent.

Monitoring

- Standard ASA monitors

Anesthetic Technique/Induction

- The majority of these procedures are done on an outpatient basis. IV propofol and lidocaine provide adequate anesthetic in most cases.
- Midazolam and fentanyl should only be given in cases of extreme anxiety or opioid tolerance or withdrawal. Administering these medications indiscriminately will increase discharge times and have little added benefit.
- Intubation is generally not necessary on most cases unless ventilation becomes an issue. Prone procedures such as ERCPs can be done without an ETT in many cases, but success depends on provider experience and pt co-morbidities with obesity and airway anatomy being a major factor.
- Airway adjuncts, esp. the nasal trumpet, maintain airway patency and help avoid the need for an ETT.

Surgical Stages

- Colonoscopy: Endoscopic passage through the sigmoid and splenic flexures tend to be the most stimulating and deepening of the anesthetic should be considered.
- Upper endoscopies: Passage through the oropharynx and dilation (if applicable) are most stimulating and laryngospasm and bronchospasm are risks, esp. in smokers, so a deeper level of anesthetic is required for this population.
- Procedures can be very short or last 2 hr depending on complexity and pt disease.

Blood Loss and Volume Concerns

- Significant blood loss is rare except for procedures involving varices where caution is advised and a type and cross may be prudent.
- Plavix and other anticoagulants may be of concern depending on the procedure.

Postoperative Considerations

- Recovery nearby, standard postop monitoring, recovery for some procedures are far longer than needed for anesthetic recovery,

Anticipated Problems/Concerns

- Postop pain control for some procedures
- Chest or abd pain may suggest procedure complication
- Coughing 2° to airway irritation with upper endoscopies

GIFT Procedure

Bernard Wittels

Risk

- Infertility affects 3 million couples in USA. 1 of every 100 deliveries is the culmination of assisted reproductive technologies.
- GIFT is the preferred technique for the most complicated, high risk, infertile women, incl those with advanced age, obesity, polycystic ovarian syndrome, tobacco use, marijuana use, early stage ovarian malignancies, and hypoplastic uterus assoc with a 46,XY karyotype.

Perioperative Risks

- Periop mortality is rare
- Obstetric-related risks
  - OHSS, follicular rupture, hemorrhage, pleural effusion, ascites, thromboembolism
    - Failed fertilization   70%
    - Multiple gestation   33%
    - Ectopic pregnancy   0.4%
    - Birth defects   2%
    - Neonatal death   1%
- Anesthesia-related risks
  - Conscious sedation: Awareness, anxiety, pain, nausea (20–80%), movement
  - TIVA: Airway obstruction, hypoxemia, hypercarbia
  - GA: Nausea (20–80%), delayed recovery (2–4 hr)
  - Spinal/epidural: Headache (0–5%),

Worry About

- Potential effects of drugs on oocyte fertilization, implantation, growth, development
- CO_2 insufflation requires hyperventilation
- Residual peritoneal CO_2 causes diaphragmatic, subscapular pain
- Laparoscopy can injure bowel, bladder, cause air embolism or subcutaneous emphysema

Overview

- Young, female outpatients have an increased risk of postop nausea, emesis.
- Laparoscopy increases ventilatory demands and may influence the choice of anesthesia.

ICD-9-CM Code 628.9 (Infertility, female)

Indications and Usual Treatment

- 1° or 2° infertility
  - Endometriosis
  - Ovulatory disorders
  - Male-factor infertility
  - Unexplained infertility
- Specific indications for GIFT
  - Advanced maternal age
  - Donor insemination failures
  - Repeat IVF failures
  - Difficult transcervical embryo transfers
  - IVF not acceptable due to religious beliefs
- Criteria
  - Ovulation (serum LH, U/S)
  - Adequate luteal phase (serum progesterone)
  - Normal endometrium (biopsy)
  - Normal TSH, T_4, prolactin
  - Tubal patency (laparoscopy or hysterosalpingogram)
  - Normal semen analysis
- Usual treatment
  - Ovarian hyperstimulation (clomiphene, hCG, GnRH analogs)
  - Chromotubation, tuboplasty
  - In vitro fertilization

ASSESSMENT POINTS

System	Effect	Assessment by Hx	PE	Test
RESP	Increased workload	Asthma, smoking, obesity	Auscultation	Pulse oximetry
GI	Adhesions	Previous abd surgery	Scar survey	
GU	Tubal patency	Previous infection, surgery		Hysterosalpingogram

Key Reference: Tsen LC. Anesthesia for assisted reproductive technologies. *Int Anesthesiol Clin.* 2007;Winter 45:99–113.

Perioperative Management

Anesthetic Techniques

- Conscious sedation….. total IV anesthesia
- Spinal, epidural and/or GA for laparoscopy or laparotomy

Monitoring

- Routine

Induction/Maintenance

- Propofol, N_2O, midazolam, fentanyl, and isoflurane do not alter success rates for pregnancy or delivery.
- Consider avoiding metoclopramide and droperidol to treat PONV.

Surgical Stages

Trocar Introduction

- Adhesions of intestines to anterior abd wall increase risk of bowel perforation.
- Traumatic trocar placement may perforate bowel bladder, blood vessels.

CO_2 Insufflation

- Increased intragastric pressure, increased CO_2 absorption requires increased ventilation (increase rate to avoid barotraumas with increased PIP)

Postoperative Considerations

- Mild abd pain after laparoscopy; ibuprofen and fentanyl usually suffice
- EBL: Minimal
- Pain score: 2–4
- Residual peritoneal CO_2 may cause subdiaphragmatic or subscapular discomfort.

Anticipated Problems/Concerns

- Excessive postop pain warrants evaluation for peritoneal trauma and bleeding.
- Unexplained hypotension and tachycardia may herald endotoxic shock and sepsis that must be diagnosed and treated emergently to avoid maternal mortality.

Heart Transplant, Adult

Wanda M. Popescu

Risk

- Incidence in USA: ~14,000 candidates/y with stage D heart failure (HF); most common Dx are ischemic cardiomyopathy and idiopathic dilated cardiomyopathy.
- ~2000 orthotopic procedures/y in USA, limited by suitable donor organ availability
- Overwhelmingly male; no unambiguous racial predominance for end-stage HF

Perioperative Risks

- Early (30-d) mortality: ~8% due to surgical technique complications; fulminant rejection or infection; reperfusion injury
- Early morbidity from nosocomial bacterial infection (*Pneumococcus* pneumonia, *Pseudomonas* sepsis); later opportunistic infection with *Pneumocystis carinii*, *Candida* spp, CMV

Worry About

- Recipient heart: Low cardiac index (evaluate the current level of inotropic support); ventricular irritability; mediastinal adhesions from prior cardiac surgery; pulm Htn
- Donor heart (allograft): Function compromised after CPB by increased pulm afterload, reperfusion injury, prolonged ischemia (decreased function after 4–6 hr), and atypical drug responses

- Mural thromboembolism pre-CPB or air embolism post-CPB from completely open heart
- Maintain complete sterility during placement of invasive monitors
- Hyperacute rejection (rare with ABO matches)
- Pulm aspiration of gastric content (all procedures are emergencies)

Overview

- Transplantation markedly improves survival of end-stage HF pts
- Techniques of orthotopic transplant (native heart replaced by donor heart in normal anatomic location) include the classic biatrial (posterior wall of both atrias are left in place) and, the more commonly used, bicaval (posterior aspect of left atrium with pulm veins is left in situ)
- Heterotopic heart transplant (recipient's heart remains in place and donor heart attached in parallel in the right thorax) rarely performed; reserved for cases of fixed high PVR (to avoid right heart failure) and donor size mismatch
- Rejection, infection, reperfusion injury, hemorrhage and stroke from air or thromboembolism are major causes of periop morbidity and mortality

ICD-9-CM Code: 425.40 (Cardiomyopathy)

Indications and Usual Treatment

- Specific indication: Stage D HF (refractory HF requiring specialized interventions) and NYHA Class IV (severely compromised status with guarded prognosis) unimproved by maximal medical Rx
- Maximal medical Rx usually incl oral inotropes, ACE, PDE III inhibitors, diuretics, antiarrhythmics
- Absolute contraindication: Fixed pulm Htn (pulm vascular resistance >3.5 Wu that does not decrease >20% with pharmacologic intervention)
- Relative contraindication: Severe pulm disease, chronic kidney failure, liver failure, malignancy within last 5 y, active infections, advanced age

ASSESSMENT POINTS

System	Effect	Assessment by Hx	PE	Test
CARDIO	Biventricular failure	Exercise intolerance Orthopnea PND	JVD Liver edge ↓	R & L heart cath
RESP	Pulm edema	Orthopnea	Rales	CXR
RENAL	Prerenal azotemia	PND, nocturia		BUN/Cr
CNS	Poor perfusion	Confusion?	Mental status	
HEPAT	Chronic congestion	RUQ fullness/pain	Liver edge	LFTs

Key Reference: Shanewise J. Cardiac transplantation. *Anesthesiol Clin North Am.* 2004;22:753–765.

Intraoperative Management

Monitoring

- Standard ASA monitors and arterial line cannula
- PA cath with long sheath (to facilitate withdrawal during cardiac anastomoses, use of caval snares); placement may be complicated by arrhythmias, TR
- TEE useful to optimize volume management, rule out mural thrombus and PFO pre-CPB; assist in maintaining stable hemodynamics pre-CPB, assist de-airing during CPB; evaluate RV and LV function and assist weaning off CPB

Airway

- Bacterial filter may be placed in anesthesia circuit to minimize nosocomial pneumonia risk

Blood Products

- Only CMV-neg blood products used for seronegative recipients, to avoid CMV sepsis
- Leukocyte-filtered or γ-irradiated blood unnecessary to avoid alloimmunization during transplant
- FFP and/or vit K may be required if on chronic warfarin therapy preop
- Significant bleeding and coagulopathy may occur in pts with prior cardiac procedures

Anesthetic Technique

- Judicious use of IV premedication
- Immunosuppressive drugs are often infused ASAP after arrival in OR
- Specialized antibiotic therapy
- Antifibrinolytic therapy initiated pre-CPB

- GA regimen should be least perturbing to precarious CV status; full-stomach precautions
- Phenylephrine, inotrope, judicious volume infusion may then be required to optimize CO

Surgical Stages

Dissection

- Cardiomegaly and/or prior cardiac surgery increase risk of RV or innominate vein laceration
- Epicardial irritability can lead to VFib
- Redo surgery is assoc with protracted pre-CPB interval
- With LV mural thrombus, cardiac manipulation can lead to systemic embolism

Definitive Surgery

- Bicaval cannulation for CPB mandatory due to atrial anastomoses; SVC pressure must be scrupulously monitored to avoid intracranial Htn
- Cardiectomy not performed until just before donor organ arrival
- After atrial, great vessel anastomoses, aortic cross-clamp removed ASAP to end ischemia; methylprednisolone 500 mg IV used to prevent hyperacute rejection

Weaning/Post-CPB Considerations

- Inotropic support: Usually required (in case of prolonged ischemic time or reperfusion injury)
- Chronotropic support: Due to heart denervation direct acting drugs are required (isoproterenol) to increase HR; alternatively pacing the heart at HR 90–110 beats/min

- Right heart failure is the most common cause of failure to wean CPB. Treatments to decrease PVR include vasodilators (nitroglycerin, sodium nitroprusside, PGE_1, prostacyclin) which may require addition of systemic vasoconstrictor, phosphodiesterase inhibitors (milrinone, amrinone) which decrease PVR and increase contractility, selective pulm dilators (inhaled NO or inhaled iloprost), adequate ventilation to prevent hypoxia and hypercarbia
- Pain management same as that following CABG

Anticipated Problems/Concerns

- Atypical responses to cardioactive drugs by denervated donor heart—e.g., indirect-acting agents (e.g., atropine) fail to produce expected cardiac effects (tachycardia); thus only direct-acting agents should be used (e.g., isoproterenol); but denervation supersensitivity to catecholamines, a theoretical concern, is NOT clinically relevant
- Persistently slow junctional rhythms lead to permanent pacemakers in ~5% of recipients
- Acute rejection is marked by low CO, arrhythmias; monitoring for rejection requires biopsies
- Chronic immunosuppression prones pts to infection and leads to the development of Htn, CAD, DM, kidney disease

Heart Transplant, Pediatric

Lena Sun

Risk

- More than 8000 heart transplants have been performed in pts under 18 y of age from 1982 to 2007

Perioperative Risks

- The highest risk for death following a transplant is within the first 6 mo of transplant. Survival is also influenced by indication for transplant (worse with CHD), donor age (worse with older donors) and the volume at the transplant center.
- At risk for rejection and developing allograft vasculopathy.
- Htn is common in post-transplant pts.

Worry About

- Psychosocial difficulties from chronic illness
- Drug interaction with immunosuppressants
- Airway problems from steroid therapy
- Rejection and abn cardiac function
- Other end, organ dysfunction incl renal and 2° malignancies
- Other co-morbid conditions, particularly Htn
- Vascular access could be a challenge
- "Denervated heart," therefore the use of direct acting agents is recommended

Overview

- Over the past 3 y, there is an average of 450 pediatric heart transplants per year. 27% of transplants are performed in infants (<1 year of age) in North America

- Increased use of induction therapy followed by maintenance to reduce early rejection. The assoc of induction therapy and lymphoproliferative disease or CMV disease has not been substantiated.
- Maintenance therapy usually consists of calcineurin inhibitor, cell cycle inhibitor and corticosteroids.

Etiology

- In infants, approx ⅔ require transplant due to CHD and the remaining needing transplant due to cardiomyopathy.
- In older children, about ⅔ requiring transplant due to cardiomyopathy and only 25% requiring transplant due to CHD.
- Retransplant occurs in 1% in infants, and 5% in older children.

ASSESSMENT POINTS

System	Effect	Assessment by Hx	PE	Test
Airway	Post-Tx may have difficult airway due to chronic steroid use	Hx of previous anesthesia	Airway exam	
CARDIAC	Possible need to have alternate cannulation site for CPB (i.e. femoral) Slow onset of drug effects due to poor cardiac function Exacerbated hemodynamic depression from sympatholytic or cardiodepressant drugs Post-Tx pts have denervated heart	Functional status Current meds Previous surgery Hx of transplant Most recent cardiac evaluation (ECHO? Cath? MRI?)	Routine cardiac exam Evaluate vascular access	ECHO Reports of recent cardiac evaluation
RESP	Recent infections Hx of reactive airway disease	Bronchodilator therapy	Routine resp exam	RSV titer if pt has active resp infection
IMMUNE (PTLD)	Post-Tx pts are at risk for lymphoproliferative diseases (PTLD)	Clinical presentation of PTLD is variable and could mimic viral illness		
Others	Any renal or hepatic system dysfunction			Creatinine LFT

Key Reference: Kirk R, et al. Registry of the International Society for Heart and Lung Transplantation: Twelfth Official Pediatric Heart Transplantation Report—2009. *J Heart Lung Transplant.* 2009;28(10):993–1006.

Perioperative Implications

Preoperative Preparation

- Careful review of Hx incl cardiologist's note and recent ECHO is very important.
- Psychosocial concerns for child with Hx of frequent hospitalization necessitate possible need for premedications.
- Depending on the procedure, SBE prophylaxis may be indicated.

Monitoring

- Routine
- Unless there are signs of rejection or other major end-organ dysfunctions, invasive monitoring is not usually needed.
- If child has difficult vascular access, this may further exacerbate poor volume status from preop NPO.

Induction

- Ascertain volume status is adequate.
- Children tolerate low heart rate poorly. Bradycardia often preceeds cardiac arrest.
- Pts for transplant have no cardiac reserve and onset of drug action may be slow due to poor function.
- Etomidate with small dose of opioids.
- Combination of benzodiazepines and opioids could lead to significant sympatholytic effects and unstable hemodynamics during induction.

Maintenance

- Remember to use only direct-acting agents in post-Tx pts.
- Infusion of opioid in combination with low dose of volatile anesthetics is usually well tolerated.

- Postop care should incl involvement of the cardiologist, appropriate pain management and possible ICU care for major surgery.

Anticipated Problems/Concerns

- Vascular access in pts who had multiple previous surgery
- Bleeding and hemostasis in pts who had previous surgery
- Donor heart function and ischemic time are important determinants on the success of the transplant
- Know all of the medications and their potential interactions
- Rejection and PTLD are two major causes for mortality/morbidity

Herniorrhaphy

Ramprasad Sripada
Vidya N. Rao

Risk

- Groin hernias: 750,000/y
- Annual risk of hernia incarceration: 2–3/1000 pts/y.
- Incidence in children: 10–20/1000 live births (4:1 M:F).
- Incidence: Groin 75% majority of hernias
  - Incisional hernias 15–20%
  - Umbilical and other ventral hernias comprising the remainder
- Gender predominance
  - Inguinal: M:F ratio: 9:1
  - Femoral: M:F ratio: 1:3
  - Abd: M:F ratio: 7:13

Perioperative Risks

- Periop mortality rare (<0.3%)
- Higher mortality/morbidity if strangulated bowel
- Risk related to co-morbidities
- Morbidity: Wound abscess, hematoma

Worry About

- Appropriateness of surgery as outpatient
- Possible strangulated bowel, sepsis
- Vagal stimulation with retraction, resultant bradycardia
- Postop urinary retention
- Spinal headache: Incidence ≤3% with 25-gauge needle

Overview

- An external hernia is an abn protrusion of intra-abdominal tissue through a fascial defect in the abd wall.
- The definitive treatment of hernia is operative repair.
- Procedure performed for repair of abd wall (epigastric, femoral, incisional, umbilical)
- Reducible hernia: Contents of sac return to abd spontaneously or with manual pressure
- Irreducible (incarcerated) hernia: Contents cannot be returned to the abd, usually trapped by a narrow neck. Incarceration does not imply obstruction, inflammation, or ischemia of the herniated organs.
- Obstructed: Lumen of a segment of bowel within the hernia sac may become obstructed; initially there may be no interference with blood supply.
- Strangulated hernia: Compromise to the blood supply of the contents of the sac (e.g., omentum or intestine) results in gangrene of the contents of the sac. The incidence of strangulation is higher in femoral than in inguinal hernias, but strangulation may occur in other hernias as well.

- Richter hernia: Uncommon and dangerous, part of circumference of bowel incarcerated or strangulated in fascial defect. strangulated Richter hernia may spontaneously reduce and gangrenous piece of intestine may be overlooked with subsequent perforation and peritonitis.
- May be uncomplicated or may be complicated with bowel contents
- Strangulated hernia with necrotic bowel can be assoc with sepsis syndrome
- May require bowel resection if necrotic
- Laparoscopic hernia repair currently performed; exact role poorly defined

ICD-9-CM Codes: 550–553.9

Indications and Usual Treatment

- Uncomplicated hernia: Elective surgery, binder, truss
- Incarcerated hernia: Urgent surgery
- Strangulated hernia: Emergent surgery
- Absolute contraindications to elective repair incl pregnancy, active infection
- Ascites repair difficult: Higher likelihood of complications
- Incarceration: 9–20%. 10% of inguinal and 20% of femoral hernias incarcerated
  - Frequent in children <6 mo
  - Incarcerated hernias can cause intestinal obstruction or strangulation and infarction, resulting in a high incidence of infection, hernia recurrence, and operative mortality, esp. in elderly pts
- In absence of signs of strangulation: Can usually be manually reduced followed by elective repair

Perioperative Implications

Preoperative Preparation

- Determine appropriateness of outpatient procedure.

Anesthetic Technique

- Local, regional, spinal, GA, or combined anesthetic technique
- Local anesthesia ± sedation preferred for appropriate cases [MAC]
- Local anesthesia permits pt to strain, cough during procedure if desired by surgeon
- Consider local wound or nerve infiltration for postop pain control.
- Laparoscopic surgery, strangulated hernia require GA. Factors that determine choice of anesthesia incl pt and surgeon preference, type of procedure performed (open or laparoscopic), hernia characteristics (recurrent, large, slider, bilateral), and the pt's ability to cooperate.

- GA for pts with questionable airways and those unable to cooperate (e.g., because of dementia) or for more challenging cases

Monitoring
- Routine
- Consider arterial line, CVP, PA cath if signs of sepsis

Airway
- Routine

Induction
- Require level of at least T8 for regional
- Local infiltration of ilioinguinal, iliohypogastric nerves

Surgical Stages

Dissection
- Depends on hernia site

Definitive Surgery
- Inguinal hernia most common: Transversalis aponeurosis, internal oblique fascia sutured to shelving edge of inguinal ligament
- Prosthetic mesh can be used for all sites to relieve tension
- Incisional hernia may require intraperitoneal approach
- EBL: 50–100 mL

Hernia Repair Options
- Open
- Laparoscopic

Postoperative Considerations
- Postop pain depends on site, use of local infiltration
- Pain score: 3 (local) –6
- Important to void before discharge if outpatient
- Consider stool softener for inguinal hernias to avoid strain

Anticipated Problems/Concerns

- Bradycardia during peritoneal retraction
- Potential for necrotic bowel
- Recurrence rates (1–10%). Nearly 40,000 inguinal hernia repairs performed annually for hernia recurrence. Nearly 90% of 1° adult hernia repairs have a prosthetic mesh implanted.
- Vascular injuries: In laparoscopic repairs, inferior epigastric, external iliac, femoral, and testicular vessels are at risk.
  - May result in intraop hemorrhage or may present as postop hematomas
  - Incidence of postop hematoma: 1 to 8%

ASSESSMENT POINTS

System	Effect	Assessment by Hx	PE	Test
CARDIO	Potential of sepsis		HR, BP	Invasive monitor
GI	Reflux, obstruction	Reflux Sx, emesis		
HEME	Coagulation DIC if necrotic bowel	ASA use		PT, PTT, fibrinogen, FSP

Key Reference: Cameron JL. *Current surgical therapy*. 9th ed. St Louis: Mosby; 2008.

Hip Fracture Repair

John G. Hagen
Meg A. Rosenblatt

Risk

- Young pts: Traumatic fracture
- Elderly pts: Femoral neck, intertrochanteric, subtrochanteric, intracapsular Fx through osteoporotic bone
- Pathologic Fx
- Incidence in USA: 340,000 Fx diagnosed and treated /y
  - 22.5-23.9/100,000 at age 50
  - 630.2-1289.3/100,000 at age 80
- By 2050 expected to exceed 500,000 in USA and 7 to 21 million worldwide
- M:F ratio: 1:4–5

Perioperative Risks

- Cardiac, CNS, accident and/or fall: Seek cause of Fx
- Periop fluid deficiency: Large volumes of blood in leg or thigh after fracture
- Geriatric pts with multiple co-morbidities

Worry About

- Fat embolism syndrome

Overview

- Commonly performed procedures
- Goal is reduction and stabilization of Fx to allow mobilization
- 30-d mortality 5–10%
- 1-y mortality 12–37%

ICD-9-CM Code: 820.x

Indications and Usual Treatment

- Nondisplaced neck Fx treated with closed reduction and percutaneous pinning
- Displaced neck Fx treated with bipolar hemiarthroplasty or THR
- ORIF with dynamic hip screws or other sliding nail fixations for inter- or subtrochanteric fracture
- Cemented or uncemented hemiarthroplasty prostheses for intracapsular Fx

ASSESSMENT POINTS

System	Effect	PE	Test
CARDIO	Hypotension 2° to hypovolemia vs. fat embolism	Tachycardia Right-sided heart failure	ECG ST-segment abn PA pressures, ECHO
RESP	Fat embolism syndrome	Tachypnea Pulm Htn	Pulm infiltrates on x-ray ABG's O_2 sat
HEME	Blood loss 2° to Fx	Orthostatic hypotension	Hct
CNS	Senile dementia vs. fat embolism syndrome	Confusion, agitation, stupor, coma, cerebral edema	Neuro assessment CT scan
GU	Fat embolism syndrome		Fat globules in urine
DERM	Fat embolism syndrome	Petechiae on chest, extremities, conjunctivae	

Key Reference: Parker MJ, Handoll HHG, Griffiths R. Anaesthesia for hip fracture surgery in adults. *Cochrane Database Syst Rev.* 2004;18(4): CD000521.

Perioperative Management

Preoperative Preparation

- Early surgery indicated in premorbidly fit pts (greater than 48 hr post-admission assoc with increased morbidity and mortality in low risk/healthy pts)
- Surgery delayed if correctable co-morbidities
- Treat preop pain: Consider femoral block, lumbar plexus catheter with single-shot sciatic block, fascia iliaca blocks, analgesic adjuvants (NSAIDs, opioids)

Anesthetic Technique

- No association between type of anesthesia and postop mortality after 30 d, spinal anesthesia assoc with reduction in postop confusion
- Increased use of vasopressors and arrhythmia assoc with neuraxial anesthesia
- Regional anesthesia reduces incidence of DVT, intraop blood loss and need for airway manipulations
- Isobaric spinal anesthesia may limit level of sympathectomy, thus hypotension
- Paramedian approach to neuraxial blocks 2° to inability to reduce lumbar lordosis
- US may improve success/decrease time to perform neuraxial blocks
- Prophylactic antibiotics mandatory

Monitoring

- Consider arterial monitoring if underlying severe Htn, pulm Dx, or hypovolemia.
- PA cath if significant cardiac disease
- Urinary drainage catheters: retention vs. UTIs

Surgical Stages

- Performed on Fx table: Allows manipulation of Fx and radiographic evaluation
- Arms frequently across chest or in overhead slings: avoid antecubital IVs
- Avoid compression injuries from perineal post
- Lateral position for hemiarthroplasty
- Dependent shoulder compresses brachial plexus: Place auxiliary roll
- Meticulous padding of pressure points
- Embolism of air, fat, or bone fragments during insertion of femoral prosthesis with assoc systemic hypotension and pulm Htn
- Aggressive warming to decrease blood loss
- EBL <100 to >500 mL

Postoperative Considerations

- Pain management
- Regional: Neuraxial (epidural), peripheral (lumbar plexus catheter)
- Opioids: IV PCA→PO
- Adjuvants: NSAIDs (PO/IV), Opioids
- Multimodal approach emphasizing reg + NSAID adjuvants > opioids
- Decreased hospitalization, increased joint ROM, increased analgesia
- Decreased opioid requirements
- Decreased urinary retention, decreased post-op ileus (N/V)
- Thromboembolic prophylaxis
- Recommended agents
  - Warfarin: INR of 2.0–3.0; <2.0 not effective in preventing VTE

- LMWH: Enoxaparin: 40 mg SQ q day; dalteparin 5,000 IU SQ q day
- Fondaparinux: 2.5 mg SQ q day, superior to enoxaparin in preventing VTE; however, long half-life, lack of easy reversibility, contraindicated in pts <50 kg and renal insufficiency, ↑ risk of bleeding in pts >65
- ASA /low-dose UFH: Not to be considered as sole agents
- Mortality rate in assoc with poorly controlled systemic disease, cognitive disorders, and absence of DVT prophylaxis
- Daily protein supplementation for malnourished pts
- Pressure ulcer prevention: Frequent turning, visual inspection, and topical duoderm treatment, pressure-decreasing mattresses
- Multidisciplinary approach using skilled medical, nursing, and paramedical care to maximize rehabilitation potential

Anticipated Problems/Concerns

- Be wary of elderly pts with normal-range Hcts.
- Fat embolism syndrome may be 2° to direct release of fatty acids, which cause capillary endothelial breakdown. Pericapillary hemorrhagic exudates are found in lungs and brain. Require supportive care, often incl mechanical ventilation, and vigilant fluid management.

Hypospadias Repair

Gee Mei Tan

PROCEDURES

Risk

- 1 in 250 live male births
- Hypospadias found in 6–8% of fathers of affected boys
- Hypospadias found in 14% of sibling of affected boys
- 7–9% assoc with cryptorchidism
- 9–16% assoc with inguinal hernia and/hydrocele
- Classification
  - 50% distal hypospadias
  - 30% mid shaft hypospadias
  - 20% proximal hypospadias

Perioperative Risks

- Complication rates
  - 5% for distal repairs
  - 10% for mid shaft repair
  - 15–20% for proximal repair
- Postop complications
  - Bleeding and/or hematoma (most common)
  - Wound infection
  - Repair breakdown
- Urethrocutaneous fistula and/or diverticulum
- Urethral and or meatal stricture and/or stenosis
- Urinary tract infection esp. if postop catheter in situ

Worry About

- Anesthesia for infants
- Postop moderate to severe pain
- May be assoc with other syndromes like Schinzel-Giedion, Smith-Lemli-Opitz, etc.
- Rarely assoc with intersex and adrenal dysfunction
- Postop bleeding, requiring re-exploration

Overview

- Incomplete fusion of the urethral folds ventrally in the midline
- Assoc of 3 anomalies
  - Abn ventral opening of urethral meatus
  - Ventral curvature of the penis (chordee)
  - Abn distribution of foreskin with a hood dorsally and deficient skin ventrally
- Usually diagnosed at newborn physical exam

- Operative time 1 hr for distal 2–3 hr for proximal repairs
- Minimal blood loss intraop

ICD-9-CM Code: 752.61

Etiology

- Multifactorial
  - Insufficient androgen production
  - Limited androgen sensitivity in target tissues of developing genitalia
  - Premature cessation of androgenic stimulation

Indications and Usual Treatment

- Correction of deformities that interferes with the function of urination and/or procreation
- Usually operated at 6–12 mo of age
- Surgical treatment dependent on classification of hypospadias.
- Usually one-stage approach for distal and midshaft hypospadias
- May require two or more stages for proximal hypospadias

ASSESSMENT POINTS

System	Effect	Assessment by Hx	PE	Test
ENDO	Intersex state with adrenal dysfunction which may lead to adrenal crisis	Family Hx of consanguinity, unexplained infant deaths, females who are infertile or have amenorrhea	Micropenis, cryptorchidism, proximal hypospadias	If high suspicion, karyotype US abd and pelvis Assessment of adrenal steroids Electrolytes, glucose
HEME	Bleeding	Recent NSAID ingestion? Family Hx of bleeding disorder?	Bruising Petechiae	Coagulation test if positive family or positive physical exam

Key Reference: Baskin LS, Ebbers MB. Hypospadias: anatomy, etiology, and technique. *J Pediatr Surg*: 2006; 41(3): 463-472

Perioperative Management

Preoperative Preparation

- May have clear fluids up to 2 hr before surgery
- Normal child does not require laboratory work.
- Mostly done as outpatient surgery
- Discuss with surgeon the need to obtain graft from other sites, e.g., buccal mucosa
- Explain risk and benefits to parents if regional analgesic technique, esp. if caudal, is used

Monitoring

- Routine ASA monitors plus temp monitor

Anesthetic Technique/Induction

- General anesthesia
- Have available thermoregulation capabilities, e.g., Bair hugger, overhead warming lights, and heating blankets
- Usually inhalational induction with N_2O/O_2/sevoflurane

- Intubate/LMA with positive airway ventilation/spontaneous breathing depending on length of operation
- May need antibiotic coverage esp. if urethral catheterization
- Discuss with surgeon regarding administration of IV ketorolac because this may increase the risk of bleeding postop.
- Supplement with regional analgesic technique:
  - Caudal for proximal hypospadias repair or distal/midshaft hypospadias repair with assoc orchiopexy/inguinal hernia repair
  - Dorsal penile nerve block, SQ penile ring block or caudal for distal or mid shaft hypospadias repair.
  - No epinephrine additive for dorsal penile nerve and SQ ring block
  - To prolong duration of caudal block, may add epinephrine or opioid (if inpatient) to local anesthetic

Surgical Stages

- Dependent on severity of hypospadias
  - Correction of chordee if present
  - Urethroplasty
  - Meatoplasty and glanuloplasty
- Reconstruction of foreskin coverage

Postoperative Considerations

- Pediatric age group at risk for N/V
- Postop pain relief with caudal 0.25% bupivaciane + epinephrine 1:200,000 at 1 mL/kg will last for about 4–6 hr. May repeat half dose at lower concentration, single shot caudal at end if surgery lasted 2 hr or more.
- If catheter in situ, may need oxybutyrin to relieve bladder spasms.
- Discharge per post anesthetic criteria

Hysterectomy, Vaginal

Charles Lin
Ryan Romeo

Risk

- Second most common female surgery after C-section
- Incidence in USA: 600,000 hysterectomies performed in 2003
- More than 120,000 vaginal hysterectomies performed in USA in 2003

Perioperative Risks

- Cystotomy: 1.5%
- Ureteric injury: <0.1%
- Vesico-vaginal fistula: <0.1%
- Bowel injury: 0.6%
- Hemorrhage causing return to OR: 3.1%
- Reoperation: 0.4%
- Transfusion: 1.8%
- Hematoma: 0.5%
- Ileus/obstruction: 0.2%
- Infection: 1.9%
- Thromboembolism: <0.1%
- ICU admission: 0.7%%
- Readmission: 1.1%

Worry About

- Indication for procedure
- Operative diagnosis
- Lithotomy positioning

- CO_2 insufflation for laparoscopic-assisted vaginal hysterectomy (LAVH)
- Possible hidden and/or unrecognized blood loss

Overview

- Preferred over abd approach because 2–4 × less risk of morbidity and mortality, though the vaginal approach is limited by pelvic adhesions, size of uterus, pelvic anatomy, and location of gynecological cancers that require abd approach
- Laparoscopic assistance offers improved surgical exposure and visibility of pelvic anatomy, and ability to remove adhesions
- Robotic assistance enables three-dimensional visualization, improved surgical articulation, and magnification
- Bilateral salpingo-oophorectomy may be performed in addition to hysterectomy in pts >45 y for ovarian cancer prophylaxis.

ICD-9-CM Codes (2010)

681.1 (Uterine prolapse); 625.3 (Dysmenorrhea); 215.6 (Uterine myxoma); 617.9 (Endometriosis); 233.2 (Endometrial hyperplasia); 182.0 (Endometrial cancer); 179.0 (Uterine cancer)

Indications

- Uterine myxoma
- Pelvic relaxation syndrome
- Pelvic pain 2° to endometriosis or adhesions
- Abn bleeding incl dysfunctional uterine bleeding
- Dysmenorrhea
- Endometrial hyperplasia
- Gynecological cancers incl uterine cancer

Contraindications

- Uterine enlargement
- Nulliparity and minimal uterine descent
- Need for oophorectomy
- Previous abdominopelvic surgery and extra-uterine surgery
- Cardiac or pulm co-morbidities complicated by CO_2 insufflation and Trendelenberg position

Usual Treatments

- Medical treatments may incl oral contraceptive pills, gonadatropin releasing hormone analogues, and prostaglandin inhibitors.

ASSESSMENT POINTS

System	Effect	Assessment by Hx	PE	Test
CARDIO	Dehydration, electrolyte abn from bowel prep	CHF, CAD, SOB, exercise tolerance	Cardiac exam	Basic chemistry
PULM	Pleural effusion or other lung pathology in cancer pts	Orthopnea, SOB, Cough	Chest exam	CXR, O_2 sat
HEME	Consider anemia in pts w/Hx of abn bleeding			CBC

Key Reference: Sokol AI, Green IC. Laparoscopic hysterectomy. *Clin Obstet Gynecol.* 2009;52:304–312.

Perioperative Implications

Monitoring
- Standard ASA monitors
- Foley catheter may be needed if neuraxial blockade is performed.
- May require arterial line and/or central venous access if significant blood loss is anticipated or if the pt has major medical co-morbidities.

Airway
- Increased aspiration risk from increased abd pressure and Trendelenberg
- May require orogastric suctioning to minimize aspiration

Anesthetic Technique
- General anesthesia is most common with standard induction.
- Spinal, epidural, combined spinal-epidural is appropriate for euvolemic pts with a simple hysterectomy
- Will need a sensory level of T8–T6
- Pencil-point needle is preferred to reduce incidence of postdural puncture headache

- CO_2 insufflation (LAVH)
- Increased risk of inadequate oxygenation and ventilation from CO_2 insufflation and increased intra-abd pressure
- Increased risk of hypotension from decreased venous return due to abd insufflations

Positioning
- Check and pad pressure points
- Shoulder abduction should be less than 90° to minimize brachial plexus injury
- Cushion area of leg that is against the stirrup to prevent peroneal nerve injury

Intraoperative
- Cervical or peritoneal manipulation can cause vagal stimulation leading to significant bradycardia. Manage by stopping surgery, deflating pneumoperitoneum and administering atropine or glycopyrollate.
- Epinephrine or vasopressin injection by the surgeon to minimize bleeding can cause Htn and dysrhythmias
- Unanticipated bleeding from trocar insertion

- Extra-abdominal insufflation with sufficient amounts may cause cardiopulmonary arrest or SQ air compromising the airway
- Volume overload is a risk when fluids are used to manage hypotension from the general anesthetic and intraperitoneal insufflation.

Extubation
- Awake

Adjuvants
- High risk of PONV can be treated with intraop ondansetron, metoclopramide, dexame-thasone

Postoperative Period
- Shoulder pain from diaphragmatic irritation by CO_2
- Increased risk of postop N/V secondary to female gender and genitourinary surgery

Hysteroscopy

Annette G. Folgueras

PROCEDURES

Risk

- Pt population incl women of all ages.
- Overall rate of complications is 0.01% for diagnostic hysteroscopy.

Perioperative Risks

- Operator technique
- Hemorrhage: 1.2%–3.5%
- Uterine perforation: 0.8%
- Bowel and/or bladder injury
- Infection
- Air or gas embolism
- Hyponatremia
- Hypo-osmolarity
- Pulm edema
- Cervical lacerations
- Nerve injury related to lithotomy position

Worry About

- Unrecognized preop acute/chronic anemia
- Potential injury related to positioning
- Potential complications related to chosen distention media

Overview

- Allows for direct visualization of uterine cavity through distension
- Typically performed in ambulatory and office-based settings
- Has allowed for reduced hospital stays, earlier recovery periods and lower postop morbidity
- Each distension media has its own inherent risks
- With appropriate monitoring, those risks can be minimized

Indications and Usual Treatment

- Abnormal bleeding
- Intra-uterine adhesions
- Endometrial polyps and submucosal fibroids
- Uterine septum
- Endometrial resection/ablation
- Sterilization
- Missed IUCD (Intra-uterine contraceptive device)
- Infertility evaluation
- Contraindicated for pregnancy, genital tract infection and uterine carcinoma

ICD-9-CM Code: 621.3 (Endometrial hyperplasia); 626 (Disorders of menstruation); 628 (Infertility, female)

ASSESSMENT POINTS

System	Effect	Assessment by Hx	PE	Test
CARDIO	Obesity/comorbidities, Trendelenburg position	Exercise tolerance, SOB, Hx of cardiopulmonary Dz	Auscultation	ECG, stress test
RESP	If obese/Trendelenburg	Orthopnea	Auscultation	O_2 sat
HEME	Chronic/acute blood loss	Fatigue, syncope	Orthostatic changes	Hgb/Hct

Key Reference: Bergeron M-E, Beaudet C, Bujold E, et al. Glycine absorption in operative hysteroscopy: The impact of anesthesia. *AM J Obstet Gynecol.* 2009;200:331.e1–333.e5.

Perioperative Management

Preoperative Preparation
- Assess co-existing morbidities
- Consider preop transfusion if pt symptomatic
- Consider pretreatment of pt with gonadotropin-releasing hormone (GnRH) agonists to reduce endometrial vascularity

Monitoring
- Routine
- If CO_2 insufflation used, monitor $ETCO_2$
- Monitor peak airway pressures if Trendelenburg position utilized.
- Avoid steep Trendelenburg position
- With significant CV disease, consider invasive monitoring because of assoc risks with use of fluid distention media.

Anesthetic Technique/Induction
- Local anesthetic: Paracervical versus intracervical block
- Monitored anesthetic care: Narcotic-propofol infusion versus bolus technique

- Regional/general anesthetic: Consider LMA unless Trendelenburg position required because of increased risk of gastric aspiration. Induction should be tailored appropriately if pt significantly anemic.
- Tailor the anesthetic to accommodate the ambulatory, office-based nature of the procedure.

Postoperative Considerations
- Monitor for excess bleeding.
- Monitor the irrigation fluid administered. If greater than 500 mL deficit, measure serum electrolytes, If greater than 1000 mL deficit, administration furosemide and measure serum electrolytes. If greater than 2000 mL deficit, terminate procedure
- Pt population prone to PONV: Recommend anti-emetic prophylaxis
- Pain score: 1–3. NSAIDs useful as an adjuvant for opioid-sparing effect and reducing PONV

Anticipated Problems/Concerns

- To help prevent gas embolization, gaseous insufflation equipment must limit flow rate to 100 mL/min and deaerate the supply tubing by flushing through with CO_2
- If glycine is used as the fluid distention media, monitor for possible electrolyte imbalance (hyponatremia, hypokalemia, hypocalcemia, and hypo-osmolarity) and development of female TURP syndrome
- If sorbitol and mannitol solution is used, there is still a risk of developing dilutional hyponatremia and female TURP syndrome.
- If dextran 70 is used, monitor for acute anaphylactic shock as well as pulm edema and coagulopathy.
- If physiologic media is used, monitor for fluid overload esp. in pts with cardiac and renal insufficiency. Typically, electrolyte imbalance not a problem.
- Altered levels of consciousness must be evaluated, incl electrolyte determination, particularly if large volumes of distending media were used

Ileostomy

Michael S. Higgins

Risk

- Relatively common procedure for adults ages 20–65 y
- There is no gender predominance, although more women receive the procedure for inflammatory bowel disease and more men for colon cancer.

Perioperative Risks

- Periop mortality is low (<1%) and is generally assoc with co-existing disease.
- Procedural morbidity incl ileus 5%, wound infection <5%, intestinal obstruction 2–3%, fistula formation 1–3%, and ostomy necrosis <0.5%.
- Higher risk in pts with strangulated bowel and cancer-related indications.
- Non-procedural risks incl: Aspiration, electrolyte abn, blood loss, postop pain, nutritional compromise, adrenal suppression from chronic steroid use, infection, and sepsis.
- Blood loss usually less than 200 cc

Worry About

- Pulm aspiration if bowel obstruction present
- Periop intravascular volume deficiency
- Electrolyte abn
- Bradycardia from vagal response due to bowel manipulation
- Hypotension and vagal response to insufflation and positioning (laparoscopic procedures)
- Anemia from chronic and acute blood loss
- Hypothermia due to prolonged procedure and radiant/evaporative losses
- Postop pulm atelectasis

Overview

- Diverting ileostomy is common procedure to manage intestinal obstruction or trauma to large bowel or lower small intestine or other intraabd process
- Pts with IBD have usually failed chronic steroid and immunosuppressant therapy and often show signs of those interventions.
- Long-term surgical risks incl disease recurrence, adhesions, kidney stones, and gallstones.

ICD-9-CM Codes: 555.9 (Crohn's disease), 556.5-556.9 (Ulcerative colitis), 560.9 (Intestinal obstruction)

Indications and Usual Treatment

- Most common indications are intestinal obstruction or perforation, abd abcess formation, intractable IBD (Crohn's and ulcerative colitis), abd cancer, adhesions, and intestinal trauma.
- Ileal disease: IBD, small bowel obstruction, volvulus, intussusception, mesenteric vascular occlusion, radiation enteritis, intestinal fistulae, small bowel tumors, Crohn's disease, trauma
- Large bowel disease: Proctocolectomy for IBD, Crohn's disease, ulcerative colitis, familial polyposis, neoplasm, trauma
- Surgical approach commonly involved laparoscopic assistance to reduce complications and length of stay
- Surgical alternatives incl both incontinent and continent ileostomy (Kock pouch)

ASSESSMENT POINTS

System	Effect	Assessment by Hx	PE	Test
CARDIO	Hypovolemia from ↓ fluid intake, diarrhea, bowel prep, third spacing during procedure, acute and chronic blood loss	PO status, vomiting, bowel prep, bleeding, UO	Poor pulses, hypotension with tachycardia, orthostatic BP, skin turgor, dry mucous membranes	BUN/Cr, UO, electrolytes, PCV
RESP	Resp insufficiency from abd distention/splinting and reduced FRC	Dyspnea Abd pain	Tachypnea, rales, absent BS, abd distention and rigidity	Pulse oximetry ABG CXR
GI	Possible ↑ intragastric pressure, volume, acidity			X-ray—dilated bowel
	Possible perforation with peritonitis	Abd pain	Peritoneal signs	
HEME/IMMUNO	Hemoconcentration from dehydration Blood loss Immune suppression from chronic steroid therapy Potential malnutrition from malabsorption Bacteremia and sepsis	GI losses Abn bleeding Hemodynamic instability	See under CV Febrile, hypotensive	PCV, plt, electrolytes PCV Cort stim Albumin, TP WBC with diff, lactate
RENAL	Possible hypokalemic, hypochloremic metabolic alkalosis with vomiting, lyte abn from lower GI losses/bowel prep, hemoconcentration Assoc renal insufficiency in elderly	Vomiting, bowel prep	See under CV	Electrolytes, ABG BUN/CR

Key Reference: Steele SR. Operative management of Crohn's disease of the colon including anorectal disease. *Surg Clin N Am*. 2007;87:611–631.

Perioperative Management

Premedication

- Consider acid reducer and oral nonparticulate antacid (full stomach or obstruction)
- Consider metoclopramide: Contraindicated if obstruction present
- Consider steroid stress dose if on chronic steroid therapy
- Consider NSAIDs to reduce incidence of mesenteric traction syndrome

Monitoring

- Consider arterial catheter if hemodynamically unstable or severe cardiopulmonary disease
- Foley catheter to monitor fluid administration and renal perfusion
- Consider CVP, PA catheter, or TEE to monitor volume status if pt has renal insufficiency or significant cardiac dysfunction.

Airway

- Generally routine; consider awake intubation, rapid-sequence or modified rapid-sequence intubation if increased aspiration risk present
- Consider preop NG tube placement and decompression prior to induction if upper obstruction and/or vomiting present

Induction

- Consider pre-induction intravascular volume expansion with crystalloid or colloid (RBCs if anemic) for hypovolemia.
- Use reduced dosage of sedative hypnotic agent if significant hypovolemia or myocardial dysfunction present.
- Muscle relaxant chosen for induction technique (RSI or routine) and perceived airway difficulty

Maintenance

- May be performed under regional, general, or combined anesthetic techniques depending on surgical approach and pt factors

- NG tube placed to suction reduces gastric distention
- Moderate muscle relaxation usually required to facilitate procedure
- Extra attention to fluid replacement often required
- Convective air and fluid warming indicated to maintain normothermia and reduce infectious complications
- Consider IV lidocaine infusion (2 mg/min) during and after procedure to reduce anesthetic requirements, improve return of bowel function and reduce LOS

Emergence

- Extubation depends on usual criteria with emphasis on normovolemia and normothermia
- Moderate postop pain; consider epidural infusion/PCA or IV opiate PCA.

Imperforate Anus Repair

Gracie Almeida-Chen
Ronald S. Litman

Risk

- Incidence: 1 in 500 (minor defect); 1 in 5,000 (major defect) live births
- High lesions (superlevator lesions, when rectum ends above levator muscles) are more common in males (2:1)
- Low lesions (infralevator lesions, when rectum ends below levator muscles) occur with equal frequency in both sexes.
- Runs equally through all racial, cultural, and socioeconomic groups.

Perioperative Risks

- The higher the anatomic relation of the terminal bowel to the puborectalis sling of the levator musculature, the greater is the incidence of assoc anomalies.
- Additional anomalies present in one-third of pts; incidence higher with supralevator lesions.
- Part of VACTERL: Vertebral defects, anal atresia, cardiac anomalies, tracheoesophageal fistula, esophageal atresia, renal anomalies, limb anomalies.
- Gastrointestinal: 10–20% have another GI lesion (e.g., esophageal atresia, intestinal atresia, malrotation, annular pancreas, omphalocele).
- Cardiovascular: 7% have assoc CV lesions.
- Vertebral defects: 6% have skeletal lesions such as spina bifida or agenesis of the sacrum; 24% have tethered spinal cord.
- Genitourinary: 25–50% with assoc GU anomalies such as urological anomalies, duplicate uterus, septate vagina, and vaginal atresia.

- Most frequent defect in female pts is vestibular fistula, followed by vaginal fistulas.

Worry About

- Abd distention from intestinal obstruction
- Accompanying congenital malformations that affect anesthetic management

Overview

- The hindgut comes in contact with the cloacal membrane during the sixth week of fetal development. At this time, the hindgut is divided into a ventral urogenital and dorsal rectal component. By the eighth week, the dorsal half perforates to the exterior. In imperforate anus, the process is arrested during this critical period.
- There are many anatomic variants of imperforate anus. Treatment and prognosis depends on anatomic classification: Supralevator (high) and translevator (low). Level of the lesion is determined by abd radiograph or perineal US.
- Most children diagnosed in the first days of life by abn findings on physical exam or failure to pass meconium; constipation plus signs of low intestinal obstruction (abd distention and vomiting) mandate careful examination of perianal area.
- Presenting forms: Absence of anal opening, inadequate caliber of anus, or an anterior malpositioning of the opening
- Evaluate for lumbosacral neurologic function. Anal wink can usually be elicited because a vertiginous external anal sphincter is present in most cases.

- A fistula communicating from the gut to the urogenital system or to the external opening is present in 90% of cases. In females, the fistula usually leads to the opening in the posterior fourchette of the vagina (in low lesions) or to the upper vagina (in high lesions). In males, the fistula leads to the raphe of the scrotum (in low lesions) or the urethra (in high lesions).

ICD-9-CM Code: 751.2

Indications and Usual Treatment

- Male infants with imperforate anus may require a transverse colostomy soon after birth for relief of obstruction.
- In female infants, a rectovaginal fistula usually prevents total bowel obstruction so that surgical treatment is not an emergency.
- Definitive corrective surgery some time in the first year of life: Posterior sagittal anorectoplasty (PSARP or Pena pull-through procedure).
- Surgery for the low type involves closure of the fistula, creation of an anal opening, and repositioning the rectal pouch into the anal opening.
- Major surgical challenge: Finding, using, or creating adequate nerve and muscle structures around the rectum and anus to provide the child with the capacity for bowel control.

ASSESSMENT POINTS

System	Effect	Assessment by Hx	PE	Test
CARDIO	Cardiac anomalies	Cyanosis, FTT	Abn heart sounds	ECHO
RESP	Tracheoesophageal fistula	Excessive salivation, drooling, cyanotic spells, coughing relieved by suctioning	Inability to pass a catheter down the esophagus into the stomach	Plain radiograph of the chest and abd reveals air or gas bubbles in the stomach and intestines that have entered through the fistula
RENAL	Renal anomalies			Renal US, voiding cystoureterogram, intravenous pyelogram
CNS	Vertebral anomalies, spina bifida, tethered cord			Lumbosacral films MRI of the spine

Key Reference: Brett CM, Davis PJ, Bikhazi G. Anesthesia for neonates and premature infants. In: Motoyama EK, Davis PJ, eds. *Smith's anesthesia for infants and children.* Philadelphia: Mosby Elsevier; 2006:521–570.

Perioperative Management

Preoperative Preparation

- Assess for co-existing anomalies.
- Invertogram: After sufficient time for a transit of gas (>12 hr after birth), the child is placed in an upside-down position for 3 min, after which a lateral view of the pelvis is obtained.
- Cardiac echo to assess for cardiac anomalies.
- Lumbosacral films to evaluate for vertebral anomalies.
- MRI of the spine to look for a tethered cord.
- Renal US, voiding cystoureterogram, and IV pyelogram to evaluate for urinary tract anomalies.

Monitoring

- Standard ASA monitoring
- Invasive monitors such as an arterial catheter and a CVP catheter generally are reserved for those with marked cardiorespiratory instability.
- Attempt to place IV catheters and pulse oximeter on the upper extremities because pt is often situated at the far end of the OR table.

- Esophageal temp probe is required. Hypothermia is likely unless precautions are taken. Use forced warm air blanket underneath or around pt during surgical procedure. Also advisable to use IV fluid warmer if available.
- Foley urinary catheter should be placed before surgery.

Anesthetic Technique/Induction

- Intubation of the trachea of infants with an apparently normal upper airway can be accomplished with a rapid sequence technique. If the anesthesiologist suspects that the upper airway will be difficult to visualize, the usual airway precautions should be followed. Supplemental support systems for the difficult airway (e.g., neonatal bronchoscopes, light wand, LMA) should be available.
- Anesthesia requirements vary depending on the severity of the abd distention and complexity of the surgery: e.g., simple perineal anoplasty, temporary colostomy, or extensive abdominoperineal repair.
- Anesthetic considerations for neonates with intestinal obstruction incl assessment of fluid status (anticipate insensible fluid loss of

7–10mL/kg/h during major portions of the procedure), correction of electrolyte disturbances, treatment of sepsis, and cardiorespiratory evaluation.
- Marked abd distension 2° to intestinal obstruction can impede diaphragmatic excursion and impair ventilation.
- Anesthesia during surgery can incl potent inhalation anesthetics, narcotics, or both. NO should be avoided because of the risk for increased bowel distention. Intermediate- or long-acting nondepolarizing muscle relaxants often improve surgical conditions at lower inhaled anesthetic concentrations. If early postop extubation is planned, narcotics should be judiciously administered, but in many cases postop mechanical ventilation is required.
- During surgery, the management of fluids, blood replacement, and electrolyte delivery is important. A major challenge is maintaining an adequate intravascular volume. The presence of radiopaque contrast agents, bowel manipulation, and peritonitis increases third-space fluid requirements. In such cases, 10 mL/kg/hr or more of isotonic saline solution or colloid is frequently

needed intraop. Monitoring UO, quality of heart tones, HR, and BP is a basic requirement to assess continuing fluid needs.

Surgical Stages

• Perineal signs in low malformations that will not need a colostomy are: Meconium in perineum, bucket-handle defect, anal membrane, and anal stenosis. These infants can be managed with a perineal anoplasty during the neonatal period with an excellent prognosis.

• High lesions require an emergent temporary diverting colostomy. After sufficient growth of the child, a pull-through procedure with a Peña posterior sagittal anorectoplasty (PSARP) is performed at 3–9 mo of age. The procedure usually begins in the prone position; some surgeons will turn the child and complete the procedure in the supine or lithotomy position. The colostomy is closed after the anoplasty has healed and any necessary 2° dilation has been completed.

• Laparoscopic-assisted anorectal pull through using laparoscopy and muscle electrostimulation (LAARP) has been developed.
• EBL: Usually 10–20 mL
• Regional anesthesia required for abd surgery: Caudal or lumbar epidural catheter preferred.

Postoperative Considerations

• Many infants require postop ventilatory support, total parenteral alimentation, CV support, and treatment of sepsis. The function and recovery of the GI system vary enormously among infants with imperforate anus and seem to be related to whether the lesion is isolated and whether the complications of total bowel obstruction have developed.

• Complications of surgery incl stricture of the anocutaneous anastomosis, rectourinary fistula, mucosal prolapsed, constipation, and incontinence.

• After surgery, followup with anal dilatation helps minimize the risk of stricture formation and helps the newly constructed canal to become functional.

• Continence can be attained in 90% if pts have low lesions.

• <50% of pts with high lesions are continent before school age, but most continue to improve and achieve continence by adolescence.

• Highest incidence of incontinence occurs in males with fistula between rectum and bladder.

Anticipated Problems/Concerns

• Constipation, incontinence
• Management of assoc CHD or other existing medical problems

Implantable Cardioverter Defibrillators (ICDs), Implantation

Nabil Elkassabany
Sanjay Dixit

Risk

• Incidence in USA: Each year 400,000 to 460,000 people die of unexpected sudden cardiac arrest (SCA).
• Over 127,000 ICDs implanted in 2008 (data from the national ICD registry).
• The average age for pts undergoing ICD insertion is 68.1± 12.8 y
• M:F percentage is 74/26.
• ICDs were inserted for 1° prevention in 78% of all pts.
• Assoc comorbidities: CAD, 66%, Htn, 74%; diabetes, 36.5%; and chronic lung disease, 22.7%.

Perioperative Risks

• Procedure related risks incl cardiac perforation, pericardial effusion, hematoma at the site of insertion, infection, lead dislodgment, hemo- and/ or pneumothorax, and death. Radiation exposure poses another hazard for the health care providers and the pt.
• Pt related risk factors: Pts requiring ICDs often have impaired cardiac function and HF which can place them at higher risk for development of periop complications.
• Anesthesia-related factors incl the risks assoc with delivering anesthesia in a remote location, usually the electrophysiology (EP) lab, and caring for pts who are sicker and have multiple co-morbidities.

Worry About

• Myocardial stunning and hemodynamic instability: Low CO, ↓ BP during defibrillation threshold testing (DFT). DFT is defined as the minimal energy necessary for successful defibrillation of induced ventricular fibrillation (VF). This is usually done at the time of the implant to ensure adequate safety margin in the ICDs ability to successfully treat this condition.

• Increase DFT: Sedative, narcotics, antiarrhythmics (class IA, B, C—incl lidocaine, propranolol, amiodarone, verapamil); halogenated hydrocarbons; hypothermia; myocardial ischemia; acidosis
• Limited access to the airway of the sedated pt because of the tight space and bulky x-ray equipments.
• Hypoventilation and hypercarbia in sedated pts.
• Side effects of antiarrhythmic medications: e.g., pulm toxicity in amiodarone
• Pts receiving anticoagulants
• Arrest and cerebral function; some authors found a negative relationship between the number of circulatory arrest periods and the EEG recovery time.

Overview

• Advances of the ICD technology resulted in the development of transvenous systems, which can be implanted using percutaneous vascular access in the EP lab, where the pt receives monitored anesthesia care (MAC).
• Components of the ICD system are the generator canister (can), and the lead, which incorporates the shocking coils as well as bipole for sensing/pacing. The programmer, a stand-alone unit, is used to communicate with the ICD via radio frequency (RF) link. The generator canister is made up of a low-voltage battery unit, capacitor, and circuitry.
• The basic function of an ICD is to detect tachyarrhythmias by determining the cycle length of the sensed signal and treat these if they fall under the category of VT or VF.
• The ICD therapies are of two types: Antitachycardia pacing (ATP), which is reserved only for tacharrhythmia that falls under the category of VT during which the device can deliver a short burst of overdrive pacing at a rate faster than the

arrhythmia. This therapy is typically painless. Shock which can be programmed anywhere from 1 Joule (J) to the the maximum device capacity (31J–41J).
• ICDs also have the capability of bradytherapy and so can serve as pacemakers.
• ICDs also have a diagnostic algorithm that can allow them to distinguish SVT events in order to minimize inappropriate therapy.

ICD-9-CM Codes: 427.1 (VTach); 427.41 (VFIB)

Indications and Usual Treatment:

• Survivors of cardiac arrest due to VF or hemodynamically unstable sustained VT after evaluation to define the cause of the event and to exclude reversible causes.
• Nonischemic dilated cardiomyopathy who have an LVEF less than or equal to 35% and who are in NYHA functional Class II or III.
• LV dysfunction due to prior MI who are at least 40 d post-MI, have an LVEF less than 30%.
• Structural heart disease and spontaneous sustained VT, whether hemodynamically stable or unstable
• Syncope of undetermined origin with clinically relevant, hemodynamically significant sustained VT or VF induced at electrophysiological study
• Nonsustained VT due to prior MI, LVEF less than 40%, and inducible VF or sustained VT at electrophysiological study (EPS)
• Unusual forms of genetically determined inherited arrhythmia syndromes such as long QT, Brugada, catecholaminergic polymorphic VT, hypertrophic cardiomyopathy, etc.

ASSESSMENT POINTS

System	Effect	Assessment by Hx	PE	Test
CARDIO	Myocardial ischemia LV dysfunction Rate, mechanism of VTach	Angina symptoms Exercise tolerance, DOE	S_3, rales	ECG, pharmacologic or exercise stress testing ECHO, cardiac cath EPS, ambulatory ECG, Holter monitor
RESP	Pt co-morbidities may incl COPD, obstructive sleep apnea (OSA), and amiodarone toxicity	Exercise tolerance, DOE		CXR, PFTs, ABGs
RENAL	Renal insufficiency		Edema	BUN, Cr
NEURO	CV disease	Stroke, TIAs	Bruits	Carotid duplex
LYTES	Reversible causes of arrythmias (VTach/VFIB)	Diuretic Rx		Serum K^+ and Mg^{2+}

Key Reference: Epstein A, et al. ACC/AHA/HRS 2008 guidelines for device-based therapy of cardiac rhthym abnormalities: Executive summary. *Circulation.* 2008;117(21):2820–2840.

Perioperative Management

Anesthetic Technique
• Monitored anesthesia care during device insertion
• Local anesthetic infiltration of the insertion site with IV sedation is employed.
• The choice of agent for sedation depends on the discretion and judgment of the anesthesia provider. Midazolam and fentanyl are commonly used.
• Induction of general anesthesia for DFT testing after insertion is completed. Commonly used drugs are propofol and etomidate. Choice and

dosage of the induction agent depend on the pre-existing myocardial dysfunction and the amount of sedation the pt received during device insertion.
• Support of ventilation and oxygenation usually provided with a portable anesthesia (mapleson) circuit if the EP lab is not equipped with an anesthesia machine.

Monitoring
• ASA standard monitors
• Invasive BP monitoring takes place if an arterial line was placed for either pt specific indication or if it is performed as part of the procedure.

Airway
• Support with a facemask attached to a portable anesthesia circuit. Airway instrumentation equipments should be readily available during sedation and before induction of general anesthesia for DFT testing.

Surgical Stages
• Surgical preparation and drapping of the operative site, usually the left pectoral region
• Infiltration of the skin with local anesthetic
• Obtaining venous access through the subclavian or cephalic vein. Confirm venous access cannulation using fluoroscopy.

- Insertion of transvenous defibrillation lead system with or without additional leads for atrial and/or coronary sinus pacing
- Creation of the SQ or submuscular pocket at the site of venous access
- Connect the lead to the generator can.
- Insert the device into the pectoral pocket.
- DFT testing of implanted ICD

Postoperative Considerations
- Blood loss and volume shifts are minimal

- Postop pain is treated with IV and/or oral narcotics, and NSAID drugs.
- Monitor your pt in the PACU until satisfying the discharge criteria established by the specific institution.
- CXR to validate lead position and rule out pneumothorax
- Restricted movement of the arm (in a sling) on side of the ICD implant for 24-48 hr

Anticipated Problems/Concerns
- Bleeding at the acces site with or without pocket hematoma formation
- Pneumothorax and/or hemothorax during venous access
- Cardiac perforation and pericardial effusion may lead to tamponade physiology.
- Failure to resuscitate from induced VF at the time of DFT testing

Inguinal Herniorrhaphy

Gregory Ginsburg
Lucinda L. Everett

Risk

- Incidence in USA: 700,000 groin hernias repaired per year
- Congenital: 1–5% of newborns, approx 10% of premature births
- Age predominance: Congenital; may manifest at any age, incl elderly
- Sex: 80–90% of adult repairs in males; incidence in congenital hernias quoted as 4–10× higher in males

Perioperative Risks

- Mortality: <0.01% elective repairs; higher in emergency cases and high risk/elderly pts
- Morbidity: Hematoma, 2–3%; infection, 1–2%; entrapment of ilioinguinal or genitofemoral nerve with neuralgia; ischemic orchitis, 0.03–0.5% in primary hernias; recurrence, 0.5–15%

Worry About

- Straining or bucking with emergence may damage repair
- Bowel obstruction with incarcerated hernia
- Apnea risk in formerly premature infants

Overview

- Groin hernias represent defect of transversalis fascia
- Classification incl location (direct hernia arises medially to the inferior epigastric vessels; indirect hernia develops at the internal ring; femoral hernia) and size; also sliding, recurrent, or incarcerated
- Chronically increased abd pressure thought to be predisposing factor, as in obesity, COPD, prostatic hyperplasia, ascites, pregnancy, constipation, colonic stenosis
- Most inguinal hernias can be diagnosed by palpation: Sensitivity and specificity of physical exam have been reported as 75% and 96%, respectively
- Ultrasound exam, or other imaging modalities such as MRI, may be useful in pts with symptoms but no physical signs

ICD-9-CM Code: 550.9

Indications and Usual Treatment

- Elective surgery versus watchful waiting. Risk of waiting is bowel incarceration and strangulation (risk is greatest soon after manifestation of hernia).
- Mesh versus nonmesh. Use of mesh generally seems to result in lower recurrence rate, although some studies have demonstrated similar (or even better) outcomes without mesh. Mesh may serve as focus for infection.
- Open versus laparoscopic repair. The laparoscopic approach results in less postop pain, but requires general ET anesthesia, exposes pt to rare complications of laparoscopic insufflation, requires longer surgical time, and is dependent on local surgical expertise. Open repair is often acheived with only local anesthesia combined with minimal sedation in adults, or alternatively may involve monitored anesthesia care, or general anesthesia via mask or laryngeal mask airway.

ASSESSMENT POINTS

System	Effect	Assessment by Hx	PE	Test
CARDIO	Ischemic heart disease prevalent in elderly	Exercise tolerance Chest pain/discomfort	Evaluate for signs of CHF	ECG >50 y or with Hx Testing for myocardium at risk if hx suggests
RESP	Obstructive pulm disease may predispose to hernia	Dyspnea, wheezing	Auscultation (forced exhalation; wheeze) Chest diameter Clubbing, cyanosis	O_2 sat CXR if infection suspected PFTs if etiology unclear or to evaluate Rx
	Postop apnea risk in ex-premature infants	Postconceptual <56 wk Hx apnea; caffeine Rx	Periodic breathing	
GI	Bowel obstruction if hernia incarcerated	N/V	Abd distention	KUB Electrolytes
CNS	Ability to tolerate procedure under local anesthesia	Orientation/cooperation	Mental status exam	
SOCIAL	Most procedures done on outpatient basis	Adequate home support for elderly		

Key Reference: Bay-Nielsen M, Kehlet H. Anaesthesia and post-operative morbidity after elective groin hernia repair: A nation-wide study. *Acta Anaesthesiol Scand.* 2008;52(2):169–174.

Perioperative Management

Preoperative Preparation

- Consider caffeine citrate, 20 mg/kg in ex–premature infants at risk for apnea
- Avoid sedatives in premature infants having procedure under spinal anesthesia
- Fluid resuscitation and aspiration prophylaxis if bowel obstruction present

Anesthetic Technique

- Local infiltration with sedation (nursing sedation vs. monitored anesthesia care) effective for open repair in adults; potentially fewer side effects than field block/nerve block
- General anesthesia with mask airway or laryngeal mask airway for open repair
- General anesthesia with ETT for laparoscopic repair (and for open repair in pt with risk factors for aspiration or in case of surgeon request for muscle paralysis)
- Rapid sequence intubation may be indicated in case of very large or obstructed hernia
- Spinal or epidural (T8) may be used for open repair; one retrospective study raises question of higher mortality in elderly pts with regional techniques
- Paravertebral block (T10–L2) for open repair

Monitoring

- Routine
- Consider postop apnea monitoring for ex–premature infants

Surgical Stages

Skin Incision

- Above inguinal ligament (open) or at site of ports (laparoscopic)

Dissection

- To identify type of hernia and vital structures

Definitive Surgery

- Management of peritoneal sac; repair of fascial defect

Postoperative Considerations

- Minimal blood loss; minimal fluid shifts unless incarcerated hernia with bowel obstruction
- Pain management: Local infiltration; nerve block; caudal (pediatric); NSAIDs
- Pain score: 4–5

Anticipated Problems/Concerns

- Potential for rare complications of laparoscopic insufflation with laparoscopic repair
- Occasional vagal response to traction (notify surgeon, consider treatment with atropine or glycopyyrolate)
- Possibility of femoral nerve palsy with leg weakness after blind ilioinguinal block
- Recurrence in 0.5–15% cases; increased risk with smoking, steroid use, and obesity

Intestinal Obstruction

David A. Rosen
Kathleen Rosen

Risk

- Operations counted in millions if all etiologies included
- Small bowel obstructions predominate by 60–80%
- Etiology of most cases is adhesions from factors such as previous surgery, inflammatory processes, and endometriosis. Other etiologies incl neoplasms, hernias ± strangulation, volvulus, foreign body, and treatment with NSAIDs.
- Race and gender predilection: None

Perioperative Risks

- Apache II scores > 8 correlate with increasing risk
- Mortality: SBO assoc with adhesions 5–10%. SBO assoc with cancer or bowel gangrene and LBO 15–28%.
- Increased risk (bowel factors): Strangulation, malignancy, high obstruction, delay in treatment >24 hr, nonviable strangulation, bowel resection
- Increased risk (general): Sepsis, CV instability (esp hypovolemia and hypotension prior to surgery), extremes of age, co-existing disease, suboptimal nutritional state

- Complication rate ~25%. Increased rate assoc with advanced age, comorbid illness, treatment delay, and previous abd surgery. Decreasing occurrence of death and complications when lesion is amenable to laparoscopic treatment.

Worry About

- Co-existing medical conditions: Esp. cardiopulmonary disease if >75 y. Bowel pathology requiring resection: Gangrene, perforation, malignancy
- Volume status: Acid-base, lytes
- Perfusion: Systemic, pulmonary, regional
- Sepsis
- Physiologic problems can persist or worsen after surgery.

Overview

- Indications for surgery: Strangulation of vascular supply or complete obstruction of lumen. Functional or partial obstructions may be amenable to conservative management.
- Pts may need aggressive management prior to surgery (see Worry About)

ICD-9-CM Code: 560.9

Indications and Usual Treatment

- Any intrinsic or extrinsic lesions that obstruct the intestinal lumen or strangulate the vascular supply require urgent surgery
- Prophylactic surgery may be indicated if an abn that predisposes to obstruction is detected.
- If Dx is uncertain, water-soluble contrast material may be used to distinguish partial from complete obstruction.
- Hemodynamic resuscitation can occur prior to surgery in virtually all cases.
- Many advocate an initial laparoscopic approach in a select pt population: Probable etiology, adhesion. Successful treatment is reported in 60–80%; of pts. Laparoscopy is not recommended for pts with malignancy, gangrene, or perforation.

ASSESSMENT POINTS

System	Effect	Assessment by Hx	PE	Test
CARDIO	Hypotension Tachycardia Poor peripheral perfusion Venous return impeded	Orthostasis, edema	BP (positional) Skin color Capillary refill Pulse quality, HR	As indicated by pre-existing disease and age as well as present condition
RESP	Restrictive defect	SOB (positional)	Resp rate/pattern, skin color Resp work/effort	ABGs, pulse oximetry
GI	Loss of fluids, lytes, or blood	I/O, vomiting (amount, description) BM (timing, character) Abd pain ± distention Prior operations	Abd scars Mass Rectal tenderness Abd girth Bowel sounds Hernias	Abd CT ± enhancement NG drainage
RENAL/ HYDRATION	↓ UO ↑ Other fluid ↓ Electrolytes	I/O	Skin turgor Dry mouth	BUN, Cr, Na^+, K^+, Cl^-, HCO_3^-, UA
IMMUNO	Contamination of GI flora, sepsis or peritonitis	Fever, chills	Temp (see above, CV and GI)	CBC with differential

Key Reference: Fevang BT, Fevang J, Stangeland L, Sorerde O, Svanes K, Viste A. Complications and death after treatment of small bowel obstruction. *Ann Surg.* 2000;231:529–537.

Perioperative Implications

Preoperative Preparation

- Restoration of intravascular volume
- Correction of acid-base and lyte abn
- Decompression of stomach
- Antibiotic coverage

Anesthetic Technique

- Usually GA
- Hemodynamic concerns mandate careful selection of anesthetic, relaxant, and analgesic medication

Monitoring

- Required: Routine + Foley catheter
- Consider: Arterial line, CVP, PAC, TEE

Induction/Maintenance

- Rapid-sequence
- CV instability 2° to volume status
- Avoidance of NO
- Muscle relaxation
- Large-bore IV access

Surgical Stages

- Laparoscopy in a selected population
- Laparotomy accompanied by more profound physiologic changes
- Large fluid shifts on opening of abd
- Tumors or mass manipulation may cause hemodynamic alterations
- Restriction of pulm function or cardiac performance 2° to placement of surgical retractors
- Release of hemodynamically active substances when the bowel is manipulated
- Relaxation until abd closed
- Body heat and fluid loss due to exposed bowel
- Blood loss ranges from minimal to significant depending on etiology
- Abd closure may be difficult or contraindicated

Postoperative Period

- Delay extubation if pulm and CV status in question
- Continued fluid and lyte abn
- ARDS a potential if large fluid volumes were required
- Pulm atelectasis, pneumonia, or aspiration
- DVT ± pulm emboli
- Infection: General or local
- Pain management may be vital to ensure deep breathing and coughing
- PCA for 3–5 d (pain score: 2–9)
- Coagulopathies
- Renal failure
- Malnutrition
- Antiemetics

Anticipated Problems/Concerns

- Hemodynamic, fluid, lyte, pulm alterations
- Sepsis

Intra-Aortic Balloon Counterpulsation (IABCP)

Jimmy Windsor

Risks

- Placed in approx 37,000 pts in USA (2004).

Perioperative Risks

- Most common risks of device placement incl injury of the femoral and iliac arteries and aorta.
  - Including dissection, perforation, pseudoaneurysm formation, and critical bleeding.
- Can be a nidus for clot formation, which causes thrombosis of the same vessels listed beforehand and vessels which supply the viscera
- Embolism also as a result of clot formation can lead to severe ischemic injuries of the leg and viscera.
- Incorrect placement can lead to ischemia of the left arm caused by left subclavian artery occlusion.
- Paraplegia results from the mechanisms listed above and physical occlusion of the artery of Adamkowitz.

Worry About

- Incorrect placement and incorrect use caused by faulty timing of balloon inflation.
- Overinflation (causing intimal damage) and underinflation (causing of the balloon, bleeding and limb and visceral ischemia.

Overview

- The device consists of a polyethylene or polyurethane balloon placed in the proximal portion of the descending aorta typically 2 cm distal to the left subclavian artery and proximal to the origin of the renal arteries. Helium is used to inflate the balloon because of its low density allowing faster inflation/deflation cycles.
- It is designed to inflate during diastole after closure of the aortic valve and the onset of isovolumic relaxation of the left ventricle and deflate near the onset of ventricular depolarization (using an electrocardiogram), anticipating ventricular systole.
- The inflation of the balloon causes a displacement of a volume of blood (equal to that of the balloon volume), typically 30 mL to 50 mL. This augments diastolic blood flow and velocity proximal and distal to the balloon and serving as a "diastolic pump." This increases vital diastolic inflow pressure and velocity to the coronary arteries, improving O_2 delivery to the myocardium and the vascular beds of other organs.
- Typically the hemodynamic response seen is an augmentation of diastolic BP. Also there is a lowering of systolic BP caused by the active deflation of the balloon that decreases afterload and increasing forward blood flow during systole. Think of it as creating a suction effect during systole "sucking" blood out of the left ventricle while the aortic valve is open.
- Other positive hemodynamic effects incl increases in stroke volume, reduction of left ventricular end diastolic pressure, left atrial pressure, pulm artery pressures, myocardial O_2 consumption and left ventricular stroke work index. Systolic BP could increase because of improvement in left ventricular systolic function and augmented coronary blood flow.

Indications

- Cardiogenic shock that is not promptly reversed with pharmacologic intervention
- Acute severe mitral regurgitation causing hemodynamic instability
- Acute ventricular septal rupture
- Unstable angina and severe coronary occlusion in pts undergoing percutaneous coronary intervention and/or coronary surgery. Mechanical support of the left ventricle as a bridge to transplant.

Contraindications

- Aortic valve insufficiency
- Aortic dissection and aortic aneurysm. Pts with thoracic aortic graft (may be considered 12 mo after graft placement.

ASSESSMENT POINTS

System	Effect	PE	Test
CARDIO	Dysrhythmias, volume status BP, bleeding, inspect distal extremities, UO	Pulses Inspect site CT (retroperitoneal bleed)	ECG CVP, PAP, PCWP, CI Doppler of limbs, ECHO

Key Reference: Turi Z. Intra-aortic baollon counterpulsation. In: Parillo JE, Dellinger RP, eds. *Critical care medicine principles of diagnosis and management in the adult.* Philadelphia: Mosby Elsevier; 2008:93–115.

Perioperative Management

- Optimal placement from the leg involves insertion below the inguinal ligament and above the bifurcation of the femoral artery.
- Optimal position is a point 1 cm to 2 cm distal to the subclavian artery (can be estimated by placing the balloon tip on the pt's chest at the angle of Louis and marking the distal portion of the catheter where insertion will take place at the femoral artery. Left radial arterial pressure monitoring can help assure that flow to the left arm is adequate. Fluoroscopy is highly recommended to assure ideal placement between the left subclavian artery and the renal arteries.
- Fluoroscopy should be used to ensure ideal position but if not available transesophageal echocardiography is an acceptable alternative.
- Size of balloon placed varies according to the pt's height with a general recommendation of a 25 cc balloon for pts less than 5 ft in height and 50 cc for pt's greater than 6 ft tall.
- The balloon diameter is general designed to inflate to 80–90% of the interak diameter of the descending aorta.
- Timing of balloon inflation and deflation is critical. The goal is to optimize afterload reduction during systole and optimize diastolic BP, flow and velocity without interference with systolic ejection.
- Early inflation results in increased afterload and the augmented pressure wave imposed on the systolic component of the pressure tracing.
- Late inflation and early deflation lead to reduced augmentaion of diastolic flow.

- Late deflation causes the augmented pressure wave to be seen extending into the systolic component of the pressure wave.
- Ideally an electrocardiogram is used for timing inflation and deflation. The descending slope of the T wave correlates with the onset of diastole and inflation and the R wave, which marks the onset of electrical systole, is used to trigger deflation.
- If an aortic pressure tracing is used then the dicrotic notch (aortic valve closure) is used to trigger inflation and end of diastole triggers deflation.
- The operating settings allow for augmentation of every heart beat (1:1) every other heart beat (1:2) and depending on the manufacturer as low as every eighth heart beat (1:8). There is probably little benefit beyond a low setting of augmentation of every fourth heart beat (1:4). These lower settings are used during the weaning process. A nonfunctional or stopped intra-aortic balloon pump should be removed within 20 min or less. Volume weaning, by slowing reducing the volume of the balloon inflation, can also be used.
- The physiologic goals during therapy with the device and the weaning process incl a cardiac index greater than 2.2 L/min/m², acceptable BP with no ongoing signs of organ under-perfusion (acceptable UO, no signs of visceral ischemia, good mental status, normal pH and other ABG parameters, with low lactate levels). Constant physiologic monitoring of pulm capillary wedge pressure, central venous pressure and pulm artery pressures is advisable (a drop in these pressures accompanied by a rise of cardiac index are good indicators that myocardial work has been decreased with the onset of therapy). Monitoring with frequent echocardiograms can also be useful.
- Unless there is a risk of major acute bleeding anticoagulation with heparin is commonly used to reduce the risk of clot formation on the balloon and in areas of stagnant or low flow caused by the insertion of the device (femoral artery). A partial thrombopastin time (PTT) of 1.5 to 2 times baseline is maintained while the device is needed and then allowed to wear off sufficiently to prevent major bleeding complications (usually 4 hr).
- Constant vigilance for signs and symptoms of major bleeding (following all hemodynamic parameters and hemoglobin levels) and limb and organ ischemia is important. Assessment of pulses in all extremities but esp. the affected limb is critical. Retroperitoneal bleeding is a potential complication that may not be evident immediately so be observant of subtle signs of ongoing bleeding. A non-contrast computerized axial tomography scan can be useful to diagnose this complication.

Anticipated Problems/Concerns

- Timing may be difficult in pts with variable heart rates such as atrial fibrillation. May be difficult to allow for adequate balloon inflation in heart rates greater then 120 beats/min (if heart rate cannot be slowed then consider augmentation of every other heart beat with a 1:2 setting).

Intussuscepted Bowel Repair

Kathleen Rosen

Risk, Pediatric

- Most common cause of pediatric small bowel obstruction
- 56/100,000 children each year
- Most common 4–9 mo
- 67% occur <1 y
- 75% <2 y
- Rare <3 mo
- M:F ratio: 3:1 overall
- Incidence increases with age
- Recurrence 3–11%
- Chronic course 5%
- 80–90% ileocolic
- 90% idiopathic
- Lead point ⅓ children >2

Risk, Adult

- 5–10% of intussusception
- < 5% adult bowel obstruction
- Majority terminal ileum
- Bowel abn common
- Male predominance overall
- Appendiceal intussusceptions more common in adult women
- Retrograde jejunal-gastric intussusceptions after gastric bypass, gastrectomy, gastrostomy tubes, or repair duodenal atresia
- Idiopathic 10%
- Colonic: Majority malignant lead point
- CT imaging reveals intussusception images in ~0.1% of scans
- Non-surgical intussusceptions >10 × more frequent than surgical
- Periop risk, pediatric: Mortality with treatment 1–3%
- Mortality 100% untreated ≤5 d
- Bowel perforation during enema

- Periop risk, adult: Morbidity and complications 25%
- Complications related to sepsis
- Strangulation risk highest with ileo-colic

Worry About

- Sign of advanced disease: Lethargy, fever, dehydration, changes in mental status, tachypnea
- Check Hct, electrolytes
- Contraindications to non-surgical reduction: Perforation, strangulation, sepsis, peritonitis, CV instability

Overview

- Intussusception: Telescoping of bowel into itself, usually distal.
- Lead point: Anatomic stimulus for invagination

Pediatric
- Acute presentation
- Clinical classic triad: Colicky abd pain, emesis, bloody diarrhea ("current jelly")
- Diagnosis: Ultrasound preferred: target sign >98 sensitive
- Abd x-ray: Crescent sign, free air
- Co-existing conditions: Henoch's purpura, cystic fibrosis, recent viral illness (URI or GI)/lymphadenopathy, nephritic syndrome
- Lead points benign: Meckel's, indwelling tube, polyps, blunt trauma, foreign body incl bezors, malrotation, Peutz-Jegher syndrome
- Lead points malignant: Lymphoma, sarcoma
- Seasonal peaks: Spring and Fall

Adult
- Chronic, more insidious presentation
- Clinical: Abd pain, changes in bowel movement, distended abd, N/V

- Diagnosis: CT most sensitive
- Colonoscopy for subacute or chronic
- Lead points malignant: Carcinoma, lymphoma, melanoma, sarcoma
- Lead points benign: Endometriosis, diverticulum, strictures, adhesions, Meckel's, celiac, Crohn's, lipoma, adenoma, heterotopic pancreas, HIV, infection

ICD-9-CM Code: 560.0

Indications and Treatment

Pediatric
- Surgical consultation regarding signs of peritonitis
- Enema reduction: Air versus liquid or contrast
- Enema perforation: ~1%
- Position: Prone
- Dx: US
- Sedation/GA lower reduction rates
- Recurrence rate: ~10%
- Surgery: Laparoscopy 1°, bowel resection increases with age
- Surgery indications: Perforation, failed enemas, pathologic lead point
- Enema reduction may be attempted for idiopathic small bowel.
- Delayed repeat enema beneficial

Adult
- Enema reduction rarely indicated
- Surgery: Laparoscopy 1°, bowel resection common

ASSESSMENT POINTS

System	Effect	Assessment by Hx	PE	Test
GI	Venous congestion Bowel edema Ischemia/infarction Perforation	Pain N/V BM + blood Diarrhea	Mass Tenderness Rectal prolapse	US CT Enema Abd x-ray
RENAL/ HYDRATION	Dehydration	Vomitting I/O	Urine amount/color Fontanelle Sunken eyes Skin turgor	Electrolytes BUN, Cr UA
CARDIO	Anemia Sepsis Shock	Lethargy Mental status Fever	Tachycardia Hypotension Pallor Capillary refill	Hgb/Hct WBC Lactate

Key Reference: Demirkan A, Yagmurlu A, Kepenekci I, et al. Intussusception in adults and pediatric patients: Two different entities. *Surg Today*. 2009;39:861–865.

Perioperative Management

Preoperative preparation
- Hydration
- Transfusion
- NG drainage
- Antibiotics for sepsis

Anesthetic technique
- General anesthesia preferred

Monitoring
- ASA routine monitors
- UO
- Invasive for sepsis or hemodynamic instability

Induction/Maintenance
- RSI
- NMB

Surgical Stages

Pediatric
- Laparoscopy 1° approach
- May need extension of incision for reduction or resection
- Resection 25%

Adult
- Laparoscopy primary approach
- May need extension of incision for reduction or resection
- Resection >90%
- Primary reanasthamosis vs. enterostomy

Anticipated Problems/Concerns

Intraoperative
- CV instability
- Sepsis
- Temp loss
- Pt age <1 y
- Restriction of ventilation: Gas insufflations versus retraction

Postoperative
- Pain
- Fluid shifts
- Infection

Joint Replacement Cementing (Methylmethacrylate Cementing)

Corinne K. Postle
Andrew K. Wong

Risk

- True incidence of bone cement implantation syndrome (BCIS) is unknown.
- BCIS primarily a problem assoc with hip replacement, although it has been described during other cemented procedures such as knee arthroplasty and vertebroplasty.
- Pt risk factors for BCIS incl pre-existing pulm Htn, and significant cardiac disease (New York Heart Association Class 3 or 4).
- Surgical risk factors for BCIS incl pathologic fracture, inter-trochanteric fracture, and long-stem arthroplasty.

Perioperative Risks

- Mortality after cemented and uncemented 1° total hip replacement (THR) is 2.3% and 1.6% respectively.
- Incidence of intraop mortality during cemented total hip replacement (THR) is 0.11%.
- DVT
- Fat embolism syndrome (resp, neurologic, cutaneous, hematologic symptoms) <1%
- Pulm embolism 1.8–3.4% (with no prophylaxis)

Worry About

- Increased PVR leading to decreased right ventricular EF, leading to reduced left ventricular EF, which leads to decreased CO
- Clinical features (may incl one or more): Hypotension, hypoxia, loss of consciousness, cardiac arrhythmias
- Pulm embolism 1.8–3.4% (with no prophylaxis)

Overview

- Methylmethacrylate (MMA) is used as a bone cement in orthopedic surgery
- Bone cement implantation syndrome (BCIS) occurs in pts undergoing cemented bone surgery, and is characterized by signs such as hypotension, hypoxia, arrhythmias, increased pulm vascular resistance (PVR), loss of consciousness, and cardiac arrest.
- BCIS can occur around the time of cementation, prosthesis insertion, reduction of the joint, or deflation of a limb tourniquet.
- Different models exist to explain BCIS, but many probably play a role.

- Monomer-mediated model: MMA monomers lead to vasodilation in vitro, but this hypothesis is not supported in vivo in animal studies.
- Embolic model: MMA undergoes an exothermic reaction and expands, resulting in intramedullary Htn which forces emboli into the circulation. Embolic debris can be composed of fat, marrow, cement, air, bone, plt and fibrin aggregates. ↑ PVR may be due to mechanical obstruction of pulm circulation, and endothelial damage that results in release of inflammatory mediators.
- Intraop emboli detected on TEE in 90–98% of THR pts, but embolization not always assoc with hemodynamic changes
- Increased embolic load with cemented versus uncemented arthroplasties

ICD-9-CM Code: 820.x (Hip fracture)

Indications and Usual Treatment

- Disabling arthritis, femoral fractures

ASSESSMENT POINTS

System	Effect	Test
CARDIO	BCIS can cause ↓ MAP, ↓ SV, ↓ cardiac output, ↑ PVR, ↑ PAP, ↓ RV ejection fraction Pulm Htn → Heart failure PFO → risk for paradoxical emboli	ECG, TEE CVP, PA catheterization
HEME	MMA activates coagulation cascade and mediates plt aggregation → ↑ thrombosis	Venography, duplex US
CNS	Confusion, stroke (from paradoxial emboli)	Baseline neuro exam
RESP	↑ Pulm pressure, pulm emboli → V/Q mismatch If pt awake, dyspnea may be early sign of BCIS	PA catheterization ABG $ETCO_2$, TEE

Key Reference: Donaldson AJ, Thomson HE, Harper NJ, Kenny NW. Bone cement implantation syndrome. *Br J Anaesth.* 2009;102:12–22.

Intraoperative Management

Monitoring
- Consider invasive monitoring in pts with baseline cardiopulmonary disease or in pts at high risk for BCIS
- CVP monitoring may aid volume optimization but changes in CVP may correlate poorly with changes in PAP in BCIS
- Increased vigilance during times at which BCIS can occur
- If BCIS occurs, consider arterial line, PA catheter or TEE to guide management (intravascular volume, RV function).
- Exhaled gas analysis: Decreased $ETCO_2$ if significant pulm embolism; increased end-tidal N_2 if air embolus
- Esophageal Doppler may detect impending BCIS earlier than standard monitors.

Surgical Stages

- Pre-cement
- THR: Insidious blood loss due to irrigation
- TKR: Tourniquet-induced Htn (tourniquet time >30–60 min)
- Maintain intravascular volume
- Consider avoiding N_2O to prevent exacerbating air embolism
- Cementing
- If GA, D/C N_2O
- FIO_2 100% to combat increased PVR from emboli
- Hypotension in BCIS may be due to decreased SVR, decreased CO, or both
- CV collapse may be treated for RV failure with inotropes, vasodilation with alpha agonists, insufficient preload with fluid

Anticipated Problems/Concerns

- If pt at high risk of BCIS or has prior Hx of BCIS, consider discussion with surgeon if pt would benefit from uncemented rather than cemented arthroplasty even though a cemented prosthesis has better long-term viability.
- If cement will be used, surgical measures may be taken to reduce risk of BCIS (i.e., medullary lavage, venting bone, etc.).
- Fat embolism syndrome (hypoxemia, petechiae, neuro change)
- Neurocognitive changes due to paradoxical emboli

Kasai Procedure

Sibi Pappachan
Franklyn Cladis

Risk

- Biliary atresia occurs in 1/10,000 live births in Japan, and 1/15,000 live births in USA
- 10–15% of pts have assoc abn referred to as Biliary Atresia Splenic Malformation Syndrome (BASM). Polysplenia, asplenia, preduodenal portal vein, situs inversus, absent inferior vena cava, intestinal malrotation, and cardiac anomalies
- Affects girls more than boys
- Affects Asians and African-Americans more than Caucasians

Perioperative Risks

- Impaired hepatic function (generally a latter manifestation): Coagulation disorders, drug metabolism
- Vitamin deficiencies (K and E) and malnutrition may result in coagulopathy

Worry About

- Preoperative: The differential diagnosis of conjugated jaundice in an infant incl choledochal cyst, inspissated bile, neonatal hepatitis, alpha 1 antitrypsin deficiency, CMV hepatitis, cystic fibrosis, and Alagille's syndrome (arteriohepatic dysplasia) in which jaundice is assoc with hypercholesterolemia, pulm stenosis, elfin facies. Also Dubin Johnson syndrome (DJS) is a rare autosomal recessive condition with normal liver transaminases, a unique pattern of urinary excretion of heme metabolites (coproporphyrins), and the deposition of a pigment that gives the liver a characteristic black color.
- Postop: Cholangitis, and cholestasis (malnutrition, pruritus)

Overview

- Surgical procedure to correct biliary atresia
- Infants present from 1–6 wk of age with persistent jaundice and acholic stools.

- The lumen of the extrahepatic biliary system is obliterated. In the most common type the destruction is in the porta hepatis.
- Dx is made with radionuclear scanning, MRI, and biliary ultrasound in 80% of cases. It is confirmed by either liver biopsy or by exploratory laparotomy.

ICD-9-CM Code: 751.61 (Congenital biliary atresia)

Indications and Usual Treatment

- Biliary atresia
- Neomycin, metronidazole and lactulose may be given 24–48 hr prior to surgery.
- Hepatic portoenterostomy (Kasai procedure) is usually performed before 4 mo of age.
- Intraop cholangiogram may be performed.

ASSESSMENT POINTS

System	Effect	Assessment by Hx	PE	Test
DERM	Jaundice	Progressive increase	Deep greenish-bronze color	Conjugated hyperbilirubinemia
GI	Cirrhosis	Abd discomfort	Firm, enlarged liver Splenic enlargement Abd distention	Hypoalbuminemia
	Ascites			
	Stools	White or clay-colored		Acholic stools
CARDIAC	CHD (pulm stenosis)	Alagille's syndrome	Murmur	ECHO
RENAL	Urine	Greenish color	Bile stained	
NUTRITIONAL	Wt loss	Poor appetite	FTT	Vitamin deficiency, abn PT/PTT
CNS	Vit E deficiency	Ataxia	Hyporeflexia Ophthalmoplegia	
HEME	Blood loss	Weakness	Bloody stool	Endoscopy for esophageal varices, anemia

Key Reference: Green DW, Howard ER, Davenport M. Anaesthesia, perioperative management and outcome of correction of extrahepatic biliary atresia in the infant: A review of 50 cases in the King's College Hospital series. *Paediatr Anaesth* 2000;10(6):581–589.

Perioperative Management

Preoperative Preparation
- Check PT, PTT, hemoglobin, and plts. Abn not common but a type and screen should be performed and blood and FFP made available
- NG tube
- Broad-spectrum antibiotics
- Consider epidural block if coagulation is normal
- Consider central line if vascular access is difficult

Monitoring
- A large bore (22–20 g) IV in upper limb
- Arterial line and central venous pressure monitors rarely used unless other co-existing conditions (pneumonia, sepsis, cholangitis, and sever cirrhosis) or redo procedure
- All pressure points need to be padded and reassessed.
- Temp monitoring: Forced warm air device, warming lamps

Anesthetic Technique/Induction
- If IV access is available, induction with an hypnotic agent like propofol (2-3 mg/kg) or pentothal (4-6 mg/kg) along with a muscle relaxant (cisatracurium 0.2 mg/kg)
- If IV access unavailable, inhalation induction with O$_2$, N$_2$O, and sevoflurane. Once adequately anesthetized, an IV catheter is inserted and muscle relaxant can be used to facilitate ET intubation. Anesthesia is maintained with O$_2$-air-isoflurane/sevoflurane mixture with IV opioids.
- Avoid the continued use of N$_2$O due to bowel distention
- An isotonic IVF (preferably 0.9% NS or plasmalyte) should be used and serum glucose should be monitored
- An epidural can be placed for postop pain provided there is no coagulopathy.

Surgical Stages

Dissection
- Right subcostal incision extended to the left
- Cholangiogram and wedge biopsy of the liver to confirm diagnosis
- Liver mobilization and resection of atretic biliary system at porta hepatis
- Preparation of jejunum for roux-en-Y
- For biliary drainage the antimesenteric side of the jejunum is sutured to the porta hepatis

Postoperative Considerations
- NG tube for stomach decompression
- Supplementation of fat and fat-soluble vitamins if there is impaired absorption due to poor bile flow
- Prednisone 2 mg/kg/d may be given for its choleretic effect

Anticipated Problems/Concerns

- Cholangitis, portal Htn, and fat-soluble vitamin deficiency
- Approx 10–30% have long-term normal liver biochemistry. 70–90% go on to require liver transplantation.

Kidney Transplantation

Arun L. Jayaraman
Tetsuro Sakai

Risk

- Incidence in USA: As of 2006, the prevalence of end-stage renal disease (ESRD) was 506,256 pts with a median age of 58.8 y.
- As of 2007, 48,773 active pts and 94,741 total pts were on the renal transplant waiting list.
- Etiologies of ESRD on the waiting list: Diabetic nephropathy, 28%; hypertensive nephrosclerosis, 22%; glomerular disease, 21%; and other renal pathologies (SLE, polycystic kidney disease, vasculitides, etc.).
- Renal transplant demographic data from 2008 indicate
  - 61.4% male; 38.6% female
  - 4.7% less than 18 y/o, 80.1% 18–64 y/o, and 15.2% 65 y/o or greater
  - 53.7% Caucasian, 24.5% African American, 14.8% Hispanic, and 7% minority (i.e., Asian, Native American, Pacific Islander, etc.)
- Of the 16,520 kidneys transplanted in 2008, 10,552 were from deceased donors and 5,968 were from living donors.
- As of 2004, the median time to transplantation was 3.3 y.
- As of 2006, the 3-mo pt survival rate post-transplant was 99.3% (living donor) and 97.9% (deceased donor).
- 1 y/5 y/10 y pt survival rates: 98%/91%/77% (living donor), 96%/83%/64% [deceased non-expanded criteria donor (ECD)], and 91%/70%/47% (ECD).

Perioperative Risks

- Cardiac events, pulm edema, hemorrhage from vascular anastomoses, infection, vascular thrombosis, and graft rejection (non-functioning)

Worry About

- Interval between last dialysis and renal transplant
  - Volume and electrolyte status (esp. serum K^+ level)
  - Coagulopathy
- Proper pt positioning
- AV graft and/or fistula
  - Pad graft and/or fistula
  - Prevent heat loss (place heat pad on graft/fistula)
  - Periodically palpate and/or auscultate to check bruit
- IV access while preserving dialysis access
- Renal metabolism and/or excretion of drugs
- Maintaining adequate allograft perfusion
  - Ischemia and/or reperfusion injury of leg and renal graft
  - Potential for rapid blood loss during reperfusion

- Antirejection regimen
- Hypotension, allergic reaction, increased bleeding and/or pulm edema may be seen with use of monoclonal anti-CD52 antibodies (i.e., alimtuzumab)

Overview

- 3–5 hr procedure
- Supine position
- Heterotopic renal graft implantation in extraperitoneal iliac fossa
  - No need for removal of recipient's kidneys
- Main anesthetic goal is to ensure graft perfusion and forced diuresis
  - Perfusion pressure (dopamine)
  - Volume expansion
  - Diuretics (furosemide and mannitol)

Indications and Usual Treatment

- Treatment of choice for ESRD (improves life expectancy and quality of life)
- Contraindications to renal transplant incl
  - Active infection
  - Continued illicit drug abuse
  - Complete thrombosis of IVC and iliac veins
  - Metastatic disease

ICD-9-CM Code: 55.69

ASSESSMENT POINTS

System	Effect	Assessment by Hx	PE	Test
PULM	Pulm edema, effusions, pulm Htn, pneumonia, OSA	SOB, DOE, orthopnea, cough	Crackles, rales	CXR, CT chest, ECHO, RHC, sleep study
CARDIO	CAD, cardiomyopathy, Htn, hyperlipidemia, PVD	Angina, claudication, CVA/TIA	S_3/S_4 murmur, JVD, carotid bruits, weak peripheral pulses, edema	EKG, ECHO, DSE, cardiac cath, carotid Doppler, ABI, C-reactive protein, daily weights
GI	Gastroparesis	Bloating, early satiety, GERD		Gastric emptying study
RENAL	ESRD (usually on dialysis)	N/V, altered mental status		Electrolytes, BUN, Cr, Cr clearance
ENDO	Hyperglycemia, hyperparathyroidism			Blood glucose, Ca, Phos
HEME	Anemia, coagulopathy, plt dysfunction	SOB, easy bleeding	Capillary refill, pallor	CBC, PT/INR, PTT, plt function assays
NEURO	Neuropathy	Numbness, orthostasis, syncope	Decreased sensation, orthostatics	Tilt table testing

Key Reference: Beebe DS, Belani KG, Anesthesia for kidney, pancreas, or other organ transplantation. In: Longnecker DL, Brown DL, Newman MF, Zapol WM, eds. *Anesthesiology.* New York: McGraw-Hill; 2008:1396–1419.

Perioperative Management

- Epidural or paravertebral catheter can be used for postop analgesia
- Coagulation status usually normal under scheduled hemodialysis
- Consider arterial line and central line with aseptic technique
- Consider pre-treatment with a non-particulate antacid (gastroparesis)
- Remember preop antibiotic prophylaxis
- Consider rapid sequence induction with cricoid pressure (full stomach/gastroparesis) using rocuronium (succinylcholine is best avoided due to hyperkalemia)
- Consider cisatracurium for maintenance (avoid pancuronium).
- Use of sevoflurane is controversial.
- Avoid large doses of morphine and meperidine.

- Maintain normovolemia or slight hypervolemia
- Adjuvants: Furosemide (0.25–1 mg/kg), mannitol (0.25–1 g/kg), and/or low dose dopamine (2–5 μg/kg/min) are often administered shortly prior to and following allograft reperfusion
- An immunosuppressant (methylprednisolone 10 mg/kg) is typically administered prior to graft reperfusion
- An induction immunosuppressant (OKT3 or alemtuzumab) may be used in the preop or intraop period.

Surgical Stages

- Lateral oblique skin incision in lower abd
- Extraperitoneal space (less fluid loss)
- Iliac vessel clamping during anastomoses (graft renal artery to iliac artery and graft renal vein to iliac vein)
- Donor ureter attached to recipient's bladder

Postoperative Considerations

- Maintain normal to elevated MAP and CVP to preserve graft perfusion.
- Chest x-ray (to R/O pneumothorax, pulm edema)
- Monitor fluid status and UO closely
- If stable, transfer to a monitored floor bed
- Potential for delayed graft function (ECD kidney)
  - May consider postop hemodialysis
  - Consider ICU transfer
- Use PCA and/or epidural or paravertebral block for postop analgesia

Knee Arthroscopy

Jonathan C. Beathe
Russell Flatto

Risk

- Incidence in USA: >1.5 million/y
- Incidence of arthroscopic anterior cruciate ligament (ACL) repair in USA: >100,000/y
- Pts primarily <60 y; related to athletic injury
- No racial or gender predominance

Perioperative Risks

- Mortality rate < 1:100,000
- Morbidity is rare
- Neurologic injury: Direct trauma, compartment syndrome, tourniquet-related, and dysfunction due to Complex Regional Pain Syndrome 1 (CRPS 1). Femoral nerve most vulnerable.
- Vascular injury more likely during meniscus repair (popliteal artery)
- Tourniquet: Temporary paralysis after prolonged inflation
- Infection (esp. with allografts)
- Deep vein thrombosis/pulm embolism rare (short procedure with early mobilization)
- Postop hemarthrosis, effusion, and synovitis
- Risk of CRPS 1 higher in women, and patellofemoral joint injuries

Worry About

- Risk of bradycardia and/or asystole following tourniquet deflation or with regional anesthesia
- Risk of PDPH in young pts
- Risk of transient neurologic symptoms (TNS) with spinal anesthesia
- Ability to discharge ambulatory pts
- Aspiration risk
- Technical problems with obese or very muscular pts

Overview

- Knee arthroscopy is one of the most common surgical procedures in the USA
- Very low periop mortality and morbidity
- Fiberoptic arthroscope is inserted through a small incision in the joint.

- Instruments are placed through additional ports after diagnostic arthroscopy to initiate repair.
- Regional anesthesia may allow for an earlier discharge, optimal surgical conditions, reduced PONV, and superior analgesia. General anesthesia will avoid risks of neuraxial anesthesia (TNS, PDPH).
- Postop pain control an issue, esp. following autograft ACL repair
- MRI diagnosis

ICD-9-CM Codes: 717.83 (Anterior cruciate ligament tear); 836.0 (Medial meniscus tear)

Indications and Usual Treatment

- Meniscectomy or meniscal repair for torn medial or lateral meniscus
- Removal of loose bodies or Baker's cyst
- Reconstruction of torn ACL or posterior cruciate ligament (PCL)
- Debridement of osteochondral defects or osteoarthritis
- Synovectomy for inflammatory arthritis

ASSESSMENT POINTS

System	Effect	Assessment by Hx	PE	Test
CARDIO	Risk of bradycardia/asystole due to tourniquet deflation, neuraxial anesthesia, emotional reaction	Hx of athletic state	Slow resting HR	ECG
HEME	Bleeding diathesis contraindication to regional anesthesia	Bleeding or easy bruising with injury or tooth extraction	Bruises	PT, APTT, plt count, bleeding time as indicated by Hx
GU	Postop urinary retention	Nocturia Hx of prior catheterization	Size of prostate	Bladder US if no void and if long-acting spinal used
CNS	Risk of bradycardia/hypotension and nausea with sight of blood/surgery	Fainting or stress with prior surgery Rx with anxiolytic medication	Visibly anxious	

Key Reference: Mulroy MF, Larkin KL, Hodgson PS, Helman JD, Pollock JE, Liu SS. A comparison of spinal, epidural, and general anesthesia for outpatient knee arthroscopy. *Anesth Analg.* 2000;91:860–864.

Perioperative Implications

Preoperative Issues

- Pt may have expectation to watch procedure
- Focus on early discharge
- Potential length of procedure

Monitoring

- Routine

Anesthetic Technique

- Local infiltration of portals + intra-articular injection of 20–30 mL 0.25% bupivacaine (often requires additional sedation). Inadequate for ACL repair or if thigh tourniquet is used.
- Femoral nerve block: Limited by tourniquet use and surgery in back of knee
- Epidural, spinal, or combined spinal-epidural: Issues incl PDPH risk, duration of surgery, rate of onset and resolution of blockade.
- Choice of local anesthetic for spinal
- Controversy exists with off-label use of preservative-free, isobaric 1.5% mepivacaine and 2% 2-chloroprocaine for spinal anesthesia, although evidence suggests they are efficacious for this procedure.
  - Lidocaine (risk of TNS)
  - Bupivacaine (rare TNS, long-acting, delays discharge)
    - Addition of fentanyl (PONV, pruritis)
- Conscious to deep sedation to GA: Consider short-acting agents (e.g., propofol/desflurane), airway concerns, PONV
- Choice depends on duration of surgery, use of thigh tourniquet, surgeon and pt preference, ease of discharge
- Induction: Infiltration, blocks, intra-articular local anesthetic usually performed 15 to 20 min before surgery
- Spinal and/or epidural: Control hemodynamic state
- GA: Consider LMA

Surgical Stages

- Multiple portals around knee
- Tourniquet: Pain may limit use if surgery is long—advantage of epidural or combined spinal-epidural
- Irrigation can distend soft tissues around knee
- Rotation of leg can stress hip joint or lumbar spine (figure 4 position)

Postoperative Considerations

- Control of pain and side effects can lead to early discharge
- PONV and sedation limit discharge, esp. after deep sedation, GA, narcotics
- Options: Intra-articular drugs, e.g., bupivacaine ± morphine
- Local infiltration of portals with bupivacaine
- Femoral nerve blocks particularly helpful after ACL repair. Requires knee brace for discharge.
- IV or PO NSAIDs reduce narcotic requirement
- Urinary retention usually not limiting factor in young pts
- Follow-up phone call helps define and treat problems.

Anticipated Problems/Concerns

- Postop back pain (with or without regional anesthesia)
- PDPH: Should be followed and treated
- Postop pain usually controlled with oral medication and hypothermia
- Late urinary retention
- TNS (can be managed with NSAIDs)
- Local anesthetic or epinephrine-containing solution: Toxicity with infiltration

Labor, Epidural Block

Lisbeysi Calo

Hosni Mikhaeil

Risk

- Incidence in USA: Approx 65% get an epidural block for pain relief during labor at hospitals that perform more than 1500 deliveries per year.

Preoperative Risks

- Edema offers technical difficulty while placing the epidural catheter.
- Obesity is another factor making epidural catheter placement a challenge.
- Hypovolemia, from significant bleeding or dehydration.
- Other causes of hypotension incl sepsis

Perioperative Risks

- No pain relief, also called block failure, occurs in about 1 in 20. Additionally another 15% experience partial failure, and have only partial pain relief.
- Intravascular injection (catheter misplacement is uncommon, less than 1 in 300) or migration (about 1 in 10,000 insertions) with possible arrhythmias and seizures. This also results in block failure.
- Catheter misplacement into the subarachnoid space (less than 1 in 1000), with possible subsequent spinal administration of large doses of local anesthetics.
- Level and degree of sympathetic blockade will determine the effect on the CV system (less incidence of hypotension in women who received 1 liter of Ringers lactate versus those who did not receive prehydration).

Postoperative Risks

- Postdural puncture headache

Worry About

- CV collapse due to accidental venous injection of the local anesthetic
- Hematomas in pts with underlying coagulopathies
- Increased incidence of instrumental delivery
- Alterations in uteroplacental perfusion and acidosis of the fetus due to the placental transfer of local anesthetics and subsequent hypoxia
- Epidural abscess in pts with sepsis
- Total spinal (high level of anesthesia) with loss of airway
- Hypoxemia and acidosis can develop in labor and cardiopulmonary resuscitation might be difficult.

Overview

- Epidural analgesia is a safe and effective way to manage pain in labor with minimal motor block.
- The decrease in uterine activity following the administration of epidural block is transient. However studies have suggested a better fetal outcome when epidural analgesia has prolonged the second stage of labor.
- Recent data suggest that there is no difference between the administration of early epidural block (dilation 3–4 cm) versus late epidural block (dilation greater than 5 cm) regarding the occurrence of dystocia or necessity for C-section (controversial). Combined epidural and spinal anesthesia does not seem to negatively influence the progress of labor, it might even speed up labor in early primiparous pts. Controversy remains regarding the effect of more concentrated local anesthetics solutions in the progress of labor.

- In the first stage of labor epidural block seems to decrease the intensity of the uterine contractions more than the frequency. Uterine activity usually returns to normal within 30 min.

ICD-9-CM Code: V22 (Pregnancy)

Indications

- Significant pain resulting in maternal stress
- Vaginal delivery of twins
- Preterm infant delivery (more control of delivery)

Contraindications

Absolute

- Patient refusal
- Coagulopathy or anticoagulant use depending on the mechanism of action and half life
- Severe hypovolemia (along with sympathectomy can cause profound circulatory collapse).
- Increased intracranial pressure
- Local infection over the insertion site
- Severe aortic stenosis or severe mitral stenosis
- True allergy to local anesthetics of both classes (amides and esters)

Relative

- Uncooperative pt
- Inability to increase cardiac output in response to sympathectomy
- Anatomic abn of the spine
- Certain neurologic diseases that can be further exacerbated by the block
- Inability to communicate with the pt
- Previous back surgery
- Significant blood loss

ASSESSMENT POINTS

System	Effect	Assessment by Hx	PE	Test
CARDIO	Aortocaval compression	Dizziness, syncope, decrease FHR	Hypotension in supine position	Assess UO provide left uterine displacement
RESP	Decreased FRC increases minute ventilation and O_2 consumption	Rapid development of hypoxemia	Tachypnea	Avoid high spinal blockade, provide supplemental O_2
CNS	Decreased MAC epidural vein distention	Exaggerated effect of local anesthetics	Sedation, increased sensory and motor block	Assess dermatomal blockade
COAGULATION	Decreased plt count abn function	Abn hemostasis	Oozing at IV site, bruising	Assess plt count fibrinogen, FSPs, check bleeding time
FETAL HR	Sensitive to maternal hypotension	Bradycardia, decreased heart rate variability	Decreased movement, HR variability, meconium	Phonocardiogram, fetal scalp blood sampling

Key Reference: Chestnut DH, et al. Does early administration of epidural analgesia affect obstetric outcome in nulliparous women who are receiving oxytocin? *Anesthesiology.* 2009;26:521–567.

Perioperative Management

Monitoring

- Noninvasive BP measurement and continuous fetal and maternal HR.
- Ensure drugs and equipment are available to access the airway.
- An obstetrician should be available to manage obstetric complications during induction and maintenance of epidural analgesia.
- Prehydration with Ringers lactate

Induction

- The uterus should be displaced left to improve maternal venous return, hypotension should be treated with additional IV boluses of crystalloid solution and/or administration of small IV doses of a vasopressor such as ephedrine (5–10 mg IV).
- The most commonly used intermediate-acting local anesthetic via the epidural route with catheter insertion is 2% lidocaine. Adding epinephrine to the solution (1:200,000) prolongs the duration of action by 40–60%.

Dilute Techniques

- Primigravida in early labor or slowly progressing multipara: Use bupivacaine 0.05–0.0625% (10 mL) by bolusing 5 mL at a time. Additive effect can be obtained with 50–100 mcg of fentanyl, or 100 mcg of hydromorphone. A continuous infusion of bupivacaine 0.0625–0.0125% with 2–3 mcg/mL of fentanyl, or 3 mcg/mL of hydromorphone at 5–15 mL/hr are good choices for maintenance. Alternatively a combined spinal-epidural provides advantages for pain control esp. in early labor. A combination of 12.5–25 mcg of fentanyl with 2.5 mg bupivacaine intrathecally may be used for induction, followed by an epidural continuous infusion of bupivacaine at 0.0625–0.0125%.
- Neuraxial analgesia in early labor does not increase the rate of cesarean delivery, and provides better analgesia. It also results in a shorter duration of labor than systemic analgesia.
- The use of pt controlled epidural analgesia with bupivacaine, 0.0625%–0.0125% + fentanyl 2–3 mcg/mL, is another possibility.

It can be given at 5 mL/hr basal rate, bolus of 5 mL with 5–6 min lockout, and 1-hr limit of 15–20 mL.

Standard Techniques

- Local anesthetic only: Induction with ropivacaine 0.2% (8–10 mL), followed by continuous infusion of ropivacaine 0.1% at 8–10mL/hr.
- Local aesthetic plus opioid: Induction with bupivacaine 0.125–0.25% (8–10 mL/hr) plus fentanyl 50–100 mcg. After epidural block is established, an infusion can be started with bupivacaine 0.625–0125% plus fentanyl 1.6–2 mcg/mL, at a rate of 8–10 mL/hr. Ropivacaine 0.1% mixed with fentanyl 1.6–2 mcg/mL, at 8–10 mL/hr can be used as well.
- The infusion can be maintained for pain relief during episiotomies and to facilitate the removal of the placenta. If a C-section is needed, the epidural block can be extended with lidocaine 2% plus epinephrine 1:200.000.

PROCEDURES

Concentrated Techniques

• Rapidly progressing multipara in first stage of labor: In these cases it is important to achieve fast pain relief. Lidocaine 1.5% or 2% can be used with epinephrine 1:200.000 (10 mL bolus) in 5 mL increments combined with fentanyl 50–100 mcg. If necessary, a continous infusion of bupivacaine at 0.0125% with fentanyl 2–3 mcg/mL at rate of 5–15 mL/hr may be initiated to maintain analgesia.

Special Situations

• For women in labor with a Hx of mild to moderate aortic or mitral stenosis, narcotics can be used alone. Fentanyl 1–4 µg/mL/hr or sufentanil 0.03–0.05 µg/mL/hr are good options in these instances.

• Second stage arrest: Low concentrations of local anesthetics preserve the urge reflex to push with minimization of the laxity of the perineal musculature. However, one must consider that better pain relief is achieved with higher concentrations of local anesthetics. Alternatively fentanyl 12.5–25 mcg with 2.5 mg bupivacaine can be used intrathecally, and can be repeated after 1.5–2.5 hr.

Anticipated Problems/Concerns

• Difficulties in placing the catheter: Obese pts, presence of edema, repetitive attempts, back pain, and paresthesias.

• Fetal compromise: Decreased uteroplacental perfusion with fetal hypoxia, neonatal exposure to opioids and local anesthetics, with dose-dependent CNS damage.

• Unwanted effects: Motor blockade, excessive relaxation of the perineum, decreased ability to push, necessity of oxytocin augmentation

• Neuraxial analgesia in early labor does not increase the rate of cesarean delivery, and it provides better analgesia and results in a shorter duration of labor than systemic analgesia.

Labor, Peripheral Blocks

Richard C. Month
Theodore G. Cheek

Perioperative Risks

- Periop morbidity/mortality from anesthetic technique: rare
- Morbidity: Accidental maternal IV local anesthetic (LA) injection. Risk of seizures, cardiotoxicity, and fetal bradycardia.

Worry About

- Accidental IV injection
- Hypotension (sympathetic nerve block)
- Fetal bradycardia (paracervical block)
- Neuropathy (nerve damage)
- Infection
- Hematoma formation (LSB)
- Total or high spinal very rare with lumbar sympathetic block

Overview

- Lumbar sympathetic block (LSB): Analgesia for the first stage of labor. Blocks visceral efferents as they join sympathetic chain.
- Paracervical block, Frankenhauser's plexus: Lower uterus and cervix—analgesia for the first stage of labor
- Pudendal block: Analgesia for the second stage of labor by blocking distribution of sacral nerves 2, 3, and 4 (lower vagina and perineum). Useful for forceps, vacuum or episiotomy.
- Perineal infiltration: Supplemental analgesia for the second stage of labor

ICD-9-CM Code: V22.2 (Pregnancy)

Usual Treatment

- Indications: Parturient in whom regional, parenteral, or other means of analgesia are not advisable (i.e., severe coagulopathy, previous back surgery, spine pathology, failed or unavailable epidural or spinal analgesia)
- LSB may accelerate both first and second stages of labor. Use with circumspection in parturients with a Hx of uterine hyperstimulation.
- Paracervical block may produce fetal bradycardia.

ASSESSMENT POINTS

System	Effect	Assessment by Hx	PE	Test
CARDIO	Hypotension (LSB) Hematoma Cardiac depression, arrest	Patient response Vessel puncture IV injection	Peripheral vasodilation Swelling Unresponsive	BP MRI ECG
CNS	Horner syndrome (LSB) Total spinal anesthesia Nerve damage	Subarachnoid injection	Eyelid droop, facial warmth Loss of consciousness Neuropathy	P exam EMG
FETAL	Bradycardia (PCB)	Fetal absorption	FHR	
INFECTIOUS	Retropsoas abscess Subgluteal abscess	Poor aseptic technique	Fever, pain	MRI

Key Reference: Richardson MG. Regional anesthesia for obstetrics. *Anesthesiol Clin North Am.* 2000;18:383–406.

Perioperative Management

Monitoring
- BP, pulse, O₂ sat, FHR

Anesthetic Technique
- Lumbar sympathetic block
  - Sitting position
  - Bilateral L1 or L2 transverse process
  - Needle advanced approx 9 cm to anterolateral surface of L1 or L2 vertebral body
  - Inject bilaterally 10 mL of local anesthetic (with or without epinephrine or narcotic)
    - Will block approx 4–6 dermatomes
- Analgesia for 2–3 hr with bupivacaine or ropivacaine
- Paracervical block
  - Modified lithotomy position
  - 3–5 mL of LA each side, Iowa trumpet (needle guide) is very useful
  - First injection: Lateral fornix of vagina at 4-o'clock position, 0.5 cm deep
  - Second injection at 8-o'clock position
  - Epinephrine with LA may increase incidence of fetal bradycardia
  - Analgesia for 2–3 hr depending on local anesthetic
- Pudendal block
  - Transvaginal approach usual with Iowa trumpet needle guide
  - Bilateral (10 mL) local anesthetic injections 1 cm posteromedial to ischial spines
  - Failure rate high and perineal infiltration often needed
- Perineal infiltration
  - Supplemental analgesia for vaginal delivery, episiotomy, forceps or vacuum delivery
  - Infiltration of several milliliters of LA into the posterior fourchette

Laparoscopy, Gynecologic

Susan Chan

Risk

- Incidence in USA: >400,000 pts undergo gynecologic laparoscopy yearly; female > male (50:1)
- Most common gyn surgical procedure

Perioperative Risks

- Mortality: 1.6–11/100,000
- CV complications (e.g., air embolus): 1–10/100,000
- Intra-abdominal complications: 1%
- Postop pain necessitating hospitalization: 0.5–2%

Worry About

- Hypercarbia, resp acidosis, hypoxemia, pulm Htn, systemic vasodilation
- Pressure of pneumoperitoneum
- Hypothermia
- Pulm: Atelectasis, decreased FRC, high peak airway pressure, CO_2 embolus
- CV: Decreased venous return, decreased cardiac output, cardiac dysrhythmia
- Gastric reflux: esp. in pts with gastroparesis, hiatal hernia, obesity, or gastric outlet obstruction

Overview

- Endoscopic technique to visualize pelvic structure
- Adhesions and endometriosis can be treated endoscopically
- A small incision below umbilicus is made to insufflate CO_2 and two or more slightly larger incisions for insertion of visualization devices and instruments

- Duration of hospital stay significantly reduced. Most performed on outpatient basis, but duration of procedure may exceed that for open technique
- Surgical complications incl misplacement of Veress needle or trocar resulting in acute hemorrhage; bowel, bladder, uterus perforation; SQ emphysema

ICD-9-CM Code: 54.21

Indications

- Tubal ligation, ectopic pregnancy, vaginal hysterectomy, PID, infertility
- Question of PID versus appendicitis

ASSESSMENT POINTS

System	Effect	Assessment by Hx	PE	Test
CARDIO	CV arrhythmia; ↓ venous return; ↑ level of stress hormones	Chest pain, SOB, Hx of CAD, DM, arrhythmia	CV exam	ECG
RESP	If pre-existing lung disease, hypercarbia, acidosis, hypoxia not tolerated well	SOB, ↓ exercise tolerance	Chest exam	O_2 sat ?ABGs
GI	↑ Intra-abdominal pressure Trendelenburg position may ↑ chance of aspiration	DM, gastroparesis, hiatus hernia, obesity, gastric outlet obstruction	Airway exam	
HEME	Minimal blood loss normally	Hx of anemia, exercise tolerance	Vital signs	?Hct

Key Reference: Leonard F, Lecuru F, Rizk E, Chasset S, Robin F, Taurelle R. Perioperative morbidity of gynecological laparoscopy: A prospective monocenter observational study. *Acta Obstet Gynecol Scand.* 2000;79:129–134.

Perioperative Management

Monitoring

- Postop course more benign than in open procedure, yet intraop period may have much physiologic derangement
- Routine with $ETCO_2$ waveform

Airway

- Increased risk of passive regurgitation and aspiration due to Trendelenburg position and increased intra-abdominal pressure. GA with ET intubation most common.
- Laryngeal mask airway satisfactory alternative in nonobese pts undergoing relatively short procedures

Anesthetic Technique

- No advantage of less physiologic stress has been shown by using regional anesthesia
- With increased intra-abdominal pressure, increased ventilatory pressures required to ventilate
- NG tube recommended to minimize gastric reflux
- Complete relaxation of abd muscle

Postoperative Considerations

- Pain score: 2–8 depending on procedure
- Potent opioid analgesics (fentanyl) most commonly used. NSAID ketorolac, 60 mg IM or IV, shown to decrease postop analgesic requirement.

Anticipated Problems/Concerns

- Hypercarbia and acidosis most common physiologic complications when CO_2 used
- SQ emphysema, pneumothorax, pneumopericardium, pneumomediastinum, gas embolism less common
- Hypothermia and cardiac arrhythmia may be due to increased ventricular irritability, decreased venous return, decreased cardiac output, hypoventilation, gas embolism, or profound vagal response.
- Blind insertion of the Veress needle or trocar assoc with injuries to hollow viscera, major vessels, abd wall vessels

Laryngoscopy

Risk

- Direct laryngoscopy is performed for most tracheal intubations and to visualize pharynx and larynx for diagnostic and/or therapeutic purposes in pts with upper airway pathology
- All age groups

Perioperative Risks

- Depends on nature of complaint and underlying disease
- Htn and tachycardia common because of pain and stimulation of airway reflexes
- Tracheal intubation is assoc with higher incidence of postextubation airway obstruction requiring reintubation compared to other approaches of airway management such as supraglottic airway devices

- Incidence of reintubation when laryngoscopy performed for upper airway pathology: 0.39%

Worry About

- CV response to laryngoscopy and tracheal intubation
- Postextubation laryngeal spasm and airway obstruction
- Difficulties encountered in re-establishing airway and ventilation

Overview

- Rigid laryngoscopy assoc with severe CV responses and increase in plasma catecholamine concentrations
- Difficult laryngoscopy assoc with difficult facemask ventilation, can cause hypoxic brain damage and death

Indications and Usual Treatment

- Routinely applied for tracheal intubation in the OR and outside of the OR
- In combination of esophagoscopy and bronchoscopy, is applied for diagnosis and staging of oropharyngolaryngeal malignant lesions

ASSESSMENT POINTS

System	Effect	Assessment by Hx	PE	Test
HEENT	Limited neck flexion/ extension. R/O unstable C-spine	Pain upon neck movement	ROM of neck, opening of mouth, pain on motion	C-spine x-ray
CARDIO	Underlying cardiac disease common in elderly	Angina, arrhythmias Exercise tolerance	Cardiac evaluation Heart sounds Pulse rate and rhythm	ECG Stress test Thallium imaging angiogram
RESP	Hx of smoking	Wheezing; coughing; SOB; exercise tolerance	Wheezing, cyanosis	CXR PFTs with flow-volume loop
AIRWAY	Tumors, infections Compression	SOB Difficulty in breathing Hemoptysis	Wheezing Use of accessory muscles	PFTs (flow-volume loop) X-rays ABGs

Key Reference: Law JA, Hagberg CA. The evolution of upper airway retraction: New and old laryngoscope blades. In: Hagberg C, ed. *Benumof's airway management.* 2nd ed. Philadelphia: Mosby Elsevier; 2007:532–575.

Perioperative Management

Preoperative Preparation

- Closely monitor pts with lower airway obstruction
- Communicate with endoscopist, as airway is shared with endoscopist
- Check equipment that may be needed in case of failed rigid laryngoscopic intubation

Monitoring

- Routine

Anesthetic Technique

- Consider slow inhalation induction of general anesthesia maintaining spontaneous ventilation if symptoms of compromised airway are present
- Short-acting IV analgesics attenuate CV response to rigid laryngoscopy

- Short-acting muscle relaxant such as succinylcholine should be considered when difficult intubation is expected.
- Ventilate with 100% O_2 before intubation is attempted.

Surgical Stages

- Pt supine with head and neck in sniffing position
- Laryngoscope is entered through right side of the mouth advancing midline until epiglottis is exposed.
- With curve blade the tip is advanced in the vallecula lifting epiglottis indirectly to expose the glottis opening. With straight blade the tip of blade is placed under the tip of the epiglottis lifting it up to expose the vocal cords.
- Steroid considered if airway is compromised or if manipulation was extensive

Postoperative Concerns

- Confirm position of the ETT by auscultation and CO_2 monitor.
- Secure the ETT with tape.
- Continue observation of airway.

Anticipated Problems/Concerns

- Unanticipated difficult or failed intubation
- Accidental extubation
- Blockage of the ETT
- Severe Htn and tachycardia in pts with CAD
- Danger of spinal cord injury in pts with unstable cervical spine
- Undiagnosed esophageal intubation will be lethal

484

Laser Surgery of Airway

Ira J. Rampil

Risk

- Incidence in USA: : 3000–5000/y
- Race and gender predominance: none
- Laryngeal papilloma is more common in children ≤4 y than adults

Perioperative Risks

- Airway compromise (preop and postop)
- Airway fires (5–70 reported/y)

Worry About

- Loss of patent airway
- Displacement or ignition of ETT
- Postop laryngospasm

- Residual NMB
- Misdirected laser beam igniting drapes
- Infection of OR personnel by vaporized but intact human papillomavirus (HPV)

Overview

- Focused, coherent far-infrared (CO_2) laser light can precisely vaporize superficial tissue lesions at a distance through free air (no contact)
- Shorter wavelength (i.e., Nd:YAG) laser light can coagulate and necrose deeper lesions

ICD-9-CM Code: 478.4 (Laryngeal polyp); 478.74 (Laryngeal stenosis)

Indications

- Many heterogeneous conditions, incl laryngeal papilloma, tracheal scarring, webs or synechiae, vascular malformations, neoplasms, idiopathic subglottic stenosis

ASSESSMENT POINTS

System	Effect	Assessment by Hx	PE	Test
HEENT	Glottic or tracheal stenosis	DOE Stridor	Mallampati exam	Indirect laryngoscopy PFTs (flow-volume loop)
RESP	Neoplasia (V/Q mismatch)	Hemoptysis	Auscultation	CT or MRI of chest ABGs

Key Reference: Rampil IJ. Anesthetic considerations for laser surgery. *Anesth Analg.* 1992;74:424–435.

Perioperative Implications

Preoperative Preparation

- Consider antisialogogue
- Eye protection for OR personnel appropriate to laser wavelength

Anesthetic Technique

- GA
- FIO_2 ≤40% to retard combustion, consider FIO_2 of 21%
- N_2O is contraindicated as it supports combustion
- Profound NMB

Monitoring

- Routine

Airway

- Use laser-safe ETTs, either commercial or smoothly wrapped with metal foil
- For surgical access, use smallest diameter tube consistent with adequate ventilation, i.e., 5.5–6.5 mm outside diameter for adults
- Jet ventilation may spread virus throughout resp tree

Maintenance

- Maintain close communication with surgeon as procedure may conclude without significant lead time.
- Be ready to emergently extubate trachea and provide mask ventilation in event of airway fire.

Extubation

- Despite suctioning, pharynx may contain blood that may promote laryngospasm.

- Some surgeons have strong preference for deep extubation following vocal cord surgery in order to avoid cough-induced glottic injury.

Postoperative Period

- Stridor, excess coughing, or bronchospasm warrants immediate investigation.

Adjuvants

- Topical lidocaine ointment on ETT and/or saline in cuff may retard ignition.
- Surgeons may place moist pledgets in airway—be sure to retrieve them.

Anticipated Problems/Concerns

- Airway fire: Clamp ETT and remove; then reintubate with new ETT

Liver Resection

Adrian Hendrickse

Risk

- Liver resection is most commonly performed as part of the management of malignant disease.
- 95% of hepatic tumors are metastatic.
- 5% are 1°, hepatocellular carcinomas (HCC) being the most common.
- Incidence: 4/100,000 but rising
- M:F ratio: 2:1
- Racial predominance: Asian

Perioperative Risks

- 1–10% mortality dependant on institutional, surgical and anesthetic expertise combined with pt co-morbidities.
- Cirrhotic pts undergoing general surgery have an increased risk of mortality assoc with male gender, high Child-Pugh score, presence of ascites, raised plasma creatinine, Dx of COPD, preop infection, preop GI bleeding, high ASA status: presence of intraop hypotension

Worry About

- Extended surgical time esp. prolonged Pringle maneuver (clamping of hilar structures)
- Need for vena-cava cross clamp
- Blood loss, adequacy of vascular access and availability of blood products

Overview

- Liver resection surgery has become more common and in many pts may be considered to be curative. This has been largely due to improvements in preop investigations, pt selection and operative technique.
- Some pts undergoing liver resection will exhibit features of chronic liver disease.
- The extended hepatectomy is usually a long case complicated by the potential for massive blood loss and fluid shifts. Hemodynamic instability from surgical interruption of the blood supply can cause significant problems.
- Segmentectomies may be performed with little physiological disturbance and resection is also possible laparoscopically.

ICD-9-CM Code: 155.0 (Malignant neoplasm of liver and intrahepatic bile ducts); 197.7 (Secondary malignant neoplasm of respiratory and digestive systems)

Indications and Usual Treatment

- Benign tumors: Hepatic adenoma, hemangioma, focal nodular hyperplasia
- Malignant tumors: Primary-HCC, cholangiocarcinoma, hepatoblastoma, angiosarcoma, lymphoma
- Metastatic: Breast, lung, pancreas, stomach, large intestine, ovary
- Other: Hydatid disease, living donor transplantation
- Depending on the nature and location, it may be possible to use radiofrequency or ethanol to ablate the lesion.
- Techniques for resection incl wedge, left lateral segment, right/left lobe and trisegmentectomies.

ASSESSMENT POINTS

System	Effect	Assessment by Hx	PE	Test
CARDIO	Possible hyperdynamic circulation if cirrhotic	Fatigue, SOB	CV exam	ECG, ECHO
RESP	Possible diaphragmatic splinting due to ascites, pleural effusions	SOB	Resp exam	PFTs, ABGs
GI	Cirrhosis, ascites	↑ Abdominal girth	Hepatomegaly	Paracentesis
RENAL	Hepatorenal syndrome	Urine production and use of diuretics		UO, BUN, Cr
HEME	Coagulopathy	Bleeding Hx		PT, PTT, TEG

Key Reference: Lentschener C, Ozier Y. Anaesthesia for elective liver resection: some points should be revisited. *Eur J Anesthesiol* 2002;19:780–788.

Perioperative Management

Preoperative Preparation
- Blood products must be made readily available.
- Coagulopathy should be corrected.
- Regional anesthesia may be inappropriate in the presence of coagulopathy or predicted extensive resection.

Monitoring
- Although massive blood loss may not be expected, it is necessary to prepare as if it were.
- Reliable, large-bore venous access must be obtained.
- Consider intra-arterial monitoring in long cases.
- Central venous access is highly desirable.
- Aim for a CVP <5 cm H_2O to reduce blood loss during dissection.
- Air embolism is a possibility if the CVP falls too low or if there is sudden hypovolemia.

Induction
- No one technique has been shown to be better than another.
- Consider a rapid sequence induction esp. in cases complicated by ascites.

- Reduced doses of drugs due to hepatic and/or renal dysfunction

Maintenance
- Careful monitoring of CVP
- Consider renal support.
- Acute normovolemic hemodilution can reduce the need for autologous blood transfusion.
- Cell saver can be used in noncancer resections.
- Prophylactic antibiotics
- Ensure normothermia

Extubation
- Delayed emergence due to abn pharmacokinetics/dynamics

Surgical Stages

Skin Incision
- RUQ with possible extension into xiphoid; upper midline; chevron

Dissection
- Upper and/or lower vena cava dissection with possible clamping for vena cava exclusion
- Hilar dissection and/or clamping (Pringle maneuver)

- Parenchymal dissection-finger fracture; coagulation devices; stapler; combination of techniques

Intraoperative Problems
- Blood loss
- Reduced venous return and subsequent hemodynamic instability from caval clamping
- Hepatic congestion from outflow clamping or elevated CVP

Postoperative Considerations
- Most pts may be extubated.
- Elective ventilation on ICU should be considered for prolonged surgery, hypothermia, continuing hemorrhage and severe blood loss.
- Pain can be difficult to control-balanced analgesia using PCA opioids, local anesthesic agents and simple analgesics can be useful.
- In pts with underlying liver disease, complications are relatively common: Bleeding, infection, ascites, hepatic and renal dysfunction.
- Consider return to the OR for excessive bleeding or bile leakage.

Liver Transplantation

Ann Walia

Risk

- Incidence in USA: ~16,000 pts on waiting list
- 6319 transplants in 2008; M:F ratio 2:1; 9.7% <18 y.
- 6070 from deceased donors and 249 from living donors
- No significant difference in 5-y. pt or graft survival with LDLT or DDLT

Perioperative Risks

- MELD score: Implemented in 2002; predictor of mortality on the waiting list; 10% decrease in wait-list mortality since implementation
- MELD score = 9.6 × Loge (creatinine mg/dL) × 3.8 8 pt Loge (bilirubin mg/dL) + 11.2 × Loge (INR) + 6.4
- Increased MELD score a/w increased need for pressors, ventilator support, and transfusions.
- MELD modifiers for HCC, HRS, PPHTN (add 20 points to calculated MELD); HCC modifier has resulted in 5-fold increase in transplantation for HCC.

- ECD is an evolving strategy to deal with donor shortage but is a/w increased PNF, delayed graft function and increased resource utilization.
- Pt survival: 1 y: 87.7%; 5 y: 74%; graft survival: 1 y: 83.4%; 5 y: 67.4%

Worry About

- Renal insufficiency, HRS Type 1 a/w increased waiting list mortality.
- Increasing CAD in recipients with additional co-morbidities like DM, Htn, increased age, valvular disease, cardiomyopathy (alcoholic, infiltrative, ischemic)
- Coagulopathy: Imbalance between procoagulants and anticoagulants; risk of thrombosis/thromboembolism
- Fluid/electrolyte and acid-base disturbances
- Pretransplant SeNa<126meq/l is assoc with 6.3–7.8-fold increased risk of death.
- Hepatopulmonary syndrome
- Portopulmonary Htn with RV dysfunction a/w increased periop mortality

Overview

- Remove native liver and replace with whole or partial new liver
- Increased CIT is a/w increased short-term mortality, ICU LOS, postop biliary complications
- Technique of hepatectomy can impact renal outcome.

Indications and Usual Treatment

- Noncholestatic cirrhosis (HCV, alcoholic, HBV, cryptogenic, postnecrotic, neoplasm)
- Cholestatic cirrhosis (Primary sclerosing cholangitis or primary biliary cirrhosis)
- Biliary atresia
- Fulminant hepatitis (drug induced, viral, pregnancy)
- Inborn errors of metabolism; amyloidosis, hemochromatosis, etc.
- Contraindications: Infection, obesity (BMI >35), portal and mesenteric thrombosis

ASSESSMENT POINTS

System	Effect	Assessment by Hx	PE	Test
CARDIO	↑ CO, CI, HR, CVP, SvO2, ↓ SVR, ↓/N/↑ PVR and PCWP, cardiomyopathy, CAD	Poor exercise tolerance, fatigue, DOE, orthopnea	↑ JVD, HJR, LE edema,	ECG, ECHO Radionuclide stress test Stress ECHO, RHC, LHC.
RESP	Restrictive pattern, atelectasis, pleural effusion, HPS (PaO2 <70 mmHg or A-a gradient >20 mmHg), PPHTN (MPAP >25 mmHg)	SOB, DOE,	↓ SaO2, BS, ↑ RR, clubbing, platypnea, orthodeoxia	RA-SaO2 (supine & standing), CXR, ABG, contrast ECHO, Tc-macroaggregate lung scanning, pulm angiography
GI	Portal Htn, varices, GI bleed, ascites, delayed gastric emptying, cholestasis	Hematemesis/malena, water retention, N/V, itching, confusion	Icterus, spider angiomata, ascites, hepatosplenomegaly	↑ Transaminases, bili, INR, ↓ Albumin, upper GI, CT scan
HEME	Anemia, ↓ plts, coagulopathy, hyperercoagulation	Bleeding diathesis, portal and mesenteric thrombosis, DVT, PE	Easy bruisability	CBC, plt count and function, INR, PT, PTT, fibrinogen, TEG
RENAL	Oliguria, HRS	Nephrotoxic drugs (NSAIDs, ABx, IV contrast) aggressive dieresis, hypotension		BUN, Cr, CrCl, urinary sodium and osmolality
CNS	Encephalopathy, ↑ ICP in ALF	Confusion, mental status changes, ↓ memory, precipitating factor	Lethargy, coma, papilledema	ICP monitor, Transcranial Doppler
INFECTION	SBP, sepsis	Onset of fever	Fever	WBC w/diff., acitic fluid exam
NUTRITION	Malnutrition, folate, Zn, vit.B & fat-soluble vit. deficiency, osteopenia			INR, albumin
FLUID/LYTES	Hypervolemia, ↑ or ↓ Na, K, glucose, ↓ Ca, Mg			Glucose, Na, K, Ca

Key Reference: Sharma P, Rakela J. Management of pre-liver transplant patients-Part 1&2. *Liver Transpl.* 2005 11(2):124–33 & 11(3):367.

Perioperative Management

Preoperative Preparation
- Assess cardiopulmonary status
- Correct severe electrolyte imbalance, esp. K+; consider dialysis if indicated.

Monitoring
- Strict asepsis for all invasive lines
- 1–2 arterial lines
- 1–2 8.5 Fr. or central lines; PA catheter (+/- SvO2), +/- TEE
- 7 or 8.5Fr. RIC
- Foley catheter

Anesthetic Technique/Induction
- GI prophylaxis
- Cautious anxiolysis
- RSI

Surgical Stages

Preanhepatic
- Replace blood loss with PRBC, factors
- Correct acidosis, electrolyte abn., treat increased glucose, consider mannitol/lasix
- Prepare for hepatectomy tech.

Anhepatic
- Piggyback: Occlusion of portal V., hepatic A.&V.

- TVO: Supra and infrahepatic IVC clamping- 60–70% decrease in preload. Pretreat with volume loading
- VVBP: Less hemodynamic changes. Increased risk of clotting in the circuit, air embolus, increased surgical time
- Increased requirement for Ca
- Correct lytes, Hb, coags in preparation for reperfusion
- Flush donor liver with saline, Albumin, blood.

Reperfusion

- Postreperfusion syndrome: Decreased MAP; severely decreased SVR, HR; increased CVP, PAP; decreased contractility; may progress to asystole; PE.
- Treat coagulopathy and electrolyte imbalance
- Worry about fibrinolysis and overcorrection of coagulopathy.

Postoperative Considerations

- Continue correcting bleeding and lytes abn.
- Consider early extubation, if appropriate.
- Watch for graft function with improving lactate, coagulopathy.

Anticipated Problems/Concerns

- Massive hemorrhage
- Cardiopulmonary events
- Hypercoagulopathy, low flow state and portal venous thrombosis; Hepatic A. thrombosis.

Liver Transplantation, Pediatric

Christopher Karsanac

Risk

- Incidence in USA: 15,807 pts are on the waiting list for liver transplantation
- 541 are under the age of 18
- Children <18 y of age underwent 483 transplantations in 2009 (OPTN data)

Perioperative Risks

- Global physiological derangements
- 2–5% mortality
- Reoperation risk of 18%

Worry About

- Encephalopathy requiring ICP monitoring
- Hepatopulmonary syndrome causing hypoxia
- Electrolyte and metabolic derangements
- Renal failure 2° to hepatorenal syndrome
- Air embolisms
- Hemodynamic instability
- Coagulopathies
- Hypothermia
- Immunosuppression
- Peripheral nerve injuries due to positioning
- Anemia
- Massive fluid shifts
- Pain scores of 10 out of 10 common

Overview

- Most common cause for pediatric transplantation is biliary atresia (~40%).
- Other pathologies incl: TPN related (15%), acute hepatic necrosis (10–15%), metabolic diseases (10%) and hepatoblastoma (3%)
- Demand out numbers supply with the added disparity of donor-recipient organ size mismatch
- Due to shortage of organs, recent increases in living-related and split-liver transplantation

Indications and Usual Treatment

- Indications for transplantation: Progressive primary liver disease, metabolic diseases of the liver, fulminant hepatic failure, hepatic tumors, or retransplantation for graft failure
- Biliary atresia is first treated with a Kasai procedure to aide in bile drainage.
- Only 10–15% of pts do not need future hepatic transplantation:
- Other pathologies are medically treated while the pt is placed on the transplant list.
- Children <12 are ranked according to their pediatric end-stage liver disease (PELD) score.
- This takes into account: Age, growth retardation, albumin, creatinine and INR
- Children 12 and older use the model for end-stage liver disease (MELD) scores.
- This uses only the bilirubin, INR, and creatinine.
- How quickly the pt receives a transplant depends on not only organ availability but also blood type, body size, and need for transplant.

ASSESSMENT POINTS

System	Effect	Assessment by Hx	PE	Test
CARDIO	Hyperdynamic circulatory state ($\uparrow$ CO, $\downarrow$ SVR), Cardiomyopathy, $\downarrow$ CO with pulm Htn	SOB, fatigue, symptoms of CHF	CV exam, anasarca	ECG, ECHO
RESP	Hypoxia 2° to pleural effusion/pulm edema, atelectasis due to ascites, $\downarrow$ FRC, V/Q mismatch, intrapulmonary shunting, pulm Htn, hepatopulmonary syndrome, subglottic stenosis 2° to previous prolonged intubation	Dyspnea, SOB	$\downarrow$ SpO$_2$, tachypnea, auscultation	CXR, ABGs
RENAL	Renal dysfunction due to prerenal azotemia Hepatorenal syndrome		UO	BUN, Cr, electrolytes, CrCl if indicated
HEME	Coagulopathy, anemia, thrombocytopenia, DIC			Bleeding time, PT, APTT, thrombin time, FDPs
CNS	Encephalopathy, abn blood-brain barrier, cerebral edema in fulminant hepatic failure	Sx of $\uparrow$ ICP		Ammonia level, $\uparrow$ ICP in fulminant failure, head CT (to R/O acute bleed)
GI	GI varicies, delayed gastric emptying		Edema	Bilirubin, serum albumin, SGOT, SGPT
FLUID, LYTE, ACID-BASE STATUS	Intravascular volume depletion Hypokalemia, hyponatremia (hyperkalemia in hepatorenal syndrome), metabolic acidosis, $\downarrow$ glycogen metabolism	Symptoms of hypoglycemia (lethargy, somnolence, irritability)		ABG, electrolytes, glucose

Key References: Bennett J, Bromley P. Perioperative issues in pediatric liver transplantation. *Int Anesthesiol Clin.* 2006 Summer;44(3):125–147.

Perioperative Implications

Preoperative Preparation

- Room preparation may take up to 1 hr: incl fluid warmers, forced air warmers, emergency drugs, blood and/or blood products, US for IV access, multiple cuffed tubes
- IV premedication as appropriate

Anesthetic Technique

- Rapid-sequence or modified rapid-sequence IV induction
- Volatile agent maintenance while avoiding N$_2$O, muscle relaxation and fentanyl 10–50 mcg/kg

Monitoring and Positioning

- Standard ASA monitors
- CVP from central line via internal jugular or subclavian plus two large-bore IVs above the diaphragm
- Right and left arterial cannulation for BP monitoring and blood specimen collection
- Consider TEE to monitor cardiac functions and air embolism
- ICP is measured if signs of encephalopathy are present
- UO (Foley cath), electrolytes, glucose, ABGs, coags, CBCs
- Forced air warmers and fluid warmers
- Supine position
- Fluid and blood requirements for the procedure
  - Normal saline and/or plasmalyte
  - Blood and FFP available in the room
  - Excessive use of crystalloids should be avoided to avoid pulm and bowel edema

Surgical Stages

Preanhepatic Phase

- Skin incision to remove recipient's liver
- Copious blood loss is possible if portal Htn or adhesions from previous surgeries
- Blood loss is replaced by PRBCs and FFP
- Frequent coagulation testing; avoid a hypercoagulable state for fear of future graft anastomosis thrombosis
- Massive blood transfusion assoc with increased citrate load, decreased calcium, increased potassium
- Hourly blood labs are a minimum; may need q15 min labs during hemodynamic instability
- UO maintained
- Maintain adequate BP with lowest CVP to decrease bleeding

Anhepatic Stage

- Starts with clamping of hepatic vessels
- IVC may be clamped (drastically decrease preload), but usually not in a "piggy back" technique
- Donor liver may decrease core temp by 1.5° or more

- Drastically decrease clearance of hepatically metabolized drugs, heavily decreased glycogen formation
- Decrease volatile, 100% FIO$_2$ and ready emergency drugs for reperfusion stage

Post Perfusion Stage

- Reperfusion of donor liver after unclamping portal vein and IVC
- Anticipate initial hemodynamic instability, dysrhythmias, lactic acidosis
- Rapid increase in K$^+$ level may cause cardiac arrest

- Split liver grafts may bleed more upon reperfusion
- Improvement in coagulation, decrease in lactic acid, and normalization of acid-base status and lytes
- Biliary system will then be constructed

Postoperative Period

- Transferred to PICU intubated
- Hepatic functions monitored and PT maintained 1.5–2.0 times normal to avoid hepatic artery thrombosis

Anticipated Problems/Concerns

- Discuss administrative timing of antirejection drugs with team prior to surgery
- Bleeding
- Portal vein thrombosis and/or hepatic artery thrombosis
- Primary graft nonfunction and/or rejection
- Renal failure
- Electrolyte abn
- Pulm complications

Lumbar Laminectomy

Moustafa Ahmed

Risk

- 2% of adult population suffer from sciatica due to lumbar disc herniation
- 90% improve with nonoperative care (6–12 wk)
- Neurologic complication range from 1–33%
- The reported success rate of lumbar disc surgery varies from 60–90%.

Perioperative Risks

- Preop mortality is low and assoc with preop co-morbidity
- Continuation or recurrence of lower back pain range from 30–40%
- Recurrent disc herniation range-from 4–8%
- Major complication such as pulm embolism, hemorrhage from major vessels injury is fatal but rare

Worry About

- Intraop blood loss
- Be aware that sudden drop in the BP may be a venous air embolism (in prone position). It is rare but possible because the venous system above the level of the heart.
- Be aware of sudden collapse of the ventilator billows after positioning the pt in prone position or during surgery may be due to accidental extubation.
- Decrease lung compliance because of chest wall and abd compression in prone position
- Complication of prone position, direct pressure over bony prominences may lead to tissue necrosis, direct pressure on the orbit may lead to

blindness due to ION, stretching or direct pressure on the nerves may lead to nerve injury, and hyperextension of the neck may lead to Horner's syndrome.
- Irreversible pyramidal tract damage during decompressive laminectomy in pts with spinal stenosis
- Epidural hematoma postop is rare but devastating if it happens, the risk increases with pts who require multilevel lumbar procedures and/or have coagulopathy. Immediate Dx and treatment of postop epidural hematoma are crucial.

Overview

- Symptomatic lumbar disc herniation assoc with sciatica occurs in approx 2% of the adult population.
- 90% of the pt cured with nonoperative care
- Acute surgical emergency occur with cauda equine syndrome when the back pain assoc with saddle anesthesia, urinary retention, and multiple nerve root involvement
- Another indication for surgery is intractable pain not improve by nonoperative care or progressive neurologic deterioration

ICD9-CM: 722.10 (Lumbar intervertebral disc without myelopathy)

Indications and Usual Treatment

- One of the most common back surgeries worldwide and still controversial among neurosurgeons and orthopedic surgeons.
- Indications categorized to four groups: degenerative, traumatic, neoplastic and infectious
- May affect one level or multiple levels, 90% of disc prolapses involve the L4-5and L5-S1 segments, decompressive laminectomy with or without fusion and/or instrumentation and fixation indicated in lumbar spinal stenosis, degenerative spondylolisthesis and/or stenosis, degenerative scoliosis and/or stenosis, lumbar vertebra fractures, tumors and low back pain
- Lumbar stenosis, either congenital-achondroplastic dwarfs and manifested as kyphosis, bulging discs and short pedicles or acquired, which is the most common form due to disc degeneration, leads to hypertrophy of both bone and ligaments, thereby compressing the neural elements.
- Recommend psychological consultation before any elective lower back surgery even when there are clinical indications especially if assoc with obvious psychosocial issues
- Nonop care: Brief period of bed rest, use of NSAIDs and active physical therapy as tolerated, the efficacy of epidural steroids or even oral steroids has not been convincingly demonstrated in randomized prospective studies, the use of Transcutaneous Electrical Nerve Stimulation (TENS) is controversial.

ASSESSMENT POINTS

System	Effect	Assessment by Hx	PE	Test
CARDIO	Decompasation	↓ Exercise tolerance—difficult to assess	Heart murmur, gallop	ECG, ?ECHO
RESP	Restrictive diaphragm or other rib cage movement	Smoking Hx, pulm disease	Lung exam—signs of failure?	PFTs if severe lung disease
CNS/PNS	Peripheral neuropathy, paraplegia, myelopathy or sensory deficit, compromised by prone position	Pain, inability to ambulate, bowel or bladder dysfunction	Sensory deficit, ?motor deficit	Preop evoked potentials, EMG, or MRI/CT
MS	Skeletal metastasis from primary cancer	Primary tumor from breast, lung, kidney, thyroid, prostate Chemotherapy Hx		?CXR, electrolytes (Ca^{2+}), bone scan
PSYCH	Chronic pain, possible substance abuse (opioids)	Multiple medications (narcotics, NSAIDs, antidepressants)		

Key Reference: McLain RF, Kalfas I, Bell GR, Tetzlaff JE, Yoon HJ, Rana M. Comparison of spinal and general anesthesia in lumbar laminectomy surgery. *J Neurosurg Spine.* 2005;2(1):17–22.

Perioperative Management

- Intravenous prophylactic antibiotics

Anesthetic Technique/Induction

- Most common practice using general anesthesia, it can be done by neuroaxial (spinal or epidural) anesthesia, the broad use of GA is not based on any scientific or clinical evidence but on surgeon preference, the arguments against neuroaxial anesthesia is airway complications in a sedated prone positioned pt and possibility for neural injury if the awake patient moves or shifts during the decompressive procedure.
- Muscle relaxant is given to facilitate intubation and muscle dissection, avoid succinylcholine if severe neurological deficit is present (paraplegia)
- TIVA is preferred with SSEPs and EMG for better monitoring

Monitoring

- Standard ASA monitors
- Monitoring for possible venous air embolism in prone position using Precordial Doppler/end-tidal N$_2$ or TEE
- Invasive monitoring such as intra-arterial and/or CVP based on associated co-morbidity and neurological deficits
- SSEPs and EMGs for neurologic monitoring especially with patient suffering from spinal stenosis

Airway

- Securing the airway is crucial since the patient is in prone position, confirm ETT position above the carina after change patient to prone position
- Be aware of facial edema and possible laryngeal edema in prolonged prone position (multiple level laminectomy), if no cuff leak consider postop ventilation for the next 24 hr

Positioning

- Patient placed in prone, lateral or in knee-to-chest position (prone-sitting frame)
- Padding all pressure points, no pressure applied to the eyes and nose during the length of surgery
- Be aware to free the male genitalia
- Maintenance Balanced anesthesia, maintaining euvolemic status to minimize facial edema and possible laryngeal swelling, if the spinal cord compromised with neurologic deficits, maintains spinal cord perfusion pressure by maintaining MAP as preoperative or higher.

Surgical Stages

Dissection

• Different technique used, posterior approach, minimally invasive techniques, mininvasive extraperitoneal approach.

• The skin incision in general is approximately 3–5 cm in the midline over the spinous process, dissection is carried through the subcutaneous fat to the lumbar dorsal fascia, midline is easily identified by palpating the groove over the spinous processes, on the side of disc prolapsed the fascia divided and the lateral spinal dissection then follows, the ligamentum flavum is gently dissected free and removed, then laminotomy is performed, the affected nerve root is swept medially and the disc fragment visualized the annulus is then incised and the fragment removed. The nerve should be inspected to be certain that no residual disk compression remains. The wound should be closed in appropriate layers.

Postoperative Considerations

• Early neurological assessment and frequent examination for early detection of any neurological deficits

• Postoperative pain can be controlled using PCA, intraoperative intrathecal morphine or placement of epidural catheter at the end of surgery before closing (can be placed by surgeon or anesthesiology)

• No postoperative orthosis is required

• The necessity and duration of activity restrictions after lumbar disc surgery is still controversial.

Anticipated Problems/Concerns

• Disease of elderly (CAD, COPD, CKD, DM)

• Postoperative neurological deterioration may be caused by extruded disc fragments, mechanical damage to nerve root, epidural hematoma, infections, epidural abscesses.

• Problems with prone positioning

• Reoperation, recurrence of lumbar disc prolapsed range from 3–12% in patients who underwent disc surgery for first time

• Remote cerebellar hemorrhage (rare)

Lung Transplantation

David McIlroy
Jonathan Hastie

Risks

- Worldwide: >2000 lung transplants per year for end-stage lung disease (bilateral:single, 2:1)
- Etiology of underlying lung disease: COPD (50%), IPF (19%), CF (17%), idiopathic PAH (5%)
- Recipient age varies with underlying lung disease, although peak presentation in sixth decade
- Co-morbidities vary with underlying disease process
  - COPD: Smoking related vascular disease
  - Cystic fibrosis (CF): Diabetes mellitus, GERD, malnutrition
  - Pulmonary arterial Htn (PAH): Typically anticoagulated with coumadin

Perioperative Risks

- Depends on underlying lung disease and other co-morbidities
- 30-d mortality: 4–15%
- Primary graft dysfunction (PGD): Incidence 10–65% depending on definition. Severe PGD assoc with prolonged mechanical ventilation, increased ICU length of stay, increased 30-d mortality and increased incidence of bronchiolitis obliterans
- Myocardial ischemia and/or infarction: Incidence not well-characterized
- Acute kidney injury: Reported incidence 50–60% within 2 wk, dialysis in up to 7.5%

Worry About

- CV instability at induction of anesthesia (esp. if pulm Htn present), pulm artery clamping (may precipitate acute RV failure) and allograft reperfusion
- Tolerance of OLV (hypoxemia) during dissection prior to pulm artery clamping
- Blood loss, hypothermia, acid-base disturbance (particularly severe resp acidosis)

Overview

- Anesthesia goals: Maintain adequate oxygenation with one-lung ventilation (OLV), minimize pulm vascular resistance (PVR), optimize coronary perfusion pressure to reduce risk of acute RV failure
- Cardiopulmonary bypass (CPB): Used in 15–40% of cases, typically due to severe pulm Htn, acute RV failure, hemodynamic instability or refractory hypoxemia

ICD-9-CM Code: 33.50 (Lung transplantation, not otherwise specified)

Indications and Usual Treatment

- Depends on underlying disease process and may vary between pts
- In general: Age <65 y, NYHA III or IV but ideally still ambulatory, 6-min. walk test >600 feet
- Contraindications: Significant non-pulm vital organ dysfunction, active infection with HIV, hepatitis B or C, active cigarette smoking or substance abuse, medical non-compliance, lack of social support
- Allocation system based on clinical urgency rather than time accrued on wait list

ASSESSMENT POINTS

System	Effect	Assessment by Hx	PE	Test
HEENT	Need to secure airway with double lumen ETT	Previous anesthesia difficulties, GERD	Clinical assessment of airway	
CARDIO	Pulm Htn with RV dysfunction +/− TR, CAD with LV dysfunction	Angina, orthopnea	Elevated JVP, peripheral edema	ECG, ECHO, dipyridamole thallium, coronary angiography, right heart cath
RESP	COPD/CF/interstitial lung disease/PAH	Functional capacity, productive cough, hemoptysis, Supplemental O_2	Bronchospasm, wheeze, hyperinflated, cyanotic	CXR, ABGs, PFTs, V/Q split function testing
RENAL	Renal insufficiency	Htn, diabetes	-	Creatinine, creatinine clearance
ENDO	Pancreatic insufficiency (CF), steroid use	Diabetes, medications	-	Blood glucose, HbA1c

Key Reference: Miranda A, Zink R, McSweeney M. Anesthesia for lung transplantation. *Semin Cardiothorac Vasc Anesth.* 2005;9:205–212.

Perioperative Management

Preoperative Preparation

- Assess pattern of underlying ventilatory defect (obstructive vs. restrictive), baseline SpO_2
- Assess co-existing morbidities, esp. pulm Htn +/− RV dysfunction, LV dysfunction, DM, GERD, anticoagulation status
- Consider epidural catheter placement (or paravertebral catheter for single lung transplant)

Monitoring

- Invasive arterial pressure monitoring and central venous access essential
- PA catheter routinely used—may guide selective use of inhaled vasodilators (NO, prostacyclin)
- Intraop TEE allows assessment of RV and LV function, intravascular volume state, patent foramen ovale (PFO), pulm venous anastomoses
- Consider depth of anesthesia monitoring (e.g., BIS)

Anesthetic Technique/Induction

- No single technique demonstrated to be superior, hemodynamic stability is the goal
- Beware gas trapping/dynamic hyperinflation/pneumothorax with PPV and subsequent hemodynamic instability or collapse
- Maintain systemic BP and coronary perfusion pressure esp. if significant pulm Htn present.
- Consider surgical presence in OR at induction if pulm Htn severe, in case emergent CPB required.
- Consider delayed/impaired equilibration between measured end-tidal concentration and blood concentration of volatile anesthetic agent.
- Ability to provide lung isolation and OLV required—bronchoscopy to confirm optimal tube placement

Surgical Stages

Dissection

- OLV required, may see refractory hypoxemia +/− hypercapnia. Consider iNO or prostcyclin if usual measures fail
- Blood and fluid loss may be significant if extensive adhesions present
- May require vasopressors and judicious IV fluid replacement to support hemodynamics

Pulmonary Artery Clamping

- Ensure PA catheter withdrawn from PA prior to clamping. Consider heparin 2500–5000 U.
- Monitor PA pressure and acute RV failure (rising CVP, distending RV, acute TR on TEE)
- May require vasopressors, inotropes, iNO to support RV function and systemic hemodynamics. Consider CPB if necessary.

Allograft Reperfusion

- Anticipate hemodynamic instability due to volume loss into new lung, washout of metabolites and pneumoplegic solution, marked systemic vasodilation.
- Anticipate systemic air from allograft which may enter right coronary artery producing acute ischemia, RV dysfunction, hypotension, and arrhythmias
- Support with vasopressors, volume resuscitation, defibrillation if required.

Postoperative Considerations

- Change to single lumen ETT if double-lumen in place. Bronchoscopy to provide pulm toilet and assess bronchial anastomoses, optimize re-expansion and V/Q matching with lung recruitment and PEEP.
- Protective ventilation to minimize volu- and baro-trauma is not well studied in humans. Animal studies suggest improved graft function with these strategies. Reduce FIO_2 as tolerated

• Early tracheal extubation if allografts function well and analgesia adequate. May reduce incidence of ventilator-induced lung injury and ventilator-assoc pneumonia.

• Epidural infusion of local anesthetic may necessitate judicious IV fluid and vasopressor support to maintain hemodynamic stability. Systemic ketamine or dexmedetomidine may be considered as adjuncts for improved postop analgesia and/or opioid-sparing effects.

• Consider PCA opiate if regional analgesia contraindicated. Caution advised with adjuvant NSAIDs, which are not well studied in this context.

Anticipated Problems/Concerns

• Intraop use of epidural local anesthesia may increase hemodynamic instability

• Difficult to maintain normothermia due to large body surface area exposed, large incision, prolonged surgical time and potential for large fluid requirements

• Controversies: Potential for anesthetic techniques to impact reperfusion injury remains unclear, e.g., fluid management, preemptive iNO. Early versus late ECMO for severe PGD

Lung Volume Reduction Surgery (LVRS)

Swaminathan Karthik
Brett A. Simon

Risk

- Severe, activity-limiting pulm emphysema; given prevalence of emphysema (2 million Americans affected with 90,000 deaths annually), the number of potential candidates for this operation is enormous.
- Average preop FEV_1 25–30% of predicted early studies had contradictory results, and variable outcomes.
- The National Emphysema Treatment Trial [NETT], a prospective randomized trial was conducted to compare medical and surgical treatments with a 5-y follow-up.

Perioperative Risks

- LVRS not recommended if FEV1 <20% and either DLCO <20% or diffuse pattern of emphysema seen on CT scan.
- In-hospital mortality: 5.5%
- LVRS most beneficial in pts with both upper lobe predominant disease and low exercise tolerance. LVRS is not superior to medical therapy if only one of these two characteristic is present.
- Highest mortality and cardiopulmonary complications occurred in pts with non-upper lobe predominant disease and good exercise tolerance.
- 25% morbidity incl prolonged air leaks, resp failure, pulm embolism, pneumonia
- Greatly increased risk of complications in pts with reactive airway disease, CAD, pulm Htn

Worry About

- Hypotension due to air trapping with controlled ventilation
- Difficulty with ventilation and oxygenation (less so) during one-lung ventilation
- Exaggerated resp depressive effects of narcotics (IV and neuraxial)
- Minimizing airway pressures and smoothly extubating spontaneously ventilating pt in OR to avoid creating or worsening air leaks

Overview

- Palliative procedure for severe, activity-limiting emphysema with 20–30% of lungs resected to reduce lung volume and reshape diaphragm and chest wall
- Bovine pericardial or Gore-Tex strips used to reinforce staple lines and reduce air leaks
- Variety of unilateral, bilateral, open, and VATS techniques used. Open, bilateral lung volume reduction via median sternotomy is the original approach. The NETT study showed no difference in mortality or morbidity between the median sternotomy approach and VATS. However, median sternotomy was assoc with longer hospital stays and higher costs.
- Benefit thought to result from improving mechanical function of chest wall and diaphragm by reducing total lung volume, combined with reduction and reshaping of lung tissue; results in increase in lung recoil at this lower volume and increased expiratory flows
- Pts typically require a great deal of attention to keep them extubated during first several hours postop
- Successful outcome requires team approach incl experienced pulmonologists, pulm rehab, thoracic surgeons, anesthesiologists, pain service, chest PT, ICU physicians. Sophisticated pulm function testing and lung imaging facilities should be available.
- Endoscopic LVRS is an evolving alternative. Methods under investigation incl one-way endobronchial valves or airway bypass stents (drug eluting-paclitaxel)

ICD-9-CM Code: 492.8 (Emphysema)

Indications and Usual Treatment

- Alternative to lung transplantation for pts with primarily pure emphysema that significantly limits their activity
- Exclusion criteria incl pulm Htn (mean PAP >35 at rest), bronchospasm, LV dysfunction, bronchitis or excessive sputum production, persistent smoking, previous thoracotomy or pleurodesis, obesity, or cachexia
- NETT pts required to undergo at least 6 wk of preop pulm rehab, with supplemental O_2 if necessary. Poor results expected if cannot perform at least 800 ft in standard 6-min walk test.
- Successful procedures typically result in 60–70% increase in FEV_1 by 3 mo sustained at least 1 y, decreased TLC and residual volume, improved exercise tolerance, and significant reductions in O_2 requirements at rest and during exercise. Data suggest improvements are sustained for at least 2–3 y.

ASSESSMENT POINTS

System	Effect	Assessment by Hx	Pe	Test
CARDIO	LV/RV dysfunction Pulmonary Htn	CHF, PND, palpitations	Peripheral edema, JVD, S_3	MUGA, as ECHO may be unreliable with COPD
RESP	Emphysema	SOB, exercise tolerance and performance with rehab, bronchospasm, sputum production	Wheezing	PFTs, CT, plethysmography, quantitative V/Q scan

Key Reference: Edwards, et al. The National Emphysema Treatment Trial: Summary and update. *Thorac Surg Clin NA* 2009;19(2):169–185.

Perioperative Management

Preoperative Preparation

- Successful completion of pulm rehab program
- Maximize bronchodilator therapy, smoking cessation, O_2 therapy, and influenza and pneumococcal vaccinations

Anesthetic Technique

- Thoracic epidural placement at ~T4 interspace for intraop and postop use; test and verify onset of segmental block prior to induction
- Minimize narcotics because of risk of resp depression
- Goal of anesthetic is to maximize possibility of extubation in OR
- Chest tubes placed to water seal only, unless suction required

Monitoring

- Arterial line required
- Consider central line for intraop infusions and postop fluid management

Airway

- Double-lumen tube required

Induction/Maintenance

- Anticipate hypotension due to air trapping with chest closed
- Ventilate with low pressures and low rates; tolerate hypercapnia if necessary
- Maintain on low-dose inhaled agent or propofol infusion
- Use of epidural depends on hemodynamic stability; consider waiting until chest open before dosing; use of straight local may require phenylephrine infusion for BP maintenance; if narcotics used, limit dose
- Continue bronchodilator therapy in OR if necessary

Surgical Stages

- Bronchoscopy: Flexible bronchoscopy
- Resection: Better side, usually right, resected first to improve tolerance of one-lung ventilation when second side resected (for bilateral procedure)
- Emergence: Consider switch to single-lumen tube, LMA, or mask while pt is deep to facilitate emergence
- Elevate head; optimize pain control; suctioning; bronchodilators for emergence
- Pts require up to 30–90 min observation, encouragement, and fine-tuning in OR prior to transport to ICU; first ABG in ICU has Pco_2 >70 mmHg in >50% of pts

Fluid Considerations

- Typically run dry
- Significant blood loss requiring transfusion unusual

Postoperative Considerations

- Make every effort to extubate in OR and avoid reintubation and ventilation; if required, use minimum pressure support without mandatory breaths if possible
- Use epidural infusion (⅛–¼% [0.0625–0.125%] bupivacaine ±1–3 μg/ml fentanyl) supplemented with non-narcotic pain relievers
- Pain score: 6–8

Anticipated Problems/Concerns

- Extremely marginal pts susceptible to even mild postop insults (pneumonia, pulm embolism, oversedation, pneumothorax, bronchospasm)
- Reintubation and mechanical ventilation assoc with high morbidity

Mastectomy

James A. Ramsey

Risk

- Overall incidence of breast cancer is 127.8 cases per 100,000 women. Median age 61.
- In 2009, 192,000 new cases w/62,000 Carcinoma in situ diagnosed
- Rates less in African-Americans, with greater mortality rates
- Age, alcohol, obesity, hormonal influences increase risk.
- BRCA1/2 genes `5–10%
- 5-y survival rates 83–90%
- Death rates 22% to 40% nationwide

Perioperative Risks

- Basically dependent on co-morbidities
- Postop complications greater in smokers, age >65, and obesity; with increased risk of failure of reconstruction in smokers, obesity, Htn.
- Usual risks of field avoidance, positioning

Worry About

- Choice of anesthesia
- Need for anxiolysis; no sedation prior to needle localization, or prior to plastic surgeon marking, if combined procedure
- Co-morbidities
- Positioning (brachial plexopathies reported)
- Field avoidance (eye protection, NIBP position, SpO_2 sensor position, IV integrity)

Overview

- Majority of procedures involve skin, SQ tissue, breast tissue; few involve muscles (true radical or reconstructive technique).
- Some surgeons concerned for long thoracic nerve integrity and may wish to use nerve stimulator (hampered by muscle relaxants).

- Anesthesia goals are to provide excellent operating conditions for surgical team, optimization of co-morbidities, pain and nausea-free PACU experience with proper anxiolysis throughout.

ICD-9-CM Code: 174 (Malignant neoplasm of female breast)

Indications and Usual Treatment

- Breast cancer diagnosed by mammography, needle aspiration, excisional biopsy.
- Less commonly, severely symptomatic fibrocystic breast disease
- Procedures range from simple lumpectomy, partial mastectomy, simple mastectomy, modified radical mastectomy, to (rarely) radical mastectomy.
- Increasingly common for plastic surgeon to be involved in closure, or first stage reconstruction procedure after mastectomy performed.

ASSESSMENT POINTS

System	Effect	Assessment by Hx	PE	Test
HEENT	Airway	Sore throat prior ops, Hx of difficult intubation	Usual A/W exam	
CARDIO	Circulatory integrity	Activity level	Examine/listen	EKG/CXR as appropriate
RESP	Ventilatory sufficiency	Smoking, bronchitis/RAD	Clinical assessment	CXR/PFTs
RENAL	Fluid balance	Use of diuretics/prior insults		BUN/Cr
CNS	Anxiolysis	Neuro-psych Hx	Behavior w/interview	
HEME	CV stability	Hx of anemia		Hct/T&S as indicated

Key Reference: American cancer society. *Breast cancer facts & figures 2009–2010.* Atlanta: American Cancer Society, Inc.; Morbidity and mortality following breast cancer surgery in women: National benchmarks for standards of care. *Ann Surg* 2007;245(5):665–671.

Perioperative Management

Preoperative Preparation

- Optimize co-morbidities; current consults with perioperative recommendations
- Initiate N/V prophylaxis, hydration, timely anxiolysis, prophylactic antibiotics, thromboembolic precautions.
- Confirm D/C of aspirin, anticoagulants, and supplements.

Monitoring

- Routine ASA; place IV in contralateral arm/neck/foot; EKG leads out of the field.
- Invasive as indicated by co-morbidities

Anesthetic Technique/Induction

- MAC: Local per surgeon with sedation as appropriate.

- Regional: Paravertebral blocks increasing in popularity; sedate
- GA: LMA v. ETT as indicated (inhalation v. TIVA)
- Full antinausea prophylaxis recommended
- Analgesic adjuncts may be helpful (celecoxib, gabapentin, pregabalin, ketorolac, ketamine, dextromethorphan, acetaminophen)

Surgical Stage

- Pt positioned with ipsilateral arm extended, may be prepped into operative field
- Axillary dissection usually follows mastectomy.
- Reconstruction may require muscle relaxants (submusculofascial tissue expander).
- Flap reconstruction requires adequate tissue perfusion (volume and pressure).

Postoperative Considerations

- Pain and nausea issues in PACU
- Adequate perfusion of flaps in closure or reconstruction (wound complications #1 morbidity)
- Attention to co-morbidities (morbid obesity correlates highest with postop complications)

Anticipated Problems/Concerns

- Prompt attention to nausea and analgesia problems may avoid admission.
- Early ambulation and return to activity will facilitate discharge.
- Psychiatric problems common postop, handle with care, provide appropriate support.

Meningomyelocele Repair

Cynthia Tung

Risk

- Incidence: 2–5/1000 live births
- Results from failure of neural tube to close; most commonly occurs along thoracic or lumbosacral region, can also occur along cervical region

Perioperative Risks

- Bacterial contamination leading to infection or sepsis
- Poor autonomic control below level of lesion, must maintain core body temp
- Potential for blood loss, hypotension
- Assoc with Arnold-Chiari malformations, hydrocephalus
- No assoc with congenital cardiac anomalies

Worry About

- Potential challenging intubation: Pt may be intubated in left lateral decubitus position or in customized supine position keeping pressure off the malformation; awake intubation for suspected difficult airway; cervical cord or brainstem compression in Arnold-Chiari malformations; difficulty with ventilation while prone or after closure of large defects.
- Hypothermia: Abn autonomic control below level of the lesion
- Pt positioning: Ensure no pressure on malformation; standard vigilance for other pressure points while prone
- Latex precautions: Tend to develop latex allergies even without repeat exposure

Overview

- Occurs at 28 d gestation, failure of neural tube to close
- Antenatal diagnosis with US or amniocentesis
- Assoc with Arnold-Chiari malformations, hydrocephalus, neurologic deficits
- Definitive treatment is surgical

ICD-9-CM Code: 741.9 (Without mention of hydrocephalus)

Indications and Usual Treatment

- Surgical repair within first day of life to prevent infection
- Defect covered to protect from infection and fluid losses prior to surgery

ASSESSMENT POINTS

System	Effect	Assessment by Hx	PE	Test
CARDIO	Congenital cardiac anomalies		Murmur, cyanosis	ECHO, pulse oximeter
RESP	Resp failure/RDS	Premature birth Location of defect; cervical, thoracic, or lumbosacral	Resp insufficiency	CXR
RENAL	Congenital anomalies		Abd exam	Abd US
CNS	Cord compression, paralysis Arnold-Chiari malformations Hydrocephalus		Neuro exam	CT/MRI US

Key Reference: Motoyama EK, Davis PJ. *Smith's anesthesia for infants and children.* 7th ed. Mosby; 2006.

Perioperative Management

Preoperative Preparation

- Assess for other congenital malformations, document any preop neurologic deficits.
- Antenatal Hx, birth Hx, other co-morbidities
- Latex precautions

Monitoring

- Depends on co-morbidities; usually standard ECG and non-invasive BP monitoring, pulse oximeter; arterial line placement based on other co-morbidities
- Adequate IV access or umbilical lines for fluid replacement and possible blood transfusion

Anesthetic Technique/Induction

- Depending on anticipated difficulty of airway, inhalation or IV induction with muscle relaxant. If awake intubation required, preoxygenate and premedicate with atropine.
- Monitor blood and fluid losses, replace as needed.
  - Small defects: Minimal volume of fluid losses
  - Large defects: Large volume of fluid losses
- Maintain body temp: Keep neonate warm prior to surgical draping and at end of procedure, use forced hot air warmer intraop, humidified gases.

Surgical Stages

- Usually minimal blood loss
- Prone position

Postoperative Considerations

- Postop apnea, CSF leakage, neurologic deficits
- Recover prone

Anticipated Problems/Concerns

- Prematurity: Resp insufficiency, apnea, cardiac anomalies
- Other congenital anomalies or co-morbidities
- Postop neurologic deficits
- Future development of hydrocephalus requiring ventriculoperitoneal shunt

Mitral Valve Replacement

Dawn M. Larson
Stephen T. Robinson

Risk

- Mitral stenosis
  - Rheumatic disease (predominant cause in adults); M:F 1:2. Less commonly systemic disease states or senile annulus calcification
  - Unrepaired 10- y survival: 15% if symptomatic, 80% if asymptomatic
  - Congenital abn of the mitral valve (children)
- Mitral regurgitation, organic
  - Dysfunction of mitral leaflets or chordae
  - Leaflet prolapse, endocarditis, rheumatic valve disease, connective tissue disorders and mitral annular calcification
- Mitral regurgitation, functional
  - Structurally normal leaflets and chordae tendineae
  - Ischemic heart disease
  - Idiopathic dilated cardiomyopathy and mitral annular calcification
  - Mitral regurgitation unrepaired 5- y survival 27–97% because of variability of causes

Perioperative Risks

- Depend on pt characteristics such as age, functional status, and other co-morbid conditions
- Mitral stenosis surgical mortality
  - Less than 5% in younger pts with few co-morbidities
  - 10–20% in elderly pts with severe symptoms and preexisting medical problems
- Mitral regurgitation surgical mortality
  - About 1% in organic causes in pts under 75 y old
  - Other circumstances mostly higher with wide variability
  - Mitral valve repair over replacement may confer survival benefit

Worry About

- Pulm vascular congestion and pulm Htn
- Right ventricular failure
- Left ventricular dilation and failure
- Postop stroke, myocardial ischemia, renal failure, CPB complications

Overview

- Mitral stenosis
  - Rheumatic MS pts frequently asymptomatic for 20 y or more
  - Typical age of presentation is 40s-50s
- Mitral regurgitation
  - Natural Hx quite variable because of multiple etiologies
  - Acute severe MR due to papillary muscle rupture has a bleak outcome without surgery
  - Chronic MR often has an initial asymptomatic period with a variable time course to LV failure and dysfunction

ICD-9-CM Codes: 394.0 (Stenosis); 424.0 (Insufficiency)

Indications and Usual Treatment

- Mitral stenosis
  - Normal valve area 4–6 cm^2
  - If valve area 1.5-2.5 cm^2, symptoms with moderate exertion
  - If valve area <1.5 cm^2, symptoms typically occur at rest
  - Symptoms incl dyspnea, palpitations (atrial fibrillation), or chest pain
- Mitral regurgitation
  - Acute MR often results in increases in left atrial pressures leading to pulm edema and biventricular failure
  - Ruptured papillary muscle is an indication for emergency surgery.
  - Severe MR with evidence of left ventricular dysfunction (EF<60%m ESLV diameter >45 mm) should be referred to surgery
  - Asymptomatic pts without LV dysfunction may be surgical candidates if the effective regurgitant orifice is >40 mm^2 or there is evidence of atrial fibrillation, VTach, or pulm Htn.

ASSESSMENT POINTS

System	Effect	Assessment by Hx	PE	Test
CARDIO	**MS**: RV failure, pulm Htn, atrial fibrillation **MR**: LV dysfunction, atrial fibrillation, VTach, pulm Htn	**MS**: Fatigue, chest pain, hemoptysis, palpitations, dyspnea, pulm edema, hoarseness **MR**: Fatigue, dyspnea, pulm edema, orthopnea, PND	**MS**: Opening snap, mid-diastolic, rumbling murmur **MR**: Pan-systolic murmur to axilla, +/- 3rd heart sound; cardiomegaly if chronic	EKG, ECHO, cardiac catheterization
RESP	Pulm vascular congestion	Dyspnea, pulm edema	Crackles	CXR, pulm vascular congestion
RENAL	Renal insufficiency due to CHF	Renal vasoconstriction, sodium and water retention	Edema	Electrolytes, creatinine
CNS	Systemic thromboembolism	Stroke, TIA	Focal deficits	Non contrast head CT, MRI

Key Reference: Gillinov AM, Blackstone EH, Nowicki ER, et al. Valve repair versus replacement for degenerative mitral valve disease. *J Thorac Cardiovasc Surg.* 2008;135:885–893, 893.e1–893.e2. Epub 2008 Mar 4. Also see http://my.clevelandclinic.org/heart/disorders/valve/mvrepair.aspx.

Perioperative Management

Preoperative Preparation

- Dental evaluation to R/O acute inflammation/infections and airway mgmt
- Optimize hemodynamics with medical management

Monitoring

- EKG for rate, rhythm, and ischemia
- Pre-induction invasive arterial pressure catheter
- Pulm artery catheter or central venous catheter
- Transesophageal ECHO

Anesthetic Technique/Induction

- Large IV access
- Maintain stable hemodynamics and rhythm; may need to defibrillate new onset AFib
- Mitral stenosis
  - Preload: Normal to slightly increased
  - Afterload: Normal
  - Heart rate: Normal, avoid tachycardia
- Mitral regurgitation
  - Preload: Increased
  - Afterload: Decreased
  - Heart rate: Mild tachycardia

Surgical Stages

Precardiopulmonary Bypass

- Maintain stable hemodynamics throughout case
- TEE to measure valve motion, pressure gradients, orifice diameters and cardiac function

Surgical Repair (minimal versus open)

- Mitral stenosis
  - Mitral valve replacement (mechanical vs. tissue)
  - Percutaneous mitral commissurotomy
  - Surgical commissurotomy
  - +/- Maze procedure if chronic atrial fibrillation

- Mitral regurgitation
  - Mitral valve replacement (mechanical vs. tissue)
  - Mitral valve repair: Often involves resection of a portion of the mitral valve leaflet and at times an annuloplasty ring

Postcardiopulmonary Bypass
- Maintain sinus rhythm (please)
- RV dysfunction
  - Systemic vasodilators (milrinone, dobutamine, isoproterenol)
  - Inhaled vasodilators (NO or iloprost)

- Maintain eucarbia or slight hypocarbia
- LV dysfunction: Inotropic support, afterload reduction, IABP

Postoperative Considerations
- Irreversible pulm Htn or LV dysfunction
- Possible atrioventricular block requiring pacing
- Renal insufficiency or failure
  - CNS events

Anticipated Problems/Concerns
- Pulm Htn and RV strain may necessitate post CPB inotropic and vasodilatory support
- Rhythm disturbances can be key
- Mitral valve replacement can result in perivalvular leak
- Mitral valve repair can result in systolic anterior motion of mitral valve with LVOT obstruction in 4–5% of pts

Muscle Biopsy for Undiagnosed Myopathy

Nathalia Jimenez
Jeremy M. Geiduschek

Risk

- Three main entities: Mitochondrial myopathy (MM), neuromuscular dystrophy (NMD) and congenital core myopathy (CM).
- The incidence of mitochondrial myopathy is 1/4000, equally distributed among males and females. For muscular dystrophies the x-linked types are most prevalent with Duchenne muscular dystrophy (DMD) being the most frequent with an incidence of 30/100,000 live born males. Core myopathies are rare with an estimated incidence of 2/100,000 live births.

Perioperative Risks

- Depends on pt's condition and 1° unknown diagnosis.
- Resp failure due to severe muscular involvement is a risk for all pts.
- CV failure and/or arrhythmias are potential risks esp. for MM and NMD pts. Cardiomyopathy is present in 25% and 35% of MM and NMD pts respectively.
- Core myopathy pts are at high risk of malignant hyperthermia (MH).
- For NMD pts, the risk for rhabdomyolysis or MH after an inhaled anesthetic is 1.1%.
- Pts with MM are not considered at risk of developing MH.

Worry About

- Resp failure
- CV failure and arrhythmias
- Metabolic crisis: Metabolic acidosis and hypoglycemia
- Hyperkalemic cardiac arrest following administration of succinylcholine
- Temp control

Overview

- MM is a group of heterogeneous inherited disorders affecting mitochondrial oxidative phosphorylation and electron transport. Brain, heart, and skeletal muscles are markedly energy dependent and are the organs mostly affected.
- The Dx of MM is made based on clinical presentation, raised levels of serum lactic acid, and positive findings in the muscle biopsy.
- NMDs tend to be diagnosed later in childhood in pts with gradual decrease of muscular function.
- 70% of pts with NMD have some degree of cardiomyopathy.
- Core myopathies usually involve only skeletal muscles. Resp involvement is due to muscle weakness and NM scoliosis. Cardiac involvement is rare and is 2° to severe restrictive lung disease.
- Core myopathies (central core, multiminicore and nemaline rod myopathies) and King congenital myopathy are the only known clinical entities assoc with MH. However, the 1% risk for rhabdomyolysis or MH in NMD pts following a volatile anesthetic warrants strong consideration for using other techniques or agents.

ICD-9-CM Code: 995.86 (Malignant hyperthermia)

Indications and Usual Treatment

- Muscle biopsy is indicated for definitive Dx.
- Many pts have a putative Dx prior to muscle biopsy based on clinical, laboratory, and genetic testing.

ASSESSMENT POINTS

System	Effect	Assessment by Hx	PE	Test
HEENT	Visual and/or hearing loss (MM) Chronic aspiration	Coughing, chocking, recurrent aspiration pneumonia	Sialorrhea	Swallow study
CARDIO	Cardiomyopathy (MM, NMD) Conduction defects (MM, NMD)	Sx CHF Palpitations	Murmur, gallop, crackles, irregular rhythm	CXR ECHO ECG
RESP	Restrictive chronic lung disease (muscular involvement/scoliosis) Reactive airway (chronic aspiration) (MM, NMD, CM)	Hypoventilation, hypoxia Ventilatory support (CPAP) Wheezing	↓ Baseline SpO$_2$ ↓ Resp effort Ronchi, wheezing	CXR PFTs ideal
GI	Chronic diarrhea (MM)	Episodes of dehydration	Hydration status	Electrolytes
ENDO/METAB	Lactic acidosis (MM) Hypoglycemia (MM)	Fasting times	Hyperventilation Lethargy	Serum lactate Serum glucose
GU	Nephropathy (MM)			BUN/Cr
CNS	Encephalopathy (MM) Seizures (MM) Ataxia (MM)	Developmental delay Poor coordination	Focal neurologic deficits	Head CT MRI
PNS	Peripheral neuropathy (MM)	Muscle weakness	Hypotonia	
MS	Hypotonia (MM, NMD, CM)	Muscle weakness	Hypotonia, scoliosis	Serum CK and K+

MM = Mitochondrial Myopathy, NMD = Neuromuscular dystrophy, CM = Central core myopathy.
Key Reference: Gurnaney H, Brown A, Litman R. Malignant hyperthermia and muscular dystrophies. *Anesth Analg.* 2009;109:1043–1048.

Perioperative Management

Preoperative Preparation

- Assess for cardiac and resp involvement.
- Avoid prolonged fasting and dehydration which can worsen acidosis.
- Administer preop anticholinergic if oral secretions are copious.

Monitoring

- Routine assuming no cardiomyopathy or CHF

Anesthetic Technique/Induction

- There is no optimal anesthetic as all carry some risk for complications. Choice should be dictated by most likely Dx. If feasible regional anesthesia may be best option. Beware central neuraxial blockade if pt has preload dependent cardiomyopathy.
- Avoid use of lactated solutions (MM).
- Avoid use of succinilcholine (DMD and CM, unclear in MM).
- Avoid volatile agents (CM and DMD).
- Prolonged propofol infusion may promote metabolic crisis. Consider avoiding completely (MM)
- All pts: Increased sensitivity to inhaled, opioid and NM agents. Titrate accordingly.

Surgical Stages

- Muscle biopsy is a short duration procedure (30–45 min) but is often combined with gastrostomy tube and MRI.

Postoperative Considerations

- Local anesthesia or regional anesthesia (peripheral nerve blocks) recommended for postop pain control.
- Continue close postop monitoring: resp function, risk of MH up to 4–5 hr after anesthesia, rhabdomyolysis and cardiac arrest described in NMD pts in postop period.
- Very careful titration of opioids in monitored setting.

Anticipated Problems/Concerns

- Risk of propofol infusion syndrome (bradycardia, metabolic acidosis, rhabdomyolysis, lipidemia) in pts with mitochondrial myopathy due to impaired fatty acid utilization.
- Risk of MH (metabolic acidosis, rhabdomyolysis, myoglobinuria, hypotension, and cardiovascular collapse) in core myopathies. Estimated risk for NMD 1.09%.

Myringotomy and Tympanostomy

Stanley L. Loftness

Risk
- Most common operative procedure in children
- Age 6 mo to 3 y is the peak incidence
- Higher incidence in children in large daycare settings
- Higher incidence of eustachian tube dysfunction in cleft palate pts

Perioperative Risks
- Trisomy 21 and other craniofacial syndromes may have smaller ear canals and be more difficult and surgery may take longer

- Sleep apnea pts may have respiratory insufficiency postop and require overnight hospitalization
- No increased morbidity with concurrent URI symptoms

Worry About
- Airway obstruction
- Laryngospasm

ICD-9-CM Code: 20.0 (Myringotomy); 20.1 (Removal of tympanostomy tube)

Overview
- Most common childhood surgery
- Airway maintenance issues in small children
- Postop pain management

Indications and Usual Treatment
- Recurrent otitis media
- Persistent middle ear fluid, glue ear
- Hearing loss
- Speech delay

ASSESSMENT POINTS

System	Effect	Assessment by Hx	PE	Test
HEENT	Airway obstruction	Trisomy 21 or craniofacial syndromes	Mallampati score	
RESP	Resp insufficiency	Sleep apnea Hx or severe snoring	Snoring and airway obstruction	Sleep Study

Key Reference: Galinkin JL, Fazi LM, Cuy RM, et al. Use of intranasal fentanyl in children undergoing myringotomy and tube placement during halothane and sevoflurane anesthesia. *Anesthesiology.* 2001;95(3):812–813.

Perioperative Management

Preoperative Preparation
- Evaluate airway with mallampati score.
- Consider preop Tylenol for postop pain relief
- Preop fever common in acute otitis and is not necessarily a contraindication to anesthesia

Monitoring
- Routine ASA monitors

Anesthetic Technique/Induction
- Mask Inhalational induction with sevoflurane, N_2O, O_2 induction

- 2.0 mcg/kg fentanyl intranasal, up to 50 mcg total dose
- Consider oral airway or LMA as needed
- Continue use of N_2O to facilitate myringotomies

Surgical Stages
- Cleaning ear canal
- Myringotomy
- Tympanosotmy tube placement
- Irrigation of middle ear
- Eardrops

Postoperative Considerations
- Transport to PACU on O_2
- PO pain meds
- Emergence agitation after sevoflurane anesthesia, decreased with intranasal fentanyl

Anticipated Problems/Concerns
- Airway obstruction when head turned for myringotomy tube placement
- Laryngospasm without IV in place
- Postop resp insufficiency

Nephrectomy/Radical Nephrectomy

Anuj Malhotra
Vinod Malhotra

Risk

- 85–90% of radical nephrectomies performed for renal cell carcinoma.
- Incidence: 51,000 cases/y. Mortality: 13,000 deaths/y.
- M:F ratio: 1.6:1
- Urban > rural
- 5–10% of lesions extend into IVC
- Simple nephrectomy: Indicated for nonfunctioning obstructed kidney, polycystic kidney, donor transplants, uncontrollable renal Htn

Perioperative Risks

- Periop mortality rare (2%)
- Periop morbidity high (15%), incl DVT, pulm embolism, atelectasis, renal dysfunction, prolonged ileus, transfusion requirement

Worry About

- Massive blood loss (injury to renal vein, vena cava, renal artery, liver, spleen)
- Pneumothorax in thoracoabdominal approach
- Hypotension in flank position with kidney rest up
- Preservation of remaining kidney function (maintain renal perfusion)

- Augmentation of kidney function for donor nephrectomy (mannitol)
- Thrombus in IVC/hepatic vein, potential for embolus
- Renal artery/vein avulsion during laparoscopic surgery

Overview

- Kidney and pedicle removed in simple nephrectomy
- Kidney, adrenal, perinephric fat, and Gerota's fascia removed en bloc in radical nephrectomy
- Monitoring requirements depend upon IVC involvement and pt co-morbidities
- Significant bleeding may occur if IVC involved
- CPB indicated if large atrial thrombus. Right heart catheterization to be avoided, echocardiography preferred for monitoring.
- Venous return impeded by tumor thrombus in IVC can lead to hypotension and falsely elevated CVP
- Pulm embolization may occur during mobilization of tumor thrombus

- Epidural analgesia for postop pain relief preferred by many if open procedure. *Note*: With vena caval obstruction, epidural veins are dilated and space is narrowed.
- Laparoscopic-assisted nephrectomy becoming more common, standard for living donor nephrectomies, assoc with shorter length of stay

ICD-9-CM Codes: 593.89 (Obstructed kidney); 189.0 (Renal neoplasm); V59.4 (Donor kidney)

Indications and Usual Treatment

- Radical nephrectomy is the most effective and commonly applied treatment for renal cell carcinoma.
- Radiation and chemotherapy are of limited value as adjuncts. Preop embolization and immunotherapy may be beneficial.
- A nonfunctioning, obstructed kidney must be removed to prevent sepsis, renovascular Htn, and dysfunction of the contralateral kidney.
- Donor nephrectomies are elective and performed in healthy subjects.

ASSESSMENT POINTS

System	Effect	Assessment by Hx	PE	Test
CARDIO	Thrombus extending into IVC and right atrium	SOB	Lower limb edema Abd wall collaterals Varicocele Murmur	MRI MRA MRV ECHO
RESP	Pulm metastases Pleural effusion Pulm embolus	SOB	Auscultation Tachycardia JVD	CXR CT ABG
HEPAT	Venous occlusion (Budd-Chiari syndrome)	Abd pain	Ascites Hepatomegaly	CT Venogram US
CNS	Brain metastasis	Altered mental status	Focal deficits	CT MRI
MS	Bone metastasis	Pain	Bone deformity Pathologic fracture	X-ray Bone scan CT PET

Key Reference: Malhotra V, Sudheendra V, O'Hara J, et al. Anesthesia for the renal and genitourinary systems. In: Miller R, ed. *Miller's anesthesia*, 7th ed. vol. 2. Philadelphia: Churchill Livingstone; 2009:2105–2134 [chapter 65].

Perioperative Management

Preoperative Preparation
- US, CT, MRI, metastatic work-up
- Cardiorespiratory, renal evaluations

Anesthetic Technique
- GA with controlled ventilation
- Combined epidural/general or epidural for postop analgesia (if CPB not indicated)
- CPB and cardiothoracic surgery available if evidence of atrial involvement
- Blood salvage if non-cancerous lesion, transfusion as needed

Monitoring
- Consider arterial line
- Consider CVP and/or right heart catheter (right heart catheter contraindicated if intra-atrial thrombus)

- Consider ECHO if IVC or atrial involvement
- Foley catheter

Surgical Stages

- Bleeding during renal dissection, renal vein and/or IVC injury, or injury to spleen/liver
- Hypotension during positioning in kidney position
- Decreased renal blood flow during insufflation for laparoscopy
- Decreased venous return during removal of IVC and/or intra-atrial thrombus
- Pulm embolus (air or thrombus) during thrombectomy
- Pleura may be entered through diaphragm
- EBL: 500–2000 mL (minimal for laparoscopic donor nephrectomy)

Postoperative Considerations
- Pain score: 5–10 for open cases
- Epidural analgesia improves resp function, shortens hospital stay. IV PCA can be used as an alternative.
- At risk for DVT or pulm embolism
- Atelectasis due to splinting
- Head and neck edema from head-down positioning
- Shorter length of stay if laparoscopic approach

Anticipated Problems/Concerns
- Blood loss, pulm embolism, pneumothorax, atelectasis

Neuroprotection

James G. Hecker
Joshua Atkins

Risk

- CNS injury can be the result of ischemia, hypoxia, stroke, hemorrhage, trauma (surgical or otherwise), or infections, drugs (incl chemotherapeutics, i.e., 'chemo brain'), toxins, neurodegeneration, sepsis, or immune/inflammatory insults.
- Procedures most commonly assoc with risks of CNS injury incl:
  - Neurosurgical resection for aneurysm, AVM or tumor
  - Spinal cord tumor
  - Thoracic or less commonly abd aortic aneurysm resection (incl TEVAR)
  - Carotid endarterectomy
  - CABG, including valve repair, aortic arch procedures, DHCA
  - Interventional neuroradiology incl thrombolysis, stents, coiling. Potentially any surgical procedure that involves massive blood loss, sitting position, or prolonged hypotension.

Perioperative Risks

- Bleeding
- Ischemia and hypoxia
- Increases in ICP
- Edema
- Cranial nerve and brainstem injury
- Epidural, subdural, or parenchymal hematoma
- Transient and permanent brain deficit
- Seizures

Worry About

- Hyper- and hypoventilation and effects on CBF
- Cerebral metabolic rate
- Hypoxia
- Hypercarbia
- ICP changes

- CNS perfusion pressure (avoid obstructed venous drainage)
- Transmural delta P across aneurysmal wall (wall stress)
- Hyperglycemia, hypoglycemia
- Co-existing DM, Htn, vascular and cardiac disease
- Hyperthermia or severe hypothermia
- Mild/moderate hypothermia is protective (controversial)
- N/V (effects on ICP)

Overview

- Refers to preventing and/or minimizing the effects of 2° or 3° injury once the initial insult has ended.
- In anesthetic practice it can also mean the ability to provide protection to the CNS (or to other organ systems as well) prior to the stressor. Anesthetic neuroprotection can incl drug delivery, gene expression, or other cellular manipulation, but also anesthetic management of physiologic variables to ensure oxygenation, ventilation, perfusion, and fluids (MAP, CBF, ICP, O_2, CO_2) appropriately matched to the clinical circumstances. Neuroprotection outside of anesthesia practice incl treatment after stroke, TBI, or SCI.
- Numerous failed human clinical trials in neuroprotection after stroke, despite animal models showing efficacy at several different targets.
- Early work focused on the possible benefit of thiopental induced burst suppression and hypothermia. Recent work has investigated multiple additional targets and pathways, incl ischemic preconditioning and identification of hypoxia inducible factors.

- Resuscitation with reperfusion recipes rather than single drugs may eventually salvage much more of the penumbra region after ischemia.

Indications and Usual Treatment

- Optimize pt CNS physiology. Sometimes trade off CMR vs. CBF for improved surgical operating conditions
- ICP vs. CBF: Optimize O_2 delivery at lowest possible intracranial volume when compliance decreased
- CMR is decreased with thiopental, propofol
- Inhalational anesthetics also decrease CMR but pose a clinical conundrum with studies showing both neuroprotective (anesthetic preconditioning) and potentially neurotoxic effects.
- Mild and/or moderate hypothermia (33.5 to 35.5 °C) probably beneficial. Level one evidence for global ischemia (witnessed cardiac arrest). Despite lack of efficacy in IHAST trial for aneurysms large clinical trials under way in Europe and Asia for TBI, stroke, ICH (controversial).

Etiology

- Relative importance of individual mechanisms in contributing to 2° injury after an initial ischemic insult probably depends on severity and location of ischemia, is multi-modal, and changes with time after injury. Proposed pathways incl excitatory amino acids, immediate early transcription factors and gene expression, translational modification and arrest, calcium regulation, membrane stabilization, mitochondrial failure, edema, free radicals, inflammatory cytokines, apoptosis, caspases, calpains, inflammation, membrane channels, endothelins, and other less obvious potential mechanisms.

ASSESSMENT POINTS

System	Effect	Assessment by Hx	PE	Test
HEENT	Airway, need for fiberoptic intubation for controlled induction, C-spine cleared if trauma	Hx of difficult ventilation or intubations, Hx of trauma	Airway exam, other head and neck injuries	CT
CARDIO	Htn, carotid or vertebral disease, cardiac failure or dysfunction, bradycardia	TIA, stroke, MI, IDDM, Htn, syncope, angina	BP, HR, peripheral edema, JVD, angina	EKG, ambulatory?, exercise tolerance
RESP	Apnea, COPD, asthma	Difficult weaning from prior intubation, Cushing reflex	Need for O_2 at rest, obesity, wheezing, rales	Able to lie flat, O_2, rarely PFTs, able to vigorously 'blow out candle', apnea
RENAL	CRI	UO		BUN/Cr
CNS	Increased ICP, neuro deficits, change in consciousness	N/V, lethargy, alert and oriented	Lethargy, focal deficits, alert and oriented, neuro exam	Neuro exam, CT, MRI

Key References: Sturgess J, Matta B. Brain Protection: Current and future options. *Best Pract Res Clin Anaesthesiol.* 2008;22(1):167–176.

Perioperative Management

Preoperative Preparation

- ICP, Licox or ventriculostomy in situ?
- CT showing edema or midline shift
- Fluid and volume resuscitated
- Mannitol, HTS, hyperventilation if ICP increased
- Avoid long-acting sedative medications
- Control airway, avoid hypoxia and hypercapnia
- Consider steroids, dilantin, H_2 blocker

Monitoring

- STD monitors plus arterial line for most cases (CVP for major vascular and sitting procedures)
- EEG, SSEP, MEP monitoring, incl in interventional radiology for coils, embolization
- Lumbar drain for surgical exposure

- Consider processed EEG in the absence of other neuromonitoring if burst suppression is a consideration

Anesthetic Technique/Induction

- Controlled induction with IV agents: Propofol (or thiopental), NMB, short duration opioids
- Attention to physiology, avoid hypoxia and hypercapnia and swings in BP avoid change in wall stress in aneurysms.
  - Intraop
  - Tight BP control
  - Brain relaxation (<1 MAC inhalational agent, consider propofol infusion)
  - Burst suppression (not convincing evidence but surgeons may request)
  - Surgical retraction can cause local hypoperfusion and postop edema

- Avoid muscle relaxation during MEP or EMG monitoring
- Maintain steady-state level of anesthesia during neuromonitoring

Postoperative Considerations

- Extubation some prefer deep, rapidly awake for neuro exam
- Older pts with delayed emergence common
- Frequently get CT scan if not able to do immediate neuro exam

Anticipated Problems/Concerns

- Postop brain edema
- Increased seizure risk (procedures involving cortex)
- Airway edema if unusual positioning (e.g., prone)

Neuroradiology

Vivian H. Porche

Risk

- CT
  - Intracranial imaging
  - Studies of the thorax and abdomen
  - IV contrast media can cause adverse reaction in 5–8% of cases
- Radiotherapy
  - External beam and intraop radiation
- Impossible to directly observe the pt; watch on closed-circuit television

Worry About

- Location of suction, O_2, and electricity
- Compromise of thoracic structures with an anterior mediastinal mass
- Severe contrast reactions
- Aspiration with oral contrast
- Hypothermia, esp. in children

Overview

- Goal: To provide an OR level of safety in the radiologic suite and in other places outside of the OR.
- Complicated by technique required
- Radiotherapy pts scheduled for a series of daily treatments over several weeks with daily anesthesia.
- CT scan pediatric pts are given oral contrast and then anesthetized.

Types of Patients

- Young children
- Pts with disorders causing uncontrolled movements
- Pts with whom communication is impossible (e.g., language barrier, obtundation, mental retardation)
- Pts who are very ill or in severe pain

Perioperative Implications

Preoperative Preparation

- Same careful preanesthesia evaluation as for any other surgical pt
- Physical exam should focus on vital signs, auscultation of the heart and lungs, and evaluation of the resp tract
- Diagnostic and laboratory studies should be directed toward concomitant illness
- Follow appropriate fasting guidelines for children and adults
- Ensure appropriate venous access, esp. for pediatric cases
- Consent is usually obtained from the adult pt prior to the procedure.
- Consent for the pediatric pt is often obtained the day of the procedure from the parents or guardian due to their work schedule or other conflicts.

- Know layout of area in advance for extra supplies, electrical outlets, and telephones

Anesthetic Technique

- Bring well-stocked anesthesia cart
- Conscious sedation, MAC, GETA or general anesthesia with spontaneous ventilation
- Again ensure a reliable venous access, esp. in young children

Monitoring

- Routine; may need to add temp
- BP, pulse oximetry, capnography, electrocardiogram

Positioning

- Airway and ventilation must be maintained
- Generally need long circuits, long IV tubing
- Watch for increasing fluid volumes in pediatric pts
- May need closed circuit telesivion with intercom if direct visualization is not possible

Post-Procedure Considerations

- Make sure to use standard discharge criteria.
- Have warm blankets available for pts after their test.

ASSESSMENT POINTS

Procedure	Patient Type	Anesthesia Type	Concerns	Monitoring	Comments
CT	Pediatric—less than 3 mo—with contrast	Deep sedation, MAC, TIVA (total IV anesthesia) or GA	Keep pt warm to prevent hypothermia (neurologic dysfunction ↑ thermoregulation problems)	BP, pulse oximeter, ETCO$_2$, ECG, consider temp monitoring	Position sedated child to avoid airway obstruction; mobile cart equipped for emergencies
	Pediatric—less than 3 mo—no contrast	No sedation—have infant suck on bottle of formula or allow to sleep	As above	No monitoring required Consider temp monitoring	As above
	Pediatric—under age 8 y, and/or mental handicap and/or contrast	Deep sedation—MAC, TIVA, or GA	If oral contrast given, treat pt as with full stomach	As above	As above
	Pediatric—over age 8 y, and/or no contrast	Often no sedation required, if required give conscious sedation, TIVA, or GA if unable to hold still	Maintain thermal stability	For conscious sedation: BP, pulse oximeter, ECG; consider temp monitoring	As above
	Adult—healthy	No sedation	If oral contrast is given, treat pt as with full stomach	None	If suspected ↑ in ICP, use caution to avoid ↑ arterial CO$_2$ or ↓ arterial O$_2$, which can further ↑ ICP
	Adult—difficulty holding still	Conscious sedation or MAC/GA	If oral contrast given, treat pt as with full stomach	BP, ECG, pulse oximeter, ETCO$_2$, FIO$_2$	Positioning of gantry or table during procedure may result in kinking or disconnection of anesthesia circuit
RADIOTHERAPY	Pediatric—esp. under age 8 y	Sedation, MAC or TIVA use short-acting, easily titratable drugs; for repeated treatments, pt needs central indwelling catheter	Temp maintenance Airway management and ventilation Positioning of the gantry during procedure may result in kinking or disconnection of the anesthesia circuit Observe pt prior to each treatment for sepsis or ↑ ICP	ECG, ETCO$_2$, pulse oximeter, BP Make sure closed-circuit TV shows pt and monitors	Immobility is the primary goal of anesthesia; using TIVA may avoid transporting agent vaporizers and other bulky equipment
	Adult	None, conscious sedation or easily titratable drugs		Same as above	

Key Reference: Porche VH. Anesthetic considerations in radiologic procedures performed outside the operating room. *Int Anesthesiol Clin* 1998;36:9–19.

Off Pump and Minimally Invasive Cardiac Procedures

Maudy Kalangie
Wendy K. Bernstein

Risk

- Increased risk with advanced age and male gender
- Family Hx of CAD
- Htn, hypercholesterolemia, diabetes, cigarette smoking

Perioperative Risk

- Operative mortality for bypass procedures is double for women compared to men
- Off-pump coronary artery bypass (OPCABPOS)
  - Mortality 0–5%
  - Pulm insufficiency 3–5%
  - Reoperation for rebleeding 1–4%
  - MI 0–4%
  - Mediastinal infection 1–2%
  - Neurologic complications 1–2%
  - Renal dysfunction 1–2%
- Minimally invasive cardiac procedures
  - Mortality 1–3%
  - Arrhythmias 10%
  - Conversion to sternotomy 4%
  - MI 0–4%
  - Reoperation for rebleeding 3%
  - Stroke 2%

- Port access cardiac surgery
  - Aortic dissection
  - Aortic valve trauma
  - Coronary sinus trauma
  - Right ventricular perforation
  - Endoaortic balloon migration can compromise cerebral perfusion

Worry About

- OPCAB
  - Multiple grafts require repeated occlusions and can affect hemodynamics.
  - Displacement of the heart, esp. for PDA and circumflex grafts cause labile hemodynamics.
  - Ischemia caused by the occlusion of the proximal coronaries must be recognized and treated early.
  - Possibility of conversion to traditional on-pump CABG
- Minimally invasive cardiac procedures
- CO_2 insufflation necessary for visualization can hinder heart filling and depress contractility

ICD-9-CM Code: 410 (Acute myocardial infarction); 414 (Coronary arteriosclerosis)

Overview

- Maintain cardiac output to sustain coronary flow
- Early recovery desired
- OPCAB
  - Goal is to provide adequate revascularization but avoid pulm dysfunction, coagulopathy, and CNS injury caused by CPB
- Minimally invasive cardiac procedures
  - Requires good communication between anesthesiologist and surgeon

Indications and Usual Treatment

- OPCAB is recommended for pts with severe vascular disease (esp. severe aortic atherosclerosis), stroke, pulm disease, and renal dysfunction.
- Surgeon preference and experience determine procedure.

ASSESSMENT POINTS

System	Effect	Assessment by Hx	PE	Test
CARDIO	Family Hx, previous MI, ventricular dysfunction, valvular dysfunction	Htn, DM, hyperlipidemia, smoking, level of activity	Murmurs, pulm rales, lower extremity edema, intolerance to lying flat	ECG, ECHO, stress testing, coronary angiography
PULM	COPD, emphysema, chronic bronchitis	Smoking Hx, use of supplemental O_2	Decreased breath sounds, sputum production	CXR, PFTs, ABG
CNS	Carotid disease	Previous stroke, TIA	Carotid bruits, residual deficits	Carotid US, carotid angiography
RENAL	Renal insufficiency, renal failure	Htn, Hx of dialysis	Pulm rales	Creatinine, potassium levels

Key References: Shroyer AL, Grover F, Hattler B, et al. On pump versus off-pump coronary surgery. *N Engl J Med.* 2009;361:1827–1837.

Perioperative Management

Preoperative Preparation

- Baseline cardiac function incl regional wall motion, right heart function, and valvular function

Monitoring

- Arterial line
- ECG monitoring particularly lead II and V5
- CVP
- PA catheter for multiple grafts and decreased cardiac function
- Continuous cardiac output monitoring
- TEE is most sensitive and specific for early detection of ischemic events
- Minimally invasive cardiac procedures
  - Right and left radial lines should be placed
  - Right radial line monitors endoaortic clamp migration
- TEE essential for placement
- Endoaortic clamp

- Venous drainage catheter
- Endosinus catheter
- Endopulmonary vent

Anesthetic Technique/Induction

- Adequate preoxygenation
- Preinduction arterial line for pts with decreased LV function
- External defibrillator pads prior to induction
- Avoid hypothermia, particularly for OPCAB
  - Heat lost cannot be restored as easily as compared to on pump procedures
  - Warm OR prior to pt arrival
  - Use warming pads/mattresses on OR table
  - Use forced air warming devices over head and exposed areas
  - Minimize time pt is uncovered
  - Warm IV fluids
  - Use fresh gas flows <2.5 L/min
- Displacement of heart or placement of stabilizing devices can cause significant decreases in BP

- Trendelenburg position
- Volume loading with a target CVP 10–12 prior to heart displacement
- Inotropes can begin for depressed cardiac function
- Worsening of existing mitral regurgitation can occur with heart displacement
- Rise in CVP and PA pressures despite stable BP may signify decompensation
- Bradycardia can occur during RCA grafting
- Pacemaker available

Postoperative Considerations

- Complete TEE examination incl function, regional wall motion abn, and valvular function should be assessed.
- Continue active warming
- Should evaluate for possible extubation after considering adequate hemostasis, stable hemodynamics, and pain control as well as attainment of extubation criteria

Office-Based Anesthesia

Patrick Guffey

Risk

- Approx 10 million cases performed in office based setting
- 10% of all surgeries
- Wide range of surgical subspecialties perform procedures in office settings
- Full complement of anesthesia agents may be utilized

Perioperative Risks

- Pt's underlying medical condition
- Procedure-specific risks
- Anesthetic emergencies without full complement of backup equipment
- Low number of trained responders
- Immediate transfer to hospital may not be available

Worry About

- Small number of trained responders for a crisis
- Emergency equipment (adequate dantrolene if triggering agents used)
- How to transfer pt to higher level of care
- Lack of oversight and little to no regulation

Overview

- Procedures performed in a physician's office with no direct connection to a hospital or ambulatory surgical center
- Anesthetic techniques range from monitored care to general anesthesia
- Allows for potential decrease in costs as compared to a hospital or surgical center
- May be useful in a setting where the majority of pts do not require anesthesia and capital equipment costs are high.

- Provides for convenience and privacy which may not be possible in a larger setting for both the pt and practitioner
- Little to no government regulation, which places onus of responsibility further on the anesthesiologist to ensure environment is appropriate for cases performed

Indications and Usual Treatment

- Procedure and anesthetic must be within the capabilities of the facility, incl complications requiring immediate response.
- ASA classification I & II for low-risk procedures
- Pt who desires privacy that cannot be provided in a larger setting
- May offer a level of convenience not possible in a hospital

ASSESSMENT POINTS

System	Effect	Assessment by Hx	PE	Test
HEENT	Difficult airway management	Hx of difficult mask or intubation, mouth or neck abn (mass, prior radiation), sleep apnea	Mallampati classification, thyromental distance, mouth opening	Transfer to higher level of care if imaging warranted
CARDIO	Poor CV function or reserve	CAD, Htn, diabetes, prior MI, TIA, heart failure. Assess exercise tolerance	Chest auscultation Assessment of pedal edema and JVD	ECG, stress test
RESP	Difficulty with ventilation and oxygenation	Asthma, COPD, active or recent URI	Chest auscultation and percussion	CXR if low suspicion, transfer if high suspicion
RENAL	Metabolic derangement	Renal failure, diuretic use		Basic metabolic panel, BUN/Cr
CNS	Postop agitation, exacerbation of pre-existing condition	Hx of Parkinson's disease, psychiatric disorders	Resting tremor, preop assessment	
GI	Aspiration and nausea	Hx of GERD, Hx of postop nausea		

Key Reference: Guidelines for Office-Based Anesthesia, Committee of Ambulatory Surgical Care. *American Society of Anesthesiologists.* 1999; Rev: Oct 2009.

Perioperative Management

Preoperative Preparation
- Complete preanesthetic evaluation by anesthesiologist
- Special attention to preparation for anticipated complications

Monitoring
- ASA standard monitors

Anesthetic Technique/Induction
- Full complement of anesthesia techniques can be utilized with preference to short acting agents.

- Consideration to regional technique for surgical or postop pain +/– sedation
- Preference to short-acting opioids (fentanyl, remifentanil) in anticipation of discharge home

Emergence
- Minimize long-acting agents during the case, consider regional anesthesia to decrease anesthetic requirements and facilitate timely discharge

Postoperative Monitoring
- Until pt is hemodynamically stable, able to void, pain controlled, and nausea resolved with ability to tolerate PO fluids

- Transfer pts to higher level of care if unable to discharge in a timely manner
- A physician should be immediately available until all pts are discharged.

Anticipated Problems/Concerns

- Rarely a pt will require hospitalization. Plans should be in place to facilitate this.
- Few, if any trained responders will be available for an intraop anesthetic complication
- PACU capabilities limited compared to surgical center or hospital. Plan for pts to be stable upon leaving operating suite.

Omphalocele Surgery

Wendy B. Binstock

Risk

- Incidence varies from 1/6000 live births
- Racial predominance: none

Perioperative Risks

- Possibility of impaired blood supply to the herniated organs
- Intestinal obstruction
- Significant heat losses
- Major fluid shifts
- Infection
- Risks due to assoc genetic, cardiac, urologic and metabolic abn

Worry About

- Blood glucose, esp. with possibility of Beckwith-Wiedemann syndrome

- Possibility of cardiac defects and CV compromise
- Possibility of resp compromise, postop ventilation difficulties
- Metabolic problems

Overview

- Congenital abd wall defects that result in herniation of the intestine into base of umbilical cord
- The herniated viscera are covered with a membranous sac: The bowel is morphologically and usually functionally normal
- Vary in size: May contain only small bowel or may contain liver, spleen, stomach, and other abd organs

- Assoc congenital anomalies (GI, CV, GU, CNS), metabolic anomalies (visceromegaly, hypoglycemia and polycythemia), syndromes (Beckwith-Wiedemann and trisomy 13 and 18), and prematurity or low birth weight

ICD-9-CM Code: 756.72

Etiology

- A failure of the gut to migrate from the yolk sac into the abd during gestation
- Amniotic sac present, although it may have been ruptured during birth or shortly thereafter

Indications

- Prompt surgical repair, either 1° or staged, depending on size

ASSESSMENT POINTS

System	Effect	Assessment by Hx	PE	Test
HEENT	Beckwith-Wiedemann syndrome: macroglossia, microcephaly		Head exam	
CARDIO	CHD: tetralogy of Fallot, ASD		CV exam	Transthoracic ECHO
RESP	If assoc with prematurity, may have immature lungs	Gestational age	Chest exam and signs of resp distress	O_2 sat If available, predelivery lecithin/sphingomyelin ratio
GI	Gastric and intestinal distention, small abd cavity		Size of omphalocele	
ENDO	Possibility of Beckwith-Wiedemann syndrome			Blood glucose
RENAL/ HEPAT	Immaturity of hepatic and renal systems possibility for ↓ hepatic blood flow and impaired renal perfusion post closure			

Key Reference: Roberts Jr JD, Romanelli TM, Todres ID. Neonatal emergencies. In: Cote CJ, Lerman J, Todres ID, eds. *A practice of anesthesia for infants and children.* 4th ed. Philadelphia: Saunders; 2009:763–765.

Perioperative Implications

Preoperative Preparation

- IV access and restoration of intravascular volume
- Fluid losses tend to be isotonic; therefore, balanced salt solutions often used (lactated Ringer's or 5% albumin)
- Multiple fluid boluses of up to 20 mL/kg of fluid is often necessary initially
- Maintain normothermia by wrapping abd in moist, warm, sterile dressing; lower body can be placed in plastic bag
- Decompression of the stomach to prevent regurgitation/aspiration
- Antibiotics to prevent sepsis

Monitoring

- Consider arterial line depending on extent of defect and ventilatory status
- Consider CVP if defect is large
- Adequate temp and glucose monitoring

Airway

- After decompression of the stomach, rapid sequence induction or awake intubation should carried out.
- ETT should be secured in a manner suitable for prolonged postop ventilation

Maintenance

- NO usually avoided
- A suitable mixture of O_2 and air to produce adequate oxygenation (Pao_2 50–70 mmHg), SaO_2 97–98% for term infants, 87–92% for preterm infants); will vary as surgeons attempt to replace bowel in abd
- Maximal muscle relaxation facilitates reduction of the eviscerated organs and bowel.
- Primary closure may lead to significant increases in intra-abdominal pressure which leads to decreased organ perfusion (intestinal, renal, and hepatic) will result in impaired organ function and altered drug metabolism and decreased ventilatory reserve due to significantly decreased diaphragmatic function and bilateral lower lobe atelectasis.
- Ability to tolerate primary closure assessed by the ability to measure BP and/or SaO_2 in the lower extremities
- Placing bowel in a silo assoc with higher infection rate

Extubation

- Postop care varies with magnitude of defect, type of repair, and assoc congenital anomalies
- Healthy pts with a small 1° closure often tolerate extubation in OR

- In pts with large defects, who undergo 1° closure postop intubation, ventilation, and maximal muscle relaxation should be continued until abd pressure results in little resp or circulatory compromise
- In pts with a large defect treated with a silo, although extubation might be tolerated, postop intubation should be continued due to repeated trips to the OR and muscle relaxation will facilitate the abd cavity accommodation of the increasing mass.

Anticipated Problems/Concerns

- Ventilatory care: Similar to that for other neonates with resp distress
- Fluid requirements: May remain high until abd venous pressure decreases, at which time fluid restriction and diuresis probably indicated
- FIO_2: Adjust to maintain a normal Pao_2
- PEEP: Appropriate levels used to increased FRC
- Nutritional status: Because bowel function is usually compromised and slow to resume, TPN requirements are often extended.
- Circulatory, renal, hepatic, and intestinal dysfunction common
- Infection: Common, esp. if silo used instead of 1° closure

Orchiopexy

W. Casey Lenox

PROCEDURES

Risk

- Premature infants: Risk is 30% for one or both testicles to be undescended
- Full-term infants: Risk is 3%
- 60% of undescended testicles found in inguinal position; 8% intra-abdominal; only 24% in the easily operable low inguinal/high scrotal position
- Progressive injury occurs when testicle is left undescended: Decreased sperm production after age 6 y, impaired hormonal production, increased risk of malignant degeneration
- Risk of malignant degeneration may not be improved following orchiopexy, but self-examination becomes more reliable

Perioperative Risks

- Periop mortality rare in term infants (<0.01%)
- Risks in ex-premature children dependent upon co-existing morbidity (e.g., bronchopulmonary dysplasia, reactive airway disease, subglottic stenosis, hydrocephalus and seizure due to intraventricular hemorrhage, GI dysfunction due to necrotizing enterocolitis, malnutrition, anemia, RV hypertrophy/failure, poor IV access)

- Operative risks of testicular atrophy or hypotrophy: 8% for those beyond external ring, 13% when canalicular, 26% for intra-abdominal locations

Worry About

- Co-morbidity assoc with prematurity
- Cryptorchidism a/w congenital anomalies in up to 4.4% of pts: Smith's lists cryptorchidism as frequent in 53 known syndromes/sequences, occasional in another 31 syndromes
- Venous air embolism, aspiration, diaphragmatic embarrassment if laparoscope utilized for repair
- Intravascular injection of local anesthetic

Overview

- Testicle(s) located and spermatic cord and accompanying vasculature freed and mobilized so that testicle can be relocated within hemiscrotum. Spermatic vessels may be sacrificed, with vasculature of vas deferens supplying collaterals.

- Operative laparoscope increasingly utilized for relocating intra-abdominal or high inguinal testicles
- Operative time: 1 hr (open, low testicular location) to 3 hr (laparoscopic)

ICD-9-CM Code: 752.5 (Cryptorchidism)

Indications and Usual Treatment

- Testicle will not descend beyond 1 y of age
- 2% risk per mo of germ-cell depletion for unoperated testes and later sperm counts/motility increased when operated on in first year of life. Average age of operations has decreased to 6–12 mo of age
- Some evidence that hCG may promote testicular descent, so this may be attempted prior to operation

ASSESSMENT POINTS

System	Effect	Assessment by Hx	PE	Test
HEENT	Subglottic stenosis		Stridor, wheezing, croup	CXR, bronchoscopy
CARDIO	Pulm Htn, PDA, RV hypertrophy	FTT	↑ S_2, murmurs	ECG Cardiac ECHO/catheter
RESP	Bronchopulmonary dysplasia, blebs	Asthma, O_2? Apnea monitor alarms Diuretics		CXR
RENAL	Nephrocalcinosis	Htn		BP, electrolytes, BUN, Cr
CNS	Intraventricular hemorrhage Seizures, hydrocephalus	Mental status Development Seizure type, frequency Ventriculoperitoneal shunt		Shunt evaluation Anti-epilepsy drug levels

Key Reference: Ritzén EM, Bergh A, Bjerknes R, et al. *Acta Paediatr*. 2007;96(5):638–643. Review.

Perioperative Management

Preoperative Preparation

- May have clear liquids up to 2 hr before induction
- No lab work necessary if otherwise normal
- If uncomplicated, may be done as outpatient procedure

Anesthetic Technique

- Combined general and regional anesthetic in open case
- Usually regular mask or laryngeal mask airway (LMA) and caudal injection of local anesthetic (1mL/kg 0.25% bupivicaine or 0.2% ropivicaine) or ilioinguinal/iliohypogastric nerve block for analgesia intra- and postop
- Combined technique in laparoscopic procedures but with trachea intubated (usually; LMA now being used by some)

Monitoring

- Routine

Induction

- Inhalational mask induction, with sevoflurance, then maintenance with sevoflurane or isoflurane and NO
- IV, then single-injection caudal placed following induction of anesthesia

Surgical Stages

Dissection

- Caudal usually not effective in blocking visceral pain that occurs with pulling on spermatic cord; may require increasing volatile anesthetic concentrations temporarily
- Possible resp compromise if laparoscopic procedure
- Minimal blood loss

Postoperative Considerations

- If 0.025% bupivacaine used for caudal, 4–6 hr of analgesia usual
- Most children need enteral opioids for 2–3 d
- Incidence of emesis postop 45%; usually self-limited

Anticipated Problems/Concerns

- Ex–premature children have an increased incidence of wheezing and desaturation intra- and postop. May need to be observed overnight.

ORIF of Hip

a Singh

Risk

- 250,000/y
- M:F ratio: 1:3
- Incidence increases with osteoporosis, fall risk, age, height, sex, arrhythmias

Perioperative Risks

- Mortality: In-hospital 10%, 30 d 14%, 1 y 30%
- Morbidity: Age, >48 hr to repair, co-morbidities, type of fx
- Most frequent periop complication: Cardiac
- Delirium: Up to 50% postop
- Fat emboli syndrome (FES): Physiologic response to fat emboli in circulation; 1% incidence; 15–25% mortality. Immediate or gradual 12–72 hr. Petechial rash (pathognomonic) 20–50%, pulm 75%, neurologic, hematologic.

Worry About

- Cardiac complications. [text obscured] alterations to O_2 supply an[d] (stress response, pain, h[y] fluid shifts, inflammatory hypercoagulable).
- Baseline anemia: May hav[e] blood loss. Blood may be hemo[...]
- Emboli: Fat, FES, DVT, c[...] syndrome

Overview

- Medical optimization versus [...] <48 hr shown to lower pain sc[...] periop complications; not overa[...] medical clearance common cau[...]

[handwritten notes obscuring text:]
Mandibular osteotomy out line – as facial bones can bleed so controlled Hypotension

Wake up T tube on to ensure Ø pain, Ø vomiting/ nausea as rubber bands have month shut so T aspiration risk if N/V

ASSESSMENT POINTS				
System	Effect	Assessment by Hx	PE	Test
CARDIO	CAD + O_2 supply/demand imbalance (HR, Htn, anemia, fluid shifts, emboli); arrhythmia as cause of fall	Angina, SOB, palpitations, LOC as cause of fall	Vital signs, pitting edema, irregular pulse, diaphoresis	12-lead EKG, telemetry, stress test, ECHO, cardiac enzymes
RESP	Hypoxemia/PE	Dyspnea, wheezing	RR, accessory muscle	CXR, ABG, continuous pulse ox
RENAL	Dehydration, UTI	Tachycardia, hypotension, altered mentation, dysuria	Vital signs, cap refill, mucous membranes	Cr, BUN, sodium, UA/culture
CNS	TIA as cause of fall; Delirium	Sensory/motor/speech deficit; Hx of LOC	Neuro deficit; mentation, fluctuating course, disorganization	DSM-IV-TR, CAM, MMSE, CT, MRI

DSM-IV-TR Diagnostic and Statistical Manual of Mental Disorders, Fourth Edition, Text Revision; CAM Confusion Assessment Method; MMSE Mini-Mental State Examination

Key Reference: Shiga T, Wajima Z, Ohe Y. Is operative delay associated with increased mortality of hip fracture patients? Systematic review, meta-analysis, and meta-regression. *Can J Anaesth.* 2008;55:146–154.

Perioperative Management

Preoperative Preparation

- Optimize co-morbidities. Abn cardiac testing rarely changes before ORIF, esp. in intermediate-risk pt. No advantage, possible worse outcome from PCI (restenosis, thrombosis from D/C antiplatelet Tx). LOC causing fall often warrants cardiac, neuro testing.
- Dehydration, hemoconcentration common; consider rehydration, pRBCs.
- Consider neuraxial with pt, surgeon, anticoagulation, expected EBL, risk of delirium, mechanism for postop follow up (pain management, catheter removal, management of complications).
- Consider Gram (-) Abx if S/Sx of UTI, to reduce implant infection.

Monitoring

- Consider A-line if preop hypoxemia, co-morbidities, expected EBL, controlled hypotension
- CVP if poor IV access, revision repair, large expected EBL, co-morbidities
- Cell saver: Leuokocyte removal filter shown to reduce transfusion of fat

Anesthetic Technique/Induction

- Regional versus GA: Reduced EBL at same MAP as GA, likely from vasodilation of venous, arterial vasculatures leads to redistribution of blood flow. Consider sedation to tolerate positioning, Fx table.

- B-blockers: Important to continue periop administration if previously taking agents. Control of heart rate important.

Surgical Stages

Dissection

- Muscle relaxation: NMBD versus neuraxial dense motor block
- Controlled hypotension: Balance risks (inadequate organ perfusion [SBP <80 mmHg 90% delirium]) versus benefits (reduced EBL, dry bone surface [improves prosthetic cementing and reduces duration of surgery]).
- Normothermia may reduce delirium, arrhythmias, low BP, bleeding, transfusion, infection, poor wound healing.

Reaming/cementing

- Cement implantation syndrome (CIS): Increased intramedullary pressures generated during implant insertion, are accentuated by cementing, and can cause emboli of fat, marrow, debris to pulm vasculature that are hemodynamically significant

Postoperative Considerations

- Pain: Intrathecal morphine; consider reduced dosage for elderly, appropriate postop monitoring. Inadequately treated pain can increase cardiac O_2 demand, stress response, delirium. Delirium also seen from opiates.

- Delirium: May be reduced with regional, early ORIF.
- DVT: Regional may reduce; low dose anticoagulant prophylaxis, SCDs, early ambulation.
- Fat emboli syndrome (FES): Clinical Dx with classic triad of hypoxemia, delirium, petechial rash. Typically presents 24-72 hr after Fx. Early immobilization, ORIF may prevent; therapy is supportive (oxygenation/PEEP/IV fluids); steroids controversial.

Anticipated Problems/Concerns

- Emboli: Fat, FES, CIS, DVT
- Delirium: Increased hospital LOS (urinary incontinence, feeding problems, decubitus ulcers), mortality, likelihood of being placed in nursing home for first time.
- Long term: 25% full recovery, 40% nursing home, 50% cane or walker, up to 30% mortality in 1 yr.

Pacemaker Implantation for Sick Sinus Syndrome

Stuart J. Weiss

Walter Bethune

Risk

- Sick sinus syndrome (SSS) affects approx 3 out of 10,000 people and is an indication for permanent pacemaker (PPM) implantation.
- Increased occurence with age, but may present in younger pts with a familial form of the disease or following surgery for congenital heart defects.
- Incidence in USA: More than 1 million people have a PPM and many tens of thousands are implanted yearly.
- SSS accounts for approx 50% of PPM implantations, or about 200 per 1 million population members per year.

Perioperative Risks

- SSS is assoc with periop brady- and tachy-dysrhythmias, with the potential for CV compromise due to myocardial ischemia or pulm edema.
- In the awake pt, symptoms can incl dizziness, light-headedness, confusion or other mental status changes, palpitations, angina, dyspnea, fatigue, headache, N/V and Stokes-Adams attacks; frank syncope due to asystole or ventricular fibrillation.

Worry About

- Previously undiagnosed or early disease (see Etiology), with modest early symptoms
- In the absence of a PPM or with PPM dysfunction, severe bradycardia or asystole may occur, esp. when increased vagal tone is present.
- Normal sinus rhythm will always recover in time; sudden cardiac death is therefore *not* an important risk in pure SSS.
- In the presence of a PPM, sustained paroxysmal tachycardia may require control with antiarrhythmic medications.

Overview

- SSS, also called sinus node dysfunction, is a group of arrhythmias presumably caused by a malfunction of the sinus node, the heart's normal 1° pacemaker.
- SSS is divided into three types: Simple sinus bradycardia, sinus arrest or sinus node block with or without sinus bradycardia, and bradycardia with paroxysmal tachycardia (i.e., tachy-brady syndrome).
- Tachycardia may be caused by atrial fibrillation and/or flutter.
- Syncope or severe lightheadedness results from prolonged sinus or atrial pauses following termination of tachycardia; atrial pause frequently caused by sinus exit block.
- Sinus or atrial pauses may rarely be up to 15 sec in duration.
- SSS may be assoc with high-degree AV block (pan-conduction defect).
- Stroke risk is increased in pts who are paced ventricularly (VVI) and thus more prone to develop atrial fibrillation with subsequent thrombus formation/propagation due to atrial stasis.
- Where once surgeons were primarily responsible for PPM implantation, the procedure now is typically performed by cardiologists. For most pts, PPM insertion is performed on an out pt basis in the cardiac catherization suite. For high risk pts however, anesthesiologists may be called upon to provide monitoring, administration of analgesics and sedatives, and resuscitation should any complications occur.

ICD-9-CM Code: 427.81

Etiology

- SSS is usually caused by degenerative, sclerotic, or fibrotic changes of the sinus node.
- SSS can be a manifestation of 1° cardiac disease; e.g., myocardial ischemia/infarction, pericarditis, cardiomyopathy.
- SSS may also be 2° to cardiac involvement by other diseases (typically infiltrative); e.g., muscular dystrophy, collagen disease, hemochromatosis, amyloidosis, metastatic disease.

Indications And Usual Treatment

- PPM placement is indicated in symptomatic pts or in asymptomatic pts who need β-blockers or antiarrhythmic drugs.
- Bradyarrhythmias are typically well controlled with PPMs, while tachyarrhythmias respond well to medical therapy. However, because both brady-arrhythmias and tachyarrhythmias may be present, drugs to control tachyarrhythmia may exacerbate bradyarrhythmia. Therefore, PPM implantation is indicated prior to implementation of drug therapy for tachyarrhythmias.
- For previously undiagnosed disease, temporary transvenous pacing may be appropriate.
- Sinus rate and atrial conduction may be enhanced by stimulation with β-adrenergic agonists (isoproterenol, epinephrine, ephedrine) and parasympathetic blocking agents (atropine, glycopyrrolate).

ASSESSMENT POINTS

System	Effect	Assessment by Hx	PE	Test
CARDIO	Bradycardia, tachycardia	PPM implantation	Low (or high) HR	ECG, electrophysiologic testing
CNS		Unexplained episodic lightheadedness, confusion, syncope		Holter CT scan

Key Reference: Pavia S, Wikoff B. The management of surgical complications of pacemaker and implantable cardioverter-defibrillators. *Curr Opin Cardiol.* 2001;16:66–71.

Perioperative Implications

Monitoring
- Basic ASA monitors; ECG, BP, pulse oximetry

Anesthetic Technique
- Conscious sedation in the cardiac catheterization laboratory
- Monitored anesthesia care in the OR
- Regional anesthesia; local anesthesia at insertion site, field block of the supraclavicular nerves, interscalene block at C4, and interscalene block at C6

Maintenance
- Volatile agents, esp. enflurane, may suppress SA function.

Extubation/Emergence
- Emergence excitation may contribute to development of paroxysmal tachycardia.

Adjuvants
- Calcium-channel blockers, esp. verapamil, are contraindicated in the absence of pacemaking capability due to risk of inducing severe bradycardia.
- With a PPM present, paroxysmal tachycardia may be treated acutely with IV verapamil; digoxin may be added for longer-lasting rate control.

Anticipated Problems/Concerns

- Severe brady- and/or tachydysrhythmias 2° to anesthetic agents or autonomic imbalance are common in the periop period. Relative parasympathetic predominance in particular may be caused, for example, by high-dose opioid therapy or by maneuvers that increase vagal tone. Hence, in the anesthetic management of pts with SSS presenting for PPM implantation, drugs such as atropine, glycopyrrolate and isoproterenol should be immediately available should a sudden decrease in HR compromise hemodynamics before the new PPM is functional.

Pancreas Transplantation

Adam J. Munson-Young
Raymond M. Planinsic

Risk

- 35,000 new type 1 diabetics diagnosed yearly
- Transplant recipients usually <55 y old
- 1200–1300 transplants annually

Perioperative Risks

- Myocardial infarction
- Hemorrhage
- Hyper/hypoglycemia
- Seizure
- Immunosuppressive therapy complications

Worry About

- CV disease
- Renal insufficiency and/or failure
- Autonomic dysfunction
- Connective tissue defects
- Pulm function
- Glucose control

Overview

- Primary indication for transplant is insulin-dependent DM (Type I diabetes)
- Pts often have co-existing ESRD
- Simultaneous kidney and pancreas (SKP) transplant done in more than 80% of cases
- Pancreatic graft survival 86% at 1 y and 53% at 10 y when done with concomitant renal transplant
- Can lead to complete insulin independence

ICD9-CM: 648.0 (Diabetes mellitus)

Etiology

- End-organ damage from longstanding diabetes
- Macrovascular atherosclerosis leading to coronary artery and PVD states
- Microvascular damage of kidneys, heart, retina, and extremities
- Autonomic neuropathy of GI, cardiac, and urinary systems
- Collagen cross-linking defects

Usual Treatment

- Type I diabetics with renal failure most common, usually SPK transplant
- 15% transplanted after renal transplant
- 10% without renal disease, but with labile and difficult diabetic state

ASSESSMENT POINTS

System	Effect	Assessment by Hx	PE	Test
HEENT	Stiff joint syndrome Atlantooccipical fixation and decreased neck extension	Neck and/or finger stiffness	Neck extension, failure to oppose palms (prayer sign), abn palm print	
PULM	Decreased elasticity Restrictive changes Decreased DLCO2 and cough reactivity		Auscultation of lung fields	PFTs
CARDIO	Accelerated atherosclerosis CAD PVD	Co-morbid risk factors Functional capacity	Assess heart rhythm and rate	ECG, exercise or pharmacologic stress, ECHO, Holter monitoring
RENAL	Chronic failure leading to dialysis Anemia	Dialysis history UO Fatigue	Conjunctiva, mucous membrane pallor; functional murmur	Electrolytes BUN/creatinine CBC
NEURO	Autonomic dysfunction Peripheral neuropathy	Orthostatic hypotension, neurogenic bladder	Decreased peripheral sensation	Sitting/standing BP; tilt table test
ENDO	Pancreatic insufficiency	Hyper- and hypoglycemia Insulin therapy		Blood glucose
GI	Diabetic gastroparesis Delayed gastric emptying Decreased lower esophageal tone	GERD NPO status		

Key Reference: Larson-Wadd K, Belani KG. Pancreas and islet cell transplantation. *Anesthesiol Clin North America*. 2004;22(4):663–674.

Perioperative Implications

Preoperative Preparation

- Aspiration prophylaxis with sodium citrate, metoclopramide, or H_2
- Consider epidural placement for intra- and postop pain control

Monitoring

- Central venous catheter for access, CVP monitoring, vasopressor administration
- Arterial catheter for BP and frequent blood sampling
- Pulm artery catheter if warranted if pt has severe cardiac disease

Airway

- Intubations in diabetics can be problematic.
- Increased risk of difficult laryngoscopy due to stiff joint syndrome

Induction

- Avoid succinylcholine with hyperkalemia
- Minimize hypo- and Htn, tachycardia in pts with CAD
- Cisatracurium or mivacurium with severe renal disease

Maintenance/Intraoperative Management

- Antibiotic coverage for streptococci and gram-negative bacilli
- Judicious fluid administration in pts with renal disease
- Immunosuppressive medication administrated intraop
- Hyperglycemia is preferred over tight glucose control
- Transplanted organ begins functioning within hours, therefore avoid giving insulin and glucose containing solutions after reperfusion for better evaluation of organ function.

Extubation

- Often done in ICU in a controlled setting.
- Minimize BP and HR extremes to avoid cardiac events.
- Avoid severe Htn to preserve vascular anastamoses.

Postoperative Period

- Immediate and late complications can incl bleeding, rejection, infection, pancreatitis, and graft thrombosis.

Parathyroidectomy

Mary A. Blanchette

Risk

- Primary hyperparathyroidism 50-100/100,000 (USA); in women >45 incidence is 1/500
- Females > males
- Caused 90% by benign adenoma; 85% by single adenoma; 2–3% by 2 or more adenomas; 10–15 % by hyperplasia (all 4 glands); <1% by carcinoma (rare)
- 10% of parathyroid hyperplasia cases may exist as part of MEN 1 or MEN 2 syndrome (MEN 2 assoc with pheochromocytoma)

Perioperative Risks

- Moderate to severe hypercalcemia (serum calcium >11.5–13 mg/dL), may cause abn in cardiac conduction, arrhythmias, Htn; muscle weakness, nausea, depressed mental status
- Periop mortality rare
- Postop morbidity incl the following risks: Hypoparathyroidism <5%, injury to recurrent laryngeal nerve/vocal cord paresis <2%, hypocalcemia <1%, neck hematoma <1%

Worry About

- Symptomatic elevated serum calcium should be treated and controlled before elective parathyroidectomy (volume expansion, correction of electrolyte abn, furosemide diuresis, bisphosphonates, calcitonin/glucocorticoids)

- Periop injury to recurrent laryngeal nerve, with resultant unilateral vocal cord (VC) paresis (hoarseness, aspiration risk). For bilateral neck procedures, risk of bilateral VC paresis and complete postop airway obstruction
- Transient or complete hypoparathyroidism, with resultant hypocalcemia
- Postop bleeding/neck hematoma, with potential for airway compromise

Overview

- Low incidence of morbidity
- 80% of 1° hyperparathyroidism caused by single benign adenoma. Localization studies incl technetium Tc-99 labeled scan, cervical US, MRI, CT scan. 60% of single adenoma cases can be removed with minimally invasive parathyroidectomy
- Many pts are asymptomatic, have elevated calciums detected incidentally on screening labs

ICD-9-CM Code: 252.0 (Hyperplasia)

Etiology

- Hyperparathyroidism results from hypersecretion of parathyroid hormone by abn parathyroid tissue
- Classified as 1°, 2°, or ectopic

Indications and Usual Treatment

- Surgery is treatment of choice for symptomatic hypercalcemia (or Ca > 11 mg/dL), also indicated if evidence of nephrolithiasis or renal impairment, decreased bone density
- Single adenoma verified by localization studies can be treated with minimally invasive surgery technique (local/MAC or GA), advantage is shorter operative time and hospital stay, lower cost, better cosmetic result, possibly less PONV and pain, (unilateral small incision/endoscopy assisted) and similar success rate to conventional parathyroidectomy
- Multiple adenoma or parathyroid hyperplasia is treated with conventional collar incision, bilateral neck exploration, all four parathyroid glands identified, diseased glands removed, part of a single gland is left, or reimplanted in forearm to preserve some parathyroid function.

ASSESSMENT POINTS

System	Effect	Assessment by Hx	PE	Test
CARDIO	Conduction abn (short QT_c; prolonged P-R intervals assoc with hypercalcemia)			ECG Serum calcium level
	Htn			NIBP
GI	Assoc with MEN1 (hyperplasia) (insulinoma/pancreas tumors, gastrinomas) hypercalcemia	Vague abd pain Dyspepsia/N/V	Abd exam	CT scan/MRI EGD/endoscopic US Serum calcium, glucose, electrolytes
CNS	Hypercalcemia effects Neuromyopathic symptoms	Depression, memory problems, lethargy		
ENDO	Hyperparathyroidism			Serum PTH by ria
RENAL	Nephrolithiasis (60–70%) Renal insufficiency	Flank pain Polyuria Polydipsia	Flank tenderness	X-ray to look for stone GFR serum, BUN/creatinine
NM	Peripheral muscle weakness	Easily fatigued	Extremity exam	Ca^{2+} level
MS	Osteitis fibrosa cystica Osteopenia	Frequent fractures Bone pain	Skeletal exam	Bone density studies

Key Reference: Grant SG, Thompson G, Farley D, van Heerden J. Primary hyperparathyroidism surgical management since the introduction of minimally invasive parathyroidectomy. *Arch Surg* 2005;140:472–479.

Perioperative Management

Preoperative Preparation

- Treat hypercalcemia: Volume expansion, diuresis accompanied by phosphate repletion
- Glucocorticoids, mithramycin, calcitonin may be used if necessary
- Review ECG for conductions abn (short QT, prolonged PR), signs LVH
- Review preop workup incl ENT surgeon's preop fiberoptic exam of larynx (confirms baseline anatomy), summary of localizing studies, CT scan. Discuss surgical plan with surgeon (minimally invasive technique vs. bilateral procedure, local/MAC vs GA)

Monitoring

- Standard ASA monitors

Airway

- Consider use of NIM EMG ETT (Xomed NIM II Medtronic) to aid surgeon in confirming location of recurrent laryngeal nerve. Monitors vocal cord tension by audible signal, with recurrent nerve stimulation by surgeon.

Preinduction/Induction

- Choices for minimally invasive technique incl local and/or MAC, GA, GA with EMG ETT
- Careful positioning important in osteopenic pts at risk for fracture. Arms at sides, neck extended with head on donut
- Protect eyes
- After induction, baseline PTH level is drawn. It's helpful to have access to hand and/or foot for blood draws intraop 50% drop in PTH level 5 min after adenoma removal confirms hypersecretory gland successfully removed.

Maintenance

- Avoid acidosis (acidosis, incl resp acidosis, will increase serum calcium level)
- Avoid muscle relaxant during maintenance if using EMG/NIM ETT, deeper anesthetic depth required to avoid bucking on ETT with tracheal manipulation.
- Expect intraop frozen sections to positively identify parathyroid tissue, and rule out carcinoma (rare).

Emergence

- Control BP, minimize coughing, bucking, or increased venous pressure in the neck to decrease the chance for postop neck hematoma.
- Evaluate immediately after extubation for signs of airway obstruction or compromise (edema, hematoma, vocal cord paresis). Increased risk of aspiration with vocal cord paresis.

Anticipated Problems/Concerns

- Potential for postop airway obstruction from intraop injury to recurrent laryngeal nerves with resultant VC paresis, neck hematoma, glottic edema
- Monitor serum calcium levels postop: Decrease will occur within 24 hr if adenoma successfully removed, calcium nadir 3–7 d. Also monitor serum phosphate, magnesium, PTH
- Untreated hypocalcemia may cause tetany, laryngospasm, seizure (treat with IV calcium)
- Chvostek's sign (facial muscle contraction with facial nerve tap) and Trousseau's sign (carpedal spasm with application of BP cuff) are classic signs warning of the potential for tetany from hypocalcemia.

Patent Ductus Arteriosus (PDA), Ligation of

Justin Lockman
Eugenie Heitmiller

Prevalence

- Full-term infants: 1/2500 live births
- Premature infants
  20% <1750 g
  50% <1200 g
  65% <30 wk gestation and RDS
- Occurs in 5–10% of all congenital heart defects (excluding premature infants)
- Risk increases with severity of neonatal RDS
- M:F ratio: 1:2

Perioperative Risks

- Periop mortality rare (approaches zero)
- Hemorrhage due to vascular injury
- Recurrent laryngeal nerve (RLN) injury
- Inadvertent ligation of aorta, pulm artery or subclavian vessels

Worry About

- Hypothermia
- Uncontrolled hemorrhage
- Vagally mediated reflex bradycardia
- Desaturation with lung retraction

Overview

- Ductus arteriosus (DA) is essential to maintaining fetal systemic perfusion
- DA functionally closes within 8 hr after birth when smooth muscle constricts in response to increased O_2 tension (from 18–28 mmHg in utero to 40–60 mmHg postnatally)
- Anatomic closure of DA with intimal remodeling and loss of smooth muscle occurs over next several days
- DA sensitivity to increased O_2 tension is diminished in preterm infant.
- Fluid overload, RDS or severe illness (e.g., acidosis, hypoxia) may re-open a functionally closed DA prior to anatomic closure.
- Patent ductus arteriosus (PDA) leads to L=>R shunt that results in:
  - Pulm overload: CHF, tachypnea, dyspnea on exertion or with feeding, atelectasis, recurrent resp infections, FTT, and feeding intolerance
- Hyperactive precordium and widened pulse pressure: Diastolic hypotension (runoff) and enhanced cardiac output from increased sympathetic tone related to fluid overload
- Rare cases of pulm Htn and R=>L shunting resulting in cyanosis of lower half of body; cardiac output may fall with PDA ligation in these pts
- Effect of PDA size on shunt flow
  - Small diameter PDA: Shunt flow usually limited by restrictive PDA diameter
  - Large diameter PDA: Flow also dependent on ratio of pulm vascular resistance to systemic vascular resistance

ICD-9-CM Code: 747.0 (Patent ductus arteriosus)

ASSESSMENT POINTS

System	Effect	Assessment by Hx	PE	Tests
CARDIO	Shunt-(usually L=>R) Diastolic runoff	Exercise intolerance	Continuous machinery murmur Hyperactive precordium Bounding palmar pulses	ECHO NIBP
RESP	CHF	Diuretic dependence	Rales/crackles	CXR
GI	Bowel ischemia	Poor feeding	Abd distension	Abd XR Hemoccult
RENAL	Renal ischemia	Poor UO	Fluid overload	Creatinine

Key References: Hermes-DeSantis ER, Clyman RI. Patent ductus arteriosus: Pathophysiology and management. *J Perinatol.* 2006;26:S14–S18.
Schneider DJ, Moore JW. Patent ductus arteriosus. *Circulation.* 2006;114:1873–1882.

Indications and Usual Treatment

- Medical management: Fluid restriction (120 mL/kg/day) and diuretics
- Pharmacologic closure for neonates: NSAIDs (indomethacin, ibuprofen) inhibit prostaglandin production and are effective in many cases.
- Surgical options for failed pharmacologic closure in neonates (usually after two doses) or for older pts with PDA:
  - Open thoracotomy (most common): Usually a clip for premature infants; otherwise ligation and division
    - Video-assisted thoracoscopic clip ligation
    - Transcatheter closure in select pts: Coil for <4 mm in diameter; Amplatzer® PDA device if >4 mm diameter

Perioperative Management

Preoperative Preparation

- Warm the OR prior to pt arrival
- Have RBC products available in the OR prior to incision
- Clear bubbles from all IV tubing
- Ensure peripheral or central vascular access large enough for red cell transfusion
- Check for assoc congenital anomalies of airway
- Pt transport is major risk for premature neonates; consider performing procedure in the neo-NICU if feasible

Anesthetic Technique

- General anesthesia

Airway

- Mechanical ventilation during procedure
- Usually two lung ventilation with single lumen ETT in infants
- One lung ventilation in select older pts

Monitoring

- Two pulse oximetry probes: Right hand (preductal) and one lower extremity (postductal) for confirmation of correct vessel ligation
- Capnography useful for detecting inadvertent pulm artery ligation or compression
- Noninvasive BP; invasive BP monitoring generally not necessary except in critically ill children
- Monitoring and maintenance of temp essential (very high surface area to mass ratio)

Induction/Maintenance

- Narcotic and/or ketamine induction preferred in neonates
- Mask induction appropriate for older children
- May require fluid resuscitation at induction because of preop fluid restriction and diuretics
- Avoid high FIO_2 if possible; this could increase shunting to pulm vasculature
- May need to check vocal cord function at end of case if at risk of RLN injury

Surgical Stages

Incision

- Thoracotomy incision; side depends on aortic arch orientation (normally left)

Dissection

- Lung retraction may produce hypoxia and hypercarbia

- Watch for vagally mediated reflex bradycardia; treat with atropine as needed

Ligation

- PDA is usually ligated (suture or clip); may or may not be surgically divided
- Although blood loss usually minimal, must be prepared for hemorrhage due to vessel injury or inadequate ligation
- Watch for intraop Htn after ligation; risk of stroke in neonates

Postoperative Considerations

- Postop CXR to check for pneumothorax
  - Many centers now use small-tube thoracostomy or no thoracostomy tube
- Optimal analgesia is essential for recovery
  - IV PCA (with or without intercostal nerve blocks)
  - Continuous neuraxial analgesia in select pts
- Neonates may require prolonged intubation and ongoing postop resp management
- Premature infants may develop postop hypotension

Anticipated Problems/Concerns

- CV collapse at ligation: Undiagnosed anomalous coronary artery or pulm Htn
- Residual ductal patency may result in intravascular hemolysis and ongoing hemodynamic symptoms
- Vocal cord/RLN palsy may occur after ligation (even after transcatheter device techniques)
- Risk of thoracic duct injury and chylothorax

Pituitary Resection, Transsphenoidal Approach

Stephen M. Rupp

Risk

- Pituitary adenoma: 14–20/100,000
- Males > females, 1:2

Perioperative Risks

- <1% immediate periop mortality
- 8–15% morbidity (transient–1 to 3 d–DI most frequent); hypopituitarism in large resections; CN II – VI damage
- Microadenomas of all types can have up to 90% cure rates in some surgical series
- 50% of untreated acromegalics die before age 50 y
- Untreated Cushing's disease has a 50% 5-y mortality

Worry About

- Increased ICP in large tumors; anemia preop
- Airway in acromegalics and Cushing's syndrome
- Intraop injection of epinephrine-containing local anesthetics to vasoconstrict nasal mucosa

(precipitate dysrhythmias or myocardial ischemia); severe Htn if β-blocker present
- Hemorrhage intraop (cavernous sinus intrusion or carotid artery injury)
- Air embolism reported
- Saddle deformity of nose postop
- Blood in airway at end of procedure
- Corneal abrasion if exophthalmos in Cushing's
- DI or SIADH postop

Overview

- Pituitary microadenoma usual indication for surgery; most common complaint is headache. Any tumor may cause hyperprolactinemia 2° to loss of tonic inhibition

Etiology

In descending order of frequency, tissue types/ most common presenting symptoms are:
- Nonsecreting adenoma/visual field defect, headache, CN II–VI may be affected by pressure
- Prolactin-secreting adenoma/amenorrhea; galactorrhea, lost libido, infertility

- ACTH-secreting tumor/Cushing's disease; obesity, Htn, LVH, diabetes, sleep apnea
- Growth hormone–secreting tumor/acromegaly, Htn, LVH, cardiomyopathy, diastolic dysfunction, diabetes, sleep apnea, hypertropic mandible/facial bones, laryngeal stenosis
- Thyrotropic adenomas (rare): Signs and sx hyperthyroidism, palpitations, tremor, wt loss, sweating

ICD-9-CM Codes: 253.0 (Acromegaly); 255.0 (Cushing's syndrome)

Usual Treatment

- Bromocriptine is first line of Rx for prolactin-secreting tumors and can suppress GH tumors
- Somatostatin analogues (octreotide, simvistatin) in thyrotropic adenomas
- Irradiation used as single treatment and surgical adjuvant in selected cases
- Surgical treatment is choice for macroadenomas (>10 mm in diameter) ± radiation later

ASSESSMENT POINTS

System	Effect	Assessment by Hx	PE	Test
HEENT	Airway in acromegalics; glottic fixation or narrowing in GH excess Airway in Cushing's	Hoarseness, sleep apnea? Tongue size, stridor/DOE?	Airway	
	CN III–VI impingement	Visual disturbance, field cut	Visual field	
CARDIO	Htn in acromegaly and Cushing's	CV status, LVH? Exercise tolerance Chest pain, sleep apnea?		ECG Hb/Hct
RESP	↓ FRC in obese	SOB, DOE		ABGs, SpO$_2$
ENDO	DM Hypercortisolism Hypopituitarism	Glucose intolerance		Glucose Thyroxine, TSH, Cortisol, Na+, Ca++
RENAL	Hypertensive or diabetic kidney disease			Cr, GFR
CNS	↑ ICP in severe suprasellar extension	Headache, N/V	Visual field	Funduscopic exam

Key Reference: Nemergut EC, Dumont AS, Barry UT, Laws ER. Perioperative management of patients undergoing transsphenoidal pituitary surgery. *Anesth Analg.* 2005;101:1170–1181.

Perioperative Implications

Preoperative Preparation

- Evaluate for significant CAD (Hx, ECG, exercise tolerance); may suffer myocardial stress from exogenous epinephrine, sleep apnea?
- Case requires oral ET tube; plan fiberoptic intubation if indicated
- Surgeon may request lumbar subarachnoid drain to manipulate CSF (inject saline or remove CSF) or inject air intraop to outline suprasellar extension and monitor progress of resection. Postop, CSF catheter may be placed to drain if CSF leak anticipated.

Anesthetic Technique

- GA required

Monitoring

- Routine + air embolism (ETCO$_2$)
- A-Line if cardiomyopathy/CHF in acromegalics/Cushing's

Airway

- In acromegalics, hypertrophy of facial bones, jaw, nose, turbinates, soft palate, tonsils, epiglottis, and larynx may occur: Mask fit/intubation may be difficult. Fiberoptic intubation may be indicated.

Induction/Maintenance

- Rapid-acting induction agent acceptable
- Maintain anesthetic with narcotic, volatile anesthetic ± N$_2$O and relaxant
- Target Paco$_2$ = 34–38 mmHg
- ± Subarachnoid drain prior to final positioning
- Surgical positioning: Semi-sitting 5–35° head-up
- Placement of tongs: Watch for adrenergic/hypertensive response
- Injection of epinephrine containing local anesthetic to vasoconstrict: Watch for dysrhythmias, Htn, myocardial ischemia
- Transnasal approach, endoscopic endo nasal more common, or nasal septal and sublabial incision (blood loss)
- Placement of transsphenoidal speculum or endoscope: Bone work, needs fluoroscopic control to ensure midline approach (high anesthetic requirement for this stage)
- Adenoma removal under direct visualization with microscope
- If suprasellar extension, surgeon may want saline or air injected: if air, D/C N$_2$O
- If lateral extension of tumor occurs, excessive bleeding may ensue from invasion of cavern-

ous sinus or carotid artery. Induced hypotension via high concentration volatile anesthetic may improve visualization and allow adequate hemorrhage control.
- Rebuilding sella turcica (part of nasal septum used)
- If CSF leak with valsalva, pack with fat pad (abd wall donor site)
- Close, EBL: 150–400 mL

Extubation

- Aim to have pt awake, comfortable, and cooperative prior to extubation
- Mouth and pharynx packed with gauze to prevent blood in stomach or airway; ensure its removal at end of case

Adjuvants

- PONV prophylaxis, be ready to Tx Htn (labetolol)

Postoperative Period

- Headache, pain score: 2–3
- Assess CN II – VI function
- Disorders of H$_2$O balance: DI or SIADH in up to 25% of cases
- DI in 8–15%, usually transient. Dx via analysis of high volume (3–6 mL/kg/h) of dilute urine

(<200 mOsm/L, specific gravity = 1.001–1.005). May require desmopressin (DDAVP) 0.1 mg po or 1 mcg SQ q4–6h if serum Na+ >145 meq/L. Replace urinary losses. If serum >320 Osm/L, replace H_2O loss.
• Delayed hyponatremia (SIADH). Serum Na+ <135 mEq/L. Confirm high urine Na$^+$ (>20 mEq/L) + euvolemia. Tx: Restrict H_2O. If Na$^+$ <120 consider slow hypertonic saline
• CSF rhinorrhea: Lumbar CSF drain to reduce CSF pressure
• If excessive packing needed to control cavernous sinus bleeding, CN II, IV, or VI compression can occur. Impingement of cavernous internal carotid can result in carotid spasm.
• If air has been injected subarachnoid, tension pneumocephalus can occur
• Hypopituitarism postop

Pneumonectomy

Paula A. Craigo

Risk

- Primarily for bronchogenic CA; median age 73 y
- <20% of non-small cell CA surgeries; lobectomy often as effective
- Benign: Mycobacteria, fungus, infection/necrosis, trauma

Perioperative Risks

- Mortality up to 12% within 30 d
- Cardiac morbidity significant
- Morbidity and/or mortality higher after right pneumonectomy, more complex procedure, some benign diseases
- Mortality for trauma and/or massive hemoptysis >35%

Worry About

- Pulm reserve and/or pulm Htn, edema, after resection
- Concomitant CV disease
- Cardiac arrhythmias common postop
- Periop thromboembolic events in 26%
- Benign diseases: Neovascularization, high-pressure bronchial system bleed; soiling of contralateral lung

Overview

- Mortality of untreated non-small cell lung CA is 100%; treatment is surgery
- Paraneoplastic syndromes not a contraindication
- Effective for drug-resistant TB
- Last resort for traumatic injury: Resection in hypovolemic shock leading to persistent high

PVR and R heart failure: Pulm vasodilators, NO may be tried

ICD-9-CM Codes: 162.2–9 (Primary lung cancer); CPT code 32.5 (Pneumonectomy)

Indications and Usual Treatment

- Non–small cell lung CA (T2) with hilar involvement, no distant mets; mainstem bronchus involvement or crossing major fissure
- T3 lesions: Plus resection of involved chest wall, diaphragm, mediastinal pleura and/or pericardium
- Sleeve pneumonectomy: resection of carina, ipsilateral lung, and bronchial tree; anastomosis of contralateral mainstem bronchus to distal trachea

ASSESSMENT POINTS

System	Effect	Assessment by Hx	PE	Test
HEENT	Recurrent laryngeal nerve involvement	Hoarseness	HEENT exam	
CARDIO	RV dysfunction due to PA Htn LV function, valvular disease Arrhythmias	Chest pain/SOB Exercise tolerance, palpitations	CV exam	ECG, possible ECHO, Doppler studies, PA catheterization
RESP	Sputum, bronchospasm; ability to tolerate loss of lung	SOB, exercise tolerance, sputum, smoking Hx	Resp exam Clubbing	Chest CT; ABGs; PFTs: FEV_1, DLco Quantitative VQ scan; VO_2max; *See note*
ENDO	Hypercalcemia; SIADH → hyponatremia; Cushing's syndrome	Somnolence, anorexia, N/V, wt loss, signs of water intoxication		Check Ca^{2+}, Na^+; SIADH → hypotonic plasma, relatively hypertonic urine, Cushing's, hypokalemic alkalosis
HEME	Anemia, polycythemia Migratory thrombophlebitis	Hx of thrombophlebitis		Hct
NM	Eaton-Lambert syndrome (E-L) Polymyositis		Muscle wasting	E-L: Sensitivity to nondep muscle relaxants

Note: Acceptable risk: DLCO >60%; FEV1 >60%predicted if no pulm Htn; quantitative V/Q scans predict postop DLCO >40% FEV, > 40% or VO_2max > 15 mL/kg/min. Test values are used to define risk to the patient to aid in informed decision-making, not as rigid limits prohibiting attempted surgical cure.

Key Reference: Slinger P. Update on anesthetic management for pneumonectomy. *Curr Opin Anaesthesiol.* 2009;22:31–37.

Perioperative Implications

Preoperative Preparation
- Bronchodilators
- If sputum: Antibiotics, hydration, mobilization
- Prophylactic digoxin not warranted

Monitoring
- Arterial line; CVP not routine intraop, but may be useful postop
- PA: Place on nonop side; fluoroscopy helpful; consider TEE

Airway
- If difficult airway or unable to intubate orally; bronchial blocker, nasal intubation
- Aspiration devastating

Induction/Maintenance
- Lateral decubitus positioning: Check ear and eye on down side, axillary roll, arm positioning
- Potent inhalational agents bronchodilate but ↓ LV function, attenuate hypoxic vasoconstriction; ↑ in Qs/Qt not clinically significant at 1.0 MAC

- Problems with one-lung ventilation techniques: Trauma, malposition, hypoxemia
- Limit intraop tidal volume, fluids (EBL <500 mL; capillary leak and loss of pulm tissue risks pulm edema)

Surgical Stages

Dissection and Surgery
- Posterolateral thoracotomy incision in 5th or 6th intercostal space for best exposure
- Vessels and mainstem bronchus evaluated for resectability; stapled
- Closure tested with positive pressure breath
- Postpneumonectomy space: Intermittent aspiration of air or special system used to balance mediastinum; excess mediastinal shift can leads to CV collapse

Postoperative Considerations
- CXR: Check mediastinum, trachea midline
- Cardiac arrhythmias >20%, usually supraventricular
- Postop pulm edema mortality up to 50%

- Pulm insufficiency
- Significant postop pain: Epidural analgesia probably most effective

Anticipated Problems/Concerns

- Hypotension from unrecognized blood loss; cardiac tamponade; MI/ischemia with low CO
- Postop pulm edema: R/O myocardial dysfunction; volume overload; treat dysrhythmias, hypoalbuminemia; atelectasis, pneumonitis
- DVT and pulm embolism common (20%)
- Persistent air leak
- Excess mediastinal shift life-threatening
- Cardiac herniation (mortality >50%); after R pneumonectomy, cardiac torsion→shock, SVC syndrome; after L resection, pericardial compression→ischemia, arrhythmias, outflow tract obstruction; RX: Full lateral with op side up; surgical emergency
- Empyema in 5%
- Bronchopleural fistula in 4%

Pregnant Surgical Patient

Ihab Kamel

Risk

- Incidence in USA: 75,000 pregnant pts/year undergo nondelivery procedures
- Most common: Trauma-related procedures, cervical suture, appendectomy, biliary tract disease–related procedures, breast biopsy, ovarian cystectomy
- Major procedures such as liver transplantation, cardiopulmonary bypass and craniotomy have been performed during pregnancy with good outcomes to the mother and fetus.
- Surgery is performed in pregnancy in about 1–2% of pts. The number is increasing due to laparoscopic procedures.

Perioperative Risks

- ↑ Maternal anesthetic risk for hypoxemia
- ↑ Maternal risk pulm aspiration due to failed ET intubation (increased mucosal vascularity and weight gain distortion of pharyngeal anatomy)
- Potential risk to fetus
  - Preterm delivery (preterm labor incidence 8–11%, higher for pelvic procedures)
  - Teratogenicity

Worry About

- Maternal airway precautions
- Gastric chemoprophylaxis
- Prevention and treatment of maternal hypoxemia
- Avoidance of aortocaval compression (after 20 wk of gestation) and hypotension (uterine blood flow is not autoregualted)
- Detection and treatment of preterm labor

Overview

- If surgery must be performed during pregnancy, 2nd trimester is preferred period, since organogenesis is complete and risk of preterm delivery relatively low
- Acute exposure to anesthetic agents has not been assoc with fetal malformations at birth
- Depressant effects of anesthetic agents are mainly of concern if fetus is delivered periop

ICD-9-CM Code: V22.2 (Pregnancy)

Indications and Usual Treatment

- Cervical suture placement for prevention of preterm delivery due to cervical incompetence (performed at 12–16 wk of gestation)
- Other procedures performed only when risks of postponement outweigh benefits of avoiding increased maternal anesthetic risk and potential fetal harm

ASSESSMENT POINTS

System	Effect	Assessment by Hx	PE	Test
HEENT	Engorged, fragile mucosa, difficult intubation		Airway exam	Mallampati class
CV	Supine hypotensive syndrome	Nausea, diaphoresis while supine	Assess for hypotension, bradycardia while supine	
RESP	↑ O_2 consumption; ↓ FRC ↑ Pao_2, ↓ $Paco_2$			ABGs (if indicated)
GI	Full stomach, decreased LES tone	Reflux symptoms		
CNS	↓ MAC, ↓ intraspinal local anesthetic requirements			

Key Reference: Naughton NN, Cohen SE. Nonobstetric surgery during pregnancy. In: Chestnut DH, ed. *Obstetric anesthesia: principles and practice*. 3rd ed. Philadelphia: Mosby; 2004:255–272.

Perioperative Management

Anesthetic Technique

- Regional anesthesia: ↓ Risk of maternal airway problems, ↑ risk of hypotension (compared with GA). Regional anesthesia might be considered the first choice where appropriate.
- General anesthesia: Inhalation agents are tocolytic—may prevent contractions in OR; however, preterm labor may occur in recovery period. Endotracheal intubation and rapid sequence induction after 14–18 wk of gestation.

Monitoring

- Viable-gestational-age fetus (18–22 wk): Consider pre-, intra-, postop fetal heart tone and uterine activity monitoring.
- Loss of beat-to-beat variability (present by 25–27 wk) is normal with anesthetics.
- Fetal heart rate decelerations are abn and should be managed by improving maternal oxygenation, raising BP and increasing left uterine displacement

- Nonviable-gestational-age fetus: Pre- and postop fetal heart tone documentation; consider pre-, intra-, and postop uterine activity monitoring
- Obstetric consultation highly recommended; pediatric notification indicated if delivery of a viable fetus is possible

Airway

- Edema and engorgement: ↑ risk of failed intubation, ↑ risk of bleeding, esp. during nasal intubation
- ↑ Risk of pulm aspiration

Induction

- Regional anesthesia: Spinal, epidural, or other block may be appropriate depending on location of surgical site
- General anesthesia: Full stomach—awake intubation vs. denitrogenation followed by rapid-sequence induction

Maintenance

- Maintain left uterine displacement

- General anesthesia: Inhalation agent—consider NO, opioid, benzodiazepine (last often avoided in 1st trimester, although acute exposure not thought to be teratogenic). Muscle relaxants—minimal placental transfer.

Extubation

- After pt awake, able to protect airway

Postoperative Considerations

- Pain: Consider IV or epidural PCA (opioids should not be withheld). Avoid nonsteroidal anti-inflamatory drugs.
- Left uterine displacement in PACU
- Document fetal viability
- Consider monitoring for preterm labor

Anticipated Problems/Concerns

- Pulm aspiration, failed intubation
- Preterm labor
- Fetal distress

Pyloric Stenosis Repair

J. Lance Lichtor
Ulrike Berth

Risk

- 1-4/1000 births
- Highest concentration in whites of northern European ancestry, lower incidence in African-Americans, rare in Asians
- M:F ratio: 4:1
- Tends to run in families (children of affected parents have higher incidence [20% of male and 10% of female descendants of mother who had pyloric stenosis])
- 2.5–5.5 times higher incidence for firstborn
- Increased incidence with types B and O blood groups
- Average age of onset is 1–2 mo, though can occur as early as first week of life and as late as the fifth month.
- Etiology unknown, increased incidence after repair of congenital abn (e.g., esophagel atresia, omphalocele, hyperplasia or agenesis of inferior labial frenulum)

Perioperative Risks

- Hypotension due to preop hypovolemia and volume shifts common
- Hypoglycemia common with postop apnea or convulsions due to cessation of IV glucose and inadequate glycogen stores
- Mortality: 0–0.5 %
- Wound infection: 5–20%

Worry About

- Fluid and electrolyte deficiency (hypochloremic metabolic alkalosis, hypokalemia) though can also be hyperkalemic
- Full stomach, risk for aspiration, despite suctioning
- Postop apnea due to immature ventilatory control
- Not a surgical emergency

Overview

- Gross thickening (hypertrophy) at circular smooth muscle of pylorus resulting in gradual obstruction of gastric outlet
- Nonbilious projectile (no projectile initially but usually progressive) vomiting occurring immediately after feeding; usually 2–4 wk; can have severe dehydration and acid-base abn
- Surgical treatment is curative
- Not a surgical emergency

ICD-9-CM Code: 750.5

Indications and Usual Treatment

- Persistent vomiting usually after or toward the end of a feed. After vomiting, infant is hungry and wants to feed again, until dehydration profound, when the infant becomes lethargic.
- Pyloromyotomy is treatment of choice
- No successful medical therapy

ASSESSMENT POINTS

System	Effect	Assessment by Hx	PE	Test
GI	Pyloric thickening	Vomiting	Olive-size mass, upper abd	US or upper GI series
HEME	Hemoconcentration		Volume status measures; orthostatic vital signs Vasoconstriction	Hct
LYTES	Dehydration Acid-base abn		Volume status measures; orthostatic vital signs; area with cold skin	Electrolytes Hypokalemia, hyperkalemia
RENAL	Alkaline urine (initial) Acid urine (late)	Persistent vomiting Volume depletion		UO

Key Reference: Allan C. Determinants of good outcome in pyloric stenosis. *J Paediatr Child Health.* 2006;42:86–88.

Perioperative Implications

- Correct electrolyte, acid-base abn and hypovolemia
- Gastric secretions are lost; therefore, hypochloremic alkalosis results
- Renal compensation through Na⁺ retention and acidic urine excretion
- Stop oral feeds, replace ECF volume, monitor K⁺

Monitoring
- Standard ASA monitors

Airway
- Risk of aspiration: Evacuate stomach contents (↑ Risk despite suctioning)
- Consider rapid-sequence induction or spinal anesthesia
- NG tube after induction

Maintenance
- Avoid narcotics: Rarely needed, prolong awakening

- Volatile anesthetic, consider desflurane (rapid awakening, decreased episodes of apnea)
- Local anesthetics using local infiltration of skin with bupivacaine (maximum dose 1 mL/kg of 0.25% bupivacaine) useful in combination with general anesthesia

Postoperative
- Apnea (continue close monitoring)
- Hypoglycemia
- Continue volume and fluid resuscitation
- Consider acetaminophen for pain control (40 mg/kg initial dose followed by 20 mg/kg every 6 hr rectally or 10–15 mg/kg by mouth every 4–6 hr for a total 24-hr dose of 100 mg/kg)

Surgical Stages

Induction
- Consider emptying stomach before induction

Skin Incision
- Abd opened through right transverse skin incision above liver edge, a right paramedian incision or three laparoscopic access sites

Dissection
- Pylorus delivered into wound (open procedure); incision through serosa and extended through the length of hypertrophic pylorus; hypertrophied muscle split bluntly

Anticipated Problems/Concerns

- Hypotension due to altered volume status
- Hypoglycemia and convulsions, possibly due to cessation of IV glucose and depletion of liver glycogen
- Severe metabolic disturbance (correct preop)
- Apnea, possibly related to cerebrospinal fluid alkalosis
- Vomiting on induction, postop vomiting if early feeds
- Wound infection not uncommon
- Duodenal perforation may occur during myotomy; not a life-threatening problem if recognized intraop

Radical Neck Dissection

Laura Cavallone

Risk

- More than half a million cases of new head and neck cancers every year worldwide
- Risk of head and neck cancers assoc with long-term smoking, alcohol abuse, and viral infection with HPV
- M:F ratio: 3:1

Perioperative Risks

- Periop morbidity and mortality assoc with multiple comorbidities
- Risk of MI, CVAs as per CV comorbidities related to smoking and/or alcohol abuse
- Risk of cranial nerves and major vessels injury, venous air embolism and pnx depend on site/level of surgery and technique used

Worry About

- Presence of tumor may affect airway patency (obstruction/compression/deviation)
- Previous radiation therapy can cause difficult airway management (edema, fibrosis)
- Long-term smoking in these pts frequently assoc with COPD
- Alcohol abuse linked to liver failure, anemia, neurologic impairment, postop withdrawal, DT
- Malnutrition

Overview

- The term radical neck dissection implies removal of all cervical lymph node groups that are ipsilateral to the cancerous lesion, from level I to V. The spinal accessory nerve (SAN), the sterno-cleidomastoid muscle (SCM) and the internal jugular vein (IJV) are also removed

- Modified neck dissections preserve SAN, SCM and/or IJV. Selective neck dissections preserve one or more lymph node groups, depending on the location of the tumor

ICD-9-CM Code: 40.40 (Radial neck dissection, not otherwise specified)

Indications and Usual Treatment

- Neck dissections are the procedures of choice to control the spreading of metastases from cancers of the upper airway, thyroid, parotid glands, and upper digestive tract
- Often are performed in combination with the resection of the 1° tumor
- Surgical defect may need repair with flap and/or skin graft

ASSESSMENT POINTS

System	Effect	Assessment by Hx	PE	Test
HEENT	Tumor impact on airway	Dyspnea, dysphagia, dysarthria	Direct and FO airway exam	CXR, CT/MRI, flow-volume loops
CARDIO	Smoking and alcohol-related co-morbidities	SOB, exercise tolerance, Hx of palpitations and/or chest pain	CV exam	CXR, ECG, stress test echocardiogram/angio
RESP	Smoking related	SOB, cough, sputum	Chest auscultation	CXR, PFTs, consider ABG
HEME	Anemia, coagulation abn	Fatigue, bleeding, easy bruising	Inspection of skin, mucosae	CBC, PT, PTT, LFTs
CNS	Alcohol withdrawal Nutritional deficiencies	Anxiety, tachycardia, diaphoresis, peripheral neuropathy	Neuro exam	Based on Hx and PE

Key Reference: Kerawala CJ, Heliotis M. Prevention of complications in neck dissection. *Head Neck Oncol.* 2009;1:35.

Perioperative Management

Preoperative Preparation

- Prepare for table rotation at 180° (head of pt 180° away from anesthesia provider) with extensions on IV lines and ventilator circuit
- 2 large-bore peripheral IVs required also considering arms tucked and 180° rotation (consider CVC if peripheral access not adequate; femoral line preferred, as neck is site of surgery)
- Prepare blood infusion set connected to fluid warmer

Monitoring

- Standard + Temperature measuring urinary catheter + A-line +/− CVC for invasive BP/CVP monitoring
- Consider minimally invasive hemodynamic monitors based on beat-by-beat derivation of hemodynamic variables from A-line waveform
- Close monitoring of NMB: Complete reversal of muscle relaxation must be obtained to allow nerve monitoring by surgeon

Anesthetic Technique/Induction

- General anesthesia with ETT inserted orally (DL or FO technique), unless elective awake tracheostomy is required to secure airway

Maintenance

- General inhalational/IV anesthesia + opioid continuous infusion (infusion pump required)
- Avoid peripheral vasoconstrictors if flap reconstruction is part of the procedure
- Cautious fluid management is recommended, better if goal directed, as guided by hemodynamic monitoring
- Administration of LMWH is suggested to prevent venous thrombosis

Surgical Stages

- Neck incision and dissecting technique may vary
- Large vessels and nerves can be damaged with risk of significant blood loss and nerve paralysis
- Occasionally carotid artery is sacrificed when invaded by tumor

- Duration: 4–8 hr (mono or bilateral). If combined with tumor resection and flap reconstruction, may take up to 20 hrs or more.

Postoperative Considerations

- Pts that have been intubated and have not had a tracheostomy during the case may be extubated immediately after surgery (esp if monolateral neck dissection) or kept intubated overnight (bilateral neck dissection, combined tumor resection/flap reconstruction)
- Pts with tracheostomy /stoma may also be allowed to wake up immediately after surgery (calm, optimal pain control) or kept sedated overnight.

Anticipated Problems/Concerns

- Preventing coughing and retching at emergence is of paramount importance to avoid straining of sutures and rebleeding.
- Adequate nutritional support, pulm toilet and treatment of potential alcohol withdrawal symptoms are critical points in the postop management of these pts.

Radical Prostatectomy (Retropubic)

Lee A. Fleisher

Risk

- 50,000 pts/y but decreasing with alternative therapies (randomized outcome data shows requires about 48 ops to save 1 life with this procedure) Often done robotically now.
- Racial predominance: None

Perioperative Risks

- Periop mortality rare (<1%)
- Increased risk of DVT, pulm embolism
- 25% risk of impotence with nerve-sparing procedure; 75% risk without nerve-sparing procedure

Worry About

- Venous air embolism
- Massive blood loss
- Nerve injury from position and surgical manipulation
- Often in flexed position with head down, increasing risk of aspiration

Overview

- Prostate, bladder, and seminal vesicles are removed
- Significant blood loss assoc with transection of dorsal vein
- Regional anesthesia may be assoc with lower blood loss and lower incidence of DVT
- Laparoscopic procedure rarely being performed
- Although autologous predonation common, becoming less widely used
- Consider hemodilution techniques to ↓ blood loss
- Myocardial ischemia ↑ if Hct <28%
- Epidural analgesia with general anesthesia and use of NSAIDs prior to operation may reduce cancer recurrence rates compared to general anesthesia and postop opioids

ICD-9-CM Code: 185.0 (Cancer of prostate)

Indications and Usual Treatment

- The following conditions should be met:
  - Isolated and localized prostatic malignancy
  - Anticipated life expectancy of ≥10 y
  - Good general health
  - Absence of indication of metastatic disease by work-up
- Robotically assisted prostatectomy becoming more common
- If co-existing disease, orchiectomy and hormonal therapy 1° treatment
- Radiation therapy has similar 5-y survival rates
- "Smart bomb" radiation therapies also have similar 5-y survival rates with less surrounding tissue toxicity than classic radiation therapy
- Proton therapy newer option without known success rate
- Herbal therapies are alternative—8 hydroxy compounds in green teas have effectiveness in experimental animal models

ASSESSMENT POINTS

System	Effect	Assessment by Hx	PE	Test
RESP	Pulm metastases	SOB	Auscultation	CXR, CT scan
MS	Skeletal metastases	Bone pain	Palpation	X-ray, bone scan, prostate-specific antigen (PSA)
RENAL	Chronic obstruction			Cr and/or BUN

Key Reference: Biki B, Mascha E, Moriarty DC, Fitzpatrick JM, Sessler DI, Buggy DJ. Anesthetic technique for radical prostatectomy surgery affects cancer recurrence: A retrospective analysis. *Anesthesiology*. 2008;109:180–187.

Perioperative Implications

Anesthetic Technique

- Can be performed under regional, general, or combined anesthetic techniques

Monitoring

- Large-bore IV lines for blood loss
- Consider arterial line depending on extent of surgery
- Consider CVP, PCWP, or TEE if co-existing disease
- Consider monitoring for air embolism
- Consider aspirin or other NSAID prior to induction

Airway

- None

Induction

- Requires level of at least T8 for regional

- Continuous regional techniques offer excellent pain management and reduce cancer recurrence rates.
- Consider blood conservation strategies

Surgical Stages

Dissection

- Steady blood loss during dissection

Definitive Surgery

- May have significant blood loss during control of dorsal vein complex
- Hypotension may develop from blood loss or air embolism
- Indigo carmine frequently given to facilitate repair—incidence of anaphylaxis after indigo carmine and disturbance of pulse oximetry
- EBL: 1000–2000 mL
- Moderate volume shifts

Postoperative Considerations

- Significant postop pain
- Epidural may lead to fewer complications
- Pain score: 4–8
- IV PCA or epidural PCA for 2–3 d; newer modalities with education are assoc with discharge on postop day 2 or 3
- May develop pulm embolism or DVT; use aspirin or other NSAID preop and continue postop daily for at least 3 wk
- May develop peroneal nerve injury from lithotomy position

Anticipated Problems/Concerns

- Air embolism may occur because of large open veins and pt position

Retained Placenta, Removal of

Emily Baird

Risk

- Incidence: 3% of vaginal deliveries in developed countries
- Risk increases with Hx of high parity, uterine injury and/or anomaly, preterm labor, and induction of labor

Perioperative Risks

- Second most common cause of postpartum hemorrhage
  - 10% mortality if left untreated
- Extraction with curettage increases risk of uterine perforation
- Umbilical cord traction may lead to uterine inversion

Worry About

- 6% of placentas requiring manual extraction are placenta accretas·
- Blood loss is often much greater than that visually estimated
- Pt is at high risk for difficult intubation and pulm aspiration if general anesthesia indicated

Overview

- 1° causes incl: Placenta adherens, myometrium underlying placenta fails to contract; trapped placenta, detached placenta is trapped behind a closed cervix; and partial accreta, a small area of accreta prevents detachment
- Significant increase in risk of postpartum hemorrhage when the third stage of labor is greater than 30 min

ICD-9-CM Code. 666-0 (Retained placenta with hemorrhage)

Indications and Usual Treatment

- Manual removal is effective in all causes of retained placenta
- Medical management may be attempted for placenta adherens and trapped placenta
  - 20% of placenta adherens respond to intraumbilical oxytocin (30 IU in 30 mL saline)
  - Trapped placenta may respond to IV (50 to 100 µg) or sublingual (1 mg) nitroglycerin
- If third stage of labor exceeds 60 min, manual exploration and extraction is indicated

ASSESSMENT POINTS

System	Effect	Assessment by Hx	PE	Test
AIRWAY	Airway edema	Snoring, stridor	MP classification	
CARDIO	Hemorrhage	EBL	BP HR	Hgb, Hct
GI	Delayed gastric emptying	NPO status		
HEME	Coagulopathy		Bleeding from puncture site	PT, PTT, plt, FSP
UTERUS	Placenta adherens Trapped placenta	3rd stage >30 min 3rd stage >30 min	Fundus soft Fundus contracted; edge of placenta palpated through tight cervical os	US

Key Reference: Weeks AD. The Retained Placenta. *Best Pract Res Clin Obstet Gynaecol.* 2008;22:1103–1117.

Perioperative Management

Preoperative Preparation

- Prepare for postpartum hemorrhage: adequate multiple large bore IV access, type and cross

Monitoring

- Standard monitors incl non-invasive BP and pulse oximetry
- Consider invasive BPs and Foley catheter if blood loss is significant

Monitored Anesthesia Care/Sedation

- May be sufficient with trapped placenta
- Analgesia achieved with 10 mg ketamine boluses (not exceeding 0.5 mg/kg) or 50 to 100 µg fentanyl
- Nitroglycerin (50 to 100 µg) provides reliable, rapid (60 sec) smooth muscle relaxation with a short duration (1 to 3 min)

Neuraxial Anesthesia

- Addition of local anesthetic through existing epidural catheter or initiation of spinal

- Provides analgesia, not uterine relaxation
- Severe hypotension may occur in the setting of a postpartum hemorrhage

General Anesthesia

- Indicated in the presence of hemorrhage or the need for additional uterine relaxation
- 1.5 MAC of sevoflurane or desflurane decreases uterine contractility by 50%
- Increased risk of difficult intubation and pulm aspiration

Surgical Stages

- Blind identification of the interface between the uterus and placenta and gentle manual dissection
- Inability to completely manually extract placenta may require curettage or laparotomy
- Hysterectomy may be required in the setting of placenta accreta
- EBL: 300 mL (uncomplicated)–10 L (severe postpartum hemorrhage)

Postoperative Considerations

- Oxytocin may be required for enhanced uterine tone following removal of placenta
- Increased risk of endometritis with manual removal of placenta
- Pain score: 5–10 depending on mode of extraction
- Postop analgesia: Epidural or IV PCA

Anticipated Problems/Concerns

- Uterine atony may lead to additional blood loss following removal of placenta
- Ergometrine, which causes a powerful, continuous uterine contraction, may close the cervix at the same time as placental detachment occurs, thus trapping the placenta behind a closed cervix

Retinal Buckle Surgery

Dhamodaran Palaniappan
Steven Gayer

PROCEDURES

Risks

- Jeopardy of vision loss
- Incidence in USA: >100,000 cases/y
- Racial predominance: None

Perioperative Risks

- Airway obstruction and resp depression from oversedation during MAC
- Blindness from increased IOP 2° to interaction of N_2O with intravitreal gas (SF_6, C3 F_8)
- Bleeding 2° to antiplatelet/anticoagulant therapy
- Increased risk for globe puncture in severe myopic pts during needle blocks

Worry About

- Oculocardiac reflex (OCR)
- IOP elevation

- Ability to tolerate hyperosmotic agents
- Intravitreal injection of gas and N_2O interaction
- Co-morbid illness (DM, HTN, CAD)
- PONV
- Pain

Overview

- Pts are often elderly with other assoc diseases
- Frequently performed as ambulatory surgery
- Degree of surgical stimulus varies significantly (minimal to intense)
- Duration of surgery is often variable and may be prolonged
- IOP reduction may be required prior to scleral buckle placement

ICD-9-CM Code: 361.9 (Retinal detachment)

Etiology

- Diabetes mellitus
- Myopia
- Eye trauma
- Marfan's syndrome
- Idiopathic

Usual Treatments

- Cryotherapy, laser photocoagulation, plombage
- Scleral buckling or banding ('Explant')
- Vitrectomy
- Intravitreal injection of oil or gas (air, SF_6, perflurocarbons)

ASSESSMENT POINTS

System	Effects	Assessment by HX	PE	Test
HEENT	Axial length of eyeball Claustrophobia Deafness	Hx of myopia	Eyeglass prescription	US globe to determine axial length
CARDIO	Htn, CAD, Arrhythmias	Exercise tolerance/angina/ palpitations	Pulse rate, rhythm/BP Auscultation for heart murmur	EKG/ECHO
RESP	COPD, OSA, Interstitial lung disease	Chronic cough Snoring, home O_2, CPAP, exercise tolerance	Chest exam Airway exam	CXR/O_2 sat
HEME	Bleeding 2° to anticoagulants/antiplatelet agents	Easy bruisability Hx of DVT	Bruise marks	PT/PTT/INR
ENDO	Hypo/hyperglycemia Autonomic instability	Glucose control/antidiabetic medications	Orthostatic hypotension	Fasting Glucose
RENAL	Impairment 2° to DM	UO		BUN/Cr

Perioperative Management

Preoperative Preparation
- Identical for local and general anesthesia
- Preop fasting as per ASA guidelines
- Anxiolysis and reassurance are crucial
- Ability to lie supine for prolonged duration

Intraoperative

Monitoring
- Routine ASA monitors

Anesthesia Techniques
- RA with MAC, GA, combined RA and GA
- RA: Peribulbar, retrobulbar, sub-tenon's block
- Often requires MAC sedation
- Peribulbar (extraconal) preferred over retrobulbar (intraconal) block if axial length of globe is unknown
- RA preferred over GA
  - Decreased requirement for periop systemic analgesia
    - Decreased incidence of OCR
    - Decreased incidence of PONV
    - Avoidance of IOP alterations 2° to airway instrumentation

MAC Sedation for RA
- Midazolam, fentanyl, remifentanil infusion
- Propofol infusion
- Dexmedetomidine infusion
- Avoid oversedation

- Use O_2 by nasal prongs monitor nasal $ETCO_2$
- Elevate drapes at head to prevent CO_2 rebreathing
- Consider forced air or active suction cannula to dissipate CO_2
- Consider precordial stethoscope

General Anesthesia

Induction
- Intravenous agents
- LMA, ETT (Oral RAE preferred for field avoidance)

Maintenance
- Inhalation agents or TIVA
- N_2O: Preferable to avoid, if used D/C 15 min before intravitreal injection of gas (air, SF_6, C_3F_8)
- Muscle paralysis: Usually not required
- Ventilation: IPPV, maintain eucapnia
- Consider IV dexamethasone for multimodal PONV prophylaxis
- Supplementary intraop sub-tenon's block provides excellent postop pain relief

Emergence
- Beware of premature emergence
- Avoid bucking or coughing and consider deep extubation (IOP)
- Consider IV NSAID for postop pain management if supplemental block not administered intraop

- Consider antiemetic prophylaxis before emergence

Postoperative Considerations
- Pain: 3-5, NSAIDs usually adequate, opioids may be required (beware of PONV)
- PONV: 5-HT3 receptor antagonists preferred
- EBL: Nil

Surgical Considerations
- OCR: Vigilant monitoring for bradycardia and asystole during insertion of RA block, intraop muscle traction
- OCR: Avoid hypercapnia and light plane of anesthesia
- OCR: Stop precipitating surgical stimulus
- OCR: Anticholinergics may be considered for rescue or persistent OCR
- IOP management: Avoid hypercapnia and light plane of anesthesia
- IOP management: Mannitol or acetazolamide may be required to decrease IOP
- N_2O: Intravitreal gases and N_2O interaction may result in expansion of bubble and subsequent retinal ischemia and blindness

Retropharyngeal and Peritonsillar Abscess Drainage in Adults

Michael F. Roizen

Risk

- Rare without other debilitating conditions, such as alcohol abuse, immune compromise, or dental disease

Perioperative Risks

- Losing airway: No perfect approach (see below), all have risks and benefits

Worry About

- Airway compromise, esp. if severe enough to cause pt to drool and lean forward

Overview

- Complications of acute tonsillitis in which the infection has spread deep to the tonsillar capsule. Pus forms between the tonsillar capsule and the superior constrictor of pharynx, and the tonsil is displaced medially. Uvula becomes edematous, marked trismus and pain occur (head usually tilted toward site of abscess).
- Local infection with systemic implications due to airway compromise and potential for sepsis. Usually a β-hemolytic strep or anaerobe.

- George Washington is believed to have died from this disease.

ICD-9-CM Code: 478.24 (Retropharyngeal abscess)

Indications and Treatment

- Depends on degree of airway compromise: Goal is 48 hr of antibiotic prior to incision and drainage

ASSESSMENT POINTS

System	Effect	Assessment by Hx	PE	Test
ENT	Can be massive swelling and edema that inhibits airway and mouth opening and access	Ability to lie flat Drooling	Airway exam Voice distortion	Lateral neck x-ray "Hot potato" voice
CARDIO	Sepsis Hypovolemia	Hx of symptoms of infection	HR BP Temp	ECG ?CVP

Key Reference: Herzon FS, Martin AD. Medical and surgical treatment of peritonsillar, retropharyngeal, and parapharyngeal abscesses. *Curr Infect Dis Rep*. 2006;8:196–202.

Perioperative Management

Anesthetic Technique

- Alternatives based on two factors:
  - Most important: How to secure airway
  - Presence of sepsis

Monitoring

- Without sepsis: Usual
- With sepsis: CVP, and consider arterial line

Airway

- Difficult choices depending on severity and judgment of individual anatomy
- Topical and awake I & D if pt can tolerate is usual first choice

- Awake trach preferable if no other easy means and sepsis does not involve that area of neck
- Awake fiberoptic risks abscess contamination or accidental I & D and severe lung infection or losing airway

Surgial Stages

Induction

- After airway secure

Surgery

- Usual I & D and return at another time for tonsillectomy, etc.
- Pus cavity and site of infection can be difficult to find

- Airway patency
- Lung infection
- Underlying problem
- Sepsis management usually easier after abscess drained

Anticipated Problems/Concerns

- Airway compromise
- Underlying illness, incl drug withdrawal

Rotator Cuff Repair

Moustafa Ahmed

Risk

- Incidence in USA: More than 250,000 rotator cuff repair performed annually
- Rotator cuff tears mainly in older pts and middle age athletes
- 20–30% incidence of asymptomatic rupture of supraspinatus tendon in cadavers >60 y
- M:F ratio: 3:1
- Smoking and obesity may consider two risk factors

Perioperative Risks

- Periop mortality is low and assoc with preop co-morbidity
- Complication assoc with regional anesthesia-ISB-like accidental injection of LA intrathecal, epidural or IV, pneumothorax and direct nerve injury.
- ISB assoc with 100% ipsilateral phrenic nerve block so pt with severe or advanced pulm disease may worsening their resp status
- Venous air embolism

Worry About

- Losing airway, since the head is partially accessible
- Venous air embolism in sitting position

Overview

- The four muscles compose the rotator cuff are subscapularis, supraspinatus, infraspinatus, and teres minor

- Subscapularis tendon sits in front, and supraspinatus, infraspinatus, and teres minor sit posteriorly to glenohumoral joint
- Rotator cuff stabilizes the glenohumoral joint through the concavity-compression effect occurring with synchronized rotator cuff contraction.
- Rotator cuff tendon injury may have adverse effects on the muscle as well.
- Rotator cuff tears caused by many factors like impingement, degeneration, and overload all may contribute in varying degrees to develop rotator cuff tears.
- Typically Rotator cuff tears start as partial tears of the undersurface or articular portion of the supraspinatus tendon (the supraspinatus insertion is relatively hypovascular, which explains the common location of rotator cuff tears), over time the partial tear can progress to full thickness tears to affect the supraspinatus, infraspinatus, and subscapularis and biceps tendons.
- Rotator cuff injury in the athlete can be divided into two categories: contact sports such as football and rugby, and sports requiring repetitive overhead activity such as tennis and baseball
- Hx and physical exam are important to diagnose rotator cuff diseases. Typical complaints are shoulder pain mainly in the lateral aspect of the arm and exacerbated by overhead activities. Positive clinical sings like painful arc sign, drop arm test, weakness in external rotation. MRI usually confirms the clinical impressions and determines the size of the tear, muscle atrophy, tendon retraction, and the quality of the remaining tissue for repair.

ICD-9-CM Code: 83.6

Indications and Usual Treatment

- The goal in the treatment of rotator cuff tear is not only to eliminate pain but also to restore normal function.
- Restoring anatomy is the 1° goal in rotator cuff repair
- Nonoperative indicated for chronic atraumatic cuff tears, noncompliant pts and medical contraindications to surgery, in this condition will consider activity modification, avoiding repeated forward flexion beyond 90 degrees, and an aggressive rotator cuff and scapular stabilizer strengthening program. NSAIDs and corticosteroid injections may provide only temporary relief of symptoms.
- Operative approach has evolved from a classic open approach, to a mini-open or deltoid-sparing to an all arthroscopic technique. The advantages in the arthroscopic approach are to decrease morbidity and hospital length of stay, ability to visualize the entire joint, preservation of deltoid muscle and decrease postop pain compared to classic open approach, biological healing of the rotator cuff tendon to the humerus estimated to require a minimum of 8 to 12 wk.

ASSESSMENT POINTS

System	Effect	Assessment by Hx	PE	Test
HEENT	If RA or connective tissue disease, may have limited ROM of head/neck	Limited ROM head/neck or neck	Airway exam	C-spine x-ray
CARDIO	If RA or connective tissue disease, may have valvular heart disease/conduction defects	Angina/PND/orthopnea Palpitations/CHF Exercise tolerance	Chest exam Exam of peripheral pulses and vital signs	ECG ECHO
RESP	If RA, may have pulm fibrosis or pleural effusion	SOB Exercise tolerance	Chest exam	CXR ABGs PFTs
HEME	Hx of NSAID use—may affect coagulation	Hx of medications, bleed/bruise	Inspection for evidence of same	
IMMUNO	If RA, may be immunocompromised	Hx of medications, infectious disease		CBC and differential

See Rheumatoid Arthritis if appropriate
Key Reference: Feeley BT, Gallo RA, Craig EV. Cuff tear arthropathy: Current trends in diagnosis and surgical management. *J Shoulder Elbow Surg.* 2009;18:484–494.

Perioperative Management

Preoperative Preparation
- Within normal complete blood count, serum electrolyte, and coagulation variables
- IV prophylactic antibiotics

Monitoring
- Standard ASA monitors
- Monitoring for possible venous air embolism in sitting position using precordial Doppler and/or end-tidal N_2 or TEE
- Securing the airway is crucial since the head is only partially accessible
- Positioning either in lateral decubitus or in beach chair position
- In sitting position be aware to keep the neck in neutral position and avoid right or left tilting to avoid occlusion of venous drainage from the head
- Pad pressure points

Anesthetic Technique/Induction
- Anesthesia is provided by ISB, GA with endotracheal anesthesia, or a combination of both.
- GA: Different induction agents based on the medical status
- ISB for preemptive analgesia intra and postop period (Interscalene block)

Surgical Stages

- Positioning either in lateral decubitus or in beach chair position, beach chair position is convenient to convert from arthroscopic to open procedure

Arthroscopic Repair
- Need multiple portals: Posterior portal, anterior, lateral, and anterolateral
- Posterior portal is located about 2 cm inferior and 2 cm medial to the posterolateral margin of the acromion within the posterior soft spot of the GH joint. The anterior portal is placed lateral to the coracoids in line with the AC joint. The lateral portal is placed 3 cm lateral to the acromion in line with the posterior border of the clavicle. An accessory anterolateral portal is created for instrumentation and suture management.
- Examination and evaluation of the GH joint and subacromial space, probing the undersurface of the rotator cuff to its insertion on the greater tuberosity to note and evaluate the location, size, and character of any tears as well the amount of cuff retraction and the quality of the tissue then subacromial decompression to increase in working space for cuff repair, avoid injury to the suprascapular nerve and vessels located 1 to 2 cm medial to the lateral edge of the glenoid.

Open Repair
- Mini-open or traditional open approach to rotator cuff repair
- Incision: Oblique over acromion, part of the deltoid muscle detached to reach rotator cuff. In mini-open repair no deltoid detachment
- After acromioplasty, visualize and mobilize the tear off the bursa, deltoid and corachohumeral ligament using blunt and sharp dissection, 1° repair of the soft tissue component followed suture anchors. Careful repair of deltoid if detached and close the wound.

Postoperative Considerations
- A sling and 30-degree abduction pillow are used for a week and placed before awakening; supervised graded passive range of motion is initiated as soon as possible
- Pain control with ISB using long acting LA
- Augmenting ISB with NSAIDs
- Inpatient may use PCA

Anticipated Problems/Concerns
- Disease of elderly (CAD, COPD, CKD, DM)
- Be aware that sudden drop in the BP may be venous air embolism
- Axillary and musculocutaneous nerve injury with open procedures and aggressive dissection

Scoliosis and Kyphosis Surgery

Chris C. Lee
Jacob M. Buchowski

Risk

- Scoliosis is defined as a spinal deformity with a Cobb angle of more than 10° in the coronal plane
- Scoliosis is present in 1–15% of adult pts and in 1–4% of adolescents where it is most commonly idiopathic (60-70%) with F:M ratio of 4:1
- Of NM scoliosis, DMD is the most common disorder with an incidence of 1/3300 male births
- Scheuermann's kyphosis occurs in 0.4% to 8.3% of the general population with male predominance

Perioperative Risks

- Risk of neurologic injury during spinal deformity surgery is <1 to 5% (more frequently in adults than adolescents) with 0.37% incidence of major neurologic complications, but can be higher with severe deformity procedures such as pedicle subtraction osteotomy (PSO) or vertebral column resection (VCR).
- Substantial blood loss (usually from surgical field, but occasionally from laceration of the greater vessels)
- Visual field defects and vision loss (0.03–0.1%)
- Intraop awareness with explicit recall (0.1–0.2%)
- Pulm embolism, incl fat embolism and air embolism (VAE)

Worry About

- Neurologic complications due to direct injury to spinal cord by compression or excessive traction, and the adjacent nerve roots by misplaced pedicle screws, or indirect injury to peripheral nerves by malpositioning or through prolonged compression
- Vascular injuries ranging from laceration of the greater vessels (with 50% mortality) to ligation of the segmental vessels
- Dural lacerations and CSF leaks with resulting cranial nerve dysfunction and/or potentially subdural hematoma
- Postop wound infection, atelectasis, pneumonia, and pneumothorax

Overview

- Most commonly coronal and/or sagittal plane deformity correction is performed through a posterior approach during which instrumentation (pedicle screws and/or hooks and rods) is placed and deformity correction is achieved through various deformity correction maneuvers.
- Occasionally, and an anterior approach may be utilized instead or in addition to the posterior approach; typically this is done through a transthoracic approach (i.e., thoracotomy), a thoracoabdominal approach, or an abd (typically retroperitoneal) approach.
- If both a posterior and an anterior approach are necessary, the procedure may be performed at the same operation or in a staged manner.

- Prepare for large blood loss (with large-bore PIVs, fast fluid infusion devices and banked PRBC immediately available)

ICD-9-CM Codes: 737.30; Scoliosis (Idiopathic) 754.2; (Congenital) 737.10; Kyphosis (Acquired) (Postural) 756.19 (Congenital)

Indications and Usual Treatment

- Scoliosis: Treatment incl nonoperative methods (brace and observation) and surgery that is indicated when the Cobb angle is >40° in the lumbar spine or >50° in the thoracic spine; other factors incl deformity magnitude, symptoms such as pain, skeletally immature vs. mature, and presence of sagittal plane deformity.
- Kyphosis: Treatment incl nonoperative methods and surgery, depending on the symptoms (pain and/or neurologic impairment), degree of curvature, and curve progression. Kyphosis >75° often warrants surgery.

ASSESSMENT POINTS

System	Effect	Assessment by Hx	PE	Test
Airway/HEENT	Difficult laryngoscopy and intubation; cervical scoliosis and kyphosis in the neurofibromatosis; scoliosis or kyphosis may limit normal movement of the cervical spine.	Hx of anesthesia and difficult airway management	Range of motion of the head and neck, body habitus, Mallampati classification	Atlanto-occipital extension, thyromental distance, length and thickness of the neck
CNS	In NM and congenital scoliosis, careful preop evaluation and documentation of neurologic status		Neuro deficits	Preop SSEP and MEP
CARDIO	High incidence of CHD and MVP (e.g., Marfan's syndrome); cardiomyopathy in Friedreich's ataxia and MD (DMD is the most common and severe form of childhood MD)	Exercise tolerance	Heart murmurs	ECG, ECHO, CXR
RESP	Restrictive lung disease with resp impairment proportional to Cobb angle (angle of lateral curvature). Both VC and TLC are decreased. If VC <40% predicted, postop ventilation usually is required.	Exercise tolerance and dyspnea	Cyanosis, clubbing, and possible rapid shallow pattern of breathing	CXR; ABG; PFT; flow-volume loops
HEME	Preop autologous blood donation and coagulation study; avoid plt inhibitors for 7-10 d before surgery	Hx of easy bruising and bleeding? Any contraindication to use tranexamic acid?		CBC, plt quantity, quality and PT/PTT/INR
GI	Regurgitation and susceptible to aspiration in pts with scoliosis of NM origin	Pt and parents' report		

Key References: Bridwell KH. *The textbook of spinal surgery.* 3rd ed. Philadelphia: Lippincott, Williams and Wilkins; 2010.; Boezaart AP. The pediatric spine and the adult spine. In: *Anesthesia and orthopaedic surgery.* McGraw-Hill, 2006.

Perioperative Management

Preoperative Preparation

- Pt should be instructed how to correctly use incentive spirometry (IS) and PCA.

- Discuss risks with pt and family concerning blindness, awareness, PE, paraplegia, MI, CVA, left intubated to ICU, etc.
- Warn pt of possibility of intraop wake-up test.

- Ask pt to practice wake-up test at home and in the preop holding area.

Monitoring

- Routine ASA monitors
- Consider arterial line

- CVP line useful to assess volume status intraop and provide TPN postop
- Spinal cord monitoring (SCM) incl SSEPs, MEPs (NMEP and TCeMEP) and EMG
- BIS monitor
- Estimate blood loss from suction canister contents, cell saver device and sponges
- Urinary catheter to assess UO and monitor core temp (normothermia is essential)
- Consider O_2 sats pulse oximetry on big toes during anterior exposure of the lower lumbar spine to assess amount of iliac artery compression

Induction/Maintenance

- Induction (either IV anesthesia or inhalation techniques) is guided by pt's airway and medical conditions.
- Consider awake fiberoptic intubation if indicated.
- Inhalational agents may interfere with SSEP or MEP monitoring.
- After adequate bag-mask ventilation, a short-acting muscle relaxant (NMBA) is administered for intubation. No NMBA is used during the operation if TCeMEP or EMG is used. Sux is contraindicated in pts with various dystrophic and myopathic conditions and spinal cord injury due to the potential for rhabdomyolysis, hyperkalemia, and cardiac arrest.
- Maintenance with TIVA (continuous infusion of IV propofol and remifentanil preferred) and midazolam 1 mg/hr. IV anesthetic agents have less effect on SSEPs or MEPs.

Surgical Stages

- **Posterior approach**
  - Pt placed prone with abd and axillae allowed to hang free. Recommend adequate padding and make sure that eyes are protected and not compressed (use an appropriate face pillow or use Gardner-Wells tongs or Mayfield head holder).

- Maintain temp using a forced-air warming device and warming IVF and blood products.
- After the spine is exposed, instrumentation is placed, and deformity correction is performed. This is then followed by decortication, bone grafting, and wound closure.
- Substantial blood loss can occur during the procedure given the large surgical area and decortications of bone.
- Adequately resuscitate the pt using blood products. Use both colloids (albumin, voluven, or hespan) and crystalloids to maintain intravascular volume and reduce postop edema.
- Monitor SSEPs or MEPs. Significant intraop neurophysiologic changes occur if SSEP amplitude decreases by 50% or latency increases >10%, or TCeMEP amplitude decreases by 75% from baseline. Systematic approach to evaluate for potential causes of neurologic injury.
- Step 1: R/O technical error or electrical interference (artifact or cautery)
- Step 2: R/O anesthesia-related factors (hypotension, hypoxemia, hypothermia, high concentrations of inhalational agents, and whether using muscle relaxant or not)
- Step 3: R/O surgical factors (modifying or removing instrumentation or distraction forces)
- Step 4: Prepare to perform wake-up test.
- At conclusion, pt placed supine. Pt should be fully awake for neurologic exam (wake-up test) prior to extubation.
- Consider postop pain management with IV PCA
- **Anterior approach**
  - Pt placed in a lateral decubitus position for a transthoracic or thoracoabdominal approach and supine for an abdominal approach. Recommend adequate padding and an axillary roll if pt is placed in a lateral decubitus position.

- After the spine is exposed, instrumentation is placed, and deformity correction is performed. This is then followed by decortications, bone grafting, and wound closure. If the thorax was violated during the surgery, a chest tube is typically placed.
- Anesthetic issues are similar during an anterior approach, except that massive bleeding can be encountered if the greater vessels are lacerated during the surgery.

Anticipated Problems/Concerns

- Soft tissue: Hematoma, seroma, skin necrosis and most commonly, wound infection. Monitor BIS and BP to make sure neither is too low (as guide to protect somewhat against blindness)
- Continued pain from either unresolved, incompletely resolved, or recurrent pain postop.
- Pulm problems incl: Atelectasis, pneumonia, and PE; postop ventilation may be required in pts with severe resp impairment or NM scoliosis.
- Neurologic compromise or deficits (acute vs. delayed): epidural hematoma or abscess, spinal cord ischemia 2° to anterior vascular injury by direct injury with spinal instrumentation or stretch or spinal artery compression after coronal and sagittal plane correction.
- GI: There are many causes of postop ileus, incl pain and the use of narcotics for analgesia, electrolyte imbalances, and manipulation of the bowel during surgery; in addition superior mesenteric artery syndrome may occur particularly in pediatric pts with extensive deformity correction.

Seizure Surgery

Judit Szolnoki
Kelly Stees

Risk

- The lifetime risk of single seizure: ~10%; cumulative lifetime incidence of epilepsy: 3% with more than half of cases beginning in childhood
- An estimated 2.5 million Americans and 30 million persons worldwide have epilepsy; ~20% of which are refractory to medical treatment.
- Although 13% of medically intractable pts are considered candidates for surgery, only 1% undergo surgery.

Perioperative Risks

- 3% or less risk of major morbidity (i.e., hemorrhage, infection, stroke, memory, language, or hemianopic visual field deficit) incurred by surgery
- Cognitive dysfunction; more profound in adults than children
- Combined morbidity and mortality for epileptogenic focus resection 5–6%, corpus callosotomy <11%, functional hemispherectomy <17%
- Infants are at higher risk for periop morbidity and mortality than any other age group.

Worry About

- Seizures and/or status epilepticus
- Loss of airway with sedation
- Increased ICP with mass lesions
- Hemodynamic instability: Acute and severe bradycardia, sinus arrest; pediatric population with age <2 y have lower autoregulatory reserves and can be at greater risk of cerebral ischemia
- Effects of specific anticonvulsant medications

Overview

- Seizure: Abn electrical activity in the brain resulting in paroxysmal change in motor activity or behavior. Focal or generalized.
- Status epilepticus is defined as more than 30 min of continuous seizure activity or two or more sequential seizures without full recovery of consciousness between the seizures.
- First surgical resection for epilepsy performed 1886
- Seizure surgery: Identify and localize epileptogenic focus, then determine whether the pt has adequate functional reserve for safe resection.
- 50–90% pts undergoing seizure surgery have significant decrease in Sz frequency or complete resolution of Sz; surgical efficacy contrasts with a 5% or less chance that additional medical therapy will render the refractory pt Sz free
- Surgical procedures: Focal resection, corpus callosotomy, hemispherectomy, and vagus nerve stimulation

ICD-9-CM Code: 790.3

Etiology

- Seizures occur in ~10% children but most are provoked by somatic disorders outside of brain such as fever, infection, head trauma, hypoxia, or cardiac arrhythmias; less than 30% of Sz in children are caused by epilepsy

- Localization-related epilepsies and syndromes are seizures that originate from a localized cortical region; generalized epilepsies and epilepsy syndromes are characterized by seizures with initial activation of neurons within both cerebral hemispheres
- Idiopathic refers to syndromes that arise spontaneously without a known cause.
- Symptomatic denotes epilepsies with an identified cause such as mesial temporal sclerosis. Lesional epilepsy refers to focal epilepsy in which a lesion is identified on neuroimaging studies that is the probable cause of seizures. Lesions incl mesial temporal sclerosis, developmental malformations, neoplasms, vascular malformations, and ischemic insults. The distinction between lesional and nonlesional focal epilepsy is particularly important in pts being considered for epilepsy surgery.

Indications

- Medical intractability is 1° reason to consider surgical therapy
- Considered appropriate when
  - Seizures persist despite an adequate trial of at least two to three appropriate anticonvulsants, alone or in combination
  - Seizures or the medical treatment for seizures significantly reduce quality of life
  - A unilateral, localized seizure focus that can be reliably identified
  - Resection of the seizure focus does not cause unacceptable neurologic deficits

ASSESSMENT POINTS

System	Effect	Assessment by Hx	PE	Test
HEENT	Facial trauma; gingival hyperplasia; wt gain or poor airway	Hx of fall with Sz	Facial bruising, etc	
RESP	Hyperventilation preop; risk of aspiration pneumonia	Review medications	Rales, wheezing	CXR ABG
GI	Liver toxicity from AEDs; increased hepatic enzyme metabolism			Liver function tests
ENDO	Bone marrow suppression, coagulopathy, plt dysfunction; metabolic acidosis/ketosis for pts on ketogenic diet hyponatremia	Bleeding, infection	Bruising	CBC, BMP, coags
CNS	Cognitive dysfunction; Sz, personality changes			CT, MRI, EEG, SPECT scan, Wada test
MS	Trauma from Sz, bone fragility from AEDs			

Key Reference: Soriano SG, Bozza P. Anesthesia for epilepsy surgery in children. *Childs Nerv Syst.* 2006;22:834-843.

Perioperative Implications

Preoperative Preparation

- Clear communication with surgeon regarding procedure and surgical approach as this will dictate anesthetic technique
- Evaluate if pt is appropriate candidate for awake craniotomy
- Determine baseline neurologic status; review preop radiographic and neuropsychological diagnostic evaluation
- Identify specific anticonvulsant regimen and potential implications for anesthetic.
  - Phenytoin: Leukopenia, anemia, hepatitis
  - Valproate: Pancreatitis, hepatic failure, coagulopathy, plt dysfunction
  - Carbamazepine: Aplastic anemia, cardiotoxicity, hypothyroidism, hyponatremia

- Felbamate: Leukopenia, liver failure, aplastic anemia
- Lamotrigine: Rash and hypersensitivity
- Topiramate: Asymptomatic nonion gap metabolic acidosis due to inhibition of carbonic anhydrase
- Ketogenic diet (high-fat, low-carbohydrate diet that promotes ketosis and used as adjuvant therapy for intractable epilepsy). Avoid carbohydrate containing medications and solutions. Monitor acid-base status and glucose levels frequently.
- Pehnytoin and carbamazepine may exhibit resistance to nondepolarizing muscle relaxants and opioids.

- Other SE include: Nephrolithiasis, electrolyte abn, nausea, paresthesias, wt changes; chronic polytherapy for refractory cases leads to drug-drug interactions
- Presence of concomitant medical problems assoc with epilepsy
- Avoid premedication with benzodiazepine unless activation of epileptogenic foci not necessary in which case it is acceptable to administer
- Preop laboratory evaluation on case-specific basis; type and cross-matched blood esp. for pediatric pts

Monitoring

- Standard ASA monitors; $ETCO_2$ via nasal cannula for sedation
- Large-bore IV access prior to surgical start, consider central venous line

- Arterial catheter for direct BP monitoring and blood sampling
- Consider PICC line for pediatric cases performed in two stages (grid and strip placements)

Airway
- Case dependent
- Risk of airway compromise due to sedation, seizure, or positioning

Maintenance
- Choice of anesthetic agent and technique based on two factors: (1) is intraop electrocorticography (ECoG) necessary and (2) should the craniotomy be performed with general anesthesia/intubation or with local anesthesia/conscious sedation
- If GA *without* ECoG, anesthetic designed to maintain suppression of seizure activity and provide optimal operating conditions
- If *intraopera*tive ECoG used, anesthetic should permit activation of ECoG: AVOID benzodiazepines, and volatile anesthetics
- Conscious sedation: Fentanyl, remifentanil, *dexmedetomidine*, benadryl intraop fluid and electrolyte management – maintain normovolemia
- Frequent monitoring electrolytes and hemoglobin esp. in infants

- Be prepared to treat
  - Seizures
  - Increased ICP
  - Venous air embolus
  - Hemodynamic instability due to arrhythmias or blood loss

Special Considerations
- Awake craniotomy: Need cooperative and motivated pt
- Grids and/or strips: Two-stage procedure. Craniotomy for grid placement; monitoring for seizures over following days or week, then return to OR for grid removal and resection of seizure focus. **AVOID** administration of NO until dura opened because intracranial air can persist for up to 3 wk following a craniotomy and NO can cause rapid expansion of air cavities and result in tension pneumocephalus. Pts can be somnolent for few days postop.
- Resection: Discussion of modality and type of neurophysiological monitoring to be used is critical, specifically ECoG and EEG.
- Corpus callostomy: Intraop EEG not required; any anesthetic regimen can be utilized. Postop lethargy and somnolence are common increasing the risk of aspiration and airway problems; leave intubated until fully awake.

- Hemisherectomy: Highest morbidity of all surgical procedures for epilepsy. Potential for large blood loss esp. in young pt population.
- Vagus nerve stimulator: Thought to inhibit seizure activity at brainstem or cortical levels. Device is placed in SQ pocket under left anterior chest wall and bipolar stimulating electrode coils are implanted around L vagus nerve. Side effects of VNS involve vocal cord paralysis, bronchoconstriction, bradycardia, and asystole.

Extubation
- Aim for rapid smooth emergence.
- Consider leaving intubated if concern for postop somnolence.

Postoperative Period
- Close observation in ICU with serial neurologic exams
- Seizures common
- PONV, fluid and/or electrolyte management, pain
- High infection risk in staged procedures

Anticipated Problems/Concerns
- Congnitive dysfunction
- New neurologic deficits
- Seizures and/or status epilepticus

Spinal Fusion

Ihab Kamel

Risk

- Incidence in USA: About 50,000 surgeries/y.
- 328,468 spinal fusions performed from 2002-2006
- Indications: Congenital, oncologic, traumatic, degenerative or infectious

Perioperative Risks

- Periop mortality rare (0–0.5%)
- Venous air embolism (VAE) can occur and produce CV collapse
- Postop neurologic deficit (0.7–5%)
- Massive blood loss possible (1–5%)
- Pneumothorax (1–5%)
- Permanent postop visual loss (POVL) is rare but devastating (0-1%)

Worry About

- Underlying pathology; scoliosis, spinal stenosis, herniated disc, trauma, infection, tumor
- Large intraop blood loss
- Difficult airway with trauma and cervical cases
- Potential for VAE
- Problems of prone position

- POVL due to ischemic optic neuropathy (Risk factors: Surgery duration >6.5 hr, and blood loss >44.7% of estimated blood volume. Intraop hypotension and anemia may contribute).
- Postop resp insufficiency

Overview

- Scoliosis is a rotational abn of spine and ribs that may be assoc with restrictive lung disease
- Unstable cervical fracture (trauma) or severe compression due to spinal stenosis or tumor lead to neurologic symptoms and the potential for difficult airway.
- Evoked potential monitoring can limit choice of anesthetic technique.
- An intraop wake-up test may be requested by operating surgeon
- Intraop VAE is possible

ICD-9-CM Code: 737.30

Indications and Usual Treatment

- Adolescent idiopathic scoliosis

Skeletally mature
  - Observation for curves <45°
  - Fusion for curves >50°

Skeletally immature
  - Observe for curves <25°
  - Braces for curves 25° -40°
  - Fusion for curves >45°

- Curves >50° or if a lesser curve with resp compromise, pain, or likelihood of progression to 50° surgery is absolutely indicated.
- Failure to correct significant curve results in a doubling of mortality for age, potential for progressive back pain, and progressive pulm dysfunction
- Spinal stenosis, herniated disc, tumor, infections
- Laminectomy is indicated to decompress the spinal cord and/or spinal nerve roots in pts with intolerable pain, progressive neurologic symptoms and weakness to prevent further progression and irreversible neurologic deficit.
- Fusion is needed to stabilize the spine after laminectomy.

ASSESSMENT POINTS

System	Effect	Assessment by Hx	PE	Test
CARDIO	Cor pulmonale possible if significant lung disease	Exercise tolerance		ECG ECHO
RESP	Pulm dysfunction occurs with significant thoracic curves		Exercise tolerance testing	PFTs corrected for height
CNS	Preop neurologic dysfunction unusual; should lead to further assessment and diagnostic tests		Complete neurologic exam	?CT ? MRI
MS		Careful exam may lead to an alternative Dx, e.g., Marfan's, Ehlers-Danlos, Goldenhar's syndromes; syrinx	Careful airway exam. Identify pts with difficult airway	CBC Blood type and cross-match

Key Reference: Ornstein E, Berko R. Anesthesia techniques in complex spine surgery. *Neurosurg Clin N Am.* 2006;17:191–203.

Perioperative Implications

Anesthetic Technique

- Performed utilizing general ET anesthesia in prone position
- Awake fiberoptic intubation for unstable cervical spine cases
- Awake fiberoptic intubation or inline stabilization for trauma cases
- Controlled hypotension used to limit blood loss
- Potential for interference with evoked potential monitoring influences anesthetic agent choice. May contribute to POVL if prolonged and assoc with anemia.

Monitoring

- Arterial line useful
- Consider CVP line to monitor volume and perhaps to treat VAE
- Somatosensory evoked potentials (SSEP) and motor-evoked potentials (MEP) are often used to monitor the integrity if the neural elements throughout the procedure.
- Foley catheter may facilitate adequate volume resuscitation

Induction/Maintenance

- Narcotics do not interfere with SSEPs or MEPs
- <1 MAC inhalation agent exerts only minimal effect on potential monitoring
- Muscle relaxants will interfere with MEP
- Consider total IV anesthethetic technique (TIVA) for maintainance
- Anticipate need for midprocedure wake-up test
- Controlled hypotension accomplished with β-blockade and IV vasodilators

Preoperative Management

- Large-bore IV lines because of anticipated blood loss
- Discuss possible complications with the pt incl POVL
- Discuss with surgeon the possibility of staging the procedure if expected to be >6 hr
- Blood availability for extensive lumbar and thoracic cases.

Surgical Stages

Positioning

- Pt positioned prone on a frame that allows abd to be free from external compression to reduce venous pressure

- Pressure points padded carefully
- Head and neck must be midline and in neutral position. There must be no pressure on ocular structures or ear cartilage.
- Shoulder abduction should be less than 90° to avoid brachial plexopathy in the prone surrender position.

Dissection/Definitive Surgery

- Prior to skin incision, surgical field is often infiltrated with dilute solution of epinephrine.
- Steady bleeding during dissection and decortication
- Hypotension may be due to blood loss or VAE
- After instrumentation in place, distraction is performed
- After distraction complete, a wake-up test may be performed
- Approx duration: 4–8 hr

Postoperative Considerations

- Pain score: 6–9
- Postop resp failure unusual but should be considered a possibility in scoliosis pts with pre-existing restrictive lung disease
- Neurologic exam after wake-up. New neurologic injury is an emergency and requires urgent removal of all hardware.
- Early postop gross check of vision

Anticipated Problems/Concerns

• Potential for massive blood loss and rapid development of hypotension

• Modest risk of VAE because of open epidural veins and prone position

• Periop neurologic injury mainly due to instrumentation. Perform postop neurologic exam.

• Occasional reports of neurologic injury in spite of normal evoked responses support considering continued use of wake-up test

• Potential for POVL, avoid anemia and prolonged hypotension. Surgeon to consider staging long (>6.5 hr) procedures. Perform a gross visual exam after emergence.

Splenectomy

Wendy K. Bernstein
Lee A. Fleisher

Risk

- No age or sex predilection

Perioperative Risks

- Mortality rate 0–3%
- Overall complication rate is 11.8% assoc with pulm complications, DVT

Worry About

- Potential for major blood loss requiring transfusion
- Trauma of pancreatic tail, stomach, lineal flexure of colon, left hemidiaphragm, left suprarenal gland, upper pole left kidney

Overview

- Spleen most commonly injured organ in blunt trauma
- Splenomegaly affects 3% of full-term newborns, and 10% of healthy children
- Splenomegaly common complication of sickle cell disease (African or Mediterranean descent)
- Splenic trauma frequently assoc with other intra-abdominal injuries

ICD-9-CM Codes: 865.10 (Splenic trauma); 289.4 (Hypersplenism)

Etiology

- Always required
  - Cancer
  - Hereditary splenocytosis (HS): Absence of specific protein in RBCs that leads to fragile cells
- Usually required
  - Idiopathic thrombocytopenic purpura (ITP)
  - Trauma S/P blunt or penetrating abd trauma requiring emergency operation (14%)
- Abscess: Uncommon
- Rupture splenic artery (complication of pregnancy)
- Hereditary elliptocytosis (rare disorder)
- Sometimes required
  - Hodgkin's lymphoma (27%): Splenectomy preferred to determine progression of disease
  - Autoimmune hemolytic disorders: Adults >50 y
  - Myelofibrosis: Bone marrow replaced by fibrous disease, splenectomy preferred for pain
  - Relief
  - Thalessemia

Usual Treatment

- Depends upon indication
- Splenorrhaphy for splenic salvage after trauma

ASSESSMENT POINTS

System	Effect	Assessment by Hx	Test
CARDIO	Cardiotoxicity, dysrhythmias, CHF	Chemotherapeutic agents—doxorubicin (dose > 550 mg/m^2)	ECG, ECHO, MUGA → determine LV function
RESP	Pleural effusions; left lower lobe atelectasis if splenomegaly; pulm fibrosis	Chemotherapeutic agents—bleomycin, methotrexate, cytarabine	CXR
GI	Hepatotoxicity	Chemotherapeutic agent—methotrexate	LFTs
HEME	Splenomegaly, cytopenia	Hematologic disease	CBC with differential Plt count Bleeding time
GU	Renal insufficiency	Chemotherapeutic agents—methotrexate, cisplatin	BUN, serum Cr UA, electrolytes
CNS	Neurologic deficits Peripheral neuropathies	Chemotherapeutic agents—vinblastine, cisplatin	

Key References: Pivalizza EG, Tjia IM, Juneja HS, Cohen AM, Duke Jr JH. Elective splenectomy in an anemic Jehovah's Witness patient with cirrhosis. *Anesth Analg.* 1998;87:529–530.
Trimmings AJ, Walmsley AJ. Anasthesia for urgent splenectomy in acute idiopathic thrombocytopenic purpura. *Anaesthesia.* 2009;64:226–227.

Perioperative Implications

Preoperative Implications

- Ensure polyvalent pneumococcal vaccine (1 mo prior to surgery, if possible; Pneumovax, Pro-Immune 23 and Menomune-A/C/Y/W-135)
- NG decompression
- Stress steroids (100 mg IV hydrocortisone q8h), if received in past
- Treat infection
- Correct abn in blood coagulation

Monitoring

- Routine
- Large-bore IV access

Airway

- Trauma pts: rule out cervical instability

Induction

- Routine

Maintenance

- Prevent hypothermia

Extubation

- Routine

Adjuvants

- Open or laparoscopic approach
- Combined general/epidural (1.5–2% lidocaine with 1:200,000 epinephrine)
- Muscle relaxants required
- Minimize sedatives: ↑ likelihood of postop resp depression

Postoperative Period

- Postsplenectomy sepsis: Due to encapsulated organisms (e.g., pneumococci)
- Booster pneumococcal vaccine 5–10 y post splenectomy

Anticipated Problems/Concerns

- Bleeding
- Subphrenic abscess
- Bronchopneumonia
- Thrombotic complications
- Atelectasis (left lower lobe)
- Complications related to underlying cause for splenectomy

Split-Thickness Skin Graft

Robert Gaiser

Uses

- Burns: 2 million people injured/y
- Wounds: Trauma, diabetic foot ulcers, postradiation skin breakdown, sacral decubitus, melanoma excision

Perioperative Risks

- Periop mortality: Rare
- Large areas may involve significant blood loss
- May be performed by plastic, general, orthopedic, and ENT surgeons

Worry About

- Airway involvement in burns that may make intubation difficult
- Blood loss if large areas to be debrided and grafted
- Pain at donor site
- Postop infection at donor or recipient site

- Nutritional status of pt
- Cleanliness of donor and recipient sites
- Suitable locations for application of monitors and IV access
- Loss of joint mobility due to scarring

Overview

- Split-thickness skin graft (STSG) consists of epidermis and only a portion of dermis. STSGs categorized as thin (0.005–0.012 in.), medium (0.012–0.018 in.), or thick (0.018-0.028 in.)
- Must consider both donor and recipient sites: Addition of epinephrine will decrease bleeding at donor site without affecting survival of STSG
- Involves the harvesting of only the epidermal layer and part of the dermis
- Since dermal cells are left in situ from the donor site, it may heal by 2° intention

- May be used in less than ideal conditions as it does not require a well-vascularized wound
- To cover granulating wound

ICD-9-CM Codes: Procedure Code: 151.00; Diagnosis Code (dependent upon location): 707.00 (Decubitus ulcer); 707.10 (Ulcer on LE); 873.40 (Ulcer on face); 884.00 (Ulcer on UE); 941.00 (Burn on face); 942.00 (Burn on trunk); 944.00 (Burn on UE); 945.00 (Burn on LE)

Indications and Usual Treatment

- Used to cover granulating wound: Tolerates less vascularity than full-thickness skin graft
- Disadvantage: Abn pigmentation, contraction
- Donor site: Any area of body incl scalp and extremities; depends on resulting skin match and appearance of the donor scar

ASSESSMENT POINTS

System	Effect	Assessment by Hx	PE	Test
DERM	Donor/recipient site	Discussion with surgeon		
HEENT	Burns or radiation	Review medical record	Airway exam	
CARDIO	Hypotensive shock, arrhythmias	Dyspnea, orthopnea	Vital signs	CXR, ECG, orthostatic vital signs
RESP	ARDS	Dyspnea, SOB, chest pain, mental status change	Chest exam	CXR ABGs
GI	Debilitated pt	Bed-bound		Albumin
HEME	Possible large blood loss			Hct
RENAL	ATN, myoglobinemia	Massive tissue destruction	Oliguria, anuria	BUN, serum Cr Cr clearance; serum/urine myoglobin
NEURO	Compartment syndromes	Hx of circumferential extremity burns	Weak pulses	Transduce compartment pressures

Key Reference: Unal S, Ersoz G, Demirkan F, et al. Analysis of skin-graft loss due to infection: Infection-related graft loss. *Ann Plast Surg.* 2005;55:102–106.

Perioperative Management

Preoperative Preparation
- Determine donor and/or recipient sites
- Stabilize hemodynamics
- IV access: Large-bore IVs if anticipate large blood loss
- Warm room and all fluids

Monitoring
- Donor and/or recipient sites limit locations available for application of monitors: Secure leads and pulse oximeter away from sites used
- May use lower extremity for BP monitoring
- Temp monitoring

Airway
- For burn or postradiation pt, determine if airway involved. Involvement of face may make intubation more difficult: Consider fiberoptic intubation/consider consultative, collaborative airway management

Induction/Maintenance
- Avoid succinylcholine, as may precipitate hyperkalemia response in pts with burns
- No generally accepted preferred agent or technique
- Regional anesthesia is an option
- Consider lateral femoral cutaneous nerve block if donor site is lateral thigh.
- If using local anesthetic, keep amount within recommended limits.

- Addition of epinephrine to local anesthetic is not contraindicated.
- Donor site assoc with significant pain; plan should incorporate means for postop pain management
- EMLA cream has been used for anesthesia for donor site
- Application of lidocaine spray to donor site ↓ postop pain
- Acute phase: Anticipate hemostatic problems if large area is to be grafted; consider electrolyte abn and volume status
- Chronic phase: Scarring may cause loss of function and difficulty with positioning of the pt

Surgical Stages
- Variety of dermatomes available to cut STSG. In general, air- or electric-powered dermatomes and free hand knife are used to cut lengthwise on extremity; drum dermatomes used sidewise across extremity.
- Width of graft determined by width setting on dermatome
- If betadine is used to prep donor area, it must be washed off to prevent sticking.
- Skin thoroughly lubricated with sterile mineral oil to facilitate graft cutting
- Advancing the dermatome flat across the skin with gentle downward pressure
- Wound cleaned with saline or betadine solution

- Surgical debridement may cause bleeding; hemostasis important for graft survival
- Graft placed on the wound, sutured around the periphery, and dressed. Main object of the dressing is to ensure contact between graft and host bed. Dressing left in place for ~7 d, at which time sutures can be removed.
- Reasons for graft failure: Inadequate graft bed (poor vascularity), hematoma, movement, infection, technical errors
- EBL: Depends on extent of grafting, minimal to 250–500 mL

Postoperative Considerations
- Pain score: 4–6
- Application of lidocaine spray to donor site reduces postop pain
- Activity level kept at a minimum for first 2 d after surgery
- Monitor CV status
- Heat loss in transfer to and from OR

Anticipated Problems/Concerns
- Blood loss may be difficult to assess and may be high; assess Hct and volume status frequently for large areas of skin grafting
- Malnutrition may lead to unexpected amounts of edema
- Hypothermia common if not assiduously avoided pre- and intratransport
- Anesthetic plan must incorporate means for management of donor site pain postop.

Stereotactic Neurosurgery

Christine E. Goepfert

Risk

- Often performed as an awake procedure, esp for DBS and brain tumor surgery
- Skill of anesthesiologist required keeping pt comfortable, responsive, and cooperative over a long period of time under optimal surgical conditions while rapidly diagnosing and treating potential complications
- Major risks: Hemorrhage, seizures

Perioperative Considerations

- Planned approach to select suitable pts, develop an anesthetic plan and deal with problems

Worry About

- Contraindications
- Coagulation disorders
  - Coagulopathies: Bleeding diatheses, iatrogenic (heparin or coumadin)
  - Low plt count: PC <50,000/mL absolute contraindication, desirable to get PC <100,000/mL

- Major complications rare: (most <1%), highest in AIDS pts and pts with multifocal high-grade gliomas, most frequent: intracerebral hemorrhage

Overview

- More appropriately called image-guided stereotactic surgery because coordinate system relates to specific points in CT/MRI/angiogram
- Most commonly used for biopsies of deep-located lesions and movement disorders, in which STN, GPi, or VIM of the thalamus are targeted
- Mechanism of beneficial effect for movement disorders not fully understood, in high-frequency stimulation interference with several points along a pathway of synchronized oscillations in incriminated neuronal circuits
- "Awake" surgery in eloquent areas
  - For electrophysiological monitoring with MER (microelectrode recording) to guide device placement (unique pattern of spontaneous firing in specific brain areas), which make anesthetics undesirable and limit the options

- To perform neurologic testing (e.g., motor testing) for tremor surgery and detect complications with an acute onset of focal neurologic deficits

Indications and Usual Treatment

- Biopsy, in areas near eloquent brain, also brain stem lesions, multiple small lesions (e.g., in some AIDS pts)
- Catheter placement for drainage of deep colloid cysts and abscesses, catheter placement for intratumoral chemotherapy, radiation brachytherapy, and hunt placement
- Placement of deep brain stimulation electrode for epilepsy, chronic pain, essential tremor
- Lesion generation for movement disorders: Parkinsonism, dystonia, hemiballismus, chronic pain, and epilepsy
- Others, infrequently evacuation of intracerebral hemorrhage, stereotatic 'radiosurgery', locating a lesion for open craniotomy, transoral biopsy of C2 lesions, and experimental or unconventional applications such as aneurysm clipping

ASSESSMENT POINTS

System	Effect	Assessment by Hx	PE	Test
COAG	PC <50,000 mL	Easy bruising, Hx of postop bleeding, anticoagulants	Petechia, bruises	Plt count
RESP	Pre-existing pulm disease, OSA	Dyspnea, apnea episodes		Auscultation, spirometry test, CXR
CNS	Ability to cooperate	Medication, appearance	Anxiety, agitation	Assessment

Key References: Poon CCM, Irwin MG. Anaesthesia for deep brain stimulation and in patients with implanted neurostimulator devices. *BJA*. 2009;103:152–165.
Lozano AM, Gildenberg PL, Tasker RR, eds. *Textbook of stereotactic and functional neurosurgery*. Vols 1&2. Springer; 2009.

Perioperative Management

Preoperative Preparation

- Multidisciplinary assessment of pt in regards to aptitude for anesthetic technique:
  - General medical condition, e.g., CV co-morbidities, rare syndromes
  - Neurologic and psychiatric history, e.g., cognitive function, claustrophobia, epilepsy
  - Failure of previous sedation, ability to cooperate e.g., due to anxiety or severe off-period dystonia
- Check medication, esp.
  - Anticoagulants: Coumadin, plt inhibitors, herbal substances; check coagulation labs, manage coagulation status
  - Antiepileptic medication, their plasma levels and potential side-effects: Liver function, (rare) cardiac toxicity, ↑ confusion and sedation
  - Antiparkinson medication: Off-symptoms (dystonia, tremors, and pain) through periop discontinuation
- Establish rapport to pt with psychological preparation and reassurance
- In awake procedures
  - Careful explanation of course of procedure, its likely duration with emphasis of restraints on pt movement, esp. the lack of ability to move the head if frame used
  - For attachment of frame short-acting drug to increase tolerance possible, but not necessary (e.g., remifentanil, possibly propofol, or low-dose midazolam) to not interfere with clinical and electrophysiological monitoring later on
  - Debrief process of surgery and esp. the use of drugs with neurosurgeons

Monitoring

- Standard ASA monitors with EKG, NIBP, SpO2 and ETCO2
- Arterial line only if medically indicated

- Airway equipment readily available, like nasal and oral airways, LMA, ETT, laryngoscope, fiberoptic endoscope, also in 'awake' surgery
- In 'awake' procedures
  - Nasal prongs (or face mask) for O2 inhalation with end-tidal capnography
  - Restricted access to head, preventing mask ventilation and laryngoscopy, potentially requiring awake fiberoptic intubation
  - Urinary catheter or sheath catheter in men to avoid restlessness due to urgency, alternatively restrictive fluid management

Anesthetic Technique in "Awake" Procedures and MAC

- Nerve blockade
  - Infiltration of local anesthetic at pin sites
  - Scalp block to anesthetize supraorbital, supratrochlear, greater and lesser occipital nerves
  - Preferably long-acting local anesthetics (e.g., ropivicaine or bupivacaine with epinephrine), add short-acting LA (e.g., lidocaine) if rapid onset desired
- Increased compliance and tolerance due to continuous communication and reassurance of pt in quiet and comfortable environment with padding, appropriate room temp, and appropriate draping
- Frame placement in LA, placement of urinary catheter and preop scanning usually well tolerated, if not contemplate MAC with short-acting, rapidly reversible drugs such as remifentanil or propofol, alternatively dexmetedomidine
- Contemplate non-sedative antiemetic, e.g., dexamethasone or 5-HT3 antagonists such as ondansetron, esp. in epilepsy surgery and deep lesions
- Supplemental O2 to decrease incidence of desaturations
- No or restrictive use of anesthetics due to electrophysiological recordings and the necessity to

judge the pt clinically: Dexmetedomidine drug of choice, avoid benzodiazepines, propofol, and opioids; titration according to pharmacologic profile as required, in MAC aim at minimally depressed level of consciousness and ability to verbally communicate
- Benzodiazepines: Midazolam in low dose prior to pinning possible; anxiolysis, amnesia; alteration of threshold for stimulation and ↓ in vigilance; paradoxical agitation
- Dexmetedomidine: Low dose reported to preserve alertness for cognitive tests, no interference with MER pattern, no impairment of motor movements like tremor and dykinesia while ↓ hemodynamic and endocrine responses to stimuli; ↓ arterial BP, ↓ ICP, maintenance of airway patency, anesthetic sparing effects
- Opioids: ↓ Vigilance, resp depression, ↓ MER; epileptiform activity in pts with epilepsy, myoclonia in high doses; remifentanil ↓ tremors
- Propofol: Short-acting and easy to titrate; ↓ tremors, ↑ dyskinesia, ↓ epileptogenic activity; changes cortical surface EEG despite the pt being fully alert; interference with mapping (D/C 15–30 min before EEG recording); unpredictable PHARM in Parkinson pts; sneezing with risk of ↑ ICP
- Prevention or treatment of arterial Htn during procedure with short-acting antihypertensives such as clevidipine (or others), also dexmedetomidine, avoid sys. BP above (preop normal BP + 20%) to ↓ risk of hemorrhage; optimal BP controversial
- Prevention or treatment of arterial Htn esp. in Parkinson pts who are positioned in a sitting position
- Small doses of propofol or midazolam for seizures
- Equipment as for GA ready to use
- Continuous vigilance

PROCEDURES

533

Anesthetic Technique in General Anesthesia

- Pts who do not require awake technique or are uncooperative due to severe dyskinesia, pain, and anxiety
- Asleep-awake-asleep variant, preferably with LMA, alternatively spontaneous ventilation with or without nasal airway or ETT to increase pt tolerance, secure the airway and use hyperventilation
- Might be started before initial frame placement and imaging or afterwards with ↑ risk for intubation difficulties, consider rigid or flexible fiberoptic intubation
- TIVA or inhalational technique comparable
- Use of drugs according to possible testing, e.g., omitting muscle relaxants for motor testing
- General considerations and precautions for craniotomies

Surgical Stages

Localization with Imaging

- In or outside the OR
- Attachment of localizing device, e.g., frame, or less frequently frameless device
- Radiological imaging: Usually MRI, or CT, to identify targets

Orientation and Targeting

- In scan suite or OR
- Orientation within the same coordinate system and evaluation of the images

Image Guided Neurosurgery

- Usually in the OR
- Via burr hole or (mini-) craniectomy
- Uni- or bilaterally
- Passing microelectrodes, biopsy needles etc. along their trajectory towards the target

- In certain awake procedures clinical testing for side effects, improvement of symptoms, and neurologic exam and/or electrophysiological recordings to fine-tune the device placement with oscilloscope and audio monitors in superimposing scaled drawings on a brain atlas at each depth
- Securing device, connection to tunneled leads to implanted generator in chest or abd, potentially performed as a second-stage surgery and closure

Postoperative Considerations

- Invariably radiologic confirmation with CT scan
- 30° head up position to improve ventilation, reduce edema and facilitate cerebral venous and CSF drainage
- Postop monitoring, usually on ICU or OU for neurologic testing, also after 'awake' procedures
- Antiparkinson medication ASAP to avoid motor fluctuation and resp problems
- Avoid sedative opioids (such as morphine or hydromorphone) for pain relief, use fentanyl or codeine instead
- Specific screening for potential CNP (cranial nerve palsies), e.g., nerve X with vocal cord palsy, worsening of OSA, which might cause breathing difficulties, increasing risk of aspiration

Anticipated Problems/Concerns

- Resp complications in "awake" procedures
  - Resp depression due to oversedation
  - Mechanical obstruction with difficulties to access the airway or shifting of the body which might require release from the frame

- LOC with resp depression due to acute intracranial hemorrhage or seizures
- Pre-existing resp depression, e.g., due to stiffness of resp muscles in Parkinson pts, restrictive pulm disease, and ↑ sensitivity to drugs
- CV complications in "awake" procedures
- Arterial hypotension during positioning (orthostasis) and induction of GA
- Higher incidence of intracranial hemorrhage with high intraop BP
- Neurologic complications in "awake" procedures
- Sudden onset of focal deficits, usually not requiring anesthesiologic intervention
  - Seizures, mostly focal, rarely tonic-clonic
  - Agitation and anxiety
  - Excessive pain and discomfort
  - Acute LOC
- Air embolism (rare)
- N/V
- Pharmacologic complications due to drug-drug interactions with antiepileptic medication, altered sensitivity to drugs in Parkinson pts, and LA toxicity
- Specific demands for skills to communicate well with pt and surgical team esp. in awake procedures and to titrate anesthetics to keep pt comfortable and communicative under optimal surgical conditions and monitoring

Strabismus Repair

Gregory Weller
Ronald S. Litman

Risk

- Incidence: 3–5%
- Most common pediatric eye surgery
- Usually idiopathic, but may be assoc with other ocular abn, NM disorders, meningomyelocele, or congenital syndromes
- Mostly pediatric pts
- In adults, often 2° to trauma

Perioperative Risks

- Surgery is elective, and usually outpatient
- Globe perforation ~1%
- Endophthalmitis 1:3000
- Retinal detachment 1:5000

Worry About

- Arrhythmias due to stimulation of oculocardiac reflex
- High incidence of PONV (>80% without prophylaxis) due to altered visual fields and oculogastric reflex

- Iatrogenic ocular injury
- Strabismus can be a sign of an as yet undiagnosed underlying myopathy

Overview

- Strabismus is the misalignment of the visual axes.
- Repair involves manipulation of extraocular muscle lengths or insertion sites to improve visual alignment.
- Adjustable sutures are sometimes placed in adults to allow for minor corrections later.
- Anesthetic goals are to provide adequate akinesia, prevention of PONV, safely manage the oculocardiac reflex, and provide sufficient analgesia.
- Oculocardiac reflex (OCR)
  - Usually causes sinus bradycardia +/- hypotension, but can lead to more serious arrhythmias (junctional, ectopic beats, PVCs, ventricular fibrillation, asystole)

  - Afferent limb: Trigeminal nerve; efferent limb: Vagal nerve
  - Initiated by pressure on globe or traction on extraocular muscles, esp. medial rectus
  - Shows tachyphylaxis: Subsequent stimulations less likely to generate response
- In past, pediatric strabismus pts thought to be at elevated risk for malignant hyperthermia, because of observed increased incidence of masseter muscle spasm, esp with succinylcholine and/or halothane. No modern evidence of this association.

Indications and Usual Treatment

- Diplopia
- Marked esotropia
- Compensatory head posture
- Surgical repair most successful when undertaken in early childhood to prevent development of amblyopia

ASSESSMENT POINTS

System	Effect	Assessment by Hx	PE	Test
HEENT	Assoc syndromes with possible difficult airway	Snoring/sleep apnea	Airway exam	
CARDIO	Assoc congenital heart disease possible	SOB, poor growth, birth, and gestational Hx	CV exam	ECHO may be indicated
RESP	Bronchopulmonary dysplasia if premature	Birth and gestational Hx	Chest exam, feeding Hx	O$_2$ saturation
GI	PONV	Past surgical history		
NM	Myopathy	Fatigue, weakness	Weakness, spasticity	

Key Reference: Hauser MW, Valley RD, Bailey AG. Anesthesia for pediatric ophthalmic surgery. In: Motoyama EK, Davis PJ, eds. *Anesthesia for infants and children.* Philadelphia: Mosby Elsevier; 2006:770–788.

Perioperative Management

Preoperative Preparation

- Assess for assoc congenital abn or co-existing morbidities
- Be aware of systemic effects of topical ophthalmic drugs
- Standard NPO guidelines
- IM atropine decreases incidence of OCR from 90% to 50%

Monitoring

- Routine
- Close attention to ECG for OCR

Anesthetic Technique/Induction

- GA for pediatric pts
- For cooperative adults, consider local + regional (peri/retrobulbar blocks)
- Oral RAE ETT required in most cases; may be performed with LMA
- Hypercarbia and hypoxia increase incidence and worsen severity of OCR
- Position and secure ETT or LMA with care: pt turned 90° away from anesthesiologist

Surgical Stages

Induction

- Sevoflurane inhalational induction for children, or propofol induction in older pts or those with IV access

- Succinylcholine, which causes sustained extraocular muscle contraction, is relatively contraindicated due to potential interference with surgeon's forced duction test
- Ondansetron, dexamethasone, metoclopramide, or droperidol (with due consideration of black-box warning), or a combination of these, for PONV prophylaxis
- Maintain adequate muscle relaxation for duration of surgical manipulation, to prevent eye injury from pt movement
- Maintenance with propofol assoc with less PONV

Strabismus Repair

- Consider pretreatment with vagolytic (e.g., atropine) to minimize OCR.
- Respond to decrease in HR >20% by asking surgeon to cease manipulation, and giving IV atropine 5–20 mcg/kg.
- Mydriatic topical agents sometimes used by surgeon. Ocular phenylephrine, esp. the more concentrated solutions, may be readily absorbed and can cause significant Htn, pulm edema, and even cardiac arrest.
  - Preferably choose parasympatholytic agents instead of phenylephrine

- Don't treat phenylephrine-induced Htn with beta-blockers, which are assoc with development of pulm edema and cardiac failure; rather treat by deepening anesthesia.
- Almost no blood loss or fluid shifts

Postoperative Considerations

- Pain is variable
- Analgesia with ketorolac, acetaminophen, or narcotics (recognizing that narcotics may contribute to PONV)
- Treat PONV with ondansetron or metoclopramide
- Usually outpatient surgery, so ambulatory practices and goals are recommended

Anticipated Problems/Concerns

- Must communicate effectively with surgeon preop regarding anesthesia plan, and intraop regarding effects of oculocardiac reflex
- PONV causes significant pt discomfort and dissatisfaction, and can lead to dehydration, delayed discharge, or unanticipated admission.

Testicular Torsion Surgery

Lyndsey Cox
Ronald S. Litman

Risk

- Incidence 1/160 males; adolescents, less commonly in neonatal period
- May follow testicular trauma or strenuous physical activity (20%)

Perioperative Risks

- Dependent only on baseline health of pt

Worry About

- N/V from severe pain and opioid administration
- Full stomach: Aspiration of gastric contents during induction of general anesthesia

- Testicular ischemia depends on time from diagnosis to surgery: 6 hr critical time frame
- Pt anxiety

Overview

- Presents as acute scrotal pain and results from twisting of spermatic cord with vascular compromise of testicle
- Temporizing treatment involves manual de-torsion by a urologist, which may alleviate ischemia, but surgical orchidopexy still required
- Often confusing diagnosis; color Doppler US considered to be test of choice

- Differential Dx incl epididymitis, orchitis, testicular appendix torsion, hydrocele, inguinal hernia, Henoch-Schönlein purpura (abd pain, hematuria, nephritis).

ICD-9-CM Code: 608.2

Indications and Usual Treatment

- Treatment is surgical de-torsion and subsequent orchidopexy; highly successful if performed within 6 hr of onset of pain
- Success less than 5% if performed after 24 hr

ASSESSMENT POINTS

System	Effect	Assessment by Hx	PE	Test
HEENT	Minimal	N/A	N/A	N/A
CARDIO	Systemic signs of severe pain	Systemic	Htn, tachycardia	Vitals assessment
RESP	Minimal			n/a
RENAL/ GU	Minimal			US can show decreased blood flow to affected testes.
CNS	Systemic signs of severe pain	Dizziness or nausea	n/a	n/a

Key Reference: Litman RS. Anesthesia for pediatric urologic procedures. In: Litman RS, eds. *Pediatric anesthesia, The requisites.* New York, NY: Harcourt Health Sciences; 2004.

Perioperative Management

Preoperative Preparation

- Thorough Hx and physical for systemic disease
- Adequate Hx and family Hx of prior anesthetics
- Consider administration of metoclopramide and oral sodium citrate as aspiration prophylaxis
- Administer IV opioids for pain and benzodiazepines for amnesia and anxiolysis

Monitoring

- Routine monitors: Electrocardiograph, noninvasive BP, pulse oximeter, temp probe

Anesthetic Technique/Induction

- Rapid sequence induction for general endotracheal anesthesia
- Spinal anesthesia also appropriate if pt prefers
- Local infiltration with minimal systemic sedation possible in selected cases
- Scrotum innervated by inferior pudendal branch (long scrotal nerve) of posterior femoral cutaneous nerve (from the sacral plexus), and the medial and lateral posterior scrotal branches of peroneal nerve (from the pudendal nerve)

Surgical Stages

- Small incision in scrotum performed
- Testis is isolated and untwisted; removed if found to be without blood flow by intraop flow Doppler study
- Bilateral orchidopexy usually performed to prevent recurrence

Postoperative Considerations

- Minimal pain after torsion corrected
- Underlying pt condition will play a larger role in determining postop care

Anticipated Problems/Concerns

- Full stomach: Risk of pulm aspiration with induction of GA
- Testicular ischemia if duration of torsion prolonged (>6–8 hr)

Tetralogy of Fallot, Correction of

Veronica C. Swanson
Norah Janosy

Risk

- CHD incidence < 1% of live births
- TOF accounts for 10–15% of total CHD

Perioperative Risks

- Operative mortality <5% for children without RV failure or pulm Atresia
- Major perioperative risk factors after repair: Major pulm artery anomaly, other major cardiac defect, very young age, increased Hct, absent pulm valve, major AP collaterals
- 85% 10-y survival with surgery
- 90% mortality by the age of 21 y without surgery

Worry About

- Degree of R → L shunt and hypercyanosis (end-organ damage)
- Arterial hypoxemia
- Venous air embolus and ↑ likelihood of paradoxical embolism
- Polycythemia and thrombotic events

- Other congenital anomalies

Overview

- Anatomic problems: VSD(s), dynamic RV outflow obstruction, aorta overriding RV and LV, RV hypertrophy
- Aberrant takeoff of coronary arteries: 5–12% of cases
- Functional problems: Bidirectional or R → L shunt, arterial hypoxemia, progressive RV dysfunction
- Cyanosis worsened by anemia, infection, stress, posture, hypercontractile states
- Pulm valve: Thickened, hypoplastic, or bicuspid
- Symptoms and urgency of correction depend on degree of pulm obstruction with resultant pressure load and RV failure, R → L shunt, and diminished pulm blood flow

- Challenge:
  - Avoid ↑ R → L shunt
  - Avoid ↓ SVR and/or ↑ RV outflow obstruction

ICD-9-CM Code: 745.2

Indications and Usual Treatment

- Increase in severity of cyanosis and polycythemia leads to early correction when possible. Exceptions: Prematurity, low birth weight, other anomalies and medical conditions.
- Severe cyanosis in first month of life may necessitate palliative systemic-to-pulm arterial shunt
- Correction often done in first year of life to avoid progressive RV failure

ASSESSMENT POINTS

System	Effect	Assessment by Hx	PE	Test
CARDIO	R → L shunt	Cyanotic spells, relation to crying or exercise	Observe for clubbing, squatting during tet spell, and cyanosis	ECHO, catheterization pulse oximetry (O_2 sat 80–90% room air)
	RV failure	Exercise intolerance, SOB, syncope	↑ JVP, tachypnea, hepatosplenomegaly (late)	ECG: RV hypertrophy, right axis deviation ECHO, CXR
	Polycythemia, prior palliative shunt	CVA (increased risk)	Neurologic exam, look for scars, absent peripheral pulses	Hct ECHO, catheterization, look at old operative reports
RESP	Decreased pulm blood flow	Exercise intolerance	Tachypnea, clubbing	Catheterization, ECHO, expect low O_2 sat
OTHER	Developmental and growth delay	Developmental and growth delay	Small size, test for developmental delay	Variety of measures
	Assoc congenital anomalies	Thorough Hx of all systems	Thorough exam of pertinent systems	Variety of tests

Key References: Samuelson PN, Lell WA. Tetralogy of Fallot. In: Lake CL, ed. *Pediatric cardiac anesthesia*. 3rd ed. Stamford: Appleton & Lange; 1998:303–314.; Lake CL. Anesthesia for patients with congenital heart disease. In: Kaplan JA, ed. *Cardiac anesthesia*, 4th ed. Philadelphia: Saunders; 1999:785–820. Breitbart R, Fyler D. Tetralogy of Fallot. In: Keane, Locke, & Fyler, eds. *Nadas' pediatric cardiology*, 2nd ed. Philadelphia: Saunders; 2006:559.

Perioperative Management

Monitoring

- Arterial catheter: If pt has a palliative systemic artery-to-pulm shunt, arterial line should go to other side
- TEE for evaluation pre- and post-repair
- Central venous line for inotropes and pressure monitoring: Scrupulous attention to avoid air bubbles in lines
- Standard ASA monitors

Airway

- Avoid excessive airway pressures (may ↑ PVR)
- Airway concern if velocardiofacial syndrome

Induction

- Premedication is important and may incl midazolam, morphine, and ketamine.
- Ketamine a good choice: Does not ↑ PVR. Also, ↑ SVR effect overshadows any ↑ in contractility (as in infundibulum), therefore improving cyanosis.
- Fentanyl a good choice: Slow HR and decreased catecholamine release.
- Sevoflurane for inhalation induction; use caution to avoid ↓ in SVR assoc with inhaled agents—less of a problem in younger pts.
- Ensure adequate hydration: Special risk in severely polycythemic children
- Anesthetic technique

- Choice of maintenance drugs should seek to avoid ↑ HR and myocardial contractility, and ↓ SVR
- Specific drug choices not important. Vigilance and responsiveness is.
- Phenylephrine diluted and ready for possible tet spells.
- Heparin drawn up in the event the tet spell does not reverse with treatment—urgent crash onto bypass.

Surgical Stages

Pre-Cardiopulmonary Bypass

- Maintain adequate preload, cardiac output, and SVR
- Severe episodic tet spells
  - Can occur at anytime, Especially at induction, incision, opening the sternum, and manipulating the heart and PAs.
  - Goal is to ↓ R → L shunt
  - May require IV fluids to increase blood volume and decrease Hct
  - 100% O_2, pulm vasodilation
  - Phenylephrine to increase SVR
  - Esmolol and deepening depth of anesthetic to decrease RV outflow obstruction
  - Avoid decrease in SVR while deepening anesthetic

- Surgical compression of aorta (reversing shunt) or crash on bypass if other steps ineffective

Post Cardiopulmonary Bypass

- Assess components of repair: Regurgitant flow through the pulm valve, residual VSD via TEE
- Assess RV function: RV pressure < or = ½ LV pressure.
- For struggling RV: Fluid load, inotropic support, afterload reduce pulm circulation (milrinone)
- The greater the RVH and RV failure preop, the higher the inotropic requirements and filling pressures postop.
- Common arrhythmias: Junctional ectopic tachycardia (JET)—cooling, overdrive pacing, ↑ depth of anesthesia, amiodarone—and heart block—temporary or permanent pacemaker.

Postoperative

- Ensure adequate RV function and low PVR
- Early extubation if possible

Anticipated Problems/Concerns

- Persistent RV dysfunction
- Persistent RV outflow tract obstruction
- Persistent VSD
- Postop bleeding
- Persistent R → L shunt (VSD)
- Most postop mortality found in pts with acute RV failure

Thoracic Aortic Repair

Christopher C. Young

Risk

- Incidence in USA: 3.4% incidence of aortic aneurysm; 26% involve thoracic aorta (TAA)
- Untreated TAA greater than 10 cm confers a 2-y survival rate of <30%; ½ of these deaths are due to aneurysm rupture
- Increased incidence with Htn
- M:F ratio: 2.9:1
- Peak incidence 50–70 y

Perioperative Risks

- Htn, coronary and carotid vascular disease
- Untreated dissection: 25–35% mortality within 24 hr, 90% in 3 mo
- Surgical repair carries 10% mortality. Causes of postop death are hemorrhage (29%); cardiac events—ischemia, MI, CHF (26%); and multi-organ system failure (22%).
- Traumatic disruption immediately fatal in 85%.

Worry About

- Elevated HR and BP promote dissection
- Acute dissection can lead to compromised blood flow (coronary, renal, splanchnic, spinal cord), pericardial tamponade, acute aortic valvular insufficiency, or bleeding
- Assoc injuries (lungs, heart, head, abd) with traumatic rupture
- Major blood loss; need for rapid transfusion intraop
- Acute dissections frequently brought for repair with minimal preop preparation

Overview

- Primary risk factors are Htn, tobacco use, and atherosclerosis
- Thoracic aortic aneurysms 2–3 × more likely to dissect than abd

- Distribution of thoracic dissections: Ascending aorta 60–70%; descending aorta 30–35%; aortic arch 5–10%

ICD-9-CM Code: 441.01 (Dissection of aortathoracic); 441.03 (Dissection of aortathoracoabdomina)

Etiology

- Aneurysm develops as vascular wall weakens from hydraulic forces (Htn) coupled with degeneration (atherosclerosis). Involves all 3 layers of aortic wall. Usually becomes symptomatic by compression of adjacent structures.
- Dissection risk factors: Htn, cigarette smoking, Marfan's, congenital anomalies (coarctation, AS), pregnancy, rheumatologic disorders, bacterial infection, syphilis. Intimal tear allows separation of intima from media and adventitia.

Location	DeBakey	Stanford
Ascending and descending aorta	Type I	Group A
Ascending aorta only	Type II	Group A
Distal to left subclavian	Type III	Group B

- Traumatic rupture occurs commonly at ligamentum arteriosum (aorta fixed at this point)

Indications and Usual Treatment

- Group A (types I and II) dissections are surgically repaired immediately via median sternotomy using cardiopulmonary bypass (CPB) and deep hypothermic circulatory arrest (DHCA)

- Group B (type III) dissections are medically managed; when operation is indicated (>10 cm diameter, progressive enlargement, or producing symptoms), left thoracotomy and one-lung ventilation employed
- Traumatic aortic dissections are treated surgically regardless of symptoms

- Endovascular stenting is gaining in popularity for elective TAA repair; this approach is assoc with fewer short term complications (myocardial ischemia, renal failure, resp complications); long-term outcomes still being assessed.

ASSESSMENT POINTS

System	Effect	Assessment by Hx	PE	Test
HEENT	SVC syndrome Recurrent laryngeal nerve compression	Dyspnea Hoarseness	JVD edema	Flow-volume loop Indirect laryngoscopy
CARDIO	Myocardial ischemia LV dysfunction Aortic root dilation Valvular disease Venous compression	Angina Dyspnea Dyspnea	S_3 gallop Friction rub Early diastolic murmur Muffled heart sounds Plethora	ECG/Echo Stress testing TTE/TEE Coronary angio
RESP	Bronchial/tracheal compression Recurrent pneumonia Pulm compression	Dyspnea Cough	Wheezing Tracheal deviation Hemoptysis	ABGs Flow-volume loop CXR Chest CT or MRI
GI	Mesenteric ischemia	Abd pain Bloody diarrhea	Tenderness	Colonoscopy Angio
RENAL	↓ Renal perfusion	Oliguria		Cr, Cr clearance
CNS	Spinal cord ischemia Carotid stenosis	Weakness Paraplegia		MRI, EMG Carotid duplex
MS		Back or chest pain		Chest CT or MRI

Key Reference: Bavaria JE, Appoo JJ, Makaroun MS, et al. Endovascular stent grafting versus open surgical repair of descending thoracic aortic aneurysms in low-risk patients: A multicenter comparative trial. *J Thorac Cardiovasc Surg.* 2007;133:369–377.

Perioperative Implications

Preoperative Preparation

- IV sodium nitroprusside with β-blockers (consider calcium channel blockade if β-blockers contraindicated)
- Preop statins and discontinuance of tobacco use if elective
- Premedication to prevent anxiety and pain
- Early, prompt reduction of shear stress (dP/dt) indicated to reduce chance of rupture

Monitoring

- Invasive arterial BP—left radial for group A, right radial for group B, and femoral or dorsalis pedis for distal aortic pressure measurement during crossclamping
- PA catheter and/or TEE
- SSEPs not consistently reliable guide to spinal cord ischemia

Airway

- Difficult airway if compression or deviation of tracheobronchial tree

- May interfere with placement of double-lumen ET tube

Induction/Maintenance

- High-dose narcotic useful to blunt intubation response
- Inhalation agent useful to ↓ myocardial contractility, provide amnesia
- Avoid N_2O during one-lung ventilation and to prevent expansion of air emboli

Extubation
- Usually keep sedated and mechanically ventilated until warmed and stable
- Neurologic status important to assess following deep hypothermic circulatory arrest
- Prevent hemodynamic response to extubation

Adjuvants
- β-blockers, nitroprusside, nitroglycerin continued periop
- Maintain adequate hydration
- Questionable renal benefit: Mannitol 0.5 g/kg well prior to crossclamping; "renal dose" dopamine, fenoldopam

- Maintenance of aortic pressure distal to cross-clamp; mild hypothermia; CSF drainage; steroids, intrathecal papaverine may limit spinal cord ischemia (5–7% incidence)

Anticipated Problems/Concerns
- Aortic cross-clamping causes ↑ LV afterload, LV wall tension, and O_2 consumption. Vasodilators useful, but distal hypotension may induce spinal cord ischemia. Vascular shunting or partial bypass during cross-clamp may overcome these effects.
- Aortic unclamping results in ↑ stroke volume but profound ↓ in SVR and significant metabolic acidosis if no shunt used. Fluid management, α-agonists (phenylephrine), and sodium bicarbonate may be useful.
- CPB and DHCA are assoc with increased rates of complications incl coagulation abn, paraplegia, CNS injury, stroke, myocardial ischemia, renal failure, and resp complications.

PROCEDURES

Risk

- Incidence in USA: 440,000/y develop hyperthyroidism +5% of pregnant females
- 1/1000 females, 1/3000 males; ~240,000 thyroid operations/y (2000–2004 data)

Perioperative Risks

- Increased risk of thyroid storm, even if pt was made euthyroid prior to surgery
- Risk of postop airway compromise
- Occasionally late tetany (usually 2–3 d postop) due to removal of, or damage to, parathyroid glands
- Mortality <0.3%
- Hypoparathyroidism 2–3%

Worry About

- Assessing euthyroid state
- Securing airway if large goiter or displaced trachea
- Postop risks of nerve injury (immediate stridor requires immediate reintubation); surreptitious bleeding (examine wound prior to PACU discharge); thyroid storm (uncommon without acute illness or 3 d postop)

Overview

- Major goal is to avoid thyroid storm; if not euthyroid prior to surgery, try to delay operation
- If emergency operation, use β-blockers and iodides to ↓ periop effects of released thyroid hormones and ↓ further synthesis and release of hormones; keep in ICU until risk of storm has passed
- Done in young adults with hyperthyroidism, or normal thyroid function with a cold nodule, or with a goiter that is bothersome physiologically o[...] psychologically
- Hyperthyroidism is an endocrinopathy wi[...] CV disease—tachycardia (commonly idiopathic if no prior Dx of hyperthyroidism), CHF, dysrhythmias (AFIB)—as major manifestation
- Other target systems of hyperthyroidism are resp and CNS (↓ drive to breathe, anxiety, psychoses) and metabolic

- If pt is ma[...]
of thyroid s[...]
ished by >[...]

ICD-9-[...]
rotoxi[...]
(Thy[...]

[...]
ou[...]
- Gon[...]

Handwritten notes:
HINTS: Thyroidect[...]
- make sure "lid" on to[...] tight if using glidescope [...] ct tends to[...] from very top to move thru [...] semi-controlled
- lean on cuff. also [...] as ct
- ALWAYS artline [...]
- hypotension
- fentanyl / Remi) for induct[...]
Propofol
Roc 5m dose as [...]
OR just as [...]
- Remi[...]

ASSESSMENT POINTS

System	Effect	Assessment by Hx	PE	Test
HEENT	Weakened tracheal rings, distorted/displaced trachea; Ophthalmopathy; Large tongue if associated with goiter or amyloidosis	Snoring, hoarseness, neck pain	Ask to vocalize "e"; examine airway and neck, look at eyes	CXR (PA and lat), lat neck films, CT scan of neck, US of neck
CARDIO	CHF, cardiomyopathies; Sinus tachycardia, mitral valve prolapse, AFib	DOE, orthostatic SOB palpitations, ↑ HR during sleep	Standard exam	Rhythm strip or full ECG
GI	Wt loss, diarrhea, dehydration	Dizziness on arising, Hx of diarrhea, constipation	Skin turgor, orthostatic VS	↑ Serum alkaline phosphatase
HEME		Mild anemia, thrombocytopenia; Agranulocytosis 2° to propylthiouracil or methimazole	Skin/mucous membranes for infection/petechiae	CBC with plt count, differential
CNS		Shaking, anxiety, emotional lability; Hypothyroid goiter assoc with slow thought processes	Reflex speed, tremor, nervousness, mental status	
METAB	Need to assess if euthyroid; Malnourished	Reflex speed, tremor, heat intolerance, fatigue, weakness; wt loss, anorexia, or ↑ appetite	Reflex speed, HR	Free T_4

Key Reference: Roizen MF, Fleisher LA. Implications of concurrent disease. In: Miller RD, ed. *Anesthesia.* 7th ed. New York: Churchill Livingstone/Elsevier; 2010: 1077–1080.

Perioperative Implications

Anesthetic Technique
- No one best technique

Airway
- Occasionally distorted anatomy 2° to goiter, tracheal ring involvement, inflammation 2° to thyroiditis
- Consider awake fiberoptic intubation
- Consider armored tube or equivalent if tracheal rings are affected

Preinduction/Induction
- Prehydrate if CV status tolerates
- Routine unless abn airway or CV system or noneuthyroid condition

Monitoring
- Temp (also place cooling blanket on OR table to treat thyroid storm if it occurs)
- Consider invasive monitoring if CV system severely affected
- If considerable head-up position, consider air embolus monitoring and therapy strategies

- If done with minimally invasive surgery, can monitor for pneumothorax with endtidal CO_2 and with portable ultrasound

Induction/Maintenance/Extubation
- Extubate with optimal conditions for reintubation

Surgical Stages

Initial Dissection
- Can approach from axilla if minimally invasive approach or robotic minimally invasive approach (majority at Cleveland Clinic for Hyperthyroidism are now done with this approach)
- Transverse collar incision if open approach
- Thyroid lobe freed from strap muscles with securing of superior thyroid vessels; these are clamped after ensuring localization and preservation of recurrent laryngeal nerve and parathyroid glands in either open or minimally invasive approach

Thyroid Removal
- Following division of middle and inferior thyroid vessels, thyroid lobe is retracted medially and liberated

Adjuvants
- Usually no requirement for NMB
- Can be done with regional: Superficial and deep cervical plexus blocks and infiltration

Postoperative Considerations
- EBL: 50–150 mL
- Pain score: 2–4
- Usually can be treated with NSAIDs or occasionally with PCA

Anticipated Problems/Concerns

- Thyroid storm is life-threatening illness manifested by hyperpyrexia, tachycardia, striking alterations in consciousness
- Bleeding can compromise airway function
- Recurrent laryngeal nerve injuries damage abductor fibers, resulting in hoarseness. Bilateral injury results in fixed narrow opening to glottis with inspiratory airflow obstruction (stridor), inability to vocalize, aspiration risk, and immediate need for tracheal intubation.

Extubation

- Usually keep sedated and mechanically ventilated until warmed and stable
- Neurologic status important to assess following deep hypothermic circulatory arrest
- Prevent hemodynamic response to extubation

Adjuvants

- β-blockers, nitroprusside, nitroglycerin continued periop
- Maintain adequate hydration
- Questionable renal benefit: Mannitol 0.5 g/kg well prior to crossclamping; "renal dose" dopamine, fenoldopam

- Maintenance of aortic pressure distal to cross-clamp; mild hypothermia; CSF drainage; steroids, intrathecal papaverine may limit spinal cord ischemia (5–7% incidence)

Anticipated Problems/Concerns

- Aortic cross-clamping causes ↑ LV afterload, LV wall tension, and O_2 consumption. Vasodilators useful, but distal hypotension may induce spinal cord ischemia. Vascular shunting or partial bypass during cross-clamp may overcome these effects.
- Aortic unclamping results in ↑ stroke volume but profound ↓ in SVR and significant metabolic acidosis if no shunt used. Fluid management, α-agonists (phenylephrine), and sodium bicarbonate may be useful.
- CPB and DHCA are assoc with increased rates of complications incl coagulation abn, paraplegia, CNS injury, stroke, myocardial ischemia, renal failure, and resp complications.

Thyroidectomy (Open or Minimally Invasive) for Hyperthyroidism

Michael F. Roizen

Risk

- Incidence in USA: 440,000/y develop hyperthyroidism +5% of pregnant females
- 1/1000 females, 1/3000 males; ~240,000 thyroid operations/y (2000–2004 data)

Perioperative Risks

- Increased risk of thyroid storm, even if pt was made euthyroid prior to surgery
- Risk of postop airway compromise
- Occasionally late tetany (usually 2–3 d postop) due to removal of, or damage to, parathyroid glands
- Mortality <0.3%
- Hypoparathyroidism 2–3%

Worry About

- Assessing euthyroid state
- Securing airway if large goiter or displaced trachea
- Postop risks of nerve injury (immediate stridor requires immediate reintubation); surreptitious bleeding (examine wound prior to PACU discharge); thyroid storm (uncommon without acute illness or 3 d postop)

Overview

- Major goal is to avoid thyroid storm; if not euthyroid prior to surgery, try to delay operation
- If emergency operation, use β-blockers and iodides to ↓ periop effects of released thyroid hormones and ↓ further synthesis and release of hormones; keep in ICU until risk of storm has passed
- Done in young adults with hyperthyroidism, or normal thyroid function with a cold nodule, or with a goiter that is bothersome physiologically or psychologically
- Hyperthyroidism is an endocrinopathy with CV disease—tachycardia (commonly idiopathic if no prior Dx of hyperthyroidism), CHF, dysrhythmias (AFIB)—as major manifestation
- Other target systems of hyperthyroidism are resp and CNS (↓ drive to breathe, anxiety, psychoses) and metabolic

- If pt is made euthyroid prior to operation, risk of thyroid storm and periop CV problems diminished by >90%

ICD-9-CM Codes: 242.9 (Hyperthyroidism [thyrotoxicosis]); 242.0 (Graves' disease); 245 (Thyroiditis); 193 (Malignant thyroid disease)

Etiology

- Multinodular diffuse enlargement (Graves' disease)
- Thyroid adenoma—toxic multinodular goiter (firm gland) later in life and almost never malignant; unilateral solitary nodule with autonomous function earlier in life almost always benign
- Cold nodules assoc with radiation therapy of other diseases as well as idiopathic
- Goiter assoc with iodine deficiency

ASSESSMENT POINTS

System	Effect	Assessment by Hx	PE	Test
HEENT	Weakened tracheal rings, distorted/displaced trachea Ophthalmopathy Large tongue if associated with goiter or amyloidosis	Snoring, hoarseness, neck pain	Ask to vocalize "e"; examine airway and neck, look at eyes	CXR (PA and lat), lat neck films, CT scan of neck, US of neck
CARDIO	CHF, cardiomyopathies Sinus tachycardia, mitral valve prolapse, AFib	DOE, orthostatic SOB palpitations, ↑ HR during sleep	Standard exam	Rhythm strip or full ECG
GI	Wt loss, diarrhea, dehydration	Dizziness on arising, Hx of diarrhea, constipation	Skin turgor, orthostatic VS	↑ Serum alkaline phosphatase
HEME		Mild anemia, thrombocytopenia Agranulocytosis 2° to propylthiouracil or methimazole	Skin/mucous membranes for infection/petechiae	CBC with plt count, differential
CNS		Shaking, anxiety, emotional lability Hypothyroid goiter assoc with slow thought processes	Reflex speed, tremor, nervousness, mental status	
METAB	Need to assess if euthyroid Malnourished	Reflex speed, tremor, heat intolerance, fatigue, weakness; wt loss, anorexia, or ↑ appetite	Reflex speed, HR	Free T$_4$

Key Reference: Roizen MF, Fleisher LA. Implications of concurrent disease. In: Miller RD, ed. *Anesthesia*. 7th ed. New York: Churchill Livingstone/Elsevier; 2010: 1077–1080.

Perioperative Implications

Anesthetic Technique
- No one best technique

Airway
- Occasionally distorted anatomy 2° to goiter, tracheal ring involvement, inflammation 2° to thyroiditis
- Consider awake fiberoptic intubation
- Consider armored tube or equivalent if tracheal rings are affected

Preinduction/Induction
- Prehydrate if CV status tolerates
- Routine unless abn airway or CV system or noneuthyroid condition

Monitoring
- Temp (also place cooling blanket on OR table to treat thyroid storm if it occurs)
- Consider invasive monitoring if CV system severely affected
- If considerable head-up position, consider air embolus monitoring and therapy strategies

- If done with minimally invasive surgery, can monitor for pneumothorax with endtidal CO_2 and with portable ultrasound

Induction/Maintenance/Extubation
- Extubate with optimal conditions for reintubation

Surgical Stages

Initial Dissection
- Can approach from axilla if minimally invasive approach or robotic minimally invasive approach (majority at Cleveland Clinic for Hyperthyroidism are now done with this approach)
- Transverse collar incision if open approach
- Thyroid lobe freed from strap muscles with securing of superior thyroid vessels; these are clamped after ensuring localization and preservation of recurrent laryngeal nerve and parathyroid glands in either open or minimally invasive approach

Thyroid Removal
- Following division of middle and inferior thyroid vessels, thyroid lobe is retracted medially and liberated

Adjuvants
- Usually no requirement for NMB
- Can be done with regional: Superficial and deep cervical plexus blocks and infiltration

Postoperative Considerations
- EBL: 50–150 mL
- Pain score: 2–4
- Usually can be treated with NSAIDs or occasionally with PCA

Anticipated Problems/Concerns

- Thyroid storm is life-threatening illness manifested by hyperpyrexia, tachycardia, striking alterations in consciousness
- Bleeding can compromise airway function
- Recurrent laryngeal nerve injuries damage abductor fibers, resulting in hoarseness. Bilateral injury results in fixed narrow opening to glottis with inspiratory airflow obstruction (stridor), inability to vocalize, aspiration risk, and immediate need for tracheal intubation.

TMJ Arthroscopy

Stephen O. Heard

Risk

- Up to 17% of population suffers from TMJ disorders
- Majority of pts aged 15–45 y
- M:F estimates vary from 1:3 to 1:9
- Initiating factors: Trauma, grinding teeth at night due to stress, adverse loading of masticatory system

Perioperative Risks

- Periop mortality exceedingly rare
- Epistaxis

Worry About

- Co-existing diseases (e.g., rheumatoid arthritis)
- Establishing and maintaining airway
- Medications

Overview

- Used to evaluate and treat pain or lack of motion in TMJ
- TMJ anatomy: Joint divided into superior and inferior articular cavities by articular disk
- Approaches: Inferolateral, posterolateral, anterolateral
- Structures to watch: facial nerve, superficial temporal branch of auriculotemporal nerve, maxillary artery, superficial temporal artery and vein, parotid gland

ICD-9-CM Code: 524.6

Indications and Usual Treatment

- Diagnosis of TMJ pain
- Surgery
  - Biopsies
  - Debridement and lavage
  - Incision of adhesions
  - Restoration of disk mobility and position
  - Instillation of medication
  - Capsular or disk attachment scarification/plication
- Usual treatment
  - Behavior modification
  - Pharmacotherapy
  - Physical therapy
  - Appliance therapy
  - Occlusive therapy

ASSESSMENT POINTS

System	Effect	Assessment by Hx	PE	Test
HEENT	Epistaxis assoc with nasotracheal intubation Mouth opening	Epistaxis, nasal polyps, occluded nostril Trismus Pain on opening mouth Headache	Airway exam incl assessment of nostril patency Clicking of TMJ Muscle spasm	
CARDIO/RESP	Arthritis can be systemic disease: restrictive pulm disease, cardiomyopathy	SOB Exercise tolerance	Auscultation of heart and lungs Inspection of legs	O$_2$ saturation, ECG or CXR (if suggested by Hx, PE)
MS	Look for other joint involvement	Arthralgias	Inspection Palpation	

Key References: Ingawale S, Goswami T. Temporomandibular joints: Disorders, treatments, and biomechanics. *Ann Biomed Eng.* 2010; 37: 976–996; Kryshtalskyj B, Weinberg S. Surgical arthroscopy of the temporomandibular joint. *Ont Dent* 1996; 73:40–42.

Perioperative Management

Preoperative Preparation
IV sedation if needed

Monitoring
- Standard

Induction/Maintenance
- After standard induction, prepare nostrils with 4% cocaine or phenylephrine and dilate with lubricated nasal airways of increasing diameter
- Nasotracheal intubation (soften NT tube in warm H$_2$O; may need Magill forceps)
- Cover eyes with moistened eye pads (possible laser use)
- Some surgeons request IV administration of dexamethasone (10 mg)

Surgical Stages

- Injection of local anesthesia: Usually 1% lidocaine with 1:100,000 epinephrine
- Incision over superior joint space, insertion of obturator and/or sheath, removal of obturator, camera attachment
- Use of helium or Nd:YAG laser
  - Protective eyewear for pt and staff
  - Wet towels surrounding operative area
  - Water readily available
- Complications (<1%)
  - Hemorrhage (usually superficial temporal artery or vein)
  - Joint damage
  - Perforation into middle cranial fossa
  - Damage to middle ear ossicles
  - Injury to auriculotemporal nerve

- Minimal blood loss
- Some surgeons inject intra-articular steroids or local anesthetics (bupivacaine 0.5% with 1:200,000 epinephrine) for anti-inflammatory and analgesic effects

Postoperative Considerations
- Pain score: 0–5
- IV or PO narcotics/anti-inflammatory medications in PACU

Anticipated Problems/Concerns

- Epistaxis with intubation or extubation
- Postextubation pulm edema reported
- IV injections of local anesthetic

Tonsillectomy and Adenoidectomy

Joana Ratsiu

Helen W. Karl

Risk

- One of the most common surgical procedures in children
- Incidence varies by region and country; continues to decrease since 1970
- Racial and gender predominance: None
- Bimodal peaks at ages 4 and 16–17
- Most available data is in pediatric pts

Perioperative Risks

- Estimates of 30-d mortality range from 1/4000 to 1/35,000, usually from hemorrhage
- Resp complications are more common when <3 y
- 2° hemorrhage is more common >10 y

Worry About

- Indication for procedure: Usually airway obstruction (81% of pts <3 y) or recurrent infection

- Assoc URI increases the risk of resp complications and bleeding
- Obstructive sleep apnea (OSA) severity (as measured by a formal sleep study or overnight oximetry) predicts the nature of periop resp complications
- Bleeding, airway obstruction, apnea, and pain postop

Overview

- Adenoidectomy and tonsillectomy usually performed together, but consideration given to the specific risk-benefit ratio for each procedure
- Bleeding may occur in first 24 hr (1°) or 7–10 d postop (2°)
- Age and co-morbidities of pts dictate postop care

- Several operative methods exist; each is assoc with different risks of postop pain and hemorrhage

ICD-9-CM Codes: 474.0 (Chronic tonsillitis); 474.1 (Hypertrophy of tonsils and adenoids)

Indications and Usual Treatment

- Obstruction of nasal or pharyngeal airway, esp. when assoc with anatomic or physiologic disturbances
- Adenotonsillectomy is currently the treatment of choice for surgical treatment of OSA in children, although there is no strong evidence to support this.
- Chronic or recurrent infection of adenoids (also ears or sinuses) or tonsils despite adequate antibiotic therapy
- Acute peritonsillar abscess

ASSESSMENT POINTS

System	Effect	Assessment by Hx	PE	Test
HEENT	Chronic nasal obstruction assoc with abn facial growth	Snoring, enuresis, speech disorders; cognitive deficits	Adenoid facies, mouth breathing, obesity	Ask child to breathe with mouth closed
CARDIO	Chronic airway obstruction may lead to pulm Htn and right heart failure	Exercise intolerance	Cardiac exam: Loud 2nd heart sound	ECHO, ECG, CXR *if positive history/exam*
RESP	Tonsillar hyperplasia may result in sleep apnea and CO_2 retention	Disturbed sleep, daytime sleepiness	Airway exam, tonsil size	Polysomnography, O_2 sat
HEME	Pts with pre-existing bleeding disorders are at greater risk of postop hemorrhage	Patient or family Hx of bleeding, bruising, or aspirin (check OTC meds)	Multiple bruises above the knees	PT, PTT, plt count, bleeding time *if positive Hx*
NEURO	Brainstem dysfunction may amplify sleep apnea with moderate tonsillar hyperplasia	Cerebral palsy, Arnold-Chiari malformation		Polysomnography, O_2 sat
SYSTEMIC	Craniofacial abn (e.g., trisomy 21, Treacher Collins may have pre-existing airway narrowing), NM disorders, mucopolysaccharidoses, obesity		General exam	

Key Reference: Hannallah RS, Brown SA, Verghese ST: Otorhinolaryngologic procedures. In: Cote CJ, Lerman J, Todres ID, (eds): *A practice of anesthesia for infants and children,* 4th ed. Philadelphia, WB Saunders, 2009.

Perioperative Management

Perioperative Preparation

- Avoid preanesthetic sedatives if Hx of sleep apnea or very large tonsils
- Consider moderate dose of anxiolytic to ease induction
- Evaluate for bleeding abn; stop meds that interfere with coagulation
- Pre- or interop acetaminophen

Monitoring

- IV prior to induction if Hx of significant airway obstruction

Airway

- Preformed RAE ETTs fit best into groove of mouth gag
- Use cuffed tubes when possible
- LMA may also be used in older children and adults

Induction

- Consider atropine (0.02 mg/kg, max 1 mg) during induction

Surgical Stages

- Placement or removal of mouth gag may dislodge or obstruct ETT

- A single intraop dose of IV corticosteroid (up to 1 mg/kg dexamethasone, max 20 mg) decreases postop vomiting
- Local infiltration with epinephrine-containing local anesthetic decreases intraop blood loss, does not improve pain control, and may increase complication rate
- Spontaneous rather than controlled ventilation offers benefit of careful titration of opioids in pts with OSA
- Suction under direct vision before extubation; emptying the stomach with an orogastric tube may reduce the incidence of emesis
- Extubation—usually when the child is awake—and recovery in lateral position with head slightly down keeps blood away from larynx
- If trachea is extubated while pt is anesthetized, recovery personnel must be very experienced in management of airway obstruction in small children

Postoperative Considerations

- EBL: Underestimated because blood may be swallowed during or after surgery
- Bleeding most common cause of morbidity. NSAIDs are effective analgesics with less N/V

than opioids and without increased risk of bleeding after tonsillectomy. Consult with the surgeon about NSAID use.

- N/V in about 60% of pts after tonsillectomy due to blood in stomach, inflammation of posterior pharynx, and/or premature oral fluid intake. Emesis more likely in those >7 y.
- If N/V is suppressed, pt may have swallowed large amounts of blood without overt evidence of bleeding. Be esp careful in such pts to consider surreptitious blood loss.
- Pain score: 3–4 after adenoidectomy; managed with acetaminophen alone in some pts
- Pain score: 7–9 after tonsillectomy; may require IV and PO opioids
- Children with OSA should receive greatly reduced doses of opioids and be admitted for overnight monitoring
- Admission for those <3 y and with assoc anatomic or physiologic abn
- Most children may be discharged day of surgery if stable, no evidence of bleeding, pain, and vomiting

Total Abdominal Hysterectomy

Ferne R. Braveman

Risk

- Hysterectomy is the second most commonly performed surgical procedure in USA (cesarean delivery is first)
- In 2003, a rate of 5.38/1000 females for benign disease (~550,000, total ~660,000 with all diagnoses)
- By age 40.9, 25% of American women will undergo hysterectomy
- Racial predominance: None
- Age: 30 + y

Perioperative Risks

- Overall mortality ~0.1%; lowest mortality in women <55 y, greatest mortality in women >75 y
- Periop morbidity rare; overall incidence of 7.5% (fever and wound infections most common)
- Reduce surgical site infection with preop (within 60 min of incision) IV antibiotics
- Recommend routine VTE prophylaxis

Worry About

- Femoral nerve injury
- Bladder and/or ureter injury
- Hemorrhage requiring transfusion
- VTE

Overview

- Choice of TAH, total vaginal hysterectomy (TVH), laparoscopic or robotic surgery made according to pelvic anatomy, uterine size, adnexal or other assoc disease (i.e., malignant versus benign)
- Technique for TAH varies according to indication for operation; may incl oophorectomy, lymph node dissection, omentectomy, or tumor debulking
- Choice of anesthetic will vary with indication for surgery as well as presence of co-existing disease

ICD-9-Codes: 826.8 (Dysfunctional uterine bleeding); 179 (Uterine neoplasm, malignant); 219.9 (Uterine neoplasm, benign); 218.9 (Uterine fibroid); 180.9 (Cervical neoplasm, malignant); 219.0 (Cervical neoplasm, benign); 220.x (Ovarian neoplasm, benign); 614.6 (Pelvic adhesions); 617.9 (Endometriosis)

Indications and Usual Treatment

- Most common indications are fibroids and dysfunctional uterine bleeding
- Indications for hysterectomy incl:
  - Uterine, cervical, ovarian cancer
  - Pelvic relaxation syndrome, fibroids, abn bleeding, endometriosis, or other benign disorders (usually via vaginal approach)
- Route of hysterectomy may be influenced by uterine or adenexal size, presence of adhesions, malignancy, pt body habitus, and surgeon skill relative to the technique
- In 2003, abd hysterectomy was performed in ~66% of cases. This percentage is decreasing rapidly as the use of robotic technology and improved surgical techniques with both laparoscopic and robotic techniques improve.

ASSESSMENT POINTS

System	Effect	Assessment by Hx	PE	Test
CARDIO	Dehydration 2° to bowel prep Blood loss from primary problem	Menorrhagia	Orthostasis	Hgb/Hct Electrolytes
RESP	Rule out effusion or metastases	SOB, bronchospasm	Auscultation	CXR ABGs ± PFTs as indicated

Key References: Brill AI: Hysterectomy in the 21st Century: Different approaches, different challenges. *Clin Obstet Gynaecol*. 2006; 49: 722–735. Chiung C, Chen G, Falcone T. Robotic gynecologic surgery: Past, present, and future. *Clin Obstet Gynaecol*. 2009; 52: 335–343. Falcone T, Walters MD: Hysterectomy for benign disease. *Obstet Gynecol*. 2008; 11: 753–767.

Perioperative Management

Anesthetic Technique

- Regional, general, or combined techniques are options. Regional and/or combined techniques allow for postop regional analgesia.

Monitoring

- Routine
- Consider arterial line, central monitoring for extensive oncologic procedure if indicated by surgical plan and/or skill or by co-existing disease

Induction/Maintenance

- GA: Abdominal manipulation makes ET intubation preferable to LMA or mask airway
- Regional anesthesia: Dense T3–T4 level necessary for pt comfort. Avoid in obese pts or those who might otherwise not tolerate high regional levels.

Surgical Stages

Incision

- Pfannenstiel or low-transverse incision: Limited access to upper abdomen
- Midline incision extending from ~4 cm above symphysis pubis to umbilicus offers greater exposure, important for oncologic procedure

Inspection

- Avoid excessive bowel manipulation
- Self-retaining retractor may be used

Dissection

- Extrafascial hysterectomy
- Intimate proximity of uterus to ureters makes ureteral identification and dissection important
- Bladder must be carefully advanced down off lower uterine segment
- EBL: <1500 mL

Postoperative Considerations

- Moderate-severe postop pain (pain score 5–7)
- Single-dose spinal opioid followed by IV PCA for 12–24 hr (36-48 hr for oncologic procedures)
- Nononcologic pts usually taking oral medication on operative day or PO day 1
- High incidence of postop N/V

Anticipated Problems/Concerns

- Older pts, obese pts and oncology pts at greater risk for DVT
- Bladder and/or ureteral damage may prolong utethral catheterization and/or hospitalization
- Recognition of femoral nerve injury may be delayed by use of regional anesthesia—consider epidural opioid analgesia without local anesthetic postop

Total Anomalous Pulmonary Venous Return Correction

Risk

- 1–3% of all congenital CV abn
- Marked male predominance

Perioperative Risks

- Periop mortality is rare (<3%)
- Symptomatic arrhythmias are infrequent
- Pulm venous obstruction
- Cyanosis, impaired systemic O_2 delivery
- Myocardial dysfunction

Worry About

- Obstructed form typically presents in neonatal period with cyanosis, tachypnea, heart failure, and alveolar edema 2° to pulm venous Htn
- May be assoc with other cardiac anomalies

Overview

- All pulm veins drain abn to right atrium (RA), directly or indirectly, via remnants of cardinal or umbilical venous system

- Classification based on anatomic ___ connection
  - Type 1: supracardiac (49%), mo___ enters left innominate vein
  - Type 2: cardiac (25%), connec___ nary sinus
  - Type 3: infracardiac (18%), distal site of connection usually below diaphragm, connecting with vessel of portal system
  - Type 4: mixed (8%), two or more sites of abn pulm venous connections
- Because venous return to RA is mixture of oxygenated (pulm veins) and deoxygenated (IVC, SVC) blood, R → L atrial shunt causes systemic desaturation; under most circumstances, this is not severe enough to cause significant hypoxemia or end-organ dysfunction
- Pulm venous obstruction results in pulm Htn, diminished pulm blood flow, and significant R → L shunting, with severe hypoxemia and heart failure in the newborn period

structed at the level of the diaphragm or ___ tus venosus
- Cardiac lesions entering the coronary sinus are rarely obstructed.

ICD-9-CM Code: 747.41

Indications and Usual Treatment

- All require surgery; anatomy, physiology, and clinical presentation dictate timing
- One of the few true congenital cardiac surgery emergencies is a case of obstructed total anomalous pulm venous return
- Institution of ECMO may be required as a temporary measure to ensure adequate oxgenation, promote systemic blood flow, and reduce myocardial O_2 demand prior to surgery

ASSESSMENT POINTS

System	Effect	Assessment by Hx	PE	Test
CARDIO	CHF	Tachycardia, cyanosis	Flow murmur	ECHO
RESP	PV obstruction	Tachypnea	Pulmonary edema	CXR
RENAL	Renal insufficiency (prerenal)	↓ UO, acidosis		BUN, Cr

Key Reference: Karamou T, Gurofsky R, Al Sukhni E, et al. Factors associated with mortality and reoperation in 377 children with total anomalous pulmonary venous connection. *Circulation* 2007:115:1591–1598.

Perioperative Implications

Anesthetic Technique
- Opioid, NMB, controlled ventilation

Monitoring
- IV, arterial line, CVP, or transthoracic atrial/PA line placed by surgeon intraop
- TEE helpful (limited by pt size, potential for airway compression)
- Placement of temporary epicardial pacing wires for potential postop use

Airway
- No unique concerns

Induction and Maintenance
- IV induction with high-dose opioid, NMB, ± benzodiazepine
- Volatile anesthetics poorly tolerated by neonates with CHF, myocardial dysfunction

Extubation
- Usually deferred until after immediate postop period

Surgical Stages

- Goals: Redirection of pulm venous drainage to left atrium and ligation of abn connection to systemic venous system

- Pulm veins normally converge to a confluence posterior to LA; correction involves creation of unobstructed pathway from pulm veins to this confluence, and ultimately to LA. Anomalous ascending or descending venous connection is ligated.
- Surgery is performed with CPB, occasionally with deep hypothermic circulatory arrest

Postoperative Considerations
- Pulm Htn poses significant risk for periop morbidity. Strategies for management incl controlled hyperventilation, inotropic support, liberal use of opioids, NMB, maintaining adequate Hct in immediate postop period. Inhaled NO as a selective pulm vasodilator can be effective in some cases; its potential to promote methemoglobinemia warrants frequent monitoring of methemoglobin levels.
- Agents most useful for inotropic support incl dopamine (3–10 μ/kg/min), epinephrine (0.03–0.1 μg/kg/min), and milrinone (0.25–0.75 μg/kg/min)
- After immediate postop period, weaning of inotropic support, ventilation, and sedation are guided by atrial and/or PA pressure monitoring, ABGs

Anticipated Problems/Concerns

- If pt has obstructed pulm veins, at higher risk for periop morbidity/mortality from pulm Htn and/or ventricular dysfunction
- Pulm Htn can result from volatile PVR, kinking at anastomotic site, impaired LV function.
- RV dysfunction resulting directly from pulm Htn can lead to decreased pulm blood flow, diminished LA-LV filling, and dramatic reduction in systemic blood flow
- Etiology of LV dysfunction incl inadequate myocardial protection or inadequate LV preconditioning due to predominant L → R atrial shunt
- Arrhythmias are infrequent, but loss of AV synchrony worsens poor ventricular function. Sequential pacing via temporary epicardial leads and/or pharmacologic management of supraventricular tachycardia is indicated.

Total Hip Arthroplasty

[handwritten: Bone cement implantation syndrome.]

Michael F. Roizen

Risk

- Incidence in USA: >200,000/y; worldwide about 700,000
- Racial predilection: None
- Very successful at restoring function

Perioperative Risks

- Risks: 0.25–2% 30-day mortality (0.7% in large VA study). Risk down 67% over 10 y
- CV collapse ? 2° to pulm emboli, embolization of fat, marrow, bone, or cement
- Thromboembolism (peripheral venous thrombophlebitis in 60+% of pts w/o prophylaxis—50+% ↓ with prophylaxis)—pulm emboli in 2–4% of pts who do not receive prophylaxis

Worry About

- Causes of Fx or arthritis or joint deterioration (? CV disease, syncope, inflam joint diseases such as RA, psoriatic CT disease, etc., that are assoc with systemic conditions)
- Periop fluid deficiency
- Hypoxia and/or hypotension on cementing
- Pulm emboli periop

Overview

- Diseased articular surfaces are replaced with synthetic materials, thus relieving pain and improving joint kinematics and function
- Assoc with high immediate morbidity, mortality 2° to volume shifts, embolization
- 1–6-d mortality assoc with pulm emboli
- Age, co-morbidities of pts dictate monitoring strategies

- Regional anesthesia and postop analgesia preferred by many to reduce blood loss, risk of thromboembolism; to increase mobility

ICD-9-CM Code: 715.9 (Osteoarthritis)

Indications and Usual Treatment

- Replacement of hip socket (acetabulum) and/or femur with alloys of metals, plastic porcelain for
  - Chronic osteoarthritis
  - Hip Fx (large amounts of blood can be sequestered around Fx site). Investigate cause.
  - Avascular necrosis 2° to steroids, infarction (e.g., sickle cell disease)
- Usual medical Rx incl NSAIDs, aspirin, chondroitin and glucosamine, exercise, calcium, vitamin D_3

ASSESSMENT POINTS

System	Effect	Assessment by Hx	PE	Test
HEENT	Arthritis can involve airway joints	Snoring	Airway exam	
CARDIO	Impairment due to age; if Fx caused by CV problem—dysrhythmia, etc. Hypovolemia if Fx, bleed into leg	CV status Hx chest pain/SOB Hx palpitations Exercise tolerance	CV exam	ECG Orthostatic BP by tilt table test
RESP	Arthritis can be systemic restrictive pulm disease/ fat emboli with Fx or with replacement of hip	SOB Exercise tolerance	Chest exam Leg exam	O_2 sat
HEME	Blood loss 2° to Fx	Orthostatic dizziness	Leg; tilt table BP	Hct
RENAL/CNS	Impairment 2° to age; if Fx, investigate cause: CNS Hx if cause of Fx is CVA, dysrhythmia, etc.	CNS Hx	CNS exam	BUN/Cr

Key References: Stevens RD, Van Gessel E, Flory N, Fournier R, Gamulin Z. Lumbar plexus block reduces pain and blood loss associated with total hip arthroplasty. *Anesthesiology.* 2000; 93: 115–121. Ibrahim, SA, Stone, RA, Han, X, et al. Racial/ethnic differences in surgical outcomes in veterans following knee or hip arthroplasty. *Arthritis Rheum.* 2005; 52:3143–3151.

Perioperative Management

Monitoring

- Volume status monitoring of blood loss a major concern—blood loss ↓ with regional anesthesia or intentional hypotension
- Consider CVP or TEE (if GA chosen), several large-bore IVs.
- Check availability of predeposited autologous and/or homologous blood; irradiate directed donor blood; erythropoietin use controversial but common to bring Hgb from below 13 (with or without autologous donation) to over 13 g/dL
- UO, HR, BP not reliable signs of intravascular volume during anesthesia or with postop epidural pain relief
- Myocardial ischemia with ECG, ST segments, even PA cath or TEE if general anesthesia
- Patient's Sx of angina or CHF may be used but may be distorted if high regional anesthesia (need T6 level for regional)

Airway

- Side operated on is usually up, so securing airway after positioning may be difficult (three approaches: posterolateral is most common, but posterior and anterior are used; minimally invasive (4 in.—[10 cm]) or less incisions versus prior 6 to 12 in. incisions (15–30 cm) common. Resurfacing, rather than replacing, now used for under 55-y-old active males with osteoarthritis and minimal underlying hip adformity after approval by FDA with metal-on-metal devices with a polished acetabular head and mated metal head ball which caps the femoral head. Less blood

loss and less risk of cement induced hypotension, but risk of femoral neck fracture and reoperation probable.
- Airway involvement with arthritis possible
- Delayed gastric emptying of acute hip fracture with pain
- Positioning often uncomfortable after 1–2 hr in pt with regional anesthesia due to pressure on side, axilla; in GA pts, pay special attention to eye-ear position
- BP can be taken in up arm (but ↓)—down arm may have altered BP

Surgical Stages

Induction

- CV instability 2° to volume status
- If regional, consider slow titration

Skin Incision

- Large incision over operated hip, leg
- Can observe wound for excessive bleeding

Dissection (see diff approaches in Airway section above)

- During dissection down to femur, acetabulum, major blood vessel can be accidentally injured, difficult to control—esp femoral, iliac vessels
- Reaming of acetabulum, then femur
- Major blood loss 2° to bone dissection
- High-pressure lavage occasionally used to prepare surfaces: Embolization of fat possible
- Use of heparin during reaming of femur ↓ risk of thromboembolism

Definitive Surgery

- Some are cemented—methacrylate produces hypotension (within 30 min)

- Increased pulm embolization (?fat, air, methyl-methacrylate monomer) that results in increased ventilation-perfusion mismatch or shunt, ↓ O_2 sat, right heart dysfunction
- Decreased myocardial contractility 2° to above
- Can anticipate, hydrate for 10–20 min prior to cementing, ↑ FIO_2, have ephedrine ready
- Duration: ~5 hr
- Fluid shift can be sizable
- Decrease emboli by cath removal of pressure on cement insertion

Closure/Postoperative Considerations

- Blood loss of 1–2 units continues—if auto-transfusion used, may have reaction to non-washed cells immediately and may not get as great a long-term boost in Hct as planned (Hcts of 30 desirable if CV disease)
- Keep warm to reduce complications and blood Tx
- Pain score: 6–9
- Pain relief via NSAIDs, PCA, or epidural (start epidural narcotics 1 hr prior to end of surgery)
- Early ambulation reduces thromboemboli

Anticipated Problems/Concerns

- Blood volume status and rapid changes due to position, onset of regional and/or general anesthesia
- Extreme age may make less able to tolerate resp insult and CV instability after cementing
- Thromboembolism and infection prophylaxis desirable
- Pain with early ambulation may be considerable

Total Knee Arthroplasty (BCIS)

Michael Urban

Risk

- Incidence in USA: >500,000 cases
- >60 y with osteoarthritis
- Rheumatoid arthritis, trauma, infection, hemophilia, hemochromatosis, pigmented villonodular synovitis, avascular necrosis, obesity

Perioperative Risks

- Mortality rare <1.0%; in hospital 0.14%, higher for simultaneous bilateral total knee replacement (SBTKR) 0.39%; risks higher in current smokers by factor of 2
- High rate of DVT >40%; reduced with pneumatic compression plus aspirin, warfarin, or low molecular weight heparin
- Pulm embolism 0.1–2.0%
- Fatal pulm embolism after tourniquet release rare
- Common orthopedic surgical procedure in morbidly obese pts with concomitant ↑ risk
- Cardiopulmonary complications: Older age, no. of co-morbidities
- Postop bone-cement implantation syndrome (fat embolism syndrome, FES) more common with SBTKR ~ SB = simultaneous bilateral
- Bleeding (major ~1%)
- Infection
- Sciatic and peroneal nerve palsies; more common with valgus deformity
- Pain

Worry About

- CV collapse with tourniquet deflation
- Postop bone-cement implantation syndrome (FES)
- Pulm emboli periop
- Intraop bleeding (popliteal artery); postop bone
- Overview
- Replacement of both tibial, femoral components of knee joint, often with methylmethacrylate cemented implants.
- Increased risk of FES with intramedullary components

- Unicompartmental knee arthroplasty may have lower periop risks

ICD-9-CM Codes: 715.26 (Osteoarthritis, knee); 714.0 (Rheumatoid arthritis)

Indications and Usual Treatment

- Pain (OA, RA)
- Avascular necrosis
- Seronegative spondyloarthropathies
- Post-traumatic arthritis
- Hemophilia arthropathy of knee

Treatment

- NSAIDs and COX-2 inhibitors
- Glucosamine and chondroitin sulfate
- Calcium, magnesium, and vitamin D_3
- Physical therapy and build up of shock absorbing muscles above and below
- Alignment of joints with shoe prostheses
- Surgical wash out of loose fragments, experimental replacement of cartilage with stem cell rebuilding, etc., are all alternatives.

ASSESSMENT POINTS

System	Effect	Assessment by Hx	PE	Test
HEENT	Arthritis involving conical spine TMJ, cricoarytenoids Sleep apnea Smoking Hx	Hoarseness, difficult intubation Pickwickian Sx	ROM of neck Morbid obesity Color of fingers	C-spine x-ray or CT scan
CARDIO	RA: Pericardial effusion, cardiac conduction abn, cardiac valve fibrosis; OA ischemic heart dz, CHF	Dyspnea, palpitations Angina PND	Murmurs; rales	ECG, ECHO
RESP	Restrictive disease, pulm effusions	Dyspnea, cough	Lung auscultation	CXR, ABGs
GI	Obesity: Full stomach	Wt gain Inability to lie flat	Observation, lying flat	
HEME	Hemophiliac arthropathy of knee	Hemophilia		PTT, PT
CNS	Cervical nerve root compression	Pain on movement, paresthesias	Extremity weakness, ↓ sensation	Lateral neck x-ray

Key References: Parmet JL, Horrow JC, Singer R, et al: Echogenic emboli upon tourniquet release during total knee arthroplasty: pulmonary hemodynamic changes and embolic composition. *Anesth Analg.* 1994; 79:940–945; Parmet JL, Horrow JC, Berman AT, Miller F, Pharo G, Collins L: The incidence of large venous emboli during total knee arthroplasty without pneumatic tourniquet use. *Anesth Analg.* 1998; 87:439–444.

Perioperative Management

Preoperative Preparation

- Treat hemophilia if present
- Pre-treatment with LMWH for pts at higher risk for DVT/PE
- Encourage smoking cessation, preop walking, and portion control
- Continue aspirin (81 or preferably 162 mg) pts with stents, Hx CVA, AFib
- Beta-blockers and statins in pts at risk for ischemic events

Anesthetic Technique

- Although no clear advantage of regional over GA, regional eliminates manipulation of airway, provides vehicle for postop pain Rx; epidural anesthesia may be extremely difficult with severe arthritis, scoliosis, or ankylosing spondylitis. Consider paramedian approach.
- Alternatively femoral / sciatic nerve blocks
- Consider GA if on LMWH

Monitoring

- Consider arterial catheter for dramatic swings in BP with tourniquet inflation, deflation
- Large-bore IV or CV catheter

- For pts with Hx of significant cardiac disease (LV dysfunction or ischemic disease) consider PA cath or TEE; embolization of fat, cement, bone marrow debris may result in significant ↑ in PA pressure without change in PAOP.
- UO, HR, BP not reliable indicators of intravascular volume status with epidural anesthesia and analgesia   ASCVD = atherosclerotic CV disease

Surgical Stages

- Supine position; attention to neck and arthritic shoulder and arms at side
- Prolonged tourniquet inflation may result in elevated BP, myocardial ischemia and/or elevated pulm artery pressure in pts with ASCVD, LV dysfunction
- Tourniquet deflation: Hypotension, tachycardia, pulm emboli with hypoxia, possible cardiac arrest. Consider hydration, ephedrine before deflation, epinephrine infusion with epidural
- EBL: Usually 100–300 mL intraop; with arterial bleeding >1000 mL

Postoperative Considerations

- Significant blood loss over the first 24 hr from surgical drain; if possible, consider autologous blood donation, erythropoietin preop controversial; cell scavenge and re-infusion

- Pain: PCEA if not on LMWH; femoral nerve block +/- catheter with infusion; NSAIDs; lyrica
- Revision TKR and SBTKR: close monitoring for 24 hr postop; blood loss, FES

Anticipated Problems/Concerns

- Pulm emboli of cement, thrombi, bone marrow debris with tourniquet deflation
- Postop bleeding with hypotension, cardiac ischemia, renal failure
- DVT, thromboembolization (ACCP recommended LMWH for 10-d, ↑ bleeding; hematoma, infection); combined therapy pneumatic compression plus apirin, warfarin or LMWH. Early ambulation.
- Fat embolism syndrome: Hypoxia, tachycardia, hyperpyrexia, thrombocytopenia, leukocytosis, mental status changes; if monitoring PA pressures, pulm artery diastolic to PAOP gradient present. Rx aimed at minimizing pulm edema while maintaining end-organ perfusion; judicious use of diuretics, O_2, blood transfusions; may progress to ARDS.
- Delirium: ↑ with advanced age, FES, pain, use of benzodiazepines

Tracheal Resection

Alex Chen
Edward A. Ochroch

Risk

• Annual incidence of 1:200,000 adults
• 2.7 new cases of malignant tracheal mass per million per year

Perioperative Risks

• Periop mortality ~2%

Worry About

• Difficult ventilation and/or impending airway collapse
• Ventilation strategy changes in different phases of the operation

Overview

• Variable surgical/airway course that is dependent on the lesion's extent, percent obstruction and location with respect to the carina and vocal cords. Surgery and anesthesia must work in congruence and share the airway
• Resection with end-to-end anastomosis depending on how many rings are involved

• >90% good long-term results may be expected with resection and end-to-end anastomosis
• PFTS (spirometry, flow volume loops: Erect and supine); characteristics of an extra-thoracic tracheal lesion: a greater decrease in inspiratory flow than in expiratory flow; a delay in reaching peak expiratory flow, a reduced peak expiratory and peak inspiratory flow, and/or an abrupt drop of expiratory flow at the end of expiration; with a fixed upper airway obstruction such, there is flattening of both the inspiratory and the expiratory phase

Etiology

• Neoplasm: Adenoid cystic CA, squamous cell CA, neurofibroma, chondroma, chondroblastoma, hemangioma, pleomorphic adenoma
• Inflammatory lesions: SLE, sarcoidosis, amyloidosis, Wegener's
• Trauma: Mostly related to ET intubation, or from tracheostomy-induced formation of granulation tissue

• Other: Tracheal webs, tracheal agenesis/atresia, tracheomalacia, idiopathic laryngotracheal stenosis

Treatment

• Irradiation: Squamous cell CA and adenoid cystic CA: Edema may critically narrow airway
• Bronchoscopy: Dilatation used in emergency situations, final therapy (injection of steroids or mitomycin C may retard the recurrence) or bridge to surgery
• Laser: Great precision with less periop edema; choice of laser determines depth of penetration
• Stents: Palliation, temporizing measure or as an adjunct to surgery to reinforce the new anastomosis
• Tracheal reconstruction: Resection and reconstruction with 1° anastomosis

ICD-9-CM Code: 519.19 (Tracheal stenosis)

ASSESSMENT POINTS

System	Effect	Assessment by Hx	PE	Test
HEENT	Stridor	Resp distress	Auscultation of the trachea, palpitation of the trachea, neck mobility	Bronchoscopy
CARDIO	CV decompensation, pulm Htn	Cyanosis, resp distress, orthopnea	Murmur, hepatomegaly, edema	ECHO, stess, cath (as indicated)
Resp	Obstructive physiology	Exercise intolerance, inspiratory stridor, expiratory wheezing (frequently misdiagnosed as asthma	Accessory muscle use, tachypnea	CXR, CT 3D recon, PFTs

Key References: Pinsonneault C, Fortier J, Donati F et al. Tracheal resection and reconstruction. *Can J Anaesth*. 1999;46:439–55. Wright,CD , Grillo HC, Wain JC et al. Anastomotic complications after tracheal resection: Prognostic factors and management *J Thorac Cardiovasc Surg* 2004;128:731–739.

Perioperative Implications

Preopative Preperation
• A clear Hx of any previous airway management needs to be reviewed
• Determine which position the pt breaths best—OR rescue
• Presurgery steroid weaning and ventilator weaning and pulm optimization
• Consent for femoral vessel cannulization for CPB in case of complete obstruction
• Set up for immediate rigid bronchoscopy should airway compromise occur
• Readily available small ETTs, fiberoptic cart, jet ventilator, thin injector and/or exchange catheters and surgeons standing by to perform a tracheostomy if necessary
• Premedication: Sedatives reserved for very anxious pts, ± an anticholinergic

Anesthesia Technique
• GA (TIVA due to open airway manipulation)

Monitoring
• Two IVs: TIVA + bolus meds, significant blood loss is rare
• Standard monitors
• Arterial line in the left arm (the innominate artery may be operatively manipulated or compressed)
• Prolonged jet ventilation will necessitate arterial CO_2 sampling
• Minimal fluid shifts: Rare need for CVP, pulmonary artery pressure/CCO Swan (TEE will impinge posterior membranous wall)

Airway
• Preoxygenation and/or denitrogenation vital prior to starting the procedure. It can take considerably longer than usual: small tidal volumes.

• The complex nature of the airway necessitates a plan discussed with the surgical team and will invariably require maneuvers to control the proximal and distal airway that may involve use of LMA, ETT or jet ventilator

Induction
• NMB may be avoided with the pt ventilating spontaneously, but PPV is rarely a problem (a longer E time is required when ventilating proximal to the stenosis)

Maintenance
• TIVA during jet ventilation

Fluid management
• Typically run dry
• Significant blood loss requiring transfusion is rare

Extubation
• Attempts should be made to extubate the pt in the OR to prevent exposure of the anastomosis to positive airway pressures

Surgical Stages

Example of an Airway Course
• After induction of GA a LMA is placed for bronchoscopy.
• After bronchoscopy the LMA is exchanged with a small-bore oral ETT that passes beyond the lesion; or ETT sits between vocal cords and lesion; or the case is started with LMA.
• Once the distal trachea is divided ventilation is by a sterile ETT and ventilator circuit passed off the field; or a jet ventilation catheter is passed into the distal trachea. The trans-oral ETT is retracted to just below the vocal cords.

• Once the stenotic lesion is excised, a jet ventilation catheter is placed though the trans-oral ETT and into the distal trachea for posterior wall repair.
• Once the posterior wall of the trachea is reapproximated, the trans-oral ETT is advanced across the suture line until the balloon is distal to the suture line. Tidal ventilation is resumed and the trachea and neck are closed.
• The ETT is removed and the LMA is placed for surgical bronchoscopy.
• If, at this point there is any concern about the repair, the pt's ability to cough and control airway secretions, a tracheostomy or a mini-tracheostomy is placed. A retention suture from pt's chin to chest is placed to prevent extension of neck and stretch of anastomosis.
• Spontaneous ventilation is allowed and the LMA is removed.

Postoperative Considerations/Complications
• Postop airway edema: Racemic epinephrine, steroids, diuretics and fluid restriction.
• Wound or anastomotic dehiscence
• Infection in <2%
• Recurrent laryngeal nerve damage
• Formation of granulation tissue and restenosis
• Tetraplegia related to postop hyperflexion of the neck

Anticipated Problems/Concerns
• Hypoxemia and/or hypercarbia
• CV compromise due to hyperinflation and auto peep seen with high frequency ventilation
• Barotrauma from the distal HFJV

Tracheoesophageal Fistula Repair

Michael J. Tobin

Risk

- 1/3000 live births
- Dx confirmed by the inability to pass a soft suction cath into stomach

Perioperative Risks

- Periop mortality low in full-term, healthy newborns; almost 100% survival
- Periop mortality approaches 15–60% in infants less than 1800 g
- Tracheomalacia
- Esophageal stricture

Worry About

- Difficult ventilation and/or hypoxemia
- Prematurity: Up to 3% assoc with TEF; consider possibility of retinopathy or prematurity
- VATER syndrome: Vertebral anomalies, anal atresia, tracheoesophageal fistula, esophageal atresia, radial dysplasia

- CHD to 25% assoc with TEF (VSD, ASD, PDA, tetralogy of Fallot), causing CV instability
- CV collapse and/or hypotension due to gastric distention or surgical compression
- Hypothermia, consequent acidosis/metabolic dysfunction

Overview

- Primary repair incl fistula ligation, esophageal anastomosis
- Four types
- Staged repair incl placement of gastrostomy tube under local anesthesia, subsequent ligation of fistula, esophageal repair when more stable

ICD-9-CM Code: 750.3 (Congenital)

Indications and Usual Treatment

- Carefully define other congenital defects
- Unstable pts: Consider staged procedure
- Premature infants: Consider staged procedure
- Gastrostomy tube placement when gastric distention compromises ventilatory status
- Passage of Fogarty cath through gastrostomy into esophagus can occlude esophagus/fistula, thus promoting ventilation of lungs

ASSESSMENT POINTS

System	Effect	Assessment by Hx	PE	Test (If Indicated)
CARDIO	CV decompensation, cyanosis, CHF	Cyanosis, tachypnea, resp distress	Murmur, cyanosis, enlarged liver, hypotension, bounding pulses	CXR, ECG, ECHO, cardiac cath
RESP	Pneumonia, subglottic stenosis	Resp distress, tachypnea, stridor	↓ Breath sounds, tachypnea, cyanosis	CXR, ABGs (if indicated), flexible fiberoptic bronchoscopy
GI	Gastric distention, assoc anal atresia or bowel obstruction	Enlarged abd Resp distress	Tympanic abd, enlarged abd	KUB series
RENAL	Dysplastic/dysfunction	Anuria	Palpation for kidneys	Créde, cath, or collect urine by bag appliance BUN/Cr

Key Reference: Andropoulos DB, Rowe RW, Betts JM: Anaesthetic and surgical airway management during tracheo-oesophageal fistula repair. *Paediatr Anaesth*. 1998; 8:313–319; Kovesi T, Rubin S. Long-term complications of congenital esophageal atresia and/or tracheoesophageal fistula. *Chest*. 2004; 126: 915–925.

Perioperative Implications

Anesthetic Technique
- GA for complete repair
- Local anesthesia for gastrostomy tube placement in staged repair

Monitoring
- Large, well-functioning IV for blood loss
- Consider art line if resp or CV problems
- Urinary catheter

Airway
- Awake intubation and/or careful rapid-sequence
- ETT positioned just above carina to avoid ventilating fistula and to ensure ventilation of both lungs: intentional right main stem intubation with subsequent slow withdrawal of ETT until breath sounds first heard on left usually ensures that ETT optimally placed
- Consider facing the bevel posteriorly during intubation to avoid direct intubation of fistula
- Monitor for kinking and/or obstruction of trachea and/or ETT by surgical traction during dissection, repair
- Monitor for complete obstruction of ETT by blood and secretions, necessitating suctioning and/or replacement
- Precordial stethoscope on left chest to monitor breath sounds intraop; accidental advancement of ETT into right mainstem bronchus may then be detected
- Subglottic stenosis may necessitate placement of smaller diameter ETT than usual

- Soft Silastic cath or esophageal stethoscope most easily placed in blind esophageal pouch before final positioning

Induction
- Healthy neonates may tolerate inhalation induction with spontaneous ventilation until chest opened when a muscle relaxant is given.
- Premature infants or those with significant resp disease may require careful mechanical ventilation, use of muscle relaxant at induction.

Surgical Stages

Dissection
- Blood loss usually minimal, although large blood vessels may be transected
- Recurrent laryngeal nerve damage may occur

Definitive Surgery
- Hypercarbia and/or hypoxemia possible from these causes: Compression or retraction of right lung, kinking of trachea and/or ETT from surgical traction, plugging of the ETT, its migration into right mainstem bronchus or fistula, preferential ventilation of fistula
- Hypotension may result from cardiac compression, hypovolemia, or blood loss
- Hypothermia may result from administration of cold IV fluids, cool ambient room, anhydrous gas administration, heating pad malfunction. Metabolic acidosis may result from hypothermia.
- Blood loss can be steady; apparently small losses can be clinically significant in newborn.

Postoperative Considerations
- Vigorous infants may be extubated at conclusion of surgery this preferred for maintenance of repair
- Premature infants and those with significant pulm disease may require continued mechanical ventilation.
- Suction caths marked to point at which they will contact repair

Postoperative Complications
- Pulm aspiration, tracheomalacia, vocal cord paralysis
- At later date, pts at risk for intubation of tracheal diverticulum that may develop at site of fistula closure
- Esophageal stricture, esophageal foreign body entrapment relatively common following repair
- Regional anesthesia may be used as a supplement to general anesthesia and may improve management of postop pain. A single-dose caudal block may be administered. Alternatively, a caudal catheter may be placed and advanced to a thoracic level for intermittent dosing.

Anticipated Problems/Concerns
- Pulm disease
- Difficulty sustaining airway, avoiding hypoxemia and/or hypercarbia
- CV compromise and/or CHD
- Hypovolemia and/or blood loss
- Hypothermia
- Prematurity

Tracheotomy/Tracheostomy and Cricothyroidotomy

Priti Dalal
Gaurang Dalal

Risk

- Most commonly performed in pts who are ventilator dependent (10%) or those with acute airway obstruction

Perioperative Risks

- Depends on the indication, degree of airway obstruction and whether emergency or elective
- Overall risk of complications is approx 6–8% for elective tracheostomy and 6.1% for elective cricothyrotomy

Worry About

- Obese pts: Technically difficult identification of landmarks, positioning and bleeding
- Pediatric pts: Short neck, high risk of misplacement of the tracheostomy tube
- Bleeding and airway fires

Overview

- The term tracheotomy is used for temporary and tracheostomy is used for permanent procedure
- May be performed as emergency or elective procedure, open or percutaneous technique
- Advantages of percutaneous tracheostomy: Smaller skin incision, less trauma, bedside procedure, less incidence of wound infection
- Goals of general anesthesia should be to avoid airway fires, optimize oxygenation and ventilation, use the lowest safe inspired O_2 concentration, position the existing ETT such that the damage to its cuff is minimized, control all bleeding points, meticulous suction

Indications and Usual Treatment

- Airway obstruction: Congenital, trauma, infection, neoplasm, foreign body
- Long-term ventilator support: For resp failure in critically care unit
- Provide tracheobronchopulmonary hygiene: facilitate frequent suctioning for secretions in pts with NM diseases, prevention of aspiration
- Planned prophylactic tracheostomy: During extensive head and neck procedures

ASSESSMENT POINTS

System	Effect	Assessment by Hx	PE	Test
HEENT	Stridor Change in voice drooling	Trauma, tumor, infection	Type of stridor in relation to breathing phase	Inspiratory – supraglottic obstruction Expiratory – subglottic obstruction Biphasic – supra and subglottic obstruction or glottis obstruction
CARDIO	Hypotension Critically ill on ICU	Invasive monitoring	Ionotrope dependence	ECG, ECHO
RESP	Dyspnea, long-term ventilation Cough	Ventilator support, increased O_2 requirements	Decreased breath sounds	ABG CXR, CT scan/MRI Fiberoptic endoscopy
RENAL	Renal insufficiency	Long term ICU stay	Depending on cause	Serum creatinine, BUN, electrolytes
CNS	Cerebral effects of hypoxia and hypercarbia	Trauma, compromised breathing	Restlessness loss of consciousness	ABG

Key Reference: Liu L, Gropper MA. Overview of anesthesiology and critical care medicine. In Miller RD. *Millers' anesthesia.* 2010. 7th edition. Churchill-Livingstone/Elsevier, p. 2859.

Perioperative Management

Preoperative Preparation

- Assess the severity of airway compromise
- Beware while transporting a critically ill pt from the ICU to the OR

Monitoring

- Standard monitoring: ECG, BP, pulse oximetry and capnography
- Arterial line in critically ill pts

Anesthetic Technique/Induction

- General anesthesia for optimal surgical condition
- Local anesthesia in pts with severe airway compromise
- Position: Supine with extended head; may be sitting semi-upright in severe airway obstruction

Surgical Stages

Dissection: Tracheostomy

- Landmark: Midway between the cricoid cartilage and suprasternal notch, site overlying the 2–3 tracheal rings, skin infiltration with lidocaine with epinephrine may help reduce bleeding
- For open tracheostomy, skin incision may be vertical or horizontal, electrocautery used to remove subcutaneous fat, thymic isthmus may

be divided, tracheal incision may be T-shaped, U-shaped or involve removal of a small anterior part of the trachea for a permanent stoma
- Before incising the trachea, be sure that the cuff is not in the way of the tracheal incision. Once trachea is opened stop ventilation, deflate the ETT cuff, withdraw the ETT carefully under direct vision until the tip is just above the tracheal stoma.
- Do not remove the ETT until the tracheostomy tube placement is confirmed.
- Confirm placement with chest rise, auscultation for breath sounds and $ETCO_2$
- Fiberoptic endoscopy is useful to assist percutaneous tracheostomy.

Cricothyroidotomy

- May be performed with the open, percutaneous or needle cricothyroidotomy techniques
- Open technique: Horizontal stab incision with 20-g scalpel, 1 cm horizontal incision above the superior border of the cricoid cartilage, insert the handle of the scalpel to widen the incision, then insert the tracheostomy tube, may be performed in 30 sec and used up to 72 hr
- Percutaneous cricothyroidotomy using Seldinger technique

- Needle cricothyroidotomy may be performed using a cannula and transtracheal jet ventilation (55 psi) commenced in case of emergency situation (cannot intubate cannot ventilate)
- Always confirm ventilation with chest rise, chest auscultation, and capnography

Postoperative Considerations

- Ventilation, critical care management
- Postoperative CXR

Anticipated Problems/Concerns

- Immediate complications: Bleeding from the thyroid gland, pneumothorax (0–4%), pneumomediastinum, injury to recurrent laryngeal nerve, esophagus, and large blood vessels
- Early complications: Increased bleeding around the tracheostomy site on emergence from anesthesia, bloody secretions, tracheitis, mucous plugs, skin infection at site
- Delayed complications: Hemorrhage (1–6 wk after procedure) may be due to tracheoinnominate artery fistula (0.6%), tracheal stenosis, tracheomalacia, trachea-esophageal or tracheocutaneous fistula, scarring, granulation tissue formation

Transjugular Intrahepatic Portosystemic Shunt (TIPS)

Zheng Xie

Risks

- Incidence in USA: Cirrhosis of the liver occurs in 3–4/1000 adults
- 26,000 deaths per year in the USA are related to cirrhosis
- >60% with cirrhosis have portal Htn and 33–98% with cirrhosis have GI varices
- Variceal bleeding occurs in 25–40%
- Portal vein thrombosis occurs 24–32% in cirrhotics and 5–10% in pts referred for TIPS

Perioperative Risks

- Technical success rate of the TIPS procedure ranges from 75% to greater than 90%
- Overall direct procedure mortality rate is <2%
- 30-d mortality rate ranges from 4 to 45%
- Rebleeding rate is 10–26% and usually assoc with shunt stenosis or thrombosis
- Postprocedural encephalopathy: 5–55%
- Fever has been reported in 10% of pts
- Child-Pugh or MELD score has been used to predict the overall survival rate
- TIPS in children and post-liver transplant pts is feasible, but with potential difficulties

Worry About

- Hypotension 2° to bleeding caused by severe coagulopathy, vein rupture or perforation of liver capsule
- CHF, cardiac arrhythmias: HB, VF, AF
- O_2 desaturation 2° to excessive sedation
- Aspiration
- Tension pneumothorax
- Mental status changes: ↑ encephalopathy postop
- Septic shock
- Unexpected difficult and lengthy procedure due to technical or anatomical reasons

Overview

- A creation of a communication between hepatic and portal veins through the liver parenchyma with an expandable metallic stent to relieve portal Htn (<12 mmHg)
- Portal Htn causes ↑ flow through the portosystemic collaterals that bypass the liver to the systemic circulation. Results in gastroesophageal varices, intestinal varices, and splenomegaly.
- Major clinical manifestations of portal Htn: Hemorrhage from gastroesophageal varices, splenomegaly, encephalopathy, ascites, death
- Main periop complications: Intra-abdominal hemorrhage, aspiration, cardiopulmonary failure, arrhythmias, worsening encephalopathy, infection, fluid and electrolyte disturbance

Etiologies

- Cirrhosis is most common cause of portal Htn in adult pts in USA. Others incl portal vein obstruction, hepatic vein thrombosis (Budd-Chiari syndrome), and hepatic veno-occlusive disease
- In infants and children, biliary atresia is the most common cause of portal Htn. Cystic fibrosis, congenital hepatic fibrosis and α1-antitrypsin deficiency can also cause portal Htn

ICD-9-CM Codes: 572.3 (Portal hypertension); 571.5 (Portal cirrhosis)

Indications and Usual Treatment

Accepted Indications
- Acute variceal bleeding not successfully controlled with medical Rx
- Recurrent variceal bleeding refractory or intolerant to conventional medical Rx
- Particularly helpful when bleeding occurs from inaccessible intestinal or gastric varices or is the result of severe portal hypertensive gastropathy

Probable Indications
- Refractory ascites, refractory hepatic hydrothorax, hepatorenal syndrome, Budd-Chiari syndrome, and veno-occlusive disease
- Acute variceal bleed while awaiting Tx

Usual Treatments
- Pharmacologic Rx to ↓ portal pressure
- Endoscopic band ligation or sclerotherapy of the varices
- Balloon tamponade, then devascularization
- Surgical portosystemic shunting

Absolute Contraindications
- Right-sided heart failure
- Polycystic liver disease
- Severe hepatic failure, unless active variceal bleeding or fulminant Budd-Chiari syndrome
- 1° pulm Htn
- Cavernous portal vein thrombosis

Relative Contraindications
- Biliary obstruction, systemic infection, and severe hepatic encephalopathy

ASSESSMENT POINTS

System	Effect	Assessment by Hx	PE	Test
NEURO	Hepatic encephalopathy (from confusion to coma)	Disturbances of awareness and mentation, personality change	Asterixis (liver flap), rigidity, hyperreflexia	EEG, ammonia level
CARDIO	Cardiomyopathy, CAD, arrhythmias (QT prolongation, Toursades, etc)	ETOH abuse, smoking Hx	Tachycardia, S_3, edema	ECG, ECHO
RESP	Atelectasis, pulm shunting, hypoxemia, hyperventilation, pulm effusion, pulm Htn	SOB, poor exercise tolerance		CXR, ABGs, PFTs, ECHO
GI	Ascites, aspiration, variceal bleeding, gastritis, ulcer	↑ Abd girth, hematemesis	Fluid wave, bulging flanks, postural tachycardia	US, paracentesis, endoscopy
HEPAT	Drug metabolism change			LFTs
RENAL	Hepatorenal syndrome			BUN/creatinine, electrolytes
ENDO	Hypoglycemia			Glucose
HEME	Anemia, coagulopathy, incl factors and plt deficiency. Resistant to activated protein C	GI bleed, recurrent TIPS stent stenosis		CBC, plt, PT/INR, PTT, thromboelastogram

Key Reference: Scher, C. Anesthesia for transjugular intrahepatic portosystemic shunt, *International Anesthesiology Clinics*, vol 47, No. 2, Lippincott Williams & Wilkins; 2009:21–28.

Perioperative Management

Preoperative Preparation
- Avoid excessive sedation to minimize aspiration risk.
- Pre-existing LBBB may require a pacemaker pre-TIPS due to the risk of RBBB during TIPS.
- PRBCs, FFP, and platelets available
- Some centers recommend correction of coagulopathy if plts <60,000 and INR >1.8
- Monitor blood glucose if hepatic failure

Monitoring
- Standard monitors; in selected cases, arterial line and central venous catheters can be added

Anesthetic Technique/Care
- Based on severity of liver disease and comorbidities and preference of institution
- Sedation and local anesthesia may suffice in some pts and is preferred in some centers
- General anesthesia preferred if pt is agitated or uncooperative from encephalopathy
- Most institutions prefer general anesthesia with ET intubation over LMA

Induction/Maintenance
- Rapid-sequence induction common if encephalopathy, abd distention, or recent variceal bleed
- Broad-spectrum antibiotic for gram-negative organisms (e.g., 1 g ceftizoxime) at start
- May be sensitive to all agents

Emergence
- Extubation after pts are awake and their protective laryngeal reflexes present

Surgical Stages

- US is performed to assess the size and patency of portal and hepatic venous systems
- Jugular and hepatic vein access and pressure measurement—right internal jugular vein approach is preferred because a straight path into the infrahepatic IVC. An angiographic catheter is advanced to the infrahepatic IVC and pressures measured. Sheath is advanced into the right hepatic vein, and both free hepatic vein pressure and wedged hepatic vein pressure are measured.
- Identification of portal vein—wedged hepatic venogram is performed with either iodinated contrast or CO_2 for portal vein localization
- Dilation and stent placement—a puncture needle is advanced to access the portal vein. The needle is removed while a guidewire is advanced to the superior mesenteric vein or splenic vein. Portal pressures are measured and a portal venogram is obtained. An angioplasty balloon is advanced to dilate the transhepatic tract. A bridging expandable stent is deployed and then dilated to 8–12 mm. Ideally, the pressure gradient following shunting should be 6–12 mmHg.
- Ultrasound within 24 hr to assess patency of the stent
- EBL: 0–3000 mL

Postoperative Considerations

- Monitor in an ICU or step-down unit for 24–48 hr due to potential for portal vein thrombus, worsening encephalopathy, sepsis, bleeding, pulm edema, and fluid and lyte disturbance
- Pain score is 7–8 in first few hours. Usually, opioid is needed only for the first few hours.

Anticipated Problems/Concerns

- Portal vein rupture and perforation of liver capsule leads to intra-abdominal hemorrhage
- Cardiopulmonary failure from sudden hemodynamic changes
- Pts with pre-existing LBBB may need pacemaker pre-TIPS due to risk of RBBB
- Encephalopathy may worsen due to ↓ hepatic portal blood flow

Transposition of the Great Arteries (TGA)

Laura K. Diaz
Alan Jay Schwartz

Risk

- Incidence: 0.02–0.05% of live births; 7–8% of all congenital cardiac defects, second only to VSD
- Most common cyanotic CHD presenting in infancy
- M:F ratio: 2-3:1.1

Perioperative Risks

- Assoc cardiac anomalies: VSD (40–45%), LV outflow tract (subpulmonic) obstruction (LVOTO) 25%, secundum ASD, aortic arch obstruction
- Systemic or pulm ventricular failure
- Pulm Htn and/or pulm vascular occlusive disease (PVOD) may develop early esp. in presence of aortopulmonary collateral vessels, large VSD
- Cyanotic pts: Polycythemia, coagulopathy
- Rhythm disturbances affecting CO
- Use of PGE$_1$ to maintain ductal patency may result in apnea, fever, vasodilation, and edema

Worry About

- Neonates with CHF, cyanosis should be evaluated for TGA.
- With intact ventricular septum (IVS), PGE$_1$ infusion is utilized to maintain ductal patency, blood mixing until balloon atrial septostomy (BAS) performed
- PVR and SVR need to be balanced to maintain optimal ratio of systemic to pulm blood flow

- Severely cyanotic pts:
  - Polycythemia may cause sludging; ↑ risk of CVAs
  - Thrombocytopenia, ↓ plasma clotting factors can be present
- Age at repair depends on assoc features. Older pts at greater risk for CHF and PVOD

Overview

- d-TGA: Concordance of atrioventricular connections and discordance of ventriculoarterial connections exists creating two parallel circulations.
- Communication between circulations must exist (PDA, ASD, VSD) at one or more levels to allow mixing and survival until surgical intervention
- Echocardiography gold standard of diagnosis
- Without intervention, 30% mortality in first wk, 45% first mo, 90% first y; anoxia, CHF 1° causes of death
- Type of surgical intervention depends on assoc presence of VSD or LVOTO
- Balloon atrial septostomy (BAS): Rashkind procedure, early corrective surgery have improved long-term outcome

Etiology

- Assoc risk: Possible maternal diabetes

Usual Treatment

- PGE$_1$ infusion utilized to maintain ductal patency

- BAS frequently performed at bedside or in cath lab to promote mixing preop
- Successful BAS may allow D/C of PGE$_1$ preop
- Palliative surgery
  - If LVOTO and VSD are present: systemic to PA shunt
  - If VSD and advanced PVOD are present, atrial switch (Mustard procedure) may be performed without VSD closure.
- Repair
  - Physiologic: Intra-atrial repair (Mustard or Senning procedure) to connect systemic, pulm circuits at atrial level with RV remaining as systemic ventricle
  - Anatomic: Arterial switch (Jatene) with coronary artery reimplantation to anatomically correct circulation by anastomosing aorta to systemic ventricle and PA to the pulm ventricle. If severe LVOT obstruction and VSD exist, VSD is closed via intracardiac baffle redirecting LV blood to aorta and RV-PA conduit is placed (Rastelli operation).
  - Timing of repair: Pts with IVS: first 1–2 wk of life to prevent reduction in LV mass. If LV regression has occurred PA band may be done before repair to prepare LV. Pts with VSD: first 1–2 mo to prevent development of CHF or PVOD.

ASSESSMENT POINTS

System	Effect	Assessment by Hx	PE	Test
CARDIO	CHF	Resp distress Poor perfusion	Rales, S$_3$, hypotension	ECHO
RESP	Pulm vascular occlusive disease	Dyspnea	Clubbing, cyanosis	CXR, cath
HEME	Polycythemia (if > 6–9 mo) Coagulopathy, bleeding Thrombocytopenia	Bleeding		CBC Coag factor levels, plt studies
CNS	CVA	Assoc with polycythemia	Focal deficit	CT or MRI

Key Reference: Fulton DR, Fyler DC. D-transposition of the great arteries. In: Keane JF, Lock JE, Fyler DC, eds. *NADAS' pediatric cardiology*. 2nd ed. Philadelphia: Elsevier; 2006:645–661.

Perioperative Implications

Preoperative Preparation

- Maintain CO with adequate HR, contractility, preload
- Maintain ductal patency with PGE$_1$ (0.01–0.05 μg/min/min) in ductal dependent pts
- Premedication rarely required; consider sedative premedication for infants >6 mo of age

Monitoring

- Arterial line may be placed after induction
- Central line or right atrial line may be used for drug infusion, pressure monitoring

Airway

- Pt may or may not be intubated preop
- Nasal ETT recommended to minimize interference with potential use of TEE

Preinduction/Induction

- Avoid ↑ PVR, can ↓ PBF, intercirculatory mixing
- PVOD present, use ventilatory interventions to ↓ PVR: ↑ FIO$_2$, ↓ PaCO$_2$
- If LVOTO present, ↑ ventilation can ↓ PVR, ↑ pulm blood flow and intercirculatory mixing
- Maintain SVR relative to PVR to maintain effective pulm blood flow and SpO$_2$

- If CHF present with VSD, ventilatory manipulations may be deleterious, due to pre-existing ↑ pulm blood flow, difficulty of maintaining systemic blood flow with failing heart
- Anesthetic induction may be accomplished with opioid or pentothal if IV line in place, otherwise inhalation induction may be used.

Maintenance

- Opioids preferred drugs for maintenance anesthesia (fentanyl 10–20 μg/kg); affords hemodynamic stability; does not depress myocardium; blunts reactive pulm Htn. May be used in concert with low doses of volatile agent.
  - In infants with TGA and IVS, O$_2$ delivery can be tenuous
  - In infants with TGA and VSD, volume overload possible
- Avoid hypercarbia and acidosis
- Pancuronium usually relaxant of choice due to vagolytic properties

Post CPB

- Maintain age-appropriate HR; keep BP low-normal range to avoid excessive bleeding
- Monitor for ischemia, dysrhythmias
- Initiate inotropic and/or vasodilator therapy for ventricular dysfunction
- TEE useful to assess for air, ventricular function, assess coronary arteries, and VSD closure

Extubation

- In ICU when pulm and hemodynamic stability present, postop bleeding controlled, pt awake

Anticipated Problems/Concerns

- Atrial switch
  - Interatrial baffle obstruction (systemic or pulm) may occur with resulting low CO or SVC syndrome; pulm venous obstruction may result in low CO, pulm edema
  - Baffle leak may allow atrial level shunting
  - Dysrhythmias ultimately seen in >60% of pts: Sinus bradycardia may require atrial pacing; junctional rhythm may require AV sequential pacing; rapid AF may require cardioversion
  - RV (systemic) dysfunction may occur if right ventriculotomy used
- Arterial switch
  - Bleeding from suture lines
  - Myocardial ischemia due to coronary reimplantation (air or kinking)
  - Inadequate LV function due to insufficient mass, ischemia, or inadequate preservation during CPB–inotropic support
  - Supravalvar pulm artery stenosis
- Rastelli operation
  - Left ventricular dysfunction or failure
  - Arrhythmias, sudden death
  - Conduit stenosis

Transposition of the Great Arteries, L Form (L-TGA)

Laura K. Diaz
Alan Jay Schwartz

Risk
- Incidence 0.5% of pts with CHD
- Male slightly greater than female incidence

Perioperative Risks
- 1–10% may have no assoc lesions and may be unrecognized until right ventricular failure occurs
- 25% of pts with no assoc defects develop CHF by age 45 y
- Assoc defects: VSD (60–80%); pulm stenosis (left ventricular outflow obstruction) 30–50%; tricuspid (left AV valve) valve abn incl Ebstein-like malformation (50–80%).
- Increasing risk of AV block, RV dysfunction, worsening TR with increasing age

Worry About
- Pts can present with CHF 2° to large VSD or severe tricuspid (left AV valve) regurgitation
- Significant cyanosis can occur in pts with LVOTO and VSD
- Increased incidence of complete heart block (2% cumulative increase/y)

- Late complications in unoperated pts: Right ventricular dysfunction, CHF
- Assoc defects such as tricuspid (left-sided) regurgitation and AV conduction abn often progress and are risk factors for mortality.

Overview
- L-TGA: Discordant atrioventricular connections and discordant ventriculoarterial connections are both present, resulting in a series circulation
- Atrial position is normal, but ventricles are inverted and aorta is anterior and lies to the left of the pulm artery.
- Dextrocardia or mesocardia exists in 25% of pts.
- In the absence of other cardiac lesions pts are physiologically corrected.

Etiology
- No known genetic predisposition

Usual Treatment
- Digoxin, diuretics, afterload reducing agents utilized in pts with CHF
- Palliative surgery
- Pulm artery banding may occasionally be performed in pts with large VSDs
- Pulm artery banding may be performed esp. in older pts prior to "double switch"(atrial and arterial) procedure to prepare the LV to accept systemic workload.
- Blalock-Taussig shunt (BTS) may be necessary in cyanotic pts with LVOTO and VSD
- Definitive surgery: Goal is to make LV the systemic pumping chamber
- For pts with no RVOTO: "Double switch" Senning or Mustard procedure/arterial switch procedure: Combined atrial and arterial switch performed to allow left ventricle to become the systemic ventricle
- For pts with VSD and LVOTO: "Double switch" Senning or Mustard procedure/Rastelli procedure: Combined atrial switch and intra-ventricular Rastelli type VSD closure and RV-PA conduit placement

ASSESSMENT POINTS

System	Effect	Assessment by Hx	PE	Test
CARDIO	CHF	Poor wt gain, FTT Resp distress Poor perfusion	Jugular venous distention Hepatomegaly S$_3$ gallop Rales Edema	ECHO CXR
	↓ Pulm blood flow	Cyanosis	Cardiac murmur Clubbing	Pulse oximetry ABG ECHO
	AV block	SOB Exercise intolerance Dizziness/syncope	Slow heart rate CHF Decreased perfusion	EKG CXR
RESP	Congestion/pulm edema	Frequent URIs Pneumonia	Rales	CXR
HEME	Polycythemia Coagulopathy Thrombocytopenia	Bleeding	Plethora	CBC Coagulation studies TEG Plt studies

Key Reference: Jonas RA. Congenitally corrected transposition of the great arteries. In: Jonas RA (ed): *Comprehensive surgical management of congenital heart disease*, London, Arnold, 2004, pp 483-496.

Perioperative Implications

Preoperative Preparation
- Preop medication useful for most pts to allay anxiety and facilitate separation
- Note preop issues with cardiac rate or rhythm

Monitoring
- Arterial line may be placed after anesthetic induction
- Central line or right atrial line may be used for drug infusions and pressure monitoring
- Pacemaker capability should be readily available

Airway
- Nasal ETT recommended to minimize interference with potential use of TEE

Preinduction/Induction
- IV or inhalation induction may be utilized.

Maintenance
- Opioids (fentanyl 10–20 µg/kg) affords hemodynamic stability and avoids myocardial depression. May be used in concert with volatile agent.
- Pancuronium usually relaxant of choice due to vagolytic properties

Post CPB
- Monitor for ischemia, dysrhythmias
- Initiate inotropic and/or vasodilator therapy for ventricular dysfunction.
- TEE useful to assess for air, ventricular function, assess coronary arteries and VSD closure.

Extubation
- Early extubation possible if bleeding, arrhythmias controlled and ventricular function is adequate

Anticipated Problems/Concerns

VSD Closure
- Worsening of tricuspid regurgitation
- Onset of AV block

VSD Closure and RV-PA Conduit
- Conduit stenosis and/or obstruction and need for replacement
- Late onset of AV block

Double switch procedure
- Atrial arrhythmias, baffle obstruction
- Bleeding
- Myocardial ischemia due to coronary reimplantation (air or kinking)

Transsphenoidal Surgery

Lauren Berkow

PROCEDURES

Risk

- Incidence of pituitary adenoma: 2.9/100,000/y
- Prevalence: 16.7% of population

Perioperative Risks

- Mortality <1%
- Morbidity 3–5% (diabetes insipidus [DI], CSF leak, carotid artery injury, visual loss, meningitis, hemorrhage)

Worry About

- Endocrine abn (panhypopituitarism, Addison, Cushing's, thyroid dysfunction)
- DI: increased UO, hypernatremia, dehydration
- Acromegaly (potential difficult mask airway and intubation, increased risk of sleep apnea)
- Increased ICP
- Intracranial hemorrhage 2° to invasion into cavernous sinus

Overview

- Resection performed through nasal, sublabial incisions with aid of microscope
- Newer techniques often use fluoroscopic or MRI guidance, endoscopic approaches, intraop hormonal assays
- Tumors may secrete hormones (GH, ACTH, TSH, prolactin) or be nonfunctional
- Tumors may compress optic chiasm, causing visual field deficits, or may abut or invade cavernous sinus

ICD-9-CM Code: 227.3 (Benign pituitary adenoma)

Indications and Usual Treatment

- Pituitary tumor without extensive suprasellar extension or hypothalamic involvement (these usually require craniotomy)
- Other options incl transcranial approach, radiation or radiosurgery, medical treatment with bromocriptine or somatostatin analogues (octreotide, simvastatin)
- Pts with acromegaly may receive preop bromocriptine or octreotide

ASSESSMENT POINTS

System	Effect	Assessment by Hx	PE	Test
HEENT	Overgrowth of chin, tongue, vocal cord paralysis, subglottic stenosis (acromegaly)	Snoring, sleep apnea hoarseness	Airway exam Stridor, facial features	Lateral neck films FOB
CARDIO	Htn, DM, CHF Obesity, ischemia	Chest pain, dyspnea Exercise tolerance	CV exam	ECG, CXR Stress thallium ECHO
ENDO	Panhypopituitarism Acromegaly ($\uparrow$GH) Cushing's ($\uparrow$ACTH) Hyperthyroidism ($\uparrow$TSH) Insulin resistance	Cold intolerance Wt gain Nervousness	Hemodynamic instability CV collapse Obesity	GH, TSH, glucose Cortisol level Dexamethasone suppression test
RENAL/ LYTES	$\uparrow$ Aldosterone (ACTH) → $\uparrow$ Na$^+$, $\downarrow$ K$^+$, metab alkalosis $\uparrow$ ADH → DI	Oliguria Thirst, polyuria	Pulm/peripheral edema Orthostasis, hypotension UO	ABGs, lytes Urine lytes Osm serum Osm

Key References: Jho H, Park I, Alfieri A. The future of pituitary surgery. *Clin Neurosurg.* 2000;47:83–98. Atkinson AB, Kennedy A, Wiggam MI, et al. Long-term remission rates after pituitary surgery for Cushing's disease: The need for long-term surveillance. *Clin Endocrinol (Oxf).* 2005;63:549–559.

Perioperative Implications

Preoperative Preparation

- Assess and document neurologic deficits, evaluate endocrine function
- Assess for possible difficult intubation and sleep apnea (acromegaly, Cushing's)
- Avoid sedation, esp. if concerns about increased ICP

Anesthetic Technique

- GA with controlled ventilation

Monitoring

- Routine monitoring plus Foley catheter to follow UO
- Consider arterial line to watch BP during local infiltration and to follow electrolytes periop
- Consider precordial Doppler, or TEE to detect VAE if head elevated >15°

Airway

- Anticipate difficult airway if acromegaly present (may require awake FOB)
- Routine oral intubation if normal airway, consider oral RAE ETT to facilitate surgery
- Packs placed in oropharynx intraop to prevent aspiration of blood and irrigating solution

Induction/Maintenance

- Similar to any craniotomy: balanced vapor, narcotic and relaxant
- Stress dose steroids, antibiotics to cover naso/oropharyngeal flora
- Minimal postop pain; avoid narcotics overdose

Surgical Stages

Incision

- Infiltration of nose and mouth with local anesthetic, cocaine may trigger Htn, tachycardia, arrhythmias

Definitive Surgery

- Watch for DI, hemorrhage from carotid artery or cavernous sinus
- Watch for venous air embolism; D/C NO if suspected

Postoperative Considerations

- Confirm oropharyngeal packing removed, potential for aspiration of blood from nasopharynx, extubate awake
- May need postop steroid replacement
- EBL variable, may be hard to quantitate
- Potential complications: CSF leak, epistaxis, sinusitis or meningitis, intracranial hemorrhage, pneumocephalus, nasal septum perforation

Anticipated Problems/Concerns

- DI 2° to lack of ADH: Increased UO, hypernatremia, increased osmolality, dehydration; treat with IVF, DDAVP as needed
- Hemorrhage from ICA or cavernous sinus can lead to herniation, CN dysfunction, death
- Watch closely for postop neurologic changes
- Addisonian crisis: Hemodynamic instability, CV collapse; treat with steroids

Transurethral Resection of Bladder Tumor

Moustafa Ahmed

Risk

- Incidence in USA: 69,000 new cases in 2008. Fourth-most common cancer in men.
- The ninth-most common cancer in women.
- The ninth-most common cause of death among cancer in American men
- Race: Whites to African-Americans 2:1, but African-Americans have mortality rates twice that of whites; whites to Hispanic 2:1, but Hispanic have lower mortality rate than whites
- Bladder cancer accounts for 3% of all cancer deaths in men and 1.5% in women
- Gender: M:F ratio: 3:1, but women have 30% mortality higher than men
- Risk factors: Smoking, age, chemical exposure, chronic analgesics abuse, artificial sweeteners, chronic cystitis (calculus, indwelling catheters, infection) pelvic irradiation

Perioperative Risks

- Periop mortality low (<1%)
- Shedding of the tumor cells
- Ureteral obstruction from tumor or tumor resection
- Less risk of absorption syndromes than during TURP
- Clinical bladder perforation and bowel injury

Worry About

- Bladder perforation
- Uncontrolled hematuria
- Peroneal and sciatic nerve neuropathy from lithotomy position
- Obturator nerve stimulation that may lead to bladder perforation

Overview

- TURBT is indicated as diagnostic and therapeutic procedures in a suspicious of bladder cancer
- TURBT is relatively simple and quick procedures (30–60 min)
- Bladder cancer can occur at any given age, but the median age is 69 in men and 71 in women and the incidence of bladder cancer increase directly with age
- Assoc with multiple co-morbidity due to late median age

ICD-9-CM Code: 57.49 (Other transurethral excision or destruction of lesion or tissue of bladder)

Indications and Usual Treatment

- Most common presenting symptoms: Painless hematuria 85% and irritative symptoms (frequency, urgency, and dysuria)
- Dx tests incl urinary microscopic cytopathology (low sensitivity for low–grade tumors but 80% sensitivity with high-grade tumors), CT with or without contrast, excretory urography only if CT is not available, cystoscopy
- Procedure: TURBT is diagnostic by stage resection and therapeutic by resection and fulguration of all grossly visible tumors
- Repetitive TURBT is common with recurrence or second opinion for muscle invasion
- Other adjuvant Rx incl periop Mitomycin C (MMC) intravesical to prevent tumor cell implant, combined intravesical chemotherapy with MMC and BCG, intravesical immunotherapy, photoradiation therapy, laser therapy, cystectomy

ASSESSMENT POINTS

System	Effect	Assessment by Hx	PE	Test
CARDIO	CAD, PV, CHF	Chest pain, SOB, palpitation, claudication, lower extremities edema	Cardiac exam JVD LE edama	ECG, ECHO, stress test
RESP	COPD	SOB, coughing	Prolonged expiratory phase, wheezing, rales	CXR, PFTs
RENAL	CKD Chronic UTI	Oliguria, hematuria, disuria, frequency, urgency	Bimanual examination of the bladder and pelvis	UA, BUN/Cr, GFR
CNS	Cerebrovascular disease, stroke	Kirkali I, Chan T.	exam	

Key References: Kirkall I, Chan T. Bladder cancer: Epidemiology, staging and grading, and diagnosis, *Urology*. 2005;66(suppl 6A):4–34. Wihlborg A, Johansen C. Incidences of kidney, pelvis, ureter, and bladder cancer in a nationwide, population-based cancer registry, Denmark, 1944-2003. *Urology*. 2010;75(5):1222-1227. Hahn RG. Fluid absorption in endoscopic surgery. *Br J Anaesth*. 2006;96:8–20.

Perioperative Management

Preoperative Preparation
- Within normal complete blood count, serum electrolyte and coagulation parameters
- Documented negative UA and culture
- Intravenous prophylactic antibiotics

Monitoring
- Standard ASA monitoring
- Invasive monitoring as CVP depending on the co-morbidity and inability to measure the UOP

Anesthetic Technique/Induction
- GA: Different induction agents based on medical status, muscle paralysis not required if the tumors on the bladder floor or dome but if the tumors at lateral bladder wall muscle paralysis is required because using electrocautery for resection may lead to stimulation of obturator nerve and subsequent bladder perforation from sudden leg contraction
- Spinal anesthesia: T10 sensory level sufficient, higher level masks. Sx of perforation of bladder. Spinal anesthesia will not prevent obturator nerve stimulation. Obturator nerve block below pubic ramus if the resection at lateral wall of the bladder.

Surgical Stages
- Dorsal lithotmy position
- Bimanual exam of the bladder is performed under anesthesia
- Actual resection time usually <30 min
- Pan-endoscopy to identify and locate the tumors as well the location of ureteric orifices
- Water used as a bladder irrigant during the procedures because of its cytolytic effects
- IV absorption of irrigating solution rare because of minimal open veins, but lengthy one may lead to absorption of water cause electrolyte imbalances, volume overload and intravascular hemolysis (hemolysis can be avoided by using mannitol, sorbitol, or glycine all are more isotonic)
- Bipolar electroresection is reported to allow transurethral resection in saline (TURIS) as well decrease the risk of obturator reflex.
- Extra or intraperitoneal bladder wall perforation is rare, small perforation of no clinical significant can be treated with bladder drainage and antibiotic postop, but a symptomatic perforation or concern of bowel injury a laparoscopic or open exploration for repair is recommended
- Avoid bladder overdistension to decrease the incidence of bladder perforation.
- Low incidence of tumor seeding after bladder perforation
- Usually minimal blood loss

Postoperative Considerations
- Pain and bladder irritation
- Occult bleeding and clot formation in the bladder
- Signs and symptoms of peritoneal irritation raise the flag of bladder perforation
- Peroneal and sciatic nerve injury from lithotomy position
- Observe for ureteral obstruction if resection near ureteral orifice

Anticipated Problems/Concerns
- Disease of elderly (CAD, COPD, CKD)
- Sudden hypotension and loss of return of irrigant suggested perforation
- Lengthy surgery with change of mental status suggest electrolytes abn and volume overload
- Occult blood loss (but bleeding and clot can be performed and may require evacuation)
- Be aware that obturator nerve stimulation occurs suddenly if NMB is gone.

Transurethral Resection of Prostate (TURP)

Basavana Gouda Goudra
Nina Singh

Risk

- Histologic evidence of BPH: 50% of men by age 50; 75% by age 80
- BPH clinically significant in 40–50% of these pts
- Approx 400,000/y performed
- Mortality 0.2%–6% (increases with age, co-morbidity)

Perioperative Risks

- Age-assoc co-morbidities (cardiac, pulm, cerebrovascular)
- TURP syndrome
- Bladder perforation, hypothermia, coagulopathy and/or DIC, septicemia
- Toxicity of irrigating fluid components

Worry About

- TURP SX: Spectrum of clinical, physiologic conditions resulting from absorption of irrigating fluid through exposed venous sinuses of surgical capsule
- Hypervolemia: 20 mL/min absorbed; average 45–60 min
- Neuraxial versus general anesthesia

Overview

- TURP SX: Related to surgeon's experience, aggressiveness with electrocautery loop, size of gland, amount of tissue removed and irrigation used; manifestations from circulatory fluid overload, water intoxication, hyponatremia, pressure and volume of irrigant, duration of resection

- Irrigating solutions: Slightly hypotonic, non-electrolyte solutions (glycine, sorbitol, mannitol); electrolyte solution can disperse electrocautery current; water hypotonicity lyses RBCs

Indications and Usual Treatment

- TURP appropriate for prostate gland volumes <40–50 mL; alternative approach if >80 mL
- Less invasive, morbidity, expensive c/w open prostatectomy
- Transurethral laser coagulation, microwave thermotherapy are new techniques that eliminate complication of hyponatremia; bipolar electrovaporization allows use of saline irrigation

ICD-9-CM Code: 600 (Benign prostatic hypertrophy)

ASSESSMENT POINTS

System	Effect	Assessment by Hx	PE	Test
CARDIO	Hypervolemia/Htn, dysrhythmia, hypotension/CHF	Angina, palpitations, SOB	BP, HR, JVD, pedal edema, crackles, murmurs	EKG, ECHO, stress test, electrolytes
RESP	Pulm edema	SOB	O₂ sat, crackles, dyspnea	CXR, ABG
GU	Hyponatremia, hypo-osmolality, ARF	CRF, DM, Htn	Pedal edema	[Na], osmolarity, Cr, BUN
CNS	Agitation, seizure, coma, death, transient blindness (glycine)	Mental status, burning smell	Mental status	Neuro exam

Key Reference: Hahn RG. Fluid absorption in endoscopic surgery. *Br J Anaesth*. 2006;96:8–20.

Perioperative Management

Preoperative Preparation

- Careful preop assessment of cardiac, pulm, renal dysfunction
- If neuraxial, R/O coagulopathy, metastasis to spine
- Preop Abx may reduce bacteremia, septicemia; prostate often colonized with bacteria, may enter blood by gland manipulation, opening of venous sinuses

Monitoring

- Standard monitors; O₂ sat may indicate fluid overload; EKG changes (up to 18% pts); assess temp to avoid hypothermia
- Amount of irrigating fluid, hydrostatic pressure, time
- Labs: Na+, osmolarity

Anesthetic Technique/Induction

- Neuraxial block (T10 sensory level) allows for neuro exam (HA, restlessness, AMS); no difference in EBL, postop cognitive function, mortality, c/w GA

Surgical Stages

- Specialized cystoscope (rectoscope) passed through urethra
- Surgical field visualized by continuous irrigation through resectoscope; distends bladder, washes out blood and tissue from field

Dissection

- Moveable electrocautery, cutting wire, loop passed through resectoscope
- Bladder perforation: Resectoscope, overdistention with irrigation; sudden hypotension, generalized abd pain; increased airway PIP

Postoperative Considerations

- Tx postop shivering; can dislodge clots, coagulopathy

- Perforations are extraperitoneal, signaled by poor return of irrigating fluids
- DIC can result from thromboplastins released from prostate into circulation; up to 6% of pts may have subclinical DIC; dilutional thrombocytopenia can develop
- TURP Sx can occur within 15 min and up to 24 hr postop

Anticipated Problems/Concerns

- Tx of TURP SX—avoidance, early recognition key; absorbed water must be eliminated; Tx of mild hyponatremia with fluid restriction, loop diuretic; if severe, <115, consider hypertonic saline (cautious use, can result in additional fluid overload, complicating management; central pontine myelinolysis)
- Seizures with benzodiazepine, thiopental; consider ETT if AMS.

Trauma

Peter Nagele
Wolfgang Voelckel

Risk

- Leading cause of death among young (1–45 y of age; >60% of all deaths)
- Incidence in USA: 1:10 (7% violent); 60/100,000 for fatal trauma (30% violent)
- Increased risk with concurrent alcohol or drug use
- 30% of trauma deaths are caused by hemorrhagic shock

Perioperative Risks

- Hemorrhagic shock, hypotension, side effects of massive transfusion
- Hypoxemia, hyper- or hypocarbia esp. in brain trauma pts
- Lethal triad of trauma: Acidosis, coagulopathy, and hypothermia
- High incidence (40–100%) of systemic inflammatory response syndrome (SIRS) in serious trauma
- Mortality after major trauma 10–25%

Worry About

- Minimize time between trauma and damage control surgery
- Full or distended stomach
- Difficult airway in combination with C-spine protection
- Extensive fluid resuscitation prior to surgery may result in increased blood loss and boost coagulopathy
- Limit hyperventilation and excessive PEEP in hypovolemic pts

Overview

- Anesthesia for trauma pts has several goals: Securing the airway and protecting the C-spine, optimizing oxygenation and ventilation, restoring and maintaining hemodynamic stability, and preventing 2° complications
- Advanced Trauma Life Support (ATLS) is the common standard for the resuscitation phase

- Pts with multiple trauma are more likely to die from hemorrhagic shock and metabolic failure than from a failure to complete operative repairs.
- Principles of damage control surgery are control of hemorrhage, prevention of contamination and protection from further injury.

Indications and Usual Treatment

- Immediate identification of hemorrhage employing US (FAST sonography) and whole body CT scan is crucial.
- Life-saving interventions such as chest tubing, emergent thoracotomy or laparotomy may be indicated in critical pts even without further workup or imaging.
- In penetrating or violent trauma pts, large vessel injury is a major concern.

ASSESSMENT POINTS

System	Effect	Assessment by Hx	PE	Test
HEENT	Direct trauma to airway; airway obstruction; maxillofacial fractures	Often clearly visible	Airway Stridor; blood or vomitus in airway; limited ability to open mouth; raccoon eyes or CSF rhinorrhea	Inspection Auscultation X-ray; CT
RESP	Chest trauma; (tension) pneumothorax; serial rib fractures; flail chest	High degree of suspicion in all major trauma	Breathing Dyspnea, distended neck veins; reduced breath sounds; SQ emphysema; cyanosis (often absent in hemorrhagic shock)	CXR, ABG, CT
CARDIO	Acute hemorrhage; shock; vascular injury; cardiac tamponade; cardiac contusion	Observed blood loss	Circulation Hypotension, tachycardia, absent pulses, diaphoresis, cold extremities, distended neck veins, UO	ECG, TTE, TEE, FAST, ABG, lactate, CT, CT angio,
RENAL	Kidney trauma; acute renal failure	Location; crush injury	Hematuria; myoglobinuria	UA; FAST
CNS	Head trauma, neck and spine injury	Unconsciousness	Disability GCS; paraplegia, pain	Head and neck CT

Key Reference: Steill IG, Nesbitt LP, et al. for the OPALS Study Group. The OPALS Major Trauma Study: Impact of advanced life-support on survival and morbidity. *Can Med Assoc J.* 2008;178:1141–1152.

Perioperative Management

Preoperative Preparation

- Have emergency release blood set up (for major trauma: 10 PRBC, 10 FFP).
- Adequate preoxygenation is paramount before induction (low O_2 reserve)
- Large-bore IV access (often a combination of central and peripheral lines) critical
- Have rapid infusion device and fluid warmer ready.
- Have emergency drugs ready (epinephrine, vasopressin, phenylephrine, norepinephrine).

Monitoring

- Standard ASA monitors plus Foley
- Invasive hemodynamic monitoring essential (arterial line); serial ABGs to assess resp and metabolic status
- Consider central venous access; CVP monitoring is of questionable relevance.
- Extended hemodynamic monitoring such as continuous cardiac output, SvO_2 and Swan-Ganz catheter may be beneficial for select group of pts. Consider TEE.
- Consider advanced coagulation monitoring (TEG, ROTEM).

Anesthetic Technique/Induction

- Have difficult airway equipment, incl a primary surgical airway, ready as well as a functional suction device.

- Airway management is usually by orotracheal intubation and manual in-line stabilization of the C-spine.
- Rapid sequence induction is standard; induction agents that maintain hemodynamic stability are preferred (ketamine, etomidate).

Fluid Resuscitation

- Consider permissive hypotension until hemorrhage control has been achieved.
- After initial resuscitation with plasma isotonic crystalloids, switch to PRBC and FFP early.
- All fluids should be warmed.
- Fluid therapy can be guided by TEE or blood lactate values, which are highly indicative for hypovolemia and inadequate tissue oxygenation.
- When coagulopathy becomes clinically relevant, consider fibrinogen concentrate and plts as needed; monitor and treat hyperfibrinolysis when needed.
- Use of buffering agents (bicarbonate) to treat metabolic acidosis is controversial.

Maintenance

- Low-dose inhalational agent may be used if hemodynamically tolerated and when brain trauma and intracerebral pressure is not a concern.
- IV anesthesia may consist of opioids and benzodiazepines.

- Consider NMDA receptor antagonist (i.e., ketamine) to reduce the likelihood of opioid-induced hyperalgesia.

Postoperative Considerations

- Controlled ventilation may be needed until hemostasis has been restored, and lung function as well as cerebral performance allow safe extubation
- Transfer multiple trauma pts to an ICU unit for further stabilization

Anticipated Problems/Concerns

- Postop multiorgan failure
- Postop mortality substantially higher in elderly pts
- Pts after damage control surgery require multiple surgeries in the following days
- Risk for intraop awareness is increased in major trauma—explain preop to family and postop to pt to reduce incidence of PTSD and nightmares.

Tubal Ligation

Jason G. Lai
Andrew M. Malinow

Risk

- 700,000 performed annually in USA as either postpartum mini-laparotomy or interval laparoscopy
- Mortality in USA is 4/100,000 tubal ligations

Perioperative Risks

- Minor risks: Infection, bleeding, bruising, abn or painful scar formation, allergic skin reaction to tape, dressings and/or latex, delayed return of bowel and/or bladder function
- Major risks: Serious bleeding, serious infection, damage to organs (uterus, fallopian tubes, ovaries, bladder, and/or ureters), damage to the intestines (perforation and/or burn injury), nerve injury, blood vessel injury, blood clots, pulm embolus, myocardial infarction, adverse reaction to medications or anesthesia

Worry About

- Postpartum: Airway; aspiration risk (administration of opioid increases the likelihood of delayed gastric emptying in the early postpartum period); hypovolemia (postpartum hemorrhage, uterine atony)
- Interval: Complications of laparoscopy (bowel laceration, vascular injury, hypercarbia, gas embolism, adverse hemodynamics, pneumoperitoneum, Trendelenburg's position, conversion to laparotomy)
- Peripheral nerve injury due to positioning on the OR table

Overview

- Tubal ligation is a permanent form of female sterilization, in which the fallopian tubes are severed and sealed or occluded to prevent future fertilization
- Occlusion methods incl:
  - Partial salpingectomy: Suture ligation of a small loop of fallopian tube and then removing the interval segment of the loop
  - Clips: Clamp the fallopian tubes, thus inhibiting blood flow and causing a small amount of scarring or fibrosis
  - Tubal rings: Similar to clips, mechanically blocking the fallopian tubes
  - Electrocoagulation/cauterization: Coagulation/burning a small portion of each fallopian tube
- Mini-laparotomy: Advantages incl lower rate of serious complication (bowel laceration, vascular injury), less technical surgical expertise required, and hospital stay in postpartum women is not extended
- Laparoscopy: Advantages incl decreased operative time, less postop pain, shorter hospital stay, and more rapid return to normal functional activities

- Local anesthetic technique under IV sedation has been described by skilled surgeons with injection of local anesthetic directly into the wound, then bathing parietal and visceral peritoneum with small volumes of lipid-soluble local anesthetic, and finally injecting the mesosalpinx before fallopian tube ligation.
- In the postpartum period, regional anesthesia (epidural or spinal) is preferred to reduce the risk of failed airway and/or aspiration
- General anesthesia (GA) with controlled ventilation avoids hypercarbia from the mechanical and chemical effects of peritoneal CO_2 insufflation during laparoscopy
- Laparoscopy may be contraindicated if the pt has a Hx of abd surgery and known, extensive intra-abdominal adhesions.

ICD-9-CM Codes: V25.2 (Sterilization); 659.40 (Grand multiparity with current pregnancy unspecified as to episode of care)

Indications and Usual Treatment

- Multiparous pt desiring sterilization
- Medical contraindication to pregnancy (appropriate advance consent must be obtained with reaffirmation at the time of the procedure)

ASSESSMENT POINTS*

System	Effect	Assessment by Hx	PE	Test
HEENT (AIRWAY)	Airway edema Abn anatomy	Difficult airway	Airway exam	
CARDIO	Hypovolemia	Hemorrhage	HR, BP (orthostatics)	Hct, plts
GI	↑ Gastric volume ↓ Gastric pH ↓ Lower esophageal sphincter tone Morbid/super morbid obesity	Heartburn Opioids during labor	Wt, BMI	
GU	Uterine atony, chorioamnionitis, endometritis, UTI Pre-eclampsia	Postpartum hemorrhage, fever, diaphoresis Headache, visual disturbances, epigastric pain, edema	HR, BP (orthostatics), foul lochia BP, proteinuria, oliguria thrombocytopenia, hemolysis, edema	Hct, plts ↑ WBC, temp UO, Hct, plts

* Postpartum

Key Reference: Practice guidelines for obstetric anesthesia. An updated report by the American Society of Anesthesiologists Task Force on Obstetric Anesthesia. *Anesthesiology.* 2007;106:843–863.

Perioperative Management

Preoperative Preparation

- Assess intravascular volume status and hydrate as necessary.
- NPO status: A pt planning to have an elective postpartum tubal ligation should have no oral intake of solid foods within 8 hr of surgery
- Postpartum pts are often given acid-aspiration chemoprophylaxis, incl nonparticulate antacid, H_2-receptor antagonist, and/or metoclopramide
- Pts with pregnancy-induced Htn and/or preeclampsia may safely receive regional anesthesia for postpartum tubal ligation provided that there is no evidence of pulm edema, oliguria, uncontrolled Htn, or thrombocytopenia; however, the clinical team should carefully weigh the risk of worsening maternal condition in a pt undergoing elective surgery

Anesthetic Technique

- Can be performed under local, regional, or GA

Monitoring

- Routine ASA monitors

Airway

- Postpartum pts may have unexpected upper airway edema esp. after a lengthy second stage of labor

Induction

- Local technique: Intraperitoneal infiltration of local anesthetic (lidocaine, ropivacaine, chloroprocaine) can be used to achieve peritoneal anesthesia suitable for mini-laparotomy and laparoscopy. Moderate-to-deep levels of IV sedation along with surgical expertise in this technique are mandatory.
- Regional (epidural and/or spinal) technique: Sensory dermatome level of T4 is often needed to block visceral pain during exposure and manipulation of the fallopian tubes.

- Clinicians debate the conventional teaching that epidural catheters placed during labor are more likely to fail with longer postdelivery time intervals to tubal ligation. In some institutions, the expected failure rate to achieve an adequate surgical level of up to 25% predisposes practitioners to remove the epidural catheter immediately after delivery and then later induce spinal anesthesia (with 10–12 mg of bupivacaine with or without spinal opioid) in pts desiring regional anesthesia. Other clinicians choose to leave an epidural catheter placed during labor in place.
- If the epidural catheter used for labor analgesia is left *in situ*: Inspect the catheter site, administer a test dose to confirm nonintravenous and nonsubarachnoid position of the catheter tip, and then extend the sensory level by injecting incremental doses (cumulative 18–24 mL) of local anesthetic with a concentration suitable for surgical anesthesia (2% lidocaine with added epinephrine 1/200,000, 3% 2-chloroprocaine, 0.5% ropivacaine)

- GA for postpartum pts: Most practitioners still use a rapid sequence induction technique with cricoid pressure and maintain anesthesia with controlled ventilation and IV anesthetic adjuvant drugs, avoiding high-inspired concentrations of volatile halogenated agent for fear of inducing uterine atony/postpartum hemorrhage
- Laparoscopic technique: Deflate the stomach before trocar insertion, obtain large-bore IV access, hyperventilate to maintain normocarbia, reassess ventilation after insufflation (peak airway pressure, minute ventilation, $ETCO_2$)

Surgical Stages
- Postpartum minilaparotomy: Small infraumbilical incision
- Interval laparoscopy: Introduction of trocars to peritoneal cavity, insufflation of CO_2, and insertion of laparoscope and instruments
- Mini-laparotomy and laparoscopy: Fallopian tubes identified and severed or occluded
- EBL: Minimal (10 mL)
- Duration of surgery: Ideally <30 min

Postoperative Considerations
- Pain: Moderate and of short duration, typically treated with parenteral opioids and oral analgesics
- Local anesthetic infiltration of the mesosalpinx or topical application of a local anesthetic to the fallopian tubes by the surgeon significantly decreases postop opioid requirements

Ureteral Reimplantation

Constance L. Monitto

Risk

- Incidence: 1–3% of healthy children; 30–50% of children with symptomatic UTIs
- Gender predominance: Female
- Racial predilection: Caucasian
- Age: Dx antenatally or in childhood, with majority of surgical procedures performed by 5–6 y of age
- Genetic factors: Unknown but suggested by 30–35% incidence in siblings, and 67% incidence in offspring of affected individuals

Perioperative Risks

- Mortality extremely rare
- Minimal periop blood loss
- Postop ureteral obstruction (caused by edema, bleeding or blood clots, bladder spasms, or ureteral ischemia) can occur; usually asymptomatic and resolves spontaneously
- Symptomatic obstruction can present with abd pain, N/V, but is usually diagnosed on postop follow-up renal US
- Disruption of bladder innervation possible, esp. with extravesical repair

Worry About

- Most pts are healthy children (ASA I-II), but some pts requiring procedure will have significant congenital anomalies (e.g., spinal dysraphism) or GU anomalies (e.g., UPJ obstruction, ureteral duplication, bladder diverticula, posterior urethral valves, bladder or cloacal exstrophy).

Overview

- Ureteral reimplantation is usually performed to treat high-grade (Grade III-V) vesicoureteral reflux (VUR), where reflux is assoc with calyceal blunting and, at times, ureteral dilatation
- Untreated VUR can result in chronic and/or recurrent UTIs, renal scarring, renal insufficiency, Htn, and impaired somatic growth; renal failure is uncommon (estimated risk <1%)

Etiology

- VUR produces retrograde flow of urine from the bladder through the ureter and, at times, into the kidney.
- Dx of VUR is generally made by renal US and voiding cystourethrogram.
- 1° VUR is a congenital anomaly resulting in development of an inadequate valvular mechanism at the ureterovesical junction.
- 2° VUR is caused by anatomic (e.g., posterior urethral valves or ureterocoeles) or functional (e.g., neuropathic bladder or bladder instability) bladder outlet obstruction.

Usual Treatment

- Most pts are initially managed medically (low-dose prophylactic antibiotics), as 70–90% of low-grade reflux will resolve spontaneously as pt grows
- Indications for surgery incl breakthrough UTIs while on antibiotics, noncompliance, increasing or severe reflux (Grades IV and V), deteriorating renal function, persistent reflux in females approaching puberty, and assoc congenital anomalies of the ureterovesical junction.
- Goal of surgery is the creation of a valvular mechanism that allows ureteral compression with bladder filling and contraction
- Open surgical techniques (ureteroneocystostomy) can be extravesical, intravesical, or combined depending on the approach to the ureter, and suprahiatal or infrahiatal depending on the position of the new submucosal tunnel in relation to the original hiatus.
- Extravesical repairs (e.g., modified Lich-Gregoir ureteral reimplantation) have a similar success rate to the intravesicular approach. They leave the bladder intact, lessening the risk of urinary contamination, bladder spasms, and hematuria, but concerns exist about disrupting bladder innervation and causing urinary retention with bilateral reimplantation.
- Intravesicular and extravesicular repairs through small suprapubic incisions (2–4 cm) can be attempted if minimally invasive surgical techniques are utilized.
- >95% success rate of open surgical correction
- Endoscopic injection of the dextranomer/hyaluronic compound (Deflux®), a closed surgical treatment of VUR, is 70–90% effective in treating low-grade reflux, but has an increased likelihood of failure with increased severity of reflux.
- While laparoscopic surgical repairs are complex and not generally employed; a pneumovesical approach to the reimplantation of ureters within the bladder has also been reported.

ICD-9-CM Code: 593.7 (Vesicoureteral reflux)

ASSESSMENT POINTS

System	Effect	Assessment by Hx	PE	Test
HEENT/RESP	Generally uninvolved	Snoring Exercise tolerance	Routine airway exam and lung auscultation	
CARDIO	Htn		Measure BP	
IMMUNE	Possible latex allergy in pts with spinal dysraphism or exstrophy	Hx of rash, hives, or anaphylaxis with latex exposure		
RENAL	Possible renal insufficiency or RTA			Electrolytes, BUN/Cr
CNS	Weakness or paralysis with spinal dysraphism	CNS Hx, incl Hx of bladder or bowel dysfunction	CNS exam Sacral dimple or hair tuft	MRI of spine

Key Reference: Khoury A, Bagli DJ. Reflux and megaureter. In: Wein AJ, Kavoussi LR, Novick AC, Partin AW, Peters CA, eds. *Campbell-Walsh urology*. 9th ed. Philadelphia: Saunders; 2007:3423–3481.

Perioperative Implications

Preoperative Preparation

- Appropriate fasting interval and premedication (e.g., rectal, oral, IM. or IV. midazolam) given pt age and level of preop anxiety

Monitoring

- Routine ECG, noninvasive BP monitoring, pulse oximetry, capnography, temp

Airway

- General endotracheal anesthesia for open procedures, while general anesthesia via laryngeal mask airway is generally sufficient when endoscopic surgery is performed

Induction

- Mask or IV induction depending on pt age, preference, and risk factors (e.g., GERD)

Maintenance

- General endotracheal anesthesia alone or a combined technique (general anesthesia with a single shot caudal or caudal and/or lumbar epidural catheter inserted following induction) are both effective intraop.
- Regional anesthesia alone is not generally advocated given pt age
- Combined techniques are not employed in pts with assoc spinal dysraphism
- Local infiltration of the skin incision can be performed before skin closure if a regional technique is not incl in intraop management.

Extubation

- Generally attempted at the conclusion of surgical procedure

Adjuvants

- Ketorolac has been shown to provide analgesia and decrease the frequency and severity of bladder spasms following ureteroneocystostomy

Postoperative Period

- Postop length of stay ranges between 1 and 6 d for open ureteroneocystostomy
- Minimally invasive surgical techniques may shorten length of stay, diminish acute postop pain, and decrease the likelihood of inducing urinary retention.
- Some minimally invasive extravesicular repairs are being performed on an outpatient basis, as are endoscopic Deflux® injections.
- Postop pain can be incisional or related to bladder spasms, and may require treatment with oral or IV opioids, anticholinergics and bladder smooth muscle relaxants (e.g., oxybutinin and diazepam), NSAIDs, and/or epidural local anesthetic/opioid infusions.
- When outpatient surgery is contemplated, pts must meet specific criteria prior to discharge, incl adequate pain control, tolerance of a regular diet, ability to void postop (or comfort with the care of an indwelling urethral catheter), and the ability to ambulate without difficulty.
- Complications of postop pain management can incl ileus, resp depression, sedation, emesis, and urinary retention.
- Postop pain/bladder spasms may persist after discharge and require treatment with oral opioids, acetaminophen, NSAIDs, oxybutynin and/or diazepam.

Ureteral Stent Placement

Gregory L. McHugh

Shawn T. Beaman

Risk

- Incidence of unilateral ureteral obstruction: acute 1:1,000; chronic 5:1,000
- Incidence of bilateral ureteral obstruction; acute 5:10,000; chronic 1:1,000
- M:F ratio: 1:1
- Performed on pts of all ages

Perioperative Risks

- Extremely low mortality (<0.1%)
- Serious complications: 4% of pts
- Perforation of ureter or adjacent visceral structures
- Renal hemorrhage requiring transfusion
- Minor complications: 10% of pts
- UTI from instrumentation of the urinary tract
- Irritative bladder symptoms
- Microscopic hematuria
- Flank or loin pain from vesicorenal reflux or stent coiling

Worry About

- Pre-existing renal insufficiency or renal failure from the underlying disease process
- Fluid retention, edema, CHF
- Delayed drug metabolism (e.g., morphine, pancuronium, vecuronium)
- Complications of bacteremia or sepsis (e.g. hypotension) in pts presenting with obstructive pyelonephritis
- N/V with assoc electrolyte and fluid disturbances in pts with renal colic
- Risk of autonomic hyperreflexia in paraplegic/quadriplegic pts who have a predilection for nephrolithiasis

Overview

- First described in 1967, modern stents are composed of polyurethane or complex copolymers
- Proximal and/or distal pigtail loops prevent migration
- Depending on the indication, stents may be temporary or indwelling, with exchange occurring every 3–6 mo

Indications and Usual Treatment

- 1° goal is restitution or maintenance of urinary drainage
- Nephrolithiasis: As an adjuvant to extracorporeal shock wave lithotripsy for large stones or as monotherapy for small stones
- Tumors: Relief of external ureteral compression from retroperitoneal or intra-abdominal malignancies
- Intra-abdominal urine leakage: Manage and bypass defects caused by trauma, surgery, or ureteral fistulas
- Congenital strictures or obstructive uropathies: Commonly in the pediatric population

ASSESSMENT POINTS

System	Effect	Assessment by Hx	PE	Test
CARDIO	Hypovolemia	Hx of N/V, orthostasis, oliguria	Orthostatic BP, mucous membranes	Electrolytes, H/H
RESP	Pulm edema	Dyspnea, anuria	Crackles, rales, peripheral edema	CXR
RENAL	Chronic renal insufficiency, acute renal failure	Renal colic pain, oliguria or anuria, recurrent UTI, hematuria or proteinuria	Flank pain, peripheral edema	Urinalysis, BUN, Cr, plasma and urine electrolytes, renal U/S, IVP
CNS	Uremia, electrolyte disturbances	Obtundation, coma, seizures	Weakness, asterixis, hyperreflexia, tetany	Serum electrolytes, BUN/Cr

Key Reference: Walsh PC, ed. *Campbell's Urology*. 8th ed. Philadelphia: Elsevier Science; 2002.

Perioperative Management

Preoperative Preparation

- Ensure NPO status, evaluate for volume and electrolyte disturbances
- Establish IV access, consider IVF if signs/symptoms of IV are present
- Anxiolysis and pain control for pt comfort; important for pts with stones

Monitoring

- Standard noninvasive ASA monitors in most cases
- Consider arterial cannulation in critically ill or paraplegic or quadriplegic pts at risk for autonomic hyperreflexia
- Rarely CVP monitoring in pts with acute volume overload or dialysis dependence

Anesthetic Technique/Induction

- General anesthesia most common. Routine induction with inhalational or IV maintenance, consider NMB given that ureters are thin and prone to injury if the pt moves or coughs during the procedure, ETT for secure airway but may consider LMA for short procedures
- Spinal anesthesia: Levels around T8 are desirable
- Epidural anesthesia: May require supplemental IV sedation

Surgical Stages

- Cystoscope insertion: Potential for pt discomfort and/or sympathetic stimulation
- Guidewire introduction into ureter with threading of stent. Fluoroscopic guidance is occasionally required; important to prevent pt movement to avoid perforation of bladder or ureter by ureteroscope
- Majority of stenting procedures are short, typically 15–45 min in duration

Postoperative Considerations

- Pain management: Usually mild discomfort, small doses of IV opioids titrated to effect, ketorolac or prazosin for relief of bladder spasm
- N/V: Not a high risk procedure, consider individual pt risk factors

Anticipated Problems/Concerns

- Lithotomy position: Risk of peroneal nerve injury
- Occasional need for percutaneous placement if endourological approach fails

Vaginal Delivery, Normal

Adrienne T. Kung
Nancy E. Oriol

Risk

- Incidence in USA: ~4 million live births per year

Peripartum Risks

- Maternal mortality ↓: 12.1 deaths/100,000 live births in 2003 compared with 607.9/100,000 in 1915
- Perinatal mortality rate also ↓ : 6.23/1000 live births in 2003
- Thromboembolism, hemorrhage, hypertensive disorders, infection remain common causes of maternal mortality and morbidity
- Decline in anesthetic-related causes noted (UK data)

Worry About

- Supine hypotension syndrome
- Difficult airway

- Co-morbid conditions: Preeclampsia, diabetes, antepostpartum hemorrhage, multiple gestation, vaginal delivery after C-section
- Fetal well-being

Overview

- Effects of maternal interventions on fetus
- Effects of maternal interventions on course of labor
- Role of anesthesiologist
  - Labor analgesia
  - Anesthetic for operative delivery
  - High-risk obstetrics
  - Newborn resuscitation
- Maternal resuscitation

ICD-9-CM Code: V22.2

Indications and Usual Treatment

- Labor analgesia
  - Lumbar epidural
  - Spinal
  - Combined spinal/epidural
  - Parenteral opioids
  - Others: Psychoprophylaxis, TENS, hypnosis, inhalational analgesia
- Operative delivery
  - Spinal anesthesia
  - Epidural anesthesia
  - Continuous spinal analgesia
  - General anesthesia
  - Local anesthesia
  - Bilateral pudendal nerve block
- Spinal/epidural anesthesia
- Neonatal resuscitation, esp. in situations of nonreassuring fetal heart tracings, meconium-stained amniotic fluid

ASSESSMENT POINTS

System	Effect	Assessment by Hx	PE	Test
CARDIO	↑ CO, ↓ SVR		BP, HR	ECHO, ECG
RESP	Edema, ↑ soft tissue	Previous GA	Airway exam	None
HEME	↑ Plasma vol > ↑ RBC mass	Sx of easy fatigue with significant anemia	None specific	CBC: Occasional ↓ plt in normal preg
HEPAT/RENAL	Significant changes if pregnancy complicated by PIH	Epigastric pain, N/V, headache	Epigastric tenderness, hyperreflexia	BUN, Cr, LFTs, UA

Key Reference: Chestnut DC. *Obstetric anesthesia principles and practice.* Philadelphia: Mosby; 2009:15–31.

Intrapartum Management

- Parturients in active labor should consider brief interview with anesthesiologist; emphasis on airway exam, previous anesthesia experience, co-morbid conditions
- Establish fetal status by cardiotocography, relevant prenatal test
- Antacid prophylaxis before any anesthetic intervention
- Establish IV access; consider preload before regional procedure; maintain left uterine displacement at all times

Monitoring

- Baseline pulse, BP, temp
- Following regional technique, monitor hemodynamics aggressively for the 1st 30 min; then at ½-hr to 1-hr intervals
- Equal attention to fetal status at induction, during maintenance of regional analgesia for labor

Labor Analgesia

Lumbar Epidural

- Local anesthetics, opioids alone or in combination; low-dose, ultra-low dose (0.04% bupiva-

caine) solutions; latter allow for consideration of ambulation during labor as incidence of motor blockade is low

- Complications
  - Hypotension
  - Inadequate analgesia
  - Dural puncture headache
  - Subarachnoid block
  - Subdural block
  - Nerve damage (rare)
- Contraindications
  - Coagulopathy
  - Infection
  - Pt refusal

Spinal

- Intrathecal drugs
- Opioids: Sufentanil, fentanyl, morphine commonly used; addition of bupivacaine 2.5 mg may improve quality, duration of analgesia but increase incidence of motor weakness
- Much ↓ incidence of spinal headache since introduction of pencil-point needles

Parenteral Opioids

- Maternal N/V, sedation
- Decreased beat-to-beat variability in FHR
- Risk of neonatal depression
- Despite low efficacy, remain most common form of labor analgesia

Anticipated Problems/Concerns

- Airway: ↑ Incidence of difficult and/or failed intubation with resultant hypoxemia, aspiration
- Water deliveries
- Aortocaval compression
- Peripartum hemorrhage
- Effect of interventions on fetus
- Postpartum neuropathy
- 20–25% of all planned normal spontaneous vaginal deliveries go to C-section

Venous Air Embolism

Thomas J. Toung

Risk

- Pts with operative field right heart gradient of >5 cm
- Probe patent foramen ovale in 25% of adult population
- Pts for laparoscopic surgery
- Incidence of VAE in children same as adults

Perioperative Risks

- Periop mortality <1%, but depends on early detection
- VAE: 40–80% in sitting, 10% in prone, 15% in supine, and 8% in lateral position
- Paradoxical air embolism (as high as 12%)
- Children suffer greater hemodynamic derangements

Worry About

- Pulm venous outflow obstruction
- CV collapse
- Paradoxical air embolism

Overview

- Lethal volume of venous air in adult: 100–300 mL (two cardiac stroke volume)
- Entrained venous air can cause
  - Right ventricle outflow obstruction
  - Paradoxical arterial embolism (coronary embolism, stroke)
- Multiorifice catheter is preferable; the tip must be placed 2 cm below the SVC-atrial junction
- 75% N_2O can increase air bubble size about 3-fold
- Sensitivity for detection of VAE: TEE > precordial Doppler > PAP and $ETCO_2$ > CVP > BP > ECG
- Mill-wheel murmurs late, catastrophic sign
- PA catheter may provide prognostic information

ICD-9-CM Codes: 958.0; 673.0 (Obstetrical)

Indications and Usual Treatment

- Operative site elevated to gain better exposure, blood drainage
- When VAE occurs
  - Notify surgeon of episode
  - Turn off N_2O
  - Gently apply bilateral jugular vein compression
  - Inflate MAST
  - Aspirate air from central catheter
  - CV support
  - Left decubitus position (Durant's maneuver)

ASSESSMENT POINTS

System	Effect	Assessment By Hx	Pe	Test
CARDIO	Patent foramen ovale	SOB	Auscultation	CXR, cath

Key Reference: Mirski MA, Lele AV, Fitzsimmons L, Toung T. Venous air embolism. *Anesthesiology*. 2007;106:164–177.

Intraoperative Management

Monitoring

- Direct arterial pressure
- Precordial Doppler
- $ETCO_2$
- Consider CVP or PAP catheter

Surgical Stages

- Dissection
- VAE mostly in beginning, closure
- Definitive surgery

- Depends on pathology
- When VAE occurs
  - Notify surgeon of episode
  - Turn off N_2O
  - Gently apply bilateral jugular vein compression
  - Inflate MAST
  - Aspirate air from central catheter
  - CV support
  - Left decubitus position (Durant's maneuver)

Postoperative Considerations

- Possible hypoxemia from pulm infarction
- Possible stroke from parodoxical air embolism
- Possible cardiac arrest from massive venous air or paradoxical air embolism

Anticipated Problems/Concerns

- Hypoxemia, ARDS (late sequelae of massive air embolism and resuscitation)
- Stroke
- MI

Ventricular Septal Defect, Repair of

Aris Sophocles
Mark Twite

PROCEDURES

Risk

- Most common form of CHD, occurring in 50% of all children with CHD and in 20% as an isolated lesion
- Incidence has increased with advances in imaging and screening of infants: Range 1–50 per 1000 live births
- Assoc with a variety of syndromes incl trisomy 21, VACTERL, CHARGE
- Familial recurrence risk in offspring: paternal VSD 2%, maternal VSD 6–10%

Perioperative Risks

- Endocarditis: Lifelong risk 18.7/10,000 pt-y in unoperated pts
- Pathophysiologic consequences depend on the size and location of the VSD and incl shunting, pulm Htn, and CHF

Worry About

Perioperative

- L→R shunts: Volume overload in left atrium, left ventricle, and pulm artery leading to CHF, increased incidence of URI, and pulm edema.
- R→L shunts: Irreversible pulm Htn, desaturation, cyanosis, and 2° erythrocytosis.
- Eisenmenger's syndrome: Assoc with arrhythmias, endocarditis, hemoptysis, and pulm artery thrombosis
- Infundibular defects are assoc with aortic insufficiency
- Paradoxical air embolism

Postoperative

- Residual or unrecognized VSD (0.7–2%) causing failure to separate from CPB, CHF, or failure to wean from mechanical ventilation
- RBBB or complete heart block (1–3%) due to damage of conducting system post repair.
- Ventricular outflow obstruction post repair

- Aortic regurgitation 2° to prolapse of aortic valve leaflet post repair
- Tricuspid valve insufficiency

Overview

- Spontaneous closure commonly occurs in muscular defects before age 5 y. Size may predict closure rate: Defects up to 5 mm rarely require surgery whereas defects 6.5 mm or larger almost always require surgery.
- Pulm Htn can be seen by age 1 y if large VSD, multiple VSDs, or PDA exists; Eisenmenger's syndrome seen in second decade of life
- Goal of surgical therapy is to prevent pulm vascular obstructive disease and to treat intractable CHF assoc with FTT
- Factors determining time of repair incl
  - Degree of L→R shunting
  - CHF unresponsive to medical therapy
  - Increased pulm vascular resistance

ICD-9-CM Code: 745.4

Etiology

- Four types based on location:
  - Type I (5–7%) subarterial beneath the pulm and aortic valves in the right ventricular outflow tract. Aortic insufficiency may occur.
  - Type II (80%) perimembranous defect in the fibrous trigone of the heart where the aortic, mitral, and tricuspid valves are in fibrous continuity.
  - Type III (5–8%) involves the inlet of the right ventricular septum immediately inferior to the atrioventricular valve apparatus. May be assoc with an endocardial cushion defect.
  - Type IV (5–20%) involves the muscular ventricular septum. Multiple (>3) VSDs are called "Swiss-cheese" defects.

Indications and Usual Treatment

- Infant and child: CHF and FTT. Infants with trisomy 21 are at particular risk for pulm Htn and should have their VSDs closed early.
- Adults: Unrepaired small defect without evidence of left ventricular volume overload require endocarditis prophylaxis and periodic follow-up. Those with left ventricular volume overload or progressive aortic valve disease usually require closure.
- Other indications for surgical closure incl infundibular defects, chamber enlargement, increasing PVR (>6 wood units/m^2 despite administration of a pulm vasodilator considered inoperable), and multiple "Swiss cheese" defects refractory to medical management.
- Medical management of symptomatic CHF incl digoxin, diuretics, and after-load reduction agents.
- Surgical closure is performed using cardiopulmonary bypass. Surgical approach depends on defect location but is usually via a right atrial approach.
- Pulm artery banding via a partial sternotomy or right thoracotomy may be used for small infants who are symptomatic, to allow for growth and easier technical repair later. Banding may also be used when there are multiple muscular VSDs and in pts at high risk for cardiopulmonary bypass.
- Transcatheter closure of VSDs has been performed as an alternative to surgery as well as intraop for difficult defects such as multiple muscular VSDs and postop for residual VSDs. Major limitation to this technique is the size of the sheath necessary for device delivery, which precludes its use in infancy.
- Heart and lung transplantation is the only option for end-stage Eisenmenger's syndrome.

ASSESSMENT POINTS

System	Effect	Assessment by Hx	PE	Test
CARDIO Small defect L→R shunt	Trivial L → R shunting	Incidental murmur found by pediatrician	Left parasternal holosystolic murmur. Smaller defects are loudest and may have a thrill.	CXR normal. ECG normal or may show mild LVH. TTE, TEE, 3D ECHO, MRI cardiac catheterization
Large defect L→R shunt	Significant L → R shunting, ↑ PAP	FTT, dyspnea, feeding difficulties, recurrent pulm infections	Harsh pansystolic murmur. Larger defects may have murmurs of constant quality that vary little throughout the cardiac cycle.	CXR: Cardiomegaly, increased pulm vascularity. ECG: Biventricular hypertrophy, notched P waves. TTE, TEE, 3D ECHO, MRI cardiac catheterization
Large defect R→L shunt or no shunt	Varying degrees of R→L shunting 2° to pulm vascular obstructive disease	Eisenmenger syndrome often cyanotic with clubbing	May not have a murmur but may have a loud pulm component of the second heart sound	CXR: Right chamber enlargement, dilated main pulm artery, loss of pulm vascularity. ECG right axis deviation, RVH TTE, TEE, 3D ECHO, MRI, cardiac catheterization

Key Reference: Minette MS, Sahn DJ. Ventricular Septal Defects. *Circulation.* 2006;114:2190–2197.

Perioperative Implications

Preoperative Preparation

- Optimal control of CHF

Monitoring

- Standard ASA monitors
- Arterial and central venous monitoring for tight control of hemodynamics
- TEE to assist with postop diagnosis of residual VSD

- Consider Swan-Ganz catheter or direct PA/LA lines for postop management of pts with elevated pulm vascular resistance

Preinduction/Induction

- Premedication
- IV induction or inhalational induction in children

Airway

- ETT. PPV may limit degree of L → R shunting

Maintenance

- Medium to high-dose opioid with NMB and an inhalational agent
- Avoid maneuvers that excessively lower PVR (hyperventilation, anemia)
- Avoid myocardial depression

Extubation

- VSD repair: Extubate in ICU when hemodynamically stable (weaned from inotropes, free of arrhythmias, normothermic, etc.)

564

- If pt with unrepaired VSD is undergoing non-cardiac surgery, extubate at end of procedure if overall condition good. Avoid worsening L→R shunting (hypoxia, pain, shivering) or worsening CHF (excess fluid administration).

Adjuvants
- If PVR is increased, a phosphodiesterase inhibitor (milrinone) or NO may be used to decrease PVR on separation from bypass.

- O$_2$, furosemide, digoxin for continued CHF
- Inotropic support often necessary
- Temporary pacemaker for heart block

Postoperative Period
- Pain management critical
- Pts with increased PVR may require continuation of pulm vasodilators and aggressive diuresis for 48–72 hr.

- Complete heart block that does not resolve by 7–10 d is treated with a permanent pacemaker.

Anticipated Problems/Concerns
- Air embolism, shunt reversal, RV failure 2° to pulm Htn
- Pts with large VSDs, CHF, or FTT, are at greatest risk and difficult to wean from bypass.

Ventriculoperitoneal Shunt

Thomas A. Moore, II

Risk

- Elevated ICP
  - Congenital (e.g., intraventricular hemorrhage, meningomyelocele, Chiari malformations)
  - Aqueductal stenosis, brain tumors, infection and trauma
  - Shunt malfunction requiring revision (can be as high as 40% of shunt procedures)
    - Assoc with Chiari malformations
    - Overproduction of CSF
    - Subarachnoid hemorrhage
- Normal ICP
  - Assoc dementia, gait disorders in elderly
- Gender predominance: None

Perioperative Risks

- Periop mortality rare
- Intracranial bleeding may occur with placement of proximal tubing

Worry About

- Prevent further elevations in ICP, which can lead to herniation syndromes
- Ventricular dysrhythmias assoc with rapid removal of CSF
- Assoc pathology

Overview

- Procedure to divert CSF from ventricles to peritoneum
- Many pts present with a previously placed external ventricular drainage devise allowing for intracranial pressure (ICP) monitoring if needed
- Proximal catheter passed into lateral ventricle through burr hole, preferably on the right to reduce risk of dominant hemisphere injury
- Distal catheter tunneled SQ; multiorificed tip placed in peritoneum

- Pts typically present signs of shunt malfunction or elevated ICP

ICD-9-CM Code: 331.4 (Hydrocephalus: acquired)

Indications and Usual Treatment

- Clinical and radiographic evidence of elevated ICP and/or shunt malfunction
- Hx of previous shunts
- Pseudotumor cerebri
- Normal-pressure hydrocephalus with demonstrated improvement in Sx with large-volume lumbar puncture
- If multiple failed ventriculoperitoneal shunts, ventriculojugular, atrial, or pleural shunt may be placed
- Hx of subarachnoid hemorrhage

ASSESSMENT POINTS

System	Effect	Assessment by Hx	PE	Test
CARDIO	Htn, bradycardia			VS
RESP	Aspiration	Vomiting	Auscultation	CXR
CNS	Herniation, seizures	Obtundation	Shunt tap by neurosurgeon	CT, EEG

Key Reference: Rekate HL. Treatment of hydrocephalus, Ch.7. Anderson RCE, Garton HJL, Kestle JRW. Treatment of hydrocephalus with shunts, Ch.8. In: Albright AL, Pollack IF, Adelson PD, eds. *Principles and practice of pediatric neurosurgery*, 2nd ed. New York: Thieme; 2008.

Perioperative Implications

Anesthetic Technique
- GA usual

Monitoring
- Routine
- Consider arterial line in cases of uncontrolled ICP, hemodynamic instability

Airway/Induction
- Normal ICP: IV or mask induction adequate
- Elevated ICP: Atropine (in children), preoxygenate, cricoid pressure, thiobarbiturate, narcotic, lidocaine, rapid-acting nondepolarizing muscle relaxant followed by hyperventilation

Maintenance
- Controlled mild hyperventilation to maintain $PaCO_2$ at 30–35 mmHg in pts with elevated ICP

- If used, maintain low levels of inhaled agent to avoid ↑ CBF, blood volume, and ICP

Surgical Stages

Positioning
- Table turned 90°, head to surgeon
- Head turned 30° from neutral, bump placed under shoulder ipsilateral to shunt

Dissection
- Small flap turned in parietal region with subsequent burr hole
- Small abd incision, enters peritoneum. Laparoscopic assistance by general surgery is becoming more common in placing the distal portion of the catheter.
- SQ tunnel tracked to pull distal catheter through; can be stimulating, assoc with ↑ anesthetic needs

Definitive Surgery
- EBL: Minimal
- Rapid decompression can be assoc with tachydysrhythmias, hypotension
- Ventriculoatrial shunts can be complicated by air embolism

Postoperative Considerations
- Pt remains flat to avoid over drainage of CSF
- Assoc with minimal pain (pain score: 2)

Anticipated Problems/Concerns
- Elevated ICP with assoc hemodynamic changes
- Shunt misplacement with continued elevated ICP and assoc hemodynamic and neurologic changes

Whipple Procedure (Pancreatico Duodenectomy)

Edward J. Norris
Anila S. Bhatti

Risk

- 32,000 cases of cancer of exocrine pancreas diagnosed annually (fourth leading cause of cancer death in USA)
- Mean: 60 y
- M:F ratio: 1.5:1
- Racial predominance: None

Perioperative Risks

- Periop mortality rate (30 d) <5%; may be as low as 1% in centers of excellence
- Major morbidity most often 2° to underlying cardiopulmonary disease, pancreatic or biliary fistula, hemorrhage, or infection
- Leak or fistula from pancreatic anastomosis is leading cause of morbidity (incidence 5–25%)

Worry About

- Massive blood loss (superior mesenteric vessels, portal vein, or vena cava injury)
- Significant fluid shifts
- Venous air embolism with injury to vena cava

- Overview
- Most commonly performed cancer-directed operation for pancreatic cancer
- Distal stomach, gallbladder, common bile duct, head of pancreas, proximal jejunum, duodenum, regional lymphatics removed
- Requires pancreaticojejunostomy, choledochojejunostomy, gastrojejunostomy
- Risk factors incl diabetes, cigarette smoking, alcohol ingestion, familial chronic pancreatitis
- Age, co-morbidities of pt will dictate periop monitoring strategies
- Significant blood loss and fluid shifts with extended Whipple resections (more extensive soft tissue, lymphatic dissections, resection of superior mesenteric vessels, portal vein if necessary)
- ~70% of tumors of head of pancreas unresectable at time of exploratory laparotomy
- Adoption of laparoscopic approach slow due to anatomic complexity of pancreatic surgery

ICD-9-CM Code: 157.0 (Cancer of pancreas)

Indications and Usual Treatment

- Following conditions should be met
  - All evidence of gross tumor can be resected
  - No evidence of distant metastatic disease or extensive vascular or retroperitoneal involvement by work-up
  - Good general health
- Palliative operations directed to relief of obstructive jaundice (cholecystojejunostomy, choledochojejunostomy), gastric outlet obstruction (gastrojejunostomy), pain (celiac plexus injection with ethanol)
- 5-y survival ~20% after curative resection
- Combined radiotherapy and chemotherapy have been shown to ↑ survival in pts with resectable, unresectable disease

ASSESSMENT POINTS

System	Effect	Assessment by Hx	PE	Test
GI	Gastric outlet obstruction	Vomiting	Abd mass	CT scan
HEPAT	Liver metastases Bile duct obstruction	Pruritus	Hepatomegaly Jaundice, hepatomegaly, palpable nontender gallbladder	CT scan Laparoscopy CT scan Bilirubin level
NUTRITION	Tumor Malnutrition	Wt loss		Total protein, prealbumin
ENDO	Tumor			Blood glucose

Key References: Sosa JA, Bowman HM, Gordon TA, et al. Importance of hospital volume in the overall management of pancreatic cancer. *Ann Surg.* 1998;228:429–438. Cameron JL, Riall TS, Coleman J, Belcher KA. One thousand consecutive pancreaticoduodenectomies. *Ann Surg.* 2006;244:10–15

Perioperative Implications

Preoperative Preparation

- Bowel prep routine, requiring rehydration
- Consider referral to high-volume center

Anesthetic Technique

- General
- Combined
  - General/lumbar epidural (narcotics)
  - General/low-thoracic epidural (local anesthesia/narcotics)
  - General/intrathecal narcotics
- Technique needs to allow for unresectability (open, close)

Monitoring

- Large-bore IV access for fluid requirements, blood loss
- Consider central venous, arterial pressure monitoring

Airway

- None

Induction

- Cricoid pressure if gastric outlet obstruction suspected
- Combined technique with low-thoracic epidural requires only moderate volume of local anesthetic (6–8 mL)

Surgical Stages

Dissection

- Small-to-moderate amount of blood loss
- Moderate ongoing fluid requirements
- Resectability determined by absence of distant metastases, extent of major vascular involvement

Definitive Surgery (Pancreatico Duodenectomy)

- Significant volume requirements; consider colloid
- Arterial anomalies can increase operative complexity.
- Isolated venous involvement requiring resection and reconstruction is well accepted.

- Blood loss can be massive with portal vein or vena cava injury.
- Restoring gastrointestinal continuity
- Moderate ongoing volume requirements; consider colloid

Postoperative Considerations

- Pain score: 5–9
- Usual hospital stay: 8–12 d
- Combined technique with neuraxial narcotics
- May develop significant fluid shifts
- May require postop ventilation and/or extended ICU stay
- Glycemic control

Anticipated Problems/Concerns

- Risk of significant fluid shifts, blood loss
- Malnutrition
- Delayed gastric emptying and/or ileus
- Leak or fistula from pancreatic anastomosis

SECTION

Drugs

ACE Inhibitors

Thai T. Nguyen

Uses

- Treatment of essential Htn, CHF, and mitral regurgitation
- Numerous studies show that ACE-I improves symptoms and quality of life as well as reduces mortality rate in elderly with heart failure and decreased LVEF.
- Decreases mortality after myocardial infarction
- Safe and effective treatment of Htn in diabetics. Strong evidence ACE-I delays the progression of diabetic renal disease.

Perioperative Risks

- Severe and prolonged hypotension in pts undergoing general anesthesia
- May increase insulin sensitivity and hypoglycemia in diabetics

Worry About

- Decrease glomerular filtration rate and not recommended in pts with renal artery stenosis
- Life-threatening angioedema involves the swelling of head, neck, and tongue
- Hyperkalemia because of decreased production of aldosterone
- Fetal anomalies and fetal and neonatal death

Overview/Pharmacology/Dose

- Captopril is available in oral dose and very effective in treating Htn
- Enalapril has to be converted by esterase in liver to the active metabolite enalaprilat
- Both captopril and enalapril are renally excreted and should be reduced in pt with renal dysfunction
- Lisinopril is absorbed as the active form and offered as once-a-day dosing

Characteristic	Captopril	Enalapril	Lisinopril	Benazepril	Fosinopril	Quinapril	Ramipril
Elimination	Renal	Renal	Renal	Renal	50% Renal 50% Hepatic	61% Renal 37% Hepatic	Renal
Onset of hypotensive action (hr)	0.25	1	1	1	1	1	1–2
Peak hypotensive effects (hr)	1–1.5	4–6	6	2–4	2–6	2	3–6
Duration of hypotensive effects (hr)	Dose related	24 (18–30)	24 (18–30)	24	24	24	>24 (24–60)
Dose (mg)	25–150, max 450	5–40, max 40	10–40, max 80	20–80, max 80	10–40, max 80	10–80, max 80	2.5–20, max 20

Drug Class

- Affects the renin-angiotensin system by blocking the conversion of angiotensin I to the active angiotensin II and delaying bradykinin breakdown and assoc prostaglandins

ASSESSMENT POINTS

System	Effect	Assessment by Hx	PE	Test
HEENT	Angioedema	Swelling of face, neck, tongue Dyspnea	Difficulty speaking, swallowing	Airway exam
	Bronchospasm		Wheezing	
CARDIO	Hypotension	Assess CV response to Rx		
GU	Renal failure Hyperkalemia	Orthopnea, dyspnea	Edema	BUN, Cr, lytes
HEME	Leukopenia, agranulocytosis	Fever		CBC with diff

Key Reference: Brabant SM, Eyraud D, Bertrand M, Coriat P. Refractory hypotension after induction of anesthesia in a patient chronically treated with angiotensin receptor antagonists. *Anesth Analg*. 1999;89:887–888.

Drug Interactions

Preoperative Period

- Assess for evidence of renal insufficiency
- Monitor for hyperkalemia
- ACE-I can be continued until the day of surgery because of the potential benefits in reducing mortality and morbidity
- Consider reducing the ACE-I dose so that hypotension can be avoided

Induction/Maintenance

- Severe and refractory hypotension that can be resistant to vasopressors such as phenylephrine, ephedrine, and norepinephrine
- Vasopressin and analogs can be useful to restore BP.
- Use of succinylcholine with elevated K^+ may be assoc with cardiac arrhythmia.

Adjuvant/Regional Anesthesia/Reversal

- Hypotensive episodes may be assoc with spinal and epidural anesthesia.

Postoperative Period

- Monitor for hypotension

Acetaminophen

Jason E. Pope

Uses

- Minor analgesic for acute, chronic, and periop pain
- First line agent in WHO analgesia treatment ladder
- First line agent in treatment of pain in pregnancy (class B), compatible with breastfeeding
- Combination therapy formulations (e.g., with opioids) as adjuvant
- Antipyretic

Perioperative Risk

- In normal therapeutic doses, well-tolerated
- Overdose assoc with hepatotoxicity, nephrotoxicity, metabolic acidosis, and hypoglycemia
- Can precipitate asthma exacerbation
- Little peripheral antiplatelet effects, although case reports of pts with acetaminophen-induced coagulopathy, randomized controlled studies demonstrated no risk
- Little anti-inflammatory effects

Pharmacokinetics/Pharmacodynamics

- Mechanism of action unclear
- Postulated mechanisms include: Inhibition of prostaglandin synthase, inhibition of cyclooxygenase isoensymes (COX-3), interaction with descending endogenous opioid pathways, interaction with L-arginine-NO-pathway (inhibits substance P–mediated hyperalgesia), augmentation of descending serotoninergic pathway, and increase in cannaboid and/or vanilloid tone.
- Selectively inhibits COX activity with low oxidant environments (i.e., endothelial cells) vs. those with high oxidant environments (plts).
- Antipyretic activity postulated to be 2° to the blockade of prostaglandin (PG) production and antagonism of prostaglandin endoperoxide H_2 synthase (PGHS) and COX centrally (hypothalamus)
- Questionable opioid-sparing effect
- It is rapidly absorbed in GI tract, mostly in the small intestine.
- Half life ($t_{1/2}$) 1.25–3 hr, peak plasma concentration 30–60 min
- Serum therapeutic levels 10–30 μg/mL
- Analgesic effect approx 6 hr
- 25% of dose undergoes first pass effect in the liver
- Approx the vast majority (90%) is metabolized by conjugation in the liver via glucoronidation and sulfate conjugation, forming non-toxic metabolites (saturated at doses greater than 150 mg/kg) and renally excreted (90–100% recovered in urine within 24 hr)
- Roughly 10% undergo oxidative metabolism via CYP2E, CYP1A2, CYP2A6, and CYP3A4 to form the potentially hepatotoxic and nephrotoxic metabolite N-acetyl-p-benzoquinoneimine (NAPQI)
- Increase in production of NAPQI attributed to P450 system induction or low glutathione levels (which normally detoxify metabolite to mercapturic acid a cysteine conjugates)
- NAPQI can covalently bind to cysteinylsulfhydral groups, causing hepatocellular (zone III) necrosis (oxidative damage, mitochondrial dysfunction)

Drug Class/Mechanism of Action/Usual Dose

- Available in oral and rectal formulations in the USA, parenteral in Europe
- In USA: 325 mg and 500 mg immediate release tablets, 650 extended-release tablets and rectal suppositories
- Maximum dose 4 g/24 hr, (although American Liver Foundation 3g/24 hr)
- Adjust dose for CrCl: if 10–50 mL/min interval q6h, if <10 mL/min interval q8h

ASSESSMENT POINTS

System	Effect	Assessment By Hx	Test
CNS	Encephalopathy, antipyretic effects, analgesia	Coma	GCS, CT/MRI (cerebral edema)
PULM	Bronchoconstriction	Labored breathing, wheeze	Increased peak /plateau airway pressure, auscultation
GI	Hepatic dysfunction	N/V, anorexia, sequella of liver failure	Transaminases, INR, bilirubin, hypoglycemia
RENAL	Renal dysfunction, acute tubular necrosis	Oliguria	BMP, Cr, UA
METABOLIC	Metabolic acidosis		Lactate, ABG

Key Reference: Mattia C, Couluzzi F. What Anesthesiologists should know about paracetamol (acetaminophen), *Minerva Anestesiol.* 2009;75:644–653.

Suspected Toxicity and Treatment

- Overdose accounts for approx 40% of acute liver failure in USA and UK
- Half of the hospitalizations for acetaminophen overdose (150 mg/kg) were unintentional
- Mean dose ingested causing hepatic failure was 24 g.
- Nephrotoxicity occurred in 1–2% of pts with acetaminophen overdose
- If suspected toxicity, don't delay giving NAC (N-acetylcysteine). Proposed mechanisms of action for antidote incl increasing glutathione stores and conjugation to NAPQI, antioxidant effects, anti-inflammatory effects, increases NO resultant microvascular perfusion
- Serum acetaminophen concentration plotted on Rumack-Matthew normogram

Symptoms

- Phase I: (0–24 hr): Asymptomatic, anorexia, N/V, malaise, subclinical rise in serum transaminases
- Phase II: (18–72 hr): Right upper quadrant abd pain, anorexia, N/V, increased transaminases levels
- Phase III (72–96 hr): Centrolobular hepatic necrosis, jaundice, coagulopathy, hepatic encephalopathy, renal failure, fulminant hepatitis, death
- Phase IV (96 hr–3 wk): Complete resolution of symptoms and organ failure

Treatment (Pediatric and Adult Populations)

- Gastric decontamination: Within 4 hr of ingestion (charcoal 1g/kg PO)
- NAC administration within 8 hr of ingestion either IV (150 mg/kg over 15 min then 50 mg/kg over 4 hr, then 100 mg/kg over 16 hr) or PO (140 mg/kg, then 70 mg/kg Q4 × 17 doses)
- Supportive measures

Perioperative Implications

- Increased periop morbidity with pts with increased liver function tests
- Pediatric population younger than 5 y have better prognosis after acetaminophen toxicity, potentially related to increased capacity
- Asthma may be co-morbid in pts with chronic acetaminophen use.
- Avoidance of anesthesia techniques that impair hepatic/renal blood flow (i.e., halothane)
- Delay elective surgery, follow hepatic function tests and renal function tests to optimize timing of surgical intervention
- Auto-regulatory curve for hemodynamic organ perfusion homeostasis may be altered by women taking acetaminophen chronically 2° to Htn
- Potential coagulopathic augmentation of anticoagulants (e.g., warafin, NSAIDS)

Drug Interactions

- CYP inducers: Barbiturates, buproprion, caffeine, carbamazepine, charcoal-broiled food, cruciferous vegetables, dihydralazine, isoniazid, phenytoin, primidone, rifampin, ritonavir, sulfinopyrazone, ethanol, isoniazid
- Questionable inhibition of glucoronidation with ranitidine, propranolol, cisapride
- Questionable potentiation of glucoronidation by estrogen-containing contraceptives
- Warfarin, NSAIDs coagulopathic effects may be potentiated by acetaminophen

Anticipated Problems/Concerns

- Pts with salicylate hypersensitivity (urticaria) have approx 11% of cross-reactivity with acetaminophen
- Long-term use has been linked to Htn in prospective studies in females, no association with males (likely related to imbalance of vasoconstrictive and vasodilatory effects of prostaglandins).
- Increased risk of toxicity with baseline hepatic dysfunction (low glutathione levels: HCV, cirrhosis, malnutrition/fasting, HIV) or CYP enzyme induction
- Asthma was found to be 63% higher among acetaminophen users than nonusers in multivariate analyses

Alkylating Agents

Victor A. Filadora, II
Mark J. Lema

Uses

- Bone marrow transplants
- Breast and bladder cancers
- Lymphomas and leukemias
- Lung, pancreas and brain cancers
- Ovarian and testicular cancers
- Multiple myeloma
- Sarcomas and melanomas

Perioperative Risks

- Increased risk of infection
- Aspiration (subsequent to N/V)
- Prolonged succinylcholine action (CTX)
- Fluid retention (HN_2)

Worry About

- Extravasation if given by IV infusion
- Prolonged bleeding (thrombocytopenia)
- Aspiration during intubation

Overview/Pharmacology

- First chemotherapy agents (1940s)
- Structurally diverse compounds
- Generate reactive, electron-deficient intermediates
- Covalently bind to DNA bases, esp. guanine, often during mitosis
- Disrupt DNA replication and transcription
- High incidence of cytotoxicity to normal, rapidly dividing cells

- Side effects (acute): 1–3 wk after therapy
- Myelosuppression (pancytopenia)
- N/V
- Sterility
- Increased risk of 2° malignancies (leukemia)
- Alopecia
- End-organ toxicities
  - CNS
  - Hepatic
  - Pulm
  - Renal
- Phlebitis

DRUG EFFECTS

Class	Name	Abbrev	Special Indication*	Adverse Effects
Nitrogen Mustards				
Mechlorethamine	Mustargen	HN_2	LM	N/V, phlebitis, hyperuricemia, potent vesicant
Cyclophosphamide	Cytoxan	CTX	LM, Brt, Bl, Lu, Ov	Decreases pseudo-ChE; myocardial toxicity, hemorrhagic cystitis
Ifosfamide	Ifex		LM, Ov, Te, Sa	Hemorrhagic cystitis, N/V, CNS toxicity, metabolic acidosis
L-Phenylalanine	Alkeran (melphalan)	L-PAM	MM	Mild N/V
Chlorambucil	Leukeran	CLR	CLL, LM	N/V, seizures
Triethylene-thiophosphoramide	Thiotepa	T-TEPA	BMT	Can ↓ pseudo-ChE, prologns succinylcholine action
Alkyl Sulfonates				
Busulfan	Myleran	MYL	CML	Pulm toxicity, N/V, seizures, mucositis, hyperbilirubinemia
Nitrosoureas				
Chloroethyl-cyclohexyl-nitrosourea	Lomustine	CCNU	LM, Brn	N/V, hepatic toxicity, pulm toxicity, renal toxicity
Bis-chloroethyl-nitrosourea	Carmustine	BCNU	LM, Brn	N/V, phlebitis, pulm toxicity
Streptozocin	Zanosar	STZ	Pa	N/V, dose-related renal toxicity
Triazenes				
Dimethyltriazenoimidazole carboxamide	Dacarbazine	DTIC	HD, Sa, Me	N/V, anaphylaxis, phlebitis, hepatotoxicity

* *CLL, CML*: leukemias; *Bl*: bladder; *BMT*: bone marrow transplant; *Brn*: brain; *Brt*: breast; *HD*: Hodgkin's; *LM*: lymphoma; *Lu*: lung; *Me*: melanoma; *MM*: multiple myeloma; *Ov*: ovarian; *Pa*: pancreas; *Sa*: sarcoma; *Te*: testicular

Key Reference: Maracic L, Van Nostrand J. Anesthetic implications of cancer chemotherapy. *AANA J.* 2007;75:206–226.

Perioperative Implications

Preoperative Preparation

- Full-stomach precautions
- Risk of infection (leukopenia)
- Adequate hydration (bladder toxicity)
- Check plt count (thrombocytopenia)
- PFT (busulfan, cyclophosphamide)
- MUGA (cyclophosphamide)

Intraoperative

- Risk of aspiration during induction
- Prolonged bleeding
- Plan for RBC transfusion (anemia)
- Maintain UO
- Reduced dose of succinylcholine (CTX, thiotepa)

Postoperative Concerns

- Risk of N/V (most agents)
- Continued fluid hydration
- Monitor cardiac/pulm dysfunction (CTX, busulfan)
- Monitor renal and hepatic function

DRUGS

Alpha-2 Adrenergic Agonists

Marco Caruso

Uses (off-label uses included)

- Treatment of hypertensive states (clonidine, guanfacine, guanabenz, alpha-methyldopa)
- Sedation in mechanically-ventilated pts (dexmedetomidine)
- Adjunct agent in general anesthesia (dexmedetomidine, clonidine)
- Sedation for awake intubation (dexmedetomidine)
- Management of withdrawal symptoms (reduction in cardiosympathetic stimulation during naloxone therapy, and abatement of alcohol, nicotine, benzodiazepine, or cocaine withdrawal symptoms) (clonidine)
- Reductions in intraocular pressure via reduced aqueous humor secretion (brimonidine, apraclonidine)
- Reductions in postop shivering (clonidine, dexmedetomidine)
- Additive in central neuraxial and perhaps (question if systemic effect) in peripheral nerve blockade (clonidine)

Perioperative Risks

- Initial phase of acute Htn mediated by postsynaptic alpha-2B vasoconstriction
- Hypotension and bradycardia mediated by postsynaptic central alpha-2A decreases in peripheral sympathetic outflow and presynaptic peripheral alpha-2A/2C inhibition of NE/EPI release
- CV collapse in hypovolemic states or other pts dependent on avoiding reductions in sympathetic tone or SVR to allow maintenance of BP (e.g., trauma pts, aortic stenosis)

Worry About

- Rebound Htn (esp. if dexmedetomidine infusions of greater than 24 hr) or any interruptions of clonidine (esp. after 18 hr or in pts taking >1.2 mg daily)
- Assoc xerostomia (which may be beneficial in awake intubation)
- Increases in half time ("context sensitivity") with prolonged infusions of dexmedetomidine. For example half time of 4 min after 10 min infusion grows to 250 min after 8 hr infusion.

Overview/Pharmacology

- Dexmedetomidine is a highly alpha-2 specific (1620:1 alpha-2/alpha-1 activity) imidazole derivative with wide-ranging effects. It binds to postsynaptic alpha-2A receptors on inhibitory neurons the CNS (predominantly in the locus ceruleus) resulting in its sedative properties (simulating natural sleep and with characteristic preservation of respiration). These effects may also be in partly due to activation of central imidazoline receptors in several brainstem nuclei. Dopaminergic modulation in the CNS via alpha-2C receptors probably plays less of a role. The sedation is non-GABAergic and thus is less prone to agitation and/or disinhibition phenomena seen with other agents such as benzodiazepines. Other central locations of alpha-2A postsynaptic agonism lead to inhibition of peripheral sympathetic outflow and are responsible for the vasodepressor and negative chronotropic/inotropic effects via stimulation of inhibitory neurons in the medullary vasomotor centers. This is added to by presynaptic alpha-2A inhibition of norepinephrine release in sympathetic nerve terminals (autoreceptor modulation) and alpha-2C autoreceptor inhibition in the adrenal medulla with net reductions in arterial tone, venomotor tone, stroke volume, and heart rate.
- An initial phase of increased SVR may occur due to postsynaptic alpha-2B agonism in sympathetic nerve terminals with enhanced norepinephrine release.
- Signal transduction is via coupling to G-protein effector systems. Activation of Gi leads to decreases in adenylyl cyclase activity (with resultant reductions in protein kinase activity), as well as increases in hyperpolarizing K^+ currents. Decreases in N-type and L-type Ca^{+2} currents are also seen and may in part be coupled to activation of Go.
- Both amnestic (not reliably seen) and analgesic properties are also ascribed to dexmedetomidine. Analgesia may occur at multiple sites. Direct presynaptic and postsynaptic alpha-2 agonism in the substantia gelatinosa may diminish substance P and glutamate release (presynaptic heteroceptor agonism) and directly inhibit second order neurons (postsynaptic agonism); thus ascending nociceptive afferent flow is reduced (in a manner with mimimal cross tolerance with opioids). Supraspinal modulation of ascending input may also occur in the CNS itself
- Clonidine is also an imidazole derivative with similar properties (220:1 alpha-2 and/or alpha-1 activity). In general its effects on the vascular system are more pronounced than those of dexmedetomidine, while its sedative effects are less significant. It has also nonetheless been used to reduce anesthetic requirements in people undergoing general anesthesia, and has been successful as an additive in central neuraxial and peripheral nerve blockade in both extending the duration, and enhancing the quality of sensory neural blockade and avoiding side effects seen with neuraxial opioids used for the same purpose.
- Dexmedetomidine undergoes extensive hepatic metabolism while clonidine is approx 50% hepatically metabolized and 50% excreted unchanged in urine

Drug Class/Mechanism of Action/Usual Dose

- Dexmedetomidine: Imidazole derivative given by IV infusion. A loading dose of 1 mcg/kg is given on an infusion pump (200 mcg ampule diluted in 48 mL saline to a final 50 mL volume with resulting concentration 4 mcg/mL) over 10–15 min, followed by an infusion of 0.2–0.7 mcg/kg/hr). Loading doses may be given over slightly longer times (20–30 min) in pts undergoing awake FOI so that response and airway patency may be continually evaluated, and peak sedation may be made to match the end of an assoc topicalization of the airway. Rates may need to be reduced in infusion over 24 hr as half life increases markedly with prolonged infusion. Elimination half life 2–3 hr. May be reversed with atipamezole.
- Clonidine: Imidazoline derivative given in dosages of 100–300 mcg orally 1–4 times daily or via transdermal patch. Elimination half life of 6–10 hr limits utility as sedative
- Guanfacine and guanabenz: Phenylguanidine derivatives with relatively long half lives (12–24 hr and 4–6 hr respectively). Functional antihypertensives rarely utilized currently.
- Alpha-methyldopa: 1–2 g daily in divided doses. Acts via its central alpha-2 agonist metabolite alpha-methylnorepinephrine. May cause positive Coomb's test or hemolytic anemia. Safe historic record for use as antihypertensive in pregnancy.
- Brimionidine and apraclonidine: Ophthalmologic agents for use topically in glaucoma
- Tizanidine: Antispasmodic used in treatment of cerebral and spinal spasticity.

DRUG EFFECTS

System	Effect	Assessment by Hx	PE	Test
CARDIO	Increased SVR Decreased SVR Decreased inotropy Decreased chronotropy	Headache, palpitations, dizziness, diaphoresis, abd pain	Pulse, BP, skin temp and turgor	ECG PA Cath TEE
RESP	Usually minimally reduced Minute ventilation and preserved CO_2 Responsivity		Hypopnea, apnea, cyanosis	Spirometry Pulse Oximetry Capnogram
CNS OTHER	Sedation Amnesia Analgesia Reduced CBF Xerostomia/antisialogogue Plt aggregation Lipolysis inhibition Insulin secretion inhibition	Ramsay sedation scale Recall Pain Dry mouth/nasal decongestion	Somnolence	BIS Blood Glucose

Key Reference: Carollo DS, Nossaman BD, Ramadhyani U. Dexmedetomidine: A review of clinical applications. *Curr Opin Anaesthesiol.* 2008;21457–21461.

Perioperative Implications

Preoperative Concerns

• Rebound Htn common in pts on clonidine who do not take their dose on the morning of surgery. Pts on clonidine have often been placed on it for refractory Htn and labile BP should be anticipated. Baroreceptor sensitivity is generally preserved.

• Clonidine has some evidence for myocardial protection in CV surgery and can be considered in pts who would benefit from but have contraindication to periop beta blockade.

• Consider adding low dose (30–70 mcg/kg) midazolam to sedation plan for awake FOI if definitive amnesia is strongly desired.

• Clonidine interaction with cimetidine (inhibition of cytochome P450 and reduction of hepatic blood flow) may lead to CNS toxicity.

Induction/Maintenance

• Slow controlled induction is preferable when not contraindicated as adjunct decreases in SVR and inotropic state may lead to severe hypotension.

• Treatment of dysrhythmias such as symptomatic bradycardia and AV block may become necessary. Use caution in treating hypotensive bradycardia with anticholinergics alone (esp. in those in whom coronary perfusion is SVR dependent). Increases in HR in a pt with catastrophically low SVR can precipitate severe myocardial ischemia (altered supply/demand ratio).

• Reductions in MAC are common in pts on clonidine and dexmedetomidine (30%–50% in most studies but wide range seen). Titration to hemodynamic variables or BIS may be useful.

Postoperative Period

• Continue to maintain clonidine use postop to reduce risk of rebound Htn.

• Rebound Htn unlikely with dexmedetomidine infusions less than 24 hr duration

Anticipated Problems/Concerns

• Postop hypothermia may be accentuated.

Aminophylline

Avery Tung

Uses

- Acute and chronic Rx for asthma, COPD
- Rx for neonatal apnea
- As 2° agent in CPR settings
- Potential for life-threatening CNS, cardiac toxicity
- Administered IV, PO, or rectally

Perioperative Risks

- Toxic levels from overaggressive use or coadministration of cimetidine/propranolol
- Increased arrhythmogenicity with pancuronium
- Increased CNS toxicity (lower seizure threshold) with ketamine or in children

Worry About

- Prolonged clearance in presence of cimetidine, erythromycin, propranolol, or in pts receiving influenza vaccines
- Enhanced clearance in smokers and pts taking dilantin, barbiturates
- Narrow therapeutic/toxic ratio
- Decreases sedative effect of propofol (but does not alter desflurane MAC)
- May alter bispectral index measurements

Overview/Pharmacology

- Methylated xanthine
- Bronchodilatory and anti-inflammatory effects
- Onset of effect within 1 hr from IV dose

- Biotransformed by demethylation in liver; renally excreted
- 7–15% excreted unchanged in urine
- Crosses placenta, found in breast milk

Drug Class/Mechanism of Action/ Usual Dose

- Methylated xanthine
- Proposed mechanisms of action incl inhibiting phosphodiesterase, antagonizing the effect of adenosine, causing catecholamine release, inhibiting cellular immune function
- Usual dosage: 4 mg/kg q 8–12 hr PO; 5–6 mg/kg IV load followed by 0.2–0.75 mg/kg/hr IV

DRUG EFFECTS

System	Effect	Assessment by Hx	PE	Test
CARDIO	Inotropy and chronotropy; ↓ in SVR, PCWP, BP	Predisposes to ventricular arrhythmia	Auscultation of heart sounds	ECG
RESP	Bronchodilation, suppression of cellular immune response	Relief of dyspnea, improvement of bronchospastic symptoms	Auscultation of chest	Peak flow, PFTs
CNS	Nonspecific CNS stimulation; stimulates central resp drive; alters BIS readings	N/V, irritability, insomnia, delirium, convulsions, stupor, coma		

Key Reference: Turan A, Kasuya Y, Govinda R, et al. The effect of aminophylline on loss of consciousness, bispectral index, propofol requirement, and minimum alveolar concentration of desflurane in volunteers. *Anesth Analg.* 2010;110:449–454.

Perioperative Implications

Preoperative Concerns

- Toxic preop blood level 2° to over-administration or coadministration of drugs that affect clearance (cimetidine, erythromycin, propranolol, verapamil, phenytoin [Dilantin])
- Potential for seizures or malignant arrhythmias if toxic levels
- Presence of underlying bronchospastic disease
- Administration via peripheral vein to avoid cardiotoxicity

Induction/Maintenance

- Can interact with halothane or pancuronium to cause ventricular arrhythmias
- Can interact with ketamine to lower seizure threshold
- Continue infusion if carefully monitoring for toxicity
- No proven effectiveness in treating intraop bronchospasm in humans
- Reduction of NMB
- Increases BIS readings

Postoperative Period

- Check plasma levels before restarting infusion if toxicity is suspected
- May be used as central resp stimulant in neonates recovering from general anesthesia

Anticipated Problems/Concerns

- Most common problems are from narrow therapeutic and/or toxic window, potential for severe CNS, cardiac toxicity.
- Pts taking aminophylline often have severe bronchospastic disease.
- Dialysis or charcoal hemoperfusion can acutely lower blood levels.

DRUGS

Amphetamines

Edgar J. Pierre
Faisal Huda

Uses

- Narcolepsy and attention deficit hyperactivity disorder (ADHD)
- Also used to treat enuresis and incontinence
- Not recommended for fatigue or wt loss
- Administered orally and effects can last for several hr

Perioperative Risks

- Chronic use can lead to decreased MAC
- Acute use can increase MAC
- Risk of Htn, tremors, hyperactive reflexes, anxiety, and delirium
- When used with thyroid hormone, diuretics, laxatives it can lead to arrhythmias or cardiac arrest.

Worry About

- Severe Htn, palpitations, confusion, dizziness, and vasomotor disturbances esp. in pts with ischemic heart disease, Htn, rhabdomyolysis, and hyperthyroidism

Overview/Pharmacology

- Causes release of catecholamine resulting in sympathomimetic toxidrome
- Schedule II drug
- Acute use can cause seizures, intracranial hemorrhage, stroke, increased cardiac output, increased heart rate, increased peripheral vascular resistance, angina pain, renal failure, and cardiac arrhythmias.
- Chronic use can cause increased tolerance, dependence, and a depletion of body stores of catecholamine. Also, wt loss and psychotic effects can occur.
- May have a small analgesic effect and can enhance the analgesia produced by opiates
- Metabolized by the liver

- Overdose is treated by supportive management, IV hydration for possible rhabdomyolysis, sedation, acidification of urine to enhance elimination, and sodium nitroprusside for severe Htn. Be sure to check core temp, obtain an EKG, and evaluate renal function.
- Benzodiazepines, often in high doses, are useful for control of agitation.

Drug Class/Mechanism of Action/Usual Dose

- Phenethylamine derivative
- Amphetamines act indirectly to release biogenic amine neurotransmitters from nerve terminals centrally and peripherally.
- Usual oral dosages
  - Narcolepsy: 5–10 mg bid
  - ADHD: 5–10 mg bid

DRUG EFFECTS

System	Effect	Assessment by Hx	PE	Test
CARDIO	Increases BP, CO, HR, SVR, arrhythmias	Hx of recent/chronic use	Vitals	EKG
RESP	Resp stimulation	Hx of recent/chronic use	Pulm exam	ABG
CNS	Increased alertness, electrical activity. Overdose: Anxiety, psychoses, seizures	Hx of recent/chronic use	CNS exam	EEG
METAB	Renal failure, lactic acidosis Dehydration	Hx of recent/chronic use	Vital signs, PE	ABG, electrolytes
Other	Mydriasis, diaphoresis, hyperthermia, decreased GI motility	Hx of recent/chronic use	Vitals, PE	

Perioperative Implications

Preoperative Concerns

- Recent, acute ingestion
- Concomitant use of MAOI
- Hx of polysubstance abuse
- Monitor BP for Htn, HR, and preop EKG for ischemia

Induction/Maintenance

- With severe Htn, may need to use alpha or beta blocker and/or vasodilators
- Chronic use will decrease anesthetic requirements
- May increase analgesic effect of opioids

- Diminished response to vasopressors from chronic abuse

Adjuvant /Reversal

- Drug interactions noted are the major concerns

Postoperative Period

- Continue to monitor CV, CNS hyperactivity, UO, body temp
- Withdrawal symptoms are non-life threatening

Anticipated Problems/Concerns

- Ask about Hx of substance abuse. Worry about concomitant use of other drugs as well.
- Ask about most recent usage due to changes in anesthesia requirements and need for further labs and/or tests.
- Possible drug interactions

Angiotensin II Receptor Blocking Drugs

Davide Cattano

Uses

- AT1-receptor antagonists or sartans, are a group of pharmaceuticals which modulate the renin-angiotensin-aldosterone system. Their main use is in Htn, diabetic nephropathy, and CHF.

Perioperative Risks

- ARBs do not inhibit ACE, they do not cause an increase in bradykinin, which contributes to the vasodilation produced by ACE inhibitors and also some of the side effects of ACE inhibitors (cough and angioedema).
- Dementia: pts who were already suffering from Alzheimer's disease or dementia, and found those subjects had up to a 50% lower chance of being admitted to nursing homes or dying if they were taking ARBs.

Worry About

- Rebound Htn if drug acutely withdrawn esp. with longer-acting agents
- Refractory hypotension in pts undergoing general anesthesia. BP responds to vasopressin agonists.
- Questionable increased risk of MI with ARBs

Pharmacology Overview

- Renin-angiotensin cascade begins with the cleavage of angiotensin by rennin, angiotensin I converted by ACE to angiotensin II, angiotensin II receptors activated by binding of angiotensin
- Clinical effects of angiotensin II (vasoconstriction, sodium/water retention, renin suppression, etc.) are mediated by the angiotensin receptor 1 (AT1)
- Blockade of AT1 receptors directly cause vasodilation, reduces secretion of vasopressin, reduces production and secretion of aldosterone, among other actions—the combined effect of which is reduction of BP.
- Three important PD/PK factors: Pressor inhibition, AT1 affinity, biological half life (example Losartan 100 mg 25–40%, 1000-fold, 6 hr or valsartan 80 mg 30%, 20,000-fold, 6 hr).
- Contraindicated in pregnancy

Mechansim of Action/Usual Dose

- The activated receptor in turn couples to Gq/11 and thus activates phospholipase C and increases the cytosolic Ca^{2+} concentrations, which in turn triggers cellular responses such as stimulation of protein kinase C. Activated receptor also inhibits adenylate cyclase and activates various tyrosine kinases.
- Available in once-a-day dosing
  - Candesartan (Atacand) 4–32 mg
  - Irbesartan (Avapro) 150–300 mg
  - Losartan (Cozaar) 50–100 mg
  - Telmisartan (Micardis) 40–80 mg
  - Valsartan (Diovan) 80–320 mg

DRUG EFFECTS

System	Effect	Assessment by Hx	PE	Test
CARDIO	Lowers BP	Assess response to Rx	BP	Monitor BP, can also have tachycardia and bradycardia with lowering BP, careful when D/C
GI	↑ in LFTs Rare reversible hepatotoxicity reported			Watch for rebound Htn, LFTs
METAB	Hyperkalemia			K^+
DERM	Angioedema reported	Ask pts for clinical Hx		
HEME	Microcytic anemia			CBC
RENAL	Can cause ARF if pts with renal artery stenosis or diffuse infrarenal stenosis			BUN/Cr
CNS		Rare headache, dizziness, fatigue insomnia		

Key Reference: Burnier M. Angiotensin II receptor antagonists. *Lancet.* 2000;355:637–645.

Perioperative Risks

- Reduced responsiveness to vasopressor, potential risk of rebound Htn in withdrawal (potential risks in general/neuron-vascular surgery).
- Potential risk of ARF in major bleeding and kidney ischemia

Induction/Maintenance

- Watch for refractory hypotension, which needs treatment with vasopressin agonist

Adjuvants/Regional Anesthesia/Reversal

- No known interactions

Postoperative Concerns

- Resumption of preop drugs for BP control if no ARF
- Only available in PO forms

Anticipated Concerns

- Recommended preop withdrawal for 12–24 hr.

Aspirin (Acetylsalicylic Acid)

Lee A. Fleisher

Uses

- People in USA consume 10,000–20,000 tons annually
- Rx for mild and/or moderate pain, fever, arthritis, prevention of myocardial infarction

Perioperative Risks

- Peptic ulcer disease
- Plt dysfunction
- Hemorrhage
- Stroke
- Interstitial nephritis
- Reye's syndrome

Worry About

- Displacement of protein-bound drugs: e.g., warfarin, sulfonylureas, thiopental, methotrexate
- Potentiation of anticoagulants
- Thrombosis 2° to aspirin withdrawal

Overview/Pharmacology

- Cyclooxygenase inhibition prevents plt aggregation and vasoconstriction
- Plt inhibition irreversible for the life of the plt
- Aspirin
  - Metabolized by liver, excreted by kidney
  - Mildly antagonizes antihypertensive medications (β-blockers, vasodilators, diuretics)
  - Displaces protein-bound drugs, increasing their effects

Drug Class/Mechanism of Action/Usual Dose

- NSAID
- Cyclooxygenase inhibitor
- Chronically taken for
  - MS pain (e.g., arthritis, neuralgia)
  - Prevention of CV events
  - Claudication
- Acutely taken for
  - Acute, mild to moderate pain (e.g., headache, myalgia)
  - Fever
  - Dysmenorrhea
- Usual dose, 325–1000 mg q3–4h for acute illnesses and pain
- 62.5–325 mg for plt inhibitor effects
- Alternatives: Acetaminophen, other NSAIDs (ibuprofen, naproxen), steroids, opioids, gold, ticlopidine, dipyridamole, pentoxifylline

DRUG EFFECTS

System	Effect	Assessment by Hx	PE	Test
RESP	Hyperventilation, resp alkalosis		Tachypnea	ABGs
GI	Gastritis	Dyspepsia		Endoscopy
	PUD	N/V, hematemesis, melena		Upper GI, x-rays, stool heme, Hgb
ENDO	Hyperglycemia, corticosteroid release			Glucose
HEME	Plt dysfunction	Bleeding, bruising	Hematomata, petechiae	Bleeding time
HEPAT	Hepatocellular damage	Nausea, anorexia	Hepatomegaly, jaundice	SGOT, SGPT, alk phos
TOXICITY				
CARDIO	Vasomotor paralysis		Hypotension	
RESP	Hypoventilation, resp acidosis		Hypopnea	ABGs
DERM	Eruptions	Pruritus	Acneiform, erythematous, pruritic, eczematoid, or desquamative lesions	
RENAL	Renal failure due to analgesic nephropathy	Oliguria, anuria	Edema, rales	BUN/Cr, UA, CXR
CNS	Headache, tinnitus, drowsiness, dizziness, diminished vision and hearing		Sweating, confusion, convulsions, coma	
ACID-BASE	Metabolic acidosis			ABGs

Key Reference: Metzler H, Kozek-Langenecker S, Huber K. Antiplatelet therapy and coronary stents in perioperative medicine—the two sides of the coin. *Best Pract Res Clin Anaesthesiol.* 2008;22(1):81–94.

Perioperative Implications

Preoperative Concerns

- D/C 1 wk prior to surgery for full reversal of plt inhibition (need only ⅓ of normally functioning plts, so if no dilution effect expected, need only 48 hr off low-dose ASA); May see hyperthrombotic state around 7–10 d, particularly in pts with coronary stents
- Continue aspirin in pts with coronary stents unless contraindicated.
- May potentiate the effects of protein-bound drugs

Induction/Maintenance

- Possible mildly exaggerated effects of thiopental

Adjuvants/Regional Anesthesia/Reversal

- May increase the risk of hemorrhagic complications of regional anesthesia. Aspirin does not contraindicate regional anesthesia, but those techniques with low potential for bleeding are preferable (e.g., spinal may be preferred over epidural).
- May increase the risk of hemorrhagic complications of invasive monitoring

Special Considerations

- A potent inhibitor of plt aggregation that can seriously impair surgical hemostasis. Most surgeons request D/C of aspirin 1 wk prior to surgery. However, if CAD or other vascular occlusive disease will be left untreated, consult with surgeon, pt's primary physician, and pt about advisability of D/C aspirin.
- Risks of regional anesthesia and invasive monitoring may be increased.
- May displace protein-bound drugs (e.g., warfarin, sulfonylureas, thiopental, methotrexate), thus augmenting their effects
- Assoc with gastritis, PUD, GI bleeding, and increased risk for aspiration of gastric contents
- Assoc with Reye's syndrome and contraindicated in febrile viral illness in children

Asthma Drugs, New

Michael Bishop
Yulia Ivashkov

Uses

- Asthma therapy is based on the recognition that it is primarily an inflammatory disease.
- There are no major changes in the last 5y in treatment of acute asthma.
- Treatment of chronic asthma incl:
  - Inhaled corticosteroids are a first-line therapy. Introduction of a selective inhaled corticosteroid ciclesonide may further minimize the adverse effects of inhaled corticosteroids (specifically, oral thrush).
  - Use of inhaled anti-inflammatory drugs such as nedocromil (mast-cell stabilizer) and cromolyn for mild persistent asthma.
  - Oral anti-leukotriene drugs zileuton, montelukast and zafirlukast
  - Recombinant humanized monoclonal anti-IgE antibody, omalizumab, for treatment of allergic asthma
- Drugs for chronic treatment have no place in the face of an acute asthma attack for which beta adrenergic agonists remain first-line therapy.

Risks

- Oral antileukotriene drugs are recommended for use in mild to moderate persistent asthma, and are less effective in asthma exacerbations, than inhaled corticosteroids. They have no direct bronchodilatory effects. They do not prevent an asthma attack in the face of airway stimulation.

- Zafirlukast and zileuton may cause drug interactions due to cytochrome P450 isoenzyme involvement (inhibition of warfarin and theophylline metabolism)
- Zileuton can cause hepatotoxicity, and requires monitoring of liver function.
- Potential safety concerns for omalizumab incl risk of development of anaphylaxis. Side effects may also incl diarrhea, vomiting, menorrhagia, and increased hematoma formation. It is given as a SQ injection once in 2 to 4 wk.

Overview

- Leukotrienes are potent bronchoconstrictors. They also cause chemotaxis, mucus secretion, edema, and eosinophilia. The anti-leukotriene modifiers prevent formation of leukotrienes from arachidonic acid via the lipoxygenase pathway.
- Zileuton inhibits the first step of the pathway: Conversion of arachidonic acid to leukotriene A4 by the enzyme 5-lipoxygenase.
- Zafirlukast and montelukast act as receptor antagonists for the cysteinyl leukotrienes, leukorienes C4, D4 and E4.
- Clinical effects of anti-leukotriene drugs are modest. The most beneficial effect was shown in pts with exercise-induced asthma and asthma assoc with allergic rhinitis. They may be used as a monotherapy in persistent mild asthma.

- Symptoms of atopic asthma may be mediated through a number of IgE-dependent mechanisms. Omalizumab is a recombinant humanized monoclonal anti-IgE antibody that markedly reduces free circulating IgE. It is used as an add-on therapy in severe persistent asthma not responding to a traditional therapy.

Perioperative Implications

- Other than the above mentioned drug interactions with warfarin and theophylline, there are relatively few implications of the drugs themselves.
- It is critical to recognize that pts on these drugs are asthmatic and that these drugs will not necessarily prevent bronchoconstriction to an acute stimulus.
- Prophylactic beta adrenergic agonists prior to surgery are indicated in pts on these drugs and are the first line of acute therapy.
- These drugs are sometimes used in an effort to lower doses of oral steroids. Pts with recent steroid tapers may be at risk during the periop period due to adrenal suppression.
- Anesthesia providers should recognize that omalizumab can be a cause of anaphylaxis.

Atorvastatin (Lipitor)

Lori Heller

DRUGS

Uses

- Synthetic lipid-lowering agent
- Selective, competitive HMG CoA reductase inhibitor (the rate-limiting enzyme of LDL cholesterol synthesis)
- Lowers LDL and triglycerides and raises HDL (the latter at high doses, e.g., 40 mg/d and over to the average 70 kg pt)
- Augments elimination of LDL and VLDL by upregulating LDL receptors on surface of hepatocytes
- Statins also modify endothelial function, decreasing inflammatory responses, and thrombogenicity, while increasing plaque stability.
- Evidence widely shows statins reduce the rates of MI, stroke, and coronary and all cause mortality in the 1° and 2° prevention settings.
- Three studies indicate it reduces incidence of age-related cognitive dysfunction.
- Also been shown to ↓ risk of first major coronary event in patients with known risk factors for CAD and normal LDL cholesterol levels

Perioperative Risks

- Clinically important side effects of all statins incl myositis (may be modified by creatine or CoQ10 administration) and liver dysfunction.
- Incidence of ↑ transaminase levels of more than 3× normal is <2%.

- LFT elevations completely reversible and resolve within a few weeks on D/C of the drug
- Severe hepatic dysfunction or cirrhosis not reported
- Assoc rarely with rhabdomyolysis in the periop period of major surgeries
- Myositis rarely seen with monotherapy. Increases significantly (to nearly 30%) when used in combination with immunosuppressives (cyclosporine, tacrolimus), azole antifungal agents (ketoconazole, itraconazole), fibrinic acid derivatives (gemfibrozil), niacin, erythromycin, clarithromycin, and fluvoxamine. Greater risk with those on higher doses of statins, > age 65 y, with baseline renal insufficiency and uncontrolled hypothyroidism.

Pharmacokinetics/Pharmacodynamics

- Antilipemic drug: Interferes with production and enhances uptake of cholesterol and its lipoprotein complexes
- Orally administered and rapidly absorbed
- Hepatic first-pass metabolism causes a low systemic bioavailability.
- Undergoes extensive metabolism to active metabolites
- Elimination of parent drug and metabolites occurs primarily in bile after hepatic and/or extrahepatic metabolism
- <2% of a dose recovered in urine

- Mean plasma elimination $T_{1/2}$ 14 hr, but $T_{1/2}$ of HMG CoA reductase inhibitory activity is 20–30 hr due to the active metabolites. As a result, drug has greater efficacy than other statins.
- Second most efficacious LDL lowering statin (26–60%)
- Unique structure, long half-life and hepatic selectivity possible explanations for increased potency
- Unlike other statins, increased dosages do not necessarily result in increased ability to raise HDL, but seems to require higher dosage to have an HDL raising effect

Drug Class/Mechanism of Action/Usual Dose

- Cholesterol lowering, statin
- Inhibition of HMG CoA reductase results in decreased synthesis of hepatic cholesterol
- Compensatory ↑ in hepatic LDL receptor production then results in an ↑ in uptake of LDL cholesterol from the circulation
- Reduces elevated total cholesterol, LDL-C, apo B, triglyceride levels and ↑ HDL-C
- Usual initial dosage 10 mg once daily. Maintenance dosage 10–80 mg once daily.
- No dosage modifications needed for renal insufficiency

DRUG EFFECTS

System	Effect	Assessment by Hx	PE	Test
HEPAT	Transaminitis	Asymptomatic		LFTs
GI	Bloating, dyspepsia	Abd pain	Abd exam	
MS	Myalgias, myositis, arthralgias, rhabdomyolysis	Muscle aches, tenderness or weakness; malaise, fever	MS exam/palpation	CPK
DERM	Rash		Inspection of skin	

Key Reference: Le Manach Y, Coriat P, Collard CD, Riedel B. Statin therapy within the perioperative period. *Anesthesiology.* 2008;108:1141–1146.

Perioperative Implications

Preoperative Concerns

- Assess for CAD and other assoc conditions such as Htn, diabetes, atherosclerotic CVD
- When possible, HMG CoA reductase inhibitors should be continued periop but with hydration and observation to avoid significant rare skeletal muscle damage.
- Based on a $T_{1/2}$ of 30 hr for its active metabolites, the drug should be D/C 3–5 d preop if such D/C is desired
- Should also be D/C in pts with symptoms suggestive of a myopathy or with other risk factors predisposing to the development of renal failure 2° to rhabdomyolysis such as hypotension, trauma, and severe acute infection

Induction/Maintenance

- No reported cases of atorvastatin assoc intraop/periop events, although other statins have been assoc with adverse events such as rhabdomyolysis and concomitant myoglobinuria and renal failure
- If surgery involves significant muscle damage in the setting of a statin, consider placement of urinary catheter for early detection of myoglobinuria and avoidance of succinylcholine.

Adjuvants/Regional Anesthesia/Reversal

- No interactions known
- Avoid grapefruit premedication if MAC proposed as grapefruit within 2 hr decreases metabolism of this statin.

Postoperative Concerns

- Relatively long elimination $T_{1/2}$ makes resumption of drug in immediate postop period unnecessary if it is D/C.
- May be at ↑ risk for cardiac event given known risk factor

Drug Interactions

- Risk of myopathy ↑ with concurrent administration of cyclosporine and erythromycin
- Antacids ↓ plasma concentrations by 35%
- Digoxin levels can ↑ by 20%

Anticipated Problems/Concerns

- Assess for CAD

Atropine

Judy G. Johnson
Neil Bhatt

Uses

- Primary indication: Treatment for reflex-mediated bradycardia
- Preop medications to reduce oral and tracheobronchial secretions
- Production of mydriasis and cycloplegia
- Biliary and ureteral smooth muscle relaxation
- Treatment of organophosphate poisoning
- Bronchodilation esp. administered as aerosol
- Treatment for organophosphate poisoning; this poisoning may cause side effects known as SLUDGE: Salivation, Lacrimation, Urination, Diaphoresis, Gastrointestinal motility, and Emesis

Perioperative Risks

- Tachycardia that may produce angina, cardiac ischemia, or CHF
- Side effects: Rapid onset of symptoms characteristic of muscarinic (cholinergic) receptor blockade
- Tachycardia
- Dry mouth
- Production of thick pulm secretions
- Blurred vision and/or photophobia
- Flushing (occasionally in infants)
- Increased body temp 2° to inhibition of sweating

Pharmacology

- Structurally resembles cocaine and has weak analgesic properties
- Competitively antagonize the effects of the neurotransmitter acetylcholine at the postganglionic sites known as muscarinic receptors.
- Muscarinic cholinergic receptors are found in salivary glands, smooth muscles of the GI and GU tract, and the heart.
- At high doses, the drug produces partial block of autonomic ganglia (nicotinic receptors)
- Parasympatholytic effects of anticholinergic drug decreasing the actions of rest and digest
- Lipid-soluble, easily pass the blood-brain barrier
- Plasma T ½ 2.3 hr
- Metabolism by hydrolysis in the liver, excreted by kidneys

Dosages (70 kg adult):

- 0.4–0.5 mg IV for intraop bradycardia
- 1–2 mg IV before reversal of muscle relaxants
- 1–2 mg IV before intrinsic sinus node dysfunction or organophosphate poisoning repeated prn
- 0.4–0.5 mg SQ, IM for control of secretions
- 0.01–0.02 mg/kg in infants and children (minimum 0.1mg)

Special Considerations

- 2–4 mg diluted with NS may be given in the ETT in absence of IV access
- For cardiopulmonary resuscitation larger doses may be necessary.

Central Anticholinergic Syndrome

- Atropine can enter the CNS and produce symptoms ranging from restlessness, hallucinations, somnolence, depressed ventilation to loss of consciousness. This syndrome can be mistaken for delayed recovery from anesthesia. Physostigmine is the specific treatment.

ASSESSMENT POINTS

System	Mechanism of Action/Effects	PE
HEENT	Decreased secretions Block sphincteric and ciliary muscles	Dry mouth/upper airways Mydriasis (Dilated pupils)
CARDIO	Block vagal effects of M_2 receptors on SA node	Tachycardia (Palpitations)
RESP	Dry airways	Thick secretions
GI	Decreased gastric acid production	Decreased peristalsis
GU	Block sphincteric muscles	Pain in lower abd (Enlarged bladder)
CNS	Toxic doses	Restlessness, disorientation, delirium
DERM	Flushing	Red body, dry skin (Possible increase of body temp)

Key References: *Goodman & Gilman's The pharmacological basis of therapeutics.* 9th ed. New York: McGraw-Hill Professional Publishing; 1996:148–15. Holzman RS. The legacy of atropos. *Anesthesiology.* 1998–07;89:241–249. *pharmacology & physiology in anesthetic practice.* 4th ed. Lippincott Williams and Wilkins; 2006:266–275.

DRUGS

Benzodiazepines (Midazolam, Lorazepam, Diazepam)

Robert I. Cohen

Uses

- Prescribed for the treatment of anxiety
- Used for conscious sedation and premedication

Perioperative Risks

- High levels assoc with hypnosis, unconsciousness, resp depression, apnea

Worry About

- Combination with opioids or other CNS depressants may result in severe resp depression, apnea, hypotension

Overview/Pharmacology

- Anxiolysis, sedation, hypnosis, muscle relaxation, anterograde amnesia, anticonvulsant
- Midazolam: Short-elimination $T_{1/2}$ (2.5 hr)
- Lorazepam: Intermediate-elimination $T_{1/2}$ (15 hr)
- Diazepam: long-elimination $T_{1/2}$ (30 hr)
- Metabolized by hepatic microsomal oxidation and glucuronide conjugation
- Diazepam has active metabolites
- Midazolam
  - IV: Peak effect in 2–4 min
  - IM: Peak effect in 30–60 min
- Lorazepam
  - IV: Peak effect in 5–15 min, painful injection, thrombophlebitis
  - IM: Peak effect in 60–90 min
  - Oral: Peak effect in 2 hr
- Diazepam
  - IV: Peak effect in 1–2 min, painful injection, thrombophlebitis
  - IM: Painful, unpredictable absorption, do not use
  - Oral: Peak effect in 30–60 min, well absorbed; food, aluminum-containing antacids delay absorption
- No clear difference in speed of recovery from diazepam and midazolam drug effect after low dose for sedation in short procedures; faster recovery from midazolam drug effect becomes more prominent after larger dose/prolonged administration
- Lorazepam provides long duration (>4 hr) of sedation and amnesia by any route of administration; do not use when rapid recovery from drug effect desired
- Prolonged use can lead to tolerance

Drug Class/Mechanism of Action/Usual Dose

- Anxiolytic, sedative, hypnotic
- Potentiation of gamma-aminobutyric acid-mediated neural inhibition
- Safe use involves careful titration to the desired effect
- Usual dosage for premedication and conscious sedation:
  - Midazolam
  - IV: 0.5–1 mg, repeated; maintenance infusion: 0.04–0.10 mg/kg/h
  - IM: 0.07 mg/kg
  - Oral: 15 mg (0.5mg/kg in children up to 20 kg)
  - Lorazepam
  - IV: 0.25 mg, repeated
  - IM: 0.05 mg/kg, max 4 mg
  - Oral: 0.5–4 mg
  - Diazepam
  - IV: 1–2 mg, repeated
  - Oral: 5–10 mg

DRUG EFFECTS

System	Effect	PE	Test
CARDIO	Decreased systemic vascular resistance and cardiac output	Arterial BP	
RESP	Central resp depression Apnea	Resp rate	Tidal volume Minute volume, capnography, oximetry
CNS	Anxiolysis Sedation Hypnosis Amnesia Anticonvulsant ↓ Cerebral metabolic rate and cerebral blood flow	Slurred speech, drowsiness, ataxia Unresponsiveness	

Key References: Reves JG, Glass PSA, Lubarsky DA, et al. Intravenous anesthetics. In: Miller RD, ed. *Anesthesia*, 7th ed. Philadelphia: Churchill Livingstone; 2010:734–742. Riker RR; Fraser GL. Adverse events associated with sedatives, analgesics, and other drugs that provide patient comfort in the intensive care unit. *Pharmacotherapy*. 2005;25:8S–18S. Maxa JL; Ogu CC; Adeeko MA; Swaner TG. Continuous-infusion flumazenil in the management of chlordiazepoxide toxicity. *Pharmacotherapy*. 2003;23:1513–1516.

Perioperative Implications/Possible Drug Interactions

Preoperative Concerns

- Elderly: Reduce dose up to 5-fold (5–10%/decade reduction)
- Cimetidine, ranitidine (microsomal cytochrome P450 inhibitors), and liver cirrhosis ↓ clearance; enhanced effect may be seen
- Smoking and enzyme-inducing drugs increase diazepam clearance.
- Renal failure increases diazepam $T_{1/2}$
- Monitor ventilation

Induction/maintenance
- Synergistic interaction with anesthesia induction agents, and opioids

Regional Anesthesia

- Possibly exacerbates resp depression during spinal anesthesia (mechanism unknown)

Anticipated Problems/Concerns

- Combination with opioids or other CNS depressants may result in severe resp depression, apnea, hypotension
- Large doses result in prolonged drowsiness and resp depression, esp. in the elderly; reversal with flumazenil
- Undesirable degree of amnesia

DRUGS

Beta-Adrenergic Receptor Antagonists (Blockers)

Roberta Hines

Uses

- Precise role in periop period (risks and benefits) still controversial
- Used in management of essential Htn
- Effective in decreasing infarct size
- Used to ↓ HR
- Available as oral and IV preparations
- Used to suppress cardiac dysrhythmias
- Value in prevention of excess SNS activity
- Must be continued periop in pts who have been taking them (Class I AHA indication)
- Reduced CV morbidity and mortality in pts with symptomatic ischemic heart disease for major surgery with periop use of β-blockers (major vascular surgery only)
- Whether one should give β-blockers periop (prophylactically) to pts with cardiac risk factors alone remains unclear

Perioperative Risks

- Nonselective blocker may precipitate bronchospasm

- May worsen or precipitate CHF in pts with ↓ LV function
- May cause hypotension, bradycardia

Worry About

- Decreased ventricular performance esp. with underlying cardiac dysfunction
- Can worsen lung disease, esp. with nonspecific blockers and Hx of COPD or bronchospasm

Overview/Pharmacology

- All β-blockers are derivatives of isoproterenol
- β-adrenergic receptor agonists classified as partial or pure agonists on basis or absence of intrinsic sympathomimetic activity
- Partial antagonists often better tolerated than pure antagonists in pts with ↓ LV function
- β-blocker may produce varying degrees of membrane stabilization in heart (detectable only at extremely high plasma concentration)
- Effective in both acute, chronic management

Drug Class/Mechanism of Action/Usual Dose

- All β-blockers bind selectively to β-receptors
- β-blockers interfere with ability of other drugs/substances with sympathomimetic activity to activate β-receptors
- Action of β-blockers negates effect of catecholamines, other sympathomimetics on heart and smooth muscle of airways, blood vessels
- Bind to β-receptor by competitive inhibition
- Exhibit selective affinity for β-adrenergic receptors
- Binding of agonists to the β-receptor is reversible
- Chronic administration is assoc with ↑ in number of β-adrenergic receptors
- Principal method of clearance hepatic, renal, or plasma hydrolysis (esmolol)
- Elimination T½ specific to individual agents, depends on dose, protein binding, route of administration (oral/IV)

DRUG EFFECTS

System	Effect	Assessment by Hx	PE	Test
CARDIO	↓ HR ↓ CO ↓ LV function ↑ Coronary vascular resistance ↓ Myocardial O₂ consumption	Relief of angina ↓ BP ↓ HR	HR BP	ECG; stress ECG
RESP	↑ Airway resistance (esp. nonselective agents)	↑ Wheezing ↑ Bronchospasm		FEV₁ ↑ Peak airway pressure
ENDO	Hyperglycemia Hypokalemia			Laboratory measurements of K⁺ and glucose
CNS	Fatigue, lethargy, peripheral paresthesia, withdrawal hypersensitivity			
OB	All cross placenta, fetal effect: Bradycardia, hypotension, hypoglycemia			

Key Reference: Poldermans D, Boersma E, Bax JJ, et al. The effect of bisoprolol on perioperative mortality and myocardial infarction in high-risk patients undergoing vascular surgery. Dutch Echocardiographic Cardiac Risk Evaluation Applying Stress Echocardiography Study Group. *N Engl J Med.* 1999;341:1789–1794.

Perioperative Implications

Preoperative Concerns

- β-blocker should be continued in periop period (in pts previously on β-blockers)
- May have value in pts with symptomatic cardiac disease preventing for major vascular surgery (Class I indication-AHA guidelines)
- Acute D/C can result in excess SNS activity that manifests in 24–48 hr

Induction/Maintenance

- Myocardial depression observed with inhaled or injected anesthetic is worsened with addition of β-blocker
- Esmolol has been assoc with profound bradycardia in presence of inhaled anesthetics

Adjuvants/Regional Anesthesia/Reversal

- Bradycardic effects often can be reversed by atropine
- Isoproterenol most effective at reversing negative cardiac (both dromotropic and inotropic) effects; but need to administer 1 dose of isoproterenol (2–25 µg/min⁻¹) to reverse negative cardiac effect
- CaCl₂ (250–1000 mg) or glucagon (1–5 mg) administered IV (adult) effectively reverses myocardial depression
- Life-threatening bradycardia may require insertion of transvenous pacemaker

Anticipated Problems/Concerns

- When β-blockers are administered in presence of anesthetic drugs they may unmask direct negative inotropic effects of concomitantly administered anesthetic; this effect results in profound ↓ in BP, CO

Bicarbonate Sodium

Priscilla Nelson
Nina Singh

Uses

- Management of hyperkalemia
- Promote alkaline diuresis (hastens secretion of salicylates, TCA; renal protective in rhabdomyolysis, transfusion reaction)
- Possible protection against contrast-induced nephropathy (CIN) in pts with compromised renal function.
- Alkalinize local anesthetics (weak bases); uncharged form can cross bilipid cell membrane to bind to Na^+ receptor (site of action) intracellularly. Decreases time to onset, minimum concentration required. Can reduce pain with SQ injection.
- Controversial efficacy in metabolic acidosis. Usually reserved for situations when pH <7.1.

Perioperative Risks and Implications

- Hypernatremia; Na^+ retaining states (CHF, pulm edema, cirrhosis) can worsen
- Hyperosmolality
- Hypercapnia

- Hypokalemia
- Other physiologic effects: Left shift in oxy-Hg curve, accelerated lactate production, CSF acidosis

Special Considerations

- Treatment for hyperkalemia is temporizing; does not reduce total body K^+
- Necessitates adequate ventilation to excrete CO_2 (produced when neutralizes H^+); otherwise, resp acidosis can result
- Metabolic acidosis: Dx and Tx of underlying cause (hypovolemia, anemia, hypoxia, uremia, sepsis) should be undertaken; $NaHCO_3$ should be viewed only as temporizing measure.

Overview/Pharmacology

- H^+/K^+ ion membrane exchanger shifts K^+ intracellularly, reducing intravascular K^+.
- Excess HCO_3^- ions are excreted renally, alkalinizing the urine.
- $Na^+ + HCO_3^- + H^+ \leftarrow \rightarrow H_2O + CO_2$ via carbonic anhydrase.

Drug Class/Mechanism of Action/ Usual Dose

- Electrolyte and alkalinizer; dosing is specific to abn being treated.
- Hyperkalemia: 1 ampule of $NaHCO_3$ (50mEq/ 50 mL) over 5 min
- Metabolic acidosis: [0.2 × weight (kg) × {desired HCO_3-measured HCO_3}] = bicarbonate dose in mEq; half of calculated dose is administered initially over 30 min; reassessment of ABG: pH, HCO_3, BE.
- Alkalinizes urine, which prevents reabsorption of TCA, salicylates, Hg, and myoglobin into renal vasculature, aiding in excretion
- Protection against CIN (unlabeled use): 154 mEq/L of $NaHCO_3$ in D5W, with an initial infusion of 3 mL /kg/hr 1 hr prior contrast bolus, 1mL/kg/hr for 6 hr post procedure.
- Local anesthetics: Typically 1 cc $NaHCO_3$: 10 cc lidocaine.

DRUG EFFECTS

System	Effect	Test
CARDIO	Acidosis can reduce inotropy, responsiveness to catecholamines. $NaHCO_3$ can exacerbate/cause CHF, edema from Na+ load	BP, cardiac output, TEE
RESP	Pulm edema; hypercapnia, requiring adjustment in minute ventilation	X-ray, ABG
CNS	AMS/increased ICP from hypercapnea, coma from hyperosmolarity	Neurologic exam
Renal	Alkalinizes urine, aiding in diuresis of toxic compounds; impaired renal function may be incapable of handling sodium load; protection against contrast nephropathy	Urine pH >7, Cr, BUN
Endocrine	Hypernatremia can reduce renin/aldosterone; hyperosmolality can increase ADH	ABG, HCO_3 levels, BMP, BNP, serum osm

Key Reference: Navaneethan SD, et al. Sodium bicarbonate in the prevention of contrast-induced nephropathy: A systematic review and meta-analysis. *AJKD.* 2009;53: 617–627.

Perioperative Implications

Preoperative Concerns

- Perform ABG, [K^+] prior to initiation of $NaHCO_3$ therapy, if possible.
- Plasma-expanding properties may make it useful in pts with HD shock.
- Consider controlled ventilation over spontaneous (LMA). If ETT in situ, evaluate if minute ventilation can be augmented to handle increased CO_2 loads.
- Digoxin: Hypokalemia ca₃n exacerbate effects.

Induction/Maintenance

- If excess $NaHCO_3$ creates alkalosis, basic drugs (opioids, local anesthetics) have increased activity due to higher non-ionized fraction crossing lipid membranes.

- Rapid bolus can cause transient fall in MAP, rise in ICP; can be alleviated by slow IV infusion.
- 100 mEq of $NaHCO_3$ produces 2.24 L of CO_2; equivalent to 10 min of CO_2 production.

Postoperative Period

- Therapy should be guided by ABG analysis of pH, HCO_3^-, BE.

Anticipated Problems/Concerns

- No convincing evidence exists that $NaHCO_3$ confers any survival benefit in cardiac arrest/VF. Should not be used routinely in CPR. Consider when prolonged VF, severe acidosis, hyperkalemia, medication overdose (TCA, salicylate).
- No convincing evidence that improves mortality when used to treat metabolic acidosis, even at pH <7.1; additionally, use is not benign; can cause hypernatremia, hyperosmolality, hypercapnia,

alkalosis, volume overload, hypokalemia, left shift oxyhemoglobin curve, CSF acidosis.
- Alternatives for buffering acidotic states are limited and have no proven advantage over $NaHCO_3$.
- Carbicarb (equimolar sodium carbonate and $NaHCO_3$) may cause very alkaline pH, local tissue injury, dysrrhythmias; vasodilator effect can reduce coronary perfusion pressure.
- THAM (tris[hydroxymethyl]aminomethane) acts intracellulary (vs $NaHCO_3$); can cause hyperosmolarity, hypervolemia; vasodilatory actions shown to reduce aortic and coronary perfusion pressures.
- Tribonate ($NaHCO_3$+THAM+phosphate+ acetate) may be more effective treating intracellular acidosis, but studies have not been done during human CPR to prove effectiveness.

Bleomycin

Victor A. Filadora, II
Mark J. Lema

Uses

- Treatment of squamous cell carcinoma
- Treatment of melanomas and sarcomas
- Treatment of testicular carcinoma
- Treatment of Hodgkin's and non-Hodgkin's lymphoma
- Sclerosing agent for malignant pleural effusion

Perioperative Risks

- Greater than 10%
  - Acute febrile reactions (25–50%)
  - Dermatologic
- 50% of pts can develop erythema, rash, striae, induration, hyperkeratosis, vesiculation, and peeling of the skin. This is predominantly seen on the palmar and plantar surfaces of the hands and feet.
- Hyperpigmentation (50%), alopecia, and nail bed changes.
- These effects are usually dose related and reversible with D/C.
  - Gastrointestinal: Stomatitis and mucositis (30%), anorexia, wt loss
- Between 1–10%
  - Dermatologic: Skin thickening, diffuse scleroderma, onycholysis, pruritus
  - Respiratory: Tachypnea, rales, acute or chronic interstitial pneumonitis, and pulm fibrosis (5–10%)
- Miscellaneous: Anaphylactoid-like reactions and idiosyncratic reactions (1% in lymphoma pts)
- Less than 1%
  - Angioedema, cerebrovascular accident, cerebral arteritis, hepatotoxicity, hypoxia, MI, Raynaud's phenomenon, renal toxicity, scleroderma-like skin changes, thrombotic microangiopathy, vomiting
- Rapidly progressive interstitial pneumonitis known to occur after general anesthesia using O_2 conc >30%, overhydrating pt

FDA Black Box Warning

- Idiosyncratic reaction: A severe reaction similar to anaphylaxis has been reported in 1% of lymphoma pts treated with bleomycin. These reactions typically occur after the first or second dose.
- Pulmonary fibrosis: The most severe toxicity of bleomycin, with risk increasing in elderly pts, those receiving >400 units total lifetime dose and possibly smokers and pts receiving concurrent O_2 therapy
- Experienced physician: Should be administered under the supervision of a physician experienced in delivering chemotherapy

Contraindications

- Hypersensitivity of bleomycin or any component of the formulation
- Severe pulm disease
- Pregnancy

Worry About

- Sustained O_2 conc >30%
- Liberal use of maintenance fluids

Overview/Pharmacology

- 1 U bleomycin = 1 mg activity of bleomycin
- $T_{1/2}\beta$ 2 hr, but if Cr <35 mL-/min exponentially ↑ $T_{1/2}$
- 70% is recovered in urine as active bleomycin

Drug Class/Mechanism of Action

- Mixture of cytotoxic antibiotics isolated from *Streptomyces verticillus*
- Cytotoxic action caused by inhibition of DNA synthesis
- Usual dose: 0.25–0.5 U/kg (10–20 U/m²) to 400 U (total dose)

ASSESSMENT POINTS

System	Effect	Assessment by Hx	PE	Test
CARDIO	Raynaud's (rare)	Color changes in fingers	Observation	
RESP	Interstitial pneumonitis (10%) Pulm fibrosis (1%)	Dose (>250 U), age (>65 y) Previous lung disease	Dyspnea, fine rales and cough, fever	PFTs (↓ TLC, ↓ VC)
GI	N/V			
HEME	(Not assoc with pancytopenia)			
DERM	Mucocutaneous toxicity (50%)	1–3 wk after start of Rx (dose 150–200 U)	Urticaria, hyperpigmentation, hyperkeratosis, alopecia	

Key Reference: McEvoy GK, ed. *AHRS 95 Drug Information*. Bethesda, MD: 600–602.

Perioperative Implications

Preoperative Period

- Assess bleomycin cumulative dose (>250 U)
- Assess age (>65 y)
- Assess previous lung disease Hx
- Ask about previous radiation to thorax
- Obtain PFTs, CXR, ABGs

Interoperative Period

- Limit delivered O_2 to <30% if adequate for O_2 sat >89%.
- Limit fluids and avoid fluid overload.
- Consider CVP monitoring.
- Consider arterial monitoring and sampling.
- Use upper limit alarm for percentage of O_2 delivery.

Postoperative Period

- Keep delivered O_2 to <30% if adequate for O_2 sat >89%.
- Limit fluids
- Corticosteroid use for pulm toxicity is controversial.

Anticipated Problems/Concerns

- Cyclophosphamide, radiation Rx (thorax) potentiates pulm toxicity.
- Cisplatin potentiates renal insufficiency.
- Vinca alkaloids (vincristine, vinblastine, VP-16) potentiate Raynaud's phenomenon.
- Mitomycin C exhibits similar properties to those of bleomycin but with milder effects.

Calcium-Channel Blockers

W. Scott Beattie
Duminda N. Wijeysundera

Uses

- Prescribed to treat Htn, angina, supraventricular arrhythmias, cerebral vasospasm, and HCM

Perioperative Profile/Risks

- A significant proportion of the surgical population come to surgery chronically taking calcium channel blockers. Many pts receive Ca^{2+}-channel blockers because of the systemic Htn, CAD or supraventricular arrhythmias. A combination of ACE inhibitors and CCB are indicated in diabetic pts with Htn. This class of drug effectively decreases myocardial O_2 demand through its effects on AV conduction, inotropy, and vasodilatation of systemic and coronary vasculature. There is also theoretic evidence of an effect on plt function but clinically this has not been demonstrated.

Worry About

- Hypotension, meta-analysis of both cardiac and noncardiac RCTs shows a 50% increase in the incidences of unplanned periop hypotension.
- Neither RCTs or nonrandomized trials have demonstrated increased incidence of CHF, or the need for inotropic support
- AV nodal block or asystole has not been demonstrated, however, there is an increased utilization of temporary cardiac pacing after cardiac surgery.

Bradycardia, requiring treatment, has been demonstrated in a frequency similar to beta blockers.
- In both cardiac and noncardiac surgery, beneficial effects have been demonstrated; acute withdrawal may precipitate acute coronary ischemia.
- Plt function is a theoretic risk, however, increased bleeding or increased transfusion requirements have not been demonstrated in meta-analysis or nonrandomized trials.

Overview and Pharmacology

- Ca^{2+} channels: Functional pores in cardiac and smooth muscle cell membranes—allow calcium to flow down an electrochemical gradient. Channels are also present in sarcoplasmic reticulum and mitochondria. Calcium is a primary generator of the cardiac action potential and intracellular events regulating muscular contraction.
- Calcium enters through voltage-dependent or receptor-operated channels. Most of the effects of calcium channel blockers is regulated by components of the L (long lasting) type receptor.
- Amlodipine is the most widely prescribed calcium channel blocker; a half life of 30–50 hr; a bioavailability of 60–90%; is predominately metabolized to inactive metabolites and excreted in urine.
- Verapamil: 90% absorbed PO, 20–35% bioavailability, onset of action 2 hr, peak effect IV PO peak effect 3–4 hr, 85% eliminated by first-pass

hepatic metabolism with elimination $T_{1/2}$ of 3–7 hr. The IV effects are almost immediate.
- Diltiazem: 89–90% PO absorption, 40–70% bioavailability, PO onset of action <15 min, peak effect 30 min, 60% metabolized by liver, remainder excreted by kidneys, $T_{1/2}$ 3.5–6.0 hr
- Bepridil: >90% absorption, >80% bioavailability, PO onset of action 2–3 hr, peak effect 8 hr, hepatic elimination with $T_{1/2}$ 26–64 hr
- Hepatic disease may necessitate decreased dosing of verapamil and other Ca^{2+}-channel blockers

Drug Class/Mechanism of Action

- Four different classes of Ca blockers:
  - 1,4 dihydropyridine (e.g., amlodipine, nifedipine, nicardipine)
  - Phenylalkylamines (e.g., verapamil)
  - Benzothiazepines (e.g., diltiazem)
  - Diarylaminopropranolamine ether (e.g., bepridil)
- Mechanisms of action: Amlodipine—blockade of voltage-dependent L-type inactive Ca^{2+}-channel receptor that has recently undergone activation and cannot open; the other 3 classes bind to specific receptors within the L-type channels,
- The dose periop use of calcium channel blockers (nicardipine, diltazen, and verapamil) should be titrated to effect.

ASSESSMENT POINTS

System	Effect	Assessment by Hx	PE	Test
CARDIO	Ischemic protection, myocardial depression, vasodilation, AV conduction slowing	Short-acting nifedipine should be avoided, due to reflex tachycardia	Hypotension, bradycardia	BP measurement, ECG, ECHO for ventricular contractility
CEREBRAL	Cerebral vasodilation and ↓ vasospasm, there is no indication of increased stroke in clinical studies	Ongoing assessment of neurologic status in pts at risk for vasospasm	Changes in neurologic assessment	Cranial Doppler or angiogram
NEURO	Potentiation of NMBs	Increased risk of aspiration if extubated with residual block	Prolonged block	Use of NMB monitor
ENDO	Nifedipine delays insulin release and ↓ serum glucose in DM; diltiazem has no effect on insulin, glucagon, growth hormone, cortisol levels	Better glucose control in DM pts on nifedipine		Blood glucose

Key References: Wijeysundera DN, Beattie WS, Rao V, Karski J. Calcium antagonists reduce cardiovascular complication after cardiac surgery: A meta analysis *J Am Coll Cardiol*. 2003;41:1496–1505. Wijeysundera DN, Beattie WS. Calcium channel blockers for reducing cardiac morbidity after noncardiac surgery: A meta-analysis *Anesth Analg*. 2003;97:634–641.

Perioperative Implications

Preoperative Concerns

- Continue chronic Ca^{2+}-channel blockers throughout the periop period to minimize ↑ BP, or ischemic syndromes
- Careful assessment of baseline hemodynamic variables
- Drug interactions: Verapamil ↑ digoxin levels; cimetidine and ranitidine ↑ serum levels of Ca^{2+}-channel blockers through ↓ hepatic blood flow

Monitoring

- Routine
- Pacing capability if assoc AV block, or CHF
- Arterial line if BP instability likely

Airway

- No special concerns

Preinduction/Induction

- Assess hemodynamics and ECG before induction

Maintenance

- Goal-directed fluid therapy may decrease incidence of hypotension
- Volatile anesthetics may potentiate vasoactive effects
- Effects of Ca^{2+}-channel blockers can be antagonized by administration of calcium or by administration of other pressor agents.

Extubation

- Check TOF if using NMBs; potentiation of succinylcholine, pancuronium, D-tubocurarine, atracurium, vecuronium have been described.

Potential for incomplete reversal of NMBs owing to interaction with Ca^{2+}-channel blockers on the postsynaptic membrane and blockade of Ca^{2+} channels in skeletal muscle.

Anticipated Problems/Concerns

- Hypotension
- Bradycardia
- AV nodal block and the increased use of temporary pacemakers
- Paradoxical aggravation of myocardial ischemia with the use of short-acting nifedipine due reflex sympathetic stimulation and tachycardia

Capsaicin

Uses

- Topical analgesic if repeatedly used in diabetic neuropathy, postherpetic neuralgia, osteoarthritis, rheumatoid arthritis, and other painful disorders
- Spray used as less-lethal force by law enforcement
- May cause apoptosis in breast and prostate cancer cells

Perioperative Risks

- None reported
- After exposure to aerosolized capsaicin, e.g., in a trauma pt restrained by police, airway irritability, coughing, and bronchospasm may occur.

Pharmocokinetics/Pharmacodynamics

- Topical effects only since very poorly absorbed from the skin.

Drug Class/Mechanism of Action/Usual Dose

- Analgesic; 8-methyl-N-vanillyl-noneamide, an agonist of temp-sensitive TRPV1 receptor.
- Selective binding to afferent C fibers in the skin causes neuronal excitation and release of substance P.
- Repetitive application causes depletion of substance P and calcitonin gene-related peptide from C fibers and eventually reduced sensitivity to pain.

- Reversible degeneration of small nerve fibers in the epidermis occurs with long-term use.
- Various creams and patches available over-the-counter and by prescription in a wide range of strengths as low as 0.025%.
- For best results, repeated application of topical capsaicin is necessary several times a day for several weeks.
- An 8% patch has been recently approved by the FDA and an injectable capsaicin product (Qutenza) is in clinical trials at the time of this writing.

DRUG EFFECTS

System	Effect	Assessment by Hx	PE	Test
DERM (topical)	Burning pain at site, possibly redness	Hx of chronic pain	Thermal allodynia at site, or hypaesthesia at site of application	
EENT (topical or inhaled)	Lacrimation, blepharospasm	Accidental exposure of topical agent to the eye; exposure to aerosol in confrontation with law enforcement.	Eye exam	
RESP (inhaled)	Extreme airway irritability, coughing and bronchospasm, and possibly death with heavy exposure.	Exposure to aerosol in confrontation with law enforcement or industrial accident.	Auscultation, pulse oximetry	

Key References: Ito K, Nakazato T, Yamato K, et al. Induction of apoptosis in leukemic cells by homovanillic acid derivative, capsaicin, through oxidative stress: Implication of phosphorylation of p53 at Ser-15 residue by reactive oxygen species. *Cancer Res.* 2004;64:1071–1078. Knotkova, H, et al. Capsaicin (TRPVI agonist) therapy for pain relief. *Clin J Pain.* 2008; 24(2)

Perioperative Implications

- None known

Drug Interactions

- None known

Anticipated Problems/Concerns

- Only moderate to poor efficacy in chronic pain syndromes, which have an anatomically superficial and localized pain generator.

- Compliance is poor because of burning sensation with application.

DRUGS

Carbamazepine

Christine E. Goepfert

Uses

- FDA-approved (since 1976) for
  - Epilepsy: Complex partial seizures; generalized tonic-Clonic seizures; and mixed seizure pattern of the above mentioned, with the exception of petit mal seizures
  - Bipolar disorder with manic or mixed episodes
  - Trigeminal and glossopharyngeal neuralgia
- Off-label use for
  - Pain syndromes, e.g., phantom limb pain, complex pain syndromes, diabetic neuropathy
  - Psychiatric disorders, e.g., PTSD, ADHD, mania, schizophrenia, bipolar disorder in remission, dementia, alcohol withdrawal
  - Other disorders, e.g., prevention of seizures, paroxysmal choreoathetosis, RLS, diabetes insipidus
- Oxcarbamazepine, a keto-analogue of CBZ
  - FDA-approved (since 2000)
  - Indicated for partial seizures

Perioperative Risks/Worry About

- PHARM: Clinically significant drug interactions
- CNS: Increased sedation, dizziness, and ataxia
- CVS: Aggravation of Htn, hypotension, CAD, arrhythmias, and AV block (rare, but potentially life-threatening)
- LAB: Higher incidence of hyponatremia, aplastic anemia, agranulocytosis, thrombo- and leukopenis as well as elevated LFTs and hypothyroidism

Overview/Pharmacology

- Pharmacokinetics/pharmacodynamics
  - Rapid oral absorption
  - Peak plasma concentrations: Tablet 2–6 hr after ingestion, suspension 1.5 hr, extended release up to 26 hr
  - Plasma protein binding: 70–80%, epoxide metabolite 50%
  - Volume of distribution Vd: Children: 1.9 L/kg; adults: 0.59–2 L/kg
  - Initial half-life values: Range from 25–65 hr, ↓ to 12–17 hr on repeated doses
  - Metabolization: To 98% in the liver:
  - Cytochrome P450 3A4 as the major isoform responsible for formation of the principle metabolite carbamazepine-10,11-epoxide (antiseizure effects), accounting for many of the dose-limiting side effects
  - Induction of its own metabolism, half-life therefore variable (autoinduction completed after 3–5 wk of a fixed dosing regimen); dose adjustment necessary 2–4 wk after initiation of therapy
  - Excreted (72% in urine, 28% in feces), largely in form of hydroxylated and conjugated metabolites, only 3% unchanged, indicating that renal insufficiency can potentially increase CBZ toxicity
- Faster metabolism in children <15 yr
- Esp. in geriatric pts neuropsychiatric symptoms with agitation, confusion, psychosis possibly due to anticholinergic and tricyclic effects of CBZ and pre-existing renal insufficiency
- No known substantial gender influence on pharmacokinetics
- Race not studied in pharmacokinetics, but differences in HLA-B genes account for the frequency of side effects like Stevens-Johnson syndrome
- Drug-drug interactions relevant for anesthesia

- Increased CBZ plasma levels with potential toxicity due to CYP3A4 inhibitors: macrolide antibiotics such as erythromycin and clarithromycin, azoles like fluconazole, metronidazole, diltiazem, verapamil, cimetidine, propoxyphene, valproate, possibly levetiracetam, acetazolamide, some antidepressants (esp SSRIs and also other tricyclics), oxybutynin, grapefruit juice
- Decreased CBZ plasma levels with potentially ↑ risk for seizures due to CYP3A4 inducers CBZ (autoinduction): theophylline, phenytoin, phenobarbital, and other barbiturates
- Increased levels of substances and risk for their toxicity due to CBZ: phenytoin, lithium (potentially fatal neurotoxic reactions), acetaminophen, theophylline (also ↓), alcohol
- Decreased levels of medications and therefore less effectiveness due to CBZ: hormonal contraceptives (frequent—potential of pregnancy), anticoagulants (e.g., warfarin), caspofungin, corticosteroids, other antiepileptics like valproic acid with the exception of topiramate, benzodiazepines (e.g., midazolam, phenobarbital) and other barbiturates, tramadol, methadone and theoretically all other opioids, muscle relaxants (doxacurium, rocuronium, pancuronium, suxamethonium, vecuronium, and, to a much lesser extent also, (cis-)atracurium and questionably mivacurium), aprepitant, statins, felodipine, neuroleptics like clozapine and, to a lesser extent, haloperidol and others, tricyclics, theophylline (also ↑)

Side effects

CNS
- Most frequent and already within upper normal range of plasma level
  - Dizziness, drowsiness, fatigue, confusion, ataxia, impaired cognition, transient diplopia, oculomotor disturbances, nystagmus, blurred vision
- Rare
  - Speech disturbances, dystonia, peripheral neuritis/neuropathy and paresthesias, depression/agitation, suicidal ideation, visual hallucinations, headache, hyperacusis, tinnitus, myalgia, isolated cases of malignant neuroleptic syndrome, activation of latent psychosis

RESP
- Less frequent
  - Pulm hypersensitivity with fever, dyspnea, or pneumonitis

CVS
- Rare (but potentially fatal) above upper range of plasma level
- CHF, edema, aggravation of Htn, hypotension syncope and collapse, aggravation of CAD/myocardial infarction, arrhythmias (esp. bradycardia) and AV block, thrombophlebitis, thromboembolism, or lymphadenopathy, edema

HEM
- Rare
  - Aplastic anemia, agranulocytosis, pancytopenia, thrombocytopenia, leukopenia, leukocytosis, acute intermittent porphyria

DERM
- Less frequent
  - Toxic epidermal necrolysis and Stevens-Johnson syndrome, erythematous rashes, urticaria, photosensitivity reactions, exfoliative dermatitis

METAB
- Less frequent
  - Fever and chills, SIADH, water intoxication with hyponatremia, hypocalcemia, altered thyroid function, primarily hypothyroidism, hyperammonemia

GIS
- Most frequent
  - N/V, gastric distress, and abd pain
- Less frequent
  - Severe diarrhea, constipation
- Rare
  - Glossitis and stomatitis, pancreatitis, abn in liver function tests, very rare cases of hepatic failure

GUS
- Rare
  - Azotemia, renal failure, elevated BUN, acute urinary retention, oliguria with elevated BP, erectile impotence

OTHER
- Less frequent
  - Allergic reactions, conjunctivitis, leg cramps

Contraindications

- Hypersensitivity to any drug with tricyclic compounds (e.g., amitryptiline, desipramine, etc.) and MAO inhibitors, higher in pts with hypersensitivity to phenytoin and phenobarbital
- Complete AV block (risk of asystole)
- Bone marrow depression (aggravation)
- Porphyria (increases porphyrin precursors)
- Pregnancy (teratogenic, malformations, pregnancy category D)
- Co-administration with nefazodone (hepatotoxicity, insufficient plasma level of nefazodone)

Acute Toxicity

- Lowest known lethal dose in a 24-year-old adult: 3.2 g, and in a 3-y-old girl 1.6 g
- First signs and symptoms appear after 1–3 hr, primarily with NM dysfunctions like seizures, coma, and resp depression; CV disturbances with arterial hypotension milder and only with very high doses (>60 g)

Drug Class/Mechanism of Action/Usual Dose

- Derivative of iminostilbene (5H-Dibenz[b,f] azepine) with a structure of a tricyclic 2° amine similar to other tricyclic compounds
- Reduces polysynaptic responses and blocks post-tetanic potentiation through stabilization of voltage-gated sodium channels protein type V subunit alpha similar to phenytoin
  - Potentiation of GABA(A) receptors
- Mild anticholinergic, central antidiuretic, antiarrhythmic, antidepressant, sedative, and NMB activity
- Very potent inducer of CYP 450 3A4 and as such significant drug-drug interactions possible with a variety of drugs used in anesthesia
- Available only oral as normal, chewable, and extended release tablets and suspension
- Usual dose range between 200 and 1600 mg/day in adults (max. 2000 mg/d), 10 mg/kg – 35 mg/kg in pediatrics
- Monitored and guided by blood level (4–12 mcg/mL)

Oxcarbazepine
- Pro-drug, activated to eslicarbazepine in the liver, converted into active metabolite 10-hydroxy CBZ
- Widely used due its markedly reduced impact on CYP450 system, esp on CYP3A4, and lower incidence of agranulocytosis and bone marrow depression while having similar seizure control

DRUG EFFECTS

System	Effect	Assessment by Hx	PE	Test
CARDIO	Heart failure	SOB, pulm edema	Auscultation	X-ray, ECHO
	AV-block	Palpitations		EKG
CNS	Sedation		Clinical assessment	
METAB	Hyponatremia	Edema, drowsiness		Electrolytes
	SIADH	Wt gain	Oliguria	↓ Na, serum hypoosmolality
HEME	Anemia/aplasia	Palor	Clinical assessment	CBC
	Thrombocytopenia	Petechias	Clinical assessment	CBC
RENAL	Renal insufficiency		Azotemia, Acute oliguria	Cr, BUN, ABG
RESP	Pneumonitis	Pulm hypersensitivity	Clinical assessment	

Key References: Lingamaneni R, Hemmings Jr HC Differential interaction of anaesthetics and antiepileptic drugs with neuronal Na+ channels, Ca²⁺ channels, and GABA(A) receptors. *Br J Anaesth.* 2003;90:199–211. Richard A, et al. Cisatracurium-induced neuromuscular blockade is affected by chronic phenytoin or carbamazepine treatment in neurosurgical patients. *Anesth Analg.* 2005;100:538–544.

Perioperative Implications

Preoperative Concerns
- Continue CBZ medication
- Check blood level to assess potential risk of toxicity, esp. in old pts with polypharmacy.
- Check for pathologic laboratory tests in mostly affected organ systems:
  - HEM: Electrolytes, leukocytes, erythrocytes, plts
  - HEP: Liver enzymes
  - REN: Kidney function with urinalysis and BUN
  - METAB: Thyroid function (TSH)
- Assess CVS: Physical capacity and ECG (arrhythmias, AV-block incl second- and third-degree block, ischemic changes, QT-prolongation)
- Assess resp in regards to pulm hypersensitivity/pneumonitis

Induction/Maintenance
- Take potential for drug-drug interactions seriously.
- Increased dosages of anesthetics very likely, concerning esp IV sedatives like thiopentone (additive effects of CBZ with propofol and ketamine, but antagonistic effects with etomidate in animal studies), midazolam and muscle relaxants (incl [cis-]atracurium) as well as opioids since their primary metabolism occurs via CYP 450 3A4

- Toxic plasma levels of CBZ possible with co-medication (e.g. macrolide antibiotics and levetiracetam) which possibly result in delayed wake-up, ↑ drowsiness, and tendency to syncope postop
- Nerve stimulator recommended to dose and titrate muscle relaxants
- Be attentive for arrhythmias, esp. bradycardia, aggravation or appearance of AV-block and cardiac ischemia as an additive effect of concomitant use of cardiodepressive drugs that are used during anesthesia
- Reckon with aggravated arterial hypo- or Htn
- Consider increased tendency to hyponatremia esp. in certain surgeries and co-administration of drugs (e.g. in craniotomies due to the administration of mannitol)
- Adjust anesthetic medications (e.g., dosage of opioids) and plan (e.g., potentially extended monitoring) according to possible pre-existing cardiac, hepatic, and renal damage
- Reckon with possibly increased risk for larygospasm and brochospasm during emergence (although rare)
- Develop anesthetic plan to facilitate early mobilization to avoid thromboembolic events

Postoperative Period
- Continue with CBZ medication; bear in mind however that change from tablets to suspension might cause higher plasma peak levels with potentially increased side effects.

- Monitor esp. geriatric pts for increased confusion/agitation, AV-block, bradycardia or SIADH
- Inform pts who take oral hormonal contraceptives about decreased safety and the need of additional safety precautions for anticonception.
- Monitor for serious and fatal dermatologic reactions, incl toxic epidermal necrolysis (TEN) and Stevens-Johnson syndrome (SJS) esp. in the presence of an inherited variant of the HLA-B gene, HLA-B*1502
- Often in pts originating from certain Asian countries (15% of the population in Hong Kong, Thailand, Malaysia, and parts of the Philippines, 10% of Taiwan and 4% in North China, but only 2–4% of South Asians incl Indians, and only <1% of people of Japan and Korea)
- HLA-B*1502 practically absent in people who are not of Asian origin (e.g. Caucasians, Native Americans, African-Americans and Hispanics)

Anticipated Problems/Concerns
- Plasma level of CBZ decreased (withdrawal syndrome with seizures) or increased (toxicity)
- Drug levels of concomitant medications altered
- Hyponatremia
- Confusion and/or agitation and activation of latent psychosis, esp. in geriatric pts
- Arrhythmias, esp. AV-block
- Increased risk for thromboembolism

Chemotherapeutic Agents

Anasuya Vasudevan

Uses

• One of the treatment modalities available to prevent cancer cells from multiplying, invading, metastasizing and killing the host; also inhibit multiplication of normal cells, therefore have a high incidence of debilitating systemic side effects.

DRUG CLASS

Class and Type	Agents	Used to Treat
Alkylating Agents		
Alkyl sulfonate	Busulfan (Myleran)	Chronic granulocytic leukemia, acute leukemia, lymphoma
Ethylenimine derivative	Thiotepa	Testis, ovary, cervix, bladder, endometrial, lung, soft tissue, bone
Metal salt	Carboplatin, cisplatin	Solid tumors, lymphoma
Nitrogen mustard (HN$_2$)	Chlorambucil (Leukeran), cyclophosphamide (Cytoxan),	Chronic lymphocytic leukemia, Non-Hodgkin's Waldenstroms macroglobulinemia
	Ifosamide, Melphalan (Alkeran), Mechlorethamine, estramustine	Trophoblastic tumors Breast, lung, ovary, testis, bladder
Nitrosourea	Carmustine (BCNU), lomustine, streptozocin	Brain tumors, lymphomas
Triazene	Dacarbazine, temozolamide	Melanomas, brain tumors
Antimetabolites		
Antifolate	Methotrexate, pemetrexed	Solid tumors, leukemia
Purine analogs	Cladribine, clofarabine, fludarabine mercaptopurine, thioguinine	Leukemias, lymphomas, osteosarcoma, ALL
Pyrimidine analogs	Azacitidine, cytarabine, decitabine, fluorouracil, decitabine, floxuridine, gemcitabine	Myelodysplastic syndromes Breast, GI, bladder, head and neck
Natural Products		
Antibiotics	Bleomycin, danurobicin, doxorubicin (Adriamycin), Mitomycin, valrubicin	Lymphomas, head and neck, testis, vulva, anus, skin cancer Acute leukemias, ovary, breast Rhabdomyosarcoma, anal carcinoma
Enzyme	Asparaginase	Wilms tumor, breast, lung, ALL
Mitotic inhibitor	Vinblastine, vincristine, vindesine, vinorelbine	Lung, brain, lymphoma
Topoisomerase inhibitors	Irinotecan, etoposide, teniposide, topotecan	Neuroblastomas
Microtubule polymer stabilizer	Docetaxel, paclitaxel	Breast, head and neck, lung
Molecularly Targeted Agents		
Monoclonal antibody	Alemtuzumab, cetuximab, rituximab, bevacizumab	B and T cell leukemia, head and neck (cetuximab), colon (cetuximab, panutumab), renal cell carcinoma, lung (bevacizumab), breast (trastuzumab, bevacizumab)
Gene expression modulators	Retinoids, rexnoids	Multiple myeloma
Interleukin 2 receptor toxin	Deneleukin, diftitox	Graft vs. host disease, APML
Receptor tyrosine kinase inhibitor	Dastinib, sorafenib, semaxanib, sunitinib, gefitinib	GI, breast, lung cancers Non small cell lung cancer (gefitinib/erlotinib), pancreas (erlotinib), renal cell carcinoma (sorafenib, sunitinib, axitinib), hepatocellular carcinoma (sorafenib)
Biological Response Modifiers		
Interferons	Interferon α-2a, interferon α-2b	Melanoma, renal cell carcinoma, multiple myeloma, kaposis, CML, mycosis fungoides, non-Hodgkins
Interleukins	Aldesleukin (interleukin 2),	
Nonspecific immune modulation	hang R.O, oprelvekin, diftitox	
Myeloid and erythroid stimulating factor	Thalidomide, lenalidomide Epoitin, filgrastim	Myelodysplastic syndrome, multiple myeloma Cytopenia
Miscellaneous Agents		
Bisphosphonates	Pamidronate, zoledronic acid	Breast cancer, cancer with bone metastasis
Methylhydralazine derivative	Procarbazine	Hodgkin's, lymphosarcoma, reticulosarcoma
Photosensitizing agent	Profimer	Lung, cholangiocarcinoma, bladder
Platelet reducing salt	Anagrelide	Chronic granulocytic leukemia, polycythemia rubra vera
Substituted urea	Hydroxyurea	Head and neck cancer, acute leukemia

(Continued)

DRUGS

Class and Type	Agents	Used to Treat
Hormones and Hormone Antagonists		
Androgen, Androgen antagonist	Fluoxymesterone	Prostate cancer
	Bicalutamide	
Estrogen, estrogen antagonist	Diethylstilbesterol	Breast cancer
Thyroid hormones	Tamoxifen	Breast
	Levothyroxine	Thyroid

Key Reference: Skeel RT. *Handbook of cancer chemotherapy*. 7th ed. Wolters Kluwer/LWW.

Mechanism of Action

• Alkylating agents: Alkylate the DNA double strands with resultant inhibition or inaccurate replication of DNA.

• Antimetabolites: Inhibit mitosis by blocking or altering the substrate and inhibit DNA synthesis.

• Natural products: Inhibit microtubular proteins with resultant metaphase mitotic arrest, some cause DNA strand breakage and arrest cell multiplication.

• Antibiotics: Antitumor antibiotics, affect the synthesis of nucleic acids.

• Enzymes: Deprive cancer cells of essential amino acids by a chemical reaction with the essential substrate, (e.g., asparginase catalyses the reaction of asparagine to aspartic acid and ammonia)

• Molecularly targeted agents (monoclonal antibodies, tyrosine kinase inhibitors etc.): Directed to inhibit/antagonize vascular endothelial growth factors or their receptors.

• Adjuvants: Interleukins (IL-2): Enhance killer cell activity, lymphocyte mitogenesis and cytotoxicity.

• Interferon α 2a, 2b: Direct inhibition of tumor cell growth and modulation of the immune response, activation of NK cells, modulation of antibody production and induction of histocompatibility antigens.

• Hormones and hormone antagonists: Inhibit tumor growth by exploiting hormone sensitive tumor receptors.

Perioperative Risks

• Cardiac: Caused by antibiotic chemotherapeutic agents. Acute toxicity: acute fulminant cardiomyopathy; chronic toxicity: cardiomyopathy and biventricular failure. Adriamycin and daunorubicin can cause acute fulminant or chronic recrudescent cardiomyopathy. Biventricular failure is dose related, increased risk when dose >550 mg/m^2 and with advancing age. Echocardiography prior to treatment with adriamycin and post if symptoms develop will help in early DX and further progression of heart failure by altering treatment regimens. High dose cyclophosphamide and busulfan can cause cardiotoxicity too. Interleukins

can cause sepsis like syndrome with vasodilatation and hypotension.

• Pulmonary: Interstitial lung disease bronchiolitis obliterans and organizing pneumonia (BOOP), and predisposition to O$_2$ toxicity. Bleomycin, busulfan and the monoclonal antibodies (Rituximab, cetuximab, bevacizumab, alemtuzumab) can predispose to interstitial lung disease. Gemcitabine can cause pneumonitis and fibrosis. Serial estimation of DLCO can help diagnose onset of interstitial lung disease at an early stage. Vincristine can cause severe bronchospasm during its administration. Carmustine and lomustine can cause delayed pulm fibrosis. Interleukins can cause pulm edema from leaky capillaries.

• Hematology: All chemotherapeutic agents cause cytopenia. Severe bone marrow depression is more frequent with alkylating agents, antimetabolites, plant alkaloids, antibiotics and nitrosoureas. Aplastic anemia, anemia, thrombocytopenia and neutropenia predispose to increased risk of infection and hemorrhage.

• Nervous system: Acute cerebellar syndrome with 5FU. Methotrexate can cause leukoencephalopathy. Vincristine can cause autonomic and PNS toxicity. Cyclophosphamide and ifosfamide can cause water retention with resultant hyponatremia and coma. High dose cis-platinum can cause ocular toxicity.

• Renal: Hemorrhagic cystitis with ifosfamide and cyclophosphamide. Methotrexate can cause renal tubular necrosis. Streptozocin can be nephrotoxic.

• Hepatobiliary: 6-Mercaptopurine, thioguanine, mithramycin and L-asparginase can be hepatotoxic.

• Immune suppression: All chemotherapeutic agents cause immune suppression from neutropenia, but the incidence is higher with alkylating agents, antimetabolites and plant alkaloids.

• Fluid and electrolytes: Interleukins cause capillary leak syndrome similar to systemic sepsis, resulting in fluid retention causing airway and pulm edema and circulatory instability. Treatment cycles of acute leukemias, lymphomas, particularly Burkett lymphoma, can be complicated by tumor necrosis syndrome due to rapid cell destruction (high sensitivity to chemotherapy).

• Endocrine: Use of steroids with chemotherapeutic agents impairs blood sugar control. Steroids can cause wt gain, truncal obesity and moon facies.

Anesthetic Implications

• Drug interactions: Prolongation of succinylcholine by inhibition of psudocholinesterase (cytoxan)

• Vincristine causes muscle wasting; therefore, risk of hyperkalemia with succinylcholine. Thiotepa can further prolong pancuronium. NSAIDs can elevate methotrexate levels. Procarbazine can exaggerate CNS depression of sedatives and analgesics, therefore consider careful titration of analgesics and CNS depressants.

• Airway: Cytopenias, particularly thrombocytopenia, can result in easy bruising and airway hemorrhage/bleeding can complicate laryngoscopy and intubation. High dose steroid regimen can result in moon facies and airway edema. Stomatitis and mucosal dryness accompanies many chemotherapy regimens predisposing to easy mucosal bruising even with gentle airway manipulation.

• Venous access: Chemotherapeutic agents cause venous sclerosis, and IV access can be difficult. Will often require a semipermanent central venous access (portacath/PICC lines).

• Pulmonary: High inspired O$_2$ concentration can cause pulm toxicity in pts treated with bleomycin. Chemotherapy induced pulm toxicity can present as restrictive lung disease.

• Renal: Chemotherapy induced impaired renal function can alter drug excretion of some active metabolites. Periop NSAIDs can worsen pre-existing renal disease. Risk of postop renal failure is high when renal function is already impaired.

• Neuropathy: Care with positioning; careful documentation of pre-existing neuropathy prior to performing regional techniques.

• Hematology: Thrombocytopenia can increase the risk of hematoma; low plt count may contraindicate neuraxial anesthesia. May require transfusions due to anemia/aplastic anemia.

• Photodynamic therapy (profimer): Pts are extremely photosensitive, will need to be in a location without bright lights.

Chloramphenicol (Chloromycetin)

Henry A. Hawney
Joseph R. Koveleskie

Uses

- Infections such as typhoid fever, meningitis (*Haemophilus influenzae, Neisseria meningitidis, Streptococcus pneumoniae*), plague (*yersinia pestis*), and rickettsiosis not treatable with other antibiotics
- Infections in pts with hypersensitivity to penicillin

Risks

- Anemia (dose dependent), aplastic anemia (dose independent)
- P450 (CYP) inhibition

- Grey Baby Syndrome (in premature infants because of the lack of liver UDP-glucuronyl-transferase)

Worry About

- Increased $T_{1/2}$ of dicumarol, warfarin, chlorpropamide, phenytoin, tolbutamide

Overview/Pharmacology

- Inhibition of protein synthesis by interfering with the incorporation of amino acids into ribosomes (inhibits 50S peptidyltransferase, bacteriostatic)
- Active against gram-positive and gram-negative bacteria incl *Salmonella typhi*, *Proteus*, and *Rickettsia*

- Decreases P450 (CYP—multiple isoforms) activity thus changing $T_{1/2}$ of P450-dependent drugs such as warfarin (see above)

Drug Class/Usual Dose

- Antibiotic for otherwise intractable gram-negative infections (e.g., salmonellosis, *Haemophilus influenzae*, meningitis)
- Usual dosage: 50 mg/kg/d IV in divided doses

Drug Effects

- Newborns who cannot glucuronide-conjugate chloramphenicol may develop abd distention, cyanosis, vascular collapse, and death (rare) known as Grey Baby Syndrome

DRUG EFFECTS

System	Effect	Test
GI	N/V	
HEME	Agranulocytosis, aplastic anemia	CBC

Key References: Chambers Henry F. *Protein synthesis inhibitors and miscellaneous antibacterial agents* (Chapter). [Chapter 46]. Brunton LL, Lazo JS, Parker KL. *Goodman & Gilman's the pharmacological basis of therapeutics*. 11th ed. http://www.accessmedicine.com/content.aspx?aID=949328. Berliner N. Clinical disorders of neutrophils. In: Andreoli TE, Carpenter CC, Griggs RC, Loscalzo J, eds. *Cecil essentials of medicine*. 6th ed. Philadelphia: Saunders; 2004:464. Murray M. Disaster preparedness. In: Barash PG, Cullen BF, Stoelting RK, Cahalan MK, Stock MC, eds. *Clinical anesthesia*, 6th ed. Philadelphia: Lippincott Williams and Wilkins; 2009:1570–1571.

Perioperative Implications/Possible Drug Interactions

- Acute prolongation of action of dicumarol, chlorpropamide
- Action: Assess clotting status
- Chronic use: Assess status of bone marrow

Anticipated Problems/Concerns

- Expect prolonged/increased action of drugs predominantly cleared via P450 (CYP) biotransformation

Cimetidine

Michael F. Roizen

Uses

- Incidence in USA: >1,000,000 plus
- Rx for ulcers, gastric reflux, gastric hypersecretion
- High levels assoc with confusional states in elderly

Perioperative Risks

- Drug interactions esp. with local anesthetics (↑ toxicity), aldomet, clonidine (CNS toxicity)

Worry About

- Decreased hepatic P450 clearance of drugs, ↓ hepatic blood flow, ↑ fentanyl, phenothiazine, β-blocker drug, lidocaine, with ↑ potential for toxicity

Overview/Pharmacology

- H$_2$ antagonist
- Cleared by renal excretion; ↓ dosage intervals to 12 hr with Cr clearance of 0–20 mL/min/1.73 m^2
- Decreased hepatic metab of drugs requiring specific cytochrome P450 (β-blocking agents, Ca^{2+}-channel blockers, theophylline, phenothiazines) or drugs requiring liver for first-pass metab (by ↓ hepatic blood flow—lidocaine, β-blocking agents)

Drug Class/Mechanism of Action/Usual Dose

- H$_2$ antagonist
- Chronically taken for ulcer Rx, prophylaxis or to raise gastric pH for prophylaxis or Rx of gastric reflux
- Acutely taken for prophylaxis against pulm aspiration and part of prophylaxis against immune or nonimmune CV effects from immune or non-immune release of H$_2$
- Usual dose: 100–300 mg bid
- Alternatives
  - Other H$_2$ antagonists; longer-acting agents have displaced much of use; now available OTC
  - Antibiotics to ↓ *Helicobacter pylori* (tetracycline + metronidazole + bismuth)

DRUG EFFECTS

System	Effect	PE	Test
HEPATIC	↓ Hepatic drug metab ↓ Hepatic blood flow		
GI	↓ Gastric acid secretion		
ENDO	Weak antiandrogenic effect; gynecomastia (men)	Gynecomastia	
GU	Renal		BUN, Cr
	Placenta—crosses placental barrier, excreted in milk		
CNS	Poor penetration to CNS; with high doses in pts, esp. with impaired renal function, assoc with disorientation to coma	CNS exam	

Key References: Lam AM, Parkin JA. Cimetidine and prolonged post-operative somnolence. *Can J Anaesth*. 1981;28:450. Sawyer D, Conner CS, Scalley R. Cimetidine: Adverse reactions and acute toxicity. *Am J Hosp Pharm*. 1981;38:188–197.

Perioperative Implications/Possible Drug Interactions

Preoperative Concerns

- Cimetidine + clonidine or aldomet assoc with CNS dysfunction
- Decreased clearance of phenothiazines, phenytoin, theophylline

Induction/Maintenance

- Fentanyl T$_{1/2}$ may be prolonged 2° to direct or indirect ↓ in hepatic BF by cimetidine

Adjuvants/Regional Anesthesia/Reversal

- Increased biologic availability of lidocaine and other local anesthetics and thus toxicity
- Increased NMB agent requirements anecdotally reported (mechanism unknown)

Anticipated Problems/Concerns

- Decreased hepatic P450 clearance of drugs, ↓ hepatic blood flow; ↑ fentanyl, phenothiazine, β-blocking drug, lidocaine potential for toxicity
- CNS dysfunction by itself (esp. in aged and those with ↓ renal function) or with clonidine and aldomet

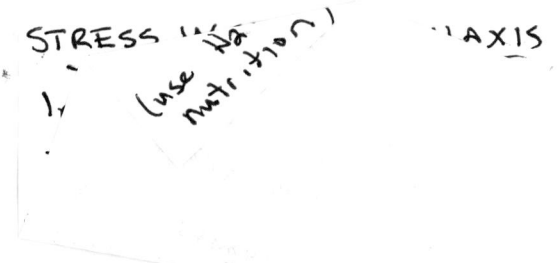

Cisplatin

Joseph F. Foss

Uses (See also Chemotherapeutic Agents)

• Pts undergoing chemotherapy for testicular, ovarian, or bladder cancer

Perioperative Risks

• End-organ damage, esp. renal and neurotoxicity

• Renal toxicity prominent, seen in 28–36% of pts after 1 dose: Effect cumulative, minimized by aggressive hydration, allowing renal function to return to baseline between treatments

• Decrease in renal tubular function is dose-related, typically occurs during 2nd wk of administration

• Hyperuricemia, hypomagnesemia, hypocalcemia, hyponatremia, hypokalemia, hypophosphatemia have been reported and are related to renal tubular damage. Allopurinol Rx reduces uric acid levels.

• Neurotoxicity happens to 85% of pts at total dose over 300 mg/m². Peripheral sensory neuropathy, hearing loss, autonomic neuropathy, Lhermitte's sign (electrical sensation running down the back and into the arms), seizures, and encephalopathy predominate.

Pharmacokinetics/Pharmacodynamics

• Reaches site of action by diffusion

• High concentrations in kidneys, liver, prostate, intestines, testes; low CNS penetration

• $T_{1/2}$ 20–30 min following bolus administration or infusion of 50 or 100 mg/m²; clearance is 15–16 L/h/m²; vol of distribution, 11–12 L/m²

• Highly protein-bound, poorly dialyzable

• Cleared renally at rate greater than that of Cr; 13–17% of parent compound excreted within 1 hr after administration

Drug Class/Mechanism of Action/Usual Dose

• Inorganic platinum-containing compound (*cis*-diamminedichloroplatinum [*cis*-DDP])

• Disrupts DNA helix, preventing duplication

• In chemotherapy of metastatic ovarian and testicular CA and advanced bladder CA, often used in combination with other drugs, particularly cyclophosphamide (Cytoxan)

• Contraindicated (relatively) in pts with pre-existing renal disease, hearing loss, myelosuppression; use of other nephrotoxic or ototoxic agents (e.g., aminoglycosides) may increase toxicity

• Must be administered IV (See the current oncology literature for dosage, administration guidelines, and protocols. Has been used in doses of 20 mg/m² for 5 d for testicular cancer, 75–100 mg/m² once every 4 wk for ovarian tumors in combination with other agents, 50–70 mg/m² for advanced bladder CA.)

• Pretreatment hydration of 1–2 L over 12 h before administration and infusion of *cis*-DDP in a dilute vol with mannitol recommended. Repeat courses usually not given until renal function returns to baseline, circulating blood elements are at acceptable levels, and audiometric and hepatic function monitoring have been completed.

DRUG EFFECTS

System	Effect	Assessment by Hx	PE	Test
HEENT	Ototoxicity (31% of pts) manifested as tinnitus or loss of hearing; more pronounced in children	Total exposure		Audiometry
CARDIO	Anaphylactic-like reactions with edema, bronchospasm reported Cardiac dysrhythmias reported	SOB after administration, palpitations	CV exam	ECG
HEPAT	Transient elevations in liver enzymes reported with use of *cis*-DDP			Hepatic transaminases
GI	N/V severe, triggered by action at chemoreceptor trigger zone of medulla	N/V within 1–4 hr up to 24 hr		
HEME	Mild–moderate myelosuppression (25–30%)			CBC
GU	Renal toxicity – typically nonoliguric with increased loss of water, electrolytes, and hypomagenesemia			BUN, Cr, electrolytes, Mg²⁺
CNS	Hearing loss, autonomic neuropathy, and encephalopathy. Seizures with high acute doses.			
MS	Peripheral neuropathies in a stocking/glove distribution with prolonged Rx of 4–7 mo	Total exposure (>300 mg/m^2)	Neuro exam	Pinprick vibration

Key References: Tomioka S, Kurio T, Takaishi K, Nakajo N. Propofol is effective in chemotherapy-induced nausea and vomiting: A case report with quantitative analysis. *Anesth Analg.* 1999;89:798–799; Siddek ZH. Cisplatin: mode of cytotoxic action and molecular basis of resistance *Oncogene.* 2003;22:7265–7279.

Perioperative Implications

Preoperative Concerns

• Determine the total exposure of the pt as most toxicities are related to total dose

• Estimate GFR from serum creatinine or post-chemotherapy studies of renal function

Adjuvants/Regional Anesthesia/Reversal

• One case report of a 14-y female pt who experienced profound nerve injury after an interscalene block with bupivicaine and epinephrine and after having had previous extensive chemotherapy which incl cisplatin (840 mg/m^2) (Hebl et al. *Anesthesia & Analgesia* (2001), 92: (1): p. 249).

Drug Interactions

• Plasma levels of anticonvulsants may become subtherapeutic with the use of cisplatin.

• ↓ Clearance of renally excreted drugs in proportion to previous damage

• Avoid aminoglycosides (increased toxicity)

Anticipated Problems/Concerns

• Should not be administered through needles or IV sets containing aluminum, which reacts with cisplatin, causing precipitation

• *Cis*-DDP and equipment used for administration should be handled as potentially carcinogenic

• May be irritating to the skin; if extravasated may cause local soft tissue toxicity

Clopidogrel Bisulfate

Ann C. Duncan
Zachary D. Bush
Lee A. Fleisher

Uses

• Indicated for reduction of atherosclerotic events in pts with known atherosclerosis confirmed by recent stroke, TIA, MI, or established arterial disease; after PCI with or without stent placement

Perioperative Risks

• Increased risk of bleeding if not D/C 5 d before surgery
• Risk of coronary events increase post stent placement if full course of post procedure antiplatelet therapy is not completed. Risk in drug-eluting stent (DES) may persist for years if clopidogrel D/C

Worry About

• Hypersensitivity reactions (rare): Bronchospasms, angioedema, and anaphylactoid reactions
• Increased bleeding intra- and postop
• Elective surgery undertaken <4 to 6 wk from bare metal coronary stent (BMS) placement

demonstrated a high occurrence of stent thrombosis. Elective surgery <365 d after DES demonstrated high rate of stent thrombosis. It is recommended to postpone elective noncardiac surgery until the course of antiplatelet treatment is completed, thus reducing the risk of bleeding complications and stent thrombosis. 5-7 d delay recommended after D/C.
• Black Box Warning: Variant alleles for the cytochrome P450 enzymes, specifically CYP2C19, have been shown to decrease the conversion of clopidogrel to its active metabolite. Poor metabolizers (mainly Caucasians/Asians) may not receive full drug benefit. Pharmacogenomic testing is available.

Overview/Pharmacology

• Inhibitor of plt aggregation. Active metabolite irreversibly modifies the plt ADP receptor, affecting the plt for its entire lifespan after exposure.

• Plt inhibition can be seen within 2 hr of loading dose (300–600 mg) of clopidogrel bisulfate with steady-state of inhibition reached between d 3 and 7 (maintenance dose 75–150 mg)
• Bleeding time and plt aggregation returned to baseline in 5 d after D/C.
• Metabolized: Liver
• Excretion: urine, feces, and breast milk

Drug Class/Usual Dose

• Antiplatelet
• Normal metabolizers: 75 mg PO daily (no effect whether taken with meals or not)
• Slow metabolizers: 150 mg PO daily

Contraindications

• Hypersensitivity to the drug or components of it
• Active pathologic bleeding such as intracranial bleeding or peptic ulcers
• CYP2C19 poor metabolizers
• PPIs diminish the antiplatelet effect of clopidogrel's active metabolite

DRUG EFFECTS

System	Effect	Assessment by Hx	PE	Test
CARDIO	Edema, Htn	MI, stroke, established PVD	Pulse, rales	ECG, BP
CNS	Headache, dizziness, pain, depression, and fatigue, intracranial hemorrhage	Intracranial hemorrhage	↑LOC	CT scan (if indicated)
GI	Abd pain, dyspepsia, diarrhea, nausea, GI hemorrhage	GI hemorrhage	Stool guaiac	Bleeding time
GU	UTI			
HEME	Anemia, purpura, epistaxis, bleeding	TTP (rare)		Bleeding time
RESP	Upper resp infections, rhinitis, coughing, bronchitis, sinusitis, pneumonia		Lung auscultation	
ENDO/METAB	Hypercholesterolemia			Cholesterol level
DERM	Rash, pruritus	Rash, pruritus	Rash, pruritus	
MS	Back pain and arthralgia, arthrosis hypoesthesia	Back pain and arthralgia		

Key References: Fleisher LA, Beckman JA, et al. 2009 ACCF/AHA focused update on perioperative beta blockade incorporated into the ACC/AHA 2007 guidelines on perioperative cardiovascular evaluation and care for noncardiac surgery: A Report of the American College of Cardiology Foundation/American Heart Association Task Force on Practice Guidelines. *Circulation.* 2009;120(21):e169–e276.

Possible Drug Interactions/Perioperative Implications

• Markedly ↑ risk of surgical bleeding if D/C <5 d. Decision to continue or D/C drug depends on risk of surgical bleeding versus risk of coronary thrombosis. Discussion between cardiologist/surgeon/anesthesiologist critical.

• Avoid use with CYP2C19 inhibitors (e.g., Prilosec)
• Use with NSAIDs increases GI bleeding risk
• Concomitant use with warfarin increases bleeding risk.

Cocaine

Zeev N. Kain
Sharon L. Lin

Risk

- Prevalence: 5 million regular users; 36 million in USA have tried drug (14% of population)
- Abuse in the OB population 7.5– 45%
- Most frequent cause of drug-related death reported by medical examiners

Perioperative Risks

- Hemodynamic instability, ↑ sympathetic discharge
- Myocardial ischemia
  - Increased myocardial O_2 demand (↑ HR, ↑ BP, ↑ LV contractility)
  - Decreased myocardial O_2 supply (↑ endothelin, ↓ NO resulting in coronary vasoconstriction)

Worry About

- CV: Htn, tachycardia, dysrhythmias, MI, cardiomyopathy, premature coronary atherosclerosis, sudden cardiac death
- Neurologic: Intracerebral bleed, seizures
- Pulmonary: Pneumomediastinum, cocaine-induced asthma, hypersensitivity pneumonitis, chronic cough, pulm edema, diffusing capacity abn
- OB: Placenta previa, abruptio placentae, premature labor, fetal distress

Overview/Pharmacology

- Cocaine is an ester local anesthetic and sodium-channel blocking drug, classified as a Class I antiarrhythmic agent
- Blocks presynaptic reuptake of norepinephrine, dopamine, and serotonin, resulting in activation of SNS
- May produce negative inotropic, chronotropic effects on heart muscle
- Impairs reuptake in brain of dopamine, serotonin, tryptophan
- Accumulation of dopamine in synaptic cleft may lead to acute euphoria, increased alertness
- Cocaine 4% topical solution is FDA-approved as a local anesthetic used on mucous membranes. Cocaine is useful for ENT surgery and for an awake fiberoptic intubation (not to exceed 3 mg/kg; 1 mg/kg is recommended)

ICD-9-CM Codes: 305.6 (Nondependent); 364.2 (Dependent)

Etiology

- Cocaine abuse
- OD during ENT surgery; ER use (part of tetracaine, epinephrine, cocaine mix)

Usual Treatment

- Supportive
- Myocardial ischemia induced by cocaine should be treated initially with O_2, sublingual aspirin, and benzodiazepines. If there is ongoing ischemia, use of nitroglycerine, verapamil, or phentolamine to reverse cocaine-induced coronary vasoconstriction may be necessary.
- β-Blockers may worsen coronary vasoconstriction and should be used with great caution if pt presents with signs of ischemia or acute cocaine toxicity.
- In management of short-lived arrhythmias, drug treatment should be avoided if possible, as antiarrhythmic agents and cocaine may have a synergistic depression of contractile function.
- For sustained hemodynamically tolerated SVT assoc with AV nodal re-entry, adenosine is safe and free of major side effects. If adenosine is unsuccessful, administration of an α-antagonist and a β-blocker in combination is likely to be both safe and effective. No reliable information on the safety and efficacy of other antiarrhythmic drugs.
- *Supraventricular or ventricular tachyarrhythmias* assoc with hemodynamic compromise require urgent DC cardioversion.

DRUG EFFECTS

System	Effect	Assessment by Hx	PE	Test
CARDIO	Htn, MI, dysrhythmias, myocarditis, cardiomyopathy, aortic dissection, endocarditis, premature coronary atherosclerosis, prolonged QT	Exposure Chest pain Palpitations	BP/HR Murmur	ECG ECHO CK-MB, troponin I & T
RESP	Pneumomediastinum, bronchoconstriction, pneumothorax, diffuse alveolar hemorrhage, pulm edema	Exposure Hemoptysis SOB	Wheezing Rales	CXR
HEME	Thrombocytopenia, enhanced plt aggregation promoting thrombus formation	Bleeding problems, vasoconstriction		Plt
OB	Preterm labor, premature rupture of membranes, abruptio placentae, spontaneous abortion, meconium-stained amniotic fluid	Exposure Uterine contractions Abd pain	Vaginal bleeding	US
GU	Rhabdomyolysis, ARF, ESRD	Exposure	Oliguria, anuria	K+, Cr, CK, urine myoglobin
CNS	Subarachnoid hemorrhage, intracerebral bleed, seizures, CVA	Headache, N/V	Neuro exam	CT scan

Key Reference: Lange RA, Hillis LD. cardiovascular complications of cocaine use. *N Engl J Med.* 2001;345:(5): 351–358.

Perioperative Implications

Preoperative Concerns

- Self-reporting of drug abuse unreliable, 35–55% deny cocaine use but have at least 1 positive urine assay
- Hx of smoking, alcohol use, positive syphilis serology, and use of other illicit drugs should alert to possibility of cocaine abuse.
- Difficult IV access due to sclerosis of peripheral veins
- Consider urine screen (reliable for only 14–60 hr after use).

Monitoring

- Routine
- Consider arterial line if Hx of acute intoxication, recent exposure

Airway

- Intranasal cocaine use may cause perforation of nasal septum, oropharyngeal ulcers, or chronic sinusitis

Preinduction/Induction

- Benzodiazepines are helpful to decrease HR and BP
- Increased anesthetic requirements possibly from acute cocaine exposure
- Usage of succinylcholine in acutely intoxicated pt may be assoc with prolonged paralysis, since cocaine is also metabolized by plasma cholinesterase
- Use ketamine with caution; it potentiates CV toxicity of cocaine.
- Spinal anesthesia possibly assoc with more frequent episodes of hypotension

Maintenance

- Myocardial ischemia may manifest as CV instability, ECG changes
- Increased catecholamine levels due to inadequate anesthesia, cocaine in blood may result in cardiac dysrhythmias.

- Temp rise, sympathomimetic effects assoc with cocaine can mimic malignant hyperthermia

Extubation

- No special issues

Adjuvants

- Ester local anesthetics and succinylcholine, which undergo metabolism by plasma ChE, may compete with cocaine, resulting in decreased metabolism of both
- Cocaine decreases seizure threshold, enhances convulsant effect of other local anesthetics.

Postoperative Period

- Myocardial ischemia
- Pain medication requirements in chronic abusers are same as for nonabusers.

Cromolyn Sodium

Gregory A. Wolff
Christopher Ciarallo

Uses

- Approved by the FDA in 1973 as the first prophylactic nonsteroidal drug available for treatment of chronic asthma
- Alternative initial maintenance therapy for mild persistent and moderate persistent asthma
- Preventative only. Not effective during acute episodes of bronchospasm
- Most beneficial for allergic-component and exercise-induced asthma
- May be beneficial in allergic rhinitis and atopic ocular diseases
- Oral formulations for the management of mastocytosis, ulcerative colitis, and food allergies

Overview/Pharmacology

- Inhibits antigen-induced degranulation of pulm mast cells, eosinophils, neutrophils, monocytes, and lymphocytes
- Prevents release of histamine, leukotrienes, and other autacoids
- Reverses and suppresses leukocyte activation
- Inhibits cough reflex
- Does not directly relax bronchial smooth muscle
- No apparent steroid-sparing effect; inferior to inhaled corticosteroids on measures of lung function and morbidity in 2006 Cochrane Review.
- Administered by inhalation route to treat asthma
- 8–10% of inhaled dose reaches lung parenchyma and is readily absorbed
- $T_{1/2}$ = 80–90 min; peak plasma concentration within 15 min
- Active drug excreted unchanged in urine (50%) and bile (50%)
- Can be taken prophylactically 15–20 min before exercise or exposure to known allergen to prevent bronchospasm

Drug Class/Mechanism of Action

- Cromolyn sodium (disodium cromoglycate) is a derivative of 2–chromone–carboxylic acid
- Direct mechanism of action in asthma is poorly defined
  - One proposed explanation is ↓ in accumulation of intracellular Ca^{2+} in sensitized mast cells
  - Another possible mechanism is Cl^- channel blockade in antigen-sensitized pulm C-fibers
- Effective in preventing degranulation of mast cells only if given prior to antigenic challenge

Usual Dose

- Cromolyn sodium for inhalation (Intal) via special nebulizer (20 mg/2 ml) or metered spray (2 puffs [1 mg/puff] 3–4 times daily for asthma)
- 4% liquid nasal spray (Nasalcrom) given as 1 spray to each nostril 3–6 times daily for allergic rhinitis
- 4% ophthalmic solution (Opticrom) given as 1–2 drops to each eye 4–6 times daily for atopic eye conditions

DRUG EFFECTS

System	Effect	Assessment by Hx	Test
RESP	Inhibition of pulm mast cell degranulation; ↓ release of histamine and leukotrienes; reverse or suppress leukocyte activation	↓ Episodes of exercise- or antigen-induced bronchospasm after chronic use	↓ Bronchial hyperactivity as measured by histamine or methacholine challenge

Key Reference: Undem BJ. Pharmacotherapy of asthma. In: Brunton LL, Lazo JS, Parker KL, eds. *Goodman & Gilman's the pharmacological basis of therapeutics*, 11th ed. New York: McGraw-Hill Medical; 2006:717–736.

Perioperative Implications/Possible Drug Interactions

- Continue administration periop. Do not D/C abruptly.
- Cromolyn sodium is of no benefit in treating an acute exacerbation of asthma.
- Adverse effects are infrequent
  - Unpleasant taste (most common)
  - Direct irritation (e.g., wheezing, coughing)
  - Dizziness, nausea, rash
  - Urticaria, anaphylaxis (extremely rare)
- No significant drug-drug interactions with cromolyn sodium are known.
- Compatible in nebulized solution with albuterol, levalbuterol, ipratropium, and budesonide
- Pregnancy Category B. No known evidence of teratogenicity.

Dexmedetomidine (Precedex)

Ori Gottlieb

Uses

- Alpha-2-adrenergic agonist
- Sedation of intubated pts in an intensive care setting
- Sedation of non-intubated pts prior to and/or during surgical and other procedures
- Anxiolytic for use during awake fiberoptic intubations and cases where monitored anesthesia care is appropriate
- May continue infusion during extubation as does not cause resp depression
- Useful in awake craniotomy which requires intact cooperative mental status
- Pediatric sedation in the NICU/PICU and for specific procedures (e.g., MRI)

Perioperative Risks

- Initially ↑ BP and ↓ HR (esp. when bolus used)

- After the delay assoc with the alpha-2 negative feedback loop, BP may drop due to a decrease in plasma norepinephrine levels

Worry About

- CV effects if bolus is used (↑ BP and ↓ HR)
- Recall: No amnestic component to its sedation
- Consider reducing dose in hepatic failure. Titrate to effect.
- Dosing in renal failure unchanged as no known active metabolites
- Education is vital as the pt will likely be more aware and/or cooperative than with other sedatives. This is esp. important in the ICU where nurses and/or physicians are used to a less cooperative mental status from sedated pts.

Overview/Pharmacology

- Imidazoline derivative with direct effect at the presynaptic alpha-2 receptors induces a drop in cAMP production by inhibitory G proteins.

- Alpha-2 specific over alpha-1 is 1600:1
- Direct peripheral postsynaptic activation causes vasoconstriction → increased BP

Drug Class/Mechanism of Action/Usual Dose

- Imidazoline derive; highly selective alpha-2 agonist
- Alpha-2 receptors in brainstem (locus ceruleus) induce less alertness or sedation
- ICU sedation: 0.2–0.7 mcg/kg/hr
- Awake FOI/MAC sedation: 0.2–1 mcg/kg/hr
- Bolus in PI labeled at 1 mcg/kg over 10 min. Beware CV effects.
- Allow 15–20 min of infusion for effect if dosing without bolus.

DRUG EFFECTS

System	Effect	Assessment by Hx	PE	Test
CARDIO	Initial ↑ BP followed by ↓ BP Bradycardia			BP ECG
RESP	None	None	SpO_2/$ETCO_2$	
CNS	Cooperative sedation Reduces MAC requirements of inhaled agents	Mental status/responsiveness	Anxiolysis	VAS
Other	Antisialagogue Analgesic adjunct	Xerostomia Patient feedback	Dry mouth	VAS

Key Reference: Riker RR, et al. Dexmedetomidine vs. midazolam for sedation of critically Ill patients: A randomized trial. *JAMA.* 2009;301:489–499.

Perioperative Implications

Preoperative Concerns
- May be used as an anxiolytic, esp. where resp depression is detrimental

Induction/Maintenance
- Bolus achieves faster sedation at the risk of ↑ BP and ↓ HR

- Infusion reduces inhaled agent requirements – useful for cases that require neuromonitoring (e.g., SSEP) where a balanced anesthetic approach desirable
- May continue infusion while extubating the pt—for more stable course
- Recommend D/C infusion 20 min prior to end of case if rapid return to baseline mental status desired

Postoperative Period
- Useful in the postop period to reduce narcotic requirements in those at risk for pulm complications (e.g., morbidly obese, obstructive sleep apnea)
- Unlike with clonidine, rapid withdrawal is not problematic.

DRUGS

Digitalis (Digoxin)

Amit Asopa
Swaminathan Karthik

Uses

- A glycoside extracted from leaves of the foxglove (digitalis lanata), available in oral and IV preparations
- Treatment of CHF, atrial fibrillation and flutter.
- Avoid in pts with ventricular extrasystole or VT, as it may precipitate VF due to increased cardiac excitability.
- Prevention of supraventricular arrhythmias following thoracotomy
- Narrow therapeutic range —2 mcg/L
- Cardiac side effects: Arrhythmias and conduction disturbances

- Noncardiac side effects: GI—anorexia, N/V, and abd pain: CNS—visual disturbances, headache, drowsiness, confusion

Perioperative Risks

- Cardiac arrhythmia (toxicity) can be precipitated by hypokalemia, hypomagnesemia, hypoxia, hypercalcemia, hypernatremia, and renal failure
- DC cardioversion can cause severe ventricular arrhythmias in pts with toxic levels
- AV block (with co-administration of β-adrenergic, Ca^{2+}-channel blocking drugs)

Worry About

- Hyperventilation can cause alkalosis leading to relative hypokalemia-toxicity.
- Renal insufficiency (decreased digoxin clearance and need for dose alteration, not appreciably removed by dialysis)

Overview/Pharmacology

- General pharmacologic effect: Positive inotropic and slowing of ventricular response

DOSING/PHARMACOKINETICS

Drug		Onset	Peak	$T_{\frac{1}{2}}$	Dose	
					Initial	Maintenance
Digoxin:	IV	5–30 min	1–3 hr	34 hr	0.5–1.0 mg	0.25 mg/d
	PO	1–3 hr	4–6 hr	34 hr	0.75–1.2 mg	0.125–0.5 mg/d
Digitoxin: PO		3–6 hr	6–12 hr	7 d	0.8–1.2 mg	0.05–0.3 mg/d

Excretion

- Digoxin: Renal, mostly unchanged; ↓ dose for ↑ Cr
- Digitoxin: Hepatic degradation

Drug Interactions

- Diuretics: ↓ serum K^+, ↑ toxicity
- Plasma levels increased by quinidine, amiodarone, verapamil, captopril, erythromycin
- Plasma levels decreased by antacids, phenytoin, metoclopramide, and cholestyramine

Treatment for Toxicity

- Due to Na^+/K^+ ATPase inhibition, hyperkalemia may be a feature and should be corrected
- Hypokalemia exacerbates toxicity and should be corrected.
- Severe bradycardia: Atropine or pacing preferred over catecholamines
- Ventricular arrythmias: Treat with lidocaine or phenytoin
- Digoxin specific Fab: Indicated for digoxin levels >10 mcg/L, life-threatening arrhythmias or uncontrolled hyperkalemia

Drug Class/Mechanism of Action

- Direct action: Inhibition of Na^+, K^+-ATPase, producing ↑ intracellular Na^+ ↓ K^+, resulting in increased intracellular Ca^{2+}, leading to positive inotropic effect.
- Decrease K^+ intracellular: slowing of AV conduction and of the pacemaker cell
- Indirect effect: Enhances release of acetylcholine at the cardiac muscarinic receptors-This slows conduction and prolongs the refractory period in AV node and bundle of his.

DRUG EFFECTS

System	Effect	Assessment by Hx	Pe	Test
HEENT			↓ JVD	
CARDIO	↓ HR, ↑ CO Arrhythmia from toxicity	↓ SOB, orthopnea Palpitations	↓ HR rate, size Irregular pulse	CXR: ↓ Heart size ECG: Any arrhythmia except AFib
RESP	↓ Congestion	↓ SOB, orthopnea	↓ Rales	CXR: ↓ Pulm edema
GI	Anorexia from toxicity			Serum digoxin >2 ng/ml
CNS	Headache, confusion from toxicity			Serum digoxin >2 ng/ml
MS	Fatigue from toxicity—and confusion brain often more affected than heart—can be cause of reversible cognitive dysfunction			Serum digoxin >2 ng/ml

Key References: Hood WB, Dans A, Guyatt GH, Jaeschke R, McMurray J. Digitalis for treatment of congestive heart failure in patients in sinus rhythm (Cochrane Review). *Cochrane Database Syst Rev.* 2004;CD002901. Eichhorn EJ, Gheorhiade M. Digoxin. *Prog Cardiovasc Dis.* 2002;44:251–266. PMID: 12007081.

Perioperative Implications

Preoperative Concerns

- Do not D/C digitalis preop. Withdrawal in heart failure pts may lead to recurrence of failure symptoms
- When changing from oral to IV therapy, dosage should be reduced by 20% to 25%.
- Correct and maintain serum K^+.
- Decreasing dose with increasing serum Cr

Possible Drug Interactions

- Decrease AV block with β-adrenergic, amiodarone and Ca^{2+}-channel blocking drugs
- Decrease dose with concurrent quinidine therapy

Anticipated Problems/Concerns

- Ventricular rate with AFib and/or AFLT is a rough bioassay for digoxin level; fast ventricular rate with AFib indicates inadequate serum level of digoxin.

- Digoxin is the only positive inotropic, antiarrhythmic (for atrial fib/flutter) drug available; drug of choice for this arrhythmia in pt with a failing heart
- Digoxin may depress CNS function in elderly more than it decreases AV nodal conduction
- Treatment of digoxin toxicity

Diuretics

Christopher Giordano
Nikolaus Gravenstein

Indications

- Prescribed for pts with Htn, CHF, elevated ICP, edema, hemoglobinuria, low intraop UO
- Mannitol *may* function as a renal preservative by free-radical scavenging and toxin dilution
- Fenoldopam is a selective dopamine-1 agonist. As a vasodilator, it lowers BP and augments renal blood flow which improves UO and GFR. It may serve as a renal protectant. Usual dose begins at 0.03 μg/kg/min titrated to effect.

Perioperative Risks

- Hypokalemia
- Hypovolemia
- Low intraop UO
- Hyperkalemia with aldosterone antagonists
- Hypomagnesemia

Worry About

- Hypokalemia, hypovolemia
- Low intraop UO if hold usual diuretic preop

- Hypokalemia provoking and/or aggravating digitalis toxicity
- Deafness with ECA (ethacrynic acid)
- Nephrotoxicity of cephaloridine is enhanced by furosemide
- End result of diuretic use is ↑ UO with net loss of H_2O and solute esp K^+, Mg^{++}
- Onset of diuresis is within 10 min after IV administration
- With exception of aldosterone antagonist and K^+-sparing diuretics, all others cause K^+ loss
- Serum K^+ <3.5 mEq/L in 15% of pts, <3.0 mEq/L in up to 10% of diuretic-treated pts
- Chronic diuretic-induced hypokalemia is less arrhythmogenic than acute, but serum K^+ <3.0 mEq/L assoc with 2-fold greater incidence of ventricular arrhythmias than K^+ >3.0 mEq/L
- Site-specific action assoc with additional effect if diuretics from 2 classes used

Drug Class/Mechanism of Action/Usual Dose

- Diuretics belong to osmotic, carbonic anhydrase inhibition, benzothiadiazide, high-ceiling (loop), K^+-sparing, or aldosterone antagonist class of drugs, based on mechanism of action
- Only osmotic and loop diuretics used intraop
- Osmotic diuretic: Mannitol—ascending loop, limits H_2O reabsorption; onset of action 5–15 min after IV dose; renal clearance
  - Usual dose: Mannitol 0.25–2.0 g/kg (give as drip and not bolus to avoid hypotension)
- Loop diuretics—ascending loop, limit NaCl reabsorption; onset of action 5 min after IV dose; $T_{\frac{1}{2}}$ 1–2 hr; duration of action 3–6 hr; renal clearance
  - Usual IV dose for 70 kg person: Furosemide: 5–40 mg (0.1–1.0 mg/kg); ECA: 25-50 mg (0.5–1.0 mg/kg); bumetanide: 0.5–1.0 mg q 2–3 h; max 10 mg/d

DRUG EFFECTS

System	Effect
HEENT	Transient (<24 hr) deafness or vertigo may follow IV rapid bolus ECA; less common after furosemide or bumetanide; rarely permanent
CARDIO	Transient ↑ in venous capacitance causes hypotension with rapid IV loop diuretic administration; acute transient ↑ in intravascular volume precedes diuresis with mannitol; vasodilation with fenoldopam
GI	Diarrhea may follow ECA use
ENDO	Hypokalemia, metabolic alkalosis
GU	Diuresis
CNS	Mannitol ↓ ICP following transient increase. The latter may be mitigated by coadministration of furosemide

Key References: Greenberg A. Diuretic complications. *Am J Med Sci*. 2000;39:10–24. Kaplan NM. The choice of thiazide diuretics: Why chlorthalidone may replace hydrochlorothiazide. *Hypertension*. 2009;54:951.

Perioperative Implications/Possible Drug Interactions

Preoperative Concerns

- In chronic hypertensive pts treated with diuretics, a significant intravascular volume contraction may exist, making them more prone to hypotension following induction of anesthesia and any acute blood loss.
- Hypokalemia: Check serum K^+, consider enhanced digitalis toxicity
- Hypomagnesemia is common in pts treated with loop or thiazide diuretics and predisposes to ventricular arrhythmias, and should be suspected when hypokalemia is noted
- Enhanced oto- and nephrotoxicity of loop diuretics are assoc with rapid administration of large IV doses and concurrent use of another

nephrotoxic drug, e.g., aminoglycoside antibiotic, another loop diuretic, and some cephalosporins, esp., cephaloridine
- Probably best to continue chronic dose through the periop period, incl day of surgery. (UO will decline if diuretic not given on day of surgery.)

Induction/Maintenance

- Intraop loop diuretic use may significantly decrease serum K^+ level with diuresis

Adjuvants

- Enhanced renal clearance of other drugs, e.g., NMB agents, provoked by diuresis is not clinically problematic

Anticipated Problems/Concerns

- Pts receiving diuretics preop should be considered volume-contracted until proven otherwise.
- Hypokalemia assoc with diuresis will be aggravated by hyperventilation, which further lowers serum K^+ an additional 0.5 mEq/L for each 10 mmHg decrease in $PaCO_2$.
- Catecholamine β effect (endogenous and/or exogenous); also lowers serum K^+.
- Low intraop UO in a euvolemic pt if ADH/stress mediated will, in authors' experience, respond to very low dose (e.g., 2–5 mg furosemide) with increased UO

Dobutamine

David C. Warltier

Indications

- Administered to pts with low cardiac output (CO) 2° to decreased right or left ventricular function assoc with HF, MI, or cardiac surgery
- Used for treatment of pulm Htn with right ventricular dysfunction
- Provocative test for Dx of CAD (e.g., dobutamine stress-echocardiography)

Perioperative Risks

- Risk of tachyarrhythmias

Worry About

- Tachycardia and tachyarrhythmias, worse at high doses
- Ventricular ectopy
- Rarely, hypotension or Htn may be observed
- Hypokalemia may occur

- May cause and/or exacerbate myocardial ischemia

Overview/Pharmacology

- Inotrope used intravenously for increasing CO simultaneous with a decrease in systemic and pulm vascular resistance
- Was considered to have relatively greater inotropic than chronotropic actions, but recent investigation does not support this contention
- β_1-agonist with lesser effect at β_2-receptors and minimal effects at α-receptors
- Increases intracellular Ca^{2+} by elevating cAMP through effects on β_1-receptors
- Increases SA-node automaticity and AV nodal and intraventricular conduction
- May cause systemic and pulm vasodilation through β_2-receptor stimulation

- Quick onset (within 2 min) and short duration (approx 2–6 min)

Drug Class/Mechanism of Action/Usual Dose

- Synthetic catecholamine
- β-adrenergic action increases adenylyl cyclase activity
- Increases CO by increasing SV and HR and decreasing SVR
- Usual dosage: 1–10 $\mu g/kg/min$ IV
- Combined use with other agents to increase cardiac output via different mechanisms (e.g., milrinone, sodium nitroprusside)
- Concurrent use of dobutamine with epinephrine may reduce efficacy of epinephrine

DRUG EFFECTS

System	Effect	Assessment by Hx	PE	Test
CARDIO	↑ HR ↑ CO ↓ PVR ↓ SVR	Relief of dyspnea	Capillary perfusion, JVD, UO, rales	Mixed venous O_2 sat, CO, PVR, SVR data

Key Reference: Petersen JW, Felker GM. Inotropes in the management of acute heart failure. *Crit Care Med.* 2008;36(suppl):S106–S111.

Perioperative Implications/Drug Interactions

Preoperative Concerns

- Assess systemic perfusion
- Monitor BP, CO, PCWP
- PA catheter essential for adequate drug titration

Induction/Maintenance

- Despite adequate CO and BP before induction, there may be a decrease in these values during induction of anesthesia.
- Therapy should be guided by measures of adequacy of systemic perfusion such as CO, mixed venous O_2 sat, and ABG tensions.

Adjuvant/Regional Anesthesia/Reversal

- Combining therapy with inotropes that are not β_1-agonists such as milrinone may provide greater than additive effects
- Improvement in cardiac output may also be achieved by adding sodium nitroprusside if SVR is high
- Excessive effect can be reversed with β-adrenergic antagonists such as esmolol
- Consider using digoxin prior to dobutamine in pts with AFIB and rapid ventricular response
- May be ineffective or larger doses required in pts receiving β-blockers

Postoperative Period

- Duration of treatment determined by assessment of cardiac function with PA catheter

Anticipated Problems/Concerns

- Sinus tachycardia can occur, and in pts with AFib, the ventricular rate may increase 2° to enhanced AV conduction.
- Pulm V/Q mismatch 2° to pulm vasodilation and loss of hypoxic pulm vasoconstriction may lead to a decrease in Pao_2
- Initiation or exacerbation of ventricular arrhythmias if myocardial ischemia present
- Contraindicated in IHSS
- Prolonged use assoc with β-receptor downregulation and theoretically reduced effectiveness

DRUGS

Dopamine

Ala Sami Haddadin

Indications

- A flexible molecule that fits into many receptors to cause direct β_1- and β_2-receptor stimulation, as well as some α-stimulation, and fits into dopaminergic receptors as well.
- Hypotension
- Cardiac failure/shock with low-to-normal SVR
- Oliguria or periods of renal stress such as vascular surgery, sepsis, cardiopulmonary bypass, and concurrent use of other vasopressors. The concept of therapeutic renal dose is now outdated.
- Bradycardia

Perioperative Risks

- Tachycardia, angina, arrhythmias
- N/V
- Vasoconstriction and Htn (possible gangrene of extremities)
- Skin sloughing and necrosis if infiltrated in SQ tissue
- Impairs T-lymphocyte function (hypoprolactinemia)
- Depression of hypoxic ventilatory drive
- Increases intraocular pressure
- Potentiates other chronotropes

Pharmacology

- Preparations: 200-, 400-, 800-mg ampules (must be diluted before IV administration). It must not be diluted in alkaline solutions.
- Endogenous central and peripheral neurotransmitter

Overview/Mechanism of Action

- Mixed indirect and direct sympathomimetic effects, by activating dopamine (DA_2 and DA_1), β- and α-adrenergic receptors in dose-dependent fashion
- Presynaptic DA_2 receptors (0.2–0.4 μg/kg/min) inhibit endogenous norepinephrine and prolactin release.
- Postsynaptic DA_1 receptors (0.5–3.0 μg/kg/min) produce vasodilation in renal, mesenteric, coronary, cerebral arteries.
- β-Adrenergic receptors (4–10 μg/kg/min) activate adenylyl cyclase and $\uparrow$ myocardial cAMP concentration, $\uparrow$ myocardial contractility, inotropy.
- α-Adrenergic receptors (>10–20 μg/kg/min) produce progressive vasoconstriction
- Metabolism: Substrate for both MAO and COMT

- $T_{1/2}$: 6–9 min (recent evidence suggests attainment of steady-state plasma concentrations may require 70–125 min)
- Marked interpatient variability in plasma concentrations

Clinical Applications

- Renal dose dopamine
  - DA_1 (1.5–3.0 μg/kg/min) selectively increases renal blood flow and inhibits tubular reabsorption (increases UO)
  - Induces diuresis, usually without changing creatinine clearance
  - Low-dose dopamine may also improve splanchnic blood flow
- Inotropic dose dopamine (~4–10 μg/kg/min) induces release of endogenous norepinephrine (~50% of total activity)
  - β_1-Adrenergic adenylyl cyclase activation increases myocardial cAMP
- Higher dose dopamine
  - In addition to effects noted above, α_1-adrenergic receptors (>10–20 μg/kg/min) are activated with progressive vasoconstriction

DRUG EFFECTS

System	Effect	Assessment by Hx	PE	Test
CARDIO	$\uparrow$ Cardiac inotropy; vasoconstrictor activity	Improved mental status, perfusion	Pulses, BP Capillary refill	$\uparrow$ Cardiac output; UO
RESP	$\downarrow$ Hypoxic drive $\uparrow$ Pulm artery pressure (PAP)	Hypoventilation	Resp rate, depth	ABGs Pulse oximetry Monitor PAP
RENAL	$\uparrow$ Renal blood flow: $\downarrow$ renal Na$^+$, water reabsorption	UO	Urine volume	Urine volume, electrolytes Cr, CrCl

Key Reference: Smit AJ. Dopamine in heart failure and critical care. *Clin Exp Hypertens.* 2000;22:269–276.

Perioperative Implications

Dopamine Infusion Issues
- Ensure adequate intravascular volume
- Consider invasive monitoring
  - Continuous arterial and PAP catheters; central venous and pulm artery occlusion pressure ("filling pressures"); thermodilution cardiac output
- UO and Cr clearance

Adjuvants
- Additional inotropes—other β-agonists (dobutamine, epinephrine, etc.) or phosphodiesterase inhibitors (milrinone or amrinone) may be needed to $\uparrow$ cardiac contractility.

Cautions
- Watch for arrhythmias
- May increase heart rate and LV wall stress excessively (dopamine >10 μg/kg/min frequently causes progressive tachycardia and $\uparrow$ diastolic ventricular filling pressure)

- Diminished response in pts with chronic CHF or active sepsis
- In cardiogenic shock, myocardial lactate may $\uparrow$
- Long-term infusions may suppress immune (T-cell) function with $\downarrow$ prolactin
- May exacerbate glaucoma
- If the pt has recently taken a monoamine oxidase inhibitor, the rate of dopamine
- Metabolism by the tissue will fall and the dose should be cut to one-tenth the usual

Related Agent: Dopexamine
- Dopexamine, a synthetic analogue of dopamine, lacks any direct α-adrenergic agonist activity, expressing only β_2-adrenergic and dopaminergic (DA_1) agonist action
  - DA_1 and β_2 arterial vasodilation reduces cardiac afterload while simultaneously increasing blood flow to the kidneys, intestines, liver, spleen
  - Dopexamine (doses between 1 and 4 μg/kg/min) significantly $\uparrow$ cardiac index while decreasing systemic and pulm vascular resistances after cardiac surgery

- HR $\uparrow$, but not SV index; thus, dopexamine combines positive inotropic, chronotropic, vasodilatory, diuretic, natriuretic properties
- Fenoldopam mesylate (Corlopam) is a pure DA_1-receptor agonist inducing selective coronary, renal, mesenteric, and peripheral arterial vasodilation. It causes a linear, dose-dependent reduction in systolic and diastolic BP (pharmacokinetic $T_{1/2}$ = 5 min); produces potent renal vasodilation and natriuretic actions (similar to dopamine), and $\uparrow$ UO even in the setting of $\downarrow$ BP. May replace renal dose dopamine. No known drug interactions with β-blockers, α-blockers, Ca^{2+}-channel blockers, or ACE inhibitors. Has the disadvantage of causing reflex tachycardia. Can cause asymptomatic T wave flattening on the ECG.
- Infusions have proven ineffective in prevention of contrast-induced nephropathy. Use with caution in pts with glaucoma. Contains sulfites.

Doxorubicin (Adriamycin) Daunorubicin (Cerubidine)

Richard I. Cook

Toxicity

- Two phases of toxicity, acute and chronic
- Acute toxicity: Cardiac (may be from direct effects of histamine)
  - ECG changes and conduction disturbances: ↓ QRS voltage; nonspecific ST changes; T wave flattening
  - Rhythm disturbances: Supraventricular tachyarrhythmias; PVCs
  - Decreased EF
- Acute toxicity: Other
  - N/V, alopecia, diarrhea, mucositis
  - Bone marrow suppression (may limit dose acutely); counts lowest about 2 wk after beginning therapy
  - Infiltrated drug with IV delivery may cause extensive tissue necrosis, requiring wide debridement
- Late toxicity: Cardiac
  - Most acute toxic cardiac effects (except ↓ QRS voltage) diminish with time
  - Late toxicity occurs weeks to months after administration; reports of onset up to 5 y after dosing
  - Effects are permanent (some indication that children may recover with time)
  - CHF unresponsive to inotropic drugs
  - Increased risk of CHF with higher doses but heart failure can occur after 1st dose
  - Risk 0.1–7% up to 550 mg/m²
  - Risk rises sharply after 550 mg/m² to 50% at 1000 mg/m²
  - Risk increased by radiation of LV, other cardiotoxic drugs, prior LV dysfunction
  - Risk greater in young children
  - Risk of CHF ↓ by divided dosing (e.g., weekly)
- Myocardial function evaluation requires measurement of EF by ECHO or MUGA (serial CXR, ECGs, systolic time intervals, and other clinical signs not reliable)
- Myocardial biopsy but not myocardial function shows characteristic changes

Perioperative Risks

- Acute: Anemia, thrombocytopenia, cardiac arrhythmias, and conduction disturbances
- Late: Cardiac contractile dysfunction (variable; may be severe)

Overview/Pharmacology

- IV chemotherapeutic agents used for wide variety of tumors
- Sensitizes tissues to the effects of radiation; used in combined chemo/radiation therapy protocols
- Excretion primarily by liver

Drug Class/Mechanism of Action/Usual Dose

- Anthracycline antibiotic chemotherapeutic agents
- Works by binding to DNA and interfering with DNA-directed DNA and RNA synthesis
- Variety of dosing regimens: Often given weekly until maximum dose is reached
- Maximum dosage ~550 mg/m² BSA; dose decreased when used in combination with other cardiotoxic drugs (e.g., cyclophosphamide) or radiation (see under Toxicity)

DRUG EFFECTS

System	Effect	Assessment by Hx	PE	Test
CARDIO	Conduction Contractile force	Exercise tolerance	Unreliable CHF signs; orthopnea, DOE, etc.	ECG ECHO, MUGA
GI	Mucositis, diarrhea		Volume indicators	
HEME	Marrow suppression	Bleeding	Unreliable	CBC with plt count

Key Reference: Allen A. The cardiotoxicity of chemotherapeutic drugs. *Semin Oncol.* 1992;19:529–542.

Perioperative Implications

Preoperative Concerns

- Some authorities insist on preop echocardiogram for any child who has received these drugs at any time in the past, although Hx assists in determining need
- Evaluation for signs and symptoms of CHF
- Expected nature of surgical trespass

Induction/Maintenance

- Issues dominated by cardiac condition

Related Drugs

- Epirubicin (Ellence) is a newer derivative of doxorubicin, with similar anesthetic-related features. It may be found as part of breast cancer chemotherapy. It *may* be slightly less cardiotoxic on a milligram basis.
- Idarubicin (Idamycin, Idamycin PFS) is a newer derivative of daunorubicin, with similar anesthetic-related features. It may be found as part of acute myelogenous leukemia chemotherapy. An oral form of idarubicin has been tested as part of long-term chemotherapy regimens.

Anticipated Problems/Concerns

- LV dysfunction periop with pulm edema
- Risk of infection in acute toxicity

Ephedrine

Dmitry Portnoy

Uses

- Treatment of hypotension resulting from sympathectomy effect of neuraxial blockade, vasodilatory and/or cardiodepressant effects of IV and/or inhalational anesthesia agents
- Acute hypotension due to undetermined shock, complete heart block (Stokes-Adams attack)
- As a pressor following overdose with ganglionic-blocking and antiadrenergic agents
- Orally, is used for allergic disorders, asthma, nasopharyngeal congestion, corysa, hay fever
- Topically, for treatment of nasal congestion, coryza, vasomotor rhinitis, acute sinusitis

Perioperative Risks

- May trigger arrhythmias, incl life threatening ventricular arrhythmias, if myocardium more sensitive to catecholamines (e.g., due to inhalational agents, particularly halothane and enflurane)
- May cause acute Htn resulting in intracranial hemorrhage and CV collapse
- Hypertensive crisis may occur if used in pts taking MAOI and TCA antidepressants
- May precipitate ischemia and chest pain in some pts with CAD
- Large doses used to maintain BP during C-section under spinal anesthesia are assoc with decreased umbilical artery pH

Overview/Pharmacology

- Naturally occurring, nonselective predominantly indirect-acting sympathomimetic at both α and β receptors (structurally similar to amphetamine but less blood-brain barrier penetration)
- Causes release of norepinephrine from the storage granules in postganglionic nerve endings (indirect effect); also has some direct effects at adrenergic receptors
- BP increases as a result of venoconstricton, improved preload and CO$_2$ and some chronotropic and inotropic effects
- May develop tachyphylaxis rapidly (by uncertain mechanism), possibly due to depletion of NE stores with repeated injections and persistent blockade of adrenergic receptors

- Metabolized slowly by MAO in liver (via conjugation, demethylation, and deamination); slow inactivation accounts for prolonged effect (10 × longer than epinephrine), T½: 3-6 hr
- Crosses placenta, enters breast milk, excreted by urine, mostly as unchanged drug
- Does not appear to compromise uterine blood flow, but large doses may cause fetal acidosis
- Variations in β_2AR genotype may explain wide variability in responses to β-agonist effect

Drug Class/Usual Dose

- Nonselective, noncatecholamine adrenergic agent with mainly indirect, and mild direct activity
- Dosage: Mix 50 mg in 10 mL (5 mg/ml) IV, titrated to desired effect
- Starting doses in adults from 5–10 mg as bolus; 0.5–5 mg/min as infusion titrated to effect
- Can also be given IM, SQ (suggested dose 0.5 mg/kg)
- Adult dose: 5–50 mg

DRUG EFFECTS

System	Effect	Assessment by Hx	PE	Test
RECEPTORS	α: + + β_1: + + β_2: +			
CARDIO	HR: + + Contractility: + + Automaticity: + + Peripheral resistance: + CO: + + Mean BP: + + PAP: + +		HR PR Mean BP	SV SVR CO PAP
RESP	Airway resistance: – – Resp stimulant: +			Airway resistance Min ventilation
VASC BED FLOW	Skin/viscera: – Muscle: + Kidney: – – Coronary: + Cerebral: +		Skin perfusion	
ENDO	O$_2$ consumption: + Blood glucose: + Blood lactic acid: NC			O$_2$ consumption Blood glucose Blood lactate
GU	Uterine relaxation; restores uterine BF in hypotension from epidural/spinal			
CNS	Mild stimulant Mild mydriasis	Anxiety, agitation		

+ minimal increase; + + moderate increase; – minimal decrease; – – moderate decrease; NC = no change

Key Reference: Kee N, Khaw WD, Tan KS, Ng PE, Karmakar FF, Manoj K. Placental transfer and fetal metabolic effects of phenylephrine and ephedrine during spinal anesthesia for cesarean delivery. *Anesth.* 2009;111:506–512.

Possible Drug Interactions

Perioperative Concerns

- Severe Htn with MAOIs, TCAs, furasolidone
- Increased risk of arrhythmias if taking digoxin
- Increased response in cocaine users
- Decreased vasopressor response with reserpine, methyldopa, guanethidine (due to depletion of NE stores in nerve endings)
- Increased response in pts receiving β-blockers
- Ephedra preparations (e.g., ma-huang, mormon tea), guarana and caffeine may lead to additive effects
- Additive effects and risk of toxicity is assoc with urinary alkalinizers

Induction/Maintenance

- As in Perioperative Concerns

Anticipated Problems/Concerns

- Myocardium sensitization to catecholamine by some inhalational agents (e.g., halothane)
- Tachyphylaxis with repeated doses
- Possibility of interactions with other drugs that affect ANS, incl herbals and cocaine
- Precipitates ischemia in susceptible pts
- Maternal tachycardia/other arrhythmias, potential fetal acidosis

Epinephrine

Ala Sami Haddadin

Uses

- Intraop: Systolic dysfunction—weaning from CPB, in critical care for CV collapse from many causes: cardiogenic (incl RV failure), distributive (incl anaphylaxis—stabilizes mast cells), obstructive shock
- Addition to local anesthesia to prolong action (1:200,000) and for hemostasis (field block)
- Nebulized racemic epinephrine for airway edema: Postop stridor or laryngotracheobronchitis in children, usually not for angioneurotic edema
- Inhalational forms for mild asthma
- Topical solutions for vasoconstriction (nasal, ophthalmic)
- Large repeated doses in cardiac arrest

Perioperative Risks

- Increased risk of dysrhythmias (limit to 1 μg/kg with halothane, 2–3 μg/kg with isoflurane, enflurane)
- May precipitate myocardial ischemia
- Severe Htn/stroke if dosed incorrectly
- Large doses may precipitate pulm edema
- Avoid topical application where reduced perfusion could lead to ischemic tissue damage

Overview/Pharmacology

- Potent β_1, β_2, β_3, α_1 and α_2 stimulant. More potent at both β- and β-receptors than norepinephrine.
- Water soluble—no blood-brain barrier penetration
- $\uparrow$ Pulse pressure at low doses because of β_2 effect
- β Stimulation causes increased intracellular cAMP
- α_1 Stimulation causes increased intracellular Ca^{2+} by G protein interaction as well as increased turnover of phosphoinositol
- α_2 Stimulation inhibits adenylyl cyclase
- Metabolized by MAO, COMT; conjugated and excreted in urine
- Biologic activity terminated principally by uptake in postganglionic sympathetic nerve terminals

Drug Class/Usual Dose

- Naturally occurring sympathomimetic
- Dosage: Depends on route and clinical situation—low, moderate, high doses
  - IV: Mix 1 mg in 250 mL (4 μg/mL); adult bolus doses for $\downarrow$ BP from anaphylaxis: 10–20 μg as starting dose, $\uparrow$ as needed
- Infusion, mainly β at 0.01–0.03 μg/kg/min, increasing α at 0.03–0.15 μg/kg/min, predominant α at 0.15–0.3 μg/kg/min. Cardiac arrest dose: 0.5–1 mg q5 min.
- Subcutaneous: 10 μg/kg for mild to moderate allergic reactions, severe asthma

DRUG EFFECTS

System	Effect	Assessment by Hx	PE	Test
RECEPTORS	α: + + (dose-dependent) β_1: + + β_2: + +			
CARDIO	HR: + +	Palpitations	HR	SV
	Contractility: + +			
	Automaticity: + +		Pulse	
	SVR ± (dose-dependent)		Perfusion	SVR
	CO: + +			CO
	Mean BP: + (dose-dependent)		Mean BP	BP
	PAP: +			PAP
RESP	Airway resistance: – Resp stimulant: +		Wheezing TV	Airway resistance Minute ventilation
VASC BED FLOW	Skin/viscera: – – Muscle: + + Kidney: – – Coronary: + Cerebral: +		Skin perfusion	
ENDO	O$_2$ consumption: + + Blood glucose: + + Blood lactic acid: + + (with infusion) Hypokalemia Serum FFA: + +			O$_2$ consumption Blood glucose Blood lactate Serum K$^+$ FFA
GU	Relaxation of uterus			
CNS	Mild stimulant Mild mydriasis	Anxiety, agitation, headache Mydriasis, arousal		

+ Minimal increase; + + moderate increase; + + + marked increase; – minimal decrease; – – moderate decrease

Key Reference: Andrzejowski J, Sleigh JW, Johnson IA, Sikiotis L. The effect of intravenous epinephrine on the bispectral index and sedation. *Anaesthesia.* 2000;55:761–763.

Perioperative Implications/Possible Drug Interactions

Preoperative Concerns

- Hypertensive crisis with MAO inhibitors
- May precipitate malignant arrhythmias
- Increased risk of arrhythmias if taking digoxin
- Response exaggerated if taking reserpine, guanethidine
- Increased sensitivity if taking cocaine, tricyclic antidepressants
- Decreased response with β-blockers
- Hypertensive, hyperthyroid pts more susceptible to pressor response
- Hypokalemia

Induction/Maintenance

- Dysrhythmias with halothane, hypocapnia potentiates this drug interaction (children are more tolerant)

Anticipated Problems/Concerns

- Myocardium sensitized to catecholamines by inhalational agents—possibility of malignant arrhythmias
- Severe Htn, possible stroke if dosed incorrectly
- Aggravates symptoms in psychoneurotic pts on emergence
- Hypokalemia, hyperglycemia
- Possibility of pulm edema
- Pre-existing α_1 blockade can cause the paradoxical phenomenon of epinephrine reversal

Epsilon-Aminocaproic Acid (EACA) (Amicar)

Frank W. Dupont

Uses

- EACA is a hemostatic agent used in the treatment of excessive bleeding assoc hyperfibrinolysis
- Indications: Hemorrhage caused by systemic hyperfibrinolysis*, surgical or non-surgical hematuria*, surgical bleeding assoc with CPB, hemorrhagic reaction to fibrinolytic drugs, bleeding in pts with hereditary blood coagulation disorders, treatment and prophylaxis in hemophiliacs undergoing dental surgical procedures, 2° prophylaxis against 2° hemorrhage following intraocular bleeding, recurrence of subarachnoid hemorrhage, hemorrhage in pts with thrombocytopenia
- Methods of administration: Oral solution, IV solution, topical, intravesical

*FDA approved

Perioperative Risks

- Increased risk of developing thrombosis in hemophiliac pts, who are concurrently treated with Factor IX concentrate or anti-inhibitor coagulant complex

Worry About

- EACA should not be used when there is evidence of an active intravascular clotting process. When there is uncertainty as to whether the cause of bleeding is primary fibrinolysis or disseminated intravascular coagulation (DIC), this distinction almost certainly must be made before administering EACA. EACA has too great a hazard to benefit ratio to be used in the presence of DIC without concomitant heparin.

Overview and Pharmacology

- EACA prevents formation of excessive plasmin, thereby inhibiting fibrinolysis
- EACA enhances hemostasis when fibrinolysis contributes to bleeding

- Primarily excreted in the urine, with 40–65% eliminated unchanged within 12 hr, approx 11% is metabolized; renal clearance is 116 mL/min; terminal elimination half-life is approx 2 hr

Drug Class/Mechanism of Action/Usual Dose

- EACA is an antifibrinolytic agent of the lysine analogue class.
- EACA binds competitively to lysine-binding sites within the plasminogen/plasmin molecule, which interferes with the ability of plasmin to lyse fibrin clots.
- The optimal dosage in the setting of CPB is undefined, but the following is a commonly used regimen in adults: Initial loading dose is 5 g IV over 1 hr, followed by a continuous infusion at 1 g/hr, maximum recommended daily dosage is 30 g
- Plasma concentrations are increased in pts with severe renal dysfunction, but no quantitative recommendations for dosing adjustments are available

DRUG EFFECTS

System	Effect	Assessment by Hx	PE	Test
CNS	Dizziness, confusion, delirium, headache, seizure		Neuro exam	
CARDIO	Hypotension, bradycardia		Vital signs	ECG
GI	N/V/D			Lytes
RENAL	Renal failure, urinary tract obstruction		Oliguria	BUN/Crea
HEME	Thrombosis	Potential causes for DIC	Evidence for paradox of simultaneous thrombosis and bleeding	CBC, PT/PTT, DIC profile
MS	Myopathy, rhabdomyolysis	Myalgia, malaise, fatigue	Muscle weakness	CPK

Key Reference: Serna DL. Antifibrinolytic agents in cardiac surgery: Current controversies. *Semin Thorac Cardiovasc Surg*. 2005;17:52–58.

Perioperative Implications/Possible Drug Interactions

Preoperative Concerns

- In the presence of hematuria originating in the upper urinary tract, EACA can cause intrarenal obstruction due to clot retention

Drug Interaction

- EACA is contraindicated in hemophilic pts who are treated with Factor IX concentrates or anti-inhibitor coagulant complex, unless the risk of thrombosis is outweighed by the potential benefit of EACA

Induction/Maintenance

- Close hemodynamic monitoring of cardiac pts because of the risk of hypotension and sinus bradycardia, particularly with rapid IV administration and in hypovolemia
- Monitor renal function in pts with renal dysfunction and consider dosage adjustments depending on clinical response and degree of renal function impairment.
- Consider transfusion of plts, FFP, and cryoprecipitate in the presence of bleeding not caused by hyperfibrinolysis

Postoperative Period

- Continue assessment of bleeding and monitoring of coagulation profiles after D/C of EACA therapy

Anticipated Problems/Concerns

- EACA should not be administered without a definite diagnosis and/or laboratory finding indicative of hyperfibrinolysis (hyperplasminemia) because of the potential for thrombotic complications in pts with DIC and underlying hypercoagulable states

Fluoxetine (Prozac)

Donald D. Koblin

Uses

- Incidence in USA: Taken by approx 5 million
- Rx for depression, obsessive-compulsive disorder, bulimia nervosa

Perioperative Risks

- May be assoc with periop anxiety
- Drug interactions with β-blockers, phenytoin, benzodiazepines, antipsychotics (may increase levels by inhibition of metabolism)

Worry About

- Suicidal behavior, psychotic or extrapyramidal reactions (rare)
- Serotonin syndrome with concomitant administration of MAO inhibitors, tricyclic antidepressants, antipsychotics, or meperidine
- Increased risk of abn bleeding

Overview/Pharmacology

- Selective inhibitor of serotonin reuptake
- Administered as racemic mixture of R-and S-enantiomers
- S-enantiomer more potent than R-enantiomer
- Active metabolites, R- and S-norfluoxetine, formed by demethylation
- Eliminated mainly through oxidative metabolism and conjugation
- Long elimination T½: 1–10 d for fluoxetine; 3–20 d for norfluoxetine
- Fluoxetine inhibits (and probably metabolized by) liver cytochrome P450 enzymes CYP2D6 and possibly CYP3A4: May inhibit metabolism, ↑ levels of β-blockers, benzodiazepines, antipsychotics
- Difficult to establish relationship between plasma conc of fluoxetine and effect, probably because these are four active compounds (R- and S-fluoxetine and R- and S-norfluoxetine) that require separate measurements

Drug Class/Mechanism of Action/Usual Dose

- Selective inhibitor of serotonin reuptake chronically taken for depression, obsessive-compulsive disorder, bulimia nervosa
- Not useful for acute administration, since full antidepressant effect may be delayed until 4 wk of treatment or longer
- Initial PO dose, 20 mg/d
- Maximal dose, 80 mg/d
- Alternatives: Other antidepressant medications

DRUG EFFECTS

System	Effect	Assessment by Hx	PE	Test
CARDIO	Bradycardia, dysrhythmia Slight BP increase	(rare)	Pulse	ECG
CNS	Extrapyramidal symptoms (rare), mania (rare), serotonin syndrome (rare)	Headache, anxiety, tremor		
ENDO	SIADH secretion (rare)			Urine specific gravity
GI	Nausea, wt loss			
MS	Serotonin syndrome (rare)	Arthritic complaints (infrequent), muscle rigidity		

Key Reference: Gram LF. Fluoxetine. *N Engl J Med.* 1994;331:1354–1361.

Perioperative Implications/Possible Drug Interactions

- Headache, anxiety, nausea are common symptoms
- May inhibit cytochrome P450 enzymes and ↑ the serum concentrations of other drugs (β-blockers, phenytoin, benzodiazepines, antipsychotics) and potentiate their effects
- Do not give to pregnant pts without assessing risk-benefit ratio

Anticipated Problems/Concerns

- Approx 7% of Caucasians lack the cytochrome P450 (CYP2D6) that probably metabolizes fluoxetine; these individuals may develop higher serum concentrations of fluoxetine and be more prone to side effects.
- Serotonin syndrome, characterized by agitation, confusion, diaphoresis, and muscle rigidity, may develop in pts who receive a combination of fluoxetine and MAO inhibitors

Folic Acid

Karen E. Iles
David W. Miller

Uses

- Prevention of folic acid deficiency
- Treat megaloblastic anemia
- Experimental treatment for major depressive disorder
- Treat folic acid deficiency caused by anorexia, chronic oral contraceptive use, chronic use of some anti-epileptic drugs, alcoholism, malabsorption diseases (e.g., sprue), bowel resection, and diverticulosis
- Reduces incidence of NTD (spina bifida) and congenital heart defects in developing fetus
- Reduces homocysteine; may have CV benefits (no evidence of such from randomized trials, but lots of anecdotal evidence)

Perioperative Risks

- Overdosage chronically increase cancer proliferation—demonstrated in epidemiologic studies and in-vitro studies with breast cancer
- Exposure to NO disrupts folic acid metabolism; repeated exposure can cause deficiency

- Supraphysiological doses (>15 mg/d), may decrease seizure threshold in pts on some anti-epileptic medications

Worry About

- Allergic reactions (rare); most to the parenteral form
- Loss of appetite, nausea, lethargy, stomach pain, insomnia
- Supraphysiological doses (>15 mg/d) increase in all symptoms listed above
- May cause seizures (>15 mg/d); higher risk in epileptics

Overview/Pharmacology

- Vitamin with close synergistic relationships with vitamin B_{12}, ascorbate, and zinc
- Very little found as folic acid in nature; converted to tetrahydrofolate (THF)
- Absorption most efficient in the jejunum
- Loss from the body is prevented by efficient enterohepatic recirculation

- Some fecal excretion; very little excreted in urine
- Alcohol decreases blood levels by interfering with enterohepatic recirculation
- THF accepts and denotes one carbon group in amino acid degradation and metabolism reactions

Drug Class/Mechanism of Action/Usual Dose

- Vitamin
- Accepts and denotes one carbon group in amino acid degradation and metabolism reactions (i.e., the synthesis of glycine from serine)
- Critical for cell division because required for purine and thymidine synthesis
- Oral and parenteral forms
- RDA 400 µg/d for healthy individuals; 600 µg/d for pregnant women
- Higher requirements (anemia, antifolate drug therapy, etc); 1 mg 1-3X/d (PO, IM, IV)
- Given as a multivitamin containing vitamin B_{12} because can mask vitamin B_{12} deficiency and accompanying neurologic damage

DRUG EFFECTS

System	Effect	Assessment by Hx	PE	Test
CARDIO	Improves O_2 delivery	Better exercise tolerance		Hgb
GI	Improves cell division	Less diarrhea	Better hydration/ absorption	
ENDO/METAB	Improves nucleic acid/protein synthesis		Wt gain	Folate level
HEME	Improves RBC synthesis	Better exercise tolerance		Hgb

Key Reference: Folic acid. In: Hunt SM, Groff J, eds. *Advanced nutrition and human metabolism.* 2nd ed. St. Paul: West Publishing Co; 1997:202–209.

Perioperative Implications

Preoperative Concerns

- Deficiency may cause anemia
- Consider general nutritional status (i.e., if evidence of poor diet, folic acid deficiency likely)
- Consider specific underlying conditions (i.e., anorexia, alcoholism, malabsorption disorders)
- Continue periop supplementation as needed

Induction/Maintenance

- Same as Preoperative Concerns
- Avoid repeated use of N_2O

Adjuvants/Regional Anesthesia/Reversal

- Same as Preoperative Concerns

Postoperative Period

- Same as Preoperative Concerns

Anticipated Problems/Concerns

- Rare allergic reactions
- Generally none in otherwise healthy pts
- May cause seizures (>15 mg/d) in seizure pts already on anti-epileptics

Gold (Auranofin, Aurothioglucose, Aurothiomalate)

Jeremy Hansen
James Duke

Uses

- Treatment for rheumatoid arthritis pts who do not respond to NSAIDs, steroids, or other disease-modifying antirheumatic drugs (DMARDs)
- Gold Rx as monotherapy dramatically decreasing 2° to preferred use of other DMARDs: e.g., methotrexate and use of biologic TNF inhibitors (infeximab and etanercept)

Risks

- Cutaneous reactions from erythema to exfoliative dermatitis (up to 30% of pts)
- Mucous membrane lesions: Stomatitis, pharyngitis, gastritis, colitis (20% of pts)
- Diarrhea is common in patients taking Auranofin (oral formulation)
- Gold deposition in dermis in dose-dependent manner, also renal tubule deposition
- Chrysiasis (gray-to-blue pigmentation of skin) possible with large cumulative doses; effect of transcutaneous Hgb saturation measurement unknown
- Proteinuria is common w/IM gold treatment (5–40%), usually resolves with cessation of treatment
- Cholestatic hepatic toxicity possible—resolves with cessation of therapy
- Interstitial pulm disease possible with gold therapy: Resolves w/cessation of treatment but is difficult to differentiate from underlying RA pulm fibrosis
- Thrombocytopenia (usually reverses with cessation of treatment)
- Bone marrow suppression possible, can progress to aplastic anemia
- Not usually administered to pregnant pts or those given antimalarials, phenylbutazone, or oxyphenylbutazone because of cumulative bone marrow suppression
- Not well tolerated by elderly (2° to underlying renal insufficiency and bone-marrow suppression)

Overview/Pharmacology

- Aurothioglucose, aurothiomalate administered IM, require close follow-up for side effects
- Auranofin administered orally, has differing pharmacokinetics, leading to potent immunosuppression and higher risk of rare side effects (thrombocytopenia, aplastic anemia)
- Oral preparation has lower incidence of common side effects, but slower elimination
- Peak serum levels from IM injection 2–6 hr
- 95% albumin-bound, also binds to macroglobulins
- Serum half-life of single 50-mg dose IM ~ 7 d
- After IM full dose, blood levels return to normal in 40–80 d; 75% of a given dose is eliminated renally, 25% fecal excretion
- Renal disease delays excretion and is a contraindication to gold administration

Drug Class/Mechanism of Action/Usual Dose

- Anti-inflammatory (disease-modifying antirheumatic drug)
- Gold compounds sequestered in phagocytic cells of reticuloendothelial system (liver, spleen, lymph nodes), and synovial membranes
- Gold suppresses phagocyte migration and has multi-modal anti-inflammatory effect (suppression of prostaglandin synthesis, C1 inhibition, lysosomal hydrolytic enzymes and elastase inhibition, B-cell inhibition)
- Administered in progressive doses (10–50 mg IM/wk, total dose not to exceed 1 g)
- Continuing therapy 50 mg IM every 2–4 wk
- Auranofin dosage 3–6 mg PO QD-BID

DRUG EFFECTS

System	Effect	PE	Test
HEENT	Glossitis, pharyngitis, (cricoarytenoid arthritis often present in RA pts)		
MSK	RA pts w/c-spine involvement (atlantoaxial subluxation) and sometimes TMJ involvement	ROM, decreased cervical range of motion and oral mouth opening	Lateral neck radiograph, neck CT, MRI
RESP	Tracheitis, pneumonitis, pulm fibrosis		CXR
GI	Hepatitis		LFTs
GU	Proteinuria, hematuria, membranous glomerulonephritis (contraindicated during pregnancy, breastfeeding)		Renal function, pregnancy
CNS	Encephalitis, peripheral neuritis	CNS exam	

Key Reference: Kean WF, Kean IR. Clinical pharmacology of gold. *Inflammopharmacol.* 2008;16:112–125.

Perioperative Implications/Possible Drug Interactions

- Severe RA; difficulty positioning on operating table
- Airway: Laryngeal arthritis, cervical instability, and pulm fibrosis; other problems of arthritis may be encountered
- Stomatitis, pharyngitis, tracheitis may make mucous membranes fragile

Drug Interactions

- None during anesthesia, but chrysiasis may interfere with pulse oximeter function

Anticipated Problems/Concerns

- Assess cervical instability and TMJ involvement in all severe RA pts (80% have upper C-spine involvement)
- Beware of renal, hepatic, and pulm dysfunction
- Lesions of skin, mucous membranes may make these tissues friable
- RA may require fiberoptic or nasal endotracheal intubation
- Hematologic problems (thrombocytopenia, leukopenia) may manifest as bleeding or postop infection

Haloperidol (Haldol)

Donald D. Koblin

Uses

- Rx for
- Psychotic disorders in ambulatory population (PO)
- Agitation caused by delirium in ICU pts (IV or IM)

Perioperative Risks

- Laryngospasm
- Extrapyramidal symptoms
- Neuroleptic malignant syndrome
- Cardiac arrest at high doses

Worry About

- May exacerbate symptoms in pts with Parkinson's disease
- Potential concern for neurotoxic metabolites
- Extrapyramidal symptoms less common with IV than PO doses

Overview/Pharmacology

- Dopaminergic antagonist
- Precise mechanism of action unknown
- Onset time: 5–20 min for IV; 30–60 min for PO
- Long (and variable) serum $T\frac{1}{2}$ (13–60 hr)
- 90–94% bound to serum proteins
- Therapeutic plasma concentration in range of 4–40 μg/L, but large variability among pts
- Clearance by hepatic metabolism
  - Metabolized to reduced haloperidol, which has ~ 10% of activity of parent drug; reduced haloperidol may be oxidized and reconverted to haloperidol
- Renal excretion of parent drug is negligible

Drug Class/Mechanism of Action/Usual Dose

- Dopaminergic antagonist

- Chronically taken for
  - Management of psychotic disorders
  - Control of tics and vocal utterances of Tourette's disorder
- Acutely taken to control agitation caused by delirium
- Usual PO dose 1–6 mg/d
- Usual IV or IM dose
  - 0.5–2 mg for mild agitation
  - 5 mg for moderate agitation
  - 10 mg for severe agitation (+10 mg/hr infusion)
- Alternatives
  - Other antipsychotic medications
  - Other antidelirium medications (e.g., physostigmine)
  - Usually for agitation caused by delirium; agitation caused by anxiety/pain can be treated with benzodiazepines/narcotics

DRUG EFFECTS

System	Effect	Test
HEENT	Laryngospasm (infrequent side effect)	
CARDIO	Hypotension or Htn, cardiac arrest (high doses)	
HEPAT	↓ Metabolism and ↑ serum concentration with hepatic disease	Monitoring of haloperidol concentrations is indicated only in pts with poor response at high doses or with hepatic disease
GI	Nausea	
ENDO	Gynecomastia	
GU	Urinary retention	
CNS	Extrapyramidal symptoms (akathisia, dystonia, tardive dyskinesia)	
MS	Neuroleptic malignant syndrome (NMS)	

Key References: Riker RR, Fraser GL, Cox PM. Continuous infusion of haloperidol controls agitation in critically ill patients. *Crit Care Med.* 1994;22:433–440.

Perioperative Implications/Possible Drug Interactions

- Encephalopathic syndrome with combined use of lithium and haloperidol
- May potentiate effects of general anesthetics and narcotics

Anticipated Problems/Concerns

- Laryngospasm infrequent but life-threatening
- Cardiac arrests reported with high (~10 mg) doses
- IV haloperidol is not approved by the FDA for routine use

- NMS may develop 1–3 d after haloperidol administration and is characterized by muscle rigidity, hyperthermia, tachycardia, altered consciousness, and elevated serum creatine kinase concentrations. A mild form of NMS may occur in as many as 1% of pts given haloperidol.

Hormone Replacement Therapy (HRT)

Edgar Pierre
Nicole D. Martin

Uses

- To treat the physiologic and physical manifestations of hypoestrogenism due to hypogonadism or primary ovarian failure
- To prevent or alleviate the signs and symptoms assoc with surgical or age-related menopause incl vaginal dryness, urogenital atrophy, irritability, depressed mood, osteoporosis, hyperlipidemia, CV disease, and vasomotor symptoms incl hot flashes
- A generic term that encompasses the use of unopposed estrogen therapy and combinations of estrogens and progestins

Perioperative Risks

- Increased risk for coagulopathy due to changes in coagulation and fibrinolytic pathways
- Within the first year of use, can cause a slight increase in coagulation factors II, VII, IX, X and XII, while decreasing the anticoagulation factors Protein C, Protein S, and antithrombin III, enhancing clot formation
- When used in combination with a progestin, may result in decreased levels of plasminogen-activator inhibitor protein-1 (PAI-1) resulting in increased fibrinolysis and prolonged bleeding

Worry About

- Increased risk of thrombosis incl DVT, pulm embolism, stroke, and myocardial infarction with estrogen replacement therapy if used without concomitant aspirin therapy (can be continued thru day of surgery for all but plastic, eye, and some neurologic operations).
- Increased risk of fibrinolysis and prolonged bleeding with combination estrogen-progestin
- Alterations in drug metabolism due to induction of various cytochrome P450 CYP isozymes
- Changes in drug distribution as a result of increased hepatic production of serum binding proteins

Overview/Pharmacology

- HRT provides low dosages of one or more estrogens, often in combination with progesterone or a chemical analogue, called a progestin.
- Conjugated estrogens and synthetic progestins have been most commonly used in HRT.
- Estrogens: A group of 18-carbon steroid compounds that occur naturally in three major forms: estrone, estradiol, and estriol. All steroids contain 4 condensed rings, designated A-D. The phenolic A ring is the principal structural feature that is responsible for selective, high-affinity binding to the estrogen receptors. As with most steroid hormones, estrogens can diffuse readily across cell membranes. Once within the cell, they bind and activate estrogen receptors that in turn up-regulate gene expression. Estrogen receptors are abundant throughout the body and can be found in the female reproductive tract, mammary glands, hypothalamus, endothelial cells, vascular smooth muscles, lung, brain, and bone.
- Progestins: A family of 21-carbon steroids that are synthetic derivatives of the 19-nortestosterone structure. Designed to have progestinic effects similar to progesterone, progestins work by binding to an intracellular progesterone receptor resulting in transcriptional activation. Physiologic actions incl endometrial proliferation, suppression of uterine contractility, mammary gland development, and thickening of endocervical gland secretions.

Drug Class/Mechanism of Action/Usual Dose

- Classified as steroid hormones, estrogens and progestins bind to specific receptors and have widespread effects on many tissues in the body.
- Various formulations are available for oral, parenteral, transdermal, or topical administration.
- To reduce the risks of HRT, lower-dose estrogen therapy regimens are preferred over high-dose therapy. The typical daily oral dose of conjugated estrogen is 0.625 mg, however, initial treatment should start at a dose of 0.3 mg/d and dose adjustments made based on clinical response. Additional available dosages are 0.9, 1.25, and 2.5 mg.
- The most commonly prescribed progestin is medroxyprogesterone acetate. It is typically given in a cyclic regimen (5–10 mg/d) or continuous regimen (2.5mg/d). Better choice is a micronized progestin (Prometrium, for example) which doesn't oppose the effect of estradiol on arterial function.

DRUG EFFECTS

System	Effect	Assessment by Hx	PE	Test
HEENT	Retinal vascular thrombosis, ↑ corneal curvature, ↑ lacrimal secretion	Changes or loss of vision, contact lens intolerance	Pale retina with cherry red macula, retinal hemorrhages	Ophthalmologic exam
CARDIO	Fluid retention, Htn improved lipoprotein profiles: ↑ HDL, ↓ LDL	Swelling and wt gain, Htn	Edema	Physical exam, BP, lipid profile
GI	Pancreatitis, N/V, gallstone formation	Abd pain, intolerance to fatty foods	RUQ or epigastric pain	Amylase, lipase, alk phos, RUQ U/S, bilirubin
HEPAT	Adenoma enlargement cholestasis	Abd pain, yellowing of skin	Hepatomegaly, jaundice	RUQ US, LFTs, bilirubin
GU	Abn uterine bleeding, changes in cervical secretions, increase in fibroid size, vaginal candidiasis	Vaginal bleeding, vaginal discharge, vaginal itching/burning	Enlarged lobulated uterus, vaginal discharge	Gynecologic exam, GYN US, KOH prep
HEME	Increased coagulation if not given with concomitant aspirin increased fibrinolysis	DVT, PE, MI, CVA Prolonged bleeding	LE swelling, SOB, CP, neuro deficits	PT/PTT, D-dimer, duplex US, CT angio fibrinogen, antithrombin III, Protein C
DERM	Chloasma, melasma, rashes, alopecia, hirsutism	Skin and hair changes	Hyperpigmenation, erythema, papules, nodules, hair changes	Dermatologic exam

Key References: Brunton L, Parker K, et al. *Goodman & Gilman's manual of pharmacology and therapeutics.* McGraw Hill Companies. 2008:993–1006.

Perioperative Implications

Preoperative Concerns

- Changes in angiotensin-aldosterone system may result in elevated BP and/or renal failure.
- Increased risk for thrombosis if not given with concomitant aspirin. Pts undergoing procedures assoc with moderate to high risk for venous thromboembolism should stop hormone therapy at least 4 to 6 wk prior to surgery. Rigorous prophylaxis for DVT must be observed in the periop period.
- The risks assoc with temporary D/C of hormone therapy incl withdrawal bleeding, hot flashes, and other menopausal symptoms.

Induction/Maintenance

- Alterations in the activity of various cytochrome P450 CYP isozymes may require dose adjustment of hepatically cleared drugs.
- HRT may induce metabolism of drugs which are glucuronidated, incl some benzodiazepines and analgesics.
- Progestin metabolite, allopregnanolone, may affect the excitability of neurons through direct modulation of the GABA-A receptors exerting hypnotic/sedative, anxiolytic, and anesthetic.

Postoperative Period

- Increased risk for thrombosis extends into the postop period. A hightened suspicion for postop DVT, pulm embolism, stroke, and myocardial infarction must be maintained. Restart or continue aspirin which should be always given concomitantly unless contraindicated.
- Activation of fibrinolytic pathways in pts using combined estrogen-progestin replacement therapy may result in postop bleeding.

Anticipated Problems/Concerns

- Coagulopathy, esp. increased risk for thromboembolism, remains a top concern for women using HRT.

Insulin Receptor Modifiers

Ponnusamy Saravanan
Subramanian Sathiskumar

Uses

- Oral anti-diabetic agents for Type 2 diabetes.

Perioperative Risks

- Hypoglycemia: Rare on monotherapy as the action is glucose mediated; caution is needed when used in combination with insulin or sulphonylureas (SUs).
- Hepatotoxicity: Though less likely with the currently available thiazolidinediones (TZDs), it is important to note that an earlier TZD (troglitazone) was withdrawn from market due to hepatotoxicity. Recommended monitoring would be liver function tests postop.
- CV risk: Increased sodium and water retention. Worsens heart failure esp. in NYHA class III and IV. Risk is higher with concomitant use of insulin.

Worry About

- Precipitation of heart failure: Volume expansion and sodium retention
- Hypoglycemia: When used in conjunction with insulin and SUs

- Hyperglycemia: Esp. when TZDs are stopped in severe insulin resistant, obese individuals

Overview/Pharmacology

- Mechanism of action
  - Highly selective agonist of PPAR-γ: alter the transcription and expression of genes involved in lipid metabolism (lipid sensing and regulation).
  - 1° site of action is adipocytes: adiposite differentiation and apoptosis. Increases the number of small adiposites leading to uptake of circulating free fatty acids (FFA) leading to decreased lipotoxicity in many tissues (β cells, liver, muscle, etc.), leading to decreased insulin resistance and increased insulin sensitivity and then to increased cellular responsiveness to insulin and insulin-dependent glucose disposal.
  - Improved β cell response to glucose but does not directly stimulate insulin secretion. Therefore hypoglycemia does not occur during monotherapy.
- Absorption
- Orally administered and well absorbed
  - Pioglitazone: Peak in 2 hr
  - Rosiglitazone: Peak in 1 hr

- Distribution: Drug and metabolites are extensively protein bound
- Excretion and clearance: The two available drugs, pioglitazone and rosiglitazone, are metabolized by different cytochrome P450 isoenzymes. No major adverse events due to interaction are reported; primarily excreted in bile, eliminated in feces
  - Pioglitazone metabolized by hydroxylation and oxidation
  - Rosiglitazone metabolized by hydroxylation and *N*-demethylation

Drug Class/Mechanism of Action/Usual Dose

- Peroxisome Proliferator Activated Receptor - γ agonists (PPAR-γ).
- Primarily works on adiposites by promoting free fatty acid uptake and storage. It also works by promoting glucose disposal in insulin sensitive tissues such as liver and muscle (indirectly).
- Dose
  - Pioglitazone: 15–45 mg/day (as once a day preparation)
  - Rosiglitazone: 2–8 mg/day (as once a day preparation)

DRUG EFFECTS

System	Effect	Assessment by Hx	PE	Test
General	↑ Body wt (ave. of 3–5 kg)	Pre-drug body wt	↑ SQ fat and ↓ visceral fat	Improved waist-hop ratio
CARDIO	↑ Fluid retention Vasodilatation Worsening heart failure, esp. in NYHA III & IV	↑ Ankle swelling	Edema	
HEME	↑ Anemia	Easily fatigued	Pallor	Hb – ↓ of up to 2–4 g
SKEL	↑ of fractures	Spontaneous fractures; low impact fractures		X-ray
ENT	Sinusitis, pharyngitis, URI	Coryza, headache, rhinorrhea		
GI	Hepatotoxicity (1:100,000)	Loss of appetite, abd pain	Jaundice, dark urine	LFTs
ENDO	Hypoglycemia (in combination with insulin and SUs)	Sweating, tremors, blurring of vision, palpitation	Tachycardia, altered consciousness	Glucose
EYES	↑ Macular edema (rare)	Blurring of vision	↓ visual acuity	Fundus exam
REPRO	↑ Ovulation (↑ chances of pregnancy in PCOS women)			

Key References: Quinn CE, et al. Thiazolidinediones: Effects on insulin resistance and the cardiovascular system, *Br J Pharmacol.* 2008;153:636–645.

Perioperative Implications

Preoperative Concerns

- Recommended to stop on the day. Drug effects can last for many days.
- Close monitoring of glucose levels due to the risk of hypo or hyperglycemia
- Though rare, measurement of liver function test and hemoglobin is recommended to R/O pre-existing anemia and hepatotoxicity.
- Careful consideration should be given when used in pts with known cardiac Hx because of the risk of heart failure and fluid retention.

Induction/Maintenance

- No drug interaction is reported
- Close monitoring of glucose levels because of the risk of hypo and hyperglycemia.
- Glucose and insulin infusion (sliding scale) is recommended.

Postoperative Period

- Close monitoring of glucose levels because of the risk of hypo and hyperglycemia
- Resume drug therapy if no problem with fluid retention or CV event once the pt is able to eat and drink normally.
- Interactions are reported with salicylates and quinalones.

Anticipated Problems/Concerns

- Resistant hyperglycemia needing large doses of insulin, esp. in obese individuals who have responded well to TZDs
- Use of beta-blockers may mask signs of hypoglycemia
- In doubt, stop or delay the resumption of TZDs.

Latest Development

- Recently, the FDA has introduced a stringent guideline for using Rosiglitazone because of the potential increased risk of myocardial infarction (MI). The European equivalent (EMEA) has suspended the drug from the market across Europe. Extreme caution is therefore required for patients on Rosiglitazone undergoing surgery.

Isoproterenol (Isuprel, Medihaler-ISO)

Ayana Cannon
Wendy K. Bernstein

Uses

• Primarily used in the treatment of bradycardia with heart block
• Temporary control of bradycardia in denervated heart transplant pts unresponsive to atropine
• Adjunct therapy in the treatment of hypovolemic, cardiogenic, and septic shock
• Treatment of Adams-Stokes attacks (except when caused by ventricular tachycardia or fibrillation).
• May be used as an inhaled aerosol to treat bronchospasm during anesthesia, asthma exacerbation, chronic bronchitis, and emphysema
• Unlabeled use as pharmacologic overdrive pacing for refractory torsades de points
• Provokes vasovagal syncope during tilt table testing
• Unlabeled use in mesotherapy for body contouring by promoting release of stored fat.

Perioperative Risks

• Isoproterenol may have a deleterious effect on an injured or failing heart by increasing myocardial O_2 demand, and decreasing effective coronary perfusion.
• May lead to myocardial ischemia, may transiently increase blood glucose levels and may induce thyroid storm in susceptible individuals
• Avoid with halothane and desflurane to reduce the potential for sensitization of the myocardium to effects of sympathomimetic amines.
• Avoid with MAOIs to prevent synergistic effects with released catecholamines.
• Administration may cause N/V.

Pharmacodynamics/Pharmacokinetics

• Synthetic sympathomimetic amine
• β1 and β2 adrenoreceptor agonist
• Route of administration may be oral, IV, intranasal, IM, intra-cardiac, or SQ.
• Effects on the CV system result from agonism on β1 receptors of cardiac muscle and β2 receptors found on arteriolar skeletal muscle. Positive inotropic and chronotropic effects on cardiac muscle lead to an increase in cardiac output with an elevation in systolic BP. Vasodilatory effects on arteriolar skeletal muscle act to lower diastolic BP.
• Relaxes bronchial smooth muscle by stimulation of β2 adrenergic receptors, however tolerance may develop with overuse of drug.
• Activates β receptors on adipocytes, resulting in release of stored fat
• Mean plasma elimination half-time is approx 2.5–5 min.
• Readily absorbed when administered parenterally or as an aerosol. Isoproterenol is metabolized primarily in the liver and other tissues by catechol-O-methyl transferase (COMT), and primarily excreted in the urine as sulfate conjugates.
• Onset of action is within 5 min, peak action is 5–15 min, and duration is 10–15 min.

Dosage and Administration

• Usual route of administration is IV infusion or bolus IV injection. Can also be given IM or SQ as well. In dire emergencies, the drug can be administered by intracardiac injection.
• Should be started at the lowest recommended dose and gradually increased to limit risk of ventricular arrhythmias
• Bronchospasm during anesthesia (adults): IV 0.01 to 0.02 mg. Repeat as necessary. INH 1–2 doses 0.08mg/Inh
• Shock and hypoperfusion (adults): IV 0.5 mcg to 5 mcg/min.
• Heart block, Adams-Stokes attacks, and cardiac arrest (adults): Bolus IV 0.02 mg to 0.06 mg as initial dose with subsequent dose range of 0.01 mg to 0.2 mg; IV infusion 2–10 mcg/min, with titration to pt response; IM 0.2 mg initial dose with a subsequent dose rang of 0.02 mg to 1 mg; SQ 0.2 mg initial dose of 0.2 mg with subsequent dose range of 0.15 mg to 0.2 mg; intracardiac 0.02 mg initial dose, with subsequent dosage and administration method dependent upon ventricular rate and rapidity with which cardiac pacemaker can take over when drug is withdrawn.

DRUG EFFECTS

System	Effect	Assessment by Hx	PE	Test
CARDIO	Tachycardia, increased contractility, increased CO, decreased SVR	Palpitations, angina	Pallor, flushing, hyper-/hypotension Tachycardia	ECG, pulse arterial blood pressure, CVP
RESP	Bronchodilation	Dyspnea	Pulm edema	Respirations, peak airway pressure
CNS	Stimulant	Headache, anxiety, weakness, insomnia	Nervousness, restlessness, tremor	
GI	Vasodilation of mesenteric beds	N\V		
ENDO	Hypokalemia Increased serum glucose			Basic metabolic panel

Key Reference: Kapoor WN, et al. Evaluation of syncope by upright tilt testing with isoproterenol: A nonspecific test. *Ann Int Med*. 1992;116:358–363.

Perioperative Implications

• Use is contraindicated in pts with myocardial ischemia, pre-existing tachyarrhythmia, angina pectoris, heart block caused by digitalis toxicity and cardiac glycoside intoxication.
• Caution is necessary when administering isoproterenol to pts with CAD, diabetes, hyperthyroidism, and sensitivity to sympathomimetic amines.

• Contains sodium metabisulfite which may cause allergic reaction and asthma exacerbation in susceptible individuals.
• Paradoxical airway resistance with repeated, excessive use of inhalation preparations.
• Animal reproduction studies have not been conducted. It is not known whether isoproterenol can cause fetal harm when administered to a pregnant woman. Excretion in breast milk is unknown. Should be given if clearly indicated.

• The safety and efficacy of isoproterenol in pediatric pts have not been established.

Lithium Carbonate (Lithobid)

Ira Padnos
Viet Nguyen
Alan Kaye

DRUGS

Uses

- For treatment of manic episodes for bipolar and some schizoaffective disorders
- Approved for maintenance therapy to help prevent episodes of mania or depression
- As an augmenting agent for antidepressants. Has also been used to treat aggression, PTSD, and, conduct disorder in children
- For neutropenia assoc with chemotherapy, HIV therapy, and other medications (acute exposure to lithium can cause leukocytosis; chronic exposure may cause aplastic anemia)
- For hyperthyroidism, e.g., Graves disease (may eventually lead to hypothyroidism)
- May be used to treat syndrome of inappropriate antidiuretic hormone secretion (causes nephrogenic DI)

Perioperative Risks

- Extremely narrow therapeutic level with desired serum levels of 0.6–1.2 mEq/L
- Interaction with depolarizing and nondepolarizing muscle relaxants causes a prolonged response, specifically with pancuronium and succinylcholine.

- Decreased dose requirement for IV and inhalational anesthetics (reduced MAC)
- Toxicity expressed by GI symptoms (nausea/vomiting), psychiatric symptoms (anxiety, insomnia, irritability, mood lability), neurologic symptoms (dizziness, headache, parasthesia, tremor), and somatic symptoms (fatigue, myalgias, chills, rhinorrhea)

Pharmacokinetics/Pharmacodynamics

- At cellular level, acts as imperfect substitute for Na$^+$, intracellular accumulation of lithium decreases phosphatidylinositides by interfering with hydrolysis of myoinositol-1-phosphate in the brain. Specific mechanism of action unknown.
- Decreases availability of norepinephrine at central adrenergic synaptic cleft because increased reabsortion into storage granules. Also interferes with calcium depolarization-mediated release of norepinephrine and dopamine centrally.
- May also inhibit ability of some hormones to activate adenylyl cyclase
- Apparent volume of distribution of 0.6–1 L/kg
- Almost complete absorption from GI tract; peak levels 2–4 hr after oral dose

- Initial distribution in extracellular fluid, subsequent accumulation in tissues
- No plasma protein binding
- Eliminated exclusively by renal excretion with a half-life of 20–27 hr after a single dose. One third to ⅔ acute dose excreted in 6–12 hr; 80% reabsorbed in the proximal convoluted tubules.
- Reabsortion is related to sodium balance. Na$^+$ depletion causes retention of lithium; increase lithium levels from thiazide diuretics, ECA, furosemide; Na$^+$ loading causes increased excretion of lithium
- Lithium clearance is 20% of creatinine clearance
- Low therapeutic index: 0.8–1.25mEq/L, toxic at levels >1.5mEq/L

Drug Class/Usual Dose

- Lithium salt
- Daily dose is individualized; requires regular monitoring of lithium levels. Usual adult dose varies: 900–2400 mg/d in 3–4 divided doses or 900–1800 mg/d in two divided doses of sustained release.

DRUG EFFECTS

System	Effect	Assessment by Hx	PE	Test
CARDIO	Therapeutic levels cause benign ST interval/T wave changes		CVS exam	ECG
	Toxicity: Malignant arrhythmias, heart block, hypotension	Dose, intercurrent illness, drugs precipitating toxicity		
ENDO	Enlarged tender thyroid; hypothyroidism rare	Neck pain, hypothyroid symptoms	Thyroid	FT$_4$E/TSH
GU	Nephrogenic DI	Polyuria, polydipsia		Urine/serum lytes/osmolality
CNS	Toxicity: Tremor, drowsiness, coma, convulsions	Dose, concomitant therapy, illnesses	CNS exam	Lithium level
	Therapeutic: May cause drowsiness, EEG slowing			
DERM	Dermatitis			

Key References: Hill GE, Wong KC. Lithium carbonate and neuromuscular blocking agents. *Anesthesiology.* 1977;46:122–126. Goodwin GM, Young AH. The British Association for Psychopharmacology Guidelines for Treatment of Bipolar Disorder: A Summary. *J Psychopharmacol (Oxf).* 2003;17(suppl 4):3–6.

Possible Drug Interactions

Preoperative Concerns

- Drugs that affect GFR or promote renal sodium wasting leads to increased lithium levels and risk of toxicity: Thiazide diuretics, ECA, furosemide, ACE inhibitors, and carbamazapine
- Increased risk of neurotoxicity: Verapamil, diltiazem, metronidazole
- Increased risk of serotonin syndrome with fluoxetine

Induction/Maintenance

- Must be aware of signs of lithium toxicity
- May have reduced requirement for inhaled and injected anesthesia

- Possibility of prolonged NM blocking effects
- Delayed recovery from barbituates reported

Anticipated Problems/Concerns

- Be aware of signs and symptoms of toxicity. Toxic levels can be decreased with osmotic diuretics (do not use furosemide), administration of saline, or dialysis.
- Renal toxicity is common with chronic lithium therapy. Nephrogenic DI is the most common manifestation. Electrolyte balance is very important.
- Hypothyroidism is the most common endocrine disorder cause by chronic lithium therapy.

- Acute exposure to lithium can cause leukocytosis; chronic exposure may cause aplastic anemia.
- Severe CV collapse; arrhythmias, heart block possible with toxicity
- Abrupt D/C of lithium does not cause withdrawal affect and can be continued soon after surgery.
- Lithium is cotraindicated in pregnancy with increased risk for cardiac anomalies (Epstein's anomaly). May be excreted in breast milk. Lithium should be avoided in first trimester of pregnancy.
- Affects response of commonly used anesthetic drugs

Magnesium Sulfate

Subramanian Sathishkumar
Sanjib Adhikary

Uses

- Hypomagnesemia and magnesium deficiency in critically ill pts
- Treatment of torsade de pointes, digoxin toxicity, atrial or ventricular arrhythmias
- Treatment of pre-eclampsia, eclampsia, prevention of seizures due to eclampsia, tocolysis
- Management of conditions with catecholamine excess (tetanus, pheochromocytoma, attenuation of stress response during laryngoscopy)
- Orally as cathartic or laxative
- Acute asthma
- Adjuvant to other agents during general anesthesia to reduce the requirements of analgesics, muscle relaxants, and hypnotics
- Controlled hypotension

Perioperative Risks

- Hypotension
- Potentiation of nondepolarizing NMB and muscle weakness in pts with high levels of serum magnesium (levels greater than 8 mEq/L^{-1})
- Inadvertent use in pts with impaired-renal function can lead to a state of hypermagnesemia; however, hypomagnesemia may increase the risk of periop arrhythmias.

Worry About

- Dose adjustment via titration is vital during simultaneous administration with muscle relaxant in pt on magnesium sulfate. One third of normal dose is sufficient for maintaining NMB.

- Magnesium deficiency is very undesirable in periop period and in critical care.
- Administration can cause decreased systemic vascular resistance (SVR) leading to hypotension in septic pts.
- Decreased responsiveness to vasopressors due to effect of magnesium on catecholamine reuptake

Overview/Pharmacology

- Magnesium is an emerging drug in anesthesia (molecule of the century); it is the fourth-most common cation in the body and second-most common intracellur cation after potassium.
- Physiological antagonist of calcium and has a fundamental role as a cofactor in over 300 enzymatic reactions.
- Conversion: 1 gram of magnesium sulfate is 4 mmol, 8 mEq, or 98 mg of elemental magnesium.
- Magnesium is available as an inorganic phosphate.
- CVS: Reduces the systemic vascular resistance in high doses. Prolongs SA node conduction time and reduces the rate of SA node impulse formation. Excess catecholamine induced vasoconstriction, arrthymogenic effects and diastolic dysfunction are attenuated by magnesium.
- Antiepileptic properties and the action on CNS are not very defined. Various postulations for neuroprotection incl cerebral vasodilatation, blood-brain barrier protection, and anticonvulsant actions.

- Potentiation of nondepolarizing blockade is due to its presynaptic action
- Studies have shown it to be a physiological and pharmacological antagonist of N-methyl-D-aspartate (NMDA) receptors in the CNS.
- Kinetics: 30% protein bound, 50% is excreted by kidneys, $T_{1/2}$ 4 hr

Drug Class/Mechanism of Action/Usual Dose

- Key actions are calcium antagonism via calcium channels, regulation of energy transfer, membrane sealing, or stabilization. Presynaptically inhibits release of acetylcholine at the NM junction.
- Emergency treatment: IV 2–4 grams (8–16 mmol) initially slowly over 20 min, followed by 10 gram (40 mmol) over next 5 hr.
- It can be given by IM route, however; it is very painful.
- Eclampsia: 4 g IV over at least 5 min followed by 1 g hr for 24 hr after the last seizure. Therapeutic levels: 4–8 mEq/L. Clinical signs of toxicity incl loss of reflexes and resp insufficiency. Assoc with development of cerebral palsy.

DRUG EFFECTS

System	Effect	Assessment by Hx	PE	Test
CARDIO	Vasodilatation, sympathetic blockade, inhibition of catecholamine release, decreased myocardial contractility after a bolus dose of more than 2.5 g	Light headedness, flushing or sensation of warmth if given in an awake pt	Bradycardia, low BP, poor peripheral and systemic perfusion due to vasodilatation and low cardiac output	Check levels CO monitoring (non-invasive and invasive)
RESP	Resp depressant effect due to NMB. Bronchodilator	Resp insufficiency Improvement in asthmatic pts	Hypoxia, hypoventilation, sedation, hypercapnea	Monitor levels, pulse oximetry, ABG
CNS	Anti epileptic, NMDA receptor blockade, potentiation of NMB	Cessation of convulsions Analgesic adjuvant Prolonged recovery from non-depolarizing blockade, muscle weakness	Postictal phase Decreased deep tendon reflexes Improvement in analgesia	Monitor levels
MS	Weakness, increased sensitivity to non depolarizing relaxants	Respiratory depression Heightened response to muscle relaxants	Weakness, lethargy, absent or reduced deep tendon reflexes (DTR)	Monitor DTR, twitch monitoring
OB	Tocolytic,	Arrests labor,	decreased uterine tone	

Key References: James MFM. Magnesium: An emerging drug in anaesthesia. *BJA*. 2009;103:465–467. Fawcett WJ, et al. Magnesium: Physiology and pharmacology. *BJA*. 1999;83:302–320.

Perioperative Implications

Preoperative Concerns

- Exaggerated hemodynamic response to induction agents and central neuraxial blockade
- Enhanced effects of CNS depressants and potentiation of nondepolarizing blockade.
- Monitoring levels is important in pt with renal failure.

Induction/Maintenance

- Dose of induction agent to be titrated as profound drop in BP can occur.
- Use of muscle relaxants to be avoided unless indicated. Use 30–40% of required maintenance dose. Succinylcholine can be safely used as it is not affected by magnesium.

- Volatile agents can compound the drop in SVR. MAC is found to be reduced by 20%.
- When central neuraxial blockade is used; careful titration of local anesthetics dose is needed.
- Vasopressors are most often required to maintain adequate mean arterial pressure (MAP) and SVR if serum levels are high.

Adjuvants/Regional Anesthesia/Reversal

- Obtunds the stress response to laryngoscopy, intraop BP control during surgery for pheochromocytoma, hypotensive anesthesia for surgeries requiring bloodless fields.
- Recent literature demonstrates magnesium a useful analgesic adjuvant (intravenously, regional anesthesia) as a part of multimodal therapy.

- Calcium is used an antidote to magnesium toxicity. However; it does not reverse the effects on the NM junction.

Postoperative Period

- Assess the reversal of NMB before extubation. Muscle weakness and resp insufficiency may warrant the need for extended ventilatory support postop.
- Risk of pulm edema

Anticipated Problems/Concerns

- Require intensive monitoring if magnesium infusion is continued postop.
- Postpartum hemorrhage due to tocolytic effect of magnesium (decreased uterine tone) if used for preterm labor
- Residual NMB and watch for resp failure

Marijuana

Joshua W. Sappenfield
Christopher T. Stephens

Uses

- Many states have passed laws to allow compassionate use of marijuana to alleviate symptoms of debilitating diseases such as pain, nausea and/or vomiting, cachexia, glaucoma, spasms, and seizures.
- Trials are under way for using cannabinoid derivatives as an aid for wt loss; and for preventing relapse of cigarette smoking and opioid abuse.

Perioperative Risks

- Bronchospasm, laryngospasm, uvular edema, pharyngitis
- Inability to filter unnecessary information and perform complex mental tasks

Worry About

- Multiple drug consumption
- Drug interactions with other intoxicants such as cocaine and ethanol or commonly prescribed medications (antidepressants, protease inhibitors, sildenafil)
- Panic reactions and acute psychosis, which is more common with oral intake
- Fetal effects if pregnant

Overview/Pharmacology

- Marijuana is rapidly titrated by inhalation with maximal effects after 2–4 hr. Oral administration within an hour peaks and has prolonged effects lasting approx 5 hr 2° to absorption in the GI tract.
- THC, the main active cannabinoid in marijuana, undergoes first-pass metabolism in the liver into active metabolites.
- The plasma elimination half-life of marijuana is 56 hr (28 hr with chronic use). Its tissue half life is about a week and complete elimination may take 1 mo with chronic use.
- Metabolites are eliminated via urinary excretion or secreted through the biliary tract.
- Cannabinoids are highly lipid soluble and accumulate in breast milk.
- Cannabinoids easily cross both the blood-brain barrier and placenta.

Drug Class/Mechanism of Action/Usual Dose

- Cannabinoid receptors are coupled to G proteins, which inhibit adenyl cyclase.
- Cannabinoid receptors are present on many peripheral and central sites, esp. the hippocampus, striatum, basal ganglia, cortex, cerebellum, and spinal cord.
- Inhalational use of marijuana is usually titrated to effect. The dose of dronabinol for appetite stimulation is 2.5–5 mg daily. Nausea 2° to chemotherapy can be as much as 5 mg/m^2, 6 times a day.

DRUG EFFECTS

System	Effect	Assessment by Hx	PE	Test
CARDIO	Hypotension Tachycardia (bradycardia with chronic use) Vasodilatation Myocardial depression with higher doses Increased myocardial O$_2$ demand Increased cerebral blood flow (decreased with chronic use)	Recent exposure Duration and amount of use Use of other recreational drugs Tobacco/alcohol Hx	Vital signs Injected conjunctiva Reduced oculomotor racking	Urine tox screen
RESP	Coughing Decreased O$_2$-carrying capacity 2° to CO intake with inhalation Bronchial dilation Increased ventilation (decreased with larger doses) Bronchitis Decreased transport of secretions Squamous metaplasia Emphysema			
CNS	Euphoria/dysphoria Lethargy Impairment of coordination Changes in perception Decreased ability to perform complex thoughts or actions Decreased nausea Dizziness Hallucinations Panic reactions Ataxia/dysarthria Confusion Amnesia Anticonvulsant/proconvulsant Schizophreniform symptoms Poor judgment Increasing cognitive impairment with chronic use Depression			
VISION	Decreased intraocular pressure Possible rebound increase in intraocular pressure with cessation Poor oculomotor tracking			
Immune	Decreased resistance to infection Impairment of macrophages			
GU	Urinary retention			
Pregnancy	Preterm labor IUGR VSD in fetus Delay in cognitive development			

Key References: Kumar R, Chambers W, Pertwee R. Pharmacological actions and therapeutic uses of cannabis and cannabinoids. *Anesthesia.* 2001;56:1059–1068.
Kuczkowski K. Anesthetic implications of drug abuse in pregnancy. *J Clin Anesth.* 2003;15:382–394.

Perioperative Implications

Preoperative Concerns

• Chronic use could lead to prolonged intoxication lasting several days 2° to storage in adipose tissue and reuptake of active metabolites in the gut.
• Pts may be sedated or have signs and symptoms of bronchitis and asthma.
• Marijuana may increase opioid effects on ventilation.

Induction/Maintenance

• May interact with medications that affect heart rate.
• Reduces the MAC and may cause pronounced myocardial depression with potent inhaled anesthetics.

• Anesthesiologists should anticipate interactions with anticholinergics, barbiturates, and depressants.

Postoperative Period

• Increased postop agitation and confusion
• Motor function and coordination may be reduced for a longer period than anticipated.
• Some pts may experience withdrawal. Signs incl restlessness, irritation, agitation, nausea, and cramping.

Anticipated Problems/Concerns

• Increased risk of having resp complications during anesthesia
• Periop agitation

• Recent use may impair pts' ability to give consent. Chronic use may lead to difficulty following postop instructions.
• Interactions with the effects of chronotropic medications
• Cannabinoids have prolonged action in pts of increasing age and pts with liver disease.
• Anesthesiologists should encourage preop discontinuance of the drug for elective cases and consider delaying elective cases with recent use.

Metformin (Glucophage)

Monique Espinosa
Albert J. Varon

Uses

- Oral antihyperglycemic drug used in the management of type 2 diabetes
- Most popular oral hypoglycemic drug in the United States and one of the most prescribed drugs overall.

Perioperative Risks

- Metformin-assoc lactic acidosis (MALA)
- Hypoglycemia (rare)

- Risk of metformin accumulation and MALA increases when there is renal impairment.

Pharmacokinetics/Pharmacodynamics

- Oral bioavailability 50–60%
- Absorbed from the small intestine
- Binding to plasma proteins is negligible
- Not metabolized
- Excreted unchanged in the urine
- Half-life is approx 6 hr, however antihyperglycemic effects last >24 hr

Drug Class/Mechanism of Action/Usual Dose

- Biguanide oral antihyperglycemic
- Decreases hepatic glucose production
- Decreases intestinal absorption of glucose
- Improves insulin sensitivity by increasing peripheral glucose uptake and utilization
- Usually dosed 500 mg twice a day
- Maximum recommended daily dose is 2550 mg

ASSESSMENT POINTS

System	Effect	Assessment by Hx	PE	Test
ENDO	Hypoglycemia	Use of other oral antihyperglycemic, decreased PO intake, alcohol consumption Elderly, debilitated, or malnourished pts, and those with adrenal or pituitary insufficiency more susceptible	Irritability, seizures, bradycardia, hypotension, resp failure	Serum glucose (<50 mg/dL)
METAB	Lactic acidosis	Presence of predisposing conditions: Disease states that increase production of lactic acid (CHF, hypoxic states, shock, septicemia) or decrease removal of lactic acid (severe liver disease, alcohol)	Non-specific Hypotension and resp failure have been reported	Serum lactate, serum bicarbonate, ABG, metformin levels
GI	Diarrhea, N/V, flatulence, indigestion, abd discomfort			
CNS	Headache			
Other	Asthenia, megaloblastic anemia			

Key Reference: Triplitt CL, Reasner CA, Isley WL. Diabetes mellitus. In: DiPiro JT, Talbert RL, Yee GC, Matzke GR, Wells BG, Posey LM, ed. *Pharmacotherapy: A pathophysiologic approach*. New York: McGraw-Hill; 2008:1205–1242.

Perioperative Implications

Preoperative Concerns

- Metformin should be temporarily D/C preop
- Metformin should be D/C at the time of, or prior to, use of IV contrast dye, withheld for 48 hrs subsequent to the procedure, and reinstituted only after renal function has been reassessed.
- Co-morbidities that may increase the incidence of MALA in pts taking metformin are renal dysfunction, heart failure, resp failure, impaired liver function, sepsis, and severe dehydration.

Induction/Maintenance

- No known drug interactions

Adjuvants/Regional Anesthesia/Reversal

- No known contraindications

Postoperative Concerns

- Metformin should be withheld in pts having postop renal complications
- Do not resume metformin until the pt is tolerating a PO diet

Drug Interactions

- Cimetidine competes for the renal tubular secretion of metformin and concomitant use leads to higher metformin serum levels.

- Other cationic drugs such as vancomycin, digoxin, procainamide, and trimethoprim may interact similarly

Anticipated Problems/Concerns

- MALA and risk factors for MALA can be assessed for (hypovolemia, hypotension, hypoxemia)
- Hyperglycemia from withholding metformin in the periop period

DRUGS

Monoamine Oxidase Inhibitors; Reversible Inhibitors of Monoamine Oxidase

J. Lance LaFleur
Krishna Boddu

Uses

- Monoamine oxidase (MAO) inhibitors are indicated for refractory depression, depression with prominent anxiety, low psychomotor activity, and severe phobias.
- Other indications incl Htn, narcolepsy, and intractable headache.

Perioperative Risks

- Hypertensive crisis
- Serotonin syndrome (central serotonergic hyperactivity) may be fatal and manifests as Htn, hypotension, resp depression, tachycardia, diaphoresis, hyperthermia, muscle rigidity, seizures, agitation, headache, and coma.

Worry About

- Side effects incl orthostatic Htn, agitation, tremor, seizures, muscle spasms, urinary retention, dysuria, paresthesias, hepatotoxicity, jaundice, sedation, vision changes, hallucinations, dryness of the mouth, and constipation.

- Hypertensive crisis can occur after ingestion of tyramine-containing substances such as red wine, cheeses, liver, beer, chocolate, fava beans, avocados, and pickled herring.
- Tyramine causes significant catecholamine release which can lead to headache, tachycardia, nausea, Htn, dysrrhythmias, and stroke.
- Adrenergic α-antagonists such as phentolamine and prazosin are useful in the treatment of tyramine-induced Htn.

Overview/Pharmacology

- MAO is an endogenous mitochondrial enzyme which inactivates neurotransmitters by deamination.
- MAO inhibitors block oxidative deamination of naturally occurring amines, which permits neurotransmitter accumulation and increased adrenoreceptor activation.
- 2 MAO isoenzymes (types A and B) differ in their substrate selectivities.
- MAO A is selective for serotonin, dopamine, and norepinephrine.

- MAO B is selective for tyramine and phenylethylamine; ineffective as antidepressants
- Nonselective (irreversible MAO inhibitors) agents: Phenelzine (Nardil), isocarboxazid (Marplan), and tranylcypromine (Parnate)
- Nonselective agents may interfere with many other enzymes
- Selective agents (reversible MAO A inhibitors): Moclobemide, broforamide, lazabemide, toloxatone, and cimoxatone

Drug Class/Mechanism of Action

- Although MAO is completely inhibited within days, antidepressant actions may require 2–4 wk (similar to other antidepressant classes)
- Phenelzine and tranylcypromine may cause a stimulant effect similar to amphetamines.
- MAO regeneration after irreversible inhibition usually occurs after several weeks.

DRUG EFFECTS

System	Effect	Assessment by Hx	PE	Test
CARDIO	Orthostatic hypotension, Htn	Dizziness, vision changes	BP, HR	Orthostatic BP, HR
GI	Hepatotoxicity, constipation	Jaundice		LFTs
CNS	Agitation, seizures			EEG

Key Reference: Tjan J, Malhotra V. *Brachial plexus block. Yao and Artusio's anesthesiology: Problem-oriented patient management.* 6th ed. Philadelphia: Lippincott Williams and Wilkins; 2008:641–645.

Perioperative Implications

Preoperative Concerns

- Avoid co-administration of MAO inhibitors and SSRIs within 6 wk to avoid serotonin syndrome
- Check LFTs as hepatotoxicity and/or hepatic enzyme inhibition may exaggerate depressant effects of opioids, benzodiazepines, barbiturates, antihistamines, anticholinergics, and tricyclic antidepressants.
- Controversy persists regarding D/C prior to elective surgery.
- Previous recommendations were cessation 2–3 wk prior to surgery, but the decision should take into consideration the pt's indication and dependence (risk of suicide).
- Effective anxiolysis to avoid sympathetic hyperactivity

Induction/Maintenance

- Consider arterial cannula for close monitoring of BP.
- Phenelzine can prolong the duration of succinylcholine by inhibiting pseudocholinesterase
- Interaction with opioids, particularly meperidine, can lead to the potentially fatal serotonin syndrome.
- Consider regional techniques to avoid opioids; morphine or fentanyl are preferred if necessary
- N₂O and volatile agents are acceptable
- Pronounced response to vasopressors and sympathetic stimulation can occur; direct-acting vasopressors of short duration at a reduced dose are preferred (such as phenylephrine at ⅓ the usual dose)
- Avoid drugs that increase sympathetic activity such as ketamine, pancuronium, cocaine, and epinephrine (in local anesthetics)

Postoperative Period

- Judicious opioid use if needed
- Use adrenergic α- or β-antagonists or direct-acting vasodilators for Htn

Anticipated Problems/Concerns

- Pain control
- Hemodynamic instability
- Timing and dosing of MAO inhibitor resumption

DRUGS

Nicotine Replacment Therapies (NRTs)

Esther Sung

Uses

- NRTs are FDA-approved devices that are effective in helping treat tobacco dependence, acting on nicotinic acetylcholine receptors to mimic or replace the effects of nicotine, the highly addictive chemical from tobacco products.
- NRTs are available OTC (gum, transdermal patch, sublingual lozenge/tablet) and by prescription (nasal spray, inhaler).
- NRTs provide only nicotine; they do not contain the carcinogens and toxic gases that are found in cigarette smoke.

Perioperative Risks

- While there is no clear evidence that NRTs increase CV risk in medically stable pts, the safety of NRTs in critically ill pts or in pts undergoing cardiopulmonary bypass surgery, esp. off-pump cardiac surgery, is questionable.
- During MRI procedures, transdermal nicotine patches that have metallic components can cause cutaneous burns if a pt wears them during the scan.
- Nicotine gum or sublingual lozenges/tablets can cause hiccups, nausea, and heartburn; this could potentially increase aspiration risk for pts undergoing general anesthesia.

Worry About

- A fatal nicotine dose for adults is around 60 mg. Individual cigarettes contain 1–3 mg of nicotine. While it is difficult to overdose solely by smoking, the use of nicotine patches, nicotine gum, or other NRTs concomitantly with tobacco smoking could place the user at risk. Make sure smoker takes off patch prior to surgery as increased skin blood flow with inhalation agents could increase absorption from skin depot or patch.
- Nicotine poisoning manifests as nausea, salivation, abd cramps, vertigo, mental confusion, difficulty breathing, increased heart rate, skeletal muscle weakness, and seizures.
- Nicotine withdrawal can create a negative emotional state, anxiety and irritability, perception of increased stress, difficulty concentrating, increased appetite, headache, and insomnia.
- Nicotine medication via NRTs is generally considered safer than cigarette smoking since exposure to toxic combustion products is averted; however, concerns exist regarding the safety of long-term nicotine exposure and its effect on CV disease, cancer, wound healing, and fetal development.
- NRTs can cause irritation to the skin or inside of the mouth.

Overview/Pharmacology

- Nicotine from NRTs is absorbed from the skin, the resp tract, or buccal mucous membranes. These methods deliver nicotine to the bloodstream more slowly than smoking.
- Nicotine's half-life is approx 2 hr. It is metabolized primarily by the liver and partly by the lungs. Cotamine, which can be a urinary marker of nicotine exposure, is the principle metabolite with ⅓ the pharmacologic activity of nicotine.
- Nicotine and its metabolites are eliminated by the kidneys and in breast milk.
- Nicotine can cause the induction of liver microsomal enzymes, resulting in faster metabolism of some anesthetics, analgesics, and sedatives.

Drug Class/Mechanism of Action/Usual Dose

- Nicotine is a highly addictive alkaloid. It is a sympathomimetic drug that stimulates autonomic ganglia and acts as a central nicotinic cholinergic agonist, thereby facilitating neurotransmitter release (i.e., dopamine, norepinephrine, serotonin, glutamate, GABA).
- A typical pack-per-day smoker absorbs 20–40 mg/day. The dose of NRTs is variable: transdermal patches (5–22 mg/24 hr); gum, lozenges, tablets (1–4 mg each); inhaler (cartridge contains 10 mg); nasal spray (0.5 mg/spray)
- Nicotine can have unpredictable effects, initially acting as a stimulant and then as a depressant.

DRUG EFFECTS

System	Effect	Assessment by Hx	PE	Test
CARDIO	↑ HR, BP, cardiac contractility; coronary and peripheral vasoconstriction	Palpitations, chest pain	Cardiac exam, heart sounds	Vital signs
RESP	↑ Ventilation (stim. of aortic and carotid body chemoreceptors)	↑ Resp rate	Resp exam, breath sounds	O_2 sat, resp rate
GI	Vomiting, diarrhea, heartburn, initial ↑ salivary secretions	Dyspepsia, nausea		
CNS	Stimulation	Initially tremor		
ENDO	↓ Insulin sensitivity, may aggravate or precipitate diabetes			Blood sugar; HbA1c
IMMUNO	May be a tumor promoter through angiogenesis, ↑ cell proliferation, and ↓ apoptosis			

Key References: Benowitz NL. Pharmacology of nicotine: Addiction, smoking-induced disease, and therapeutics. *Ann Rev Pharmacol Toxicol.* 2009;49:57–71.
Stead LF, Perera R, Bullen C, Mant D, Lancaster T. Nicotine replacement therapy for smoking cessation. *Cochrane Database Syst Rev.* 2008;(1):CD000146.
Warner DO. Perioperative abstinence from cigarettes: Physiologic and clinical consequences. *Anesthesiology.* 2006;104:356–367.

Perioperative Implications

Preoperative Concerns

- With respect to postop pulm complications, it is likely that the longer the duration of preop abstinence from smoking, the better. There is insufficient evidence to suggest increased risk during the first weeks of quitting smoking. Pts should be advised to quit smoking as early as possible before surgery.
- Pts may experience anxiety, irritability, increased stress, and/or headache from nicotine withdrawal in addition to the uneasiness and nervousness from surgery itself. A preop anxiolytic or maintenance of nicotine supplementation via transdermal patch in medically stable pts should be considered.
- Nicotine gum or sublingual lozenges/tablets may cause dyspepsia and nausea. Those pts using these forms of NRTs may have increased aspiration risk for general anesthesia.

Induction/Maintenance

- Pts who are smokers or receiving NRTs may experience resistance to some anesthetic or analgesic agents as a result of increased metabolism from induced hepatic enzymes.
- Nicotine is a sympathomimetic agent and also has effects on autonomic ganglia. Smokers receiving nicotine patches preop have been observed to show exaggerated increases in heart rate after tracheal intubation. NRTs may have hemodynamic effects that may need to be addressed in the periop period.
- While NRTs have been deemed safe in medically stable pts, they may be assoc with worsened outcome in critically ill pts or in pts undergoing cardiopulmonary bypass surgery, esp. off-pump cardiac surgery.

Postoperative Period

- Smoking contributes to acute physiologic effects such as increased sympathetic tone, lung inflammation, and tissue hypoxia as well as long-term pathophysiologic changes such as atherosclerosis and COPD, placing these pts at higher risk for postop complications.
- Nicotine withdrawal should be considered as a cause of postop agitation or anxiety.

Anticipated Problems/Concerns

- NRTs have proven to be both safe and effective in treating tobacco dependence in medically stable pts, even in those with smoking-related diseases. While more studies are needed, current evidence suggests that NRTs can be valuable tools to manage tobacco dependence in the periop period.
- Use of NRTs in the periop period is far preferable to continued smoking per most experts in the field.

Nitric Oxide (NO), Inhaled

Warren M. Zapol

Uses

- Children: Acute or chronic pulm Htn assoc with persistent pulm Htn of newborn (PPHN), meconium apiration, CHD, and congenital diaphragmatic hernia
- Adults: Acute or pulm Htn assoc with ARDS, pulm embolism

Perioperative Risks

- Methemoglobinemia (esp. breathing >20 ppm NO)
- NO_2 and peroxynitrite formation

Worry About

- Methemoglobinemia; measure metHb, esp. for infants, within 6 hr and then every 24 hr
- Measure inhaled NO and NO_2 levels continuously
- Do not give if high NO_2 levels (>2 ppm)

- Do not allow NO to stagnate in ventilator or breathing circuits; it slowly converts to toxic NO_2 gas
- High inhaled NO levels may inhibit plt aggregation
- In severe heart failure, reducing PVR with NO may raise LAP
- Rebound pulm Htn during NO withdrawal

Overview/Pharmacology

- Inhaled NO activates guanylate cyclase in lung vessels, airways, and increased cGMP levels, causes selective pulm vasodilation
- Very rapid and avid binding with RBC Hgb inactivates NO and thereby prevents systemic vasodilation
- NO is metabolized to nitrate and nitrite and is excreted in urine

- Supplied as stock gas of ≤1,000 ppm by vol NO in nitrogen or other inert gas
- Inhaled NO is mixed with O_2–containing gas immediately before breathing via intratracheal catheter, ventilator, mask, or nasal prongs

Drug Class/Mechanism of Action/Usual Dose

- N=O is a free radical with short $T_{1/2}$ in aqueous solutions (~17 sec)
- It combines with ferrous-heme ring of guanylate cyclase, and thereby stimulates the conversion of GTP to cGMP; cGMP reduces intracellular Ca^{2+}, causing smooth muscle relaxation and modulates other cell functions by regulating gene expression; cGMP is broken down by phosphodiesterases
- Usual inhaled NO dose is 0.1 to 20 ppm by vol

DRUG EFFECTS

System	Effect	PE	Test
RESP	↓ PVR		↓ PAP ↑ CO
	↑ Gas exchange	Skin color	↑ Pao_2 ↑ Sao_2 ↓ $Paco_2$

Key Reference: Clark RH, Kueser TJ, Walker MW, et al, for the Clinical Inhaled Nitric Oxide Research Group. Low-dose nitric oxide therapy for persistent pulmonary hypertension of the newborn. *N Engl J Med.* 2000;342:469–474.

Perioperative Implications

- Check for heart failure; do not use in severe heart failure (e.g., PCWP >25 mmHg) or with pulm venous disease (e.g., pulm vein stenosis, pulm veno-occlusive disease). Use of inhaled NO in these settings can cause severe pulm edema with hypoxemia and decreased lung compliance. Some pts with mild left heart dysfunction (diastolic dysfunction) may also develop worsening pulm edema with iNO.

Monitoring

- **Must monitor**
  - Inhaled NO, NO_2 levels
  - metHb levels
- Consider monitoring
  - PA pressure
  - RV ECHO
  - ABGs, SpO_2

Induction/Maintenance

- Inhale 0.1–20 ppm in ARDS (usual dose: 5–15 ppm) Initiate therapy with a higher dose (usually 20 ppm) in the setting of ARDS with moderate or severe pulm Htn, and lower doses (5–10 ppm) to reduce intrapulmonary shunt (e.g., ARDS).
- In persistent pulm Htn of newborn, begin therapy at 20 ppm, and progressively reduce the dose to 5 ppm or less with improved oxygenation (e.g., FIO2 <0.60) and PAP by echocardiogram. Inhaled NO therapy should not be initiated without first optimizing lung volume, ventilation, cardiac performance, and systemic BP.
- Ideal doses need better definition but lower doses are most effective for improving oxygenation by matching ventilation and perfusion, and higher doses to treat pulm Htn. Failure to respond in term infants with PPHN may reflect underlying lung developmental abn or structural (anatomic) heart disease.
- Give as little NO as possible to reduce oxidant burden of lung.

Adjuvants

- Phosphodiesterase inhibitors (e.g., sildenafil) increase sensitivity and duration of the dilatory effect of inhaled NO, but must be used with caution as they can cause systemic hypotension.

Postoperative Period

- Slowly wean from NO over hours if possible watching for abrupt worsening of oxygenation or pulm Htn with the D/C of NO ("rebound" effects).

Anticipated Problems/Concerns

- Beware rapid D/C of inhaled NO; reactive pulm vasoconstriction and hypoxemia, RHF may ensue. These effects may not be seen while reducing doses, but may be dramatic with D/C of iNO therapy, and can even occur after D/C low doses of NO.
- Do not allow NO stock tanks to deplete
- Provide NO freshly mixed in O_2-containing gas for manual ventilation even when briefly disconnecting from ventilator for suctioning or moving pt.
- If inhaled NO does not reverse hypoxemia despite mechanical ventilation with PEEP, high-frequency oscillatory ventilation, etc., ECMO may be required.

Nitroglycerin

Lee A. Fleisher

Uses

- Rx for pts with angina
- CHF
- In MI, ↓ infarct size
- Prinzmetal's angina
- Can be given as patch, paste, PO, sublingually prn
- Uterine relaxation
- May be beneficial in reducing postop morphine usage for pain management

Perioperative Risks

- Development of hypotension
- Drug rash (rare)

Worry About

- Severe hypotension, esp. with regional anesthesia

Overview/Pharmacology

- Used for both chronic Rx and acute management
- Prophylactic nitroglycerin not shown to ↓ incidence of intraop MI
- Tolerance to drug from prolonged IV infusion or continuous patch can occur.
- Metabolized by reductive hydrolysis in liver
- Rapidity of onset, duration of action directly related to method of administration
  - SL: Onset 1–2 min, duration <1 hr
  - Oral: Peak effect 60–90 min, duration 3–6 hr
  - Paste: Onset 60 min, duration 4–8 hr
  - Patch: Duration up to 24 hr
- Prolonged use can → tolerance (↓ effectiveness)
- Nitroglycerin paste and/or patch may have uneven absorption intraop

Drug Class/Mechanism of Action/Usual Dose

- Organic nitrate
- Activates guanylate cyclase; ↑ cGMP levels in smooth muscle, other tissues; increases NO
- Usual dosage:
  - SL: 0.4 mg prn
  - Paste: 1/2"–1"
  - Isordil: 5–30 mg q 6 h
  - IV: 0.5–2.0 $\mu g/kg/min$
- Bolus for uterine relaxation (slow 50 μg; may repeat × 1 with caution if has regional anesthesia actively causing sympathectomy)

ASSESSMENT POINTS

System	Effect	Assessment by Hx	PE	Test
CARDIO	Vasodilation of veins > arteries Redistribution of coronary blood flow	Relief of angina	BP	PCWP
RESP	Decreased pulm vascular resistance			PCWP
GU	Uterine (smooth muscle) relaxation			
CNS	Dilation of meningeal arterial vessels	Headache		

Key Reference: Zvara DA, Groban L, Rogers AT, et al. Prophylactic nitroglycerin did not reduce myocardial ischemia during accelerated recovery management of coronary artery bypass graft surgery patients. *J Cardiothorac Vasc Anesth*. 2000;14:571–575.

Perioperative Implications

Preoperative Concerns

- Assess volume status
- Consider monitoring:
  - BP (arterial catheter)
  - PA catheter (may give useful information if nitroglycerin infusion used)

Induction/Maintenance

- May interact with other induction agents to cause hypotension
- Ideally should be given IV because of uneven absorption intraop (binding sites on tubing)
- Effective means of alleviating myocardial ischemia intraop
- Has been used prophylactically as bolus during induction
- Anesthetic agents may mimic beneficial effects of nitroglycerin

Adjuvants/Regional Anesthesia/Reversal

- Agents that can result in hypotension may be exacerbated by nitroglycerin

Postoperative Period

- Pts on chronic nitroglycerin may benefit by resumption of agent
- Can give as patch or paste after rewarming of pt

Anticipated Problems/Concerns

- Tolerance to nitroglycerin manifests by ↓ hemodynamic effects; a function of dose, frequency of administration
- Many inhalational agents and opiates have some aspect of hemodynamic effects of nitroglycerin—e.g., venodilation, ↓ O_2 demand

DRUGS

Nonsteroidal Anti-Inflammatory Drugs (NSAIDs)

Todd A. Schultz

Risks

- Incidence in USA: 100 million NSAID prescriptions are written per year; 17 million Americans using NSAIDs daily
- 2 subclasses: Nonselective (COX1 and 2) inhibitors and selective COX2 inhibitors (coxibs).
- Have analgesic, anti-inflammatory, and antipyretic properties.

Indications

- NSAIDs are the first step in the WHO analgesic ladder, typically considered drugs of choice for mild to moderate pain.
- Can be taken OTC or prescribed for chronic somatic pain states (e.g., arthritis) and rheumatologic disorders
- Also given IV, IM, and PO postop as part of a multimodal treatment regimen for acute pain

Worry About

- Plt dysfunction
- Renal insufficiency
- Drug interactions
- Allergic reactions

- Effect on bone growth
- Gastric bleeding
- Possible increased risk of thrombotic/CV events with long-term use

Overview/Pharmacology

- Most NSAIDs are weak acids (pKa 3–5) of diverse chemical structure and half-lives.
- Well absorbed from the stomach and intestinal mucosa.
- Highly protein bound (>95%), usually to albumin.
- Work by inhibiting cyclooxygenase, which is a key enzyme in the synthesis pathway of prostaglandins
  - Leads to a ↓ in prostaglandin synthesis, therefore decreasing the inflammatory response as well as the sensitizing effect of prostaglandins on nociceptors (both central and peripheral).
- Two isoforms of the COX enzyme have been identified.
  - COX-1: Expressed constitutively in most cell types and has an essential role in functions such as gastric protection, plt aggregation, renal function

- COX-2: Traditionally considered to be induced by tissue injury/inflammation, now known to be constitutively expressed in some tissues (e.g., brain and/or kidney).
- Undergo liver metabolism to inactive metabolites, which are then excreted by the kidney
- Have a low abuse potential but also possess a ceiling analgesic effect

Drug Class

- Traditional or nonselective NSAIDs are both COX-1 and COX-2 inhibitors
- Have several different subclasses
  - Salicylate (salsate, diflunisal, and choline magnesium trisalicylate)
  - Proprionic (ibuprofen, ketoprofen, naproxen, fenoprofen)
  - Indole (indomethacin, sulindac, tolmetin)
  - Fenamate (mefenamic, meclofenamate)
  - Mixed (piroxicam, ketorolac, diclofenac)
- Coxibs are selective COX-2 inhibitors.
  - Only celecoxib is commercially available.

ASSESSMENT POINTS

System	Effect	Assessment by Hx	PE	Test
CARDIO	Htn, HF, thrombotic events	Worsening SOB	BP, edema, rales, chest pain	
RESP	Nasal polyps, rhinitis, dyspnea, bronchospasm, angioedema	In asthmatics	Wheezing	
HEPAT	Hepatitis	N/V, anorexia	Jaundice	LFTs
GI	Gastropathy (can be asymptomatic), GI bleeding, esophageal disease, pancreatitis	Hx ulcers, heartburn		Stool heme, Hgb, upper endoscopy
HEME	↑ Bleeding	Easy bruising/bleeding	Pallor	Bleeding time, Hgb
DERM	Urticaria, erythema multiforme, rash			
GU	Renal insufficiency, sodium/fluid retention, papillary necrosis, interstitial nephritis		BP, edema, wt changes	↑ K+/BUN/Cr, ↓ UO, biopsy
CNS	Headache, aseptic meningitis, hearing disturbances	Cognitive dysfunction, somnolence, confusion		CSF

Key Reference: McQuay HJ, Moore A. NSAIDs and Coxibs: Clinical use. In: McMahon SB, Koltzenburg M, eds. *Wall and Melzack's textbook of pain.* 5th ed. Philadelphia: Elsevier; 2006:471–479.

Perioperative Implications

Preoperative

- Preop nonselective NSAID use has been assoc with increased intraop blood loss due to plt inhibition.
  - Unlike aspirin, NSAID plt inhibition is reversible, common practice is to hold the NSAID for a period of 5 half-lives before surgery (e.g., ibuprofen 1 d, naproxen 5 d).
  - Coxibs do not affect plt function and therefore do not need to be held.
- NSAIDs displace albumin-bound drugs and can potentiate their effects (e.g., warfarin).

Regional Anesthesia

- According to ASRA consensus guidelines, NSAIDs do not significantly increase the risk for spinal hematoma in pts undergoing neuraxial anesthesia.
- The use of NSAIDs alone should not interfere with the performance of neuraxial blocks or the timing of neuraxial catheter removal.

Intraoperative

- Intraop administration of NSAIDs has been shown to cause a slight increase in the need for

reoperation in surgeries at high risk for postop bleeding (e.g., tonsillectomy/CABG).
  - Decision to administer an NSAID should consider the need for improved analgesia, pts ability to achieve hemostasis, and the risk of postop bleeding inherent to the surgery.
- May exacerbate asthma, esp. in pts with a Hx of NSAID-induced bronchospasm, angioedema, urticaria, or rhinitis.

Postoperative

- NSAIDs can be resumed while cautiously monitoring for GI bleeding/renal dysfunction, avoid resumption in seriously ill pts.
- Risk of adverse effect on renal function the same for both non-selective NSAIDs and COX-2 inhibitors.
  - Use caution when initiating therapy in pts with pre-existing heart/kidney disease, use of loop diuretics, or loss of blood volume > 10%.
- Both the nonselective NSAIDs and coxibs have been implicated in potentially inhibiting bone healing.
  - May be prudent to avoid in cases where bone formation is esp. crucial (e.g., spinal fusion).

Anticipated Problems/Concerns

- All NSAIDs have risk of gastropathy, ulcers typically asymptomatic before episode of GI bleed.
  - Risk with coxibs is ~50-60% less than nonselective NSAIDs, but still present.
  - Concurrent treatment with PPI or misoprostol may further decrease risk.
- All NSAIDs may carry an increased risk of CV events esp. if used with aspirin (one NSAID may antagonize benefit of another) with chronic use.
  - Significantly increased risk with COX-2s rofecoxib/valdecoxib led to withdrawal from market
  - For most pts, the increased risk is small and a risk/benefit analysis should be undertaken before continuing long-term use.
- Can exacerbate and/or induce CHF in susceptible pts.
  - Risk is nearly equivalent to that of NSAID induced gastropathy.
- Can lead to an increase in BP, esp. in pts with pre-existing Htn.

Nutritional Support

Amir Baluch
Alan Kaye

Risk

- Up to 40% of pts may be undernourished on admission to hospital and two-thirds of all pts lose wt during hospital course.

Perioperative Risks of Malnutrition

- Decreased resp, cardiac, skeletal muscle mass, strength
- Decreased visceral protein mass, altered GI mucosal barrier
- Altered humoral, cell-mediated immunity
- Altered neutrophil function
- Increased pulm, thromboembolic complications
- Pts with protein-calorie malnutrition have ↑ risk for postop cardiac, noncardiac complications
- Increased risk for nosocomial infections and decreased wound healing
- Increased risk for multiple organ failure
- Increased length of hospital stay

Worry About

- Hypo- or hyperglycemia, depending on additives to TPN
- Decreased ability to secrete insulin in malnourished pts
- Increased free fraction of certain protein-bound drugs with low albumin levels
- B-12 and/or folate deficiency leading to anemia
- Higher rates of infection with TPN
- Excess carbohydrate administration via TPN may lead to increased CO_2 production and increased difficulty in weaning from ventilatory support and hepatic steatosis. ("fatty liver")
- Excess fat administration via TPN may lead to hyperlipidemia, decreased immune function, and reduced reticuloendothelial function.

Overview

- Nutritional risk index (NRI) = 1.519 × serum albumin (g/L) + [0.417 × (current wt/usual wt) × 100]. (Malnutrition defined as NRI <100; severe malnutrition defined as NRI <83.5.)

- Preop nutritional support for 5–7 d may result in ↓ in infectious complications in severely malnourished pts

TPN Composition

- Fluid: 30 mL/kg/d, additional losses
- Calories: 25–30 Kcal/kg/d
- Glucose: 3.0–5.0 g/kg/d
- Fat: 1.0–1.5 g/kg/d
- Protein: 1.5–2.0 g/kg/d
- Additives:
  - Multivitamins in the form of balanced formula should be provided daily.
  - IV formula requires addition of vitamin K, 2 mg/d
  - Trace elements should be given daily to pts with GFR >20 mL/d; magnesium: 15–20 mg/d; zinc: 15–20 mg/d. (Requirement for replacement is based on serum level.)

Special Formulas

- Modified amino acid formula is more efficient in restoring positive nitrogen balance, ↓ ureagenesis, and ↑ support of protein synthesis

ASSESSMENT POINTS

System	Effect	Assessment by Hx	PE	Test
MS	>10% loss of body wt over 6 mo	Hx of renal, hepatic dysfunction Hx of short gut	Muscle wasting ↓ Triceps and skinfold thickness, ↓ mid-arm circumference	Alb <2.5 g/dL Total lymphocyte count <1500 cells/mm³

Key References: The VA Total Parenteral Nutrition Cooperative Study Group. Perioperative total parenteral nutrition in surgical patients. *N Engl J Med.* 1991;325(8):525. McWhirter JP, Pennington CR. Incidence and recognition of malnutrition in hospital. *BMJ.* 1994;308:945–948.

Preoperative Concerns

Monitoring

- Daily monitoring of wt, electrolytes, magnesium.
- Weekly monitoring of zinc, liver function tests, PT/PTT.
- Nutritional variable: Prealbumin and transferrin better indicators of nutritional status due to their shorter half life compared to albumin. Failure to improve or maintain adequate levels usually represents inadequate nutritional support, intercurrent systemic inflammatory response, or advanced organ failure.

Induction/Maintenance

- TPN is usually continued intraop
- Monitor glucose
- Malnutrition may predispose a pt to having a higher risk for pseudocholinesterase deficiency, use succinylcholine with caution.

Adjuvants

- For morbidly obese pts use ideal wt for calculation of TPN requirement.
- For severely underweight pts use 1/2 difference between pt's ideal wt and actual wt.

Anticipated Problems/Concerns

- Caloric and glucose overload can result in hyperglycemia and hepatic dysfunction.
- Fat overload can result in WBC dysfunction, and infectious complication, and increased CO_2 production.

Oral Contraceptives

Tracey L. Stierer

Uses

- Prevention of pregnancy
- Treatment of the following
  - Dysmenorrhea
  - Metorrhagia/Fe deficiency anemia
  - Acne
  - Endometriosis
  - Functional ovarian cyst
  - Hyperandrogenism and/or polycystic ovarian disease
  - Premenstrual syndrome and/or premenstrual dysphoric disorder
  - Perimenopausal vasomotor symptoms
  - Mittleschmerz

Perioperative Risks

- Hypercoagulability increased risk of venous and arterial thrombosis when given without concomitant aspirin, esp in blood Type A+ women

Worry About

- Thromboembolic events—increased relative risk of 2.7 (without aspirin)

- Hyperkalemia (drospirenone and/or ethinyl estradiol)
- Treatment failure and/or pregnancy. "Typical user" failure rates reported as high as 9%. Preop beta-HCG assay may be indicated in sexually active pts.

Overview/Pharmacology

- Oral preparations of synthetic estrogen, progestin generally well absorbed
- Metabolized by the liver and excreted in urine and feces

Drug Class/Mechanism of Action/Usual Dose

- Estrogens
  - Mestrol
  - Ethinyl
  - Estradiol
- Progestins
  - Norethindrone
  - Norgestrel
  - Norethindrone acetate
  - Ethynodiol diacetate
  - Levonorgestrel

- Norgestimate
- Desogestrel
- Drospirenone
- Prometrium
- Combination estrogen and progestin drugs inhibit ovulation by negative feedback effect on the hypothalamus; altering normal pattern of gonadotropin secretion by the anterior pituitary; cervical mucus thickens, and is unfavorable to sperm even if ovulation occurs. Classified as
  - Monophasic: Same ratio of progestin and estrogen in each pill
  - Biphasic: Two phases of altered progestin and estrogen ratio
  - Triphasic: Progestin and estrogen ratio varied in three phases
- Progestin only agents act directly by inhibiting ovulation or creating thick cervical mucus impenetrable to sperm.
- First and second generation progestin only drugs have a lower risk of thromboembolism. Third generation progestins carry 6-9–fold increase of VTE similar to the risk during pregnancy if given without concomitant aspirin.

DRUG EFFECTS

System	Effect	Assessment by Hx	PE	Test
CARDIO	Htn ↑↑ Thromboembolic events Arrhythmia due to hyperkalemia Altered lipid/cholesterol profile	Hx of MI or CVA Hx of DVT/PE Palpitations	BP Deep vein exam	Venous Doppler Serum K⁺ Serum lipid cholesterol levels
GI	May exacerbate gallbladder disease	Hx of jaundice/cholestasis during pregnancy		↑ Bilirubin, US, and ERCP
HEPATIC	↑ Incidence of hepatic adenoma and hepatocellular cancer			

Key References: Blanco-Molina A, et al. for the RIETE investigators: Venous thromboembolism in women using hormonal contraceptives. *Thromb Haemost.* 2009;101:478–482. Chalhoub V, Edelman P, Staiti G, Benhamou D. Oral contraceptives and hormone replacement therapy: Management of their thrombembolic risk in the perioperative period: *Ann Fr Anesth Reanim.* 2008;27(5):405–415.

Perioperative Implications

Preoperative Concerns

- Consider D/C of combination oral contraceptives and third generation progestin only OCs 1 mo prior to major surgery if administered without aspirin and adding barrier method or adding aspirin, for surgery with anticipated prolonged period of immobilization.

- Must weigh OC cessation with the risk of unwanted pregnancy or termination. In addition consider risk of anesthesia and surgery to pregnant woman and fetus, incl possible teratogenicity and spontaneous abortion.

Induction/Maintenance

- Consider thromboprophylaxis on an individualized basis judged according to additional genetic and acquired risk factors.

Postoperative Period

- Surveillance for DVT and PE. Restart aspirin.
- Early mobilization, resume agents 2 wk after surgery or mobilization.

DRUGS

Oral Hypoglycemics

Jyotsna Rimal

Uses

- Oral hypoglycemics are used for Type II DM or non-insulin dependent diabetes mellitus (NIDDM) not controlled by diet or wt loss where cells are resistant to secreted insulin.
- Main classes of agents:
  - Insulin secretagogues: Sulfonylureas, meglitinides, dipeptidyl peptidase-4 inhibitors (DPP-4)
  - Insulin sensitizers: Biguanides and thiazolidinediones
- Others: Alpha–glucosidase inhibitors
- Diabetes is the leading cause of blindness, kidney failure, and non-traumatic amputations, and a leading cause of arterial diseases such as stroke, memory loss, impotence, and myocardial infarctions.
- Prevalence of diagnosed and undiagnosed diabetes in the USA, all ages, 2007 is 23.6 million; 17.9 million are diagnosed and 5.7 million are undiagnosed. Expected to increase to 60+ million by 2030.
- Total diabetic pts in USA of which 50.6% only on oral hypoglycemics. Estimated diabetes costs in the USA in 2007 total: $174 billion (direct and indirect).

Perioperative Risks

- Sulfonylureas: Hypoglycemia, N/V, cholestatic jaundice, allergic skin reaction, agranulocytosis, aplastic anemia (pt with G6PD deficiency), hemolytic anemia, alcohol-induced flushing with chlorpropamide, SIADH with chloropamide and tolbutamide, potentially teratogenic effects
- Meglitinides: Hypoglycemia
- Dipeptidyl peptidase-4 inhibitors (DPP-4): Hypoglycemia
- Biguanides: Metformin: lactic acidosis, nausea and/or vomiting, diarrhea, anorexia, metallic taste
- Thiazolidinediones: Edema, hepatitis
- Alpha-glucosidase inhibitors: Diarrhea, flatulence

Worry About

- Sulfonylureas: may be potentiated by the following agents: NSAIDs, warfarin, salicylates, azole antifungal drugs, MAO inhibitors, beta-blockers, sulfonamides, phenylbutazone, ethanol, probenecid, chloramphenicol
- Meglitinides: Azole antifungals, clarithromycin, gemfibrozil causes increase in plasma concentration of meglitinides (Repaglinide-Prandin) causing hypoglycemia.
- Metformin: Cimetidine causes an increase in the plasma concentration of metformin, decreased absorption of vitamin B_{12} and folate.
- Thiazolidinediones: Hepatitis, water retention in pts with NYHA Grade III and IV heart failure.
- Alpha-glucosidase inhibitors: An episode of hypoglycemia should be treated with monosaccharides-glucose tablets, since the drug prevents the absorption of polysaccharides.

Overview/Pharmacology

- Sulfonylureas
  - First generation: Tolbutamide, acetohexamide, tolazamide, chlorpropamide
  - Second generation: Glibenclamide (glyburide), glipizide
  - Third generation: Glimeperide (amaryl)
  - Clearance: Metabolized by the liver and excreted in the urine
- Meglitinides: Repaglinide (prandin), nateglinide (Starlix)
  - Clearance: Metabolized by the liver and excreted urine /feces
- DPP-4 inhibitors: Sitagliptin (Januvia), saxagliptin (Onglyza)
  - Clearance: Metabolized by liver and excreted in the urine (80%)
- Biguanides: Metformin, glucophage, riomet, fortamet, glumetza
  - Clearance: The drug does not bind to plasma proteins and is excreted unchanged in the urine.
- Thiazolidinediones: Rosiglitazone (Avandia), pioglitazone (Actos)

- Clearance: Metabolized by the liver and excreted in urine (Avandia), bile (Actos).
- Alpha-glucosidae inhibitors: Acarbose (Precose), miglitol (Glyset)
- Clearance: Acarbose metabolized in the GI tract and minimal renal excretion, miglitol excreted 95% in urine

Drug Class/Mechanism of Action/Usual Dose

- Sulfonylureas: Triggering insulin release by direct action on the K-ATP channel of the pancreatic beta cells
- Dose: Acetohexamide: 500–700 mg daily, chlropropamide: 250–375 mg daily, tolazamide: 100–250 mg daily, tolbutamide: 250–3000 mg daily
- Glyburide: 5–20 mg daily, glipizide: 5–20 mg daily
- Glimepiride: 2–8 mg daily
- Meglitinidines: Action similar to sulfonylureas but at a different binding site
- Repaglinide (Prandin): 0.5–4 mg with meals, nateglinide (Starlix): 60–120 mg q 8 hr
- DDP-4 inhibitors: Sitagliptin (Januvia), saxagliptin (Onglyza): Increases insulin secretion and delays gastric emptying
- Sitagliptin (Januvia): 50–100 mg daily, saxagliptin (Onglyza): 2.5–5 mg daily
- Biguanides: First line of drug for type II overweight /obese with normal renal function. Lactate uptake by the liver is diminished and because lactate is a substrate for hepatic gluconeogenesis, hepatic glucose production decreases. Metformin: 500–1000 mg q 12 hr
- Thiazolidinediones: They improve the way cells in the body respond to insulin by lowering insulin resistance. Rosiglitazone (Avandia): 4–8 mg daily, pioglitazone (Actos): 15–30 mg daily
- Alpha-glucosidase inhibitors: Competitive inhibitors of enzymes needed to digest carbohydrates at the intestinal brush border.
- Acarbose (Precose) 50–100 mg q 8 hr, miglitol (Glyset) 50–100 mg q 8 hr

ASSESSMENT POINTS

System	Effect	Assessment by Hx	PE	Test
CARDIO Thiazolidinediones	Water retention	SOB	Edema	CXR
RENAL Metformin	Lactic acidosis	Tiredness, dysrhythmia	Tachypnea	Lactate
ENDO Sulfonylureas Meglitinides DPP-4 inhibitors	Hypoglycemia	Altered mental status, convulsion, coma	Sweating, tachycardia	Blood glucose

Key Reference: Stumvoll M, Goldstein BJ, van Haeften TW. Type 2 diabetes: Principles of pathogenesis and therapy. *Lancet*. 2005;365(9467):1333–1346.

Perioperative Implications

Preoperative Concerns

- Generally withhold sulfonylureas, meglitinides and dipeptidyl peptisade-4 inhibitors on the day of surgery to avoid hypoglycemia.
- Hold metformin on the day of surgery because complications or alterations in renal function arising intraop may potentiate the risk of development of lactic acidosis (very rare risk).
- Type II diabetics usually not prone to ketoacidosis.

- Blood sugar measurement required before surgery to control hyperglycemia with regular insulin and dextrose solution.

Induction/Maintenance

- Hypoglycemia should be treated with IV dextrose solution.
- For uncontrolled intraop hyperglycemia use insulin drip with frequent blood sugar measurements.

Postoperative Period

- Avoid hypoglycemia

- Blood sugar measurements required frequently, use regular insulin to control hyperglycemia as needed until pt able to resume oral agents.

Anticipated Problems/Concerns

- Sulfonylureas, meglitinides, and dipeptidyl peptidase may cause significant hypoglycemia if given to NPO status pt.
- Metformin may increase the risk of lactic acidosis.
- Sulfonylureas may be potentiated by various other drugs as listed above.

Penicillins

Lucy Waskell

Uses

• Prescribed for pts with infections by sensitive organisms, primarily *Pneumococci* and those in genera *Streptococcus, Staphylococcus, Neisseria, Pseudomonas, Proteus, Haemophilus*, etc., used as prophylaxis for subacute bacterial endocarditis (penicillin G benzathine)
• Can be administered PO, IM as regular or slow-release repository form, or IV

Worry About

• Hypersensitivity reactions (0.7–4%): rash, fever, bronchospasm, vasculitis, serum sickness, exfoliative dermatitis, Stevens-Johnson syndrome, angioedema, anaphylaxis
• Hyperkalemia when penicillin G potassium is administered IV (1.7 mEq K$^+$/1 × 10^6 units penicillin G), esp. if administered rapidly
• Plt dysfunction, defective hemostasis after ticarcillin, and penicillin G
• Rare bone marrow depression, granulocytopenia, hepatitis
• Headaches, seizures after 1 dose of 5 MU of penicillin G procaine
• Clearance lower in neonates and infants
• After PO ingestion, nausea and diarrhea, rarely *Clostridium difficile* pseudo-membranous colitis

Overview/Pharmacology

• Used to treat wide spectrum of infectious diseases
• Many penicillins are acid-labile (pH2 destroys antibiotic); often not administered orally
• Actively and rapidly excreted by renal tubule
• T$_{1/2}$ of penicillin markedly increased in anuria
• Dosage should be decreased in renal failure.
• Other organic acids, e.g., probenecid, can compete at the renal tubule for excretion, prolonging the T$_{1/2}$ of the antibiotic
• High concentration in urine
• Ampicillin and amoxicillin often administered with β-lactamase inhibitors such as clavulanate and sulbactam.

Drug Class/Mechanism of Action/Usual Dose

• Penicillins are organic acids consisting of a β-lactam ring to which is attached a side chain and a thiazolidine ring; they inhibit bacterial cell wall synthesis primarily by inhibiting the transpeptidase reaction that is essential for bacterial cell wall synthesis
• Dose and route of administration depend on penicillin used and severity of disease treated

DRUG EFFECTS

Drug	Absorption After Oral Dose	Resistance to Penicillinase	Dose IV	Antimicrobial Spectrum	Side Effects
Penicillin G	Poor: ~1/3 of dose; take on empty stomach	No	1–10 MU q 4–6 hr	*Streptococcus, Neisseria*	↑ K$^+$ (1.7 mEq K$^+$/1 × 10^6 units Pen G); >20 1 × 10^6 U/day can cause seizures; inhibits plt aggregation
Penicillin V	Moderate 2–5> Pen G	No	0.5 gm q 6 hr PO	Like Pen G	K$^+$ salt
Dicloxacillin	Good (30–80% of dose on empty stomach)	Yes	0.5–1 gm PO q6h	*Staphylococcus aureus*	90–95% bound to albumin; not removed by dialysis
Ampicillin	Good; take on empty stomach	No	1–2 g q6h (250–500 mg q 6 hr PO)	*gm + cocci*, gm neg, *H. influenzae, E coli, P. mirabilis*	
Amoxicillin	Good (better absorption than Ampicillin)	No	0.75–1.5 g PO q8h	Like ampicillin	
Ticarcillin	Poor	No	50–75 mg/kg q6h	*Pseudomonas, Enterobacter, Proteus (indole +)*	CHF 2° to Na$^+$ overload; 5 mEq Na$^+$/g; low K$^+$ 2° to obligatory cation excretion with anion; ↓ in plt aggregation
Piperacillin	Poor	No	2–6 g q8h	*P. aeruginosa, Enterobacter*, some *Klebsiella*, other *gm negatives, gm + cocci, L. monocytogenes*	Same as ticarcillin: 2 mEq Na$^+$/g
Mezlocillin	Poor	No	1.5–4.5 g q6h	*Pseudomonas, Enterobacter, Klebsiella sp.*	2 mEq Na$^+$/g

Key Reference: Petri WA. Penicillins, cephalosporins, and other β-lactam antibiotics. In: Brunton LL, Lazo JS, Parker KL, eds. *Goodman & Gilman's the pharmacological basis of therapeutics.* 11th ed. New York: McGraw-Hill, Medical Publishing Division; 2006:1127–1154.

Perioperative Implications

Preoperative Concerns

• Is pt allergic to any penicillins? What exactly happens when the drug is taken (rash vs. anaphylaxis)?
• If pt on large doses of penicillin G, ticarcillin, or piperacillin, are serum electrolytes normal?
• Hemostasis, esp. plt aggregation, may be inhibited by the antibiotics.
• If pt has renal insufficiency or failure, dose of antibiotic should be q12h or less frequently.

Induction/Maintenance/Postoperative Period

• Penicillins should have no effect on induction or maintenance unless allergic reaction occurs; no known interactions with any anesthetic agents.

Anticipated Problems/Concerns

• Relate to administration of large amounts of Na$^+$, K$^+$, and organic anions (acids). Possible bleeding problems due to plt dysfunction.

Phencyclidine (PCP)

Davide Cattano

Uses

- DEA Schedule I drug of abuse with no present medical indications
- Street terms for phencyclidine: Angel dust, supergrass, killer weed, embalming fluid, rocket fuel, wack, ozone
- Common routes of administration: Smoking (often laced in marijuana cigarettes), oral ingestion; less common is IV injection.

Risk

- Psychosis, seizures, anticholinergic type syndrome
- Experimentally PCP causes irreversible brain damage, per excitotoxicity, with the typical bull's eye neuronal cell and vacualization

Perioperative Risks

- Aggressive and/or psychotic behavior, Htn, stroke, hyperthermia, rhabdomyolisis, aspiration

Worry About

- Kidney failure, aspiration, malignant Htn, prolonged action

Overview/Pharmacology

- Effects due to parent compound, highly lipid soluble, pK_a of 8.6, peak effects 15 min when smoked and 2 hr by ingestion, distribution 4 hr, elimination up to 48 hr. Metabolites are active and are described in elimination time up to weeks in chronic users.
- Metabolized in the liver; urinary excretion of metabolites at low doses, excretion of free drug at high doses, only small fraction of the drug excreted unchanged.
- Produces an acute state of intoxication lasting 4–6 hr but may produce a chronic state of psychosis that can last for up to several days. With low-moderate doses, acute intoxication incl staggering gait, slurred speech, nystagmus, numbness of extremities, sweating, catatonic muscular rigidity, blank stare, changes in body image, disorganized thought, drowsiness, apathy, anterograde amnesia, possibly aggressive behavior

- With moderate-high doses elevated HR and BP, hypersalivation, sweating, fever, repetitive movements, muscle rigidity on stimulation
- With high doses, anesthesia, stupor, coma, convulsions can occur.

Drug Class/Mechanism of Action/Usual Dose

- Arylcyclohexylamine
- Acts at the *N*-methyl-D-aspartate receptor as a noncompetitive antagonist, but weak dopamine, serotonin, and noradrenergic agonist.
- Experimentally PCP-induced desphorylation of ERK ½ and Akt and dephosphorylation of GSK3-beta (activation) that is prevented by lithium.

ASSESSMENT POINTS

System	Effect	Assessment by Hx	PE	Test
CARDIO	Tachycardia, Htn	Quantification, chronicity, acuity of drug exposure	Vital signs Diaphoresis	Blood, urine toxicology screens
RESP	Tachypnea vs. depression	Concurrent drug exposure (e.g., alcohol)	Resp rate Sat O_2%	
CNS	Psychosis, coma, convulsions, analgesia	Pupils, speech, reflexes		
ANS	Hypersalivation vs. dry mouth, hyperthermia		Observation, temp	

Key Reference: O'Brien CP. Drug addiction and drug abuse. In: Hardman JG, Limbird LE, eds. *Goodman & Gilman's The pharmacological basis of therapeutics.* 9th ed. New York: McGraw-Hill Professional Publishing; 1996:574–575.

Perioperative Implications/Possible Drug Interactions

Preoperative Concerns

- No elective cases if pt has potentially taken PCP within 72 hr
- Steps to increase elimination of PCP from body (hydration and diuretics are supportive measures)
- Appropriate premedication (Lorazepam, clonidine/dexmedetomedine)

Induction/Maintenance

- Ketamine contraindicated (cross-tolerance) unless used cautiously to treat addiction and/or withdrawal symptoms (rare, descalating doses); probably avoid NO and isoflurane.
- Not selective beta blockers with alpha effects (labetalol)
- Clonidine and dexmedetomidine

Postoperative Period

- Psychosis (acute vs. withdrawal), rhabdomyolisis, anticholinergic syndrome
- Precaution with muscle relaxant reversal

Anticipated Problems/Concerns

- Phenothiazines, anticholinergics, acidification of urine
- There is no withdrawal, but addiction tolerance is common.

Phenothiazines

Eric Schnell

Uses

- Phenothiazines share a tricyclic core functional group and have multiple clinical applications.
- Phenothiazine neuroleptics such as chlorpromazine are used in the treatment of schizophrenia and psychosis.
- Phenothiazine antihistamines such as promethazine and prochlorperazine are highly effective antiemetics.
- Chlorpromazine can effectively treat uncontrollable hiccups and acute migraine headaches.

Perioperative Risks

- Severe extrapyramidal symptoms may arise from phenothiazines' antidopaminergic activity.
- Tardive dyskinesia may result from long-term use and may be irreversible.
- Contraindicated in Parkinson's disease; may worsen tremor and Parkinsonism
- Autonomic dysfunction may result from phenothiazines' sympatholytic and anti-cholinergic effects.

- Cardiac conduction defects and arrhythmias may occur with acute or chronic dosing, most commonly manifesting as a long QT interval.
- Side effects of sedation and delirium may be particularly notable in postop period.
- Accidental arterial injection or venous extravasation of promethazine can cause tissue necrosis.
- Neuroleptic malignant syndrome is a potentially fatal reaction to phenothiazines involving hyperthermia, rhabdomyolysis, tachycardia, and arrhythmias.

Pharmacokinetics/Pharmacodynamics

- Phenothiazines undergo hepatic metabolism; use caution in pts with hepatic dysfunction.
- Inactive metabolites excreted in bile/urine; pharmacokinetics rarely affected by renal failure
- Phenothiazines are highly protein-bound (>90%).
- Prochlorperazine and promethazine have clinical half-lives of approx 4–8 hr after IV administration.

Drug Class/Mechanism of Action/Usual Dose

- Phenothiazines antagonize many receptors, incl dopamine receptors (primarily D_2), muscarinic receptors, serotonin receptors, α_1 adrenergic receptors and H_1 histamine receptors
- Phenothiazine neuroleptics mediate their antipsychotic effects by blocking mesolimbic D_2 receptors, but D_2 blockade in striatum causes extra-pyramidal side effects
- Phenothiazine anti-emetics are potent H_1 histamine antagonists and exert antimuscarinic and anti-D_2 dopaminergic activity at the chemoreceptor trigger zone.
- Promethazine is used at doses of 6.25–25 mg IV/IM q4–6h, IV doses given in diluted form slowly into well-functioning large-vein IV
- Prochlorperazine is used at doses of 2.5–10 mg IV/IM/PO q4–6h (max 40 mg/d), 25 mg PR q12h

ASSESSMENT POINTS

System	Effect	Assessment by Hx	PE	Test
ANS	α_1 Adrenoceptor blockade, antimuscarinic action		Orthostatic hypotension, tachy/bradycardia	Orthostatics
CNS	Extrapyramidal symptoms Neuroleptic malignant syndrome Sedation Decreased seizure threshold	Acute or chronic Muscle cramps, delirium	Akathisia, tardive dyskinesia Rigidity, tachycardia, hyperthermia, arrhythmias Lethargy, delirium	CK, K^+, uric acid EEG
CARDIAC	Conduction defects: Long QT, ventricular and supraventricular arrhythmias	Can cause sudden death	Tachycardia, bradycardia, or irregular rate	EKG
PULM	Resp depression	May potentiate opioids	Low resp rate	SpO_2, ABG, $ETCO_2$
VASC	Tissue necrosis (promethazine)	Arterial injection or tissue extravasation	Gangrene	
HEME	Leukopenia, agranulocytosis	Usually in chronic dosing only		CBC

Key Reference: Schatzberg AF, Nemeroff CB. *The American psychiatric publishing textbook of psychopharmacology.* 3rd ed. Washington, DC: American Psychiatric Publishing; 425-441.

Perioperative Implications

Preoperative Concerns
- Obtain baseline EKG for all pts taking chronic phenothiazines to assess cardiac conduction and QT interval.
- Neuroleptic malignant syndrome may present in pts undergoing chronic treatment, but may be precipitated by other antidopaminergic agents such as metoclopramide.

Induction/Maintenance
- Autonomic insufficiency may contribute to profound intraop hypotension.

Adjuvants/Regional Anesthesia/Reversal
- Treat extrapyramidal side effects with diphenhydramine, benztropine, or benzodiazepines.
- Neuroleptic malignant syndrome is treated with bromocriptine, dantrolene, and aggressive hydration/monitoring.

Postoperative Concerns
- Clinically significant resp depression if given to pts <2 yo or those with pulm disease, esp. if combined with opioids
- Arrhythmias and prolonged QT
- Increased risk of sedation and delirium in elderly pts

Drug Interactions
- Increased risk of extrapyramidal symptoms if given with other antidopaminergic medications (typically metoclopramide)
- May increase concentration of other hepatically metabolized (CYP2D6) drugs (some beta-blockers and tricyclic antidepressants)

Anticipated Problems/Concerns
- Assess mental status, resp status, and CV function after administration, particularly in early postop period

DRUGS

629

Phenoxybenzamine

Michael F. Roizen

Uses

- Incidence in USA: 3,600/y
- Rx for preop pheochromocytoma; occasionally, chronic Rx of pheochromocytoma, sympathetic hyperactivity states, carcinoid syndrome, benign prostatic hypertrophy (BPH)

Perioperative Risks

- Drug interactions: Sometimes requires very high doses of α-adrenergic agents to produce vasoconstriction
- Vasodilation, orthostatic hypotension accentuated in hypovolemic pts

Worry About

- Occasionally assoc with confusional states
- Assoc with fatigue and prolonged sedation
- Drop attacks on preop standing to urinate

Overview/Pharmacology

- α_1-Blocker (relatively selective $\alpha_1 \gg \alpha_2$) by covalent (irreversible) binding to a receptor; compensatory response calls for production or availability of more (spare) receptors
- Effect develops slowly; peak effect not attained for 2 hr after IV or 4 hr after oral administration
- Absorption from GI tract incomplete
- Renal excretion of 50% in 12 hr, 80% in 24 hr

- $T_{1/2}$ of effect over 24 hr, effects accumulate for at least 4–6 d
- High lipid solubility at body pH

Drug Class/Mechanism of Action

- α_1-Blocker agent (a haloalkylamine)
- Chronically taken
  - Decreased α_1 effects in pheochromocytoma
  - High doses inhibit release of H_2 serotonin (occasionally used in carcinoid syndrome)
  - Ameliorate or prevent Raynaud's phenomenon
- Vasodilator for chronic treatment of CHF (occasionally)

DRUG EFFECTS

System	Effect	Assessment by Hx	PE	Test
HEENT	Vasodilation of mucous membranes of nasopharynx; miosis	Nasal congestion	Mouth breathing	
CARDIO	Antihypertensive agent Postural hypotension, reflex tachycardia ↑ CO	Orthostatic dizziness	Orthostatic VS	Hct ECG
GI	↑ Intestinal motility, causes diarrhea	Orthostatic hypotension		
ENDO	Stimulates insulin release ↑ Presynaptic norepinephrine release (blockade of presynaptic α_2 receptors inhibiting release of norepinephrine)			
GU	↑ Blood volume, Na⁺ retention inhibits contraction of vas deferens	Impairs ejaculation		BUN, Cr electrolytes
CNS	Depression, sedation, fatigue Extrapyramidal symptoms rarely N/V, motor excitability rare		CNS exam	

Key Reference: Kinney MA, Narr BJ, Warner MA. Perioperative management of pheochromocytoma. *J Cardiothorac Vasc Anesth.* 2002;16:359–369.

Perioperative Implications/Possible Drug Interactions

- See also Pheochromocytoma in Diseases section and Adrenalectomy for Pheochromocytoma in Procedures section

Preoperative Period

- Ensure not hypovolemic
- Interaction with methyldopa (Aldomet): Urinary incontinence
- Preop treatment: Major goal to avoid pheochromocytoma crisis; pre- and intraop goals of management of extra-adrenal surgery same as for adrenal surgery. If pt not on α-blocker before surgery, try to delay until appropriate degree of α-

blockade. Increased dose of phenoxybenzamine by 10 mg bid to qid every third day until appropriately blocked. Judge appropriate level of blockade by:
- No BP readings higher than 165/90 mmHg (even during psychologic stress) for 48 hr before surgery
- Orthostatic hypotension present, but BP on standing should not be lower than 80/45 mmHg
- ECG free of ST-T changes due to cardiomyopathy
- Absence of other signs of catecholamine excess and presence of blockade effects such as nasal stuffiness

Induction/Maintenance

- Can produce ↑ sedation, ↓ anesthetic requirements by ⅓ (not studied but anecdotally reported)

Muscle Relaxants

- No interactions known

Regional Anesthesia/Reversal

- No interactions known

Anticipated Problems/Concerns

- May need very high doses of vasopressors to ↑ vascular resistance, BP in pt taking large doses
- CNS dysfunction by itself

DRUGS

Phenylephrine (Neo-Synephrine)

Arvind Rajagopal
Kenneth J. Tuman

Uses

- Prescribed mainly as nasal decongestant or ophthalmically for mydriasis Rx, capillary decongestion
- Reliable vasopressor in treatment of hypotension
- Prolongs local anesthetic duration in regional anesthesia
- Available as parenteral IM/IV and various ophthalmic and/or nasal preparations

Perioperative Risks

- Risk of Htn increases left heart work; may precipitate myocardial ischemia, MI
- Infusions to augment systolic BP ↑ incidence of myocardial ischemia in pts undergoing carotid endarterectomy
- Increased pulm vascular resistance, right heart work
- Bradycardia may occur (usually not severe) related to baroreceptor reflex
- Decreased renal, splanchnic blood flow
- May ↑ uterine artery vascular resistance, ↓ uterine artery blood flow in pregnant pts
- Systemic absorption of topical preparations may cause Htn, headache, tremulousness, myocardial ischemia

Worry About

- Increase preload, afterload may worsen LV failure in pts with LV dysfunction
- Raised PA pressures may worsen RV dysfunction
- May ↓ renal blood flow

Overview/Pharmacology

- Direct α_1-agonist activity causes systemic and PA vasoconstriction, resulting in ↑ impedance to forward flow, ↑ BP
- Rapidly metabolized by MAO
- IV duration less than 5 min
- May terminate supraventricular tachycardia by vagal reflex from baroreceptor stimulation
- Increased SVR during CPB
- Increased perfusion pressure to vital organs in hypovolemic pts until vol restored, CPR
- May be used in conjunction with nitroglycerin to elevate coronary perfusion pressure in hypotensive pts with myocardial ischemia
- Decreasing right to left shunts in pts with cyanotic spells (tetralogy of Fallot)
- Vasopressor of choice in hypertrophic cardiomyopathy, systolic anterior motion of mitral valve and aortic stenosis, when ↑ inotropy or tachycardia undesirable

- Advantageous in catecholamine-depleted pts (chronic cocaine or amphetamine abuse), or in pts on tricyclic antidepressants or MAO inhibitors, when indirect vasopressors are unpredictable

Drug Class/Mechanism of Action/Usual Dose

- Synthetic noncatecholamine activates predominantly α-adrenergic receptors (postsynaptic, heart, iris), triggers release of intracellular Ca^{2+}, resulting in smooth muscle contraction
- Differs structurally from epinephrine only in lacking 4-hydroxyl group on benzene ring
- Usual adult dosage
  - IV bolus: 50–100 μg
  - IV infusion: 20–200 μg/min/70 kg
  - Ophthalmic solutions: 2.5–10%
  - Supraventricular tachycardia dose: 150–800 μg titrated to ↑ BP

ASSESSMENT POINTS

System	Effect	PE	Test
HEENT	Mydriasis without cycloplegia ↓ Production of aqueous humor		
CARDIO	Vasoconstriction of veins and arteries ↑ Systolic and diastolic BP ↓ HR	BP HR	PCWP ECG
RESP	↑ PVR		PCWP, PAP
RENAL	↓ Renal blood flow	UO	BUN, Cr

Key Reference: Dellinger RP, Levy MM, Carlet JM, et al. Surviving sepsis campaign: International guidelines for management of severe sepsis and septic shock: 2008. *Intensive Care Med.* 2008;34:17–60.

Perioperative Implications

Preoperative Concerns

- Assess LV function and Hx of CAD
- Consider arterial catheter if phenylephrine infusion anticipated (carotid endarterectomy, relative hypovolemia)
- Assess renal function (Cr)
- For nasal intubations, phenylephrine can be used as a nasal vasoconstrictor in a mixture with 3–4% lidocaine

Induction/Maintenance

- Monitor ECG for signs of ischemia due to increased ventricular work or coronary artery spasm
- May ↓ hepatic blood flow due to α-adrenergic-mediated vasoconstriction of portal venous vasculature

Adjuvants/Regional Anesthesia/Reversal

- Duration may be prolonged in pts on MAO inhibitors
- Side effects with ophthalmic use occur within 20 min; usually self-limited
- 2.5% nasal, ophthalmic solutions recommended in infant and elderly populations or in pts with CAD

Anticipated Problems/Concerns

- Small doses can be titrated in a parturient when a β-adrenergic agonist is undesirable
- Can be titrated slowly to avoid overshoot (with resultant Htn)

- Can be used when severe hypotension presents immediate danger to compromised myocardium or other end organ (e.g., brain)
- With a failing heart, increasing afterload and preload may ↑ left-sided filling pressures enough to precipitate pulm edema

Phenytoin

Bozena R. Jachna

Indications

- Management of generalized tonic-clonic (grand mal) and complex partial seizures
- Prophylaxis against seizures after trauma or surgical intervention
- Treatment of ventricular arrhythmias, esp. those assoc with digitalis or tricyclic antidepressant toxicity
- Treatment of prolonged QT interval
- Treatment of epidermolysis bullosa and chronic pain syndromes

Overview/Pharmacology

- Drug of choice for status epilepticus
- Treatment for acute and chronic seizures
- Onset of action: 30–60 min
- Protein binding >90% in adults
- Elimination half-life: 22 hr
- 95% hydroxylated and conjugated in liver with glucuronic acid for renal excretion
- Therapeutic range: 10–20 mcg/mL

Drug Class/Mechanism of Action/Usual Dose

- Hydantoin derivative
- In the CNS, helps to limit nerve impulse generation thereby limiting seizure focus spread by
  - Decreasing influx of Na^+ ions across cell membranes in the motor cortex
  - Decreasing presynaptic Ca^{++} release
  - Decreasing extracellular K^+ concentration
- In the heart works to limit re-entrant arrhythmias by:
  - Prolonging the effective refractory period and suppressing ventricular pacemaker automaticity
- Shortening action potential for status epilepticus (IV and PO dosages are the same)
  - Pediatric: Loading dose—15–20 mg/kg in single or divided doses, then 5mg/kg/d in divided doses
  - Adult: Loading dose—10–15 mg/kg, then 5–6 mg/kg/d in three divided doses
- For treatment of cardiac arrhythmias: 1.5 mg/kg IV every 5 min for maximum dose of 15 mg/kg or 1.5 g

Perioperative Risks

- Hypotension, bradycardia, cardiac arrhythmias and/or collapse with rapid IV administration (likely due to propylene glycol vehicle)
- Venous irritation and/or pain
- Decreased efficacy of muscle relaxants

Concerns

- Pts with renal failure, jaundice, or other causes of hypoalbuminemia may exhibit phenytoin toxicity
- Increased P450 clearance may cause decreased effectiveness of certain drugs: Antibiotics, oral contraceptives, procainamide, and oral anticoagulants

DRUG EFFECTS

System	Effect	Assessment by Hx	PE	Test
HEENT	Nystagmus at toxic levels, > 20mg/mL		Gingival Hyperplasia with chronic use	
CARDIO	Hypotension, bradycardia, cardiac arrhythmias with rapid administration		Vital signs, monitoring	
PULM	Resp depression		Saturation, resp rate monitoring	
DERM	Rash; Stevens-Johnsons syndrome (rare)			
GI/LIVER	Constipation, vomiting, nausea, hepatitis: increased hepatic drug metabolism; toxicity in low albumin states; avoid or limit Ethyl alcohol use	GI irritation if not taken with food		Albumin
HEME	Folic acid depletion, hyperglycemia, leukopenia, thrombocytopenia, agranulocytosis			CBC with differential
RENAL	Toxicity in uremic pts			BUN/Cr
CNS	Ataxia, diplopia, drowsiness, lethargy, coma, nystagmus, mood changes		CNS exam	

Key Reference: Phenytoin in University of Maryland Medical Center Medical Encyclopedia. 2009-downloadable at www.umm.edu/ency/article/002632.htm.

Perioperative Implications

Preoperative Concerns
- Pts with renal, liver disease or decreased nutritional states can increase level of free phenytoin

Induction/Maintenance
- Rapid administration of phenytoin may cause hypotension, bradycardia, arrhythmias. Administer at rate of less than 50 mg/kg/min
- Larger doses of nondepolarizing muscle relaxants may be required
- Shorter duration of nondepolarizing muscle relaxants
- Concern with too rapid administration of vehicle (depending on vehicle)

Contraindications

- Hypersensitivity to phenytoin, other hydantoins
- Pregnancy: Phenytoin crosses the placenta resulting in congenital malformations—the "fetal hydantoin syndrome"—which results in wide-set eyes, a broad mandible, and finger deformities
- Lactating states, enters breast milk
- Isolated cases of malignancies: Neuroblastomas have been reported

Phenytoin Syndrome

- Fever
- Rash
- Psychiatric changes, slurred speech, dizziness, insomnia
- Tremor
- Constipation
- Hepatitis
- Rarely seen: SLE-like syndrome, lymphadenopathy, Stevens-Johnson syndrome, blood dyscrasias, lymphoma, coarsening of facial features, hypertrichinosis

Physostigmine, Eserine

Jeffrey S. Shiffrin

Uses

- Central anticholinergia; for diagnosis and treatment. Hx of anticholinergic ingestion and/or exposure: (atropine, scopolamine, belladonna, jimson weed, toxic mushrooms, tricyclics, phenothiazines, antihistamines, benzodiazepines, opiates, inhalation anesthetics, propofol, GHB)
  - "Blind as a bat": Mydriasis and loss of accommodation
  - "Dry as a bone": Urinary retention and dry mucus membranes
  - "Hot as a hare": Hyperthermia from loss of sweating
  - "Red as a beet": Cutaneous vasodilitation to counteract hyperthermia
  - "Mad as a hatter": Fluctuating consciousness, delirium, disorientation, decreased social restraint, slurred speech, in-coordination, hallucinations, phantom behaviors, coma, paranoia during recovery
- Postop delirium, from agitation to excessive somnolence
- Glaucoma, ciliary muscle contraction = miosis = facilitates outflow of aqueous humor
- Treatment for antimuscarinic xenobiotic toxicity (a chemical compound that is foreign to a living organism, ex: benzodiazepines, tricyclics, antihistamines, jimson weed)
- NMB reversal (neostigmine better choice as it avoids central CNS effects)
- Hereditary ataxias
- Alzheimer's disease (may improve STM but not used clinically)
- Analgesia (decreases morphine consumption postop)

Perioperative Risk

- Cholinesterase inhibition = Excess acetylcholine. Can lead to 3 sets of problems: Analogous to organophosphorous compound poisoning, a cholinergic crisis (basically the opposite from anticholinergia syndrome above)
  - Muscarinic cholinergic (parasympathetic) over-stimulation (DUMBELS)
    - D = Defecation, diarrhea, diaphoresis, GI distress
    - U = Urination
    - M = Miosis
    - B = Bronchorrhea, bronchospasm, bradycardia
    - E = Emesis (nausea)
    - L = Lacrimation
    - S = Salivation
  - Nicotinic cholinergic excess (continuing depolarization of motor endplate leading to fasciculations at low dose and progressive weakness at high dose)
  - CNS (anxiety, confusion, tremors, seizures, resp depression, coma)

Worry About

- Reactive airway disease
- Peripheral vascular disease
- Diabetes
- Bowel or bladder obstruction
- Pre-existing intraventricular conduction delay, long Qt
- Pre-existing AV block
- Pregnancy (Class C)
- Sulfite allergy (contains sodium bisulfite preservative)

Overview/Pharmacology

- Physostigmine is a parasympathomimietic carbamate derived from the beans and/or seeds of an aquatic leguminous plant (calabar or ordeal bean). Used in the Old Calabar region of Nigeria as part of the Esere witchcraft ritual (believed to test the guilt or innocence of a person accused of a crime)
- Characterized and named Physostigma venenosum balfour in 1857 by John Balfour
- Active alkaloid isolated and called physostigmine by Jobst and Hesse 1864, and independently by Vee and Leven 1865 who named it eserine.
- Reversibly binds cholinesterase (AchE) thus inhibiting acetylcholine degradation and increasing synaptic acetylcholine.
- Tertiary amine structure allows penetration of blood brain barrier.
- Prototypical carbamate insecticide
- Early medical use by 1935 as miotic agent for glaucoma pts, myasthenia gravis treatment, atropine antidote, and reversal agent for curare induced paralysis.

Drug Class/Mechanism of Action/Usual Dose

- Physostigmine is a tertiary amine and a competing substrate for cholinesterase enzymes, thus decreasing the breakdown of acetylcholine.
- 1.5 mg given over 60 min = Vd 2.4+/− L/kg; t1/2 16.4+/−3.2 min; peak plasma conc 3+/−0.5 ng/mL; clearance 0.1 L/min/kg.
- Inhibition of plasma cholinesterase within 2 min of infusion start. Half-life of plasma cholinesterase inhibition = 83.7+/−5.2 min.
- For glaucoma: Not commonly used due to systemic absorption and side effects. Replaced by other agents. Physostigmine ointment placed 1–3 times daily. Physostigmine solution 0.25%, 0.5% used 1–4 times daily while holding pressure over medial canthus/tear duct to minimize absorption.
- For reversal of central anticholinergia: Pysostigmine salicylate (antilirium) 1 mg/mL; dose = 0.04 mg/kg or 1–2 mg IV/IM. IV given slowly, no more that 1 mg/min every 20–60 min as effective and necessary, or until side effects develop.

DRUG EFFECTS

System	Effect	Assessment by Hx	PE	Test
EYES	Constriction pupil	Glaucoma topical application	Miosis, conjunctival hyperemia	Decrease IOP, red eye
CARDIO	Bradycardia/tachycardia Vasoconstriction/vasodilation, decrease cardiac contractility	Variable depending on CNS vs. peripheral effects and use of other meds (ganglionic blockers, alpha and beta blockers)	Slow or irregular HR, asystole, or tachycardia, Htn, or hypotension	ECG, BP
RESP	Bronchoconstriction Bronchorrhea		Wheezing Secretions, "frothing at the mouth"	Auscultation
GI	Parasympathetic stimulation, abd cramps		Diarrhea, defecation	
GU	Bladder stimulation		Urination	
CNS	Excess acetylcholine	Somnolence, delirium, coma		

Key References: Taylor P. Anticholinesterase agents. In: *Goodman & Gilman's the pharmacological basis of therapeutics.* 11th ed. 2006:[chapter 8]. Howland MA. A13 Antidotes in depth: Physostigmine salicylate. In: *Goldfrank's toxicologic emergencies.* 8th ed. 2006. Physostigmine salicylate in AHFS Drug Information. 2009. Bruns JJ. Toxicity, anticholinergic. In: http://emedicine.medscape.com/article/812644. Pratico C, et al. Drugs of anesthesia acting on central cholinergic system may cause post-operative cognitive dysfunction and delirium. *Med Hypotheses.* 2005;65:972–982. Lepouse C. Emergence delirium in adults in the post-anaesthesia care unit. *BJ Anaesthesia.* 2006;96:747–753. Beilin B, et al. Continuous physostigmine combined with morphine-based patient-controlled analgesia in the postoperative period. *Acta Anaesthesiol Scand.* 2005;49:78–84. Cook B, Spence AA. Post-operative central anticholinergic syndrome. *Eur J Anaesthesiol.* 1997; 14(6):664-665.

Perioperative Implications

Preoperative Concerns

- Scopolamine, antihistamines, benzodiazepines (esp. in elderly) Can contribute to central anticholinergia.
- Use of jimson weed (belladonna) or hallucinogenic mushrooms
- Interaction with vasopressors (possible Htn tachycardia).
- Long Qt or AVB (increases chance for asystole).
- Tricyclic antidepressant use (asystole has occurred in treatment of tricyclic overdose).

Induction/Maintenance

- **Not** used

Postoperative Period

- Many if not all anesthetics can cause anticholinergic signs and symptoms.
- Differential diagnosis: Metabolic (hyper/hypoglycemia, electrolyte imbalance, sepsis, MH, NMS); respiratory (hypoxia, hypercarbia); neuro (CVA, seizures); psychiatric (narcolepsy, psychosis); iatrogenic (residual NMB, bladder distension, prolonged anesthetic effects/sensitivity).

Anticipated Problems/Concerns

- Physostigmine can be very effective in reversing excessive sedation or agitation assoc with anticholinergia. However, anticholinergia is usually self-limited and is a diagnosis of exclusion; although confirmed by a positive response to physostigmine. Also, physostigmine side effects are unpredictable and can be severe (asystole, seizures). In general, they are limited to exaggerated parasympathetic effects: N/V, stomach pain, salivation, urination, defecation, miosis, inability to focus, lacrimation, sweating, bronchospasm, bronchorrhea, dyspnea, bradycardia or tachycardia, hypotension or Htn, irregular pulse, muscular twitching; but weakness, seizures, collapse, coma, pulm edema, death (i.e., cholinergic crisis) can occur.
- Avoid in pts receiving other cholinergic agents (methacholine, bethanehol)
- Avoid in pts receiving depolarizing NMBs (succinylcholine)
- Atropine is the antidote for physostigmine overdose and central cholinergic symptoms.
- Glycopyrrolate is the antidote for peripheral cholinergic excess.

Prilocaine (Citanest)

Ramprasad Sripada
Vidya N. Rao

Indications

- Infrequently used local anesthetic in USA, still used extensively in Germany
- Administered either as an injection local anesthetic 4% (with or without epinephrine) or topically as EMLA, a **eutectic** mixture of 2.5% prilocaine and 2.5% lidocaine
- Widely used for anesthesia and analgesia during circumcision. Newborns at higher risk for toxicity and methemoglobinemia
- Percutaneous anesthesia with EMLA for venipuncture, ulcer debridement, and skin graft harvesting
- Liposuction
- Painless treatment of hydrocele

Perioperative Risks

- Toxicity from excessive dose
- Hypersensitivity reaction
- Methemoglobinemia

Worry About

- Metabolism to *o*-toluidine, which causes Hgb to be reduced to methemoglobin

Overview/Pharmacology

- 2–Propylamino-o-propionotoluidide
- Pharmacokinetics: $T_{1/2} \alpha$ 0.5 min; $T_{1/2} \beta$ 5 min, Vd_{ss} 261 L; $T_{1/2} \gamma$ 1.5 hr; clearance rate 2.84 L/min (distributed at rapid rate from blood to tissue)

Drug Class/Mechanism of Action/Usual Dose

- Intermediate-acting amide local anesthetic (less readily metabolized than esters); this ↓ in metabolism ↑ risk of adverse reactions
- Permeates nerve's axon membranes and equilibrates there and in axoplasm, depending on drug's pK_a (8.0), hydrophobicity of base and cation specificity, and concentration. Hydrophobicity measured by octanol:buffer partition coefficient of base: 129, making it moderately hydrophobic.
- Binds to local anesthetic sites on voltage gated Na^+ channels. A conformational change of receptor prevents opening of channel during activation; axon potentials cease to be propagated. Onset, recovery from blockade limited by diffusion of local anesthetic molecules into/out of nerve membrane and axoplasm.
- Prilocaine is dealkylated in the liver by mixed-function oxidases. About 75% in liver; the most rapidly metabolized of amides.
- Excreted in kidney; perhaps some kidney metabolism
- Low protein-binding capacity leads to ↑ clearance rate

Drug Effects

- Addition of epinephrine does not affect block duration, a result of vasodilating action of prilocaine
- Contraindicated in pts with G6PD deficiency
- Its increased volume of distribution reduces its CNS toxicity, making it suitable for IV regional blocks
- It must not (DO NOT!!) be used on mucous membranes or abraded skin, as rapid absorption may result in systemic toxicity.

Toxicity

Methemoglobinemia

- Dose-response relationship exists between amount of prilocaine and methemoglobinemia (occurs with ≥600 mg, >8 mg/kg). Occurrence related to chemical structure: Prilocaine has one less methyl group in benzene ring than lidocaine; metabolism in liver results in formation of o-toluidine, which oxidizes Hgb to methemoglobin. In healthy persons, methemoglobinemia usually is not a problem.
- Methemoglobinemia is significant when methemoglobin exceeds 10% of total Hgb (shift to left with less release of O_2). Cyanosis observed; methemoglobinemia of concern if anemic or pregnant (when maternal transfer leads to methemoglobinemia of fetus).
- Methemoglobinemia is more common in neonates due to decreased resistance of fetal hemoglobin to oxidant stresses and the immaturity of enzymes in the neonate that convert methemoglobin back to the ferrous state.
- Treatment: If spontaneous reversal does not occur, IV injection with 1–2 mg/kg of 1% methylene blue solution (tetramethyl-thionine chloride)

Other Toxicity

- CNS, CV systems; generally 4–7 × the amount producing convulsions → CV collapse
- Toxicity assoc with >400 mg (>8 mg/kg)
- Intercostal injection leading to higher blood levels than with epidural

DRUG EFFECTS

Indication	Conc	Drug Dose	Onset	Duration
Minor nerve block	1%	50–200 mg	10–20 min	60–120 min, up to 180 with epinephrine
Major nerve block	1–2%	400–600 mg	10–20 min	180–300 min
Epidural	1–3%	150–600 mg	5–15 min	120–180 min

ASSESSMENT POINTS

System	Effect	Assessment by Hx	PE	Test
HEENT	Toxicity	Metallic taste, tinnitus		
CARDIO	Pulm vasoconstriction Systemic vasodilator Neg inotrope Neg chronotrope			↑ PAP ↑ PVR ↓ SVR ↓ CO ECG: ↑ P-R, ↓ QRS
CNS	Toxicity: More sensitive than CV	Shivering, twitching, tremors in face, extremities, progressing to tonic-clonic seizure	Twitching, hyperreflexia possible Resp depression	
PNS	Block nerve transmissions		Loss of sensation and motor function	
MS	IV may augment NM blocker (both depolarizing and nondepolarizing)			Nerve stimulator: ↓ Twitch height

Key References: Soderberg L, Dyhre H, Roth B, Bjorkman S. Ultralong peripheral nerve block by lidocaine:prilocaine 1:1 mixture in a lipid depot formulation: Comparison of in vitro, in vivo, and effect kinetics. *Anesthesiology.* 2006;104:110–121.
pseudo-lysosomal storage disease caused by EMLA cream. *J Inherit Metab Dis.* 2004;27:507–511.

Possible Drug Interactions

- In large doses, blocks NM transmission; in smaller doses, enhances NMB from nondepolarizing and depolarizing NM blockers
- Acidosis, hypercarbia, hypoxia may potentiate neg chronotropic, inotropic actions

Preoperative Considerations/Induction/Maintenance

- Routine

Anticipated Problems/Concerns

- EMLA cream = eutectic mix of 5% lidocaine + prilocaine base for topical cutaneous anesthesia. EMLA applied under occlusive bandage for 45–60 min to obtain effective cutaneous anesthesia. EMLA cream produces anesthesia to a maximum depth of 5 mm. The efficacy of this combination lies in the fact that the mixture of prilocaine and lidocaine has a melting point less than that of either compound alone; existing at room temp as oil that can penetrate intact skin. Guidelines are available to calculate maximum amount of cream that can be applied and area of skin covered.
- EMLA → methemoglobinemia when large amounts used in children, particularly in newborn
- Methemoglobinemia if >600 mg given or given to anemic or pregnant pts

Procainamide (Procan, Procanabid, Pronestyl)

Mia Kang
Jeffrey M. Berman

Uses

- Treats recurrent or sustained hemodynamically stable monomorphic VT (MVT) (IIa/C)/(IIa/C)*
- Treats focal atrial tachycardia in hemodynamically stable pts (IIa/C)
- Treats recurrent atrial flutter (only in combination with AV-nodal-blocking agent) (IIb/A)
- Treats SVT during pregnancy

Perioperative Risks

- Potential for hypotension 2° to ganglionic blockade more likely than myocardial depression
- Nausea in pts on oral procainamide (related to levels of N-acetyl procainamide?)
- Chronic use can cause lupus-like syndrome; 25–50% of pts develop rash, small-joint arthralgias positive ANA. Resolves with cessation or administration of N-acetyl procainamide

Worry About

- Ventricular dysrhythmias if plasma concentration of NAPA >30 μg/mL

- QT_c prolongation
- CNS toxicity
- Procainamide-induced lupus syndrome
- Bone marrow aplasia in 0.5% of pts; may be fatal, mechanism unknown
- Hypokalemia may exacerbate toxicity.
- Avoid use in pts with myasthenia gravis, may exacerbate symptoms

Overview/Pharmacology

- Analog of procaine
- Na^+ channel blocker (intermediate recovery)
- Decreases automaticity, increases refractory periods, slows phase 4 depolarization
- Highly lipophilic but no relationship between drug properties and volume of distribution
- Major metabolite N-acetyl procainamide (NAPA) does not block Na^+ channels but equipotent in prolonging action potentials
- Rapid hepatic conjugation by N-acetyl transferase ($t_{1/2}$ = 3–4 hr) to active metabolite NAPA

- Renal excretion of unchanged drug as well as NAPA ($t_{1/2}$ = 6–8 hr)
- Procainamide and NAPA have different pharmacologic effects so sum of concentrations should not be used to guide therapy
- Slow acetylators more likely to develop lupus, symptoms; often resolve with administration of NAPA

Drug Class/Mechanism of Action/Usual Dose

- Class IA antiarrhytmic; Na^+-channel blocker
- Marked slowing of conduction by blocking of sodium channels (SA node and intraventricular conduction)
- IV loading dose: 1 g IV given at 20 mg/min (up to 17 mg/kg); IV maintenance 2–4 mg/min IV;
- Narrow therapeutic window: Therapeutic plasma levels: procainamide 4–10 mcg/mL, NAPA 15–25 mcg/ml
- Toxic level: Procainamide >10 mcg/mL

DRUG EFFECTS

System	Effect	Assessment by Hx	PE	Test
CARDIO	Slowing of conduction	Assess for clinically symptomatic bradycardia, heart block, CHF	Auscultation of heart sounds, ECG	Continuous ECG monitoring
RESP	Lupus-related pleuritis or pneumonia	Assess for dyspnea	Auscultation of lung fields	O_2 sat monitoring
CNS	High plasma concentrations may cause confusion/disorientation and/or seizures; rarely muscle weakness	Evaluate regimen, pt compliance	Monitor blood levels of procainamide and NAPA	Neurologic assessment

Key References: Blomström-Lundqvist C, et al. ACC/AHA/ESC guidelines for the management of patients with supraventricular arrhythmias—executive summary: A report of the American College of Cardiology/American Heart Association Task Force on Practice Guidelines, and the European Society of Cardiology Committee for Practice Guidelines (Writing Committee to Develop Guidelines for the Management of Patients with Supraventricular Arrhythmias.). *J Am Coll Cardiol.* 2003;42:1493–1531. Zipes DP, et al. ACC/AHA/ESC 2006 guidelines for management of patients with ventricular arrhythmias and the prevention of sudden cardiac death: A report of the American College of Cardiology/American Heart Association Task Force and the European society of Cardiology Committee for Practice Guidelines (Writing Committee to Develop Guidelines for Management of Patients with Ventricular Arrhythmias and the Prevention of Sudden Cardiac Death). *Circulation.* 2006;114:e385–e484.

Perioperative Implications

Preoperative Concerns

- Hx of arrhythmia, ischemic or structural heart disease
- Ventricular function
- Plasma concentration of procainamide
- May be used to treat contractions in pts with myotonic dystrophies; should be continued periop

Induction/Maintenance

- Caution with drugs that slow cardiac conduction (e.g., other Na channel blockers, beta-blockers)
- Use of other Na^+ channel blockers
- LA toxicity with major conduction blocks
- Arrhythmias with high plasma concentration
- Myocardial depressive effect worsened by hyperkalemia
- Potentiates activity of NMBs

Postoperative Period

- Toxicity
- Arrhythmias caused by slowed conduction

Anticipated Problems/Concerns

- Monitor for clinical signs of toxicity: Torsades, heart block, arrhythmias, confusion, lupus syndrome
- Not well tolerated for long-term control of atrial tachycardias because of dosing regimen, complications
- In renal pts: Concentrations of procainamide and NAPA may rise to toxic levels => reduce dose, monitor levels of both

*The first number and lower-case letter refer to the ACC/AHA system of classifying guidelines while the upper-case letter refers to the level of evidence.

DRUGS

Propylthiouracil—Antithyroid Drugs

Michael F. Roizen

Uses

- Incidence in USA: 5% of pregnant women, plus 480,000/y develop hyperthyroidism
- Rx for hyperthyroidism, goiter associated with hyperthyroidism
- Definitive Rx to control hyperthyroidism in anticipation of spontaneous remission
- Rx for hyperthyroidism in conjunction with ^{131}I or ^{125}I to hasten recovery while awaiting effects of radiation therapy
- Rx for hyperthyroidism to control disorder in preparation for surgery

Perioperative Risks

- Side effects of drug: Hypothyroidism (see Hyperthyroidism or Hypothyroidism in Diseases section); liver failure esp. in pts with liver transplants; be careful in pregnancy.

Worry About

- Agranulocytosis (less than 0.5% of treated pts develop this side effect)

Overview/Pharmacology

- Antithyroid drug: Absorbed within 20–30 min; effect begins to ↓ in 2–3 hr (methimazole $T_{1/2}$ estimated to be 6–13 hr)
- Drug and metabolites cleared by renal excretion
- Antithyroid drugs cross placenta, can be found in breast milk

Drug Class/Usual Dose

- Antithyroid drug: Interferes directly with synthesis of thyroid hormones by preventing incorporation of iodine into tyrosyl residual thyroglobulin; inhibits coupling of iodotyrosyl residues to form iodothyronines by inhibiting peroxidase enzyme

- Depletes pre-formed hormone over time; only then do clinical effects become noticeable ($T_{1/2}$ of thyroid hormones is >3 d in circulation)
- Other useful antithyroid Rx drugs incl those inhibiting conversion of less active T_4 into more active T_3, such as propranolol; methimazole, carbimazole do not appear to do so with anti-β-blocker effect (e.g., propranolol and others); those that inhibit release of pre-formed thyroid hormone (e.g., iodine). Also temporarily inhibits synthesis and ↓ vascularity of thyroid glands.
- A thioureylene

Chronic Rx Uses

- Decreased hyperthyroidism and thyrotoxicosis
- Decreased goiter size in hyperthyroidism

Acute Rx Uses

- Relieves symptoms of hyperthyroidism while waiting for ^{131}I or ^{125}I to take effect

DRUG EFFECTS

System	Effect	Assessment by Hx	PE	Test
HEENT	Goiter shrinkage; occasionally goiter develops if hypothyroidism occurs	Snoring, hoarseness, neck pain	Ask pt to vocalize "e"; examine airway, neck	Check CXR (PA, lat), lat neck films; if needed, CT scan of neck
CARDIO		Assess CV response to Rx		Rhythm strip or full ECG if CV system is involved by either Hx or PE
GI	Rare hepatotoxicity			SGPT, SGOT
HEME	Mild anemia, thrombocytopenia; agranulocytosis as toxic reaction to propylthiouracil or methimazole (0.05–0.12% of pts)	Hx of sore throat or fever often heralds agranulocytosis	Skin/mucous membranes for infection/petechiae; purpura if at risk	CBC with plt count; differential leukocyte count
DERM		Rare depigmentation of hair		
MS		Pain/stiffness in joints (rare side effect)		
GU	Placenta—crosses placental barrier and is excreted in breast milk			
CNS		Headache, paresthesia rare side effects. Shaking, anxiety, emotional instability are signs that hyperthyroidism not yet controlled.	Reflex speed, tremor, nervousness, mental status	
ENDO	Need to assess if euthyroid	Refer to all other systems, esp. reflex speed, tremor, heat intolerance, wt loss, fatigue, weakness, anorexia, ↑ appetite	Reflex speed; HR	Free T_4 level if unable to assess if euthyroid by Hx, PE

Key References: Earling PA. Thyroid disease. *Br J Anaesth.* 2000;85:15–28. Nayak B, Burman K. Thyrotoxicosis and thyroid storm. *Endocrinol Metab Clin North Am.* 2006;35:663–686.

Possible Drug Interactions

Preoperative Period

- Assess euthyroid state (see table)
- Fairly certain sign that remission may have occurred is ↓ in size of goiter

Induction/Maintenance

- No interactions known

Adjuvants/Regional Anesthesia/Reversal

- No interactions known

Postoperative Concerns

- Resumption not necessary if surgery to correct hyperthyroidism successful
- Be careful in pts with Hx of liver disease, pregnant or breastfeeding

- Short $T_{1/2}$ makes resumption in nonthyroid surgery necessary ASAP, or give medication IV

Anticipated Problems/Concerns

- Assess for hyperthyroidism, agranulocytosis

Pyridostigmine Bromide

J. Lance LaFleur
Krishna Boddu

Uses

- Therapy for myasthenia gravis (MG) which is caused by decreased postsynaptic acetylcholine (ACh) receptors
- Antagonism of nondepolarizing neuromuscular blocking drugs (NMBD)
- Therapy for glaucoma
- Therapy for atony of GI and urinary tracts

Perioperative Risks

- Muscarinic effects on GI, resp, and CV systems
- Prolonged response to succinylcholine if administered shortly afterward by inhibition of pseudo-cholinesterase and ↑ postsynaptic depolarization
- Paralysis may be prolonged by excessive doses which can produce a depolarizing NMB

Pharmacology

- Oxydiaphoretic (acid-transferring) inhibitor of acetylcholinesterase (AChE)
- Transfers a carbamate group to AChE and forms a covalent bond at the esteratic site
- Quaternary ammonium ion which is poorly lipid soluble; does not effectively penetrate GI tract or blood-brain barrier (no CNS side effects)
- Onset is 10–15 min (versus 5–10 min for neostigmine); duration is 4 hr (similar to neostigmine)
- 20% as potent as neostigmine
- Renal excretion accounts for ~75% of elimination
- Very large volume of distribution with extensive tissue storage
- Oral bioavailability is 7.6 +/- 2.4%

Drug Class/Mechanism of Action/Usual Dose

- Reversibly inhibits AChE which increases the concentration of ACh at the motor endplate
- May be administered PO, IV, or IM
- Dose is 0.1–0.4 mg/kg IV

DRUG EFFECTS

System	Effect	Assessment by Hx	PE	Test
CARDIO	Bradyarrhythmias, hypotension	Presyncope, angina, confusion	HR, BP, orthostasis	ECG
RESP	↑ Secretions, bronchospasm	Dyspnea, wheezing	Auscultation	PFTs
GI	↑ Secretions, ↑ motility, spasms	Diarrhea, abd pain	Palpation	Electrolytes

Key Reference: Barash PG, Cullen BF, Stoelting RK. *Clinical Anesthesia*. 5th ed. Philadelphia: Lippincott Williams and Wilkins; 2006:297–300, 848.

Perioperative Implications

Preoperative Concerns

- In MG pts, skeletal muscle response to repetitive impulses is augmented by increased availability of ACh
- Chronic administration in MG pts may alter effects of NMBD, and some may consider omission or reduction of morning dose on the day of surgery.

Induction/Maintenance

- While nicotinic effects are desirable, muscarinic effects should be attenuated by an anticholinergic (typically glycopyrrolate 0.05 mg per 1 mg of pyridostigmine)

Postoperative Period

- Incidence of recurarization in renal pts is not ↑ as clearance of both AChE inhibitors and NMBD is similarly affected.
- MG pts taking >750 mg/d have ↑ potential for resp insufficiency
- Myasthenic and cholinergic crises may occur after periop alterations in AChE inhibitor therapy.

Anticipated Problems/Concerns

- If maximal dose of pyridostigmine (0.4 mg/kg, or 20 mg in adults) fails to antagonize the residual blockade, it is not advisable to redose the AChE inhibitor as this may lead to further motor weakness.
- Causes of inadequate antagonism incl profound blockade, resp acidosis, hypokalemia, hypermagnesemia, hypothermia, verapamil, and antibiotics such as aminoglycosides and polypeptides.

Quinidine

Brian McClure
Kathryn Dorhauer

- See Also Procainamide

Uses

- Used in the treatment of ventricular arrhythmias (hemodynamically stable wide complex tachycardia) or supraventricular arrhythmias (i.e., AFib/flutter, PAT, WPW) for the conversion to and maintenance of a normal sinus rhythm.

Perioperative Risks

- Plasma levels >2 μg/mL results in prolongation of the PR interval, QRS complex, and QT interval which may lead to life-threatening ventricular arrhythmias (i.e., torsades de pointes). Acidosis, hypomagnesemia, and hypokalemia increase risk of adverse events.

Worry About

- High plasma levels assoc with hepatic and renal disease because quinidine is metabolized by the liver and subsequently excreted by the kidney (dose must be reduced and plasma levels followed)
- Thrombocytopenia possible 2° to drug-plt complexes that cause the production of antibodies
- N/V/D occur in approx ⅓ of people
- Decreasing plasma levels in assoc with rifampin, phenytoin, barbiturates
- Increasing plasma levels in assoc with amiodarone, cimetidine
- Causes serum levels of digoxin to increase to toxic levels

- Not recommended in incomplete AV block because quinidine may lead to complete AV block or sudden cardiac death
- May cause significant hypotension due to its effects on both resistance and capacitance vessels, causing a decrease in systemic pressure and preload (esp. IV)

Overview/Pharmacology

- Dextroisomer of quinine and thus also has antimalarial and antipyretic effects
- Quinidine blocks the fast inward sodium channel, which leads to a prolongation of phase 0 of the cardiac action potential and therefore a decreased heart rate
- Well absorbed from GI tract (80% bioavailability) and peak plasma concentrations occur in 60–90 min with effects lasting 6–8 hr (up to 12 hr with extended release formulations)
- Elimination through kidneys, 20% unchanged, 80% after hepatic metabolism through hydroxylation to an inactive metabolite
- 90% bound to plasma proteins
- Serum concentration should be monitored to fit narrow therapeutic range: 2–5 μg/mL
- Interacts with drugs that alter hepatic enzyme function, other highly protein-bound drugs
- Urine alkalinization leads to decreased excretion

- It has anticholinergic properties, which may lead to increased HR in people with NSR
- When used for supraventricular tachycardia must be used in conjunction with an AV nodal blocking agent (e.g., digoxin, CCB, beta blocker) in order to prevent a paradoxical increase in the ventricular response (1:1 conduction)

Drug Class/Mechanism of Action/Usual Dose

- Class IA antiarrhythmic (use-dependent Na⁺-channel blocker which causes prolongation of the cardiac action potential and is responsible for effectiveness in tachyarrhythmias)
- Dosage
  - Quinidine gluconate (324 mg tabs): 648–2592 mg divided bid or tid
  - Quinidine gluconate IM form: 400–2400 mg daily
  - Quinidine sulfate (200 mg, 300 mg, 300 mg ER tabs): 400–4000 mg divided bid or tid
  - Quinidine is rarely administered IV due to peripheral vasodilation and myocardial depression, which can lead to severe hypotension
  - Doses must be titrated to the individual based on plasma levels and EKG findings
- Alternatives: Other class IA drugs (e.g., procainamide, disopyramide, cibenzoline, pirmenol)

DRUG EFFECTS

System	Effect	Assessment by Hx	PE	Test
CARDIO	↑ QRS duration, vagolytic cardiac/peripheral α blockade, negative inotropic, ↓ conduction velocity	↑ HR Dyspnea Syncope	↑ HR, ↓ BP, JVD, Abnormal S₃ Bradycardia, asystole	CXR ECG (3° AV block)
GI	Diarrhea (18%), nausea (18%)	α Blockade		
HEME	Thrombocytopenia		Mucosal bleeding	Plt count
CNS	Headache (13%), dizziness (8%), tinnitus, blurred vision, tremor			Quinidine serum concentration
MISC	Drug-induced SLE, anaphylactoid reactions, aggravation of asthma (caution)	Rash Joint pain Mucosal swelling	CV collapse	

Key Reference: RuDusky BM. Quinidine as an antiarrhythmic. *Chest.* 2001;119:1617–1619.

Perioperative Implications/Possible Drug Interactions

Preoperative Preparation

- ECG should be closely monitored when initially starting quinidine. Consider serial measurements of QRS duration and QT interval on the ECG to prevent arrhythmias; QRS should be <140 ms or <50% increase from baseline
- Quinidine will cause increased plasma levels of warfarin and digoxin; monitor levels closely and ↓ dosage to prevent toxicity.
- Decrease dose in hypoproteinemia, liver failure, and renal failure

Induction/Maintenance

- Possible ↓ in hepatic metabolism of halogenated agents
- ↓ Levels of plasma proteins after CPB augment free fraction of drug

Adjuvants/Regional Anesthesia/Reversal

- Quinidine may ↑ muscle weakness in pts with myasthenia gravis, ↓ effect of anticholinesterases, enhances NMB and may lead to recurrence of skeletal muscle blockade in immediate postop period.
- Quinidine can enhance the effects of vasodilating, negative inotropic, sinus node depressant agents (e.g., β-blockers, verapamil, rauwolfia alkaloids, bretylium) leading to severe hypotension or syncope.
- Concurrent administration of other class IA drugs, amiodarone, or phenothiazines ↑ risk of torsades de pointes
- Quinidine has attenuates effects of anticholinergic drugs

Anticipated Problems/Concerns

- Quinidine contraindicated when ventricular arrhythmias assoc with or caused by QT prolongation (risk of torsades)
- Usually administered orally due to adverse effects assoc with parenteral routes
  - IM injection very painful
  - IV routes cause vasodilation and myocardial depression, esp. when rapidly infused. D/C if hypotension persists.
- Must weigh risk-benefit ratio in each pt due to proarrhythmic qualities of quinidine even when plasma levels in therapeutic range; may actually have increased mortality.

DRUGS

Riboflavin (Vitamin B$_2$)

Lynn A. Fenton

Other Names

- Flavin, flavine, lactoflavin, riboflavine, vitamin G.
- The name riboflavin comes from ribose (the sugar that forms part of its structure) and flavin, the ring-moiety that imparts the yellow color to the oxidized molecule.

Etiology/Sources

- Organic: Leafy green vegetables, milk, cheese, kidneys, legumes, tomatoes, yeast, mushrooms
- Synthetic: Water-soluble B-complex vitamins and vitamin B$_2$ preparations.

Indications/Uses

- Riboflavin is required for a wide variety of cellular processes in humans and animals.
- Taken orally for the prevention of common deficiency with general nutritional deficiency (malnutrition, starvation, chronic alcoholism) and for preventing migraine headaches.
- Also used in the treatment of alcoholism, ariboflavinosis, acne, burning feet syndrome, burns, canker sores, carpal tunnel syndrome, cataracts, congenital methemoglobinemia, eye fatigue, glaucoma, lactic acidosis induced by NRTI (antiretroviral) drugs, multiple acycloenzyme A dehydrogenase deficiency, liver disease, memory loss (incl Alzheimer's disease), RBC aplasia, sickle cell anemia, and ulcers.
- Riboflavin is also used to increase energy levels, boost immune system function and athletic performance, slow aging, promote healthy reproductive function, and to maintain healthy hair, skin, mucous membranes, and nails.

Perioperative Risks

- Excessive intake causes increased excretion of unchanged riboflavin in the urine.
- Deficiency causes anemia, neuropathy, and more friable lip tissue and oral/tongue mucosa.
- Use caution with tape and pressure at or near facial, nasal areas if seborrhea is present.

Anticipated Problems/Concerns

- Riboflavin is likely safe when taken orally, no toxic effects have been reported.

- During pregnancy, it is likely safe when used at the RDA of 1.4 mg/d.
- When lactating, it is likely safe when used at the RDA of 1.6 mg/day.
- Adequate phosphorus must be given along with riboflavin and other vitamins when refeeding starved pts to prevent depletion of phosphate stores and energy of cells.
- Exposure to light can destroy vitamin B$_2$.

Overview/ Mechanism of Action/ Pharmacology

- Component of the electron transfer chain in mitochondria, oxidative metabolic coenzymes.
- Absorbed from upper GI tract by specific transport mechanism involving phosphorylation of an enzyme to FMN by the enzyme flavokinase.
- Central component of cofactors FAD and FMN and is therefore required by all flavoproteins.
- Like other B vitamins, riboflavin plays an important role in energy metabolism and for the metabolism of fats, ketone bodies, carbohydrates, and proteins.
- Distributed to all tissues, but little stored and the rest is excreted unchanged in the urine.

ASSESSMENT POINTS

System	Effect of Deficiency	Assessment by Hx	PE	Test
HEEENT	Sore throat, cheilosis, glossitis, corneal vascularization, cataracts	Burning tongue, soreness in mouth and throat	Red, fissured lips; blue-red tongue with edematous surface—"cobblestone tongue"	Urinary excretion of <50 mcg/24 hr of riboflavin
HEME	Anemia			Reticulocytopenia, normochromic normocytic anemia
DERM	Seborrheic dermatitis of face, dermatitis of arms and trunk	Burning, itching eyes	Rough, sharkskin appearance of nose	
PNS	Neuropathy		PNS function exam	

Key Reference: Jellin JM, Gregory P, Batz F, Hitchens K, et al. *Pharmacist's Letter/ Prescriber's Letter Natural Medicine Comprehensive Database.* 3rd ed. Stockton, CA: Therapeutic Research Faculty; 2000:899–901.

Drug Class/ Usual Dose

- Water-Soluble B-Complex Vitamin; RDA For adults is 0.6 mg/1000 kcal/d diet.

Possible Drug Interactions/Perioperative Implications

- Aspirin: Concomitant use with riboflavin may cause gastric intolerance.
- Beta-blockers: Theoretically, concomitant use with riboflavin may enhance migraine prevention without increasing adverse effects.
- Nucleoside reverse transcriptase inhibitor (NRTI) drugs: Riboflavin is reported to reverse lactic acidosis caused by these antiretroviral drugs.
- Probenecid: Decreases riboflavin absorption.

- Propantheline: Delays and increases riboflavin absorption
- Drug influences on nutrient levels and depletion:
  - Antibiotics: Can destroy normal GI flora, which can cause decreased production of B vitamins.
  - Metoclopramide: Concomitant use can decrease riboflavin absorption in the GI tract.
  - Oral contraceptives: By an unknown mechanism the use of oral contraceptives can reduce serum vitamin B$_2$ levels. The need for supplementation has not been adequately studied.
  - Phenothiazines: Use of phenothiazines can increase urinary vitamin B$_2$ excretion and reduce serum vitamin B$_2$ levels.

- Probenecid: Inhibits dietary riboflavin absorption.
- Propantheline bromide: Delays and increases supplemental riboflavin absorption.
- Absorption depends on flavokinase activity, which in turn depends on thyroid hormone status and is inhibited by TCAs and chlorpromazine.
- Preop normochromic normocytic anemia in a nutritionally depleted pt responds to riboflavin administration.
- Boric acid poisoning induces riboflavin deficiency.

Rifampin

Gaurav Rajpal
Manuel C. Vallejo

Uses

- Antibiotic therapy for TB (incidence (9.4/100,000/y) and *Neisseria meningitidis* infection (incidence 4.6–10/100,000/y)
- Used in the treatment of opioid-induced pruritis assoc with the cholestatic jaundice of malignancy
- Administered PO or IV
- 10% of pts receiving rifampin develop chemical hepatitis; 16 deaths/500,000 receiving drug

Perioperative Risks

- Hepatic dysfunction, most likely in presence of pre-existing liver disease and when used in combination with other hepatotoxic agents like isoniazid

- Decreased duration of action of narcotic and barbiturates due to P450 (CYP2D6) enzyme induction
- Pts receiving antiarrhythmic therapy, digoxin, theophylline, phenytoin, or glucocorticoid therapy may need increased doses of these drugs due to enzyme induction

Overview/ Pharmacology

- Complex macrocytic antibiotic
- H_2O-soluble at acidic pH; inhibits gram-positive and many gram-negative organisms, incl *E. Coli, Pseudomonas, Proteus, Klebsiella, N. meningitidis, H. influenzae, M. tuberculosis*
- Increases in vitro activity of streptomycin and isoniazid
- Eliminated by biliary clearance with significant enterohepatic circulation

- $T_{1/2}$ of 1.5–5 h, increases with hepatic dysfunction

Worry About

- Induces hepatic microsomal (P450, CYP2D6) activity, decreases $T_{1/2}$ of hepatically metabolized drugs
- Theoretical increases risk of halothane hepatitis
- Hemolytic anemia, thrombocytopenia (rare)

ASSESSMENT POINTS

System	Effect	Assessment by Hx	PE	Test
OVERALL		Fatigue, drowsiness, dizziness, ataxia, confusion, weakness		
HEENT	Secreted in saliva, tears		Orange sputum, tears, conjunctiva, sweat	
GI	Hepatic dysfunction (rare with normal pre-Rx hepatic function)	N/V	Jaundice	Elevated transaminases
HEME	Thrombocytopenia, hemolytic anemia	Bruising/ bleeding		Plt count, Hgb/Hct, microscopic exam
RENAL	Interstitial nephritis, ATN, renal failure (with high doses)		Orange urine	Cr clearance, light chain proteinuria

Key Reference: Dilger K, Hofmann U, Klotz U. Enzyme induction in the elderly: Effect of rifampin on the pharmacokinetics and pharmacodynamics of propafenone. *Clin Pharmacol Ther.* 2000;67:512–520.

Perioperative Implications/ Possible Drug Interactions

Preoperative Concerns

- Decrease duration of action of benzodiazepines, narcotics, barbiturates due to hepatic (P450, CYP2D6) enzyme induction
- Adequacy of pre-existing drug regimens should be verified (see Special Considerations)

Induction/ Maintenance

- Decreased narcotic and analgesic efficacy: barbiturates, methadone, diazepam, midazolam; β-blockers have increase clearance, decrease duration of action
- Halothane metabolism increases with increased risk of hepatotoxicity

Adjuvants/ Reversal

- Mycobacteria quickly develop resistance when rifampin used alone; administer with isoniazid and/or streptomycin

Special Considerations

- Risk of hepatic dysfunction periop ↑ by pre-existing hepatic disease
- Delays oral absorption of ASA
- Decreases $T_{1/2}$ requiring ↑ doses to maintain adequate therapeutic levels: Digoxin, digitoxin, quinidine, propranolol, metoprolol, verapamil, coumadin, theophylline, phenytoin, prednisone, cortisol, cyclosporine, oral hypoglycemic agents, ketoconazole, fluconazole
- Can precipitate opioid withdrawal symptoms in an opioid dependent pt because of enhancing the hepatic enzymatic metabolism of opioids

Drug Class/Mechanism of Action/Dose

- Rifamycin antibiotic family
- Inhibits DNA-dependent RNA polymerase in bacteria and mycobacteria; nuclear eukaryotic RNA polymerase not affected

- Administered for chemoprophylaxis of meningococcal infections, with β-lactams for *staphylococcus* endocarditis, osteomyelitis, for methicillin-resistant *S. aureus* infections; and in conjunction with isoniazid and streptomycin for active TB
- Usual dose: 600 mg qd: pediatric dose 10 mg/kg qd, PO or IV
- Possible interaction of rifampin with 5HT3 and opioid system as well as mediators of itching is proposed. Dose 300 mg bid IV
- Should be administered 1 hr before or 2 hr after meals PO

Anticipated Problems/Concerns

- 10% on therapy may develop hepatitis; pts with pre-existing liver disease are at higher risk
- Rifampin induces microsomal enzyme activity in liver, results in ↓ efficacy, duration of action of hepatically metabolized drugs

DRUGS

Serotonin: Agonists, Antagonists, and Reuptake Inhibitors

David F. Stowe

Indications

- Serotonin (5-hydroxytryptophan, 5-HT) not given as a drug
- Partially selective receptor *agonists* (used mostly for Rx of acute migraine headaches)
    - Sumatriptan (Imitrex) 5–20 mg nasal, 25–100 mg/d PO mg
    - Naratriptan (Amerge) 2.5 mg/d PO
    - Rizatriptan (Maxalt) 5 mg/d PO
    - Zolmitriptan (Zomig) 5 mg nasal, 2.5 mg/d PO
    - Metoclopramide (Reglan) 5–15 mg qid PO, 2–10 mg IV (Rx for GERD, gastroparesis, N/V)
- Partially selective receptor 5-HT$_3$ antagonists (used for Rx of N/V)
    - Dolasetron (Anzemet) 12.5 mg IV or 100 mg PO 30–60 min before emergence to prevent postop N/V or before chemoRx
    - Ondansetron (Zofran) 4–8 mg tid PO to prevent N/V due to emergence or emetogenic chemoRx treatment
    - Granisetron (Kytril) 10 μg/kg IV, 1 mg/bid PO, TD patch (Sancuso) for prevention of N/V due to chemoRx; for postop N/V
    - Palonosetron (Aloxi) 0.25 mg IV 30 min before chemoRx
- Selective serotonin reuptake inhibitors (SSRIs) (all used PO for Rx of major depression and personality disorders)
    - Citalopram (Celexa) 20–40 mg/d PO
    - Escitalopram (Lexapro) 10 mg/d PO
    - Fluoxetine (Prozac) 20–80 mg/d PO
    - Fluvoxamine (Luvox) 25–50 mg/d PO
    - Paroxetine (Paxil) 20–50 mg/d PO
    - Sertraline (Zoloft) 50–200 mg/d PO

Perioperative Risks

- Sumatriptan: Not for pts with IHD, angina, Prinzmetal's angina, severe Htn
- Metoclopramide: Not for pts with pheochromocytoma, on MAOIs; may worsen mental depression; effect antagonized by narcotics
- SSRIs can cause serotonin syndrome (hyperthermia, muscle rigidity, myoclonus, rapid mental change) if given in the presence of MAOIs; may increase coumadin, digitalis effects by reducing plasma protein binding; increased suicide risk <24 y age

Worry About

- Sumatriptan and other 5-HT agonists: pts taking these may have exacerbation of anginal Sx
- Ondansetron, granisetron, etc: chemoRx pts may exhibit ↑ N/V during anesthesia
- SSRIs: Serotonin syndrome: concomitant use of MAOIs, displacement of other drugs highly bound to plasma protein (digoxin, antianginals, betablockers, tricyclic antidepressants) increased bleeding with coumadin, so monitor prothrombin time

Overview/Pharmacology

- Serotonin secreted 90% by enterochromaffin cells of GI tract; released into plasma by unclear mech, neuronal stimuli; some taken up, much is stored in plts; 5-HT receptors on vascular endothelium stimulate release of NO to promote vasodilation, but receptors on vascular smooth muscle promote vasoconstriction. Excess release involved in carcinoid syndrome, due to enterochromaffin cell neoplasm. As an amine neurotransmitter, serotonin also secreted, stored, released by raphe nuclei in brainstem (serotonergic neurons).
- Serotonergic neurons diffusely innervate most regions of CNS; with other neurotransmitters is involved in modulating mood, depression, anxiety, migraine headache, sleep, appetite, temp regulation, perception of pain and itch, regulation of BP
- Abn in secretion or receptor activation likely underlie mental depression, migraine headache, sensitivity to pain, sleep pattern, and central BP control. In CNS, 5-HT receptor activation increases K$^+$ conductance to promote membrane hyperpolarization, → mostly inhibitory action. As CNS neurotransmitter, 5-HT modulates effects of other monoamine transmitters—e.g., norepinephrine, dopamine, and other transmitters such as ACh, glycine, GABA. Inhibition of 5-HT reuptake elevates mood, normalizes behavior.

ASSESSMENT POINTS

System	Effect	Assessment by Hx	PE	Test
CARDIO	Htn, IHD (agonists)		BP	
	ECG: Longer P-R and QT$_c$ intervals (antagonists)			
	Hypotension (SSRIs)			
	Serotonin syndrome (SSRIs)	MAO drug interaction	BP, CNS	Drug levels
	Altered drug levels (SSRIs)	Dysrhythmias, bleeding	Bleeding	
ENDO	Carcinoid syndrome (↑ 5-HT)	Diarrhea, abd pain, asthma, flushing, hyperglycemia, PAT, SVT		5-HT, kallikreins
HEME	Leukopenia (antagonists)			CBC
CNS	Psychosis, depression, altered mood, Sz disorder	Mental disorder	CNS evaluation	Drug levels

Key Reference: Lacasse JR, Leo J. Serotonin and depression: A disconnect between the advertisements and the scientific literature. *PLoS Med.* 2005;2:e392.

Perioperative Implications

- Avoid narcotics in pts with carcinoid syndrome (surgery or 5-HT antagonists usual Rx for carcinoid tumor)
- Use caution in giving metoclopramide; pt must not be taking MAOIs—e.g., isocarboxazid (Marplan), phenelzine (Nardil), or tranylcypromine (Parnate)
- Check pt's drug profile if Hx of migraine; ↑ risk of coronary vasoconstriction with sumatriptan
- Check pt's drug profile if Hx of schizophrenia; may have low WBC count if taking clozapine
- Check pt's drug profile if Hx of major depression; if taking coumadin or digitalis, levels may be ↑.

Sildenafil Citrate

John G. Augoustides
Lee A. Fleisher

Indications

- Treatment of erectile dysfunction (Viagra)
- Sildenafil (Revatio) is used to improve the ability to exercise in people with pulm arterial Htn
- Oral sildenafil is used as part of multimodal management of severe periop pulm Htn and right ventricular dysfunction in clinical settings such as:
    - Heart transplantation
    - Pulm Htn assoc with CHD
    - Pulm Htn assoc with mitral valve disease

Perioperative Risks

- None for elective surgery based on $T_{1/2}$
- Drug may still be present in emergent surgery

Worry About

- Potentiation of vasodilating agents
- Hx of coronary ischemia or congestive heart failure
- Severe hepatic impairment

Overview/Pharmacology

- Sildenafil citrate was discovered by accident during testing as a treatment for heart disease.
- Terminal $T_{1/2}$ 4–6 hr
- Total protein binding 96%, also distributed in tissues
- Bioavailability 41%
- Metabolized in liver via the cytochrome P450 isoenzymes, 3A4 (major route) and 2C9 (minor route)
- Active *N*-desmethyl metabolite
- Peak plasma concentration 60 min
- Excreted via feces (80%), kidney (13%), and semen (<0.001% of a dose)
- Metabolism may be delayed after a high-fat meal and in pts with liver disease
- Contraindicated in pts with hypersensitivity to sildenafil products and pts taking nitroglycerin or other organic nitrates
- Precautions: Anatomic deformities of the penis, conditions predisposing pts to priapism, bleeding disorders or active peptic ulceration, retinitis pigmentosa or other retinal abn, coronary ischemia or CHF, multidrug antihypertensive regimens
- Excretion in breast milk is unknown

Drug Class/Mechanism of Action

- Potent and selective inhibitor of phosphodiesterase type V (PDE V)
- PDE V isoform is responsible for breaking down cyclic guanosine monophosphate (cGMP) in corpus cavernosum. cGMP relaxes smooth muscle to cause local vasodilatation and swelling of corpora as they fill with blood.
- With sexual arousal, NO is produced in cavernosal tissue to stimulate the secretion of cGMP.
- Sildenafil inhibits PDE V, causing 35% increase in cGMP levels.
- Sildenafil inhibits PDE V in the lung, thus increasing cGMP levels in the lung to cause pulm vasodilatation and improvement in pulm Htn.

Usual Dose

- Supplied in 100-mg, 50-mg, 25-mg tablets
- May be taken 0.5–4 hr prior to sexual activity
- Dose ranges from 25–100 mg, with a maximum frequency of once-a-day orally
- Dose adjustments required in pts with severe renal and hepatic impairment
- For geriatric pts (>65 y), starting dose should be 25 mg

ASSESSMENT POINTS

System	Effect	Assessment by Hx	PE
HEENT	Activity on PDE VI (PDE VI is important for phototransduction in the retina)	Transient disturbance of blue-green color discrimination	
CARDIO	Dilatation of systemic blood vessels	Transient drop in BP, flushing, Hx of nitrates	Low BP
GI	Relaxation of lower esophageal sphincter	Dyspepsia, diarrhea	
CNS		Headache, dizziness	
RESP	Mucosal vasodilatation	Nasal congestion	

Key Reference: Schwartz BG, Kloner RA. Drug interactions with phosphodiesterase-5 inhibitors for the treatment of erectile dysfunction or pulmonary hypertension. *Circulation.* 2010;122:88–95.

Perioperative Implications

- Risk primarily related to emergent cases based on $T_{1/2}$
- Caution with the concomitant use of hypotensive agents
- Precautions to prevent reflux and regurgitation
- Pts on regular sildenafil for pulm vasodilation will have significant pulm Htn that is often assoc with significant underlying lung disease and right ventricular dysfunction.
- Pts on regular sildenafil for pulm vasodilation may require aggressive periop management of severe pulm Htn to maintain adequate cardiac output. Adequate pulm vasodilatation may require periop therapy with IV inodilators such as milrinone and/or inhaled selective pulm vasodilators such as NO or prostacyclin.

Drug Interactions

- Concurrent use of nitrates may cause hypotension.
- Drug interactions with cytochrome P450 inhibitors (e.g., ketoconazole, erythromycin, and cimetidine) can be expected, and during concomitant therapy a lower dose is suggested.

Statins

Frederic T. Billings, IV
Bernhard Riedel

Uses

- Incidence in USA: Estimated 20 million
- Primary indications include:
  - Hyperlipidemia: Hydroxymethylglutaryl coenzyme-A (HMG CoA) reductase inhibitors (statins) are powerful drugs for lowering low-density lipoprotein (LDL) cholesterol and certain brands—atorvastatin in high doses and rosuvastatin—increase healthy HDL cholesterol.
  - 1° and 2° prevention of CV disease: CV benefits (reduction in myocardial infarction and stroke) in pts with hypercholesterolemia. Benefits also in normocholesterolemic pts with elevated markers of inflammation (e.g., C-reactive protein (CRP).
  - 2°, less robustly proven, benefits: Decreased risk of sepsis, venoembolic disease, osteoporosis, cancer, and dementia; blood pressure reduction; renal function preservation; reduced morbidity in heart failure.

Perioperative Risks

- Myopathy: Incidence among nonoperative chronic statin users is 2–11% for myalgias, 0.5% for myositis, <0.1% for rhabdomyolysis. Incidence increased in severe renal insufficiency (CrCl <30 mL/min).
- Hepatic dysfunction: Incidence of persistent elevations in aminotransferases is 0.5–3%, and 0.1% for >10-fold increase in alanine aminotransferase. Reversible following D/C.
- Incidence of myopathy and transaminitis increased when cytochrome P-450 3A4 inhibitors, incl cyclosporine, tacrolimus, azole antifungals, fenofibrates, protease inhibitors, and macrolide antibiotics are used concomitant with those statins that are extensively metabolized by cytochrome P-450 3A4 (lovastatin, simvastatin, and to a lesser extent atorvastatin).
- Lipophilic statins may be associated with more adverse events than hydrophilic statins

Overview/Pharmacology

- Statins inhibit the reduction of HMG CoA to mevalonate, the rate-limiting step in cholesterol biosynthesis. Statins primarily inhibit hepatocyte cholesterol synthesis and increase LDL receptor transcription and hepatic LDL cholesterol uptake. Consequently, statins reduce systemic concentrations of LDL cholesterol by 25–55%. Plasma HDL cholesterol levels may rise by 8–10% with atorvastatin and rosuvastatin.
- The reduction in intracellular isoprenoid synthesis, which reduces prenylation of small GTPases (e.g., Rac, Rho), and may mediate the beneficial pleiotropic (non-lipid lowering) effects of statins. These effects include atherosclerotic plaque stabilization, inflammation reduction, reversal of endothelial dysfunction (through eNOS upregulation), decreased thrombogenicity, reduced reactive O_2 species generation (through NADPH-oxidase assembly inhibition). Improved survival occurs primarily in pts with elevated serum CRP levels. The statin-induced reduction in serum CRP concentration occurs unrelated to lipid levels at baseline or during therapy.
- Statins are orally administered once daily and peak plasma concentrations achieved in 1–3 hr.
- The hepatic cytochrome P-450 system metabolizes most statins to active and inactive metabolites, and statins are primarily excreted in bile.

PHARMACOKINETICS

Statin	Dose (mg)	Elimination Half-life, hrs	Protein Binding	Solubility	Cytochrome P-450 Isozyme	Active Metabolites	Renal excretion, %
Atorva–	10–80	15–30	80–90	Lipophilic	3A4	Yes	2
Fluva–	20–80	0.5–2.3	>99	Lipophilic	2C9	No	<6
Lova–	20–80	2.9	>95	Lipophilic	3A4	Yes	10
Prava–	10–40	1.3–2.8	43–55	Hydrophilic	–	No	20
Rosuva–	5–40	19	88	Hydrophilic	2C9	No	10
Simva–	10–80	2–3	94–98	Lipophilic	3A4, 3A5	Yes	13

SIDE EFFECTS

System	Effect	Presentation	PE	Test
HEPAT	Transaminitis	Asymptomatic	None	LFTs
MS	Myositis	Myalgia, cramps, aches	Muscle tenderness	Creatinine kinase

Key References: Schouten O, Boersma E, Hoeks SE, et al. Fluvastatin and perioperative events in patients undergoing vascular surgery. *N Engl J Med.* 2009;361:980. Durazzo AE, Machado FS, Ikeoka DT, et al. Reduction in cardiovascular events after vascular surgery with atorvastatin: a randomized trial. *J Vasc Surg.* 2004;39:967. Poldermans D, Bax JJ, Kertai MD, et al. Statins are associated with a reduced incidence of perioperative mortality in patients undergoing major noncardiac vascular surgery. *Circulation.* 2003;107:1848.

Perioperative Implications

- Pts with coronary disease or a coronary disease risk equivalent (DM, symptomatic carotid artery disease, peripheral arterial disease, abd aortic aneurysm, chronic kidney disease, or multiple risk factors that confer a 10-y risk of CHD greater than 20%) should receive statin therapy. As such, pts on statin therapy should be examined preop for coronary and peripheral vascular disease.
- Concern for statin accumulation and muscular and hepatic side effects among pts receiving major surgery led the ACC/AHA/NHLBI to recommend short-term periop statin administration cessation in 2002. Periop observational studies, however, have not assoc statin use with an increased risk of myopathy or rhabdomyolysis. In fact, preop cessation of statin therapy was assoc with significant CV harm in pts undergoing cardiac and major vascular surgery.
- Two randomized trials and large observational studies suggest pleiotropic effects of statins improve outcomes in the periop period for major cardiac and vascular surgery.
- In the DECREASE III trial, 497 vascular surgery pts were randomly assigned to either 80 mg of extended release fluvastatin daily or placebo at least 30 d before the procedure and continued for at least 30 d after surgery. The 1° endpoint of myocardial ischemia, within 30 d of surgery, occurred significantly less often in the fluvastain group (10.8 vs. 19.0 percent; hazard ratio 0.55, 95% CI 0.34–0.88). The 2° endpoint of the composite of death from CV causes and myocardial infarction also occurred significantly less often in the fluvastatin group (4.8 versus 10.1 percent; hazard ratio 0.47, 95% CI 0.24–0.94). There was no evidence of an increase in skeletal muscle or hepatic injury in the fluvastatin group.
- Among percutaneous coronary intervention pts, statin therapy administered 12 hr pre-catheterization reduced composite of myocardial ischemic events and death in several placebo controlled RCTs. Another RCT (ARMYDA) reported that 7 d of preop atorvastatin reduced post cardiac surgery atrial fibrillation and hospital length of stay.
- The non-lipid lowering (i.e., pleiotropic) effects of statins originate from improved endothelial function and reduced inflammation. In rodent and cell models, statins increase NO availablility, reduce reactive O_2 species generation, and reduce circulating markers of inflammation (interleukin-6, P-selectin) within 6-18 hr.
- Statin therapy is recommended as early as possible before surgery for pts undergoing elective major vascular surgery who have not been receiving a statin. Statin therapy should not be discontinued in the periop period in statin-using pts.
- Physician-scientists hope pleiotropic effects of statin therapy will provide periop protection for heart, brain, and kidney, but as yet, sufficient data is lacking.

DRUGS

Steroids

Michael Danekas
Karene Ricketts

Uses

- Replacement therapy for pts with structural or functional disorders of the adrenal cortex, pituitary, or hypothalamus
  - Adrenocorticosteroids for Addison's disease (primary adrenocortical insufficiency), for 2° or 3° adrenocortical insufficiency, and for congenital adrenal hyperplasia
  - Sex hormones for deficiency (as in 1° hypogonadism and postmenopause) and for contraception
- Glucocorticoids are used to treat
  - Inflammation: Crohn's disease, ulcerative colitis, asthma, arthritis, airway and cerebral edema, spinal cord injury, glomerulonephritis
  - Immunological disorders: Rheumatic disorders, skin disorders (for example eczema), allergic reactions, nephrotic syndrome, anti-rejection post transplantation
  - Cancer
- Antenatal glucocorticoid therapy in women at risk for preterm delivery reduces the incidence of neonatal RDS, intraventricular hemorrhage, necrotizing enterocolitis, sepsis, and neonatal mortality by approx 50 percent.
- Glucocorticoids are used to establish the diagnosis and cause of Cushing's syndrome (the dexamethasone suppression test).
- Glucocorticoids may also be used as an anti-emetic agent in the periop period.

Perioperative Risks

- The underlying condition warranting the use of steroids may carry its own inherent risks in the periop period.
- Long-term corticosteroid therapy induces adrenal insuffiency (inability to mount an adequate stress response to surgery), osteoporosis (increased risk for fracture), impaired wound healing, increased risk of infection, increased friability of skin and other tissues (mild pressure may cause skin ulceration, tape may tear skin, sutures may not hold), cushingoid body habitus (central obesity, buffalo hump, puffy and/or moon face may create a difficult airway), Htn, peptic ulcers, and psychoses.
- Oral contraceptives can increase risk for thromboembolism, thrombophlebitis, Htn, myocardial infarction, and cerebral thrombosis if aspirin is not used concurrently. These adverse effects are most common among women who smoke.

Worry About

- Fluid and electrolyte disturbances
  - Hypo- and/or Htn and myocardial events
  - Adrenal insufficiency
  - Hyperglycemia
- Possible difficult airway with cushingoid body habitus

Overview/Pharmacology

- Steroids are lipids formed of a sterane core with varying functional groups and states of oxidation that alter their physiological effects.
- Steroid hormones incl the sex hormones (androgens, progestins, and estrogens) and the hormones of the adrenal cortex (adrenocorticosteroids and the adrenal androgens). Adrenocorticosteroids are further differentiated into two classes: glucocorticoids and mineralocorticoids.

Drug Class/Usual Dose

- Dosing of steroids will vary depending on biologic potency, pharmacokinetic properties, disease process, concurrent medications, route of administration, and type of surgery.
- Mineralocorticoid
  - Fludrocortisone: 0.05–0.2 mg/d (oral adult physiologic replacement)
- Glucocorticoid
  - Hydrocortisone: 20–30 mg/d (oral adult physiologic replacement), 100 mg bolus followed by 200–300 mg/d (IV adult stress dose), 1–2 mg/kg/dose (IV pediatric stress dose)
  - Cortisone: 25–35 mg/d (oral adult physiologic replacement)
- Antenatal glucocorticoid treatment for accelerating fetal lung maturity:
  - Betamethasone (two doses of 12 mg given IM 24 hr apart)
  - Dexamethasone (four doses of 6 mg given IM 12 hr apart)

DRUG EFFECTS

System	Effect	Assessment by Hx	PE	Test
CARDIO	**Excess:** Htn, premature CAD **Deficit:** Hypotension, decreased response to vasoconstrictors	Headache, chest pain, SOB, diaphoresis, poor exercise tolerance Postural Sxs, syncope	Blood pressure, auscultation Orthostatic VS	EKG, ECHO
RESP	Decreased airway reactivity	Decreased use of rescue inhalers, decreased SOB and cough	Decreased wheezing	Spirometry
CNS	Changes in mood/behavior, brain excitability, insomnia, psychosis	Symptoms of depression, personality change, insomnia, psychosis	Mental exam	
GI	Decreased Ca^{2+} absorption Gastritis, PUD, pancreatitis	Abd pain, GI bleed, N/V	Abd pain	Total serum calcium EGD, CT scan
ENDO	Central redistribution of body fat Increase blood glucose, insulin resistance Adrenal insufficiency Increase free fatty acids	Wt gain Polydipsia, polyuria Lethargy	Obesity, buffalo hump, moon facies, supraclavicular fat, thin extremities Refractory hypotension	Glucose, insulin levels Lipid panel
RENAL	**Excess:** Positive Na^+ balance, increased extracellular fluid, Ca^{2+} excretion, hypokalemia, alkalosis **Deficit:** Na^+ wasting, decreased extracellular fluid, hyperkalemia, acidosis	Fluid retention	Edema	Lytes, ABG, BUN/Cr
MS/DERM	**Excess:** Muscle wasting/myopathy Osteoporosis/osteonecrosis Skin thinning, acne, striae, alopecia, hirsutism, edema **Deficit:** Weakness, fatigue Hyperpigmentation	Muscle wasting, weakness Hx of pathologic fractures/bone pain Skin/hair changes Fatigue, weakness Skin darkening	Decreased muscle strength, bulk and tone Bone pain	X-ray, bone density
HEME	**Excess:** Polycythemia, decreased lymphocytes, increased polymorphonuclear leukocytes, immunosuppression **Deficit:** Anemia	Increased infections Fatigue	Signs of infection Pallor	CBC, differential

Key References: Welsh GA, et al. *The surgical patient taking glucocorticoids*. UpToDate; 2009. Brunton LL, Lazo JS, Parker KL. *Goodman & Gilman's The pharmacological basis of therapeutics*. 11th ed. New York: McGraw-Hill; 2005.

Perioperative Implications

Preoperative Concerns

- Correction of fluid, electrolyte, and metabolic disturbances
- Evaluation for hypo- and/or Htn, CAD and/or myocardial events, and DM and/or hyperglycemia
- Airway evaluation (for upper airway obstruction from excess facial tissue or edema, Mallampati, mouth opening, degree of neck extension with buffalo hump or cervical arthritis, obesity, dentition)
- Adequate IV access given superficial blood vessels and friability of tissues
- Co-morbid conditions

Induction/Monitoring/Maintenance

- No specific anesthetic drug or technique has advantages in a pt on steroids; however, hemodynamic instability may occur if standard dosing is used in a hypovolemic pt.
- Induction agents, maintenance, and monitoring should be tailored to the co-morbidities of the pt and the surgical needs.
- Consider avoiding etomidate, which can inhibit adrenocorticosteroid production for up to 8 hr

- Monitor for hypo- and/or Htn, hyperglycemia, myocardial events, fluid and electrolyte disturbances
- Administer stress doses of glucocorticoid to any pt who has clinical Cushing's syndrome or any pt who has received more than 20 mg/d of prednisone or its equivalent (16 mg/d of methylprednisolone, 2 mg/d of dexamethasone, or 80 mg/d of hydrocortisone) for more than 3 wk in the past year:
    - For minor surgery: Usual steroid dose (no extra supplementation required)
    - For moderate surgical stress: In addition to usual steroid dose, administer hydrocortisone 50 mg IV on induction and 25 mg 8 q for 24 hr, then resume baseline dosing
    - For major surgery: In addition to usual steroid dose, administer 100 mg of IV hydrocortisone on induction and 50 mg every 8 q for 24 hr, then taper dose by half per day to baseline dosing
- Careful positioning and padding of pressure points (important because pts on steroids are predisposed to osteopenia and/or skin friability)

- Strict attention to sterile technique and periop antibiotics (pts on steroids are at increased risk for infection 2° to immunosuppression)
- Steroids can prolong the effect of muscle relaxants; therefore, ensure adequate strength prior to extubation.

Postoperative Period

- Monitor for hypo- and/or Htn and myocardial events
- Monitor for signs of adrenal insufficiency (hypotension)
- Continue exogenous steroid administration postop. Pts should revert to their baseline dose within 48 hr of surgery unless their clinical condition warrants otherwise.
- Consider compression devices to prevent venous thrombosis in nonambulatory pts (esp. smokers taking oral contraceptives who are not receiving concomitant aspirin)

Anticipated Problems/Concerns

- Fluid, electrolyte, and metabolic disturbances
- Adrenocortical suppression

Tacrolimus (FK-506)

Aisling Conran

Indications

• Rescue of 1° immunosuppressant Rx following liver, lung, heart, pancreas and limb transplant
• Approx candidates: 3000 liver and 9000 kidney transplants in USA; 15,000 living liver, 50,000 kidney transplant recipients chronically receiving immunosuppressants
• Has been used to suppress the inflammation assoc with ulcerative colitis

Preoperative Risks

• Htn: Ca^{2+}-channel blockers may be effective in treating tacrolimus-assoc Htn, but care required. Interference with tacrolimus metabolism may necessitate a dosing reduction
• Nephrotoxicity: Do not administer concurrently with cyclosporine; administer cautiously with other potentially nephrotoxic drugs, e.g., aminoglycoside antibiotics

• Hypersensitivity may occur with IV formulation; pts should be monitored for 30 min after injection
• May result in opioid-induced hyperalgesia

Worry About

• Drug is metabolized by cytochrome P450 (3A) enzyme system. Other medications that inhibit or induce this enzyme may affect tacrolimus drug levels.

Overview/Pharmacology

• General effect: Macrolide antibiotic with potent immunosuppressive properties, often used for rescue therapy in liver transplant pts with rejection refractory to other immunosuppressants
• Tacrolimus metabolized by liver; metabolites primarily excreted in bile; elimination T$_{1/2}$ of 8.5 hr prolonged with hepatic dysfunction
• Ca^{2+}-channel blockers, cyclosporine, erythromycin, antifungal agents, metoclopramide may ↑ blood levels of tacrolimus as function of P450 inhibition
• Anticonvulsants (carbamazepine, phenobarbital, phenytoin), rifampin may ↓ blood levels of tacrolimus 2° to induction of cytochrome P450 system
• Adverse effects requiring dose adjustments incl nephrotoxicity, neurotoxicity, alterations in glucose metabolism, infection, or susceptibility to malignancy

Drug Class/Mechanism of Action/Usual Dose

• Macrolide antibiotic, highly protein bound (>75%), binds primarily to albumin and/or α$_1$-glycoprotein
• Tacrolimus binds to calcineurin, blocking production of interleukin-2, thereby inhibiting further T-lymphocyte proliferation, immunosuppression
• Dosing: IV 0.05–0.1 mg/kg/d; PO 0.15–0.3 mg/kg/d in 2 divided doses

DRUG EFFECTS				
System	Effect	Assessment by Hx	PE	Test
GENERAL	Hypersensitivity, rash	Observe 1/2 hr; have epinephrine 1:1000 available		
CARDIO	Htn		BP/HR	
RESP	Pleural effusion, dyspnea			
GI	Diarrhea, N/V, constipation, abn liver function, anorexia, abd pain			LFTs
RENAL	Abn kidney function, oliguria			BUN, Cr
ENDO	Hyperkalemia, hypokalemia, hyperglycemia			K$^+$, glucose
HEME	Anemia, leukocytosis, thrombocytopenia			CBC
CNS	Headache, tremor, insomnia, paresthesias, mental status changes, circumoral numbness		Preop neuro exam	

Key Reference: Siniscalchi A, Piraccini E, Miklosova Z, et al. Opioid-induced hyperalgesia and rapid opioid detoxification after tacrolimus administration. *Anesth Analg.* 2008;106:645–646.

Perioperative Implications

Preoperative Preparation
• Continue all immunosuppressants through periop period
• Monitor levels: Therapeutic range 5–30 ng/ml; maintenance level 5–10 ng/mL

Monitoring
• Consider frequent NIBP or arterial catheter.

Induction/Maintenance
• Inducers of P450 system incl phenobarbital, phenytoin, isoniazid; some volatile anesthetics may result in ↑ metabolism of tacrolimus

Possible Drug Interactions
• Ca^{2+}-channel blockers, cyclosporine, erythromycin, antifungal agents, metoclopramide may ↑ blood levels of tacrolimus as function of P450 inhibition

• Anticonvulsants (carbamazepine, phenobarbital, phenytoin), rifampin may ↓ blood levels of tacrolimus 2° to induction of cytochrome P450 system
• Adverse effects requiring dose adjustments incl nephrotoxicity, neurotoxicity, alterations in glucose metabolism, infection, and susceptibility to malignancy

Anticipated Problems/Concerns

• Hypersensitivity may occur with IV formulation

Terbutaline

Mohammed Minhaj

Uses

- Prescribed for pts with bronchospasm caused by asthma, bronchitis, or emphysema
- Effective for acute asthmatic attacks, COPD
- Used as tocolytic for preterm labor (not FDA-approved for this and use in preterm labor has declined over the last decade)

Perioperative Risks

- Complications incl
  - Tachyarrhythmias
  - Hypokalemia
  - Hyperglycemia
  - Rebound hyperkalemia has been described in OB pts who have terbutaline D/C

Worry About

- Tachycardia/palpitations
- Pulm edema (unclear mechanism: myocardial failure vs. noncardiogenic etiologies)
- Hyperglycemia
- Hypokalemia

Fetal side effects are increased fetal heart rate and neonatal hypoglycemia.

Overview/Pharmacology

- Used for both acute bronchospasm, chronic management of COPD
- Tachyphylaxis possible with prolonged use
- 7–14% of delivered aerosol reaches circulation
- ⅓ SQ dose metabolized in liver to inactive sulfate conjugates
- Metabolites I and II, unchanged drug excreted in urine

Onset/Duration

- SQ
  - Onset: Significant ↑ in FEV_1 in 15 min, peak 30–60 min
  - Duration: 1.5–4 hr; $T_{1/2}$ 3–4 hr
- IV (not FDA-approved route)
  - Onset: Immediate; $T_{1/2}$ 3–4 hr
- PO
  - Onset: Significant improvement in FEV_1 in 60–120 min
  - Duration: At least 4 hr
- Metered dose inhaler/nebulizer
  - Onset: 5 min; peak, 1–2 hr
  - Duration: 3–4 hr

Drug Class/Mechanism of Action/Usual Dose

- β_2-agonist (thought to be more specific for β_2 receptors)
- β_2 stimulation ↑ adenylyl cyclase conversion of ATP to cAMP; this effect → cell hyperpolarization, ↑ inward Ca^{2+} flux, → relaxation of bronchial, uterine, vascular smooth muscle

Usual Dose

- SQ: 0.005–0.01 mg/kg to a max 0.25 mg/dose; inject every 15–20 min as needed
- PO: 5 mg tid; reduce to 2.5 mg tid if side effects occur. Not to exceed 15 mg/24 hr
- Metered dose inhaler: 2 inhalations every 4–6 hr (200 μg/actuation)
- Nebulizer: 0.01–0.03 mL/kg (1 mL = 1 mg); minimum = 0.1 mL, maximum = 2.5 mL; dilute in 1–2 mL N/S
- IV (not FDA approved) for tocolysis: IV 2.5–10 mcg/min; increased every 10–20 min. Maximum dosages from 17.5–30 mcg/min described.

DRUG EFFECTS

System	Effect	Assessment by Hx	PE	Test
CARDIO	Tachycardia, Htn, hypotension, arrhythmias, ↓ SVR	Palpitations	↑ HR; irregular rhythm, BP; rales	ECG
RESP	Bronchodilation	↓ Dyspnea	↓ Wheezing	O_2 sat, PFT, PEF
GI	Nausea	Nausea		
ENDO	Hyperglycemia, hypokalemia*	Polydipsia, polyuria	Dehydration	Blood glucose, serum K^+
CNS	CNS stimulation	Insomnia, anxiety, hyperactivity, drowsiness, headache	Tremor	

*Plasma hypokalemia is due to intracellular transport of K^+. Hypokalemia is seen most often with IV terbutaline Rx for preterm labor. K^+ supplementation rarely required, serum levels usually normalize within 3 hr of D/C of infusion.

Key References: Lam F, Elliott J, Jones JS, et al. Clinical issues surrounding the use of terbutaline sulfate for preterm labor *Obstet Gynecol Surv.* 1998;53(11 suppl):S85–S95.; Cuneo B, et al. Atrial and ventricular rate response and patterns of heart rate acceleration during maternal–fetal terbutaline treatment of fetal complete heart *Block Am J Cardiol.* 2007;100:661–665.

Perioperative Implications

Preoperative Concerns

- Evaluate the disease being treated: Asthma, preterm labor
- For asthmatic pts, consider administering inhaled β_2-agonist before inducing anesthesia
- For pts in preterm labor, assess fetal well-being: FHR, wt, indices of lung maturity, etc.
- Evaluate VS, esp. HR, BP; R/O CHF
- Assess volume status (avoid excess hydration in obstetrical pts as it could increase the risk for pulm edema)
- Lab studies to check: Glucose, K^+

Induction/Maintenance

- Increasing CO may prolong inhalation induction
- Intraop bronchospasm possible with inhaled or IV terbutaline; absorption after SQ injection possibly unreliable
- Tachycardia possible 2° to the effects of the drug, not necessarily as a result of light anesthesia

Anticipated Problems/Concerns

- Increased HR, decreased SVR possibly not tolerated well by pts with CAD, mitral or aortic stenosis
- Usually assoc with hypokalemia, but rebound hyperkalemia in pts has been described in pts who have terbutaline therapy D/C.
- Pulm edema may be a result of myocardial failure or of a noncardiogenic etiology.

Tetracyclines

Alan Kaye
Amir Baluch

Uses

- Administered PO (most common), IV (fewer side effects), IM (rare, painful), topical (eyes only)
- Original broad-spectrum antibiotic with activity against gram-positive and gram-negative bacteria; species of *Chlamydia, Rickettsia, and Mycoplasma* (in adults); and some protozoa. One of few agents active against organisms without cell walls. Resistance ↑ worldwide.
- Secondary uses: Alternative drugs in the treatment of syphilis, tx of resp infections caused by susceptible organisms, prophylaxis against infection in chronic bronchitis, tx of leptospirosis, and in the tx of acne.
- Selective uses
  - Tetracycline used for the tx of GI ulcers caused by *Helicobacter pylori.*
  - Doxycycline for Lyme disease, the prevention of malaria, and the tx of amebiasis.
  - Minocycline for meningococcal carriers
  - Demeclocycline for the management of pts with ADH-secreting tumors.
- Incidence in USA: 20 million doses/y

Perioperative Risks

- IV tetracycline frequently → thrombophlebitis, lessens efficacy of oral contraceptives

- Decrease dose with age
- Decrease dose in those with poor renal/hepatic functions as tetracycline accumulates in such pts, and can lead to hepatic toxicity (instead in pts with renal dysfunction use doxycycline which has an unchanged elimination half-time in such pts)
- Barbiturates may ↓ $T_{\frac{1}{2}}$ β; tetracycline will ↑ cone of digoxin, warfarin. Pts may exhibit GI distress, even *Clostridium difficile* colitis.

Worry About

- Tetracycline (esp. 1st generation) absorbed poorly if given within 3 hr of di-/trivalent cations (Ca^{2+}, Al^{3+}, Mg^{2+}, Fe^{2+}, Bi^{3+})
- The possibility of tetracycline-resistant bacterial enteritis as well as GI distress limit the oral dose of these antibiotics
- Doxycycline should only be administered orally or by IV

Overview/Pharmacology

- Two generations: First (e.g., tetracycline); second (e.g., doxycycline)
- Classified as bacteriostatic (newest ones possibly bactericidal)
- First generation $T_{\frac{1}{2}}$ β 6–12 hr; excreted in urine, feces

- Second generation more lipophilic, greater V_d, recirculation, $T_{1/4}$ β 16–18 hr; doxycycline excreted 90%+ in feces; safe for anephric pts
- Adjust dose with age, impaired renal/hepatic functions
- PO uptake in duodenum (esp. first generation); peak level, 2 hr; IV peak level, 1 hr

Drug Class/Mechanism of Action/Usual Dose

- Original broad-spectrum antibiotic
- Effective against *Rickettsia, Mycoplasma, Chlamydia, Borrelia*, spirochetes, some fungi
- Local irritant (sclerotherapy)
- Normal dose: Impairs bacterial protein synthesis; binds via a Mg^{2+} bridge to single active site of 30 S subunit of bacterial ribosome; prevents binding of aminoacyl tRNA to the mRNA-ribosome complex. Without this codon–anticodon interaction, peptide chain formation cannot proceed.
- Inhibit collagenase (osteoarthritis), tumor-induced angiogenesis (chemoRx)
- Usual dose: Doxycycline, 100 mg PO bid

ASSESSMENT POINTS

System	Effect	Assessment by Hx	Test
HEENT	Children: Brown teeth; risk greatest from second trimester to age 8 y		
CARDIO	Frequently causes thrombophlebitis ↓ Tumor-mediated angiogenesis		
HEPAT	Rare toxicity, esp. with ↑ dose, IV route, preg; usually reversible with drug cessation	Hepatitis	LFTs
GI	Irritation, distress, esp. PO, ↑ dose may → superinfection (*S. aureus* or *C. difficile*) Disturbances in the normal flora lead to candidiasis (oral and vaginal)	Mild N/V, severe colitis	
HEME	May inhibit/suppress antibody production, leukotaxis, complement system		
GU	May aggravate uremia in susceptible pt; crosses placenta, excreted in breast milk		BUN
CNS	Penetrates CNS; may ↑ ICP during Rx, esp. in infants	Vision change, headache	
	Doxycycline and minocycline: Vestibular problems (dizziness and vertigo), esp. in women; reversible	Dizziness, nausea	
DERM	Phototoxic skin reaction, esp. 1st generation		
MS	↓ Bone growth in preemies, ↓ collagenase in joints		

Key References: Chopra I, Hawkey PM, Hinton M. Review: Tetracyclines, molecular and clinical aspects. *J Antimicrob Chemother.* 1992;29:245–277. Stoelting RK. *Pharmacology and physiology in anesthetic practice.* Philadelphia: Lippincott-Raven; 2006. Trevor AJ, Katzung BG, Masters SB. *Katzung & Trevor's review of pharmacology.* New York: McGraw-Hill Medical; 2007.

Perioperative Implications

Preoperative Concerns
- May ↑ digoxin levels, higher prothrombin time if pt on warfarin

Possible Drug Interactions
- Methoxyflurane, tetracycline may → renal failure
- Barbiturates may ↓ T½β

Reversal
- May augment nondepolarizing NM blocker

Anticipated Problems/Concerns

- Although resistance is rising, drugs remain useful antibiotics, with nonantibiotic indications increasing
- Contraindicated in pregnancy and childhood

Thyroid Supplements

John M. Murkin

Uses

- Incidence in USA: >3 million chronic users
- T_4 prescribed for pts with chronic hypothyroidism
- T_3 used in myxedema coma
- T_3 successfully used as rescue therapy for cardiogenic shock post-CPB
- T_3 reported as favorably administered to brain-dead donors before organ harvesting for heart, heart-lung transplantation; N.B. prophylactic T_3 no benefit in recent randomized trials
- T_4 generally administered PO; T_4 and T_3 can be administered IV

Perioperative Risks

- Drugs (amiodarone, lithium, herbal supplements, catecholamines, radiopaque contrast media), cirrhosis, renal failure, sepsis, operation (CPB) can induce euthyroid sick syndrome (reduced peripheral conversion of T_4 to T_3); may precipitate myxedema coma
- Amiodarone, a potent class III anti-arrhythmic drug, is an iodine-rich compound with a structural resemblance to T_3 and T_4 and causes substantial iodine overload which may produce either thyrotoxicosis or hypothyroidism with continued administration.

Worry About

- T_4 or T_3 can aggravate Sx of myocardial ischemia

Overview/Pharmacology

- Hypothyroidism (overt) estimated at 0.5–3.8% of adults, ↑ with age (over 15% of women at age 60+)
- Post-thyroidectomy <30% of pts euthyroid at 10 y due to inadequacy or D/C of therapy
- Reversal of clinical Sx of chronic hypothyroidism, including myocardial effusions, requires 2–4 mo Rx
- $T_{1/2}$ for T_4: 7 d, T_3: 1.5 d
- T_4 relatively inactive prohormone undergoing monodeiodination in liver, kidney to biologically active T_3

ICD-9-CM Code: 244.9

Drug Class/Mechanism of Action/Usual Dose

- Thyroid hormone replacement Rx
- T_3 binding to specific membrane receptor proteins augments membrane transport activity, mitochondrial oxidative phosphorylation, protein synthesis
- Extranuclear effects of T_3 occur in min, ↑ myocardial mitochondrial and transmembrane transport activity
- Nuclear effects of T_3 occur within 0.5–1.0 hr, involve transcription, translation of myocardial enzymes, contractile proteins
- Direct effect of T_3 ↓ arterial smooth muscle tone
- Usual dosage of T_4 is 0.15 mg/d PO
- Acute Rx: T_4, 0.3–0.5 mg by slow IV infusion followed by 0.1–0.15 mg/d, or T_3, 0.005–0.01 mg IV

DRUGS

ASSESSMENT POINTS				
System	Effect	Assessment by Hx	PE	Test
CARDIO	Chronotropy, inotropy, ↓ SVR Arrhythmogenesis	Less fatigue Palpitations	HR, reflexes	FT_4E, TSH, ECG
RESP	Restoration of hypoxic, hypercapnic ventilatory drive			
GI	↑ Protein synthesis; enhanced hepatic, renal clearance/excretion functions		Normal skin turgor	
ENDO	Thermogenesis	Reversal of cold intolerance	Skin warm to touch	

Key Reference: Kohl BA, Schwartz S. Surgery in the patient with endocrine dysfunction. *Anesthesiol Clin.* 2009;27:687–703.

Perioperative Implications/Possible Drug Interactions

Preoperative Concerns

- Thyroid hormones ↑ breakdown of vitamin K–dependent clotting factors—can alter coag status
- Chronic amiodarone therapy may produce hyper- or hypothyroidism

Induction/Maintenance

- Exaggerated Htn, tachycardia can occur with agents such as ketamine, exogenous catecholamines incl ephedrine, epinephrine; in pts on both acute and chronic thyroid hormone replacement

Adjuvants/Regional Anesthesia/Reversal

- Anticholinergics with minimal CV effects, e.g., glycopyrrolate, preferred over atropine
- Caution in the presence of spinal anesthesia; T_3 administration may produce aggravated hypotension

Postoperative Period

- Cirrhosis, sepsis, renal failure, surgery may all ↓ peripheral conversion of T_4 to T_3 (euthyroid sick syndrome), precipitate hypothyroidism

Anticipated Problems/Concerns

- In critically ill pts, T_3 replacement can produce detrimental increases in O_2 requirements (esp. myocardial), protein catabolism without improving mortality rates

Tissue Plasminogen Activator

Sunil Mahbubani
Alan D. Kaye Amir Baluch

Uses

- Used for thrombolysis during Rx of pulm embolism, stroke, and myocardial infarction. Best used within 3 hr of incident or 6 hr if injected via. artery directly into the site of occlusion and after exclusion of intracranial hemorrhage via CT scan
- Rapid clot lysis by t-PA offers advantages in comparison with streptokinase.
- May be used in combination with other antico-agulants such as heparin and aspirin. Also may be combined with with β-blockers, morphine, nitro-glycerin, and plt IIb/IIIa blockers

Perioperative Risks

- Increased bleeding during surgery; if severe, possible need for blood transfusion, fresh frozen plasma, cryoprecipitate, and plt infusion therapy
- Intraop Htn may increase the risk of intracra-nial hemorrhage (about 1%)
- Incomplete restoration of coronary flow and persisting thrombogenicity may lead to cardiac instability and risk for periop infarction

Worry About

- Invasive procedures; damage to blood ves-sels during vascular access procedures can cause severe bleeding—esp. at non-compressible sites, e.g., subclavian vein. Increased risk of develop-ing large hematomas that may damage surround-ing tissues via mass effect (e.g., ulnar nerve during arterial cannulation).
- Minor bleeding at venipuncture sites

Overview/Pharmacology

- Thrombolytic agent; natural t-PA is produced by vascular endothelial cells and is naturally released from the endothelium in response to venous occlusion, physical activity, stress, or vaso-active medications.
- Accelerates the conversion of plasminogen bound to fibrin, to plasmin, resulting in fibrinoly-sis as the site of clot
- t-PA (alteplase) is commercially produced using cDNA for natural t-PA, transfected into a mam-malian cell line
- Initial thrombolytic response is seen within 30 min when given IV. $T_{1/2}$ ~5 min; elimination $T_{1/2}$ ~30–50 min. Eighty percent cleared from plasma within 10 min of stopping a standard infusion and clearance is via the liver.

- Plasminogen activator inhibitors, also released by endothelial cells, oppose t-PA action and may be a factor in preventing uncontrolled fibrinolysis.

Drug Class/Mechanism of Action/Usual Dose

- Thrombolytic agent. Binds to fibrin threads of a thrombus, converts enmeshed plasminogen to plasmin which initiates localized fibrinolysis. For this reason, unlike streptokinase, t-PA can be considered fibrin specific; t-PA lacks effect on cir-culating plasminogen thereby limiting systemic effects.
- In myocardial infarction, usual dose for pts 70 kg or more is a front-loading protocol, with 100 mg t-PA being given IV by bolus and infusion over 90 min, with heparin
- Amount of salvaged myocardium is directly related to the time until the occluded artery is reopened. GUSTO I investigators showed 84% patency within 6 hr of front-loaded t-PA.
- More rapid lysis, less systemic fibrinolysis, and few if any anaphylactic reactions when compared to streptokinases—but t-PA is more expensive
- In ischemic stroke, IV t-PA dose is lower; hepa-rin is not used

ASSESSMENT POINTS

System	Effect	Assessment by Hx	PE	Treatment
CARDIO	Bleeding from vascular puncture sites	Hematoma Check for retroperitoneal bleed in presence of femoral puncture	Hgb	Manual compression Rarely is blood transfusion necessary
	Severe bleeding during surgery	Check if heparin or plt IIb/IIIa blockers are being given	Hgb Plts APTT	Transfusion of blood, FFP, cryo Factor VIII and plts may be needed, consider using TEG to guide therapy
	Effects of ancillary treatment	Check for ongoing β-blocker, nitroglycerin, or morphine treatment		D/C if necessary; however, β-blockade has considerable benefit with little risk in most pts
	Reperfusion arrhythmias	Can occur on restoration of blood flow to ischemic myocardium	CV stability	Antiarrhythmics
CNS	Intracranial hemorrhage	Signs of stroke or raised intracranial pressure	Neurologic assessment Urgent CT, MRI	Supportive BP control (risk is increased in presence of heparin)

Key References: GUSTO Investigators. An international randomized trial comparing four thrombolytic strategies for acute myocardial infarction. *N Engl J Med.* 1993;329:673–682. Schellinger PD, Fiebach JB, Mohr A, et al. Thrombolytic therapy for ischemic stroke-a review. Part I-Intravenous thrombolysis. *Crit Care Med.* 2001;29:1812–1818.

Perioperative Implications

- Danger of bleeding with central line placement, arterial cannulations
- Risk of hypotension on anesthetic induction with adjuvant nitroglycerin infusion

- Severe Htn may predispose to or excacerbate hemorrhagic stroke
- Residual thrombus is highly thrombogenic, posing risk of rethrombosis
- Regional anesthesia should not be used with caution

- Increased need for transfusions
- Check neurologic function preop and postop

Tranexamic Acid

Philip L. Kalarickal
Charles J. Fox
Adam M. Kaye

Indications

- To prevent bleeding due to fibrinolysis after surgery or trauma (cardiac surgery with and without cardiopulmonary bypass; liver transplantation; orthopedic incl spine; GU surgery; peripartum hemorrhage). Can be diagnosed clinically or via laboratory tests (prolonged thrombin time, reduced fibrinogen levels, increased d-dimer levels, classic teardrop shape on thromboelastography).
- For short-term use (2–8 d) in hemophilia and von Willebrand disease pts to reduce or prevent hemorrhage and to reduce the need for replacement therapy during and following tooth extraction.
- To treat 1° menorrhagia, gastric and intestinal hemorrhage, urinary tract bleeding, recurrent epistaxis, and hereditary angioneurotic edema. The drug also inhibits induced hyperfibrinolysis during thrombolytic treatment with plasminogen activators.
- Used in pts with hemophilia or those receiving anticoagulation, about to undergo oral surgery.

Perioperative Risks

- Side effects of drug: Nausea, diarrhea, vomiting, and abd pain are the most common adverse effects (approx 30% with oral use)
- Giddiness has been reported
- Hypotension (if the drug is injected too rapidly)

Worry About

- Potential for thrombotic complications 2° to the inhibition of fibrinolysis.

Overview/Drug Class

- A synthetic lysine analogue. Prevents plasmin formation and therefore fibrinolysis by occupying plasminogen's lysine-binding site for fibrin.
- Has a structure similar to that of lysine, and reversibly binds to lysine-binding sites for fibrin on plasminogen, thereby blocking the binding of plasminogen to fibrin. Plasminogen acitvators are located on the fibrin clot. Without localized binding of plasminogen to fibrin, it cannot be converted to plasmin.
- Because fibrinolysis requires plasminogen (and plasmin) binding to fibrin, fibrinolysis is inhibited.
- A competitive inhibitor of plasminogen activation and at much higher concentrations, a noncompetitive inhibitor of plasmin. Suppresses fibrinolysis by inhibiting activation of plasminogen.
- Other antifibrinolytic medications incl epsilon-aminocaproic acid (lysine analog) and aprotinin (serine protease inhibitor).
- Reductions in mortality rates with TXA doses of 4.5 grams to 6 grams daily for 5 to 7 d (in most studies) produced statistical significance between TXA and placebo.
- TXA was assoc with reductions in mortality of 5%-54% in pts with upper GI bleeding compared with placebo. Meta-analysis indicated a reduction of 40%.

- Administered either PO 25 mg/kg every 6–8 hr or IV 10 mg/kg 6–8 h beginning the day prior to surgery
- Absorption after oral use is 30–50%; bioavailability is not affected by food.
- An antifibrinolytic concentration of drug remains in serum up to 7–8 hr.
- The protein binding to plasminogen is approx 3% at therapeutic plasma levels; it does not bind to serum albumin.
- The $T\frac{1}{2}$ of elimination when administered orally is 120 min.
- Urinary excretion is the main route of elimination via glomerular filtration.
- Overall renal clearance is equal to overall plasma clearance, and >90% of the dose is excreted unchanged in 24 hr.
- Pts with renal insufficiency should have their doses reduced according to creatinine clearance. Only a small fraction of tranexamic acid is metabolized.
- TXA is 6 to 10 times more potent in terms of binding to plasminogen/plasmin than epsilon aminocaproic acid (EACA).
- Concurrent administration of heparin does not influence the activity of TXA.
- Pharmacokinetic properties: Maximum plasma concentrations of TXA can be attained within 3 hr after an oral dose. Elimination after IV administration is triexponential, and over 95% of each dose is eliminated unchanged in the urine.

DRUGS

ASSESSMENT POINTS

System	Effect	Assessment by Hx	PE	Test
HEENT	Retinal degeneration is assoc with prolonged use; incidence 25–100% and dose-dependent (animal studies)	Visual changes	Ophthalmologic exam in pts receiving tranexamic acid >4 or 5 d	Visual acuity Visual field Color vision Eyeground
CARDIO	Hypotension (with rapid infusion)	Mental status changes, nausea	BP monitoring, heart rate, ECG	
RENAL	Reduce dose in pts with renal insufficiency			BUN/Cr, CrCl
GI	Nausea, diarrhea, vomiting, abd discomfort			
OB	Category B There are no well-controlled studies in pregnant females	Crosses placenta and appears in cord blood at concentration equal to that in maternal blood		
IMMUNO	Male mice receiving tranexamic acid up to 5 g/kg/d have been found to develop leukemia			

Key References: Stewart D, Marder VJ. Therapy with antifibrinolytic agents. In: Coleman RW, Marder VJ, Clowes AW, George JN, Goldhaber SZ, eds. *Hemostasis and thrombosis: basic principles and clinical practice.* 5th ed. Philadelphia, PA: Lippincott, Williams & Wilkins; 2006:1173–1193. Drummond JC, Petrovitch CT, Lane TA. Hemostasis and transfusion medicine. In: Barash PG, Cullen BF, Stoelting RK, Cahalan MK, Stock MC, eds. *Clinical anesthesia.* 7th ed. Philadelphia, PA: Lippincott, Williams & Wilkins; 2009:389–405.

Perioperative Implications

Airway
- No interactions known

Preinduction/Induction
- If given IV, inject slowly to avoid hypotention

Maintenance
- No interactions known

Emergence
- No interactions known

Adjuvant/Regional Anesthesia/Reversal
- No interactions known

Contraindications
- Acquired defective color vision: Prohibits measuring one endpoint of toxicity
- Subarachnoid hemorrhage: Cerebral edema and cerebral infarction may be caused by tranexamic acid in pts with subarachnoid hemorrhage.

Active Thromboembolic disease
- Caution in the setting of disseminatred intravascular coagulation (DIC), in which inhibition of fibrinolysis may aggravate the hypercoagulable state
- Reduced dose in renal insufficiency

Anticipated Problems/Concerns
- Potential for increased thrombotic events.

Trimethaphan

Tor Sandven
Stephen Robinson

Uses

- Production of controlled hypotension during surgery to reduce bleeding into the surgical field
- Rapid reduction of BP in the treatment of hypertensive emergencies.
    - Acute dissecting aortic aneurysm, particularly when pre-existing conditions make β-blockers a relative contraindication
    - Emergency treatment of pulm edema in pts with pulm Htn assoc with systemic Htn
- May serve as an alternative to sodium nitroprusside for pts who are resistant to this drug, or can be mixed with nitroprusside to decrease risk of cyanide toxicity from nitroprusside
- May serve as a cost efficient alternative to nicardipine or clevidipine

Perioperative Risks

- High doses may cause profound hypotension and, rarely, resp arrest
- QRS prolongation has been seen during treatment
- Tachycardia, angina, or syncope may occur without warning
- Due to trimethaphan's ability to cross the placenta, its ganglionic blocking effects may decrease GI motility in the fetus, resulting in meconium ileus or neonatal paralytic ileus
- CNS exam limited by production of mydriasis

Worry About

- Contraindicated in pts with shock, anemia, hypovolemia, uncorrected resp insufficiency, or neonates at risk for paralytic or meconium ileus
- Orthostatic hypotension; may cause severe hypotension
- Difficult to obtain as no longer manufactured for use in USA

Overview/Pharmacology

- Rapidly acting ganglionic acetylcholine blocker, onset 1–3 min
- Peak response 5–10 min
- Duration of action: 10–15 min for single dose
- Affects both parasympathetic and sympathetic pathways
- Renally excreted, mostly unchanged
- Most side effects are due to parasympathetic blockade and respond to dose reduction or D/C
- Cardiac output may increase in pts with CHF, or decrease in pts with normal heart function
- Tachyphylaxis may occur during continuous IV infusion

Drug Class/Mechanism of Action/Usual Dose

- A short-acting ganglionic blocking agent
- Prevents stimulation of postsynaptic receptors by competing with acetylcholine for these receptor sites
- Hypotensive effect is primarily through sympathetic blockade by lowering SVR
- Hypotensive effect is also mediated through direct vasodilation and histamine release (esp. at higher rate of administration)
- Usual adult dosage
    - For controlled hypotension during surgery: Initial: IV infusion, 3 to 4 mg per min, adjusted according to response; Maintenance: IV infusion, 0.3 mg to 6 mg per min.
    - For hypertensive emergency: Initial: IV infusion, 0.5 mg to 1 mg per min, adjusted according to response; maintenance: IV infusion, 1 to 5 mg per min.
- Pts on concommittent antihypertensive medications require lower doses

ASSESSMENT POINTS

System	Effect	Assessment by Hx	PE
HEENT	Mydriasis with cycloplegia	Visual changes	
CARDIO	Vasodilation, tachycardia, hypotension, ↓SVR	Angina, syncope	Orthostatic hypotension
RESP	Rare resp arrest (uncertain etiology)		
GI	↓Secretions, ↓tone/motiliy	Dry mouth, Paralytic ileus, constipation, N/V/D, reflux	
GU	Bladder atony ↓Potency	Oliguria or anuria, incomplete emptying, Erectile and ejaculation dysfunction	UO
CNS	Less increase in ICP compared to other vasodilators 2° to preserved cerebral autoregulation		
OB	Crosses placenta, may cause ↓fetal GI motility causing meconium or paralytic ileus		

Key Reference: Taylor P. Agents acting at the neuromuscular junction and autonomic ganglia. In: Hardman JG, Limbird LE, eds. *Goodman and Gillman's The Pharmacological Basis of Therapeutics.* 10th ed. New York: McGraw-Hill Professional Publishing; 2001:210–211.

Perioperative Implications

Preoperative Concerns
- Assess Hx of CAD, check baseline EKG
- Assess volume status
- Consider arterial line if trimethaphan infusion anticipated

Induction/Maintenance
- May prolong block from succinylcholine or non-depolarizing neuromuscular blockers

- For controlled hypotension during surgery it is recommended that infusion be stopped prior to wound closure
- Monitor EKG for signs of ischemia due to decreased cardiac perfusion from hypotensive state

Postoperative Period
- Mydriasis from drug may interfere with neuro checks for postop neurosurgery pts
- Risk for paralytic ileus is increased when drug infusion continued for longer than 48 hr

- Pts continued on trimethaphan infusions postop should be monitored in the ICU
- Oral antihypertensives should be instituted and timethaphan D/C as soon as pt can take oral medication and BP has stabilized.

Anticipated Problems/Concerns
- Not ideal for prolonged infusions as tachyphylaxis may develop within first 48 hr of therapy, although this may be attenuated by concommitent use of a diuretic

Vitamin B$_{12}$ (Cyanocobalamin)

John K. Stene

Indications

- Incidence in USA: 16 million, esp. in elderly 5% under 55; 10% 55 to 64; 10 to 15% of 65 to 74, and 24% of 74 to 80 year olds. 75% of those over 64 with this do not have anemia or even RBC abn.
- Prescribed for pernicious anemia
- Lack of gastric secretion of intrinsic factor → malabsorption of vitamin B$_{12}$; therefore IM route preferred. Strict vegetarian diet–induced deficiency state; responds to oral supplementation.
- Until you reach midlife, you probably get all the B$_{12}$ you need from food (unless vegetarian). But sometime around are 50, the stomach begins making less of the digestive fluids and intrinsic factor needed to absorb B$_{12}$. Pts are also almost certainly low on B$_{12}$ if taking a heartburn med called a proton pump inhibitor for a long time, which seriously diminishes B$_{12}$ absorption.
- Also assoc with *Helicobacter pylori* infection, chronic alcohol ingestion, and pancreatic exocrine deficiency condiditons

Worry About

- Permanent neurologic injury (classic combined system disease with paresthesias, balance problems with loss of position and vibratory sense, and lack of myelination in long tracts, in long-term deficiency states)
- Interactions and neurologic injury with folate, methionine synthetase inhibitors, N$_2$O, which can produce rapid neurologic deterioration

Overview/Pharmacology

- Vitamin B$_{12}$ binds to intrinsic factor (gastric glycoprotein from parietal cells) in GI tract, is absorbed from ileum, bound to transcobalamin II in plasma for transport to tissues. Approx 3 μg of cobalamin secreted into bile/d.
- Excess vitamin B$_{12}$ admin ↑ urinary excretion
- Vitamin B$_{12}$ enzymatically converted to two active forms: deoxyadenosylcobalamin, methylcobalamin
- Deoxyadenosylcobalamin is a cofactor for mitochondrial mutase enzyme that catalyzes L-methylmalonyl CoA to succinyl CoA.

- Methylcobalamin is cofactor in methionine synthetase reaction (a methyl group is transferred from 5-methyltetrahydrofolate to homocysteine to form methionine and tetrahydrofolate), pivotal in normal synthesis of purines, pyrimidines, and a number of methylation reactions through formation of N-adenosylmethionine

Drug Class/Mechanism of Action/Usual Dose

- H$_2$O-soluble B vitamin complex
- Cyanocobalamin administered IM or deep SQ route in doses of 1–1000 μg
- Oral dose to 80 μg can be administered with purified intrinsic factor; 1 U binds 15 μg of cyanocobalamin
- Need glycoprotein (intrinsic factor 60,000 MW) produced by gastric parietal cells for its absorption
- RDA: 2 μg/d for adults
- Vitamin B$_{12}$ is a quiet, conscientious type: doesn't get much hype, yet works overtime to keep your brain, your immune system, and your ticker in tip-top shape, even protects against Alzheimer's, depression, strokes, and vision loss.
- Therapeutic 100 μg SQ every month

ASSESSMENT POINTS

System	Effect	Assessment by Hx	PE	Test
GI	Achlorhydric or gastrectomy pts at risk; assoc with atrophic glossitis	Burning and tingling of mouth	Small, slick, glistening tongue	Schilling test (for vit B$_{12}$ absorption)
HEME	Megaloblastic anemia	Apathy, lassitude, fatigue	Pale skin, mucous membranes, esp. nailbeds, palmar surfaces	Peripheral blood smear: Macrocytic hyperchromic RBCs Bone marrow: Megaloblasts, megakaryocytes Plt count
CNS	Degeneration of dorsal, lateral columns of spinal cord	Numbness, tingling in extremities, difficulty walking	Loss of vibration, vibration, position sense; ataxia, Romberg's sign, muscle flaccidity	Plasma B$_{12}$ <150 pM suggests B$_{12}$ deficiency
PNS	Neuropathy	Paresthesias, dysesthesias of lower extremities		

Key References: Hillman RS. Hematopoietic agents: Growth factors, minerals, and vitamins. In: Hardman JG, Limbird LE, eds. *Goodman & Gilman's the pharmacological basis of therapeutics.* 9th ed. New York: McGraw-Hill Professional Publishing; 1996:1311–1340. Andres E, Noel E, Goichot B. Metformin-associated vitamin B$_{12}$ deficiency, *Arch Intern Med.* 2002;162:2251–2252.

Perioperative Implications/Possible Drug Interactions

- Folate admin reverses megaloblastic anemia but does not prevent (may precipitate) spinal cord degeneration.
- N$_2$O oxidizes vitamin B$_{12}$, reduces activity of methionine synthetase

- Effect of N$_2$O can be reversed by large doses of folic acid

Anticipated Problems/Concerns

- Scavenging waste anesthetic gas prevents OR personnel from developing vitamin B$_{12}$ deficiency states due to prolonged exposure to N$_2$O.

- Extensive interaction between folate and vitamin B$_{12}$ makes it imperative that pernicious anemia be treated with B$_{12}$ at same time as folate to prevent CNS degeneration.

Warfarin (Coumadin)

Indications

- Management of thromboembolic disorders: For prophylaxis, Rx, and prevention of recurrence of thromboembolic event incl DVT, pulm embolism, thrombosis of grafts. Prevention of arterial emboli assoc with prosthetic heart valves, nonvalvular AFib, acute MI. Prevention of MI, stroke, and recurrent MI. Rx for antithrombin III, protein C, protein S deficiency
- Newer indications: After angioplasty, for pts who have had coronary graft thrombosis when taking only ASA or ASA and dipyridamole
- Number of individuals receiving the drug: Unknown

Perioperative Risks

- Hemorrhage (minor to major life risk)
- Purple-toe syndrome, or warfarin necrosis
- Teratogenicity in pregnancy (decreases synthesis of vitamin K–dependent clotting factors by fetus)

Worry About

- Major drug interactions
- Multiplicity of drugs affecting action of warfarin. List extensive, continually expanding (see later). Be concerned with other drugs that potentiate bleeding (e.g., antiplatelet agents, ASA, NSAIDs); and drugs that displace warfarin from protein-binding sites or ↑ or ↓ vitamin K levels.

Overview/Pharmacology

- General effect: Anticoagulant with dose-dependent effect on coagulation

Pharmacokinetics/Pharmacodynamics

- Warfarin is a racemic mixture of R and S isomers (R-warfarin; S-warfarin)
- Racemic warfarin absorbed rapidly from GI tract, reaches max plasma conc in 90 min, has T½ of 36–42 hr; time to peak effect 36–72 hr; duration after D/C 2–5 d at least

- In circulation, bound to plasma proteins, accumulates in liver. R-warfarin metabolites excreted in urine; S-warfarins eliminated in bile.
- Warfarin resistance or ↓ warfarin effect: When warfarin absorption from GI tract impaired from malabsorption syndromes, concurrent use of liquid paraffin laxatives, cholestyramine resin, or excessive amounts of certain antacids (e.g., Mg trisilicate)
- Vitamin K intake ↑ through diet or administration of vitamin K IM or IV
- With induction of hepatic enzymes, increasing metabolism of warfarin. Enzyme inducers incl anticonvulsants, barbiturates, primidone, carbamazepine, antimicrobials (e.g., griseofulvin, rifampin, nafcillin, ethanol) and smoking
- Increased warfarin effect, or warfarin sensitivity
- Drugs displacing warfarin from albumin ↑ its bioavailability (NSAIDs, ASA, phenytoin sodium, oral hypoglycemic agents, sulfa drugs, nalidixic acid, estrogen, miconazole)
- Deficiency of vitamin K enhances; occurs with malabsorption syndromes and during administration of liquid paraffin laxatives, and clofibrate; after long-term use of oral antimicrobials that deplete intestinal bacterial source of vitamin K. Large doses of vitamin E antagonize action of vitamin K; anabolic steroids, danazol impair synthesis of vitamin K–dependent clotting factors; olestra removes vitamin K.
- Metabolism blocked by phenytoin, chloramphenicol, erythromycin, clofibrate, TCAs, cimetidine, sulfinpyrazone, sulfamethoxazoletrimethoprim, thus increasing warfarin effect. Disulfiram (Antabuse) significantly slows metabolism.
- Certain cephalosporins have a warfarin effect themselves—thus contraindicated.

- Elderly, febrile, debilitated pts and those with hepatic dysfunction, hyperthyroidism, or heart failure may have increased warfarin effect.

Drug Class/Mechanism of Action/Usual Dose

- Interferes with synthesis of 6 vitamin K–dependent proteins involved in coagulation sequence: Factors II, VII, IX, X; proteins C and S. Before these proteins are released into circulation, they undergo reactions converting glutamic acid residues to carboxyglutamic acid residues and require presence of reduced form of vitamin K.
- Inhibits cyclic interconversion between reduced form of vitamin K and its 2,3-epoxide (vitamin K epoxide)
- Defective clotting factors lacking "carboxyl tail" are produced, impairing coagulation
- Factor II has $T_{1/2}$ of 48 hr; requires 3–4 d before drops to level when PT significantly prolonged
- Nonurgent need for anticoagulation: Adult with average body mass, 5 mg/d PO prolongs PT to 1.5 × control value in 36–48 hr; if not achieved by third day, daily dose may be adjusted by ↑ or ↓ of 2.5 mg; goal: PT = 1.5–2 × control. Increases bleeding complications when PT is 2.5× control. Once anticoagulation stabilized, warfarin dose should be adjusted to maintain INR of 2–3 for all indications, except mech prosthetic cardiac valves, which require higher level of anticoagulation.
- More urgent need: Heparin anticoagulation first; start warfarin, 10 mg for 2 d

ASSESSMENT POINTS

System	Effect	Assessment by Hx	PE	Test
GI	Vit K deficiency may result from a poor diet, extrahepatic biliary obstruction, malabsorption, sterile gut	GI bleeding Tarry stools Hematemesis	Wt:height ratio (BMI)	Hct Fecal occult blood
ENDO	Vit K deficiency Hyperthyroidism, hypermetabolism potentiate warfarin effect		Malnourished	PT/PTT INR
GU	Diuresis, pregnancy ↓ effect; warfarin teratogenic			PT/PTT INR
MS	Arthritis pain medications that affect plts—e.g., ASA, NSAIDs— potentiate bleeding			

Key Reference: Enneking FK, Benzon H. Oral anticoagulants and regional anesthesia: A perspective. *Reg Anesth Pain Med.* 1998;23:140–145.

Perioperative Implications/Possible Drug Interactions

Preoperative Concerns

- Anticoag: Consider Rx with vitamin K (oral, IM, IV, SQ: 2.5–5 mg/70 kg) or FFP (15–20 mL/kg)
- Monitor this drug: PT, INR

Possible Drug Interactions

- Regional: Risk of spinal or epidural hematoma when performing a regional when pt is anticoagulated. Risk theoretically ↑ with anticoagulant. Epidural catheter thought to be assoc with greater risk of spinal or epidural hematoma if no measur-

able anticoagulant effect from warfarin (e.g., PT nml), but if receiving warfarin, not known if risks of spinal or epidural hematoma significant.

Anticipated Problems/Concerns

- Bleeding most likely complication due to further depletion of clotting factors during surgery; factor depletion may follow massive transfusions or with development of DIC
- If anticoagulation reversed preop with large doses of vitamin K, warfarin resistance possible initially; thrombosis a risk in this setting

- If anticoagulation reversed with administration of FFP, anticoagulation more easily achieved postop, but infectious risks are a concern.
- Preop dose of warfarin can be restarted with oral fluids; when risk of thromboembolism is considered esp. high (as in pts with recurrent pulm emboli undergoing pelvic surgery) or delay of more than 48 hr anticipated before warfarin can be restarted, postop heparin infusion appropriate.

Alternative Medicine

Androstenedione

Adam M. Kaye

Alan Kaye

Overview

• Growing sales trend of 20–30% in USA for both medical and nonmedical use of anabolic-androgenic steroid (AAS)
• Available since 1996 as an OTC nutritional supplement
• Estimates that 10% of anabolic-androgenic steroid (AAS) users are teens
• Estimate that 4.9% of male and 2.4% of female adolescents in USA have used legal androgenic/anabolic steroids
• Current estimates indicate that there are as many as 3 million anabolic-androgenic steroid (AAS) users in USA
• Surveys among community wt trainers attending gyms and health clubs indicate that AAS use is between 15% and 30%.
• As a major precursor to testosterone that is available without a prescription, it is purported to increase strength and athletic performance.
• Used to ↑ endogenous testosterone production to enhance athletic performance and recovery from exercise, to keep RBCs healthy, and to heighten sexual arousal and function
• Popularity related to society's preoccupation with sustaining the male libido.

Medical Use

• Testosterone replacement therapy
• Treatment of hypogonadal men
• Age-related sarcopenia
• HIV-related muscle wasting
• Increase in bone mineral density
• Prevention of age-related frailty and falls

Perioperative Risks

• Coagulopathy
• Polycythemia

Pharmacology/Mechanism of Action

• As a member of a group of compounds known as anabolic-androgenic steroids (AAS), these synthetic derivatives of testosterone are thought to possibly restore sex drive and boost muscle mass.
• Testosterone enters the cell by passive diffusion and is converted by 5α-reductase to 5α-dihydrotestosterone, which binds to intracellular androgen receptors.
• It ↑ protein anabolism and ↓ protein catabolism. Nitrogen balance is improved only when there is sufficient intake of calories and protein.
• It stimulates the production of RBCs by enhancing the production of erythropoietic stimulating factor.
• Supplementation of androstenedione in the setting of a rigorous 12-wk resistance-training program resulted in a return of baseline levels of testosterone levels and significant increases in estrone and estradiol levels. No increase in measurable lean body mass or muscular strength when compared with placebo.
• Androstenedione is produced in the gonads and adrenal glands of both male and females.
• It is synthesized from dehydroepiandrosterone and then converted to testosterone by the enzyme 17 β-hydroxysteroid dehydrogenase or to estrone by the aromatase enzyme complex.

DRUG EFFECTS			
System	Effect	Assessment by Hx	Test
CARDIO	↓ HDL, atherosclerosis	Angina	ECG, cholesterol
GI	Cholestasis, hepatocellular tumors, hepatitis, nausea		Liver enzymes, bilirubin
HEME	Polycythemia, chronic usage, Suppression of clotting factors, sodium and water retention	Easy bruising	PT, PTT Lytes
CNS	Depression, anxiety, behavioral changes, headache		

Key Reference: Broeder CE, Quindry J, Brittingham K, et al. The Andro project. *Arch Intern Med.* 2000;160:3093–3204.

Usual Dose

• Androstenedione is a direct precursor of testosterone and estrone in both males and females; it might ↑ testosterone levels.
• Marketing claims for increased strength, greater fat-free mass, and improved libido; recommended doses of 100–300 mg/d or 50–100 mg twice daily taken 1 hr before exercise or upon awakening.

Contraindications

• Males with carcinoma of the breast, prostate gland
• Women who are or may become pregnant
• Pt with serious cardiac, hepatic, or renal disease

Adverse Effects

• Several AAS-induced CV concerns reported incl Htn, left ventricular hypertrophy (LVH), impaired diastolic filling, arrhythmias, erythrocytosis, altered lipoprotein profile, and thrombosis.
• AAS-induced elevations in liver enzymes (alanine- and aspartate-aminotransferases)
• Dermatologic chances such as acne, striae, alopecia, and hirsutism are possible results induced by the action of the AAS on the skin and sebaceous glands.
• Endocrine and/or reproductive effects incl a dose-dependent depression of levels of luteinizing hormone and follicle-stimulating hormone due to the negative feedback loop of the hypothalamic-pituitary-gonadal axis.
• Feminization (gynecomastia) in males due to the aromatization of exogenous testosterone to estrogen metabolites.
• Male users may have their endocrine suppression lead to hypogonadotrophic hypogonadism, testicular atrophy, sperm morphology, infertility, and changes in libido.
• Female-specific side effects of AAS incl hirsutism, increased facial hair, voice deepening, clitorial hypertrophy, oligomenorrhea, reduced breast tissue, and male-pattern baldness.
• Restoration of hypothalamic-pituitary homeostasis, endogenous testosterone, and spermatogenesis may take between 3 and 12 mo after using AAS.

Perioperative Implications

• Retention of sodium, chloride, potassium, calcium, inorganic phosphate, and water
• N/V, rarely hepatocellular neoplasms and hepatitis
• Suppression of clotting factors II, V, VII and X; bleeding in pts on concomitant anticoagulant therapy
• Polycythemia
• Increased serum cholesterol, ↓ HDL
• Pts with osteolytic lesions or who are semi-ambulatory may develop nephrocalcinosis.
• In geriatric pts, high risk of prostate hypertrophy and prostate carcinoma

Possible Drug Interactions

• Metabolic effects of androgens may ↓ blood glucose level and insulin requirements.
• Androgens ↓ levels of thyroxin-binding globulin, resulting in ↓ total T_4 serum levels and ↓ resin uptake of T_3 and T_4
• Might interfere with androgenic or estrogenic drug therapy

Key Reference: Leder BZ, Catlin DH, Longscope C, et al: Metabolism of orally administered androstenedione in young men. *J Clin Endocrinol Metab* 2001; 86:3654–3658.

β-Sitosterol

Adam M. Kaye
Alan Kaye

Uses

- CHD and hypercholesterolemia
- Benign prostatic hyperplasia and prostatitis
- Gallstones
- Enhances sexual activity
- Prevents colon cancer
- Boosts immune system
- Topically for treating wounds and burns
- Migraine headache, chronic fatigue syndrome, and symptoms of menopause
- Asthma, allergies, bronchitis, SLE, and alopecia

Overview

- β-Sitosterol is one of the major plant sterols found in humans. It's chemical structure is similar to that of cholesterol with an ethyl group added at position 24.
- β-Sitosterol is available in many nonprescription supplements and with dietary plant consumption.

- With a low absorption rate, it inhibits intestinal absorption of cholesterol by competing for limited space with cholesterol in mixed micelles and also accelerates the esterification rate of the lecithincholesterol acyltransferase (LCAT) enzyme
- In benign prostatic hyperplasia, it binds to prostatic tissue, inhibits prostaglandin synthesis in the prostate, and has anti-inflammatory activity.
- Enhances proliferative responses of T cells in vitro
- Inhibits colon cancer growth in vitro
- Alternative for pts seeking modest reductions in LDL-C (<15%)

Pharmacology

- The reduction of dietary cholesterol available to the body may be due to inhibition of absorption in the intestine.
- Large amounts of dietary β-Sitosterol may displace cholesterol during absorption and increase fecal excretion.

- Inhibition of 5 alpha-reductase prevents the conversion of testosterone to dihydrotestosterone (DHT). This reduction of androgens may reduce prostatic hyperplasia in the same manner that finasteride (Proscar) does.

Usual Dose

- For hypercholesterolemia, usual dosage is 800 mg–6 g before meals; for severe cases up to 15 g
- For benign prostatic hyperplasia and prostatitis, 60–130 mg tid
- About 175–200 mg is consumed daily in typical diet

Contraindications

- Sitosterolemia, which is an inherited lipid storage disease with ↑ absorption of cholesterol and β-sitosterol from diet. Elevated liver β-sitosterol competitively inhibits cholesterol catabolism, which will lead to hypercholesterolemia.

ASSESSMENT POINTS

System	Effect	Assessment by Hx	PE	Test
CARDIO	CAD	Angina MI		ECG
RESP	Asthma	Wheezing	Wheezing	

Key Reference: Wong NC. The beneficial effects of plant sterols on serum cholesterol. *Can J Cardiol.* 2001;17:715–721. *J Am Diet Assoc.* 2002;102:1807–1811.

Perioperative Implications

- Obtain adequate Hx to determine indication, since may have significant co-morbidity
- No known periop implications

Side Effects

- May cause N/V, indigestion, gas, diarrhea, or constipation
- Interactions: Ezetimibe (Zetia) may reduce absorption of β-sitosterol
- Antihyperlipidemic drugs such as atorvastatin (Lipitor), cholestyramine, and gemfibrozil have additive effects in lowering cholesterol level

- Pravastatin (Pravachol) can lower the blood level of β-sitosterol
- Incresed risk of deficiency of fat soluble vitamins. β-Sitosterol may reduce absorption and blood level of α- and β-carotene and vitamin E.
- Erectile dysfunction and loss of libido have been reported in pts on β-sitosterol.

ALTERNATIVE MEDICINE

Blue Cohosh (Caulophyllum Thalictroides)

Ravish Kapoor
Berend Mets

Uses

- Orally used for inducing labor
- Orally used as an abortifacient
- Orally used an emmenagogue
- Orally used as an antispasmodic

Risk

- Ingestion of the leaf or seeds can lead to severe toxicity.
- Case reports document seizures, renal failure, and resp distress after use.
- Avoidance is advised in diabetic pts due to concern for hyperglycemia
- Reports of stroke, aplastic anemia, acute MI and CHF in infants following maternal use
- Should not be used by women with estrogen-sensitive conditions or cancers, and in pts with diarrhea

Perioperative Risks

- Coronary artery vasoconstriction that can lead to myocardial ischemia

Worry About

- Differentiating from black or white Cohosh, which have other physiological effects
- Product safety and efficacy profiles differ among manufacturers
- Usage in pregnancy due to concern of uterine stimulation, teratogenicity, and neonatal multisystemic complications
- Usage in pts with diabetes, Htn, or acute Hx of tobacco use

Overview/Pharmacology

- Several alkaloids and saponins are considered responsible for the pharmacological effects
- Anagyrine, *N*-methylcytosine, and taspine are constituents identified likely to be teratogenic
- *N*-methylcytosine acts similarly to nicotine, which can increase BP, stimulate the small intestine, and produce hyperglycemia in the developing fetus.

Etiology

- *Berberidaceae* or *Leonticaceae* family
- Listed in the *United States Pharmacopeia* 1882–1905 as a labor inducer
- Typically the dried rhizome/root parts are used

ASSESSMENT POINTS

System	Effect	Assessment by Hx	PE	Test
HEENT	Mucous membrane irritation	Complaints of oral irritation	Oral mucosa exam	----------
CARDIO	Ischemia, Htn, Tachycardia	Complaints of angina, dyspnea, or palpitations	Cardiac exam	EKG ± ECHO
GI	↑ Gastrointestinal motility, abd cramping	Changes in bowel movements (i.e., frequency, consistency, etc.), abd discomfort	Abd exam	----------
ENDO	Hyperglycemia	Fatigue, polydipsia, polyuria, vision changes, wt loss	Visual acuity exam	Blood glucose
OB/GYN	Uterine stimulation, estrogenic effects	Changes in contractions or menstruation	OB exam	Biophysical profile US, LH levels

Key References: Finkel RS, Zarlengo KM. Blue cohosh and perinatal stroke. *N Engl J Med.* 2004;351:302–303.Wright IM. Neonatal effects of maternal consumption of blue cohosh. *J Pediatr.* 1999;134:384–385.

Perioperative Implications

Preoperative Concerns
- Reliable self-reporting of use by pts
- Enhanced hyperglycemia in diabetics
- Can be assoc with coronary vasocon-striction

Monitoring
- Use of standard ASA monitors
- Intraop blood glucose level

Airway/Maintenance
- No known effects

Preinduction/Induction
- Coronary vasoconstriction

Adjuvant
- May accentuate the response to vasopressors
- May attenuate effectiveness of antihypertensive medications
- Possible drug-drug interactions due to inhibitory effects on hepatic enzymes

Postoperative Period
- Monitor CV status (i.e., BP, pulse, etc.) and blood glucose levels

Carnitine

Renyu Liu
Dajin Sun

Uses

• Treatment of 1° carnitine deficiency and deficiency 2° to complications of several inborn errors of metabolism, such as organic acidemia and fatty acid oxidation defects in children and adults, and acquired medical or iatrogenic conditions such as valproate and zidovuline treatment, cirrhosis, chronic renal failure on dialysis, etc.
• Treatment of valproic acid poisoning and/or overdosing and prevention of valproic acid-induced hepatotoxicity.
• Used for attention-deficit/hyperactivity disorder (ADHD), erectile dysfunction and male infertility, cardiomyopathy, PVD, CHF, chronic cardiac dysrhythmias; senile dementia, metabolic nerve diseases, in HIV infection, tuberculosis, myopathies, renal failure anemia, neuropathy, and neuropathic pain, etc. However, additional studies are needed to confirm these benefits.
• L-carnitine can effectively block the neuronal apoptosis caused by inhalational anesthetics in the developing rat brain. Clinical applications of this finding are unknown.

Perioperative Risks

• These are related to carnitine deficiency rather than carnitine itself.
• Hypoglycemia, lactic acidosis, and muscle weakness related to carnitine deficiencies and D/C of carnitine supplement
• Case report indicated that pts with carnitine deficiencies may develop symptoms similar to those assoc with propofol infusion syndrome when large doses of propofol are used.

Worry About

• Individuals with L-carnitine deficiency should continue this medication as scheduled preop to avoid acute hypoglycemia, lactic acidosis etc. IV carnitine or dextrose-containing solutions may be needed for fasting individuals with L-carnitine deficiencies.

Overview/Pharmacology

• Carnitine (3-hydroxy-4-trimethylamino-butyric acid or β-hydroxy-gamma-N-trimethylaminobutyrate) is a quaternary ammonium compound biosynthesized from the amino acids lysine and methionine.
• It exists in two stereoisomers: L-carnitine, biologically active form and D-carnitine, the biologically inactive form that may be harmful.
• About 75% comes from the diet, particularly from red meat and dairy products. Endogenous synthesis combined with high tubular re-absorption is enough to prevent deficiency in healthy people. Thus, carnitine deficiency is uncommon in the healthy and well-nourished adult population.
• Most of the body's carnitine is stored in skeletal muscle, but it is also found in other high energy demanding tissues such as those in the myocardium, liver, and adrenal glands. Carnitine is excreted in urine. Thus, carnitine and its metabolite may accumulate in renal failure pts.

Pharmacokinetics

• Formula — $C_7H_{15}NO_3$
• Mol. Mass — 161.199 g/mol
• Bioavailability — <10%
• Protein binding — None
• Metabolism — Slightly
• Half life — 15 hrs
• Excretion — Urine (>95%)

Drug Class/Usual Dose

• Carnitine is available both as a prescription drug and as a food supplement.
• Pregnancy: Category B. Studies in bacteria found no evidence of mutagenicity. No human data is available. Carnitine occurs naturally in human breast milk.
• Dosing: The usual supplementation dose is 2–6 g/d for a period ranging from 10 d to 10 wk. For infants and children, recommended dosage is between 50 and 100 mg/kg/d in divided doses with a max of 3 g/d. IV L-carnitine is used for treatment of lactic acidosis and cardiomyopathy 2° to L-carnitine deficiency. The recommended dosage is a 50 mg/kg bolus injection over 2–3 min, followed by an equivalent dosage over the next 24 hr (divided every 3–4 hr). Subsequent dosages would be based on responses.
• Overdosage: There have been no reports of toxicity from L-carnitine overdosage. Oral doses of 15 g/d have been well tolerated.

ASSESSMENT POINTS

System	Effect	Assessment by Hx	PE	Test
CNS	Seizures (rare)	Oral or IV L-carnitine. A reliable description of a witnessed seizure	Seizure activity Post-seizure state Signs of other injuries	Rule out other etiology
GI	N/V/D	Oral or intravenous L-carnitine. It is important to differentiate between overdose vs. deficiency		Blood carnitine level, serum glucose, lactic acid
DERM	Body odor	Oral or intravenous L-carnitine	Odor	

Key References: Alesci S, et al, ed. *Carnitine: The science behind a conditionally essential nutrient*. The New York Academy of Sciences; 2004. Berardi RR, et al, ed. *Handbook of Nonprescription drugs*. 4th ed. American Pharmacists Association; 2004. Steiber A, Kerner J, Hoppel C. Carnitine: a nutritional, biosynthetic, and functional perspective. *Mol Aspects Med.* 2004;25:455–473.

Possible Drug Interactions

• Carnitine has not been thoroughly tested for interactions with other herbs, supplements, drugs, or foods.

• L-carnitine might decrease the need for certain drugs such as glycosides, digoxin, diuretics, beta-blockers, channel blockers, hypolipidemic (cholesterol-altering) drugs, and nitro derivatives.

• L-carnitine might increase the effects of warfarin (Coumadin) and heparin.

Anticipated Problems/Concerns

• None

Chitosan

Joan Spiegel

Uses

- Excellent hemostatic agent
- Antibacterial properties useful for periodontal disease
- Pharmaceutical sustained-release drug carrier (chitosan glutamate)
- Wt loss agent (modest)
- Decreases cholesterol and triglycerides and increases (improves) HDL:total cholesterol ratio
- Cleaning petrochemical spills
- Water purification agent

Risk

- None known

Perioperative Risk

- None known

Worry About

- Theoretical inhibition of absorbtion of fat soluble vitamins A, D, E and K

Overview

- Chitosan is a naturally occurring marine polysaccharide fiber derived from a common byproduct of shellfish processing. (Chitosan is the de-acetylated form of chitin, a sugar from the shells of crustaceans).
- Recently, ingenious medical applications have been developed which use chitosan as a pharmaceutical drug carrier effectively encapsulating various anti-inflammatory and chemotherapeutic agents allowing it to function as a moiety for safe sustained release.

Etiology

- Chitosan is a completely indigestible fiber source with the ability to electrostatically attract and bond with negatively charged dietary lipids thus prohibiting their absorption.
- The hemostatic activity of chitosan is from an ionic interaction between the positively charged chitosan polymer and the negatively charged cell membrane of the red blood cell, and works irrespective of the presence of fibrin.

DRUG EFFECTS

System	Effect	Test
CARDIO	Improved cholesterol	Lipid profile
HEME	Improved hemostasis	None
GI	Stomach upset, steatorrhea, loss of fat soluble vitamins	None

Key References: Koide S. Chitin-Chitosan properties, benefits and risks. *Nutrition research*. 1998;18:1091–1101. Felt O, et al. Chitosan: A unique polysaccharide for drug delivery. *Drug Dev Ind Pharm*. 1998;24:979–993.

Perioperative Implications

- None known or studied

Red Yeast Rice (Cholestin)

Chris Broussard
Scott Gardiner
Charles Fox
Adam M. Kaye

Uses

- Hypercholesterolemia
- Prevention of coronary events, stroke, and TIA
- Treatment of dyslipidemia in statin intolerant pts
- Prostate and colon cancer

Perioperative Risks

- Obtain adequate Hx to determine indication for taking red yeast rice

Worry About

- Chemical composition of red yeast rice is not controlled by the FDA, and may vary by manufacturer.
- Relatively contraindicated in liver disease. Hepatotoxicity is worsened in combination with other hepatotoxic drugs.

Overview

- Prepared by growing red yeast (monascus purpureus) on rice to produce a red product
- Contains 10 mevinic acids incl monacolin K, also known as lovastatin
- Popular in Asian countries
- Available in several preparations in USA

Drug Class/Mechanism of Action/Usual Dose

- HMG-Co-A reductase inhibitor
- Inhibits conversion of HMG-Co-A to mevalonic acid, an early precursor of cholesterol
- Usual dose 600–2400 mg daily

ASSESSMENT POINTS

System	Effect	Test
CARDIAC	Reduces VLDL, LDL and triglyceride levels	VLDL, LDL, HDL, triglycerides
HEPAT	Rare hepatocellular damage and cholestasis	AST, ALT
MS	Rare myopathy, myalgia, and rhabdomyolysis	CPK

Key Reference: Becker DJ, Gordon RY, Halbert SC, French B, Morris PB, Rader DJ. Red yeast rice for dyslipidemia in statin-intolerant patients. A randomized trial. *Ann Intern Med.* 2009;150:830–839.

Perioperative Implications

Preoperative Concerns

- Lovastatin has been designated as pregnancy category X by the FDA. Red yeast rice should be avoided in pregnancy and lactation.

Preinduction/Induction

- Succinylcholine is contraindicated in myopathies assoc with elevated serum creatine phosphokinase (CPK) values.

ALTERNATIVE MEDICINE

Chondroitin Sulfate

Angela Zimmerman
Michael F. Roizen

Uses

- The consensus of expert and industry opinions supports the use of chondroitin sulfate (CS) for improving symptoms and stopping, possibly reversing the degenerative process of osteoarthritis.
- CS is relatively free of side effects when used at the recommended daily dosage, at least for short periods of time, and thus offers an attractive alternative to traditional treatments mainly consisting of NSAIDs.
- As CS has gained in popularity, researchers have recognized the need to conduct more scientific studies to validate or refute its efficacy, as well as its safety.
- Most trials testing the efficacy of CS have demonstrated significant improvement of pts' OA, although the level of improvement continues to be debated, and is about the level of placebo in recent trials at about 60% gaining significant pain relief in trials too short to show joint remodeling.
- Its common partner, glucosamine, has resulted in significant reduction in moderate and severe pain over 24 wk greater than placebo and NSAIDs, and either CS or itself alone.

Perioperative Risks

- No known significant complications of CS and no known anesthetic implications. Use cautiously in pts with shellfish allergy. Worsening of previously well-controlled asthma has been reported. CS has a structural similarity to heparin and may need to be reconsidered in certain health conditions where heparin is contraindicated.

Overview/Pharmacology

- Major component of extracellular matrix and important in its role in forming proteoglycans of which it is a part. The tightly packed and highly charged sulfate groups of CS generate electrostatic charges that provide much of the resistance of cartilage to compression. Loss of CS from the cartilage is a major cause of OA.
- Oral CS is a less than perfectly absorbed nutritional supplement for the treatment of OA.

- Shown to have activity and capable of ↑ proteoglycan synthesis in articular cartilage; mechanism of action may be related to local inhibition of interleukin 1β.
- CS usually takes 1 mo to exert any effect, with maximum benefits seen after 4 wk of therapy; conversely, benefits are sustained for 1–2 mo after D/C of therapy.

Drug Class/Usual Dose

- CS is a glycosaminoglycan found in the proteoglycans of articular cartilage.
- Currently manufactured from natural sources (shark and/or beef cartilage or bovine trachea)
- Dose is 400 mg three times daily or 600 mg two times daily, by mouth (18 yr and older)
- Most studies have tested doses of 1–2 g CS daily, although a higher dose has not clearly been linked to a greater effect.
- Optimal dose when used in combination with glucosamine is not clear.

ASSESSMENT POINTS

System	Drug Effect	Assessment by Hx	PE	Test
MS	Anti-inflammatory effect, slows joint degeneration	Pt assessment of pain scores	Joint tenderness and function	Joint narrowing on x-rays
GI	Low incidence of nausea and diarrhea	Subjective reports of nausea and diarrhea		

Key Reference: Vangsness Jr CT, Spiker W, Erickson J. A review of evidence-based medicine for glucosamine and chondroitin sulfate use in knee osteoarthritis. *Arthroscopy.* 2009;25(1):86–94.

Perioperative Implications/Drug Interactions

- None

Chromium

Lee A. Fleisher

Uses

- Body building (ineffective)
- May aid in glycemic control of type II DM and gestational DM
- Hyperlipidemia
- Hypoglycemia—reactive
- Obesity

Perioperative Risks

- Risks minimal
- Chronic ingestion assoc in one case with thrombocytopenia, hepatic dysfunction, renal dysfunction

Worry About

- Nephrotoxicity

Overview

- A trace mineral
- Improves glucose tolerance in type II DM and gestational DM (in some studies)
- Shown to ↑ insulin sensitivity and ↓ serum triglycerides
- Shown to alleviate symptoms of reactive hypoglycemia
- Popular as wt loss and body building supplement, but effect not supported in clinical trials

Drug Class/Mechanism of Action/Usual Dose

- Hypothesis: In normal functioning, it ↑ circulating insulin, results in binding of chromium to peripheral, insulin-sensitive tissue; ↑ insulin receptor number and activates insulin receptor kinase
- Usual dosage recommended: 50–200 μg/d
    - Available orally or IV
    - Taken as supplement of 200–1000 μg/d
- Mixed results in randomized clinical tests

ASSESSMENT POINTS

System	Effect	Test
RENAL	Nephrotoxicity	Cr
ENDO	Insulin sensitivity	Glucose

Key Reference: Hummel M, Standl E, Schnell O. Chromium in metabolic and cardiovascular disease. *Horm Metab Res.* 2007;39(10):743–751.

Perioperative Implications

- No known interaction

Cranberry

Dmitry Portnoy

Uses

• Many cranberry juice consumers are aware of a beneficial link between cranberry juice and urinary tract and of valuable polyphenol activity
• Most common as alternative agent for prevention of UTIs
• Also, believed to be beneficial for prevention of upper GI ulcers, reducing the risks of CV disease and improving oral hygiene
• Native Americans and Early American sailors used cranberries for treating wounds and blood poisoning, urinary illnesses, diarrhea, diabetes, and as antiscorbutic agent

Perioperative Risks

• A few case reports suggested possible interaction with warfarin resulting in prolonged INR and bleeding. Subsequently, two small randomized controlled trials could not confirm clinically significant enhancement of anticoagulation.

Worry About

• Theoretical risk of oxalate urinary stone formation (if large volumes consumed daily)
• Contentious issue of interaction with anticoagulation effect of warfarin

Overview/Pharmacology

• Cranberries are a fruit native to New England and belong to the *Vaccinium macrocarpon*
• The most popular form for consumption is the cranberry-juice cocktail, containing about 27% cranberry juice, sweetener, water, and vitamin C
• Also available as juice concentrate, tablets, or capsules

• Cranberries consist of 90% water and various organic substances such as quinic acid, malic acid, and citric acid as well as glucose and fructose.

Drug Class/Mechanism of Action/Usual Dose

• Increased concentration of hippuric acid and increased acidification of urine
• Inhibits bacterial adherence to mucosal surface by at least two kinds of inhibitors: fructose and proanthocyanidins
• Fructose and proanthocyanidins in cranberries inhibit type I–fimbriated *Escherichia coli* adhesion
• Cranberry products reduced the incidence of UTIs in women at 12 mo

ASSESSMENT POINTS

System	Drug Effect	Assessment by Hx	PE	Test
HEENT	Reduces dental plaque, periodontal and gum disease	Toothache	Dental exam	
CARDIO	Improves ability of LDL to resist oxidative stress (antioxidation)			ECHO of arteries
GU	Prevents UTI; stone formation	Frequency and urgency and painful urination	Cloudy urine, low back pain	UA culture of urine

Key Reference: Guay DRP. Cranberry and Urinary Tract Infections. *Drugs.* 2009;69:775–807.

Perioperative Implications

Preoperative Concerns
• Hx of recurrent UTI, possible urolithiasis, the need for antibiotics

Induction/Maintenance
• Routine monitoring
• Consider antibiotic coverage if UTI is present

Postoperative Concerns
• Immediate resumption not necessary

Anticipated Problems/Concerns

• Assess for UTI, antibiotic use, urolithiasis, anticoagulation status

ALTERNATIVE MEDICINE

Creatine

R. Blaine Easley

Uses

- **Medical:** Historically used to lower cholesterol and treat rare conditions of heart failure due to creatine deficiencies; has proposed benefits to decrease myalgias and myositis with statins
- **Fitness:** ↑ Usage over past decade to ↑ muscle mass and enhance physical performance. Initially used by professional athletes, now used as nutritional supplement in almost all areas of exercise fitness (in both casual and competitive athletes).
- **Incidence:** Unknown incidence in population

Perioperative Risks

- Unknown. Theoretical problems in pts with impaired renal function. Potential for drug interactions, though no definitive studies (see Possible Drug Interactions below)

Worry About

- Hypovolemia and/or dehydration if inadequate nutrition

Overview/Pharmacology

- Commercially available as creatine citrate, creatine monohydrate, and creatine phosphate
- Creatine exists intracellularly in skeletal muscle, cardiac muscle, brain, and testes as creatine phosphate, otherwise called phosphocreatine. Phosphocreatine contains a high-energy phosphate bond, used for short, intense muscle activity via the phosphagen energy system.
- Studies in animal and human subjects have demonstrated ↑ of cellular phosphocreatine levels in skeletal muscle following creatine ingestion. Few studies demonstrating ↑ in muscle strength or endurance.
- Recent randomized trials have shown neither increased strength nor increased stamina
- Increase in muscle mass is thought related to increase in intracellular H_2O content brought about by influx of phosphocreatine into myocyte.

- Creatine is eliminated from the body by renal excretion as creatinine, the anhydrous form of creatine.
- Creatine is usually ingested dissolved in fluid.
- Use creatine to ↑ muscle mass and performance. (Special concern should be paid to athletes desiring wt loss, i.e., wrestlers, gymnasts, body builders, football players, in examining renal function.)

Drug Class/Usual Dose

- Creatine is classified as a nutritional or dietary supplement; therefore, it is unregulated by the FDA.
- Typical usage: Initially 20–25 g ingested daily for 5–7 d, followed by 5–10 g daily for 10–12 wk. However, some individuals take higher dosages continually.

ASSESSMENT POINTS

System	Effect	Assessment by Hx	PE	Test
CARDIO	Hypovolemia/hypotension	Exposure	BP/HR	Lytes

Key Reference: Shao A, Hathcock JN. Risk assessment for creatine monohydrate. *Regul Toxicol Pharmacol*. 2006;45:242–251.

Possible Drug Interactions

Preoperative Period

- Because of the assoc risk of hypovolemia/dehydration in pts using creatine, there are theoretical problems when used with the following classes of medications: diuretics, H_2 antagonists (e.g., cimetidine), NSAIDs, probenecid, and trimethoprim, or when taken near the time of exercise.

Induction/Maintenance

- No known interactions. May need bolus of intravascular fluids and careful attention to BP at time of induction.

Adjuvants/Regional Anesthesia/Reversal

- No known interactions. Consider pro/cons of NSAID usage intraop, esp. if no assessment of renal function.

Dandelion

Shu-Ming Wang
Kimberly M. King

Uses

- Rx for liver disease (e.g., liver congestion, bile duct inflammation, hepatitis, gallstones, and jaundice)
- Rx for kidney disease
- Rx for fluid retention
- Rx for diabetes with specific hypoglycemic effects
- Less commonly used for mastitis, heartburn, boils, and fevers, among other uses
- Dietary supplement as a source of vitamins and minerals (leaves contain the highest concentration of vitamin A at 14,000 IU/100 g raw) in addition to vitamin D, vitamin B complex, vitamin C, iron, silicon, Mg, Na, K, zinc, manganese, copper, and phosphorus

Perioperative Risks

- No clinical trial to date on hemodynamic instability
- No clinical trial to date but may potentially cause bleeding 2° to ↓ the clotting

Worry About

- If used in combination with prescription diuretic drugs, effects of either or both drugs may be enhanced, leading to a hypovolemic state.
- Multiple minerals in dandelion may ↓ systemic absorption of PO-administered drugs (e.g., ciprofloxacin, famotidine, and esomeprazole)
- Too much vitamin A

Overview/Pharmacology

- 1° effect in relieving dyspepsia disorder is caused by taraxerol.
- Stimulation of bile release by the liver and gallbladder, hence, improving both bile flow (choleretic effect) and release (cholagogue effect)
- Diuretic activity comparable to that of furosemide has been demonstrated in mice; however, because dandelion replaces potassium lost through diuresis, metabolic complications occur only rarely.
- Insulin, a polysaccharide fiber composed of long chains of fructose-containing molecules contained in the plant, may act to buffer fluctuations in blood sugar levels.

Usual Dose

- Root used for general tonic and mild liver remedy up to tid
  - Dried root: 2–8 g by infusion, or decoction
  - Fluid extract: 4–8 mL
  - Tincture, alcohol based: Not recommended 2° to high dosage required
  - Juice of fresh root: 4–8 mL
  - Powdered solid extract: 250–500 mg
- Leaf preparations used for diuretic effects tid
  - Dried leaf by infusion: 4–10 g
  - Fluid extract: 4–10 mL

Toxicity

- Generally considered one of the safest medicinal plants used
- May be potentially toxic because of the high content of K, Mg, and other minerals, and vitamin A

ASSESSMENT POINTS

System	Effect	Assessment by Hx	PE	Test
CARDIO	Hypovolemia	Orthostasis, polyurea, polydipsia	↓ Skin turgor, hypotension, tachycardia, orthostasis	Orthostatic BP, HR
GI	↑ Gastric secretion	Diarrhea		
RENAL	Prerenal failure	Polyurea, polydipsia	As for CV	BUN/Cr
METAB	Hypoglycemia	Lightheaded, clammy, shaky	Sweaty	Blood glucose

Key Reference: Pizzorno Jr JE, Murray M. Taraxacum officinale (dandelion). In: *A textbook of natural medicine* 2nd ed. London: Churchill Livingstone; 1999:979–982.

Perioperative Implications

Preoperative Concerns
- Unknown effects in pediatric and pregnant pts
- Rely on pt self-report

Monitoring
- Routine

- May require fluid bolus if there is an indication of hypovolemia and UO

Regional Anesthesia
- Not clear but can potentially affect plt function

Emergence/Extubation
- No known complications to date

Postoperative Period
- Continue to assess volume status and treat accordingly
- Potentially increased bleeding

Dehydroepiandrosterone (DHEA)

Amir Baluch
Alan Kaye

USES

- Unproven benefits and uses:
  - Adrenal insufficiency
  - Aging, slowing
  - Alzheimer's disease
  - Anorexia nervosa
  - CV disease
  - Chronic fatigue
  - Chron's disease
  - Depression
  - Diabetes
  - Heart failure
  - Obesity
  - Osteoporosis
  - Perimenopause issues incl increasing bone mineral density and for vaginal atrophy
  - Sexual dysfunction
  - Sleep disorders
  - SLE
  - Well-being

Perioperative Risks

- Single case report assoc DHEA with cardiac arrhythmias and immune suppression
- May induce insulin resistance
- Unknown effects on periop stress response, adrenal and cardiac function

Concerns

- Cardiac arrhythmias occur rarely, even with large doses
- Diabetics may be prone to hyperglycemia
- Unknown coagulation and vasoconstriction/dilation effects

- Marketed as a dietary supplement because DHEA can be manufactured from natural sources, such as soy and wild yam. However, many of these products, depending on source and metabolism, are not converted into DHEA in humans and are not recommended or preferred.

Pharmacodynamics

- Hepatic, adrenal gland, testes, and in minute quantities, the brain endogenously produce
- Hepatic metabolism, urinary excretion with a 12-hr half-life
- Steroid hormone produced by adrenals, interconverted to testosterone, estrone, estradiol, androsterone
- Considered a prohormone, so effects similar to those of anabolic steroids.
- Increased protein synthesis in skeletal muscle, however, increase in serum testosterone or enhancement of strength during resistance training is controversial. A placebo-controlled, randomized clinical trial reported in the *New England Journal of Medicine* in 2006 found that supplementation in the elderly had no significant beneficial effects on body composition, physical performance, insulin sensitivity, or quality of life.
- Inhibits glucose-6-phosphate, which theoretically accounts for postulated antiatherogenic properties.
Key Reference: Fukui M, Kitagawa Y, Nakamura N, et al. Serum dehydroepiandrosterone sulfate concentration and carotid atherosclerosis in men with type 2 diabetes. *Atherosclerosis*. 2005, 181(2): 339–344.

- By decreasing serum cortisol levels, may cause early activation of the anterior cingulate cortex (ACC) 2° to neuronal recruitment of the steroid sensitive ACC that may be involved in pre-hippocampal memory processing, thereby improving memory.
- DHEA levels decrease with CHF, oxidative stress, aging, and cancer
- May have apoptotic affect in some cancer lines but also shown to stimulate hormone-producing tumors.

Overview

- Popularized after a New England Journal report that high levels correlated with fewer cardiac events (Rancho-Bernardo study); later, not found so in larger Rancho-Bernardo study
- FDA categorized DHEA as unapproved drug in 1985; reclassified as dietary supplement by 1994
- Banned by NCAA, the National Football League, and Olympics
- Contraindicated in breast, ovarian, and prostate cancers
- May cause hirsutism, acne, headache, insomnia, wt gain, alopecia, deepening of voice and abn menses in women, or gynecomastia in men
- No data indicate benefit greater than long-term risk

Usual Dose

- 25–50 mg/d for angioedema
- 50 mg tid for CV disease
- 30–90 mg/d for depression, memory improvement, or cognition
- 200 mg/d for SLE

DRUG EFFECTS

System	Effect	Hx Assessment	PE	Test
HEENT	Hirsutism			
CARDIO	Anabolic steroids assoc with sudden cardiac arrest, Htn; DHEA rarely causes arrhythmias	Determine chronic and acute dose and duration of self-administration; palpitations	HR	Preop ECG for chronic or excessive use, may show ventricular hypertrophy
GI	Anabolic steroids assoc with hepatitis, cholestatic jaundice			
HEME	Inhibits plt aggregation in vivo Antiglucocorticoid actions		Ecchymoses	Bleeding time; Preoperative glucose for diabetics
DERM	Increased acneiform dermatitis			
GU	Hypogonadism with anabolic steroids, prostate tumor growth	Prostate exam		PSA
CNS	Anabolic steroids may cause aggressiveness; DHEA binds to NMDA, sigma, GABA receptors	↑ Pituitary tumor growth		ACTH

Key References: Nair KS, Rizza RA, O'Brien P, et al. DHEA in elderly women and DHEA or testosterone in elderly men. *N Engl J Med*. 2006;355:1647–1659.
Tworoger SS, Missmer SA, Eliassen AH, et al. The association of plasma DHEA and DHEA sulfate with breast cancer risk in predominantly premenopausal women. *Cancer Epidemiol Biomarkers Prev*. 2006;15:967–971.

Possible Drug Interactions

Preoperative Period
- Insulin resistance, check preop glucose
- Synergism with corticosteroids

Induction/Maintenance
- Unknown effects of inhibition of steroid synthesis if combined with etomidate, or immunosuppressives for transplantation

Postoperative Concerns
- Unknown effects on stress response

Anticipated Problems
- Unpredictable CV effects

Echinacea (American Coneflower, Purple Coneflower: *E. Angustifolia, E. Purpurea, E. Pallida*)

Kirk Lalwani

Uses

- Purported immunostimulation; the prevention and treatment of resp tract infections.
- As an adjuvant in the treatment of other bacterial, viral, or fungal infections of the urinary and resp tract.
- Antiinflammatory action when used topically for conditions such as eczema, psoriasis, and herpes simplex.
- Promotes wound healing when used topically, i.e., in leg ulcers and burns.
- As an adjuvant for cancer therapy, and in the treatment of the chronic fatigue syndrome.

Perioperative Risks

- No known drug interactions or toxicities.
- No known sedative, CV, or coagulation effects relevant to anesthesia.

Worry About

- Immunostimulation may counteract the effect of steroids and immunosuppresant drugs in transplant recipients and pts with autoimmune disease.

Overview

- The most common side effects are GI symptoms, allergic reactions, and rashes.
- Allergic reactions are more common in atopic individuals and individuals with a Hx of sensitivity to the Asteraceae-Compositae family of plants (ragweed, chrysanthemums, marigolds, daisies etc.), and can be serious.
- Echinacea may exacerbate autoimmune diseases such as MS, SLE, rheumatoid arthritis, AIDS, tuberculosis, and pemphigus vulgaris.
- Echinacea may inhibit Cytochrome P450 (CYP 1A2, 3A4) enzymes, altering levels of drugs metabolized by these enzymes.
- Tachyphylaxis may occur with prolonged, uninterrupted use.

Drug Class/Mechanism of Action/Usual Dose

- Increases phagocytosis and lymphocyte activity, possibly by release of tumor necrosis factor (TNF), interlukin-1 (IL-1), and interferon.

- Anti-inflammatory activity by inhibition of cyclooxygenase and 5-lipogenase.
- Promotes wound healing by protecting Type 3 collagen from free radical damage and inhibiting bacterial hyaluronidase
- Concentration of active ingredients varies widely according to species and preparation used.
  - 1–3 mL of the fluid extract or cold-pressed juice of plant (or root) three times daily.
  - 1 gm of powdered root three times daily (capsules, tablets)
- Echinacea appears to modestly inhibit cytochrome P450 1A2 (CYP1A2), and to induce hepatic cytochrome P450 3A4 (CYP3A4), but inhibit intestinal CYP3A4 (opposing effects).

DRUG EFFECTS

System	Effect	Test
IMMUNE	Immunostimulation, anti-inflammatory activity	Phagocytic activation, IL-1 and TNF activity
HEPAT	P450 CYP1A2 inhibition	Caffeine clearance test

Key Reference: Charrois TL, Hrudey J, Vohra S. Echinacea: *Pediatr Rev.* 2006;27(10):385–387.

Perioperative Implications

- Possible antagonism of antirejection drugs used following bone marrow or organ transplantation

Ephedra (Ma-Huang)

Bracken J. De Witt

Uses

- Ephedra is a plant that contains a variety of ephedrine alkaloids, incl ephedrine and pseudoephedrine.
- Dietary supplements containing ephedra were marketed in the USA as agents that may aid in wt reduction and energy enhancement. Ephedra may be used in the manufacture of methamphetamine.
- Several governmental agencies inquired into the safety of ephedra and regulated the use of dietary supplements containing ephedra in response to reported pt adverse reactions. A 2004 U.S. ban on the sale of ephedra-containing supplements currently continues.
- Some supplements have marketed "ephedrine-free" or legal ephedra products, in which the ephedra is replaced with other herbal stimulants such as bitter orange.
- Ephedra-containing substances are also known as ma-huang, Mormon tea, squaw tea, and herbal ecstasy.

Perioperative Risks

- Risks assoc with an ↑ in the sympathetic nervous system activity and dysrhythmias and Htn

Worry About

- Lethal cardiac arrhythmias, Htn, myocarditis, MI, angina, ↑ thermogenesis
- Hemorrhagic and/or ischemic stroke, subarachnoid hemorrhage, cerebral vasculitis, seizures
- Bronchial dilation, acute hepatitis
- Preterm labor

Overview/Pharmacology

- Mechanism of action is via increases in sympathetic stimulation
- Ephedrine is an indirect-acting sympathomimetic that exerts its effects mainly by stimulating release of norepinephrine.
- Other ephedrine alkaloids in ephedra have direct-acting effects on both α- and β-adrenoceptors
- Ephedra is often packaged with guarana-derived caffeine, which may synergistically augment adrenergic stimulation.

Drug Class/Mechanism of Action/Usual Dose

- Works via stimulation of sympathetic nervous system

ASSESSMENT POINTS

System	Effect	Assessment by Hx	PE	Test
CARDIO	Arrhythmias, Htn, myocarditis, MI, angina thermogenesis	Chest pain	BP ↑ Temp	BP/HR ECG, cardiac enzymes Temp probe
GU	Acute hepatitis			LFTs
CNS	Stroke, subarachnoid hemorrhage, vasculitis, seizure	Decreased mental status Headache	Neuro exam	CT, vascular biopsy, EEG
PULM	Bronchial dilation			PFTs

Key Reference: Ang-Lee MK, Moss J, Yuan CS. Herbal medicines and perioperative care. *JAMA.* 2001;286:208–216.

Perioperative Implications

Preoperative Period

- Ephedra may produce adverse pt reactions with medications such as MAO inhibitors, digoxin, cold medications containing ephedrine, diuretics, and antihypertensives
- Assess preop BP, HR, and ECG
- Consider as a potential cause of preterm labor

Preinduction/Induction Period

- Control hemodynamics before induction
- Observe ECG for arrhythmias

Maintenance Period

- Response to ephedrine may be hampered 2° to tachyphylaxis; therefore, control hypotension with direct-acting adrenergic agonists, like phenylephrine

- Ephedra may interact with volatile anesthetics (e.g., enflurane) to promote dysrhythmias

Postoperative Period

- Assess postop BP, HR, and ECG for CV changes

Evening Primrose

Leila L. Reduque

Uses

• Evening primrose oil (EPO) is obtained from the seed of the plant species *Oenothera biennis*
• EPO is also known as fever plant, huile d'onagre, king's cureall, night willow-herb, scabish, and sundrops
• EPO may be used as a food supplement for the essential fatty acids linoleic acid (LA) and γ-linolenic acid (GLA).
• Infusion of the whole plant has been used for asthma, GI disorders, whooping cough, and as a sedative pain killer
• EPO had been licensed in Britain for treatment of atopic eczema and cyclic and noncyclic mastalgia; but the license was withdrawn upon a conclusion that there was not enough evidence of effectiveness.
• Other uses for EPO incl PMS, psoriasis, MS, hypercholesterolemia, rheumatoid arthritis, Raynaud's phenomenon, Sjögren's syndrome, postviral fatigue syndrome, asthma, and diabetic neuropathy, without solid evidence it is effective but with recurrent anecdotal evidence of beneficial outcomes.

Perioperative Risks

• EPO may cause an $\uparrow$ risk of temporal lobe epilepsy in schizophrenic pts being treated with epileptogenic drugs (e.g., phenothiazines)
• EPO may cause a $\downarrow$ in blood clotting

Worry About

• Obstetrics: Orally administered EPO may be assoc with an $\uparrow$ in the incidence of prolonged rupture of membranes, oxytocin augmentation, arrest of descent, and vacuum extraction

Overview/Pharmacology

• EPO is a rich source of the essential fatty acids LA and GLA. These essential fatty acids are involved in prostaglandin biosynthetic pathways.
• DGLA, a metabolite of GLA, is a precursor of both the inflammatory prostaglandin series via arachidonic acid (AA), and the less inflammatory series (PGE_1)
• Actions of PGE_1 incl anti-inflammatory, immunoregulatory, and vasodilatory properties, inhibition of plt aggregation and cholesterol biosynthesis, hypotension, and elevation of cyclic AMP
• GLA has been shown to have a favorable effect on the DGLA:AA ratio. The $\uparrow$ in AA is smaller and less consistent when compared with the $\uparrow$ in DGLA. This is beneficial because DGLA leads to the less inflammatory prostaglandin series PGE_1.

• GLA is not normally obtained from the diet. The body relies on the metabolic conversion of LA to GLA. This conversion is rate limiting in the production of GLA. It has been shown that there is a reduced rate of conversion of LA to GLA in several clinical situations incl aging, diabetes, CV disorders and high LDL cholesterol concentrations, high alcohol intake, viral infections, cancer, nutritional deficits, atopic eczema, and premenstrual syndrome. Dietary supplementation of GLA, via EPO, bypasses the rate-limiting conversion step and has a beneficial effect on the ratio of inflammatory to less inflammatory prostaglandin synthesis.

Drug Class/Mechanism of Action/ Usual Dose

• Dose of EPO is specific for each condition being treated, e.g., the EPO dose for atopic eczema is 6–8 g for adults or 2–4 g for children. These doses of EPO are based on standardized products containing 8% GLA. EPO may be swallowed directly, mixed with milk or another liquid, or taken with food. The clinical response is usually seen after 3–4 mo of continuous use.

DRUG EFFECTS

EPO studies are in a preliminary phase; its effects have been proved only in animal models. The effects mentioned here have yet to be proved in humans.

System	Effect
CARDIO	Inhibits the $\uparrow$ of serum total cholesterol + VLDL + IDL + LDL cholesterol concentrations in the presence of excess cholesterol in the diet
	Serves as an antioxidant in hyperlipemic states. Reduces oxidative stress by inhibiting lipid peroxidation and reinforcing the glutathione-dependent antioxidant defense system.
GI	Has anti-ulcer and cytoprotective effects on experimentally induced gastric lesions
HEME	Reduces plt aggregation when subject fed an atherogenic diet
DERM	May be used for Rx of atopic eczema. Treatment of atopic eczema with EPO is controversial. Clinical studies have been equivocal on whether symptoms of atopic eczema benefit from EPO.
	May be used for the treatment of limited scleroderma, or CREST syndrome. Clinical studies have been equivocal in relation to fatty acid placebos but have shown qualitative improvement in symptoms of Reynaud's phenomenon.
GU	Has been used for PMS and to help reduce frequency of nighttime hot flashes during menopause. Treatment is controversial because clinical studies have not shown a clear benefit of EPO for PMS and menopause.
	Has been shown to be no better than fatty acid placebo or topical NSAIDs for treatment of mastalgia
	Has been used by many midwives to hasten cervical ripening in an effort to shorten labor and $\downarrow$ incidence of postdate pregnancies. One retrospective study showed that EPO does not shorten gestation or $\downarrow$ length of labor. Moreover, it was found that EPO may be assoc with above-mentioned adverse effects on labor.
CNS	Significantly reduced headache in women with PMS. Pts given both EPO and fish oil had fewer symptoms assoc with headache, such as depression and fatigue.
	Animal studies suggest EPO may be useful in the treatment of diabetic neuropathy, although the exact physiological mechanism remains to be demonstrated.
IMMUNO	In pts with mild RA, EPO has been shown to improve morning stiffness, and there was also improvement in the Ritchie articular index for each pt. Pts with severe RA did not exhibit improvement.
	Although not scientifically proved, EPO has been taken by asthmatics to gain the anti-inflammatory effects of PGE_1.

Key Reference: Stonemetz D. A Review of the clinical efficacy of evening primrose. *Holist Nurs Pract.* 2008 22:171–174.

Perioperative Implications

Preoperative Concerns

• EPO may cause an $\uparrow$ risk of developing temporal lobe epilepsy, specifically in pts taking known epileptogenic drugs such as phenothiazines. Seizures have not been seen in pts not taking phenothiazines.

Preinduction/Induction
• No known interactions

Maintenance
• No known interactions

Postoperative Period
• No known interactions

Fish Oil

Dennis A. Patel
Orlando J. Salinas
Alan Kaye

Uses

- Active ingredient for brain and retinal health (more than 40% of brain and retina is structural fat) is DHA (more than 50% of fat in brain and retina is DHA)
- Decreases arrhythmias and deaths related to
- Important component for cell signaling
- Data from MIDAS trial indicate restoration of memory to that of 3.5 y younger with 900 mg of DHA (about 3 gm of fish oil) a day in pts with minimal cognitive dysfunction
- Data from trial in non-breastfed infants indicate better IQ by about 16 points in babies formula fed with 20 mg of DHA per day compared to those fed in formula without DHA
- To ↓ plasma concentrations of triglycerides. Reduces elevated VLDL and chylomicrons, causes slight ↑ in HDL. To ↓ risk of death from CAD and to ↓ risk of stroke.
- Lowers BP (minimal)
- Decreases the risk of arrhythmias
- Myocardial reinfarction prevention
- Beneficial antithrombogenic from EPA (DHA has no anticlotting effect) and anti-inflammatory effects from DHA or EPA
- Management of collagen vascular diseases (lupus, psoriasis, Raynaud's phenomenon). Symptomatic improvement in rheumatic disease.
- May prevent immunologic injury in pts with IgA nephropathy; to retard renal function loss.

May benefit renal transplant recipients treated with cyclosporine. Significant beneficial effects on diabetic nephropathy and macroangiopathy.
- Beneficial in chronic and severe mental disorders (bipolar disorder, depression)
- To reduce inflammatory Sx assoc with inflammatory bowel diseases
- Other uses: Dysmenorrhea, kidney stones, diabetic neuropathy, gout, migraine headaches, male infertility, osteoporosis, multiple sclerosis, cancer-related cachexia, reduce modestly cataract risks, may improve risk of depression

Perioperative Risks

- Risks of long-term use not known. Variable ↑ in bleeding time if given EPA (not a risk from DHA) .

Worry About

- Coagulation disorders, greater than 3 grams per day can inhibit blood coagulation and potentially reduce plt aggregability and increase risk of bleeding.

Overview/Pharmacology

- Omega-3 fatty acids: Eicosapentaenoic acid (EPA) and docosahexaenoic acid (DHA)
- Also known as cod liver oil, marine oils, menhaden oil, N-3 fatty acids, N3-polyunsaturated fatty acids, omega 3, Omega-3 fatty acids, PUFA, salmon oil, W-3 fatty acids, algael DHA

- Dietary supplements available in capsules or oil by brand names: Coromega, Solgar Omega 3 700, Nature Made, Spring Valley, Bounty, Barleans, LifeFitness DHA, NatureMade DHA and others
- Fish oil and DHA supplements are not regarded as drugs and are not regulated by the FDA medication rules except for Lovaza.
- Fish oils produce biologic effects on prostaglandins, thromboxanes, and leukotrienes; ↑ TXA_3 levels and ↓ TXA_2 levels stimulate the formation of prostaglandin I_3, moderately reduce formation of TXB_2 in plt, inhibiting aggregation and adhesion
- Results in reduced plt aggregation (EPA) and vasoconstriction (DHA)
- Recent studies show small increase in LDL levels with large doses
- Improves large artery endothelium-dependent dilation of hypercholesterolemics (both EPA and DHA) without affecting endothelium-independent dilation
- Reduces blood viscosity by ↑ RBC deformability
- Substantial ↓ of triglyceride levels; variable effects on cholesterol levels

Drug Class/Usual Dose

- Not clear: Usual dosage is 2–9 g/d of fish oil or 20mg per year of life up to age 45 (900 mg) where dose stays constant (DHA)

ASSESSMENT POINTS

System	Effect	Assessment by Hx	PE	Test
GI	Abd distention, belching, halitosis, heartburn, flatulence, diarrhea			
HEME	Prolongs bleeding time, inhibits plt aggregation (EPA only)	Anticoagulant Rx, fatigue, weakness, bleeding problems	VS	Bleeding time, Hct
ENDO	Mild glucose intolerance in pts with NIDDM			FBS

Key References: Fish consumption, Fish oil, Omega-3 fatty acids, and cardiovascular disease. *Circulation*. 2002;106:2747–2757.
Yurko-Mauro K, et al, Beneficial effects of docosahexaenoic acid on cognitive function in age-related cognitive decline. *Alzheimers Dementi*. 2010;6(6):456-464.

Perioperative Implications

Preoperative Concerns

- May reduce blood clotting and increase risk of bleeding (not an effect of DHA alone)—can switch pts on 3 gm of fish oil a day to 900 mg of DHA a day with perhaps same anti-arrhythmic and brain function preserving effects—half-life variable depending on preparation, ideally pt having surgery or pain procedure should be off fish oil 7 d, allowing enough time for fish oil–induced blood thinning effects to be gone, but switch to DHA at same time.

Induction/Maintenance
- No interactions known

Adjuvants/Possible Drug Interactions
- Caution if receiving heparin, warfarin, dipyridamole, ticlopidine, sulfinpyrazone, or aspirin
- Fish oil can reduce vitamin E levels. Caution with herbals that have antiplatelet and/or anticoagulant constituents (angelica, clove, danshen, garlic, ginger, ginkgo, Panax ginseng, red clover, turmeric, willow, and others) with EPA, not DHA.

Anticipated Problems/Concerns

- Assess for possible adverse effects on the coagulation system
- Rare side effects incl: Abd pain with cramps, blurred vision, diarrhea, dizziness, fatigue, headache disorder, nausea
- Now medical-grade fish oil is available (Lovaza), which reduces indirect risk of mercury polychlorinated biphenyls, dioxin, and dioxin-related compounds, as does DHA from algae (algael DHA).

Garlic (Allium sativum)

Lara Bonasera

Uses

- Administered orally and topically as a powder, oil, tablet, and raw clove. Allicin is pharmacologically active component.
- Potential beneficial activity as an antihyperlipidemic (conflicting results in recent clinical trials), antimicrobial (*Microsporum canis*, sporotrichosis, tinea pedis), antiplatelet (via ↑ thromboxane levels), fibrinolytic, antioxidant (↑ catalase and glutathione peroxidase), antidiabetic, and vasoprotective agent (i.e., antihypertensive and agents to protect elastic properties of the aorta)
  - *Note*: These indications are not FDA approved, but garlic is generally recognized as safe (GRAS). Interpretation of data must take into account publication bias (preferential publication of positive findings).

Perioperative Risks

- Increased bleeding diathesis

Worry About

- Major drug interactions: Anticoagulants, antidiabetic agents, ASA, NSAIDs, plt inhibitors, herbs (danshen, dong quai, feverfew, ginger, ginkgo biloba, ginseng, horse chestnut), thrombolytic agents

Overview/Pharmacology

- Intact cells of garlic bulbs contain allinin, an odorless, sulfur-containing amino acid. Crushed garlic causes the enzyme allinase to convert allinin to allicin—a potent antibacterial agent that is odoriferous and unstable. Ajoenes, a self-condensation product of allicin, has antithrombotic activity. Fresh garlic releases allicin in the mouth during the chewing process. Dried garlic preparations lack allicin but contain allinin and allinase; they should be enteric-coated so they pass through the stomach into the small intestine where allinin can be enzymatically converted to allicin. Allicin is unstable in oil. Allinase is inactivated by heat (cooking) and acid.

- Potency can vary substantially among manufacturers.
- Dosage: No clear consensus, but dosage varies with reason for use. Hypercholesterolemia/arteriosclerosis: German Commission E recommends 4 g/d (1.5–2 average-sized garlic cloves) fresh garlic; or at least 5000 μg of allicin or chewing one garlic clove daily. Extract standardized to 1.3% allicin is recommended. Htn or antibacterial effect: 2.5 g/d, or 1 clove or 300 mg of extract.
- Treatment should be evaluated over a 3–6-mo period to determine efficacy. *M. cania*, sporotrichosis, tinea pedis, oral dosage: 2–5 mg of allicin extract/d; topical dosage: sliced cloves or garlic extract (ajoenes) 2–3 times/d to lesion for 1–2 wk.
- Usual dosage is 300 mg of extract, 2–3 times/d, standardized to at least 1.3% allicin (equivalent to approx 3 g or 1 fresh clove daily)

ASSESSMENT POINTS

Moderate daily consumption has no effects on normal individuals. Effects not seen with cooked garlic.

System	Effect	Assessment by Hx	PE	Test
CARDIO	Reduced BP, reduced LDL cholesterol			BP Lipid profile
RESP		Halitosis; sulfuric odor		
ENDO	Hypoglycemia	Insulin, oral hypoglycemic use		FSBG
HEME	Bleeding	Anticoagulant use, coagulopathy, dysfunctional plts, bleeding disorders	Hematomas; poor surgical hemostasis	Prolonged PT (INR) Pit Hgb/Hct
GU Low dose	Enhanced peristalsis	>5 cloves/d Dyspepsia, eructation, pyrosis (heartburn), flatulence		
Large doses	Inhibited peristalsis; possible reduction in stomach cancer	Constipation		
CNS	Spontaneous spinal epidural hematoma	Headache, paralysis	Neuro exam	CT scan
ALLERGY/IMMUNO	Allergic reaction	Garlic oil contact dermatitis	Facial/tongue swelling	

Key Reference: Gardner CD, Lawson LD, Block E, et al. Effect of raw garlic vs. commercial garlic supplements on plasma lipid concentrations in adults with moderate hypercholesterolemia: A Randomized clinical trial, *Arch Intern Med.* 2007;167:346–353.

Perioperative Implications

Perioperative Concerns/Possible Drug Interactions

- High consumption may cause significant antiplatelet activity; ASA, NSAIDs, other plt inhibitors, thrombolytic agents, or certain herbs may cause risk of bleeding, but no clinical data are available
- Hypoglycemia may be ↑ for individuals receiving antidiabetic agents

Monitoring

- Preop PT (INR), blood glucose levels

Airway

- Malodorous breath and skin

Preinduction/Induction

- No special concerns

Maintenance

- Monitor blood glucose levels

Extubation

- No special risks

Adjuvants

- No special risks

Postoperative Period

- Theoretical ↑ risk of bleeding and hypoglycemia

Anticipated Problems/Concerns

- See Postoperative Period
- Pts who are avid garlic consumers should not double up doses to make up for missed doses while undergoing surgery
- If on coumadin postop, should be warned against heavy consumption

Ginger (Zingiber officinale)

Sanup Pathak
Wei Pan

Uses

- Ginger ranks 18th in herbal supplement sales
- Has long been used in Ayurvedic and Chinese medicine for a wide variety of conditions incl arthritis, rheumatism, constipation, indigestion, nausea, vomiting, motion sickness, and diabetes
- In vivo human studies show ginger effective in management of pregnancy assoc and postop N/V
- In vivo animal studies show ginger has significant anti-inflammatory, anti-thrombotic, hypotensive, glucose-lowering, and lipid-lowering effects
- In vitro studies show ginger has significant antioxidant, antitumorogenic, anti-inflammatory, antiviral, and antimicrobial effects

Perioperative Risks

- No toxic or unpleasant side effects reported in human studies with therapeutic doses
- High doses may prolong bleeding time due to inhibition of thromboxane synthetase and stimulation of prostacyclin
- High doses may lower BP

Worry About

- Potential additive or synergistic effects with antiplatelet agents, heparin, or warfarin, which may increase bleeding risks
- Potential hypotensive effect

Overview/Pharmacology

- Pungent constituents: Gingerol, shogaol, gingerdiols, vanilloids, and diarylheptanoids
- Plasma concentration curve defined by a two compartment model with a terminal half life of 7.2 min and a total body clearance of 16.8 mL/min/kg
- 92.4% serum-protein binding with elimination by the liver and gut flora

Mechanism of Action

- Anti-5-HT$_3$ mediates anti-emetic effects
- Direct cholinergic agonist of post-synaptic M$_3$ receptors and inhibitor of pre-synaptic muscarinic autoreceptors: May mediate GI prokinetic effects.
- Cyclooxygenase and lipooxygenase inhibition: Mediates anti-inflammatory and anti-thrombotic effects by decreasing levels of thromboxane B$_2$, prostaglandin E$_2$, and leukotrienes
- Inhibition of cytokine and chemokine induction in vitro: Mediates anti-inflammatory effects
- Insulin sensitization mediates hypoglycemic and lipid-lowing effects
- Calcium channel inhibition mediates decrease in BP
- Vanilloid mediates induction of apoptosis: Anti-tumorogenic effects
- Antioxidant effects may be hepatoprotective and nephroprotective

Usual Dosage/Indications

- Dosage: The total daily dose typically 1–4 g with an onset of anti-emetic effect within 25 min with duration up to 4 hr.
- Doses as high as 15 g/day are well tolerated in human trials.
- Indications
  - May be used to prevent pregnancy-assoc and postop N/V. Indications for post-chemotherapy N/V are less clear.
  - May be used to alleviate dyspepsia and loss of appetite
  - May have anti-inflammatory and anti-thrombotic effects
  - May be useful as an insulin sensitizer
  - May be useful in decreasing serum lipid and cholesterol levels
- Contraindications
  - Must be carefully used in combination with antiplatelet drugs, warfarin, or heparin due to potential for increased bleeding risks

ASSESSMENT POINTS

Systems	Effects	Assessment by Hx	PE
CARDIO	Animal studies: Hypotensive Positive inotropic effect by increase in Ca efflux across sarcoplasmic reticulum		BP/HR
GI	Increases gastric and intestinal motility Promotes gastric, bile, and salivary secretions Antiemetic May be hepatoprotective		
PULM	Antitussive		
HEME	Inhibits thromboxane synthetase Acts as a prostacyclin agonist	Hx of herb use Symptoms of bleeding Antiplatelet agents, heparin or warfarin	
CNS	Animal studies: Prolongs duration of anesthesia induced by sodium hexobarbital Antipyretic through prostaglandin inhibition		

Key References: Ali B, et al. Some phytochemical, pharmacological and toxicological properties of ginger: A review of recent research. *Food Chem Toxicol.* 2008;46:409–420. Grzanna R, et al. Ginger—An herbal medicinal product with broad anti-inflammatory actions. *J Med Food.* 2005;8:125–132.

Possible Drug Interactions

Preoperative Period

- Possible interaction with antiplatelet agents or warfarin

Induction

- May potentiate hexobarbital
- May potentiate hypotension

Postoperative Concerns

- May increase bleeding complications

Anticipated Problems/Concerns

- May increase bleeding complications when used with antiplatelet drugs, warfarin, or heparin
- May consider avoiding use in the presence of gallstone conditions
- May potentiate periop hypotension

Ginkgo

Kiarash Paydar
Gary Fiskum

Uses

• Used for its antioxidant and polyphenol properties, improvement of cognitive performance in demented pts with Alzheimer's disease or vascular dementia, and improvement in symptoms of intermittent claudication, Raynaud's phenomenon and acrocyanosis. Evidence for effectiveness debated
• Used in pts with macular degeneration, sexual dysfunction, symptoms of vertigo, depression, anxiety, and vitiligo
• Also used but ineffective in prevention of age-related memory impairment, dementia, and altitude sickness

Perioperative Risks

• Increased risk of bleeding and drug interactions
• Lack of safety data in certain populations. Therefore, not recommended for use in pregnancy, breastfeeding, and children younger than 12 y of age.
• Commonly reported side effects incl N/V/D, headache, and bleeding

Worry About

• Spontaneous bleeding can occur due to the inhibition of plt aggregation

• Risk of bleeding is further increased if combined with antithrombotic drugs (aspirin, NSAIDs, clopidogrel, dipyridamole), anticoagulant drugs (heparin, warfarin, enoxaparin), and other herbal medicines known to increase bleeding (ginger, garlic, ginseng)
• Can decrease the effectiveness of anticonvulsants (valproate, carbamazepine)
• May enhance the effects of MAO inhibitors (phenelzine, selegiline, tranylcypromine) and increase the risk of serotonin syndrome when taken with SSRIs.
• Interactions have also been reported with calcium channel blockers, trazadone, acetylcholinesterase inhibitors, blood glucose lowering medications, insulin, erectile dysfunction drugs, and thiazide diuretics.

Overview

• Gingko (Ginkgo Biloba) is one of the oldest tree species and is one of the most common supplements used worldwide.

Drug Class/Mechanism of Action/Usual Dose

• Active elements responsible for gingko's medicinal effects incl gingko flavone glycosides and terpine lactones, both obtained from dry leaves of the tree.

• Extracts standardized to contain 24% to 27% ginkgo flavone glycosides and 6% terpines, are commonly found in 40–80 mg oral capsules and recommended TID.
• Gingko has a wide range of properties. Hemodynamic effects incl antagonism of plt activating factor (PAF), lowering serum fibrinogen levels, stimulation of endotheliums derived relaxing factor (EDRF), facilitating prostacycline release and inhibiting nitric oxide.
• CNS effects are mainly attributed to its antioxidant characteristics. Decreasing superoxide release and acting as a scavenger of free radicals results in prevention of hypoxic brain tissue damage and improvement of cerebral metabolism. O_2 utilization in the brain may be improved and age-related changes in the animal hippocampus may be prevented.
• Additional studies have indicated that gingko reversibly inhibits MAO-A and MAO-B, inhibits acetylcholinesterase, and decreases adrenal benzodiazapine receptors.

ASSESSMENT POINTS

System	Effect	Assessment by Hx	PE	Test
HEENT	↑ Ocular blood flow	Bleeding	Mucosal bleeding	
CARDIO	Vasodilation		BP/HR	
HEME	Inhibition of platelet aggregation	Bleeding, bruising	Mucosal bleeding Petechiae	
GI	N/V/D			
CNS	↑ Cerebral blood flow Headache	Headache		
DERM	Contact dermatitis	Exposure	Rash	

Key References: Maclennan KM, Darlington CL, Smith PF. The CNS effects of Ginkgo biloba extracts and ginkgolide B, *Prog Neurobiol.* 67:235–257.
Saper R. *Clinical use of Ginkgo Biloba.* UpToDate; 30 September 2009. www.uptodate.com/patients/content/topic.do?topicKey=~Hv3PN7JVcVB1t.

Perioperative Implications

Preoperative Concerns

• Outside of the potential increased risk of bleeding, periop concern with gingko intake revolves around drug interactions.
• Minimal data on effects in pregnancy, breastfeeding, and pediatrics
• Many pts do not account for alternative medicines when asked for medication lists by their physician.
• Inhibition of plt aggregation can result in significant intraop bleeding, thus D/C gingko at least 36 hr before elective surgery is recommended.

Monitoring

• Routine

Airway

• Avoid nasal intubation to minimize intranasal bleed

Preinduction/Induction

• Avoid excessive hypotension with induction agents, because gingko's subtle vasodilatory effects can further decrease BP and gingko's effects on the adrenal receptors minimizes a normal stress response. Hence, prolonged and excessive hypotension can jeopardize vital organ perfusion.

Maintenance

• Side effects can be amplified with concomitant use of interacting drugs. Such concerns incl bleeding, hypotension, seizures, sedation, serotonin syndrome, and cholinergic crisis.

Extubation

• No known concerns

Postoperative Period

• Avoid administering classes of drugs that may interact and potentiate the effects of gingko as previously mentioned.

Ginseng

Devi Mahendran
Swaminathan Karthik

Uses

- Ginseng has been used for more than 2000 years in Chinese herbal medicine for a variety of proposed health benefits.
- Used as an adaptogen, it is believed to increase the body's resistance to stress and fatigue.
- Reputed to have antioxidant properties
- Reputed to have antihyperglycemic properties. (Some studies have shown Asian ginseng may lower plasma glucose.)
- Used as a stimulant to enhance physical, sexual, and mental performance (it has not been easy to quantify these effects, because scientific studies have not returned consistent results).
- Thought to stimulate the immune system, and to have anticancer properties

Perioperative Risks

- Ginseng has the ability to lower postprandial blood glucose in both pts with diabetes type 2 and non-diabetic pts. This effect may lead to unintended hypoglycemia, particularly in pts who have fasted prior to surgery.
- Ginseng may promote bleeding in surgical pts. Ginsenosides (the active ingredient) in American ginseng has been shown to inhibit plt aggregation. Studies in laboratory rats show prolongation of the coagulation time of thrombin and activated partial thromboplastin. One study suggests that the antiplatelet activity of panaxynol, a constituent of ginseng, may be irreversible in humans. Given these findings, it may be prudent to recommend that pts D/C ginseng use at least 7 d prior to surgery.

Worry About

- The development of hypoglycemia, esp. in diabetic pts taking insulin or oral antihyperglycemic agents
- May have additive effects when used with corticosteroids and may intensify the side effects of corticosteroids
- May lead to development of headache, tremors and manic episodes when used in pts receiving MAO inhibitors such as phenelzine
- Interferes with the pharmacodynamics and drug level monitoring of pts taking digoxin and may increase digoxin levels. The underlying mechanism is unclear.
- May increase the risk of surgical bleeding due to its antiplatelet effects and inhibition of the coagulation cascade
- Ginseng taken together with anticoagulants or with aspirin or other NSAIDs may increase the risk of bleeding.
- Ginseng may have estrogen-like effects and should be avoided in pregnant or breastfeeding women and in children. Avoid the use of ginseng in pts with hormone sensitive conditions, such as breast cancer, uterine cancer, or endometriosis.
- Consumption of ginseng can increase and/or decrease BP. Caution should be used in those with Htn or low BP.

Overview

- The term ginseng refers to several species of the genus *Panax* and comprises a family of plants (American ginseng, Asian ginseng, Chinese ginseng, Korean red ginseng, *Panax* ginseng: *Panax spp.*, incl *P. ginseng C.C. Meyer* and *P. quinquefolius L.*, excluding *Eleutherococcus senticosus*).
- Dietary supplements are typically derived from American ginseng *(Panax quinquefolius)* or Asian ginseng.
- Siberian ginseng *(Eleutherococcus senticosus)* is a different genus and does not contain the ingredients believed to be active in the two forms used in supplements.
- Ginseng can be taken as fresh or dried roots, extracts, solutions, capsules, tablets, sodas, and teas, or used as cosmetics.

Drug Class/Mechanism of Action/Usual Dose

- The active ingredients in American ginseng are panaxosides (saponin glycosides). The active ingredients in Asian ginseng are ginsenosides (triterpenoid glycosides).
- Most of the pharmacological actions of ginseng are attributed to the ginsenosides that belong to a group of compounds known as *steroidal saponins*.

DRUG EFFECTS

System	Effect	Test
CARDIO	Tachycardia, palpitations, Htn with other cardiac stimulants, edema	HR, BP
HEME	Decreases effectiveness of warfarin, inhibition of coagulation cascade	INR, PT, PTT
NEURO	Excessive use: Somnolence, hypertonia, nervousness, and excitability mania in pts on phenelzine	
ENDO	Hypoglycemia	Blood glucose
REPROD	Mastalgia, postmenopausal bleeding	Hct

Key References: Yuan CS, et al. American ginseng reduces warfarin's effect in healthy patients. *Ann Intern Med.* 2004;141:23–27. Sotaniemi EA, et al. Ginseng therapy in non–insulin–dependent diabetic patients. *Diabetes Care.* 1995;18:1373–1375. Scaglione F, et al. Efficacy and safety of the standardized ginseng extract G 115 for potentiating vaccination against common cold and/or influenza syndrome. *Drugs Exp Clin Res.* 1996;22:65–72.

Perioperative Implications

Preoperative Concerns
- Check coagulation studies, monitor blood glucose

Monitoring
- Standard

Induction
- No specific concerns

Airway
- No specific concerns

Postoperative concerns
- Monitor blood glucose level, monitor for signs of excessive postop bleeding

Glucosamine Sulfate

Holly Munnis
Anthony Passannante

Uses

- For pain assoc with osteoarthritis (OA), particularly of the knee
- IBD
- Other inflammatory disorders such as rheumatoid arthritis, psoriasis

Perioperative Risks

- No convincing evidence of increased periop risk due to glucosamine therapy
- No known significant interactions with commonly administered anesthetic drugs

Worry About

- Increase in INR in pts on warfarin who initiate glucosamine therapy, or increase glucosamine dose

Overview

- Classified as a food additive, not FDA regulated, made from crustacean skeletons
- As monotherapy, little consistent evidence of therapeutic effect
- Side effect profile indistinguishable from placebo and better than NSAIDs
- In combination with chondroitin may prolong the time to total knee replacement in those with severe OA

- High oral bioavailability with substantial first pass metabolism, freely diffusable with a 28–58 hr half life

Drug Class/Mechanism of Action/Usual Dose

- Glucosamine is a component of the extracellular matrix of articular cartilage.
- Recommended oral dose is 1500 mg qd, may have anti-inflammatory effects
- The mechanism of action of glucosamine is unknown, presumably aids in cartilage repair

DRUG EFFECTS

System	Effect	Test
COAG	May potentiate warfarin	PT/INR if pt on warfarin
ENDO	No consistent effect	Glucose if otherwise indicated

Key References: Knudson JF, Sokol GH. Potential glucosamine-warfarin interaction resulting in increased international normalized ratio: Case report and review of the literature and Medwatch database. *Pharmacotherapy.* 2008;28:540–548. Albert SG, et al. The effect of glucosamine on serum HDL cholesterol and apolipoprotein A1 levels in people with diabetes. *Diabetes Care.* 2007;30:2800–2803. Vangsness Jr CT, Spiker W, Erickson J. A review of evidence-based medicine for glucosamine and chondroitin sulfate use in knee osteoarthritis. *Arthroscopy.* 2009;25:86–94. Bruyere O, et al. Total joint replacement after glucosamine sulphate treatment in knee osteoarthritis: Results of a mean 8-year observation of patients from two previous 3-year, randomised, placebo-controlled trials. *Osteoarthritis Cartilage.* 2008;16:254–260.

Perioperative Implications

- Glucosamine therapy has no significant periop anesthetic implications. No need to interrupt therapy for a surgical procedure, no reason to modify an anesthetic plan due to glucosamine, and there is no urgency with regards to restarting therapy postop.

Glycine

Ted Strickland
Keith E. Hude

Uses

- Glycine is an inhibitory neurotransmitter in the brainstem and spinal cord.
- Glycine and GABA receptors may mediate the effects of inhaled anesthetics.
- It is a nonessential amino acid sold as a natural sugar substitute, a sedative, an antacid; to promote muscle growth, ↓ Sx of BPH, as an polyphenol, and antipsychotic.
- Glycine 1.5% used as a nonhemolytic irrigation solution during TURP.
- Antagonists of glycine binding to NMDA receptor complex are used as anticonvulsants.
- Attempts to use glycine and other NMDA agonist in schizophrenia have had little success.
- Intrathecal glycine is not different than placebo in CRPS treatment.

Perioperative Risks

- TURP syndrome incidence is 0.5–8% and mortality rate is 0.2–0.8% up to 25% in severe TURP syndrome.
- Glycine metabolized to ammonia can lead to hyperammonemic encephalopathy.

Worry About

- Glycine irrigation is contraindicated in pts with anuria.
- TURP syndrome is thought to be due to hyponatremia, hypo-osmolality, and elevated glycine levels due to absorption of irrigation fluid. Onset from 15 min after starting irrigation up to 24 hr postop. Manifestions likely related to the glycine load incl myocardial depression, hemodynamic changes, and visual disturbances. Other Sx incl burning sensations in the face, N/V, weakness, confusion, seizure, coma.
- Glycine irrigation should be used with caution in pts with CHF.

Overview/Pharmacology

- Smallest amino acid. Glycogenic. Major inhibitory neurotransmitter.
- Glycine is inhibitory on ligand-gated, strychnine-sensitive Cl–channel receptors but excitatory on strychnine-insensitive NMDA receptors where it is a cofactor for activation of the NMDA receptor by L-glutamate.
- Glycine metabolism: Primarily transamination to serine, and deamination to ammonia which is converted to urea and excreted by the kidneys. A portion of absorbed glycine is excreted unchanged by the kidneys.

Drug Class/Usual Dose

- Glycine 1.5% solution is used as an irrigation solution during endoscopic procedures, esp. TURP. It is nontoxic, has a refractive index close to that of water, and is nonhemolytic despite a hypotonic osmolality of 200–220 mOsm/L.
- Homeopathic use for BPH at 780 mg/d × 2 wk and then 390 mg for the next 3 mo.
- Glycine 30–60 g/day improves negative symptoms of schizophrenia.
- NMDA receptor allows influx of Na^+ and Ca^{2+}. Overstimulation of this channel leads to Ca^{2+} overload in neurons, which has been shown to be neurotoxic. Glycine antagonists at the NMDA receptor potentiate GABA receptor-mediated events, resulting in ↑ Cl^- conductance, leading to membrane hyperpolarization and neuroprotection. Glycine site antagonists ↓ the release of excitatory amino acids, such as glutamate, which are known to potentiate cerebral ischemic injury.

Possible Drug Interactions

- Clozapine, haloperidol, olanzapine, risperidone

ASSESSMENT POINTS

System	Effect	Assessment by Hx	PE	Test
CARDIO	T wave depression or inversion, increased long-term risk of MI Htn or hypotension may occur in TURP syndrome	Homeopathic use or glycine 1.5% irrigation		BP, HR, ECG
HEME	Antagonists assoc with aplastic anemia	Homeopathic glycine use	Skin/mucous membranes for infection/petechiae	CBC, peripheral smear, bone marrow Bx
GU	Metabolites oxalate and glycolate may produce renal failure	TURP with glycine irrigation or homeopathic use		Chem 7
GI	Gastric antacid			
CNS	Glycine accumulates in cells, which ↑ cerebral edema, hyponatremia, hypotonicity, and direct toxicity account for neurologic Sxs in TURP syndrome Encephalopathy through ammonia metabolite ↓ Negative Sx of schizophrenia	Headache, N/V, visual changes, seizure, weakness, encephalopathy, lethargy	Mental status, visual acuity, strength	Serum, Na serum osmolality
PULM	Pulm edema (↓ with spinal anesthesia)	TURP	SOB, wheeze, frothy sputum	CXR, SpO_2

Key Reference: Hawary A, Mukhtar K, Sinclair A, Pearce I. Transurethral resection of the prostate syndrome: Almost gone but not forgotten. *J Endourol.* 2009;23:2013–2020. FDA Professional Drug Information. Glycine. www.drugs.com/pro/glycine.html.

Perioperative Implications

Preoperative Period

- Elicit recent Hx of glycine use as homeopathic treatment.
- Anuria is a contraindication to use of glycine irrigation. Caution in oliguric pts.

Induction/Maintenance

- No known interactions with homeopathic doses of glycine.
- If pt is using glycine as a homeopathic antipsychotic, affect/mental status may be problematic given underlying disease and side effect profile of drug.

- Risk of TURP syndrome. Be aware of degree of blood loss and amount of irrigation used. If regional anesthetic used, monitor for symptoms of glycine toxicity: N/V, visual changes, weakness. Also monitor for hemodynamic instability; ECG changes, hypo- or Htn.
- With intraop onset of TURP syndrome, surgery should be terminated as soon as possible.

Postoperative Concerns

- TURP syndrome may occur within 15 min of beginning irrigation or as late as 24 hr postop. Monitor for signs of changing mental status, hemodynamic instability, seizures.
- Seizures, if caused by glycine activity on NMDA receptors, could be treated with NMDA receptor antagonists or glycine antagonists. Mg^{2+} exerts a negative effect on NMDA receptors and Mg^{2+} may be low after TURP, so a trial of Mg^{2+} therapy may be warranted.

Goldenseal (Hydrastis Canadensis)

ALTERNATIVE MEDICINE

Lynn A. Fenton

Other Names

• Eye balm, eye root, goldenroot, golden seal, goldsiegel, ground raspberry, Indian dye, Indian plant, Indian tumeric, jaundice root, orange root, Sceau D'Or, tumeric root, Warnera, wild curcuma, yellow Indian paint, yellow paint, yellow puccoon, yellow root

Etiology/Sources

• Goldenseal is a native, North American herb (*f. Ranunculaceae*); rhizome and root used.

Indications/Uses

• Goldenseal (GS) is considered POSSIBLY SAFE for short-term, appropriate use.
• GS may be purchased in salve, tablet, bulk powder, or tincture forms.
• Oral: Used for treating gastritis, peptic ulcers, colitis, atonic dyspepsia with hepatic Sx, jaundice, anorexia, UTIs, menorrhagia, dysmenorrhea, gonorrhea, postpartum and internal hemorrhage, cancer, conjunctivitis, tinnitus, catarrhal deafness, earaches, malaria, nasal congestion, upper resp tract inflammation, canker sores, and sore gums.
• Topical: Used for eczema, itching, acne, dandruff, ringworm, herpes labialis, and wounds.
• Goldendseal has been used orally to create false negative urine tests for several illicit drugs.

• Investigational uses: Antineoplastic and anti-HIV treatment.
• Historical uses: Native American Indians have used GS for multiple medicinal purposes and for the production of a yellow dye.

Perioperative Risks

• Prolonged use can cause digestive disorders, constipation, excitatory states, hallucinations, and occasional delirium.
• Side effects of drug (large doses): Mucocutaneous irritation, GI tract upset (N/V), cardiac and uterine contractility, bradycardia, cardiac damage, vasoconstriction/Htn, spasms, neonatal jaundice, hyperbilirubinemia, and death.
• See section on Perioperative Implications/Drug and Herbal Interactions.

Anticipated Problems/Concerns

• Not to be used by pregnant or lactating women (UNSAFE), neonates (UNSAFE), children (LIKELY UNSAFE), in pts with CV disease, seizure disorders, or coagulation problems, or when used orally in high doses or long-term (LIKELY UNSAFE).

Overview/Mechanism of Action/Pharmacology

• Compounds: Isoquinoline alkaloids are the main bioactive constituents. The chief alkaloids are berberine, hydrastine, and (–)-canadine (no information available).

• Berberine: Thought to act intraluminally; exerts antimicrobial activity against numerous bacteria, fungi, and protozoa; blocks adhesion of bacteria to epithelial cells to inhibit intestinal secretory responses to cholera and *E. coli* toxins; may increase effectiveness of insulin; may act as a vasoconstrictor to decrease uterine bleeding.
• Hydrastine: At low doses is hypotensive agent; at higher doses is a peripheral vasoconstrictor.

Drug Class/Usual Dose

• Oral doses: 0.5–1 g tid of the dried root or rhizome × 1 wk.
• Liquid extract: (1:1, 60% EtOH) – 0.3–1 mL TID × 1 wk.
• Tincture: (1:10, 60% EtOH) – 2–4 mL tid × 1 wk.
• Oral rinse and topical solution: 6 g dried root/150 mL H_2O tid – qid × 1 wk.
• LD50 of *berberine* in humans is reported to be 27.5 mg/kg.
• Doses in excess of 500 mg of *berberine* (or 8–100 g of dry root depending on the *berberine* concentration) can lead to significant toxicity.

ASSESSMENT POINTS

System	Effect	Assessment by Hx	PE/Test
CARDIO	Htn Hypotension Bradycardia Inotropic effect	CV response to Rx	HR, BP, ECG
PULM	Resp failure	SOB, DOE	Wheezing/SaO$_2$, ABG, CXR
GI	Mucosal irritation	N/V, diarrhea	Turgor of mucous membranes/ check Hct and serum lytes for evidence of dehydration, metabolic disturbances
GU	Oxytotic Diuretic	Abortion Polyuria	Uterine US, tocometry Urinary electrolytes
ENDO	Increase effectiveness of insulin	Hypoglycemic SNS, Sx Tachycardia, Hypotension Hypokalemia	CBG, serum glu and K$^+$ HR, BP, ECG
CNS	CNS stimulation Central paralysis	Muscle spasms, excitatory state, hallucinations, seizures, occasional delirium	EMG, EEG
HEME	Hemostatic	Oppose anticoagulation	INR, PTT

Key Reference: Jellin JM, Gregory P, Batz F, Hitchens K, et al. *Pharmacist's letter/Prescriber's letter natural medicines comprehensive database.* 3rd ed. Stockton, CA: Therapeutic Research Faculty; 2000:504–506.

Perioperative Implications/Possible Drug-Herb Interactions

• Acid-inhibiting drugs: Might increase stomach acid thereby interfering with antacid-type meds.
• Antihypertensive agents: Vasoconstrictive action of *hydrastine* might interfere with BP control.
• B vitamins: Prolonged use can decrease B vitamin absorption.

• Barbiturates: May potentiate barbiturate-induced sleep time.
• Bilirubin (BR): May increase BR levels (*berberine* increases total and unbound BR).
• Heparin or coumadin: Can inhibit anticoagulant effects due to *berberine*.
• Highly protein-bound drugs: *Berberine* can displace highly protein-bound drugs.

• Sedative drugs and herbs: Concomitant use of drugs/herbs with sedative properties may enhance the therapeutic (additive effect) or adverse effects.

Licorice (Glycyrrhiza Glabra)

R. Blaine Easley

Uses

- Incidence in USA: One of the top ten herbal medications
- Medical: Historically used to improve immune function and treat a variety of conditions incl PUD, duodenal ulcers, cough and/or bronchitis, atherosclerosis, chronic fatigue syndrome, various cancers, AIDS, and Addison's disease. Most recently a study has demonstrated its effectiveness in relieving postop sore throat.

Perioperative Risks

- Unknown. Theoretical problems in pts with impaired renal function, Htn, chronic liver disease, cardiac arrhythmias, and hypertonia.
- Potential for drug interactions. Pseudohyperaldosteronism has been produced experimentally in healthy subjects taking >100 g/wk.

Worry About

- Pseudohyperaldosteronism: Documented mineralocorticoid effects that result in fluid retention, hypernatremia, hypokalemia, and edema
- Hypertension: Direct effects on vascular smooth muscle tone independent of mineralocorticoid properties
- Vasospasm and/or headache: Case reports of cerebral artery spasm causing severe headache, visual disturbances, and potential ischemia have recently been published.

- Hypokalemia and/or muscle weakness: Chronic usage related to hypokalemic myopathies, muscle cramps, and skeletal muscle spasms
- Arrhythmias: Rare side effect, but more worrisome in pts with Hx of arrhythmias requiring medication (e.g., digoxin)
- Paresthesias: Numbness in extremities may be a sign of licorice toxicity

Overview/Pharmacology

- Licorice is the common name given to various substances derived from the plant root *Glycyrrhiza glabra* (Spanish licorice). This plant is a perennial that grows 3–7 ft high and originated from Europe and Asia. Also called sweet root and licorice root.
- Glycyrrhizin and/or glycyrrhizic acid (the glucoside form) and glycyrrhetininic acid (the glycoside form) are the most important substances or metabolites found in licorice. The roots also contain coumarins, flavonoids, volatile oils, and plant sterols.
- Licorice and its components are metabolized and excreted by the liver and kidneys.
- Mineralocorticoid effects of licorice, via glycyrrhetininic acid, result from the inhibition of 11-β-hydroxysteroid dehydrogenase (an enzyme that normally inactivates cortisol by converting its C11 alcohol to a ketone). Excess glucocorticoids then bind to mineralocorticoid receptors and produce a mineralocorticoid response, as evidenced by ↑ sodium retention and Htn. Thereby, licorice ingestion creates a syndrome of hyperaldosteronism characterized by hypernatremia, Htn, hypokalemia, and suppression of the renin-angiotensin system.
- Glycyrrhetinic acid also inhibits 15-hydroxyprostaglandin dehydrogenase and prostaglandin reductase. These two enzymes are important in the metabolism of prostaglandin E and F_2, perhaps explaining licorice's immunologic benefits, effects on reducing cough and/or bronchospasm, protection of gastric mucosa, and benefit by decreased plt aggregation.

Drug Class/Usual Dose

- Made from peeled and unpeeled dried root compounded and sold as powders, dry extracts, and liquid extracts. Some preparations such as deglycyrrhized licorice (DGL) have removed harmful compounds. Unfortunately, preparation and advertising of these compounds is unregulated by the FDA.
- Licorice is taken in the following manner
  - Dried root: 1–5 g PO tid, up to 6 wk (indication: general use)
  - Extract: (1:1 preparation) 2–5 ml PO tid, up to 6 wk (indication: general use)
  - DGL extract: 1.5–3 g/d for peptic ulcer
  - DGL extract: 380–760 mg PO 20 min before meals for peptic ulcer

ASSESSMENT POINTS

System	Effect	Assessment by Hx	PE	Test
CNS	Headache Visual changes Paresthesia	Exposure/use of licorice	Visual acuity Sensory exam	Neuro consult, possible MRI
CARDIO	Hypovolemia Hypervolemia Htn Arrhythmia	Exposure/use of licorice	BP/HR, consider orthostatics	ECG rhythm strip
GI	Black stools (rare) Laxative effect	Report of loose, dark stool	Abd exam	Stool guaiac
HEME	↓ Clotting (rare)	Bleeding problems	Plts, PT/PTT	
ENDO	Hyperglycemia Hypernatremia Hypokalemia	Exposure/use of licorice Wt gain, ↑ Urination		Serum chemistries

Key References: Kaye AD, et al. Herbal medicines: Current trends in anesthesiology practice—A hospital survey. *J Clin Anesth.* 2000;12:468–471.
Agarwal A, et al. An evaluation of the efficacy of licorice gargle for attenuating postoperative sore throat: A prospective, randomized, single-blind study. *Anesth Analg.* 2009;109:77–81.

Possible Drug Interactions

Preoperative Period

- Multiple adverse drug interactions reported in pts using licorice preparations and prescription medications. Licorice can interfere with the function of hormone supplements (e.g., birth control pills), oral hypoglycemic agents, and corticosteroids. Electrolyte imbalances and GI symptoms can be worsened by usage of licorice with diuretics and laxatives. Digoxin usage and licorice-induced hypokalemia can be potentially arrhythmogenic.
- Electrolyte abn of hypokalemia, hypernatremia, and metabolic alkalosis should be sought and corrected before surgery in high dose frequent users.
- Pt should be instructed to D/C use of the herbal medicine approx 2 wk before elective surgery.

Induction/Maintenance

- No known interactions with licorice metabolites. However, pseudohyperaldosteronism should be considered and anesthetic management directed at the problems of hypokalemia, Htn, and fluid status. Placement of an arterial line and/or central venous line should be considered in symptomatic pts. (See Hyperaldosteronism [secondary] in Diseases section.)

Adjuvants/Regional Anesthesia/Reversal

- No known interactions. Consider pros and cons of NSAID use intraop, esp. if no assessment of renal function. Careful attention to neurologic exam and/or paresthesias before initiation of regional technique.

Emergence/Extubation

- No known interactions. Acute topical administration has been used to prevent postop sore throat without adverse effect. However, hypokalemia with or without a Hx of muscle weakness could potentially modify nondepolarizing muscle relaxant response.

Postoperative Concerns

- Failure of resolution of preop symptoms attributed to licorice use with D/C of licorice-containing compound should prompt investigation of other causes.
- Continued monitoring of fluid and electrolyte status. If problems with hypokalemia continue, despite potassium supplementation, then consider potassium-sparing diuretics (e.g., triamterene), a competitive aldosterone antagonist (e.g., spironolactone), and investigating other causes.

Melatonin (*N*-Acetyl-5-Methoxytryptamine, Bevitamel, Vitamist, Melatonex)

Ori Gottlieb

Risks

- May interact with other CNS-acting medications such as hypnotics, sedatives, or psychotropics
- Contraindicated during pregnancy and when breastfeeding
- May cause excessive somnolence
- Not recommended in infants and children due to insufficient data
- Not FDA controlled—quality/potency may vary
- The use of animal-source melatonin products is not recommended due to the risk of viral contamination or infection.

Overview/Pharmacology

- Secretion modulated by enzymes secreted by hypothalamus in response to dark
- Exogenous routes of administration: Oral tablets, capsules, lozenges, teas, sprays
- Unlike endogenous melatonin, oral doses undergo first-pass hepatic metabolism with a bioavailability of 30–50%
- Crosses the blood-brain barrier
- The mean elimination $T_{1/2}$ is 45 min. Only 0.01% of melatonin is excreted unchanged in urine.

- Pharmacologic tolerance to melatonin has not been described
- Alcohol may potentiate side effects

Usual Dose

- Taken 1–2 hr before usual sleep time
- Significant individual dose variation
  - Insomnia: 0.3–3 mg PO q.p.m.
  - Insomnia with depression: 5–10 mg PO q.p.m.
  - Jet lag: 3–6 mg PO q.p.m.—on the destination's sleep schedule; may require up to 5 nights
  - Tinnitus: 3 mg PO q.p.m.
  - Circadian disruption/blindness
  - Adults: 5–7 mg PO q.p.m.
  - Children: 2.5–7.5 mg PO q.p.m.

Uses

- Regulates sleep-wake cycles
- Rx for jet lag, shift work, depression
- Use as antineoplastic, and anticonvulsant is under investigation
- Questionable benefit in treating breast cancer and migraines
- Categorized as a nutraceutical

Endogenous Actions

- Secreted by the pineal gland in response to the absence of photic stimuli (known as the 'Darkness Hormone')
- Reduces the body's core temp in preparation for sleep
- Secretion peaks during the pediatric years and decreases with age
- In some way, melatonin is involved in reproductive function. Receptors found in reproductive tissues.
- Endogenously produced melatonin may have a significant role in deferring a number of free radical-related diseases and some pathophysiological changes assoc with aging.

Exogenous Actions

- Resets the body to the environmental clock and allows pts to normalize physiologic and behavioral sleep patterns
- Used commonly as a preventive and therapeutic anti-jet lag agent
- Useful in individuals with poor circadian synchrony such as the visually impaired

ASSESSMENT POINTS

System	Effect	Assessment by Hx	Test
CNS	Drowsiness, prolonged sedation	Hx of sleepiness	
CARDIO	Palpitations SOB		ECG

Key References: Naguib M, Samarkandi AH. The comparative dose-response effects of melatonin and midazolam for premedication of adult patients: A double-blinded, placebo-controlled study. *Anesth Analg*. 2000;91:473–479. Kain Z, et al. Preoperative melatonin and its effects on induction and emergence in children undergoing anesthesia and surgery, *Anesthesiology*. 2009;111:44–49. Samarkandi A, et al. Melatonin vs. midazolam premedication in children: A double blind, placebo controlled study, *Eur J Anaesthesiol*. 2005;22:189–196.

Perioperative Implications

- May be used as a preop anxiolytic agent. Comparable anxiolysis to midazolam without amnestic effect. Questionable effects in the elderly.

- Studied in children as a premedicant; shown to be comparable to midazolam but with faster recovery and a lower incidence of postop cognitive impairment and delirium.

- Melatonin ↑ benzodiazepines binding to receptor sites, enhancing activity
- Methamphetamine users may also be taking melatonin to offset the insomnia brought on by the drug.

Nutraceuticals

Amir Baluch
Alan Kaye

Risks

• Approx 64% of pts have taken or are taking a neutraceutical agent.
• Incidence in USA: More than 50% take dietary supplements and in a study of over 1000 outpatients, approx 33% were using herbals at the time of surgery or pain procedures.
• 31% use herbal drugs in combination with prescriptions
• 48% use them with OTC drugs
• Up to 70% of pts do not inform the physician about use of these products at the time of routine anesthetic preop assessment.
• Some of these agents have the potential to cause serious drug interactions, incl bleeding, prolonged sedation, and hemodynamic instability periop.

Perioperative Risks

• Hemodynamic and/or CV instability or collapse
• Increased risk of bleeding (in particular many of the "G" herbals and EPA [not DHA] component of fish oil, so not a problem for people supplementing with algael DHA)
• Potential for prolongation of anesthetic and barbiturates
• Electrolyte imbalance and/or renal dysfunction
• Abn thyroid function

Worry About

• Oversedation from prolonged effects of barbiturates
• Hemodynamic instability

• Unexplained bleeding, particularly in pts on anticoagulants and/or antifibrinolytics
• Bradycardia or tachycardia
• Myocardial infarction, stroke
• Liver toxicity and immunosuppression

Overview/Pharmacology

• Particular concern regarding specific herbs and/or supplements

DRUG EFFECTS

Name	Common Uses	Possible Side Effects/Drug Interactions
Creatine	Endurance/strength, bodybuilding	Exacerbation of pre-existing renal dysfunction
Echinacea	Common colds, coughs	May cause hepatotoxicity or increase barbiturate duration
Ephedra (Ma-Huang)	OTC diet aids	Severe intraop hypotension; arrhythmias; enhanced sympathomimetic effects with MAOI; Htn with oxytocin
Feverfew	Migraine prophylactic	Inhibition of plt activity with ↑ bleeding, ↑ hemodynamic instability
Garlic	↓ BP and lipids; antioxidant and antithrombolytic	May potentiate warfarin; will see increased INR (PT), hypotension
GBL/GHB	Bodybuilding, sleep inducement, wt loss	GHB is "date rape" drug; may cause death, seizures, vomiting, bradycardia, slowed breathing, prolonged anesthetic
Ginger	Antinauseant	May ↑ bleeding time, hemodynamic instability
Ginkgo biloba	Circulatory stimulant	May enhance bleeding with anticoagulants or antithrombotics, decrease effectiveness of barbiturates
Ginseng	Energy-level enhancer, antioxidant	Tachycardia, Htn, mastalgia, postmenopausal bleeding, potential for ↑ bleeding with warfarin, hypoglycemia, Htn
Goldenseal	Diuretic	Works as an aquaretic (no sodium excreted); may worsen edema/Htn
Kava-Kava	Anxiolytic	Potentiates barbiturates and benzodiazepines; portion of kava can cause liver toxicity and liver failure
Licorice	Gastric/duodenal ulcers	May cause ↑ BP, hypokalemia, edema; contraindicated with chronic liver conditions, renal insufficiency
St. John's wort	Mild/moderate depression	May prolong anesthesia (anecdotal); pseudoephedrine, MAOIs, SSRIs should be avoided; can potentially interact with meperidine and cause serotoninergic crisis
Triax metabolic accelerator (Triax)	Wt loss aid	Contains potent thyroid hormone; may cause heart attacks, strokes; altered thyroid function
Valerian	Mild sedative or anxiolytic	May potentiate barbiturates, and other gabbaergic sedatives
Vitamin E	Antioxidant, anticlotting agent	↑ BP in Htn pts with too high a daily dosage (400 IU/d); ↑ bleeding; may worsen vitamin K deficiency; may ↓ thyroid hormone levels

Key References: Miller LG. Herbal medicinals: Selected clinical considerations focusing on known or potential drug-herb interactions. *Arch Intern Med.* 1998;158:2200–2211. Kaye A, Baluch A, Hoover J. Herbal supplements and nutrients in anesthesiology. In: Meckling KA, ed. *Nutrient: Drug interactions*. Boca Raton, Fl: Taylor and Francis Group, Publishers; 2006. Kaye AD, Clarke AC, Sabar R. Herbal medicines: Current trends in anesthesiology practice–a hospital survey. *J Clin Anesth.* 2000;12:468–471.

Perioperative Risks

• The American Society of Anesthesiologists (ASA) recommends that all herbal medications be D/C 2–3 wk prior to elective surgery, because it takes 5–6 half lives for an agent to leave the body, and these substances lack uniform uptake, distribution, and elimination as they are not considered drugs by the Food and Drug Administration.

ALTERNATIVE MEDICINE

Phytosterols

Lee A. Fleisher

Uses

- Naturally occurring in human diet
- Used as a supplement, esp. in margarines, to reduce cholesterol levels
- May also possess anti-inflammatory, antipyretic, antineoplastic, and immune-modulating properties
- Some recent evidence questions the beneficial effect of phytosterols and potential for increased CV risk

Perioperative Risks

- None known

Worry About

- Pts may be taking phytosterols because of hypercholesterolemia and occult CAD

Overview/Pharmacology

- Phytosterols (incl plant sterols and stanols) are natural components of edible vegetable oils such as sunflower seed oil and, as such, are natural constituents of the human diet.

- It is difficult to incorporate free sterols into edible fats and/or oils because of their insolubility, whereas sterols esterified to fatty acids are more fat soluble.
- In the intestine, most sterol esters are hydrolyzed to free sterols as part of the normal digestive process.
- Plant stanols are hydrogenation products of the respective plant sterols, e.g., campestanol and/or campesterol and sitostanol and/or sitosterol, and are found in nature at very low levels.
- Enrichment of foods such as margarines with plant sterols and stanols is one of the recent developments in functional foods to enhance the cholesterol-lowering ability of traditional food products.
- May reduce the absorption of some fat soluble vitamins. Randomized trials have shown that plant sterols and stanols lower blood concentrations of β-carotene by about 25%, concentrations of α-carotene by 10%, and concentrations of vitamin E by 8%.

Drug Class/Usual Dose

- Consumption of plant sterols and plant stanols lowers blood cholesterol levels by inhibiting the absorption of dietary and endogenously produced cholesterol from the small intestine, and the plant sterols and/or stanols are only very poorly absorbed themselves.
- This inhibition is related to the similarity in physicochemical properties of plant sterols and stanols and cholesterol and may be related to two mechanisms:
  - The greater the amount of plant sterols and/or stanols, the lower the solubility and perhaps the greater the amount of cholesterol precipitated. Cholesterol in the crystalline form cannot be absorbed.
  - Competition for space in mixed micelles
- Being marketed in new margarine formulations

ASSESSMENT POINTS

System	Effect	Assessment by Hx	PE	Test
CARDIO	Hypercholesterolemia	CAD, angina	Chest pain	ECG
GI	Malabsorption of some vitamins			

Key Reference: Weingärtner O, Böhm M, Laufs U. Controversial role of plant sterol esters in the management of hypercholesterolaemia. *Eur Heart J.* 2009;30(4):404–409.

Possible Drug Interactions

- No known drug interactions

Anticipated Problems/Concerns

- None known

Pseudoephedrine

Uses

- An OTC sympathomimetic commonly used as a nasal decongestant or for opening obstructed eustachian ostia
- Used in the symptomatic treatment of reactive airway disease; however, appears to be ineffective as a bronchodilator
- Also used for treatment of ejaculatory dysfunction, and as a starting material for illicit drug manufacturing
- Abuse and addiction to OTC stimulants does occur, particularly in those with eating disorders or erratic work hours such as truck drivers. Assoc with myocardial injury and withdrawal symptoms in this setting.

Perioperative Risks

- Concern about the coadministration of other sympathomimetic agents because of the possibility of additive effects and increased toxicity

- Pressor effects of pseudoephedrine are more pronounced in
  - Hypertensive pts
  - Pts taking β-adrenergic blocking drugs
  - Pts taking serotonin/norepinephrine reuptake inhibitors (SNRIs)
- May ↑ heart irritability
- MAO inhibitors, by increasing the quantity of NE, potentiate pseudoephedrine's indirect pressor effects; infrequently, a hypertensive crisis may result
- May also reduce the antihypertensive effects of reserpine and methyldopa

Overview/Pharmacology

- Acts directly on α- and, to a lesser degree, β-adrenergic receptors. Has an indirect effect by releasing NE from its storage sites.
- α-Adrenergic effects result from the inhibition of the production of cAMP by inhibition of the enzyme adenylyl cyclase, whereas β-adrenergic effects result from stimulation of adenylyl cyclase activity

- Acts directly on α-receptors in the mucosa of the resp tract producing vasoconstriction, therefore shrinking mucous membranes, reducing edema and congestion
- May relax bronchial smooth muscle by stimulation of β-adrenergic receptors, but this effect is not consistent
- Readily and completely absorbed; elimination is predominantly renal and pH dependent

Drug Class/Dose

- Direct and indirect sympathomimetic
- $T_{1/2}$ 6 h for standard preparation and 12 h for extended release
- Adults and children >12 y of age: 60 mg q 4–6 h with a maximum dosage of 240 mg/d
- Children 6–11 y of age: 30 mg q 4–6 h with a maximum dosage of 120 mg/d
- Children 2–5 y of age: 15 mg q 4–6 h with maximum dosage of 60 mg/d
- Children <2: No FDA approved dosing

DRUG EFFECTS

System	Effect	Assessment by Hx	PE	Test
CARDIO	Htn, dysrhythmias, cardiac irritability	Palpitations	BP/HR	ECG
HEENT	Mucosal vasoconstriction Reduction of vol of nasal mucosa Drainage of sinus secretions, opening of obstructed ostia	Nasal congestion Head stuffiness	Absence of hyperemia of nasal mucosa	
NEURO	Nervousness, excitability, restlessness, dizziness, weakness, insomnia, headaches, drowsiness		Tremors, anxiousness	
GU/RENAL	Urinary retention	Difficulty voiding, emptying bladder completely	Tachycardia, Htn	Bladder US, postvoid residuals
GI	N/V		Abd tenderness	

Key References: Kanfer I. Pharmacokinetics of oral decongestants. *Pharmacotherapy.* 1993;13:116S–128S. Werler MM. Teratogen update: Pseudoephedrine. *Birth Defects Res A Clin Mol Teratol.* 2006;76:445–452.

Perioperative Implications

Preoperative Concerns

- Oral administration of usual doses to normotensive pts usually produces minimal effects
- Htn, tachycardia in those sensitive
- Those with concomitant hyperthyroidism, ischemic heart disease, or prostatic hypertrophy may be more at risk
- May ↑ the irritability of the heart muscle and result in multifocal PVCs
- May be teratogenic; avoid use in pregnant pts if possible; avoid use in breastfeeding women
- Geriatric pts may be esp. sensitive

- Overdose may cause hallucinations, CNS depression, seizures, and death

Monitoring
- Routine

Induction
- Increased absorption of pseudoephedrine with antacid administration

Airway
- Improvement of airway edema and congestion related to mucosal hyperemia is often seen

Maintenance
- Careful administration/titration of other sympathomimetic drugs

Regional Anesthesia
- Pts may be more prone to urinary retention with regional techniques that block sacral roots.

Postoperative Concerns
- Resumption of drug should not pose particular problems once vital signs are stable.

Anticipated Problems/Concerns

- Caution in administering other sympathomimetic agents
- β-Adrenergic blocking drugs may ↑ pressor effect
- Antihypertensive effects of reserpine, methyldopa may be diminished

Psyllium, Bulk-Forming Laxatives (Plantago Isphagula, Plantago Ovata)

Amar Setty
Abraham C. Gaupp

Uses

- Chronic constipation (requires adequate hydration)
- Diarrhea (bulk-forming agent)
- IBS
- Management of hemorrhoids
- Regulates the effluent for pts with colostomies
- Cholesterol-lowering agent for mild hypercholesterolemia

Perioperative Risks

- Allergic reaction (rare) from ingested or inhaled powder
- Do not use if vomiting, intestinal obstruction, abd pain, nausea, or fecal impaction is present
- Do not give other oral drugs for 2 hr before or after psyllium

Worry About

- Stenosis or obstruction of esophagus or GI tract
- Adequate hydration
- Constipation, impaction, or obstruction can result without adequate hydration
- Loss of diabetic control (use sugar-free preparations in diabetics)
- Decreases absorption of oral medications

Overview/Pharmacology

- Psyllium causes retention of water, which ↑ fecal bulk (expands 8–14 × normal size in water). This provides a mechanical stimulus for peristalsis and the rate of bowel transit.
- Effective within 12–24 hr
- Maximum effect after several days

- May stabilize postprandial glucose levels in NIDDM
- Other names
  - Trade names: Metamucil, Hydrocil, Fiberall, Citrucel
  - Herbal names: Psyllium seed, black; psyllium seed, blonde

Drug Class/Usual Dose

- Daily dose 10–30 g total in divided doses PO
- Available in powder, wafer, cereal, capsules, chewable pieces
- Must be taken with adequate fluid

DRUG EFFECTS

System	Effect	PE	Test
ENDO	Altered blood sugar	Symptoms of hyperglycemia/hypoglycemia	Glucose
GI	If not consumed with adequate fluid, esophageal/intestinal impaction and obstruction	Dysphagia, odynophagia, inability to swallow, abd pain and distention	Imaging studies
CARDIO	↓ Cholesterol levels		Cholesterol profile
RESP	Inhalation-induced allergy/asthma	Exposure	Wheezing, skin rash, itching, hives
GU	Unknown effect on pregnancy and lactation		
DERM	Emollient		Dermatitis, pruritus

Key References: Blumenthal M, et al, eds. *The complete German commission E monographs: Therapeutic guide to herbal medicines.* Boston: American Botanical Council & Integrative Medicine Communications; 1998. Sierra M, Garcia JJ, Fernandez N, et al. Therapeutic effects of psyllium in type 2 diabetic patients. *Eur J Clin Nutr.* 2002;56:830-842.

Perioperative Implications

Preoperative Concerns
- Underreported due to impression that agent is not a drug
- Inquire into use of other herbal drugs
- Possible decrease in absorption of oral drugs
- Concern with hypovolemia

Monitoring
- Routine
- Consider NG tube

Airway
- None

Induction
- Hypotension a concern if hypovolemic

Maintenance
- Hypotension a concern if hypovolemic

Extubation
- None

Postoperative Period
- Worry about constipation postop if chronic use is not continued postop (can be added to almost any smoothie as long as can take smoothies and water)

Pyruvate

Alethia Baldwin

Uses

- Orally, used for wt loss, improving exercise endurance, hyperlipidemia, antioxidant protection, and inhibiting tumor growth
- Topically, pyruvic acid used for signs of aging skin and photohyperpigmentation
- Inhaled as sodium pyruvate may act as an anti-inflammatory agent to improve some chronic lung diseases (in prelim clinical trials)
- Intracoronary infusion, used to improve hemodynamics in pts with CHF due to dilated cardiomyopathy

Risks

- Available OTC without regulation
- Orally large doses, >6 g/d, can cause GI symptoms incl abd discomfort, bloating, gas, and diarrhea
- Topically, applying pyruvic acid as a facial peel can cause an intense burning sensation. Apply in adequate ventilation because the vapors have been reported to cause resp irritation.
- One child receiving IV pyruvate for restrictive cardiomyopathy died.
- There is insufficient reliable studies or evidence about the effectiveness of pyruvate for most uses.

Worry About

- Possible hypoglycemia via blood glucose extraction into muscle cells and decreased insulin resistance
- May potentiate inotropic effects of catecholamines and phosphodiesterase inhibitors
- Insufficient data about safety in pediatrics, pregnancy and lactation, and pts with liver and kidney disease

Overview/Pharmacology

- Anionic form of the three-carbon organic acid, pyruvic acid
- Present in red apples (~450 mg), red wine and dark beer (~75 mg), and cheeses.
- Serves as a biological fuel, converted to acetyl-coenzyme A, which enters the Krebs cycle and is metabolized to produce ATP aerobically
- Anaerobically energy is obtained when pyruvate is formed as an end-product of glycolysis and then reduced to lactate
- Known for infomercial with Steve Garvey where drug effects were misrepresented and resulted in $10 million settlement against the company

Mechanism of Action

- Increases contractile function of heart muscle
- Increases generation of ATP and ATP phosphorylation potential
- Reduces free radical production, increases lipid oxidation, and decreases carbohydrate oxidation resulting in greater loss of fat mass
- In combination with dihydroxyacetone, increases arm and leg exercise endurance
- Topically exfoliates the surface layers of skin
- Repairs injured mitochondria to inhibit tumor growth by suppressing the Warburg effect
- Up-regulates NO that can kill viruses, infections, and tumors and reduce inflammation in lungs

Usual Dose

- Oral: For wt loss, 22–44 grams/d as a supplement to a low-cholesterol, low-fat diet with exercise
- Topical: For aging skin, a 50% pyruvic acid peel applied once weekly for 4 wk

DRUG EFFECTS

System	Effect	Test
CARDIO	↓ Pulm artery pressure and pulm vascular resistance	PA cath calc., ECHO, heart cath
	↓ Pulm capillary wedge pressure	"
	↓ Heart rate	ECG, "
	↑ Cardiac output and cardiac index	"
	↑ Left ventricle ejection fraction	"
	↑ Inotropy and lusitropy	"
	↓ Plasma cholesterol and LDL	Chol, LDL
ENDO	↓ Insulin resistance	Glu, lytes
	↑ Levels of thyroxine	TFT
	↑ Resting metabolic rate	Calorimetry
IMMUNE	Anti-inflammatory and anti-oxidant	Poss. CBC

Key Reference: Hermann, et al. Improved systolic and diastolic myocardial function with intracoronary pyruvate in patients with congestive heart failure. *Eur J Heart Fail.* 2004;6:213–218; PDR Health: *Pyruvate.* http://170.107.206.70/drug_info/nmdrugprofiles/nutsupdrugs/pyr_0218.shtml.

Perioperative Implications

Preoperative Concerns
- Reliable self report of drug use and amount
- Check labs for glucose level

Monitoring
- Routine

Airway
- No special concerns/considerations

Preinduction/Induction
- No special concerns other than considerations of co-morbidities

Postoperative Period
- Routine

ALTERNATIVE MEDICINE

S-Adenosyl-L-Methionine (SAMe)

Adam M. Kaye
Alan Kaye

ALTERNATIVE MEDICINE

Uses

- Anti-aging, anti-disease therapeutic agent
- May protect against hepatotoxic effect of certain drugs (e.g., alcohol, acetaminophen, phenobarbital, and steroids)
- Depression, anxiety, premenstrual syndrome (PMS)
- Heart disease
- Liver disease, cirrhosis, intrahepatic cholestasis, disorders of porphyrin, and billirubin metabolism
- Osteoarthritis, tendinitis, bursitis, chronic low back pain
- Dementia, Alzheimer's disease, Parkinson's disease
- MS, migraine, seizure, spinal cord injury
- Chronic lead poisoning
- Disorder of porphyrin and bilirubin metabolism
- Chronic fatigue syndrome (CFS)
- Intellectual enhancement, attention deficit-hyperactivity disorder (ADHD)

Perioperative Risks

- N/V, flatulence, diarrhea, irregular or accelerated HR
- Anxiety

Overview/Pharmacology

- SAMe is produced endogenously by adenosine triphosphate (ATP) activation of methionine that is produced by the body from dietary protein.
- SAMe is required in numerous transmethylation reactions involving nucleic acids, proteins, phospholipids, amines, and other neurotransmitters. The synthesis of SAMe is linked with folate and cyanocobalmin metabolism, and deficiencies of both these vitamins have been found to reduce CNS SAMe concentrations.

- May improve methylation by different mechanisms in several neurologic and psychiatric disorders
- Is well tolerated with oral use and free of serious side effects. The oral supplement was developed in the 1970s and has been touted as a multipurpose treatment ever since.
- Exogenously administered SAMe has a low bioavailability due to rapid first-pass metabolism by the liver
- Peak plasma concentration in 3–5 hr
- $T_{1/2}$ 100 min
- Excreted in urine and feces
- Crosses the blood-brain barrier
- Metabolized to homocysteine, which is re-methylated to form methionine, which can form more SAMe
- Tosylate salt has 1% oral bioavailability
- Butane disulfonate salt has 5% oral bioavailability

Mechanism of Action

- Contributes to the synthesis, activation, and metabolism of hormones, neurotransmitters, nucleic acid, proteins, phospholipids, and some drugs
- SAMe crosses the blood-brain barrier and is involved in transmethylation and folate and monoamine metabolism as well as in membrane function and neurotransmission.
- SAMe plays a role in more than 100 biochemical reactions: increases levels of serotonin, dopamine, norepinephrine, phosphatides, proteoglycans.
- Improves intrahepatic cholestasis. SAMe supplementation seems to improve hepatic function and reverse imbalances of various enzymes. In liver disease deficiencies of methionine adenosyl transferase (MAP) often leads to reductions in cysteine and choline which can lead to depletion of glutathione. SAMe restores levels of glutathione, decreases inflammation and increases methylation of DNA.

- Stimulates articular cartilage growth
- Relieves joint pain possibly due to analgesic or anti-inflammatory effects. Possibly stimulation of articular cartilage growth and repair as a result of chindrocyte proteoglycan synthesis. May antagonize tumor necrosis factor–alpha (TNF-alpha) which may be beneficial in arthritic pts.
- Antidepressant effect is probably due to ↑ serotonin turnover and elevated dopamine and norepinephrine levels or due to alteration of cellular membrane fluidity, which facilitates signal transduction across membranes and ↑ the efficiency of receptor-effector coupling.
- In liver disease, it restores the biochemical factors that are depleted.
- In AIDS myelopathy, it replenishes depleted endogenous SAMe.

Usual Dose

- For depression, 400–1600 mg PO/d or 200–400 mg IV/d to speed the onset of tricyclic antidepressants
- For osteoarthritis, 200 mg tid PO or 400 mg IV
- For alcoholic liver disease, cirrhosis, or intrahepatic cholestasis, 1200–1600 mg PO or 800 mg IV/d
- For AIDS myelopathy, 800 mg IV/d for 14 d
- For fibromyalgia, 800 mg PO/d

ASSESSMENT POINTS

System	Effect	Assessment by Hx	PE
GI	N/V, diarrhea	GI complaints	KUB
MS	Osteoarthritis	Stiff joints	ROM

Interactions

- Additive serotonergic effects and serotonin syndrome-like effects with antidepressants incl SSRIs
- Due to serotonergic properties, the following should be avoided with SAMe due to the risks of serotonin syndrome–like effects: dextromethorphan (Robitussin DM, other cough syrups), meperidine (Demerol), pentazocine (Talwin), tramadol (Ultram), sumatriptan (Imitrex) and other 5-HT$_{1B/1/D}$ receptor agonists.

- Additive side effects like hyperthermia, agitation, confusion, coma when used with MAO inhibitors
- Other side effects may incl dry mouth, nausea, gas, diarrhea, headache, anxiety, nervousness, restlessness, and insomnia.
- Large doses of SAMe may cause mania (abn elevated mood). People with bipolar disorder (manic depression) should not take SAMe because it may worsen manic episodes.

Contraindications

- Pts taking MAO inhibitors or within 2 wk of their D/C
- Concurrent use with antidepressant drugs incl MAOIs could result in additive stimulatory effects. Agitation, tremor, insomnia, nervousness, irregular or accelerated heart rate are theoretical concerns.

Saw Palmetto

Joan Spiegel

Uses

- Benign prostatic hypertrophy
- Urinary tract inflammation (prostatitis)
- Underactive bladder
- Male and female pattern baldness
- Aphrodisiac
- Breast augmentation

Perioperative Risks

- No established interactions with anesthetic agents

Worry About

- Saw palmetto has been implicated in hepatitis, cholecystitis, bleeding diatheses, conduction defects, and erectile dysfunction. No studies confirm these effects.
- Unsubstantiated pharmacological effects increasing action of benzodiazepines.

Overview

- Saw palmetto extract is an extract of the fruit of *Serenoa repens* from the American dwarf palm tree. Saw palmetto's active ingredients incl fatty acids, plant sterols, and flavonoids.
- Saw palmetto has hormonal (estrogenic) effects, as well as direct inhibitory effects on androgen receptors. There are possible anti-inflammatory effects (from the berries of the plant).
- Saw palmetto has not been evaluated by the FDA.
- Saw palmetto is possibly ineffective for its intended use—BPH (NEJM, 2006).

Etiology

- Mechanism of action: Saw palmetto exhibits antiestrogenic and antiandrogenic effects by inhibiting the actions of 5-alpha reductase enzyme (thereby preventing the conversion of testosterone to dihydrotestosterone (DHT)—a cause of BPH and baldness).

Possible Drug Interactions

- Any medication that alters male sex hormones should not be taken with saw palmetto. Examples incl finasteride and flutamide.
- Drugs that effect coagulation should also not be consumed with saw palmetto: Coumadin and anti-inflammatory agents (clopidogrel, ibuprofen, aspirin).
- Because saw palmetto may have hormone-like effects, it may make oral contraceptives less effective, raising the risk of unplanned pregnancy.
- Tannins in saw palmetto may interfere with iron absorption.
- Tinctures may contain large amounts of alcohol and cause N/V when taken with metronidazole or disulfiram.

DRUG EFFECTS

	Effect	Test
GI	Occasional upset, hepatitis, and cholecystitis (very rare)	LFTs
HEME	Bleeding, iron deficiency	None, iron studies, Hb
GU	Improved urinary symptoms (conflicting data)	None
ENDO	Breast enlargement (unproved) Prevent hair involution due to DHT (unproved)	None

Key Reference: Serenoa repens. *Altern Med Rev.* 1998;3:227–229. Bent S, Kane C, Shinohara K, et al. Saw palmetto for benign prostatic hyperplasia. *NEJM.* 2006;354:557–566.

Perioperative Implications

Preoperative Concerns

- Self reporting of other herbal supplements
- Unknown effects in children, interference with birth control, and in lactating mothers

Intraoperative Concerns
- None known

Postoperative Period
- Routine

Soy

Richard M. Layman
Jorge Aguilar

Uses

- Soy is used to prevent or treat high LDL cholesterol, menopausal symptoms, osteoporosis, memory problems, Htn, breast cancer, and prostate cancer.
- Human and rodent studies support the hypothesis that soy-based phytoestrogens may decrease age-related diseases (CV disease, osteoporosis), prevent obesity, lower cholesterol, and favorably alter glycemic control; however, further research is required.

Perioperative Risks

- None known

Worry About

- Minor stomach and bowel problems such as nausea, bloating, and constipation are possible.
- Allergy to soy, though rare, can occur.

- Soy's possible role in breast cancer was uncertain, but lack of role becoming clearer. Women who have an increased risk of developing breast cancer used to be particularly concerned about using soy, but recent data show no increase (and even a decrease in) breast cancer risk from large soy consumption. Genistein is a potent inhibitor of protein-tyrosine kinase, which may attenuate growth of cancer.

Overview

- Phytoestrogens are plant-derived compounds with a structure and function similar to estradiol.
- Isoflavones, a class of phytoestrogens, have the highest concentration in soybeans and act as an estrogen receptor (ER) agonist or antagonist.
- The two major isoflavones found in soy are genistein and daidzein. As with estrogens, these isoflavones may affect glucose and lipid metabolism.
- Dietary soy may inhibit atherosclerosis by mechanisms yet unknown.

Drug Class/Mechanism of Action/Usual Dose

- Soy protein isolate (SPI) 2 mg/d - 80 mg/d PO
- Soy isoflavones 10–150 mg/d PO

Mechanism of Action

- Inactive isoflavone glycosides (genistein and daidzein) are hydrolyzed by bacterial β-glucosidases in the intestinal wall to the active forms. The phenolic ring on soy isoflavones promotes binding to estrogen receptors (both α and β) located on multiple organ systems. Health benefits may occur via selective ER modulation (SERM) activity.
- Dietary soy improves insulin sensitivity by increasing glucose uptake preferentially in skeletal muscles.

DRUG EFFECTS

System	Effect	Test
CNS	Potential cognitive improvement Suppressed levels of allodynia and hyperalgesia	Cognitive testing
CARDIO	May inhibit development of atherosclerosis May lower LDL levels	HDL, LDL, Cholesterol levels
GI	N/V and bloating may be possible	
GU	Reduces menopausal hot flash severity and decreases vaginal dryness[5] Higher rate of endometrial hyperplasia, though evidence is conflicting Concern with use in women diagnosed with or at risk for breast cancer No definitive effect on female endocrine function	
ENDO	Inhibits adipose tissue deposition and stimulates lipolysis Lowers glucose and insulin plasma levels No effect on glucose in humans	Glucose Insulin plasma levels
HEME	Allergic reactions incl anaphylaxis may occur.	

Key Reference: Cederroth CR, Nef S. Soy, phytoestrogens and metabolism: A review. *Mol Cell Endocrinol.* 2009;304:30–42.

Perioperative Implications

Preoperative Concerns
- None known

Intraoperative Concerns
- According to the package insert for propofol, a contraindication for use is a known hypersensitivity to any of propofol's components. Propofol is a 10% soybean emulsion; therefore, an allergy to soybeans is a contraindication to propofol administration.

Postoperative Concerns
- None known

References

1. Baker MT, Naguib M. Propofol: The challenges of formulation. *Anesthesiology.* 2005;103(4):860–876.
2. Cederroth CR, Auger J, Zimmermann C, Eustache F, Nef S. Soy, phyto-oestrogens and male reproductive function: A Review. *Int J Androl.* 2009;32:1–13.
3. Cederroth CR, Nef S. Soy, phytoestrogens and metabolism: A review. *Mol Cell Endocrinol.* 2009;304(1–2):30–42.
4. Gleason CE, Carlsson CM, Barnet JH, et al. A preliminary study of the safety, feasibility and cognitive efficacy of soy isoflavone supplements in older men and women. *Age Ageing.* 2009;38(1):86–93.
5. Low Dog T. Menopause: A Review of botanical dietary supplements. *Am J Med.* 2005;118(12B):98S–108S.
6. Munro IC, Harwood M, Hlywka JJ, et al. Soy isoflavones: A safety review. *Nutr Rev.* 2003;61(1):1–33.
7. Nagarajan S. Mechanisms of anti-atherosclerotic functions of soy-based diets. *J Nutr Biochem.* 2009; In Press.
8. NIH/US Dept. Health and Human Services. Soy: Herbs at a glance. 2008 March.
9. Shir Y, Campbell JN, Raja SN, Seltzer Z. The correlation between dietary soy phytoestrogens and neuropathic pain behavior in rats after partial denervation. *Anesth & Analg.* 2002;94:421–426.
10. Zhao C, Wacnik PW, Tall JM, et al. Analgesic effects of a soy-containing diet in three murine bone cancer pain models. *J Pain.* 2004;5(2):104–110.

St. John's Wort (Hypericum Perforatum)

Theodore G. Cheek

Uses

- More than 3% of presurgical pts report using St. John's wort
- Taken mainly for depression, although pts may take for a variety of reasons incl anxiety, viral and bacterial infections, menstrual cramps, HIV, cancer, chest congestion, hemorrhoids, skin wounds, and burns.
- May be as effective as low-dose first-generation tricyclic antidepressant for treating mild depression
- Most integrative medical specialists will use every other alternative first due to drug interactions; this is at best a third-line medication. Others such as S-adenosyl-L- methionine are equal to or more effective and without undesirable drug interaction side effects

Worry About

- Drug interactions: May prolong sedative effects of other drugs incl anesthetics and sedatives. Case reports of severe hypertensive response to vasopressors such as ephedrine or phenylephrine in pts taking St. John's wort
- Induces cytochrome P450 enzymes; and promotes metabolism and decreased blood levels of warfarin, cyclosporine, digoxin, Ca²⁺-channel blockers and steroids; even renders birth control pills and menopausal drug therapies ineffective (watch for unplanned and sometimes unwanted pregnancies due to this effect)
- Serotonin-like syndrome (Htn, tachycardia, agitation, restlessness)
- Unpredictable effects due to lack of strict regulation

Overview/Pharmacology

- Classified as a dietary supplement and not subject to FDA drug regulation; pharmacologic activity can be unpredictable and highly variable in different preparations. Marketed PO 300 mg hypericum extract (0.3% hypericin) tid.
- Contains many complex chemicals, but hypericin and hyperforin are responsible for the antidepressant effects
- Absorbed within 40 min of oral administration
- Mainly metabolized by the liver and cleared by renal excretion; elimination $T_{1/2}$ 43 hr

Mechanism of Action/Usual Dose

- May act as a nonspecific reuptake inhibitor of serotonin, norepinephrine, and dopamine
- Appears to work differently from conventional antidepressants
- MAO inhibition reported in early studies. Not confirmed in follow-up studies.
- Usually taken as a capsule consisting of the plant extract; typical dosage is 300–500 mg of hypericum extract tid

ASSESSMENT POINTS

System	Effect	Assessment/by Hx	PE	Test
HEENT	Photosensitivity			
CARDIO	Rarely, Htn, tachycardia, and serotonin-like syndrome	Dosage taken; also taking SSRI	BP/HR	ECG
GI	Nausea			
DERM	Rarely, rash			
CNS	Restlessness, fatigue, antidepression			

Key Reference: Skidmore-Roth L, ed. *Mosby's handbook of herbs and natural supplements*, 3rd ed. St Louis: Mosby; 2006:957–963.

Perioperative Implications

Preoperative Period

- Hx can incl dose, duration, and preparation taken and the reasons for its use
- Well advised to D/C preop at least 1 wk in advance for the drug to be cleared from body.
- May see as much as a 50% decreased effect of warfarin. Consider alternatives to warfarin.
- Can decrease digoxin levels, possibly by induction of a P-glycoprotein transporter
- Serotonin-like syndrome, esp. when combined with an SSRI, tricyclics, or MAOIs

Induction/Maintenance/Emergence

- May prolong anesthesia via potentiation of central effects of inhaled agents, sedatives, and opioids.

Anticipated Problems/Concerns

- Effects may be variable among different preparations due to lack of standardization.
- Anticipate decreased effects of certain drugs such as warfarin, cyclosporine, beta blockers, Ca²⁺-channel blockers, steroids, and digoxin.
- May prolong the sedative effects of anesthetics
- Watch for serotonin-like syndrome (Htn, tachycardia, agitation, restlessness)

Valerian (Valeriana officinalis)

Richard M. Layman
Lisa Caplan

Uses

- Insomnia (present in virtually all herbal sleep aids)
- Anxiety
- Depression
- Htn
- GI hyperactivity
- Headaches
- Muscle spasms
- Benzodiazepine withdrawal

Perioperative Risks

- Potential for valerian withdrawal exists if acute cessation after chronic high-dose administration occurs. This withdrawal can present as delirium, tachycardia, and diaphoresis.
- Chronic high dose valerian has been linked with cardiac failure and emergence delirium.

Worry About

- No direct drug interactions are reported.
- Valerian may act synergistically with sedative anesthetics leading to prolonged emergence.
- Valerian could potentiate medications such as barbiturates, benzodiazepines, opioids, antidepressants, and alcohol.

Overview

- Valerian is a native herb of temperate regions whose name is believed to be derived from the Latin word "valere," meaning to be healthy or strong. It has been used for centuries as a sleep aid by Greeks, Romans, Chinese, American Indians, and Europeans.
- Prior to the introduction of barbiturates to the U.S. National Formulary, valerian was indicated for treatment of unrest and nervous sleep disturbance. It has since been dropped from the U.S. National Formulary.
- Valerian contains many constituents working synergistically, incl volatile oils, valepotriates, monoterpene alkaloids, and furanofuran lignans.
- Volatile oils: These oils give valerian a pungent odor due to the release of isovaleric acid. The sesquiterpene skeleton present on volatile oils such as valerenic acid, valeranone, and kessyl glycol is a proposed primary source of pharmacological effects. These components have been shown to act on the amygdaloid body in the brain, and inhibit GABA breakdown thus leading to sedation.
- Valepotriates: Valepotriates have a furanopyranoid monoterpene skeleton which can be found in glycosylated forms known as iridoids. The compounds have been shown in mice and cat experiments to decrease spontaneous motility after oral administration.

Mechanism of Action/Usual Dose

- Produces dose-dependent sedation and hypnosis mediated mainly through $GABA_A$ receptor, the adenosine A_1 receptor, and recently noted, the $5-HT_{5a}$ receptor.
- Tablets: 300–400 mg PO 30 min to 1 hr prior to sleep.
- Tea: 1 cup of boiling water over 1 to 2 teaspoons (2–3 g) of the root and infuse for 10 to 15 min. May drink up to 2 cups daily.
- Tincture: 2 to 6 mL (½ to 1 teaspoon) up to three times daily.

DRUG EFFECTS

System	Effect	Test
CARDIO	High output cardiac failure Hypotension Arrhythmias Dilates coronary arteries	Rule out other causes of high output cardiac failure: Sepsis, beriberi, cardiac shunt, or Paget disease. EKG, ECHO
HEPAT	CYPA 4 inhibitor Hepatotoxicity	Baseline LFTs
CNS	Sedation Hypnosis Anticonvulsive Headache Restlessness Hallucinations Ataxia	Sleep studies: May improve sleep latency and slow wave sleep EEG
GI	Nausea Intestinal irritability	Decrease dose or stop ingestion.
MS	Muscle relaxation	

Key References: Harmony G, Indu V, Doraiswamy M. Cardiac complications and delirium associated with valerian root withdrawal. *JAMA.* 1998;280:1566–1567. Tesch BJ. Herbs commonly used by women: An evidence based review. *Am J Obstet Gynecol.* 2003;188:S44–S55. Ang-Lee MK, Moss J, Yuan C. Herbal medicines and perioperative care. *JAMA.* 2001;286:208–216. Gooneratne N. Complementary and alternative medicine for sleep disturbances in older adults. *Clin Geriatr Med.* 2008;24:121–138.

Perioperative Implications

- Valepotriate component of valerian may alkylate DNA, which could be potentially cytotoxic or carcinogenic. It has been recommended that valerian not be used in pregnancy or while breastfeeding.
- Cessation of valerian consumption prior to surgical intervention should be made on an individualized basis. If a 2-to 3-wk taper is not feasible, then pts should continue taking valerian. Benzodiazepines can be used to treat withdrawal symptoms should they develop.

SECTION V

Tests

Autonomic Function

Thomas J. Ebert
Matthew J. Rowan

Risk
- No risks assoc with most tests
- IV atropine and cold pressor test are mildly unpleasant; atropine may cause arrhythmias

Overview
- Measuring BP and HR are inexpensive.
- Equipment costs for manometer and isometric handgrip, minimal
- Simple bedside tests incl orthostatic stress, deep breathing, Valsalva maneuver, cold pressor or a slightly more involved test incl atropine administration, and isometric handgrip give valuable information on autonomic function.
- Multiple tests are usually performed; presence of two or more abn results indicates some degree of autonomic dysfunction

- Very sensitive quantitative tests delineate severity of disorder, system (e.g., cardiovagal, vasomotor, sudomotor), distribution (pre- vs. postganglionic), and level affected
- Autonomic dysfunction is assoc with ↑ periop CV and cardiorespiratory instability, spontaneous cardiac ischemia, malignant arrhythmias, and cardiac arrest.

ICD-9-CM Codes: 337.0 (Autonomic nervous system disorder); 337.1

Indications
- Pts with symptoms of autonomic failure (e.g., intolerance to standing, bladder and/or sphincter disturbances, impaired sweating) may have autonomic failure due to 1° causes such as Shy-Drager syndrome, or disorders such as DM, chronic alcoholism, chronic renal failure, advanced age, vitamin deficiency (e.g., B_{12}), HIV infection, or prescription drugs (e.g., TCAs)
- Diabetic autonomic neuropathy is the most common autonomic neuropathy characterized by both CV and pseuodomotor autonomic dysfunction

Additional Tests
- Additional tests incl plasma catecholamines, atrial vasopressor protein, pancreatic polypeptide determinations in response to standing or other maneuvers to resolve site of lesion, and responses to α_2-adrenoceptor agonist for peripheral denervation supersensitivity.

ASSESSMENT POINTS

Test	Method	System	Abnormal Response
Orthostatic stress	Pt supine 10 min; then stands or is tilted 80° head up; BP measured at 2 min	Sympathetic	↓ in SBP by >20 mm Hg ↓ in DBP by >10 mm Hg
30:15 Ratio	From continuous ECG strip; ratio of longest R-R interval (~30th beat) to shortest R-R interval (~15th beat) after assuming standing position	Parasympathetic	<1.03 (<1.01 if >65 y)
Deep breathing	Difference between mean HR at max inspiration and mean HR at max expiration for 6 breathing cycles over 1 min	Parasympathetic	<10 bpm if <40 y <5 bpm if >65 y
Valsalva maneuver	Pt blows into manometer to maintain intrathoracic pressure at 40 mm Hg for 15 sec; ratio of highest HR during blowing to lowest HR during first 20 sec after release of intrathoracic pressure; repeat for reproducibility. Same maneuver with directly measured arterial pressure	Parasympathetic Sympathetic	<1.2 (<1.15 if >65 y) BP does not exceed baseline after release of blowing
Atropine	1.8 mg IV over 3 min	Parasympathetic	HR does not change by >20 bpm
Cold pressor	Immerse hand in ice water for 1 min	Sympathetic	SBP ↑ by <20 mm Hg at peak (1 min) HR ↑ <10 bpm
Isometric handgrip	Isometric contraction at 30% max strength for 3 min	Sympathetic	↑ DBP by <10 mm Hg after 3 min

Key Reference: Hilz MJ, Dütsch M. Quantitative studies of autonomic function. *Muscle Nerve*. 2005;33:6–20.

Perioperative Implications

Preoperative Preparation
- Gastroparesis: Consider premedication with agents to ↑ gastric motility (e.g., metoclopramide), and ↓ consequence of aspiration (e.g., antacids, H_2 blockers)
- Abn sensitivity to anesthetic agents and apneic tendencies: Minimize narcotics or benzodiazepines as premedication; monitor intensively periop
- Orthostatic hypotension treated by volume expansion, which may cause supine Htn

Monitoring
- Consider arterial line

Induction
- Consider rapid-sequence induction
- Consider etomidate
- Titrate agents with CV and resp effects

Maintenance
- Aggressively treat blood loss, keep well hydrated
- Denervation supersensitivity: Unexpected Htn responses to adrenoceptor agonists used to treat hypotension; if vasopressors are required, use direct-acting agents; indirect-acting agents have unpredictable effects.

- Impaired temp regulation may require active warming
- Consider controlled ventilation

Postoperative Care
- Increased risk of hypotension, hypothermia, apnea
- Peripheral neuropathy may be assoc with requirement of less analgesic; use narcotics with caution

TESTS

692

Chest X-Ray

Muhammad B. Rafique

Risk

• Radiation dose is small (0.02 mSv) and so is radiation risk (cardiac CT gives radiation of 300–800 chest x-rays).
• The risk from misinterpretation could be significant.

Overview

• It is the most frequently performed radiographic study in the USA.
• The cost is <$250 (incl equipment, execution, and interpretation).
• Most common used views are PA and lateral; portable CXR is almost always AP view.

• CXR can evaluate the pt for the heart, lungs, pleurae, tracheobronchial tree, esophagus, thoracic lymph nodes, thoracic skeleton, chest wall, and upper abdomen diseases (both acute and chronic).
• Cardiomegaly if cardiothoracic (CT) ratio >0.5. Fluid overload if increased perihilar markings both cardiac and noncardiac.
• Consolidation could be pneumonia; hyperinflation, increased radiolucency and flattened diaphragm indicate COPD.
• Lobar atelactasis is opaque; absent lung markings and mediastinal shift is tension pneumothorax
• Trachea or esophageal FB could be visible; tracheal FB may show air trapping.

Indications

• Cardiothoracic procedures
• ASA guidelines recommend considering CXR if there is recent resp tract infection, Hx of smoking, COPD, and cardiac disease.
• Trauma and airway and/or esophageal foreign body.
• Intubated, CVL, and chest tube in place

ASSESSMENT POINTS

Aspect of Test	Positive Result	Confounding Factors	Dx Information
Cardiac shadow	CT ratio >0.5	Inspiratory film, when↑ perihilar markings present cardiac silhouette could be difficult to determine	Cardiomegaly, CHF
Perihilar markings	1-Increased markings in one area or whole lung fields 2-Absent lung markings in one area or whole field	1-Underexposed film, female breast tissue 2-Over exposure	1-CHF, fluid overload (e.g. renal failure, excess fluid administration, etc.) 2-Pneumothorax
Diaphragmatic placement	Flattened hemidiaphragms	Improper posture, splinting due to pain	Extent of COPD, extent of air trapping from exacerbation of reactive airway disease or FB
ETT and lines			Proper position of ETT, CVL, and chest tubes is confirmed.

Key References: Chen M, Pope T. *Basic Radiology*. McGram-Hill Medical; 2004:21–118. Practice advisory for preanesthesia evaluation. A report by the American Society of Anesthesiologists Task Force on Preanesthesia Evaluation. *Anesthesiology*. 2002;96:485–496.

Perioperative Implications

• CHF: Further evaluation with EKG, echo may be needed; consider invasive monitoring with arterial line, CVP monitoring, may consider PA catheter or TEE. Judicious use of fluids and minimize myocardial stress.
• COPD: Further evaluation with PFTs could be necessary; may consider invasive monitoring. Avoid interscalene block (hemidiaphragm paralysis).

• Reactive airway disease: Check for oral steroid therapy; if so, stress dose may be indicated. Avoid intubation or if necessary to intubate ensure adequate depth to avoid bronchospasm.
• Maintain spontaneous breathing in case of airway FB.

Special Considerations

• In pts with advanced COPD avoid depressing intrinsic resp drive; consider epidural for postop pain control. Consider delaying elective surgery if an acute exacerbation.
• Arrangements for ICU bed if pt's condition or surgical procedure (e.g., thoracotomy, lung resection) warrants.

TESTS

Diagnostic 12-Lead ECG

Martin J. London

TESTS

Risk

- None except misinterpretation

Sensitivity/Specificity

- Varies according to specific clinical indication, population. For rhythm and conduction disorders, 100% sensitive. Sensitivity of Q waves for autopsy-proven MI is 33–62%, with a specificity of 88–98%. Sensitivity, specificity of ST-T changes on resting ECG for myocardial ischemia in absence of clinical Sx are low.

Overview

- Cost: $15–$50 with physician charges
- ECG assesses myocardial ischemia, MI, rhythm and conduction disorders (intrinsic myocardial disease), electrolyte and metabolic disorders, and medical/systemic effects (extrinsic disorders).

- Appropriate, cost-effective starting point for more extensive, costly evaluation of cardiac diseases
- Predictive value, cost-effectiveness of preop 12-lead ECG are controversial. Incidence of ECG abn ↑ with age, concurrent medical illness (esp. Htn, CAD, diabetes).

Indications

- Known or suspected (i.e., multiple risk factors or abn on Hx or PE) CAD
- Major surgery regardless of clinical Hx in pts with known or at high risk for CAD or other cardiac disease.

- Specific age recommendations for screening are no longer considered appropriate given lack of specific benefit with regards to periop outcomes. However many centers still routinely screen males over 40, females over 50.

Additional/Alternative Tests

- Exercise treadmill testing with or without thallium imaging, static or stress ECHO, dipyridamole or adenosine thallium imaging, coronary angiography to diagnose CAD, ischemia
- Holter monitoring for arrhythmias, conduction defect, ischemia

ASSESSMENT POINTS

Disorder	Positive Result	Confounding Factors	Dx Information
Myocardial ischemia	ST-segment depression >1 mm Deep T-wave inversion	Baseline ST-T wave changes BBB (esp. LBBB) Digoxin/drug effects Abn autonomic tone Q waves ↑ ST segment due to pericarditis Intracranial pathology	ST-segment changes correlate poorly with site of CAD Magnitude of depression weakly related to severity
Myocardial infarction	New Q waves ≥40 msec, ampl >25% of R wave ↑ ST during acute stage Poor R wave progression	Q waves in V_1 and aVL or isolated inferior leads may be normal BBB (esp LBBB)	Q waves are sensitive and specific indicators
Rhythm disorders	Abn timing of P wave, QRS or absence of normal P wave and P-R interval		Depends on chronicity, Rx, hemodynamic consequences Atrial dysrhythmias usually less dangerous than ventricular Atrial fibrillation assoc with increased risk periop stroke
Conduction disorders	Axis deviation PR >120 msec QRS >100 msec J point elevation	Body habitus Digoxin hypothermia Antiarrhythmics	LAFB—usually benign LPFB—likely myocardial or conduction damage RBBB—usually benign LBBB—more likely assoc with CAD and/or impaired ventricular function J point elevation inferior or lateral leads >0.1 mm assoc with increased risk long-term cardiac death
Metabolic disorders	Hypokalemia—flattened T waves, ST ↓ Hyperkalemia—peaking T waves, wide QRS Hypocalcemia—lengthen QT_c interval Hypercalcemia—shorten QT_c interval	Other nonspecific changes	Chemistry Laboratory
LV hypertrophy	Multiple criteria Sum $V_1 + V_5$ ≥35 mm	Body habitus, age, and race influence specificity	Assoc with severe Htn or aortic stenosis

Key Reference: Tikkanen JS, et al. Long-term outcome associated with early repolarization on electrocardiography. *NEJM.* 2009;361:2529–2537. 10.1056/NEJMoa0907589.

Perioperative Implications

- Q waves diagnostic of prior MI assoc with elevated risk of postop cardiac morbidity
- Number of Q waves on ECG tracing negatively correlated with the ejection fraction
- LBBB more likely assoc with significant CAD and impaired ventricular function than RBBB. However, intraventricular conduction delay, with very wide and bizarre QRS morphology, may have similar significance as LBBB.

- Nonspecific ST-T–wave changes, T-wave flattening/inversion, and QT-interval prolongation markedly influenced by autonomic tone and common in the early postop period

Special Considerations

- Accuracy of computerized interpretation varies among manufacturers
- Sensitivity and specificity of ECG are poor following cardiac surgery

- Newer forms: These incl computerized vectorcardiography and late- and mid-QRS signal-averaged electrocardiography utilizing a different lead system (the Frank Lewis XYZ leads) and signal-averaging techniques. Their periop value is currently unknown although recent data suggests that abn spatial QRS-T angle is a strong predictor of cardiac death in high-risk medical pts.

Dibucaine Number (Atypical Cholinesterase)

James E. Heavner

Risks

• Requires a serum sample for in vitro testing. Risks assoc with blood sample collection (i.e., venipuncture) incl pain, bruising, infection, and/or syncope.
• Periop risks of not receiving the test or misinterpretation of test: prolonged muscle paralysis and apnea following succinylcholine (SCH) or mivacurium (MIV). Possible ↑ risk of toxicity of ester-linked local anesthetics.

Overview

• Cost: Approximately $50
• Dibucaine number is used to determine if a pt has a genetically determined form of atypical cholinesterase (BHCHE; butyrylcholinesterase, benzoylcholinesterase, acylcholine acylhydrolase, plasma ChE, pseudo-ChE, serum ChE) that is resistant to dibucaine inhibition. There are a number of phenotypes and genotypes of serum ChE, incl the normal gene, dibucaine-resistant genes, fluoride-resistant genes, and the silent gene. The silent gene has no ChE activity when in the homozygous state; the dibucaine and fluoride-resistant forms have reduced ChE activity.

VARIENTS OF BUTYRYLCHOLINESTERASE

Name	Abbreviation	Description
Usual	U	Normal
Atypical	A	Reduced activity, dibucaine resistant
Fluoride resistant	F	Reduced activity, fluoride resistant
Silent	S	No activity
H	H	Approx 10% reduced concentration
J	J	Approx 33% reduced concentration
K	K	Approx 66% reduced concentration

Key Reference: Levano S, Ginz H, Siegemund, et al: Genotyping the butyrylcholineesterase in patients with prolonged neuromuscular block after succinylcholine. *Anesthesiology* 2005; 102:531–535.

• Dibucaine number usually is done to determine the etiology of prolonged muscle paralysis and apnea after SCH or MIV administration. It is indicated before SCH, MIV, or ester-linked local anesthetic administration to pts with confirmed or suspected familial Hx of atypical ChE or prior to readministration of SCH to pts who had prolonged apnea after SCH. ChE rapidly hydrolyzes SCH, MIV, and ester-linked local anesthetics at rates depending on the agent (procaine, rapidly; tetracaine, 25% the rate of procaine).
• A multitude of alternative methods for determination of dibucaine numbers have been developed since 1957, when the original test was reported. Distinction between normal and heterozygous enzyme may be difficult by some tests.

• If serum ChE activity is measured and is normal, there is no indication to check for dibucaine or fluoride-resistant forms of ChE.
• Dibucaine and fluoride sensitivity testing confirm or rules out a genetic cause of low ChE activity.
• Laboratories are starting to do cholinesterase gene sequencing instead of testing for dibucaine number and fluoride number. The cost for doing gene sequencing is similar to the cost of doing number determination.

Pathophysiology

• Normal ChE is sensitive to inhibition by dibucaine, whereas the dibucaine-sensitive homozygous variant is resistant
• Only pts homozygous for the atypical ChE variant will have a significant prolongation of muscle paralysis and apnea
• Inherited forms of abn ChE are present in ~4% of the general population.
• Homozygous atypical variant occurs in <1/1500 humans.

ASSESSMENT POINTS

Variant	Approx Duration of SCH-Induced NMB	Dibucaine Number (% Inhibition of Enzyme Activity)	Incidence
Homozygous	5–10 min	70–80	
Heterozygous	20 min	40–60	1/480
Homozygous atypical	60–180 min	20–30	1/3200

Key Reference: Levano S, Ginz H, Siegemund, et al. Genotyping the butyrylcholinesterase in patients with prolonged neuromuscular block after succinylcholine. *Anesthesiology*. 2005;102:531–535.

Perioperative Implications

• Avoid use of, or use cautiously, SCH, MIV, or ester-linked local anesthetics in pts confirmed or suspected to be homozygous for atypical ChE.

Dipyridamole Thallium Imaging

Lee A. Fleisher

Risk

- In pts with CAD, risk of MI and death 1/100,000

Sensitivity and Specificity

- Sensitivity: 70–80%
- Specificity: 80–90%
- Pos predictive value: 20–50%
- Neg predictive value: 85–99%

Overview

- Cost: $1200–$1500, depending on laboratory
- Test to assess presence of coronary artery stenosis in pts unable to exercise

- Dipyridamole used to dilate normal coronary arteries, resulting in flow heterogeneity
- Thallium taken up by viable myocardial cells
- Obtain stress and at-rest images
- Areas of myocardial necrosis demonstrate fixed defect
- Areas at risk demonstrate reversible defect
- Able to quantify area at risk

ICD-9-CM Code: 414.0 (Coronary atherosclerosis)

Indications

- Dx of CAD in pts unable to exercise
- Quantification of area at risk for ischemia

Tests

- Holter monitoring for silent ischemia
- Dobutamine thallium imaging
- Dobutamine stress ECHO
- Coronary angiography
- Coronary calcium score
- Coronary CT scan

ASSESSMENT POINTS

Aspect of Test	Positive Result	Confounding Factors	Dx Information
CV thallium imaging	Reversible defect	Breast artifact	Area of myocardium at risk
	Fixed defect	Delayed imaging or reinjection needed to determine if severe ischemia or scar present	Area of old scar or severe ischemia
	LV dilation		LV dysfunction
Lung imaging	↑ Lung uptake		LV dysfunction
ECG	ST-segment changes	Baseline abn	Indicates dipyridamole results in myocardial ischemia— ↑ risk
Sx during test	Chest pain	Multiple causes	May be ischemia or nonspecific cause

Key Reference: Fleisher LA, Beckman JA, Brown KA, et al. 2009 ACCF/AHA focused update on perioperative beta blockade incorporated into the ACC/AHA 2007 guidelines on perioperative cardiovascular evaluation and care for noncardiac surgery. *J Am Coll* Cardiol. 2009;54:e13–e118.

Perioperative Implications

- A reversible defect suggests the presence of a critical coronary artery stenosis; larger defects are assoc with a greater area at risk and a higher incidence of periop cardiac morbidity.

- Increased lung uptake or LV dilation identifies those pts at risk for LV dysfunction with ischemia.
- Fixed defects represent old scar and are assoc with reduced function and increased long-term risk.

Special Considerations

- Pts with fixed defects may require reinjection or 24-hr delayed imaging to differentiate scar from severe ischemia.

TESTS

Dobutamine Echocardiography

Don Poldermans

Risk

- The incidence of potentially life threatening complications (i.e., cardiac rupture, acute MI, cerebrovascular accident, ventricular fibrillation, and sustained ventricular tachycardia) of dobutamine echocardiography and alternative tests
  - Dobutamine echocardiography 1:475
  - Exercise stress testing 1:1100
  - Dipyridamole echocardiography 1:1400
  - Dipyridamole scintigraphy 1:1600
- Dobutamine induces myocardial ischemia, contraindications are: Symptomatic severe aortic stenosis, unstable coronary syndromes, obstructive hypertrophic cardiomyopathy, and acute aortic dissections.

Sensitivity/Specificity

- Sensitivity for detection of CAD: 85–90%
- Specificity for detection of CAD: 80–85%
- Positive predictive value (for *any* periop event): 25–45%
- Positive predictive value (for a *hard* event): 15–25%
- Negative predictive value: 95–100%

Overview

- Cost: $600–$900
- Dobutamine infused in incremental doses to ↑ HR and contractility (e.g., myocardial O_2 demand)
- Normal response is dose-dependent improved wall thickening motion at every stage

- Resting wall motion abn suggests prior infarction
- Stress-induced wall motion abn indicates current ischemia

Indications

- Assessment of left ventricular function, heart valve abn, and stress-induced myocardial ischemia, all major determinants of adverse postop cardiac outcome. Myocardial ischemia is defined by the numbers of affected segments and the HR at which ischemia is induced; markers of the extent and severity of CAD.

Tests

Recommendations on Stress Testing Prior to Surgery	Class	Level of Evidence
High-risk surgery		
Stress testing is recommended in pts ≥3 clinical risk factors	I	C
Stress testing may be considered in pts <2 clinical risk factors	IIb	B
Stress testing may be considered in intermediate-risk surgery	IIb	C
Stress testing is not recommended in low-risk surgery	III	C

Class I Conditions for which there is evidence for and/or general agreement that the procedure or treatment is beneficial, useful, and effective.
Class II Conditions for which there is conflicting evidence and/or a divergence of opinion about the usefulness/efficacy of a procedure or treatment.
Class IIa Weight of evidence/opinion is in favor of usefulness/efficacy.
Class IIb Usefulness/efficacy is less well established by evidence/opinion.
Class III Conditions for which there is evidence and/or general agreement that the procedure/treatment is not useful/effective, and in some cases may be harmful.

ASSESSMENT POINTS

Test	Positive Result	Confounding Factors	Diagnostic Information
Wall motion analysis	Resting abn Induced abn Multiple abn	Cardiomyopathy, LBBB β-blockers; image quality Cardiomyopathy	Prior MI Ischemia Multivessel disease /left main
ECG	ST-segment depression	Baseline abn Low sensitivity	Ischemia
Symptoms	Chest pain	Nonspecific; multiple causes	Angina or other causes

Key Reference: Poldermans D, Hoeks SE, Feringa HH. Pre-operative risk assessment and risk reduction before surgery. *J Am Coll Cardiol.* 2008;51:1913–1924.

Perioperative Implications

- A normal stress ECHO confers favorable prognosis, very low risk of periop morbidity (*high* negative predictive accuracy)
- Inducible wall motion abn identifies pts at ↑ risk for periop event; but many pts with positive test can still undergo surgery without serious complications (e.g., MI or death low positive predictive accuracy), provided optimal medical therapy is prescribed (e.g., beta-blockers, statins, and aspirin) and administered in immediate periop and operative periods.

- Identifying high risk depends on extent of abn wall motion, and HR at which the abn develops, on top of clinical factors (e.g., Hx of MI, CHF, diabetes, stroke, renal disease, and angina)
- Pts with resting wall motion abn (e.g., prior MI) but no signs of inducible ischemia at intermediate risk

Exercise Stress Testing

Walter Bethune

Stuart J. Weiss

Risk

- Mortality risk of EST is <0.01%.
- Risk of inducing a myocardial infarction (MI) with EST is 1%.

Sensitivity/Specificity

- Accuracy of exercise ECG testing is dependent on the pretest probability of coronary heart which reflects pt gender, age, coronary risk factors, and the characteristics of the chest pain.
- Overall sensitivity is 68%; sensitivity for multi-vessel disease is 81%. Sensitivity is reduced when exercise workload is submaximal.
- Overall specificity is 77%; specificity for multi-vessel disease is 66%.
- Negative predictive value for periop cardiac events is 90–100%.
- Positive predictive value for periop cardiac events is 6–67%.

Overview

- Cost: $100–$300, depending on lab
- Exercise stress testing (EST), is a less invasive diagnostic test to:
  - Evaluate the extent of coronary artery disease (CAD)
  - Permits stratification of pts who are deemed to be at intermediate risk for periop cardiac events.
  - Assess a pt's functional capacity.
  - Determine the effects of treatment or to determine an appropriate exercise prescription for cardiac rehabilitation.
- EST attempts to induce coronary ischemia by the stress of vigorous exercise (treadmill) while detecting ischemia by monitoring the ECG and pt's vital signs.
- Exercise-induced ST-segment elevation in a previously non-infarcted territory, profound ST-segment depression, fall in exercise systolic BP and low exercise capacity (inability to achieve greater than 85% of predicted maximal HR during treadmill exercise testing) are assoc with a poor prognosis and also with multi-vessel CAD.
- In pts who cannot exercise nor have abn on the baseline ECG that interfere with interpretation, pharmacologic stress testing and alternative ischemia imaging techniques are used. (see Tests)

Indications

- Evaluate pts with angina to assess likelihood of CAD.
- Evaluate pts with palpitations to detect arrhythmias.
- Provide a prognostic estimate of the risk of a periop cardiac event.
- Provide an objective estimate of functional capacity.
- Determine a safe level of exercise for pts who are considering beginning a new exercise regimen or who require cardiac rehabilitation after an myocardial infarction.

Contraindications

- Acute myocardial infarction within 48 hr
- Unstable angina not yet stabilized with medical therapy
- Uncontrolled arrhythmia having possible hemodynamic compromise (e.g., ventricular tachycardia)
- Symptomatic severe aortic stenosis
- Aortic dissection
- Pulm embolism
- Pericarditis

Additional/Alternative Tests

- EST may be inappropriate for risk assessment or diagnosis of coronary disease in pts having an abn ECG at baseline (>1 mm depression, LBBB, paced ventricular rhythm or pre-excitation syndrome [WPW])

- Pharmacologic stress testing with dobutamine: Often used when a pt has bronchospastic lung disease (asthma or severe COPD), severe carotid stenosis, second or third degree atrioventricular block or unable to perform exercise protocol. Dobutamine mimics exercise stress physiology by increasing HR, increasing contractility, and decreasing systemic afterload.
- Pharmacologic stress testing with adenosine or dipyridamole: Often employed in pts with poorly controlled Htn, glaucoma, or a LBBB. These agents are coronary vasodilators that result in hyperemia to detect differences in coronary flow reserve between stenosed and normal vascular territories.
- Myocardial perfusion imaging: IV administration and subsequent radiologic imaging of a radioactive tracer (e.g., thallium-201 or 99-technetium) is taken up by healthy myocardial cells but not by infracted, ischemic, or under perfused tissues. The areas of reduced tracer uptake appear as relative perfusion defects.
- Echocardiography: Can be performed to supplement both EST and pharmacologic stress tests. Echocardiography provides useful additional information about ventricular function, areas of ischemia and valvular heart disease.
- Holter monitoring: Preop ambulatory ECG monitoring enables the detection of significant ischemic ECG changes, the duration and severity of which have been correlated with periop cardiac morbidity in vascular surgery pts.
- Coronary angiography: Remains the gold standard for definitive Dx and specific anatomic characterization of coronary disease.

TEST

Pretest Probability of Coronary Heart Disease In Patients With Chest Pain According to Age, Gender, And Symptoms

Age	Nonanginal Pain		Atypical Angina		Typical Angina	
	Men	Women	Men	Women	Men	Women
30–39	4	2	34	12	76	26
40–49	13	3	51	22	87	55
50–59	20	7	65	31	93	73
60–69	27	14	72	51	94	86

The probability values are expressed as the percent of patients with significant coronary artery disease on angiography.

Combined data from Diamond GA, Forrester JS. *N Engl J Med*. 1979;300:1350; and from Weiner DA, Ryan TJ, McCabe CH, et al. *N Engl J Med*. 1979;301:230.

Perioperative Implications

- High risk of periop cardiac morbidity and mortality is predicted by profound ST-segment ECG changes, poor exercise capacity (<4 METs), exercise-induced drop in BP or exercise-induced angina.
- Low periop cardiac morbidity is predicted by the absence of the findings listed above.
- Intermediate results may require additional noninvasive testing (i.e., exercise myocardial perfusion imaging and/or echocardiography) to more accurately estimate prognosis.

Special Considerations

- EST is less accurate in pts who fail to achieve 85% of age-predicted maximum HR.
- Diagnostic accuracy of EST also depends on the pretest clinical risk estimate.
- Interpretation of EST results requires integration of all information acquired during the test. Although often reported as simply positive or negative based on the presence or absence of exercise-induced ECG changes suggestive of ischemia, this over-simplification can be misleading.

- Additional imaging modalities (echocardiography or myocardial perfusion) and pharmacologic challenge (dobutamine, adenosine, or dipyrimadole) increase the diagnostic specificity and sensitivity.

Flow-Volume Loops

Peter Rock
Kathleen Davis

Risk

- Virtually no risks associated with flow-volume loops (PFTs)
- Risk from bronchodilator use and misinterpreting data

Sensitivity/Specificity

- Flows depend on pt factors, incl body size (ht, wt); habitus; gender; age; ethnicity. The 95% confidence interval incl values 20–30% above and below mean for given healthy population. This wide range of normal values limits interpretation of PFTs; interpretation of PFTs critically depends on prior probability of disease. The Dx of COPD does not usually require PFTs; it is based on clinical criteria. Results within given pt reproducible to within 5% or less in cooperative subjects. Repeated measurements of PFTs over time are sensitive to changes in health or disease status. Some pts with confusing Hx and physical findings may need PFTs to diagnose lung disease.

Overview

- Cost variable $250–650 (State of Maryland Health Services Cost Review Commission)
- Flow-volume loops show relationship between airflow, with max effort starting from position of either max inspiration or exhalation, and volume (exhaled or inspired, respectively)
- Accuracy, interpretation of PFTs highly dependent on pt cooperation, pt effort; results must be reproducible to be valid

Indications

- Confirm Dx of suspected obstructive lung diseasex
- Suggest presence of restrictive lung disease
- Intra- versus extrathoracic obstructions

Tests

- CT images of sites of airway obstruction

ASSESSMENT POINTS

Test	Positive Result	Confounding Factors	Dx Information
Measurements suggest OLD (obstructive lung disease)	Flow-volume loops show exaggerated upward concavity of descending limb of flow-volume curve with ↓ peak flows, ↓ volume; inspiratory flows relatively preserved		Causes of OLD: acute (asthma), chronic (bronchitis, emphysema), or related to upper airway lesions
Measurements suggest RLD (restrictive lung disease)	Flow-volume loops show preservation or ↑ of peak expiratory flow but ↓ volume; flow-volume curve has normal shape but reduced in all dimensions; inspiratory flows relatively preserved		Suggest RLD
Measurements suggest central airway obstruction (flow-volume loops)	Predominant ↓ in expiratory flow with relatively normal inspiratory flow; expiratory flow curve often has plateau (same flow at all lung volumes) rather than downward bowing normally seen Predominant ↓ in inspiratory flow with relatively normal expiratory flow Proportional ↓ in inspiratory and expiratory flows	Flow-volume loops have role in screening, but confirmation of location, size of lesion may be obtained from imaging studies—e.g., CT of chest	Variable intrathoracic obstruction: Pleural pressure variations during inspiration, exhalation influence magnitude of obstruction so it is less during inspiration, indicating that site of lesion is in thorax (e.g., tracheal tumor) Variable extrathoracic obstruction: Pleural pressure variations during inspiration and exhalation influence magnitude of obstruction so that it is less during exhalation, indicating that site of lesion is in upper airway (e.g., laryngeal tumor) Fixed central obstruction (e.g., tracheal stenosis): Pleural pressure variations during inspiration and exhalation do not influence magnitude of obstruction

Key Reference: Gold WM. Pulmonary function testing. In: Mason RJ, Murray JF, Nadel JA, eds. *Textbook of respiratory medicine.* 4th ed. Philadelphia, Elsevier; 2005:671–733.

Perioperative Implications

- Flow-volume loops can distinguish intrathoracic from extrathoracic lesions (see Mediastinal Masses in Diseases section for intrathoracic lesions)

TESTS

HIV Testing

Richard Silverman

Tests for Antibodies

• Antibody testing is the most efficient and routine method.

• After a person becomes infected with HIV, an antibody response is detectable within 2–8 wk (average of 25 d) in 97% pts. There is a chance that some people have a longer window period of seroconversion. Therefore if there is a definitive risk event, pts should get retested in 6 mo as in rare cases it may take that long for antibodies to develop.

• Routine testing is based on antibody detection using the enzyme-linked immunosorbent assay (ELISA) or enzyme immunoassay (EIA). In these tests the pt's serum is diluted and applied to a plate which has HIV antigens attached. If the pt has anti-HIV antibodies they will attach. The plate is then washed and covered with a 2° antibody with an enzymatic function that binds to human antibodies. The plate is again washed and finally a substrate, which reacts with the 2° antibody with the enzymatic function is added producing a catalytic change in color or fluorescence.

• The Western blot is a confirmatory test when the initial antibody testing is positive. False positives are sometimes seen in pts who have other infections, particularly hepatitis. The procedure takes cells that may be infected, lysing them and applying the proteins to a a gel to which electric current is passed. Naturally each protein band has a different velocity. The proteins are separated out and then applied to a membrane with antibodies similar to the ELISA test. The specific viral bands that are sought are for the GAG, POL, and ENV gene products. It is possible to have an indeterminate result. These people should be re-tested 1 mo later.

• Rapid point of care testing tests for antibodies using immunoassay technique. False positives are possible if the test is administered too early and antibodies are not formed. Although highly specific, false positives are possible with co-existing illness.

Tests for Antigen (the actual HIV virus particle)

• p24 test uses monoclonal antibodies. When p24 antigen is present it sticks to the antibody and the enzyme linked antibody causes a color change. The test is generally positive from about 1–3 wk following infection. Once the pt starts to produce their own antibodies, the p24 will usually be negative although they are infected. Later in the course, the p24 will once again be detectable if the disease is untreated.

• Nucleic acid amplification tests (NAAT or HIV PCR or viral load) are quantitative measurement of the HIV RNA. The test looks for and amplifies a 142 base sequence of the HIG GAG gene. Nucleic acid–based tests are used to test donated blood. Since these are costly tests they are first screened using a pooled sample of 18–20 units at a time. If a pool is positive the individual units are then tested. In addition, these types of tests are used clinically in conjunction with CD4 counts to monitor the progress of HIV pts.

• PCR tests uses RNA extracted from the plasma and is treated with reverse trsnscriptase to create cDNA. The polymerase chain reaction is then applied to amplify, hybridized, and then enzyme link identified.

• Quantiplex method centrifuges the virus, releases the RNA and bound with oligonucleotides with an enzymatic reaction.

• The results of these exams report the number of HIV copies in copies/milliliter. A low viral load of 40–500 copies/mL indicates the HIV is not reproducing. Undetectable levels does not imply cure, but rather it means the levels of circulating RNA are below the detectable amounts. The HIV will still persist in cells and tissues throughout the body.

Monitors

• CD4 and CD8 lymphocyte counts are important markers in monitoring immune function in pts with HIV. CD4 cells also known as T-helper cells identify, attack, and destroy infectious agents. HIV virus attaches to the CD4 cells, enters them and either replicates thus killing the CD4 cell or lies dormant. Eventually with unchecked infection the CD4 cell count declines. Once the CD4 count is less than 200cells/mL a person is said to have AIDS. The 200 level was selected as it correlates with increased likelihood of contracting opportunistic diseases. Sometimes the CD4 count is expressed in absolute numbers as above or as a percentage of lymphocytes or as a ratio to CD8 cells.

Risks

• There are no known risks of testing except for possible false positive or false negative.

Indications

• Recent advances in antiviral therapy whereby mother to fetus transmission can be blocked suggests routine testing of all pregnant mothers. While this is not current practice is certainly has gained support.

Perioperative Precations

• Positive state should be transmitted to OR and other staff so appropriate universal precautions can be vigorously maintained.

TESTS

Liver Function Tests (LFTs)

Megan Graybill

Harendra Arora

Risk

- No risk with testing other than misinterpretation of data or misdiagnosis
- False-positive results, esp. with routine testing not guided by Hx/physical.
- Abn values can be due to causes unrelated to the liver; tests may be normal even in severe disease.

Overview

- Costs
  - Alanine aminotransferase (ALT), aspartate aminotransferase (AST), lactate
  - Dehydrogenase (LDH), gamma glutamyl transpeptidase (GGT), alkaline
  - Phosphatase (AP), total bilirubin, direct bilirubin, albumin: $11–$40 each
  - 5'nucleotidase (5NT): $30–$50
  - Prothrombin time (PT): $8–$49
  - Multiple chemistries often available as panel $17–$49
- Liver function tests is somewhat misleading because most do not directly indicate hepatic fuction.

- Can be classifed as markers of hepatocellular injury, cholestasis, excretory function, and biosynthetic capacity.
- Patterns of abn are more accurate than individual tests and can guide additional testing.
- Aminotransferases (ALT and AST) are released when the hepatic cell membrane is injured and are sensitive indicators of hepatic injury; ALT is more specific to liver than AST.
- Sudden decline in elevated ALT/AST combined with worsening of bilirubin and prolongation of PT indicates acute liver failure and poor prognosis.
- Markers of cholestasis (intrahepatic or extrahepatic obstruction to bile flow) incl AP, GGT, and 5NT. AP may be elevated due to non-hepatic causes; concurrent elevation of GGT and 5NT can be used to confirm hepatic origin.
- AST/ALT ratio >2, GGT/AP ratio >2.5 are suggestive of alcoholic liver disease while AST/ALT ratio >1 suggests cirrhosis of any cause.
- Differentiation of bilirubin fraction (total – direct = indirect) helps suggest cause: Elevated unconjugated (indirect) occurs with increased production or impaired uptake and conjugation; elevated conjugated (direct) occurs with impaired excretion or obstruction.
- Extrinsic clotting pathway factors are normally synthesized by the liver in quantities that exceed requirements for normal coagulation, thus prolongation of PT may not be present in mild-moderate synthetic dysfunction.

Indications

- Noninvasive screening for liver disease, suggesting a general category of disease as a cause of abn results
- Monitoring disease progression or reflecting severity of liver disease (i.e., Child-Pugh score uses albumin, PT, bilirubin to predict survival)

Additional Tests

- Imaging: US, CT, MRI, magnetic resonance cholangiopancreatography (MRCP)
- Invasive studies: Cholangiography, endoscopic retrograde cholangiopancreatography (ERCP), liver biopsy
- Viral hepatitis serologies, immunologic markers (i.e., antimitochondiral antibodies in 1° biliary cirrhosis), indocyanine elimination, lidocaine metabolism (MEGX)

ASSESSMENT POINTS

Test (Normal Result*)	Significance	Abnormal Response	Extrahepatic Sources
ALT (10–55 U/L)	Hepatocellular injury	Mild ↑ nonspecific; marked ↑ in extensive damage (acute viral, toxic hepatitis, or shock liver)	Most specific for liver injury
AST (10–40 U/L)	Hepatocellular injury		Myocardium, skeletal muscle, kidney, brain, pancreas, lung, leukocytes, erythrocytes
LDH (<250 U/L)	Hepatocellular injury	Transient ↑↑ with shock liver; persistent ↑ in malignant infiltration	Myocardium, skeletal muscle, kidney, brain, erythrocytes
AP (45–115 U/L)	Cholestasis	Slight ↑ nonspecific; ↑↑ in cholestasis and infiltrative disease (i.e., metastasis)	Bone growth or ↑ turnover in bone disease states; pregnancy (placental origin)
GGT (<30 U/L)	Cholestasis	Most sensitive indicator of biliary tract disease; poor specificity	Widely distributed in many tissues. induced by ethanol and drugs (i.e., anticonvulsants, warfarin)
5NT (<11 U/L)	Cholestasis	Can be used to confirm hepatic source of ↑ AP	Widely distributed but serum ↑ specific for hepatic origin
Bilirubin (<1.0 mg/dL)	Excretory function	Mild-moderate ↑ in many disease types; ↑↑ in obstructive, viral, alcoholic, drug-induced, or congenital disease	Hemolysis, hematoma resorption, muscle injury
Albumin (3.5–5.0 g/dL)	Biosynthetic capacity	Low in chronic disease, long half-life (20d); not a reliable indicator of acute disease	↓ In burns, enteropathy, malnutrition, fluid retention, nephrotic syndrome, etc.
PT (10.9–12.5 sec)	Biosynthetic capacity	Sensitive indicator of acute hepatic dysfunction due to short half-life of Factor VII.	Prolonged with warfarin therapy, vitamin K deficiency (may result from obstructive jaundice and ↓ uptake), consumptive coagulopathy

* Normal values may change depending on assay method.

Key Reference: Ahmed A, Keeffe EB. Liver chemistry and function tests. In: Feldman M, Friedman LS, Brandt LJ, eds. *Sleisenger & Fordtran's gastrointestinal and liver disease.* 8th ed. Philadelphia: Saunders Elsevier; 2006:1575–1586.

Perioperative Implications

- Periop morbidity and mortality increased with acute or chronic liver disease
- Impaired hepatic function has implications for metabolism and elimination of some anesthetic drugs.

- Hypoalbuminemia results in diminished drug-protein binding, alters pharmacokinetics and pharmacodynamics of many commonly used drugs.
- Progression to overt liver dysfunction after surgery may occur if poor preop hepatic reserve.

- Serum aminotransferases may increase postop due to manual hepatic manipulation, ischemic injury, or exposure to anesthetic drugs.

Pregnancy Testing

Rebecca Twersky
Clinton Steffey

Ethical/Legal Considerations

- Who to test: All female pts of childbearing age versus selected populations
- If pt refuses after risks explained, should they be required to sign a waiver to legal rights relating to undetected pregnancy?
- Individual state legislature regarding rights of adolescents to keep results private from family
- Routine testing may create pt trust issues
- Important to protect the physician from unwarranted litigation

Risk

- Risk to pt is false positive or false negative test or misinterpretation
- Increases risks in anesthesia, surgery in pregnant women of spontaneous abortion, low birth wt, and premature labor, and may be cognitive dysfunction of offspring if repeated anesthetics (see SafeKidsAnesthesia.org at IARS site)

Overview

- Cost: Numerous tests available; cost varies, both to pt and to institution. Average cost to pt
  - Urine hCG: $5– $25
  - Serum hCG: $15–$85
- Importance of ruling out pregnancy before surgery
- Preop tests should be done or required on a selective basis for purposes of guiding and optimizing periop management

- hCG is a glycoprotein secreted by developing placenta shortly after fertilization; hCG molecule comprises two noncovalently bonded, dissimilar subunits, namely, α, β. The α subunit is structurally similar to α subunit of FSH, LH, TSH. Therefore, there is a high degree of cross-reactivity with these hormones. In contrast, the β subunit of hCG is structurally distinct, displaying differing immunologic specificities.
- β hCG detectable in maternal blood and urine 8–9 d post conception
- Positive test can be analyzed as follows:

Week after LMP	Concentration (in mIU)
3	0–50
4	3–426
5	19–7,340
6	1,080–56,500
7–8	7,650–229,000
9–12	25,060–228,000
17–24	4,060–65,400
25–40	3,640–117,000

Test Indications

- Pts should be offered, not required, pregnancy testing unless there is a compelling medical reason to know the pt is pregnant.
- To diagnose pregnancy in periop period; to quantify gestation
- Medical Hx alone often unreliable, esp. in adolescents

Recommendations

- Age <13: No pregnancy test unless indicated by history
- Age 13 until 1 y after last menses: Preop pregnancy test should be offered to all pts

ASSESSMENT POINTS

Pregnancy Test Technique	Sensitivity	Specificity	Test Duration	Postconception Age 1st Positive
IRMA (immunoradiometric assay) more sensitive	150 mIU/mL	No cross-reactivity to LH, FSH, or TSH	30 min	18–22 d
IRMA less sensitive	1500 mIU/mL	Same as above	2 min	25–28 d
ELISA (enzyme-linked immunosorbent assay) more sensitive	25 mIU/mL	Same as above	80 min	14–17 d
ELISA less sensitive	50 mIU/mL	Same as above	5–15 min	18–22 d
RIA (radioimmunoassay)	5 mIU/mL	Cross-reactivity with LH (0.5%), FSH (0.2%)	4 hr	10–18 d
Fluoroimmunoassay	1 mIU/mL	No cross-reactivity to LH, FSH, or TSH	2–3 hr	14–17 d
Urine pregnancy test	25–50 mIU/mL	Same as above	1–5 min	>22 d

False positives/negatives can occur with any of the above tests secondary to confounding factors including phantom hCG, pituitary hCG, exogenous hCG, trophoblastic neoplasms, nontrophoblastic neoplasms, molar pregnancy, ectopic pregnancy, hydatidform mole, and delivery or abortion within a few weeks.

For borderline results, repeat test in 48 hr (hCG doubles); correlate hCG with LMP, PE, US

Key Reference: Steffey CS, Twersky RS. Is routine preoperative pregnancy testing necessary? In: Fleisher LA, ed. *Evidence-based practice of anesthesiology*. 2nd ed. Philadelphia; Saunders; 2009:28–32.

Perioperative Implications

- 1–2% of pregnant women undergo surgery for reasons unrelated to parturition.
- Literature is inadequate to determine whether or not anesthesia causes harmful effects on pregnancy.
- Intraop concerns incl the effect of surgery and anesthesia on the developing fetus from teratogenic effects of medications, maternal physiologic changes (hypoxia and/or acidosis), and changes in uteroplacental blood flow
- Numerous studies on fetal outcome post surgery, post anesthesia demonstrate ↑ incidence of spontaneous abortions, LBW, esp. if surgery performed in first trimester
- No ↑ incidence of congenital anomalies (even with N_2O), although recent concern with doubling of behavioral abn and cognitive dysfunction

if repeated anesthesia exposure prior to age 3 y (see SafeKidsAnesthesia.org at IARS)
- If possible, local or regional anesthesia used in first trimester
- During first trimester, thiopental, muscle relaxants, narcotics, propofol safely used
- Use of benzodiazepines, N_2O, inhalation agents more controversial

TESTS

Renal Function Testing

Solomon Aronson

Risk

• No risk assoc with serum- or urine-derived renal function testing save inappropriate Rx based on misleading data or data misinterpretation

Overview

• Cost
  • Urine indices
    Basic analysis (SG, pH): $6–$12
    Lytes (Na⁺): $8–$56
    Cr: $10–$29
    Osm: $16–$46
  • Serum chemistries
    BUN: $8–$29
    Cr: $8–$29
    Lytes (Na⁺): $8–$56 (29)
    Osm: $16–$46
  • Combination indices
    Cr clearance: $60–$75
    Free water clearance: $90
    Fe Na⁺: $120

• Advanced biomarkers of renal tubular cell damage
  • Urinary glutathione S-transferase (GST)
  • β-N-acetyl-β-d-glucosaminidase (NAG)
• Test to predict periop renal function reserve, predict or Dx renal morbidity during high-risk surgery (trauma, vasc, cardiothoracic) in pts at high risk for renal failure (preop renal insufficiency, low CO syndrome, etc.)

Test Indications

• Urine formation begins with glomerular ultrafiltration and progresses to tubular reabsorption and tubular secretion. All anesthetic agents have the potential to alter renal function by altering BP and cardiac output so that renal blood flow is redistributed. This redistribution is accompanied by sodium and water conservation and decreased urine formation. Dx, evaluate extent of renal tubular function, GFR in pts to assess periop risk and/or morbidity.

Additional/Alternative Tests

• A plain KUB film may be used to identify renal disease with hematuria, pain, and/or fever to R/O trauma
• US to discriminate renal masses (cyst versus mass), locate obstructive nephropathy source
• Doppler US can facilitate finding cause of allograph dysfunction when evaluating renal flow following transplant
• Renal flow scan (^{99m}Tc-DTPA) also useful for RBF analysis esp when comparing one kidney with the other
• Renal angio can be used to visualize medium and/or small artery anatomy.
• Alternatives to above may incl MRI and contrast US.

ASSESSMENT POINTS

Test	Positive Result	Confounding Factors	Dx Information
Urinalysis	Hematuria (>1–2 RBC) Pyuria (>4 WBC) Cellular cast Proteinuria (> 3 +)	Multiple causes	Glomerular disease, free Hgb or myoglobinuria, UTI, interstitial nephritis, pyelonephritis, glomerular disease
Urine Na⁺	<20 mEq >40 mEq	Hormonal secretion (ADH, aldosterone), Na⁺-avid states (CHF, cirrhosis), saline infusion, diuretics, dopamine	Prerenal azotemia sensitivity 50% (PPV 50%), ATN sensitivity 55% (PPV 50%)
Urine Osm	>500 mOsm/kg H₂O <350 mOsm/kg H₂O	Proteins, glucose, mannitol, dextran, diuretics, advanced age, temp extremes	Prerenal azotemia sensitivity 30% (PPV 60–90%), ATN sensitivity 80% (PPV 65–95%)
Serum Cr	>2 mg/dL >20% increase postoperative	↑ N balance, tissue breakdown, basal metabolism, diet, activity, hepatic disease, hematoma, GI bleeding, drugs	Assoc with ↑ risk of postop renal insufficiency, LOS, and cost of care after CABG surgery when >1.4 mg/dL Nml variant or ↓ renal function reserve GFR ↓ by >50%
Fe, Na⁺, urine$_{Na}$ plasma$_{cr}$/ Urine$_{Cr}$ plasma$_{Na}$	<1% >1%	Vol depletion Diuretic, ATN, CHF, cirrhosis, high salt intake, saline infusion	Only helpful after ATN Does not allow prediction
Free water clearance: Urine vol (urine Osm × Urine vol/plasma Osm)	> – 20 mL/hr	See urine Osm	Indicator if pending renal dysfunction not predictive
Cr clearance: Urine$_{Cr}$/Plasma$_{Cr}$	<25 mL/min	Changing hydration states, inaccurate vol collection, nml day-to-day variation	Predicts ↑ periop renal morbidity, renal failure

PPV = positive predictive value.

Key Reference: Thakar CV, Arrigain S, Worley S, Yared JP, Paganini EP. A clinical score to predict acute renal failure after cardiac surgery. *J Am Soc Nephrol*. 2005;16:162–168.

Perioperative Implications

• Periop renal failure following high-risk procedures has a reported incidence of 0.1–50% depending on population analyzed and methods used to define renal failure; is assoc with a reported mortality of 20–90%
• Periop renal failure accounts for half of all pts requiring acute renal dialysis
• No simple, inexpensive test adequately determines renal function

• Cr clearance appears to be most efficient test to estimate renal function reserve at this time
• Isolated changes in serum Cr have been shown to be predictive of ↑ morbidity and cost of care after CABG surgery

Special Considerations

• ATN accounts for nearly 70% of cases of periop renal failure

• Inadequate RBF is most common underlying cause for periop renal morbidity
• Serial determination of Cr clearance currently most sensitive test for predicting onset of periop renal dysfunction
• AKIN criteria and RIFLE criteria utilize renal function indices to predict severity of acute renal dysfunction.

Spirometry

Peter Rock
Kathleen Davis

Risk

- Virtually no risks assoc with spirometry PFTs; risk can occur with use of bronchodilators or misinterpretation of data

Overview

- Cost: Variable: $250 spirometry; $300 diffusing capacity for CO; $650 lung volumes (State of Maryland Health Services Cost Review Commission)
- Spirometry is relationship between exhaled volume (starting from position of maximum inspiration) with maximum effort (as forceful as possible—i.e., forced) and time. Quotient of FEV in first sec of exhalation (FEV_1) and FVC (known as $FEV_1\%$) may be used to define obstructive lung disease and to suggest restrictive lung disease (see table following)
- PFTs reflect airway resistance, elastic properties of lungs, chest wall
- Airway resistance not measured by PFTs; presence of increased airway resistance inferred from decreased expiratory airflow; assumes max effort was made by pt
- Accuracy, interpretation of PFTs highly dependent on pt cooperation, pt effort. Results must be reproducible to be valid.

- FEV_1, FVC expressed as percentage of predicted normal values, which may not be appropriate at extremes of wt
- Max mid-expiratory flow rate ($FEF_{25-75\%}$: forced expiratory flow between 25% and 75% of FVC) is most sensitive to airflow obstruction in peripheral airways, where chronic diseases of airflow originate
- Peak flow determinations are inexpensive and noninvasive and can be used to assess changes in baseline in pts with bronchospasm

Sensitivity/Specificity

- Lung volumes, flows depend on pt factors, incl body size (ht, wt); habitus; gender; age; ethnicity; 95% confidence interval incl values 20–30% above and below mean for given healthy population; this wide range of normal values limits interpretation of PFTs
- Interpretation of PFTs critically depends on prior probability of disease.
- Dx of COPD does not require PFTs and is based on clinical criteria but PFTs may be necessary in some pts with unclear H&P. Results within a given pt reproducible to within 5% or less in cooperative subjects.
- Repeated measurements of PFTs over time sensitive to changes in health or disease status (FEV & VC reliably reflect change over time)

Indications

- Confirm Dx of suspected obstructive lung disease
- Dx reversible component of obstructive lung disease
- Dx change from baseline status in pts with asthma
- Dx unsuspected or occult bronchospasm or response to Rx of bronchospasm
- Suggest presence of restrictive lung disease
- Dx resp cause of SOB

Additional/Alternative Tests

- Helium gas dilution measures total lung capacity
- Body plethysmography measures airway resistance, absolute lung vol
- Diffusing capacity for CO (DLco) measures ↓ surface area for transfer of gases from alveoli to pulm capillaries; useful for predicting outcome of lung resection
- Exercise testing used to define relative contributions of resp, CV systems to development of dyspnea
- CT images sites of airway obstruction

ASSESSMENT POINTS

Test	Positive Result	Confounding Factors	Dx Information
Measurements suggestive of OLD	FEV_1/FVC ~0.8 1) FEV_1/FVC = 0.66–0.8 2) FVC < predicted 1) FEV_1/FVC = 0.5–0.65 2) FVC < predicted 1) FEV_1/FVC < 0.5 2) FVC < predicted	Requires pt's cooperation, max effort, measurements must be reproducible	Normal ratio Mild OLD Moderate OLD Severe OLD Causes of OLD: Acute (asthma), chronic (bronchitis, emphysema), or related to upper airway lesions
Measurements suggestive of *reversible* OLD	↑ In FEV_1 *and* FVC of at least 15% with administration of inhaled bronchodilator		Lack of response to inhaled bronchodilator does not exclude reversible airway obstruction in pts with severe obstruction
Measurements suggestive of RLD	FEV_1/FVC >0.85 *and* FVC < predicted	Requires lung vol measurement to confirm	Suggests RLD, incl NM disease; chest wall disease (kyphoscoliosis); infiltrative or destructive interstitial diseases (interstitial fibrosis, ARDS); space-occupying lesions; or pleural disease
Measurements suggestive of mixed OLD/RLD	FEV_1/FVC ~0.8 *and* FVC < predicted or significantly ↓ VC assoc with ↓ FEV_1/FVC ratio	When mixed defect considered, lung volume determination must be made	Suggests presence of two processes—e.g., COPD and NM disease, or COPD and tumor; sarcoidosis

Key Reference: Gold WM. Pulmonary function testing. In: Mason RJ, Murray JF, Nadel JA, eds. *Textbook of respiratory medicine*. 4th ed. Elsevier; 2005:671–733.

Perioperative Implications

- Routine use of PFTs not indicated; consider PFTs if Dx of obstructive lung disease not possible on clinical basis

- Peak flow during max exhalation useful as simple bedside test to follow response of bronchospasm to Rx. Peak flow determined primarily by diameter of large airways; is ↓ in moderate-to-severe obstruction.

Transesophageal Echocardiography (TEE)

Ramprasad Sripada

Risk

- Esophageal injury or bleeding, vocal cord paralysis, dysrhythmias, hypotension, seizures, cardiac arrest (occur in less than 3% of exams) Mortality rate (0.01–0.03%)
- Minor injuries: Lip injuries (13%), hoarseness (12%), dysphagia (1.8%), ET intubation (0.3%), bradycardia (0.2%), dental injuries (0.1%)
- Bacteremia (0–4%), little evidence that pts experience clinical consequences
- Resp complications more frequently in awake examinations (0.1–4%) or in small children (2%), whose membranous trachea is easily compressed by the probe
- Hemodynamic compromise may be more common in small children.
- No evidence that anticoagulation increases risk of bleeding during TEE.
- Erroneous interpretation, distraction from other anesthetic duties (unknown incidence)

Overview

- Cost: $300–$500/pt use
- Imaging technique utilizing US to examine structure, function of heart, great vessels, to gain information on blood flow within these structures
- US crystals mounted on gastroscope inserted into esophagus/stomach; placed behind heart
- Tomographic images constructed from intensity of reflected signals, analyzed electronically, converted to image by echoscanner
- Flow from frequency shift between emitted and reflected US using Doppler equation

Equipment

- Esophageal probe: Single-plane, transverse images; biplane, transverse, longitudinal images; multiplane, transverse to longitudinal to transverse images (180°)
- Echoscanner: Analyzes reflected echoes, generates images or flow tracings
- Recorders: Hard copy, videotape, or digital

Indications

- Cardiac Indications
  - Cardiac function: Esp. useful to assess preload, systolic, diastolic function
  - Ischemia: Regional wall motion abn, defined as changes in wall thickening, wall motion, indicative of ischemia
  - Valvular function: valvular abn identified using imaging, Doppler exam; intraop assessment allows ↑ use of valve repairs rather than replacements, vascular route placement of replacement valves
  - Aortic disease: TEE is the gold standard for Dx of aortic disease dissection; used by some to select cannulation site for A-cannulae to ↓ risk of emboli
  - CHD: TEE allows assessment of adequacy of valve repairs intraop
  - Cardiac devices: Placement of intracardiac devices and monitoring of their position during port access and other cardiac surgical interventions

Non-cardiac Indications

- Assess: Volume status, ventricular function, valve pathology, pericardial effusions, constrictions
- Monitor: Ischemia, assessment response to therapy
- Rapid Dx; trauma, pericardial pathology, hemodynamic instability and hypoxia
- Aorta: Endovascular stent, aortic dissection, aortic plaque
- Heart transplant: Right heart function

Contraindications

- Absolute
  - Extensive esophageal or gastric disease, esophagitis, strictures, advanced carcinoma, surgery.
  - Unstable cervical spine: Neck, flexion to introduce the probe a sure way of 'pithing' a pt with a fractured odontoid peg, or severe atlanto-axial subluxation
- Relative
  - Esophageal varices, Zenker's diverticulum, Barrett's esophagus
  - Postradiation: Mediastinal irradiation therapy
  - Upper airway disease, very tenuous airway
  - Poor dentition, recent dental surgery
  - Pt hasn't fasted for 4 to 6 hr

Complications

- Esophageal tear and/or perforation, Mallory-Weiss tear related to TEE, bleeding from esophageal varices, esophageal and/or gastric erosion
- Burns, electrical shock
- Swallowing difficulties, dysphagia and/or odynophagia
- Skin staining, damage of oropharynx, dental
- Airway obstruction, tracheal extubation, mainstem intubation, vocal cord paralysis, bronchospasm, desaturation and resp distress
- Sedation in awake pts: Aspiration or apnea
- Other complications: Htn, hypote-nsion, angina, vascular compression, bradycardias due to vagotonia, AV block, tachyarrhythmias (atrial or ventricular)

Training

- Development of competence in TEE requires acquisition of numerous cognitive and technical skills; a period dedicated to intensive training under direct supervision of expert is highly recommended.
- Advanced periop TEE certification since 2003
- Basic perioperative TEE certification 2010

TESTS

V/Q Scan (Nuclear Ventilation-Perfusion Scintigraphy)

William Bradford
Robert Kyle

Risk

- Essentially the same for CXRs and IV access
- Small exposure to radiation from the radioisotope which is gone in 2–3 d and should be avoided in pregnancy and breastfeeding as well as those with allergies to radioisotope.
- Pulm embolism, the most common reason for ordering a V/Q scan, has an incidence of 94,000 cases annually in the USA.

Sensitivity/Specificity

- For evaluation of pulm embolism, the sensitivity of a high-probability (PE present) scan is 77.4% (95% CI 69.7%–85%) while the specificity of a very low probability or normal (PE absent) scan finding is 97.7% (95% CI 96.4-98.9%)

Overview

- Cost: $800 to $1000 for CPT reimbursement (CPT code 78580, 78585); Total cost per test to hospital is roughly $250 to $350 per pt
- Nuclear medicine test to evaluate the flow of blood (perfusion) through the lungs and the flow of gas (ventilation) through the lungs
- The ventilation scan has radioactive tracer gas (^{133}Xe, ^{127}Xe, ^{81m}Kr, ^{99m}Tc) inhaled into lungs with bright spots being where gas is ventilated and dark spots where gas is not.
- The perfusion scan has radioactive tracer substance (^{99m}Tc MAA) injected into a vein where it travels to the lung and shows up as bright where blood is being perfused and dark where it is not.

Indications

- Evaluation of disturbances between ventilation and perfusion incl pulm embolism, non-thrombotic emboli, lung cancer, intravascular disturbances (tumor, fat, parasite), pulm stenosis/arteritis, COPD, pneumonia and for performance quantification pre- and post- lung lobectomy/pneumonectomy surgery

Additional Tests

- It is common to have a routine two-view CXR before receiving a V/Q scan
- Chemistries, cultures, and blood counts are not routine; however, may be helpful in further ruling in or out a disease process.

ASSESSMENT POINTS

Interpretation involves looking for mismatch for ventilation>perfusion, ventilation=perfusion and ventilation<perfusion by comparing tracer brightness of ventilation images to perfusion images
Interpretation for pulmonary embolism

High Probability

At least 2 large (>75% of a segment) segmental perfusion defects without corresponding ventilation or CXR abn

1 large and at least 2 moderate segmental (25–75% of a segment) perfusion defects without corresponding ventilation or CXR abn

At least 4 moderate segmental perfusion defects without corresponding ventilation or CXR abn

Intermediate Probability

1 large and less than 2 moderate segmental perfusion defects without corresponding ventilation or CXR abn

Single moderate mismatched defect with normal CXR findings

Corresponding V/Q defects and CXR parenchymal opacity in lower lung zone

Corresponding V/Q defects and small pleural effusion

Low Probability

Multiple matched V/Q defects, regardless of size, with normal CXR findings

Corresponding V/Q defects and CXR parenchymal opacity in upper and middle lung zone

Corresponding V/Q defects and large pleural effusion

Any perfusion defects with substantially larger CXR abn

Defects surrounded by normally perfused lung (Stripe sign)

More than 3 small (<25% of a segment) segmental defects with a normal CXR

Nonsegmental perfusion defects

Very Low Probability–Up to 3 Small Matching Segmental Perfusion Defects with Normal CXR

Normal

No perfusion defects and perfusion outlines the shape of the lung seen on CXR

Key Reference: Sostman HD, Coleman RE, Newman GE, DeLong D, Paine SS. Evaluation of revised criteria for ventilation-perfusion scintigraphy in patients with suspected pulmonary embolism. *Radiology.* 1994;193:103–107.

Perioperative Implications

Preoperative Preparation

- Management of anesthesia for pts with V/Q abn is to support vital organ function and to minimize anesthetic-induced myocardial depression
- If operation is not emergent and not aimed at correction of V/Q abn, strong consideration should be made to postpone operation to allow correction of V/Q abn if possible.
- Not uncommon for pts with severe V/Q mismatch to arrive in OR intubated and mechanically ventilated, often with high FIO_2.
- May be necessary to support cardiac output with inotropic drugs incl catecholamines to increase myocardial contractility or phosphodiesterase inhibitors to increase myocardial contractility and vasodilate pulm arteries

Monitoring

- Monitoring of intra-arterial pressure and cardiac filling pressures often necessary if V/Q mismatch severe
- Right atrial filling pressure can be a guide to optimize IV fluid administration

Induction

- Must avoid any accentuation of arterial hypoxemia, systemic hypotension, and pulm Htn

Maintenance

- Can be maintained with any drug or combination of drugs that avoid significant myocardial depression
- Nitrous oxide not a likely selection due to often high FIO_2 requirement as well as its potential to increase pulm vascular resistance worsening the perfusion of the lungs

- Maintenance of NMB should be done to minimize histamine release.

Postoperative Care

- Often significant hemodynamic improvements are made post embolectomy or operations aimed to correct V/Q abn.
- Postop care should aim to continue supporting vital organ function and minimize cardiac injury which may incl remaining intubated or pressor support.

EVAR= endovascular Aneurysm Repair